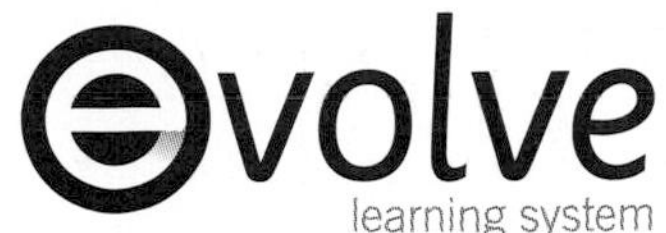

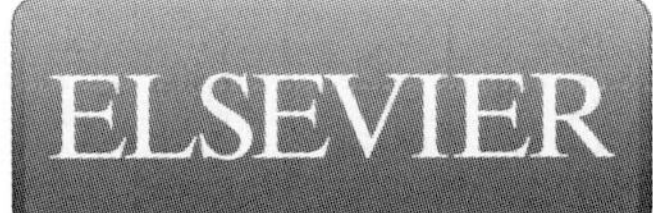

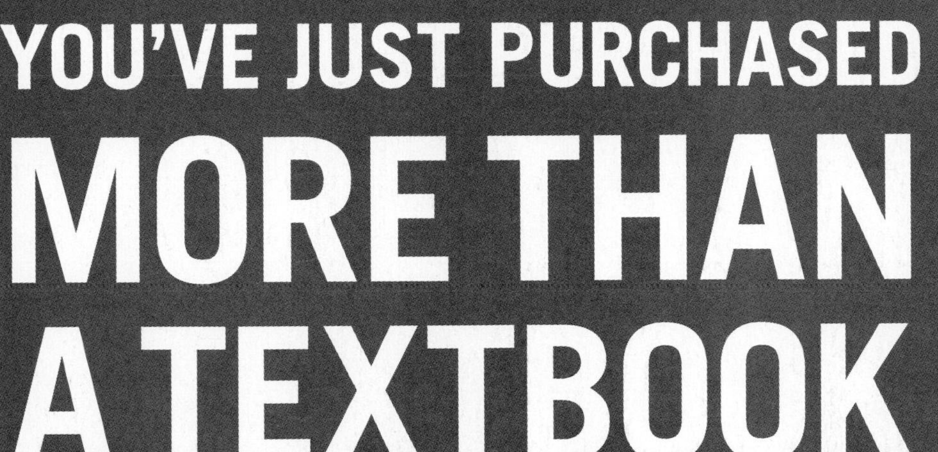

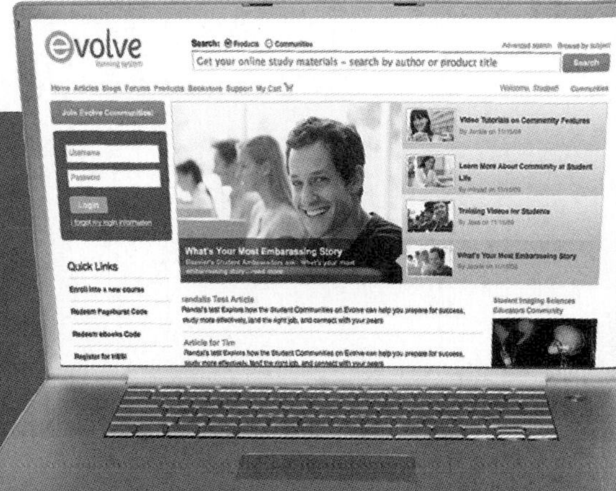

ACTIVATE THE COMPLETE LEARNING EXPERIENCE THAT COMES WITH YOUR BOOK BY REGISTERING AT

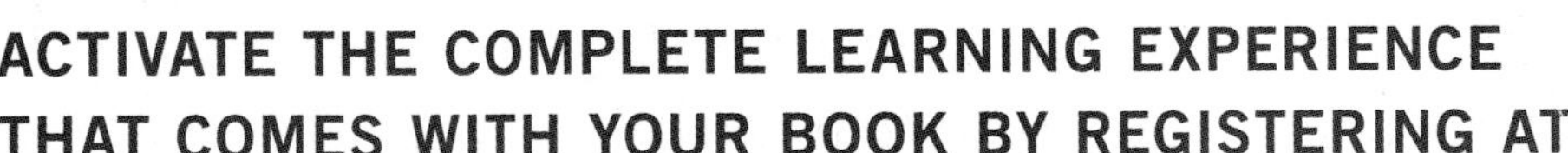

Evolve Student Learning Resources for Dennison: Pass CCRN!, Fourth Edition, offer THE FOLLOWING FEATURES:

- **Over 1000 additional review questions** with answers, rationales, test-taking strategies, and suggested references
- **Randomized questions** to let you create customized practice exams
- **Self-assessment quizzes** allowing you to select questions by body system, with immediate feedback for answers

GETTING STARTED

1. Login Instructions: For detailed instructions, please visit the How To section of the Evolve homepage at http://evolve.elsevier.com/student
2. Username & Password: If you do not have an existing Evolve account, you will be able to create one during the registration process.
3. Access Code: The first time you access the product, you will need the access code located inside the front cover of Pass CCRN!® When you are prompted, enter the code exactly as it appears in Pass CCRN!®

REGISTER TODAY!

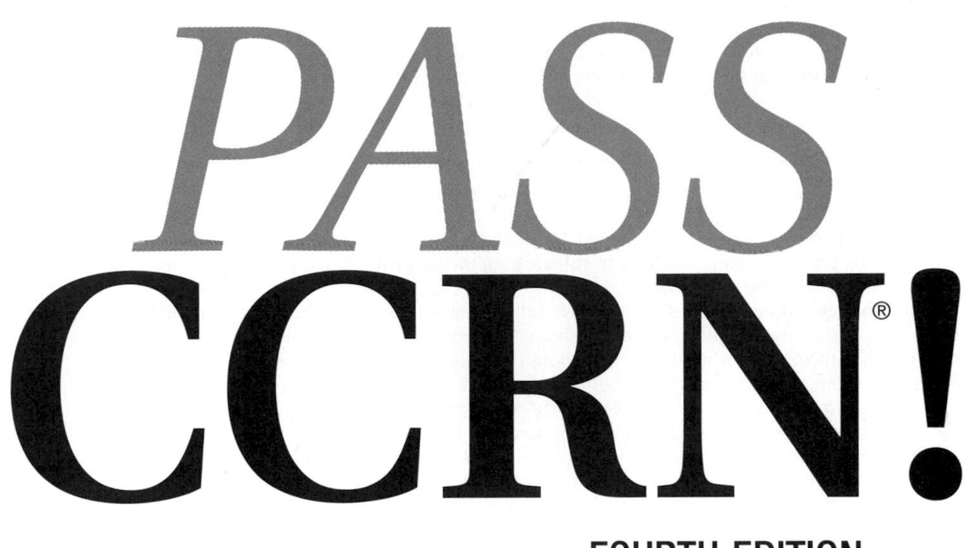

FOURTH EDITION

Robin Donohoe Dennison, DNP, APRN, CCNS, CEN, CNE
Associate Professor
Georgetown University
Washington, D.C.

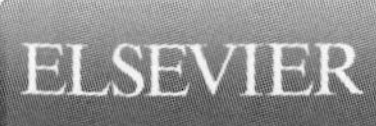

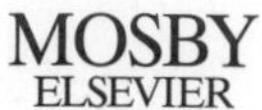

3251 Riverport Lane
Maryland Heights, Missouri 63043

Pass CCRN®! ISBN: 978-0-323-07726-2

Notices

Knowledge and best practice in this field are constantly changing. As new research and experience broaden our understanding, changes in research methods, professional practices, or medical treatment may become necessary.

Practitioners and researchers must always rely on their own experience and knowledge in evaluating and using any information, methods, compounds, or experiments described herein. In using such information or methods they should be mindful of their own safety and the safety of others, including parties for whom they have a professional responsibility.

With respect to any drug or pharmaceutical products identified, readers are advised to check the most current information provided (i) on procedures featured or (ii) by the manufacturer of each product to be administered, to verify the recommended dose or formula, the method and duration of administration, and contraindications. It is the responsibility of practitioners, relying on their own experience and knowledge of their patients, to make diagnoses, to determine dosages and the best treatment for each individual patient, and to take all appropriate safety precautions.

To the fullest extent of the law, neither the Publisher nor the authors, contributors, or editors, assume any liability for any injury and/or damage to persons or property as a matter of products liability, negligence or otherwise, or from any use or operation of any methods, products, instructions, or ideas contained in the material herein.

Library of Congress Cataloging-in-Publication Data

Dennison, Robin.
Pass CCRN! / Robin Donohoe Dennison. - 4th ed.
p. ; cm.
Includes bibliographical references and index.
ISBN 978-0-323-07726-2 (pbk. : alk. paper)
I. Title.
[DNLM: 1. Critical Care-Examination Questions. 2. Critical Care-Outlines. 3. Critical Illness-nursing-Examination Questions. 4. Critical Illness-nursing-Outlines. 5. Nursing Assessment-Examination Questions. 6. Nursing Assessment-Outlines. WY 18.2]
616.028-dc23

2012041668

Executive Content Strategist: Tamara Myers
Senior Content Development Specialist: Tina Kaemmerer
Publishing Services Manager: Deborah L. Vogel
Senior Project Manager: Bridget Healy
Design Direction: Paula Catalano

Printed in the United States of America
Last digit is the print number: 9 8 7 6 5 4 3 2

Clinical Consultants

Karen Allard, **MSN, RN, ACNS-BC, CCNS**
Critical Care CNS
UC Health University Hospital
Cincinnati, Ohio

Marylee Bressie, **DNP, RN, CCRN, CCNS, CEN**
Registered Nurse
Providence Hospital
Mobile, Alabama

Lori A. Catalano, **JD, MSN, RN, CCNS, PCCN**
Christ Hospital
Cincinnati, Ohio

Madelyn Danner, **MS, RN, CCRN, CEN, CNE**
Associate Professor
Harford Community College
Bel Air, Maryland

Anita Dempsey, **PhD, APRN, PMHCNS-BC**
Assistant Professor
Wright State University
Dayton, Ohio

Maurice Espinoza, **MSN, BSN, CNS, CCRN**
Clinical Nurse Specialist
Adult Critical Care
University of California, Irvine
Irvine, California

Wendi Kai Fox, **BSN, RN**
Staff Nurse/Charge Nurse NSICU
UC Health University Hospital
Cincinnati, Ohio

Daniel J. Mueller, **BSN, RN**
Registered Nurse
O'Fallon, Missouri

Betty Nash, **MSN, RN, CCRN**
Associate Professor
School of Nursing & Allied Health
Bluefield State College
Bluefield, West Virginia

Jill Roberts, **RN, MNSc, ACNP**
Trinity Mother Frances Hospitals and Clinics
Tyler, Texas

Brenda Shelton, **MS, RN, CCRN, AOCN**
Clinical Nurse Specialist
The Sidney Kimmel Comprehensive Cancer Center at Johns Hopkins
Baltimore, Maryland

John J. Whitcomb, **PhD, RN, CCRN, FCCM**
Assistant Professor
School of Nursing
Clemson University
Clemson, South Carolina

REVIEWERS

Janice E. O'Neil, MSN, APRN, NP/CNS
Clinical Nurse Specialist, Critical Care
The Nebraska Medical Center
Omaha, Nebraska

Scott Carter Thigpen, DNP, RN, CCRN, CEN
Associate Professor of Nursing
South Georgia College
Douglas, Georgia

Kathleen S. Whalen, PhD, RN, CNE
Assistant Professor of Nursing
Loretto Heights School of Nursing
Regis University
Denver, Colorado

This fourth edition is dedicated to my teachers and my students. I have had the pleasure and honor of learning from some dedicated and talented teachers as well as my students in both academic and professional development settings. Angelo and Cross (1993) contend that "teaching without learning is just talking" as they discuss the need for student engagement, but I feel that this statement has another profound meaning. While I have learned much in a learner role, I feel that I have learned so much more through the deliberate process of teaching and interaction with motivated learners. So I express my profound appreciation and dedicate this edition to all of you who have attended my CCRN® review courses and my students at the University of Cincinnati and Georgetown University. I am honored to have learned from you.

PREFACE

Welcome to *Pass CCRN®!* and congratulations—you have chosen the most up-to-date, comprehensive review of critical care nursing available on the market today. If you are a registered nurse planning to take the CCRN® examination for certified critical care practice offered by the American Association of Critical Care Nurses (AACN) Certification Corporation, this book is the tool that you need to prepare for the examination with confidence.

Information in this text is organized according to the latest CCRN® examination blueprint, which is summarized inside the back cover for quick reference. This test plan, issued by the AACN Certification Corporation, identifies the content areas tested and the percentage of the examination devoted to each. Only content included in the test blueprint is covered in this book, eliminating extraneous information that can be distracting. The book also offers an array of learning activities to help you understand and retain key concepts. In fact, more than 1000 additional multiple-choice questions are provided on the Evolve website so that you can practice your test-taking skills in a format that simulates the examination itself.

I have written this book for nurses who are preparing to take the CCRN® examination. Having taught exam-preparation seminars for the last 25 years has helped me learn what information will best equip nurses to sit for the examination and has familiarized me with the strengths and weaknesses of current exam-preparation books on the market. My goal is to provide a pertinent content review, fun but challenging learning activities, realistic practice questions, and comprehensive mock examinations that reflect the content and complexity of the CCRN® examination.

Content Review

Pass CCRN®! uses a succinct outline format that makes the information easy to read, understand, and remember. Illustrations and tables further explicate and clarify content, highlight key concepts, and enhance written explanations. This fourth edition includes many new concept maps to illustrate the pathophysiology of critical care conditions to aid understanding of the linkage between pathophysiology and clinical presentation.

This edition of *Pass CCRN®*! offers significantly revised content throughout the book along with a new chapter on behavioral/psychosocial. Critical care pharmacology is integrated throughout the book in this edition. Also, new sections have been added to remain consistent with the current blueprint.

Coverage of each body system begins with a brief review of anatomy and physiology. This refresher lays the foundation for introducing more complex topics in the areas of assessment, intervention, and evaluation. Assessment includes health history, physical examination, diagnostic studies, and system-specific assessment methods. For example, the cardiovascular chapter discusses hemodynamic monitoring and electrocardiography, the pulmonary chapter covers interpretation of arterial blood gases, and the neurology chapter presents intracranial pressure monitoring. The format varies for the Multisystem, Professional Caring and Ethical Practice, and the Behavioral/Psychosocial chapters due to the nature of the content in those sections.

Pathologic conditions listed on the CCRN® blueprint are included in the content review. Each condition is first defined, followed by separate sections that explore Etiology, Pathophysiology, Clinical Presentation, including subjective, objective, and diagnostic, and concludes with Collaborative Management, which includes medical and nursing management.

Learning Activities

Sometimes we learn best when information is organized and accessed in unfamiliar ways—that's the principle at work behind the diverse learning activities in this book. Every chapter features a range of question styles, including matching, fill-in-the-blank, comparison, case studies, and crossword puzzles to test comprehension and improve recall for readers with a variety of learning styles.

You won't be asked to complete a crossword puzzle or a matching exercise when you take the CCRN® examination of course, but doing so helps you learn and retain an astonishing amount of information. It also makes your study sessions more enjoyable, encouraging you to stick to the timetable that you have set for yourself. I hope that working through these activities, many of which are new to this edition of the book, will be a pleasurable way to review terminology, anatomy and physiology, and pharmacology.

Practice Questions and Examinations on the Evolve Website

Another great way to study is to use the practice questions and examinations on the Evolve website. It contains more than 1000 review questions written in a format that represents the actual CCRN® examination. The practice examinations have been thoroughly updated to reflect the percentages set forth for each content area on the most recent test blueprint and current practice.

The Evolve website offers two modes: a quiz mode in which practice questions are arranged by body system and a test mode that offers realistic practice CCRN® examinations. The quiz mode allows you to select topic areas in which you need additional review and create quizzes that target those areas. The practice-test mode, on the other hand, replicates the actual CCRN® exam as closely as possible. This timed mode draws questions from all content areas in the number and proportion called for in the latest CCRN® exam blueprint. The program will reshuffle the questions randomly (but retaining the correct percentages in each content area) to create as many practice tests as you like. Both modes are self-scoring. Instant rationales are given to explain which answer is correct and why it is the best answer among the possible choices. Test-taking strategy tips are provided as appropriate to show you how to think through the questions if you are not sure of the content. Both of these features will boost your confidence and make you a better test taker on the important day of the CCRN® examination. Analyzing your performance on several practice exams will help you focus your final preparation on your weakest areas.

Other Helpful Features

Appendix A is a list of abbreviations and acronyms used in this book and common in critical care. Each term is always spelled out in the text the first time it is used, but this appendix will help you identify abbreviations later if you don't remember them. Appendix B lists laboratory studies important in the care of critically ill adults, including the normal range of values for each. I recommend that you study this list just before taking the exam since you are expected to know common normal laboratory values. Appendix C is a list of formulae commonly used in the evaluation of critically ill patients.

This book is not a comprehensive critical care textbook, nor is it intended to be. Instead, I've focused selectively on the information likely to be covered on the CCRN® examination. I believe *Pass CCRN®!* is the only book you need to prepare for the examination, but if you would like an additional text to strengthen your knowledge of particular areas, I recommend *Critical Care Nursing: Diagnosis and Management*, by Linda D. Urden, Kathleen Stacy, and Mary Lough, published by Elsevier.

Critical care nursing has never been more exciting. For those of us who thrive on this challenge, keeping up with new research and clinical developments is a continual test of our mettle. CCRN® certification is a prestigious credential for those of us who specialize in critical care nursing. I am confident that, if you study this book and use the Evolve website to practice your test-taking skills, you will pass the examination.

I would love to hear from you about your success with the examination, how this book helped you, and how you feel it could be even more useful. E-mail me at rddennison@aol.com or write to me at the following address:

Robin Donohoe Dennison, DNP, APRN, CCNS, CEN, CNE
c/o Nursing Editorial
Elsevier
3251 Riverport Drive
Maryland Heights, MO 63043

I believe that this book will be your most valuable resource in preparing for the CCRN® examination. Good luck!

Robin Donohoe Dennison

Acknowledgments

As I mentioned recently to Tamara Myers, who manages Elsevier's critical care nursing books, I have been fortunate to have a great team for this edition. In addition to the pleasure of working with Tamara, who must be the kindest and most patient editor alive, my developmental editor, Tina Kaemmerer, and my production editor, Bridget Healy have been an absolute pleasure to work with through the long and arduous process of getting this updated version available to you.

I also thank the many clinical consultants who critically reviewed each chapter from last edition and made suggestions for changes for this edition. I also appreciate the clinical consultants who critically reviewed every practice question and suggested revision and rewrite to make this current and consistent with the CCRN examination.

Finally, once again, I thank my husband and the love of my life, R. Russell Dennison, Jr. His love and support have helped me realize personal and professional goals and this fourth edition is yet another manifestation of his encouragement. I am truly blessed.

CONTENTS

PASS **CCRN®!**

The Critical Care Certification Examination

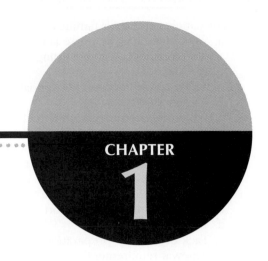

Certification

Definition

Process by which a nongovernmental agency (e.g., American Association of Critical-Care Nurses [AACN]) validates an individual nurse's qualification and knowledge for practice in a defined functional or clinical area of nursing; this validation is based upon predetermined standards of practice (AACN, 2010)

Purpose

1. Assurance of competence
   a. Competence is "the application of knowledge and the interpersonal, decision-making, and psychomotor skills expected for the nurse's practice role, within the context of public health, welfare, and safety" (National Council of State Boards of Nursing, 1996, page 5)
   b. Continued competence refers to the maintenance of adequate knowledge and skills for safe ongoing practice that occurs after the initial demonstration of competence at the time of licensure (National Council of State Boards of Nursing, 1996)
2. Protection of consumers (Kaplow, 2011)
   a. Licensure
      1) Indicates a minimum level of knowledge
      2) Granted by a governmental agency (e.g., state board of nursing)
      3) Usually renewed annually or biannually
   b. Certification
      1) Indicates an expert level of knowledge
      2) Granted by a nongovernmental agency (e.g., nursing specialty organization)
      3) Usually renewed every 3-5 years

Benefits of Achieving CCRN® Certification

1. For the nurse
   a. Self-satisfaction and validation of your knowledge and clinical judgment in your chosen nursing specialty
   b. Recognition and respect of others
   c. Professional challenge and motivation to update and maintain your knowledge base
   d. Career mobility: national certification is as prestigious in one state as another
   e. Clinical advancement and promotion
      1) Most critical care unit nurse managers encourage their nursing staff to become certified, and the majority prefers to hire certified nurses over noncertified nurses when other qualifications are equal (Stromborg et al., 2005).
      2) Certification is often recommended or required for promotion up a clinical career ladder.
   f. Financial remuneration
      1) Some hospitals offer a bonus for CCRN® certification.
      2) Some hospitals offer an hourly differential for CCRN® certification.
      3) Some hospitals prefer certified nurses for clinical or administrative promotion.
      4) Most hospitals reimburse the nurse for the expense of taking the test if a passing score is attained (Teal, 2011).
   g. Certified nurses are more likely to feel empowered (Fitzpatrick, Campo, Graham, and Lavandero, 2010).
   h. Continued practice in critical care: Some hospitals require CCRN® certification to continue to practice in critical care settings.
2. For the institution
   a. Assurance to the general public that the nurse is competent
   b. Evidence of excellence for marketing and awards such as Magnet Recognition Program by the American Nurses Credentialing Corporation (ANCC), AACN Beacon Award for Critical Care Excellence, or Malcolm Baldridge National Quality Award
   c. Financial incentives from insurance carriers
   d. Improved retention of nurses (Fitzpatrick et al., 2010)

3. For patients and their families
   a. Assurance that the nurse is currently competent and knowledgeable regarding critical care nursing
   b. Improved patient safety (Kendall-Gallagher and Blegen, 2009)
   c. Improves competence in detecting signs and symptoms of complications and initiating prompt intervention (Cary, 2001)
4. Perceived barriers (Teal, 2011; Altman, 2011)
   a. Cost of the examination
   b. Fear of testing and/or failure
   c. Lack of institutional support
   d. Lack of rewards
   e. Lack of time for preparation and maintenance of renewal requirements
   f. Lack of experience

The Synergy Model

The Synergy Model serves as the organizing framework for the certification examinations offered by the American Association of Critical-Care Nurses Certification Corporation (AACN, 2010). (Figure 1-1)

Definition of Synergy

"[A]n evolving phenomenon that occurs when individuals work together in mutually enhancing ways toward a common goal" (AACN, 2010)

Core Concept

The needs or characteristics of patients and families influence and drive the characteristics or competencies of nurses.

1. Nursing practice should be based on the needs of the patient and family.
2. Patients with more complex needs require nurses with advanced knowledge and skills.
3. The desired result is optimal outcomes for the patient, the nurse, and the system.

Assumptions

1. Patients are biologic, psychological, social, and spiritual entities who present at a particular developmental stage.
2. The patient, family, and community all contribute to providing a context for the nurse-patient relationship.
3. Patients can be described by a number of characteristics.
   a. Resiliency: the capacity to return to a restorative level of functioning using compensatory coping mechanisms; the ability to bounce back quickly after an insult
   b. Vulnerability: susceptibility to actual or potential stressors that may adversely affect patient outcomes
   c. Stability: the ability to maintain a steady-state equilibrium
   d. Complexity: the intricate entanglement of two or more systems (e.g., body, family, therapies)
   e. Resource availability: extent of resources (e.g., technical, fiscal, personal, psychological, social)
   f. Participation in care: extent to which the patient and family engage in aspects of care
   g. Participation in decision making: extent to which the patient and family engage in decision making
   h. Predictability: a summative characteristic that allows one to expect a certain trajectory of illness
4. Nurses can be described in a number of dimensions.
   a. Clinical judgment: clinical reasoning, which includes clinical decision making, critical thinking, and a global grasp of the situation, coupled with nursing skills acquired through a process of integrating formal and experiential knowledge

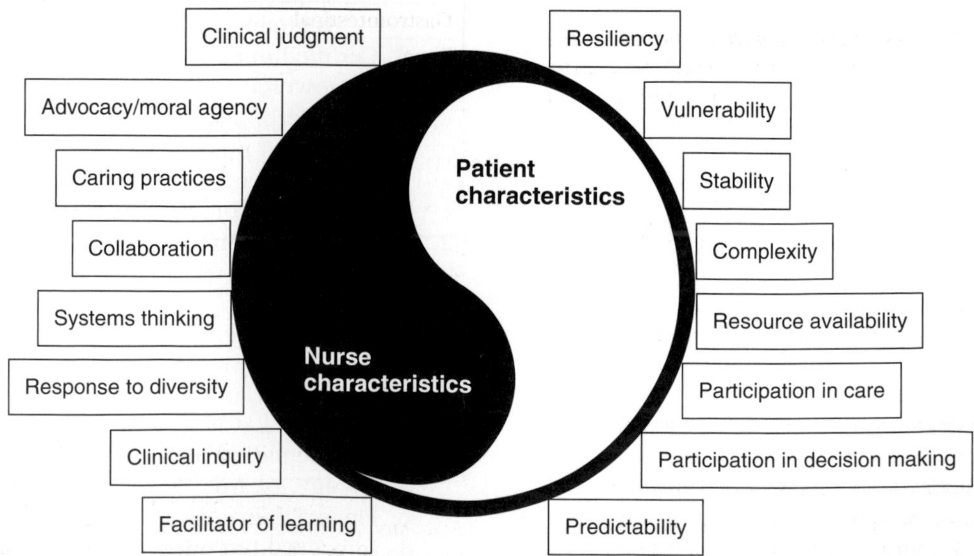

Figure 1-1 The Synergy Model with patient and nurse characteristics.

b. Advocacy/moral agency: working on another's behalf and representing the concerns of the patient, family, and community; serving as a moral agent in identifying and helping to resolve ethical and clinical concerns within the clinical setting
   1) Nurses are expected to read, understand, and observe the American Nurses Association Code of Ethics which is available at *http://nursingworld.org/ethics/code/protected_nwcoe629.htm*
c. Caring practices: the constellation of nursing activities that are responsive to the uniqueness of the patient and family and that create a compassionate and therapeutic environment, with the aim of promoting comfort and preventing suffering
d. Collaboration: working with others in a way that promotes and encourages each person's contributions toward achieving optimal and realistic patient goals; collaboration involves intradisciplinary and interdisciplinary work with all colleagues
e. Systems thinking: the body of knowledge and tools that allow the nurse to appreciate the care environment from a perspective that recognizes the holistic interrelationship that exists within and across health care systems
f. Response to diversity: the sensitivity to recognize, appreciate, and incorporate differences into the provision of care
g. Clinical inquiry or innovator/evaluator: the ongoing process of questioning and evaluating practice, providing informed practice, and innovating through research and experiential learning
h. Facilitator of learning as patient/family educator: the ability to facilitate patient and family learning

5. A goal of nursing is to restore a patient to an optimal level of wellness as defined by the patient.

While this model serves as the theoretical model for the CCRN® examination, you are not tested regarding knowledge of the synergy model or terminology; you are tested on application of the model.

The Adult CCRN® Examination

Basic Information about the CCRN® Examination

1. Critical care is considered to be at the most acute end of the critical care continuum; patients in critical care
   a. Are unstable and complex
   b. Require intense resources such as staffing, monitoring, and supplies
      1) Frequently require invasive hemodynamic monitoring, intravenous medication titration, and mechanical ventilation
   c. Require persistent nursing vigilance
2. The test is designed to evaluate your understanding of the common body of knowledge needed to function effectively in a critical care setting.
   a. The test consists of 150 multiple-choice questions to be completed within three hours; 25 of these items are not scored but are test items for the development of future exams.
   b. The questions relate to patient problems unique to critical care and to nationally recognized practice with the focus being on clinical decision making rather than memorization and recall.
3. Blueprint for the CCRN® examination (Table 1-1)
   a. The blueprint identifies the categories tested and the percentage of questions in each category.
   b. The blueprint is based on a Role Delineation/CCRN® Validation Study conducted by the AACN in 2003; in essence, this study identified tasks, knowledge, and experiences required of a registered nurse practicing in a critical care setting and what should be on the examination.
   c. The blueprint identifies what percentage of questions is in each area as well as what disease entities are on the examination.
      1) NOTE: This book includes only content and disease entities that are on the blueprint and the examination; although it may be important to understand myxedema coma, it is not on the blueprint, not on the

Table 1-1 Blueprint for the CCRN® Examination Indicating Distribution of Questions on Each Section

Clinical Judgment	**80%**
Cardiovascular	20%
Pulmonary	18%
Neurology	12%
Multisystem	8%
Gastrointestinal	6%
Renal	6%
Endocrine	5%
Behavioral/Psychosocial	4%
Hematology/Immunology	2%
Professional Caring and Ethical Practice	**20%**
Advocacy/Moral Agency	3%
Caring Practices	4%
Collaboration	4%
Systems Thinking	2%
Response to Diversity	2%
Clinical Inquiry	2%
Facilitatory of Learning	3%

The sum of these percentages is not 100 due to rounding.
From American Association of Critical-Care Nurses. (2010). Certification exam handbook. Retrieved July 11, 2010, from *http://www.aacn.org/WD/Certifications/Docs/certexamhandbook.pdf*

examination, and not in this book; focus on what is on the blueprint and the examination.

Cognitive Levels of Questions

1. Knowledge questions require you to remember previously learned information.
2. Comprehension questions require you to understand the information.
3. Application questions require you to use information.
4. Analysis questions require you to break down information into its component parts and recognize commonalities, differences, and interrelationships.
5. Synthesis questions require you to put parts of information together to form a new conclusion.
6. Evaluation questions require you to judge the value of information.
7. Questions on the examinations are distributed across these cognitive levels but the majority of the questions are at the application and analysis levels (AACN, 2010).

Distribution of Questions Related to the Nursing Process

All phases of nursing process are included on the examination.

Passing Score

1. The passing score for these examinations is approximately 70%.
2. About two thirds of nurses taking the CCRN® examination for the first time pass the exam; nurses retaking the test for recertification have a higher passing rate.

For more specific information about the examinations, the application and application process, and the testing process, download the Certification Examination Handbook at *http://www.aacn.org/WD/Certifications/Docs/certexamhandbook.pdf*

Plan for Passing the CCRN® Examination (Figure 1-2)

Permission to Take the Examination

1. Requirements (AACN, 2010)
   a. Current unrestricted RN license in the U.S. or in any of its territories that use the NCLEX® for RN licensure
   b. Clinical practice in critical care: 1750 hours within the previous two-year period with 875 of the hours accrued in the most recent year preceding application to take the examination
      1) CCRN® certification is a clinical credential and you must maintain a clinical practice to maintain your certification.
      2) Eligible hours are those spent caring for adult patients in a critical care setting; examples include intensive (or critical) care units, cardiac care units, combined ICU-CCUs, medical and/or surgical ICUs, trauma critical care units, neurologic critical care units, or critical care transport.

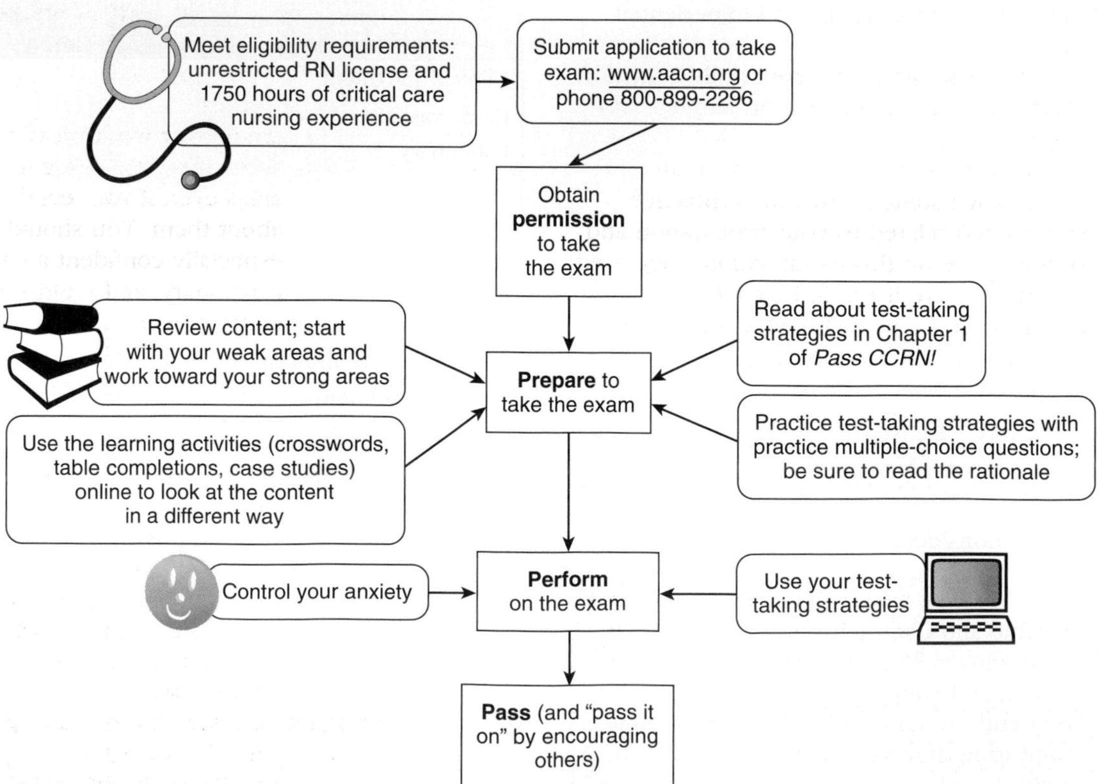

Figure 1-2 Plan for Passing the CCRN® Examination.

3) Other settings may also be considered "critical care" depending on the characteristics of the patient population cared for in the setting; AACN can assist you in determining your eligibility to take the exam.

c. BSN is not a requirement: Although the American Nurses' Credentialing Corporation (ANCC) requires a BSN to sit for some of its certification examinations, the AACN Certification Corporation is not a member of the American Nurses' Credentialing Corporation and does not require a BSN to sit for the CCRN® examination.

2. To obtain an application, contact the AACN Certification Corporation
   a. Website: *http://www.aacn.org/DM/Certifications/CertificationCenter.aspx?type=certificationcenter*
   b. Phone: (800) 899-2226
   c. Email: certcorp@aacn.org
3. After completion of the application process, approval to take the exam is received by mail; you must schedule testing within the next 90 days.
   a. Computer-based testing is available most weekdays year-round; a pencil and paper version is available only once a year at the location of the AACN National Teaching Institute.
   b. The computerized form of the test is administered by Applied Measurement Professionals (AMP) at their testing centers nationwide.

Preparation for the Exam

1. Be positive!
   a. Avoid negative self-talk; "I'll never pass this exam" can be a self-fulfilling prophecy because you begin to believe it.
   b. Practice positive self-talk.
      1) Write down some affirmations (positive statements) related to your preparation and performance on this examination; suggested affirmations are listed in Box 1-1.
      2) Say these and other affirmations that you have written over and over again throughout your preparation time; say them like you believe them and you will!
      3) Record your affirmations on audiotape and play them often; play them in the car, while you walk or do dishes, or any other time when you can listen and repeat them.
2. Schedule the examination.
   a. Complete the application and send it to the AACN Certification Corporation.
   b. You will be sent an authorization letter indicating that you meet the requirements to take the examination, along with instructions on how to schedule the examination.
      1) Call the testing service to schedule your examination date and time; you must schedule the examination within 90 days of the date printed on your authorization letter.
      2) This flexibility in scheduling allows you to avoid scheduling conflicts between the examination and major life events such as a family wedding, graduation, or birth.
      3) Schedule the time of the examination according to when you do your best thinking or are most productive: Schedule for morning if you are a lark or afternoon if you are an owl.
   c. DO SCHEDULE THE EXAM so that you have a target date; you can reschedule up to 4 business days prior to the scheduled test day if something comes up that interferes with your ability to complete the examination on the scheduled day.
3. Prepare for the test.
   a. Establish a realistic schedule for your preparation; 1-2-hour time slots are probably the most helpful.
      1) Study examination content: Plan to review a system per evening, day, or weekend, depending on how much time you have left before the examination.
         a) Set priorities.
            i) Study your weak areas first.
            ii) Study the large percentage content areas even if you feel confident about them: You should feel especially confident about cardiac, pulmonary, and multisystem content because these three areas constitute 57% of the examination.
         b) Review content using this review book.
            i) Highlight areas that you do not feel confident about; you may need to refer to more comprehensive critical care texts or articles when you need additional clarification.
            ii) Complete the learning activities at the end of each chapter to consolidate your knowledge by looking at the information in another way.
         c) Practice using your test-taking skills by doing practice questions.
            i) In addition to looking at the answer, read the rationale;

Box 1-1 Affirmations

I understand the information important for this examination.
I am a knowledgeable critical care nurse.
I feel prepared for this exam.
I am an excellent test-taker.
I will pass this exam.

remember that the question may not be written exactly the same as the practice question, but the concept may be on the examination.

ii) If you still do not understand why you missed the question, refer back to the section in this book or a critical care text to understand why the correct answer is better than your answer.

iii) In addition to looking at the answer and the rationale, read the test-taking strategy; this information will help you identify how to approach a similar question to which you do not know the answer.

iv) Analyze why you missed a question; consider:

(a) Did you not know the content? Study this content again.

(b) Did you misread the question? Slow down and read the question more thoroughly.

(c) Did you misread the options? Slow down and read all of the options and select the best one.

(d) Did you miss an important element such as age, diagnosis, or parameter? Again, slow down and read the question carefully; mentally highlight the critical points in the case study that you feel are important.

(e) Did you read into the question?

(i) Do not assume information that is not given; take the question at face value.

(ii) Do not assume that the question is intended to "trick" you, there are no "trick" questions on the practice exam questions on the website associated with this book or on the CCRN® exam.

d) Study in a quiet place with minimal distractions.

i) Turn off the television, radio, and stereo; let the answering machine and voice mail pick up phone calls.

ii) Avoid getting too comfortable; sit upright at a desk or table so that you can spread out your study materials; avoid trying to study while in bed or a recliner.

iii) Ensure adequate lighting.

iv) Reading, repeating, and writing are methods that improve remembering.

v) Use margins to write down memory joggers or additional thoughts.

b. If you like study groups, organize a study group of nurses who are also preparing for the CCRN® examination.

1) Include only members who will fulfill their obligation to participate.

2) Establish guidelines for the group.

a) When will you meet?

b) What will you do at the meetings?

i) A selected member may present essential content related to his or her specific area of interest.

ii) Members may collect resource materials related to the specified content area and distribute them to fellow members.

iii) Members may discuss review questions related to the specified content area.

c) What are the group members' expectations?

c. Create memory joggers.

1) Almost everyone knows "On Old Olympus' Towering Tops A Fin And German Viewed Some Hops" to remember the 12 cranial nerves; establish others that help you identify things that you have trouble remembering.

d. Remember case study links: For example, you remember a patient with a triglyceride level over 2000 mg/dL who developed acute pancreatitis, and then ARDS helps you remember that a major risk factor for acute pancreatitis is hypertriglyceridemia and that a major complication of acute pancreatitis is ARDS.

4. Take a practice test one week before the examination; use this test to identify weak areas for final study time.

a. Analyze which categories (systems) are your weakest and strongest.

b. Analyze which cognitive level question is the most difficult for you.

c. Analyze which component of the nursing process is most difficult for you.

5. Final preparations

a. Don't cram the night before the examination; cramming usually just decreases your self-confidence and increases your anxiety.

b. Go to bed at your usual time; if you go to bed early, you probably won't go to sleep anyway and will just worry about the test.

c. Do not consume alcohol or other sedating drugs the night before or the day of the examination.
d. Choose comfortable clothes that allow layering so you can remove or add clothing in response to the room temperature; wear bright colors (e.g., yellow, red, hot pink, orange) to project a more optimistic image.
e. Take a watch, a sweater, tissue, and hard candy; don't forget your glasses if you wear them.
f. Eat a healthy but light meal before the examination; avoid simple carbohydrates such as a doughnut or Danish pastry; rather eat peanut butter on whole wheat toast or an egg sandwich to sustain you through the exam.
g. Be sure to take two forms of identification with one of them being government-issued photo identification that contains a signature.
h. Make sure that you know where the testing site is located and how long it will take to get there considering traffic at the time your test is scheduled; getting lost or just having to rush to arrive on time, causes anxiety and may affect your performance.
i. Plan to arrive 15 minutes before your scheduled appointment; if you arrive later than 15 minutes after the scheduled testing time, you may not be admitted.
j. Take the time to visit the restroom before you check in.

Performance During the Examination

1. Control of anxiety
   a. Remember that some anxiety increases your performance; panic does not.
   b. Feeling adequately prepared decreases anxiety; take the time to prepare for this examination, including practicing your test-taking strategies.
   c. Use visualization: See yourself receiving your passing score.
   d. Use deep breathing and/or progressive muscle relaxation.
      1) Deep breathing is performed by putting your hand below your costal margin and breathing deeply enough to raise your hand; focus on your breathing instead of anything else.
         a) Use this method at any time during the examination when you feel frustrated or stressed.
      2) Progressive muscle relaxation is performed by contracting a group of muscles and then relaxing it: leg, leg, arm, arm, back, face.
         a) Use this technique in the car before you go in to take the examination and at any time during the examination when you feel tense.
   e. Use meditation or prayer depending on your religious beliefs: These techniques are also helpful in verbalizing your goals and desires.
   f. Don't let a memory lapse or a difficult question affect your attitude or throw you into panic mode; move on to the next question to which you are likely to know the answer.
2. Instructions are given at the beginning of the examination; take the time to read the instructions carefully.
3. Test-taking skills
   a. Reading questions thoroughly
      1) Mentally highlight key points as you read the question.
         a) Age and gender of the patient
         b) Setting: prehospital, emergency, critical care, progressive care, home care
         c) Medical diagnosis and other coexisting diagnoses
         d) Time frame in relation to admission, trauma, surgery, pain, medication, visitation
      2) Look for qualifying words such as:
         a) *All, most, some, few, none*
         b) *Always, usually, frequently, seldom, never*
         c) *First, last*
         d) *Best, worst*
         e) *Most, least*
         f) *Smallest, largest*
         g) *Acute, chronic*
         h) *Partial, total*
         i) *Early, late*
         j) Answers that include global answers such as *all, always, never,* or *none* are seldom the correct answer.
      3) Pay particular attention to negative words such as *not, except, contraindicated, inappropriate.*
      4) Read all the options as well as the stem.
      5) After you read the stem, answer the question without looking at the options; if your answer is there, it's probably right; however, still go ahead and read all options—there may be one better than your answer.
   b. Choosing the correct answer
      1) Make sure that you understand what the question really is; answer *the* question, not just *a* question.
      2) Always choose the best answer; even if there are two answers that you consider correct, choose the one that best answers the question being asked.
         a) If more than one option appears correct, look for the most comprehensive option.
      3) Assumptions
         a) Do not assume information that is not given; the only assumption is an ideal situation unless the question indicates otherwise.
         b) All important information is included.
            i) Do not read into the question such as "maybe she's a diabetic" or

"maybe he has COPD"; if information is important to the question, it would be included
   c) Included information is probably important.
      i) Extraneous information is not usually included, so if the case study or question gives you information that you feel is extraneous or superfluous, ask yourself why this information was given and how it is important to this situation.
4) Answer questions according to national standards of care and national guidelines rather than regional, local, or specific physician's practices.
5) Select options that are therapeutic based on evidence and show respect and acceptance for the patient and the family; eliminate options that are based on tradition rather than science and options that are inappropriate, disrespectful, or punitive.
6) Repetition of a word or a synonym of the word in the stem and an option may help you to identify the correct answer.
7) If the answers are numbers or number ranges, the extremes are less likely to be the correct option than the middle number or number range.
8) This exam is computerized and answers are random; therefore, C is no more likely to be the correct answer than A, B, or D; also, there are no patterns to the answers, so don't look for one.

c. Answering priority questions
   1) Priority one is always whatever must be done to prevent death; always follow the ABC order: airway, then breathing, and finally circulation.
   2) Priority two is whatever must be done to prevent disability or serious complication; consider this D for disability.
   3) Priority three is pain or discomfort; if nothing in the case study or question could cause death or disability, pain should be considered the priority.
   4) Actual problems always take precedence over potential problems; for example, actual hypoxemia takes precedence over potential oxygen toxicity.
   5) If there are two potential problems, the priority is the one that is more likely to cause death or disability.

d. Answering questions where the answers have multiple answers (also referred to as multiple/multiples)
   1) If the option has more than one answer (such as x and y or even w, x, y, and z), both or all of the answers must be correct for the option to be correct.
   2) Elimination works well with this type of question; if there is one answer in the option that is incorrect, that option may be eliminated.

e. Guessing
   1) Don't leave any question blank; unanswered questions are counted as incorrect so you should never not answer a question even if you must guess.
   2) You are not penalized for guessing, but it should be used only as a last resort.
   3) First eliminate any choices that you can; it is better to guess between two choices than to guess between four.
      a) Eliminate clearly wrong answers.
      b) Eliminate any response that has no relationship to the question.
      c) Eliminate similar options that say essentially the same thing because they cannot both be correct.
      d) *All, always, never, none,* or *only* options are usually incorrect.
   4) If you cannot even eliminate to two, then look for the option that is different from the others; for example:
      a) Three antibiotics and an antifungal, choose the antifungal option
      b) Three beta-blockers and a calcium channel blocker, choose the calcium channel blocker
      c) Three very specific and one very comprehensive option, choose the comprehensive option
   5) If you are unsure of your answer and want to look at it again:
      a) Go ahead and answer it with your first impression.
      b) Click on "mark" at the bottom of the screen so that you can go back to it at the end of the exam.
      c) At the end of the exam, the computer allows you to go back to these marked items and review them.
      d) Review the question again during this review process and see if there is something in the question that changes your answer about the correct answer.
      e) Once you are set on the correct answer you want to submit for that question, "unmark" it and then continue to the end of the examination.

f. Changing answers
   1) You may have been told to never change answers and you should not change an answer unless you have a good reason for changing it; one good reason is that you missed a negative qualifier, such as *not, except,* or *contraindicated*, when you read it the first time.
   2) If may be helpful to change answers in a different color when doing a practice test;

then evaluate how many you changed from wrong to right and how many you changed from right to wrong.
   a) If you change more from wrong to right, you most likely miss questions because you don't read them thoroughly so when you realize that you misread a question, then by all means change your answer.
   b) If you change more from right to wrong, don't change your initial answer (unless you realize in this case that you had misread the question) because first impressions tend to be correct more often.

g. Answering math questions
   1) Math questions are usually drug calculations, such as dopamine in micrograms per kilogram per minute, but could be other critical care calculations.
   2) You are allowed to use the computer calculator and you are provided with scratch paper and pencil.
   3) Recheck your math if you have time.

h. Maintaining concentration
   1) Write down things such as formulae, normal values, and toxic levels that you are afraid that you might forget on your scratch paper before you do the first question.
   2) Change your process of reading the case study, the question, and the options.
      a) Read the options in reverse order from option *d* to option *a*. Use this action especially when you suspect that option *a* or *b* is the correct option.
      b) Make this change every 25 to 50 questions OR
         i) When you are physically tired, mentally anxious, or lose your concentration abilities
         ii) When you come to the easier or the more difficult questions
   3) Rephrase the question rather than rereading the same question over and over.
   4) Use three slow deep breaths to regroup and get refocused at any time.
   5) Sign out and go to the restroom and splash water on your face if you are losing your ability to concentrate, but remember that the clock does not stop during this time.

i. Budgeting your time
   1) If you are a slow test-taker, you may run short on time but more likely you will run out of mental energy because concentration for a 2-3-hour period is very difficult.
   2) You should try to be at least halfway through the examination in 75 minutes; this halfway point will leave you some time to recheck your math and go back to the marked items.
   3) One helpful technique to save time is to read the question (at end of case study) and then go back and read the case study; since we frequently read the case study, then the question at the end of the case study, and then reread the case study, this technique saves you time by knowing what you are looking for in the case study.
   4) Do not be distressed by people finishing before you; we all take examinations at different speeds, and the others may not even be taking the AACN Certification Corporation examinations because several exams are given at the same place and same time.

Pass and Pass It On

1. Test Results: You will be given your test results at the completion of computerized testing and within 6-8 weeks by mail for pencil and paper testing.
2. If you pass
   a. Use your new credential proudly.
      1) You should display your credential on your hospital name badge.
      2) You should proudly write it after RN when you sign your name; CCRN® is not written with periods so, for example, it is written as Your Name, RN, CCRN.
   b. Pass it on by encouraging others to become certified; offer to tutor, mentor, and share study materials to assist your colleagues to become certified too.
3. If you fail, try again!
   a. Reasons for failing the examination
      1) Knowledge deficit
         a) Prepare to take the examination even if you feel that you are an experienced critical care nurse because we all have our chosen areas of interest and our weak areas.
         b) Use this book to review the content for the examination and complete the learning activities at the end of each chapter.
         c) Take a practice examination 1 week before the examination to identify your weak areas; use your final study time focusing on those weak areas.
      2) Testing errors
         a) Practice using your test-taking skills with the questions on the CD-ROM included with this book, and pay close attention to both the rationale and the test-taking strategy included with each question.
         b) Use the learned test-taking strategies during the CCRN® examination.
      3) Test anxiety and negative thinking: Believe in your ability to pass the exam and control your anxiety with prayer, meditation, deep breathing, and/or progressive relaxation.

b. You will likely do better the next time because the fear of the unknown is now gone and you know clearly what your weak areas are from the score breakdown that was given to you as you left the testing site.

4) Prepare by focusing on your weak areas and then reapply to take the test again.

Maintaining Your CCRN® Certification

Certification as a CCRN® is for a 3-year period.

Recertification

Recertification is achieved by providing evidence of continued practice (432 hours over the 3-year period with 144 of those hours accrued in the year prior to recertification) and retaking the examination or submitting the appropriate information about your continuing education and professional activities for review for renewal.

LEARNING ACTIVITIES

CHAPTER 1

1. What are your personal reasons for becoming CCRN® certified?
   a. ______________________________
   b. ______________________________
   c. ______________________________

2. List your top five life priorities for the next year. Is CCRN® certification on this list? What is the ranking for CCRN® certification?
   1st ______________________________
   2nd ______________________________
   3rd ______________________________
   4th ______________________________
   5th ______________________________

3. Prioritize this list from 1 (least comfortable) to 10 (most comfortable). Use this list to schedule your preparation with 1 being first and 10 being last.

Knowledge Area	Comfort Level
Cardiovascular	
Professional caring and ethical practice	
Pulmonary	
Neurology	
Multisystem	
Gastrointestinal	
Renal	
Endocrine	
Behavioral/Psychosocial	
Hematology/immunology	

4. Describe your plan to prepare for the CCRN® examination.
   a. Identify how many study days you have until the day that you have scheduled your examination.
   ____
   b. Decide if content review, case studies, or practice questions are the most effective method for you.
   ____
   c. Set up a schedule for your study with your weakest content areas scheduled early.
   ____

5. Explore the AACN website (www.aacn.org) focusing on the Certification tab.

6. List three new test-taking strategies that you have learned from this chapter and will use while taking the CCRN® examination.

a. ______________________________

b. ______________________________

c. ______________________________

Web Resources	
Website Address	**Resources Available**
www.aacn.org	Complete blueprint Application Information about the Synergy Model
http://nursingworld.org/ethics/code/protected_nwcoe629.htm	ANA Code of Ethics
www.robindennison.com	Free presentation on preparing for and performing on the CCRN exam

The Cardiovascular System: Physiology and Assessment

CHAPTER 2

Selected Concepts in Anatomy and Physiology

General Information about the Cardiovascular System

1. The cardiovascular system is a continuous, fluid-filled elastic circuit with a pump.
2. The cardiovascular system provides communication between all body parts through transportation of oxygen, nutrients, hormones, water, enzymes, vitamins, minerals, buffers, leukocytes, antibodies, and wastes; these functions maintain dynamic equilibrium to maintain homeostasis.
3. The cardiovascular system consists of the heart and vascular system.

The Heart

1. Bioelectrically driven, muscular, four-chamber organ that provides forward propulsion of blood into the vascular system
2. Size of a closed fist: usually approximately 9 cm wide and 12 cm long; weighs approximately 4 g/kg of ideal body weight
3. Lies in the mediastinum between the sternum (anterior) and the spine (posterior) with two thirds of the heart to the left of the midline and one third of the heart to the right of the midline (Figure 2-1)
4. Shaped like a blunt cone
   a. Apex
      1) Inferior, anterior, and to the left
      2) Normally at fifth left intercostal space (LICS) at the midclavicular line (MCL)
      3) On the upper surface of the diaphragm
   b. Base
      1) Superior, posterior, and to the right
      2) Normally at level of second intercostal space
5. Layers of the cardiac wall (Figure 2-2)
   a. Pericardium: maintains the heart in a stationary position
      1) Fibrous
         a) Loose-fitting, white fibrous layer
         b) Acts as a barrier against infection and neoplastic invasion
      2) Serous
         a) Parietal layer: lines inner surface of fibrous pericardium
         b) Visceral layer: lines the surface of the heart; synonymous with epicardium
      3) Pericardial space
         a) Located between the parietal and visceral layers of the serous pericardium
         b) Contains 10-30 mL of lubricating fluid
            i) Protects the heart against friction and erosion
            ii) Provides a well-lubricated sac in which the heart moves during contraction
   b. Epicardium: synonymous with visceral layer of serous pericardium
   c. Epicardial fat
      1) Thin layer of adipose tissue between the visceral pericardium and the epicardium
      2) Increased in obesity
      3) May increase risk of coronary artery disease
   d. Myocardium
      1) Largest portion of the cardiac wall
      2) Consists of the following:
         a) Specialized conduction fibers
         b) Interlacing cardiac muscle fibers
   e. Endocardium
      1) Consists of the following:
         a) Connective tissue
         b) Elastic fibers
         c) Endothelial cells
            i) Form a smooth surface for blood contact
            ii) Deter clot formation
      2) Contiguous with the lining of the great vessels
      3) Lines the heart chambers and valves
6. Cardiac skeleton
   a. Composed of continuous dense connective tissue
   b. Located at the base of the heart and in the interventricular septum

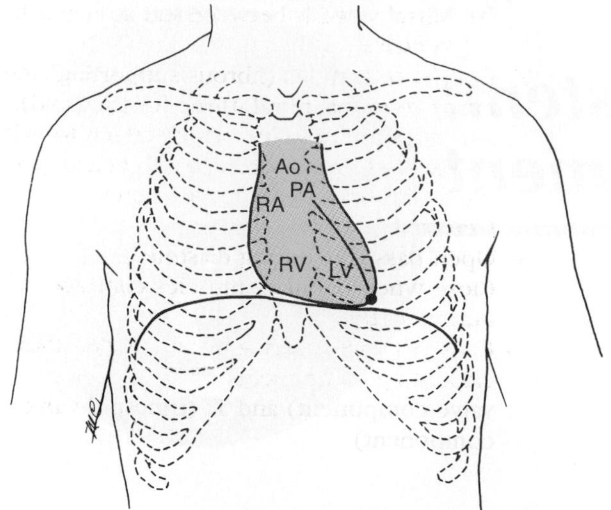

Figure 2-1 Location and orientation of the heart chambers and great vessels within the thorax. *Ao,* Aorta; *PA,* pulmonary artery; *RA,* right atrium; *RV,* right ventricle; *LV,* left ventricle. (From Price, S., & Wilson, L. [2003]. *Pathophysiology: Clinical concepts of disease processes* [6th ed.]. St. Louis: Mosby.)

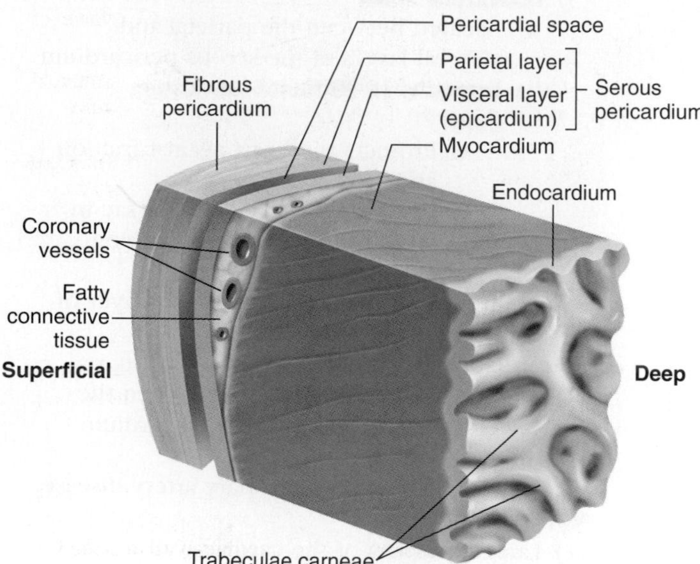

Figure 2-2 Layers of the cardiac wall. Note the fibrous pericardium, the parietal and visceral layers of the serous pericardium, the pericardial space between the two layers of the serous pericardium, the myocardium, and the endocardium. The visceral layer of the serous pericardium is also referred to as the epicardium. (From Patton, K. T., & Thibodeau, G. A. [2010]. *Anatomy & physiology* [7th ed.]. St. Louis: Mosby.)

c. Serves as the point of origin and insertion for cardiac muscle fibers
d. Supports the heart valves; includes the four valve rings (annuli)

7. Cardiac chambers (Figure 2-3)
   a. Atria
      1) Located posterior, superior, and to the right of the corresponding ventricles
      2) Contain the interatrial septum to divide left and right atria

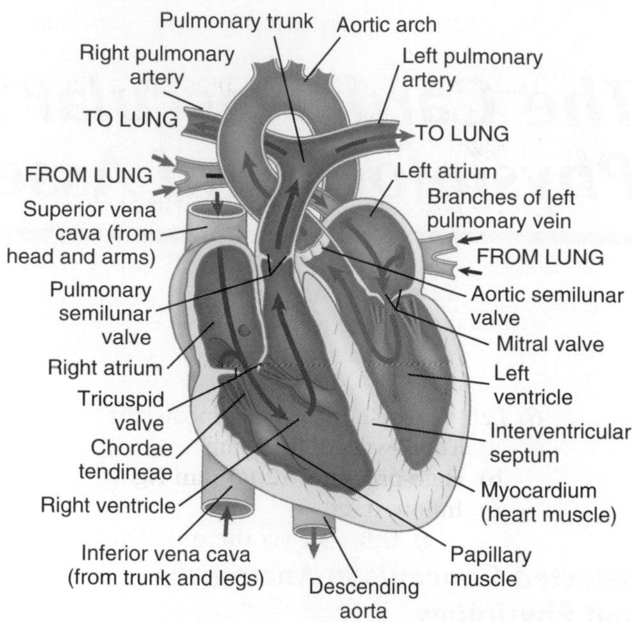

Figure 2-3 Cardiac chambers and the structures that direct blood flow through the heart. Arrows indicate path of blood flow through chambers, valves, and major vessels. (From McCance, K. L., & Huether, S. E. [2010]. *Pathophysiology: The biologic basis for disease in adults and children* [6th ed.]. St. Louis: Mosby.)

      3) Contain the trabeculae to divide atria and ventricles
      4) Thin-walled, low-pressure chambers
         a) Right: 2 mm thick, 2-6 mm Hg pressure
         b) Left: 3 mm thick, 8-12 mm Hg pressure
      5) Act as reservoirs and booster pumps for the ventricles
         a) Passive ventricular filling: 70-75% of ventricular filling is passive as blood falls through the atrium into the ventricle
         b) Active ventricular filling: 25-30% of ventricular filling is active as the atrium contracts at the end of ventricular diastole
      6) Right atria
         a) Inflow tracts
            i) Superior vena cava
            ii) Inferior vena cava
            iii) Coronary sinus
            iv) Thebesian veins
         b) Outflow tract: through the tricuspid valve to right ventricle
      7) Left atria
         a) Inflow tracts: four pulmonary veins (only case of veins carrying oxygenated blood)
         b) Outflow tract: through the mitral valve to left ventricle
   b. Ventricles
      1) Located anterior, inferior, and to the left of the corresponding atria
      2) Contain the interventricular septum to divide the left and right ventricles

3) Contain the trabeculae to divide atria and ventricles
4) Act as pumps receiving blood from the atria and pumping blood into the great vessels
5) Right ventricle
   a) Thin-walled: 3-5 mm
   b) Low-pressure pump: 25/5 mm Hg
   c) Inflow tract
      i) Right atria via the tricuspid valve
      ii) Thebesian veins
   d) Outflow tract: pulmonary artery (only case of artery carrying deoxygenated blood)
6) Left ventricle: positioned posterior
   a) Thick-walled: 8-15 mm
   b) High-pressure: 120/5 mm Hg
   c) Inflow tract
      i) Left atria via the mitral valve
      ii) Thebesian veins
   d) Outflow tract: aorta

8. Cardiac valves (Figure 2-4)
   a. Purpose: maintain unidirectional flow
      1) Permit antegrade flow; narrowing of the valvular orifice preventing normal antegrade flow is referred to as *stenosis*
      2) Prevent retrograde flow: inadequate closure of the valvular orifice allowing retrograde flow is referred to as *regurgitant, incompetent,* or *insufficient*
   b. Structure of cardiac valves (Figure 2-5)
      1) Flexible, fibrous tissue
      2) Rings of connective tissue support the valves
   c. Atrioventricular (AV) valves: tricuspid and mitral valves
      1) Located between atria and ventricles
         a) Tricuspid valve is between right atria and right ventricle.
         b) Mitral valve is between left atria and left ventricle.
      2) Consist of annulus (fibrous supporting ring), cusps (two for mitral, three for tricuspid), and papillary muscles, which attach to valve cusps by chordae tendineae; the cusps are joined for 0.5-1.0 cm at the annulus (referred to as a *commissure*)
      3) Open passively during diastole
      4) Close when papillary muscles contract during systole
      5) Cause the first heart sound, S_1, when they close; two components of S_1: M_1 (mitral valve component) and T_1 (tricuspid valve component)

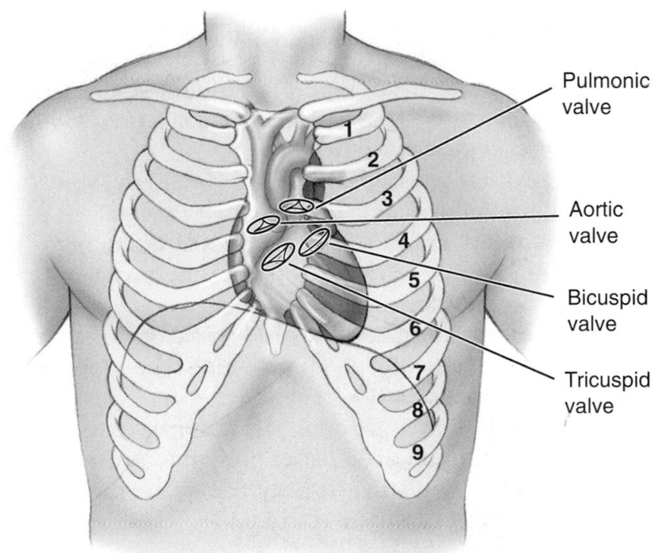

Figure 2-4 Location of the cardiac valves. (From Herlihy, B. [2011]. *The human body in health and illness* [4th ed.]. St. Louis: Saunders.)

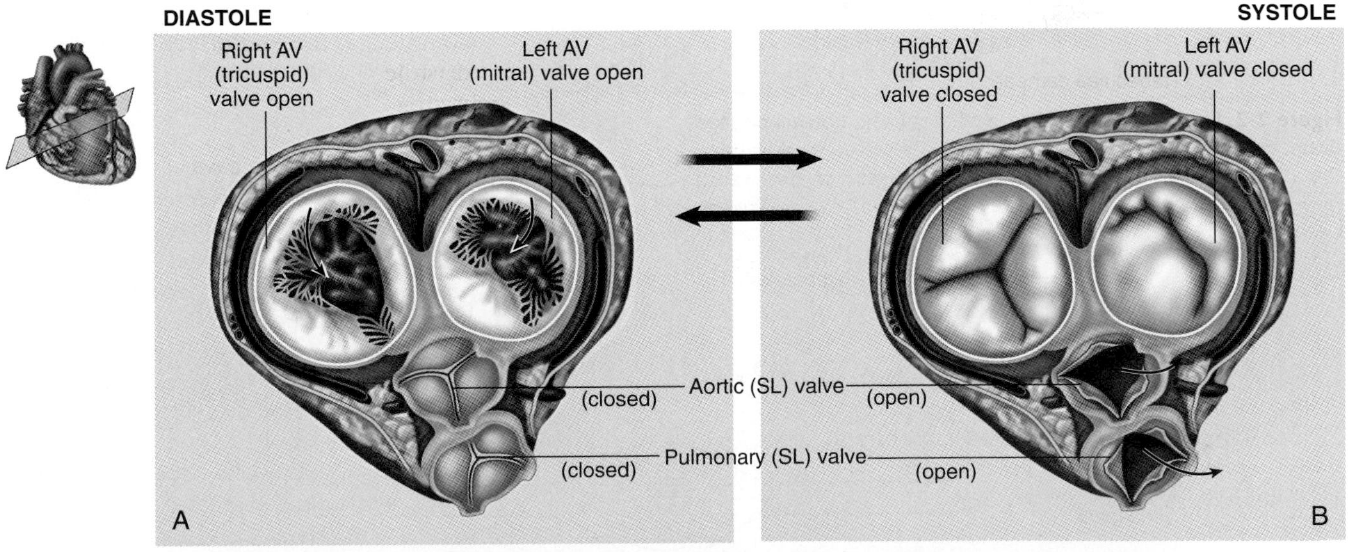

Figure 2-5 Structure of the cardiac valves, viewed from above. **A,** Ventricular diastole when semilunar valves are closed and atrioventricular valves are open. **B,** Ventricular systole when atrioventricular valves are closed and semilunar valves are open. (From Patton, K. T., & Thibodeau, G. A. [2010] *Anatomy & physiology* [7th ed.]. St. Louis: Mosby.)

d. Semilunar valves: aortic and pulmonic valves
   1) Located between ventricles and great vessels
      a) Pulmonic valve is located between the right ventricle and the pulmonary artery.
      b) Aortic valve is located between the left ventricle and the aorta.
   2) Consist of annulus and three cusps
   3) Function by pressure gradients: pushed open with systolic and closed with diastole
   4) Cause the second heart sound, S_2, when they close; two components of S_2: A_2 (aortic valve component) and P_2 (pulmonic valve component)

9. Pathway of blood through the heart and the vascular system: venae cavae (superior and inferior) → right atrium → tricuspid valve → right ventricle → pulmonic valve → pulmonary artery → pulmonary capillary bed → pulmonary veins → left atrium → mitral valve → left ventricle → aortic valve → aorta → arteries → arterioles → capillaries → venules → veins → venae cavae (Figure 2-6)

10. Coronary vasculature
   a. Coronary arteries are the first branch off the aorta, immediately outside the aortic valve.
   b. Coronary arteries lie on the epicardium, but branches penetrate through to the myocardium and subendocardium.
   c. The myocardium receives 5% of cardiac output and extracts 65-80% of oxygen in the blood even at basal rate.
      1) Blood flow through the coronary arteries is determined almost entirely by local autoregulation in response to the metabolic needs of the myocardium.
      2) Myocardial blood flow is increased by dilation of the coronary arteries.
   d. Coronary artery perfusion
      1) Effect of cardiac cycle
         a) The left ventricle is perfused primarily during diastole due to compression of musculature around intramuscular vessels during systole.
         b) The right ventricle is perfused throughout the cardiac cycle, but perfusion is greater during diastole.
      2) Effect of aortic pressure
         a) The pressure in the aorta immediately outside the aortic valve (referred to as *aortic root pressure*) is significant in coronary artery filling pressure.
         b) Coronary artery perfusion pressure (CAPP) is equal to the diastolic BP minus the pulmonary artery occlusive pressure (PAOP) (previously known as *pulmonary artery wedge pressure* or *pulmonary capillary wedge pressure*); normal CAPP is 60-80 mm Hg.
      3) Myocardial oxygen consumption (Figure 2-7)
         a) Determinants of myocardial oxygen demand include the following:
            i) Heart rate
            ii) Preload
            iii) Afterload
            iv) Contractility
         b) Determinants of myocardial oxygen supply include the following:
            i) Patent arteries
            ii) Diastolic pressure

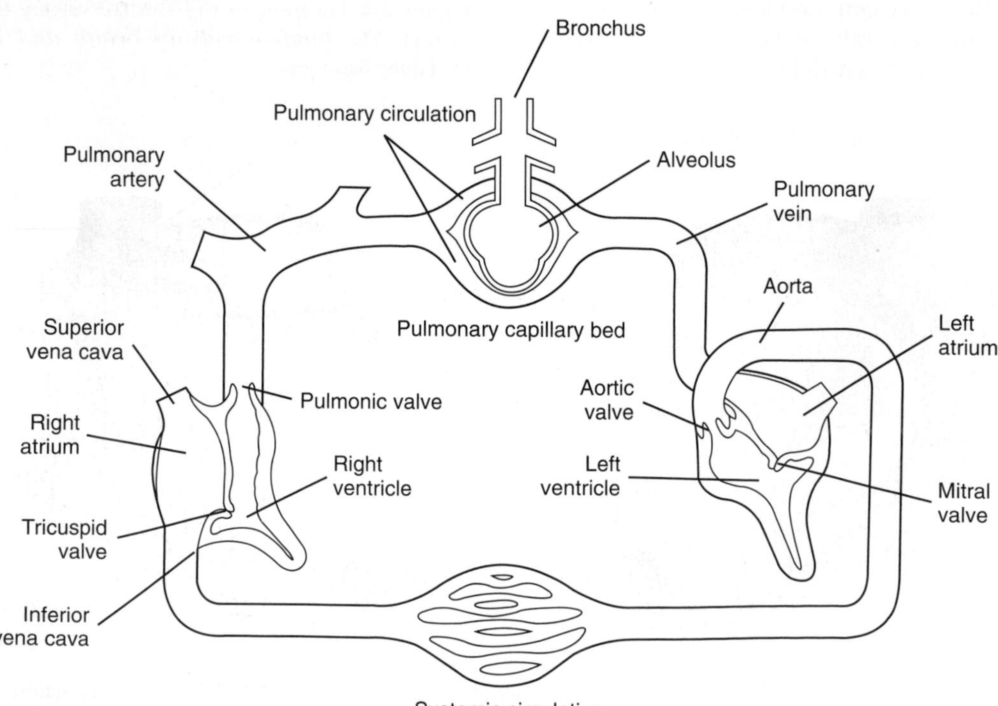

Figure 2-6 Pathway of blood through the heart and the vascular system. (Courtesy Edwards Lifesciences, Irvine, CA.)

iii) Diastolic time
iv) Oxygen extraction
(a) Hemoglobin (Hgb)
(b) Arterial oxygen saturation (SaO_2)
c) Imbalances between supply and demand cause ischemia; prolonged imbalance causes infarction.

e. Coronary arteries and distribution (Figure 2-8)
1) Coronary arteries are end (i.e., terminal) arteries supplying a specific area of myocardium; blockage of a coronary artery therefore results in ischemia or infarction
a) Partial or temporary occlusion results in ischemia
b) Complete or permanent occlusion results in infarction
2) Left coronary artery before bifurcation is referred to as the *left main coronary artery;* the left main coronary artery divides into left anterior descending and left circumflex arteries.
a) Left anterior descending (LAD) coronary artery supplies the following:
i) Anterior left ventricle
ii) Anterior two thirds of the interventricular septum
iii) Apex of left ventricle
iv) Bundle of His and bundle branches
b) Left circumflex coronary artery (LCA) supplies the following:
i) Left atrium
ii) SA node in 45% of hearts
iii) AV node in 10% of hearts
iv) Marginal (or obtuse marginal) branch supplies the following:
(a) Lateral left ventricle
(b) Posterior left ventricle
3) Right coronary artery (RCA) supplies the following:
a) Right atrium
b) SA node in 55% of hearts
c) Left posterior hemibundle (dual blood supply: LAD and RCA)
d) AV node in 90% of hearts
e) Marginal branch supplies:
i) Lateral right ventricle
ii) Inferior right ventricle
f) In RCA-dominant hearts (approximately 80% of hearts), a branch of RCA referred to as the *posterior descending artery* supplies the following:
i) Anterior right ventricle
ii) Inferior wall of left ventricle
iii) Posterior left ventricle
iv) Posterior one third of septum
4) Collateral circulation

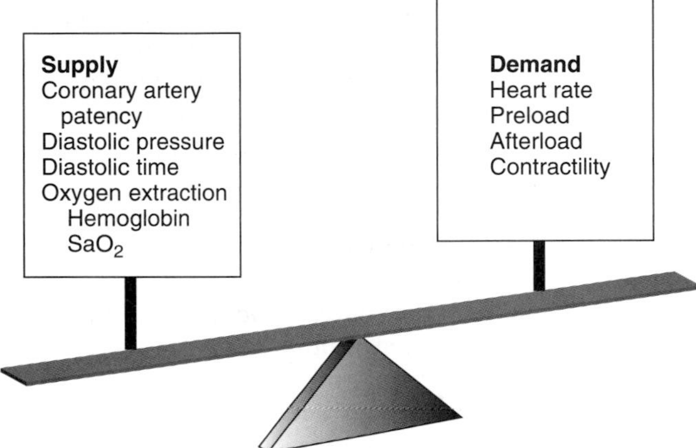

Figure 2-7 Factors affecting myocardial oxygen supply and myocardial oxygen demand.

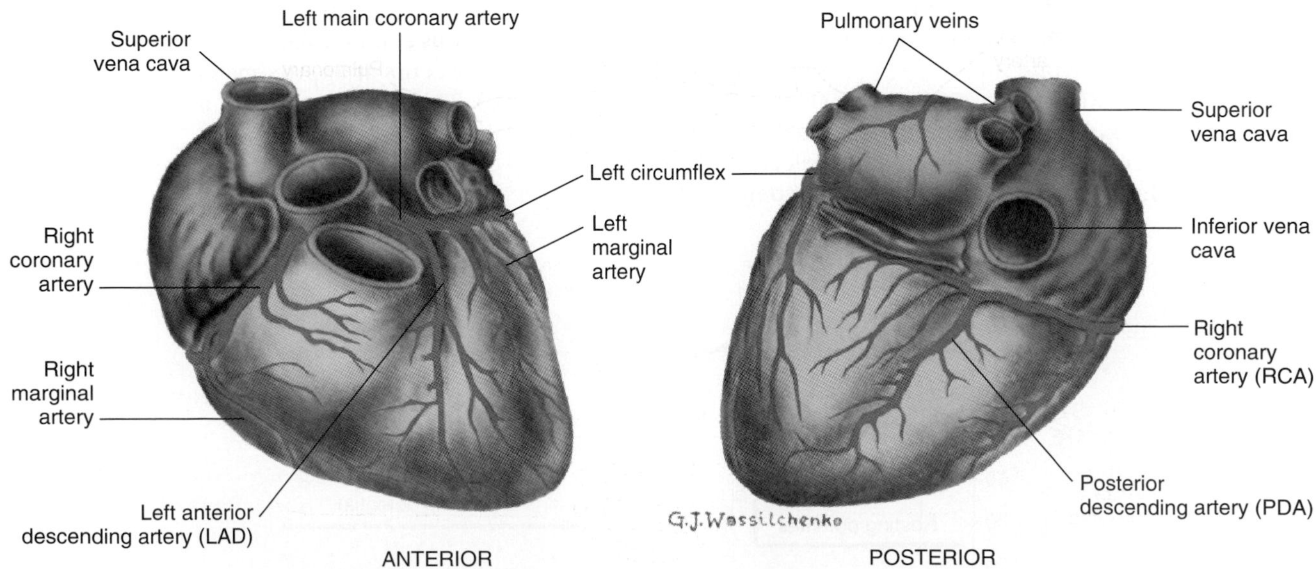

Figure 2-8 Anterior and posterior views of the coronary artery circulation and major vessels. (From Urden, L., Stacy, K., & Lough, M. [2010]. *Critical care nursing: Diagnosis and management* [6th ed.]. St. Louis: Mosby.)

a) Consists of interarterial vessels that connect, or anastomose, with each other
b) Factors that foster development of collateral flow include: anemia, hypoxemia, and arteriosclerosis (gradual occlusion)

f. Coronary veins
1) Most coronary veins empty into the coronary sinus, which empties into the right atrium.
2) The thebesian veins drain some of venous blood from myocardium directly into the right atrium, right ventricle, and left ventricle rather than through the coronary sinus; this venous blood emptying directly into the left ventricle accounts for a normal physiologic shunt because it slightly decreases oxygen saturation.

g. Lymph vessels
1) Main cardiac channel empties into the pretracheal node and then into the right lymphatic duct.
2) Drainage system is facilitated by cardiac contraction.

11. Electrophysiology and the conduction system
a. Types of cardiac cells
1) Pacemaker cells
2) Electrical conducting cells
3) Myocardial muscle cells

b. Properties of cardiac cells
1) Automaticity: ability of certain cardiac cells to initiate impulses regularly and spontaneously
2) Excitability: ability of the cardiac cells to respond to a stimulus
3) Conductivity: ability of cardiac cells to respond to a cardiac impulse by transmitting the impulse along cell membranes
4) Contractility: ability of the cardiac cells to respond to an impulse by muscle contraction
5) Rhythmicity: ability of the cardiac cells to spontaneously generate an action potential at a regular rate

c. Action potential of myocardial cells (Figure 2-9)
1) Phase 4: resting membrane potential
a) This phase coincides with isoelectric line between T wave and QRS complex
b) Electrical charge within the cell is –80 to –95 mV.
c) Negativity is maintained by the sodium-potassium pump.
i) An active transport system requires energy to pump sodium out of the cell and potassium into the cell.
ii) When cellular energy (i.e., adenosine triphosphate [ATP]) supplies are low, such as during shock, this resting membrane potential cannot be maintained and irritability occurs.

2) Phase 0: rapid depolarization of the cell
a) This phase coincides with QRS.
b) It occurs when a stimulus is applied to the cell.
c) Cell membrane permeability to sodium increases significantly so that sodium rushes into the cell (influx) and potassium begins to move out (efflux).
d) If the stimulus is strong enough to reach a critical level known as the *threshold potential* (approximately -60 to -70 mV), then the cell responds entirely and depolarization occurs.
e) This phase is referred to as the *sodium* (or *fast*) *channel.*
f) Class I antidysrhythmic agents (e.g., procainamide, quinidine, lidocaine) block the influx of sodium into the cell, thereby preventing the achievement of threshold potential and depolarization.

3) Phase 1: brief, partial repolarization
a) Sodium channels close
b) Potassium efflux continues

4) Phase 2: slowing of the repolarization causing a plateau
a) This phase coincides with ST segment.
b) Calcium influx keeps the cell isoelectric but still depolarized as potassium efflux occurs at approximately the same rate.
c) This plateau allows a more sustained contraction.
d) This phase is referred to as *calcium* (or *slow*) *channel.*

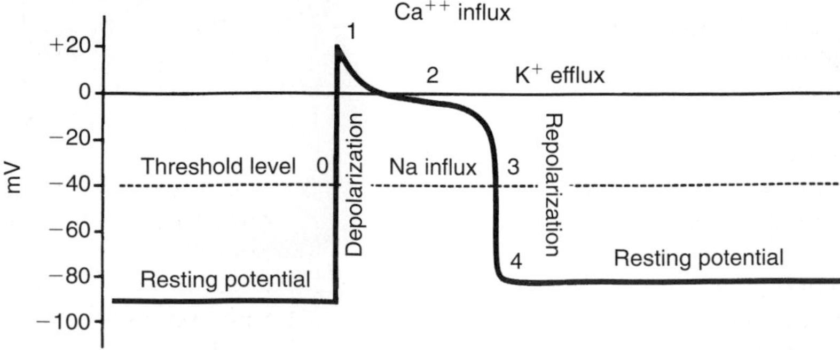

Figure 2-9 Action potential of a nonpacemaker cell. (From Urden, L., Stacy, K., & Lough, M. [2010]. *Critical care nursing: Diagnosis and management* [6th ed.]. St. Louis: Mosby.)

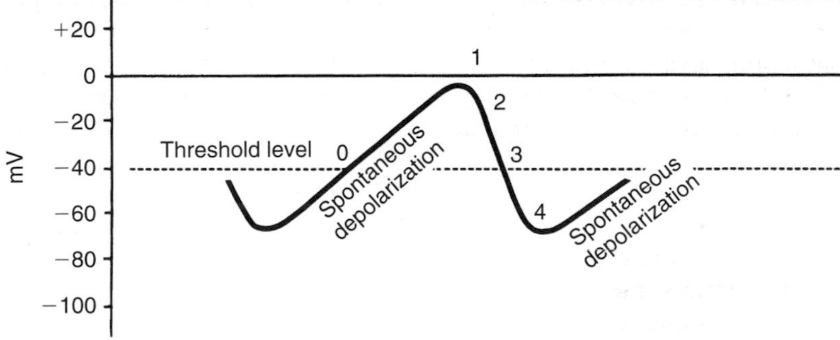

Figure 2-10 Action potential of a pacemaker cell. (From Urden, L., Stacy, K., & Lough, M. [2010]. *Critical care nursing: Diagnosis and management* [6th ed.]. St. Louis: Mosby.)

e) Class IV antidysrhythmics (calcium channel blockers [e.g., verapamil, diltiazem]) block the movement of calcium and prolong repolarization and refractoriness.

5) Phase 3: sudden acceleration in the rate of repolarization
   a) Potassium movement accelerates during this phase; potassium efflux occurs at the beginning of phase 3 to exceed the influx of calcium and potassium influx occurs at the end of phase 3.
   b) Repolarization is completed.
   c) Class III antidysrhythmics (e.g., amiodarone, ibutilide, dofetilide) block the movement of potassium during this phase and prolong refractoriness.
6) Phase 4: resting membrane potential

d. Action potential of pacemaker cells (Figure 2-10)
   1) Pacemaker cells have the property of automaticity.
   2) They demonstrate slow diastolic depolarization due to a time-dependent leak of sodium into the cell.
   3) When enough sodium has entered the cell that threshold potential is reached, spontaneous depolarization occurs.
   4) Rate of diastolic depolarization determines intrinsic rate of pacemakers.
      a) Sinoatrial (SA) node: 60-100 times per minute
      b) Atrioventricular (AV) junction: 40-60 times per minute
      c) Purkinje fibers: 20-40 times per minute

e. Refractoriness (Figure 2-11)
   1) Absolute refractory period
      a) No matter how strong the impulse is, the cell cannot be depolarized during this period.
      b) This period correlates with the period of time from phase 0 through midphase 3 on the action potential and from the QRS complex to the peak of the T wave on the ECG.

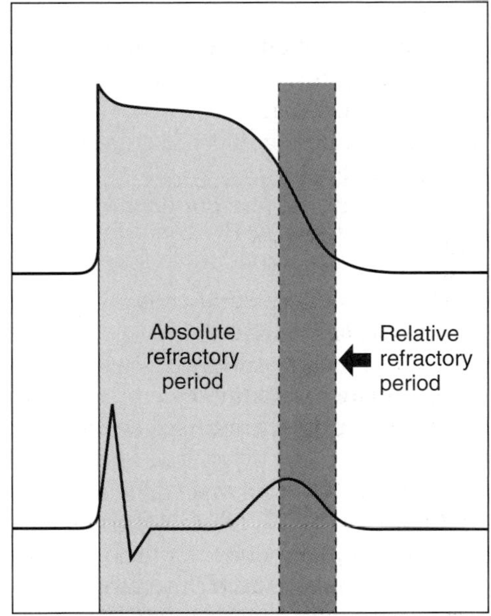

Figure 2-11 Absolute and relative refractory periods correlated with the myocardial cell action potential and with ECG tracing. (From Urden, L., Stacy, K., & Lough, M. [2010]. *Critical care nursing: Diagnosis and management* [6th ed.]. St. Louis: Mosby.)

   2) Relative refractory period
      a) If the impulse is strong enough, the cell may respond but may respond abnormally (e.g., R-on-T may cause ventricular tachycardia or ventricular fibrillation).
      b) This period correlates with late phase 3 of the action potential and the descending limb of the T wave on the ECG.
   3) Effective refractory period: the absolute refractory period plus the relative refractory period.

f. Conduction system (Figure 2-12)
   1) Sinoatrial (SA) node
      a) Functions as the natural pacemaker of the heart because it has the fastest intrinsic rate (60-100 times per minute)

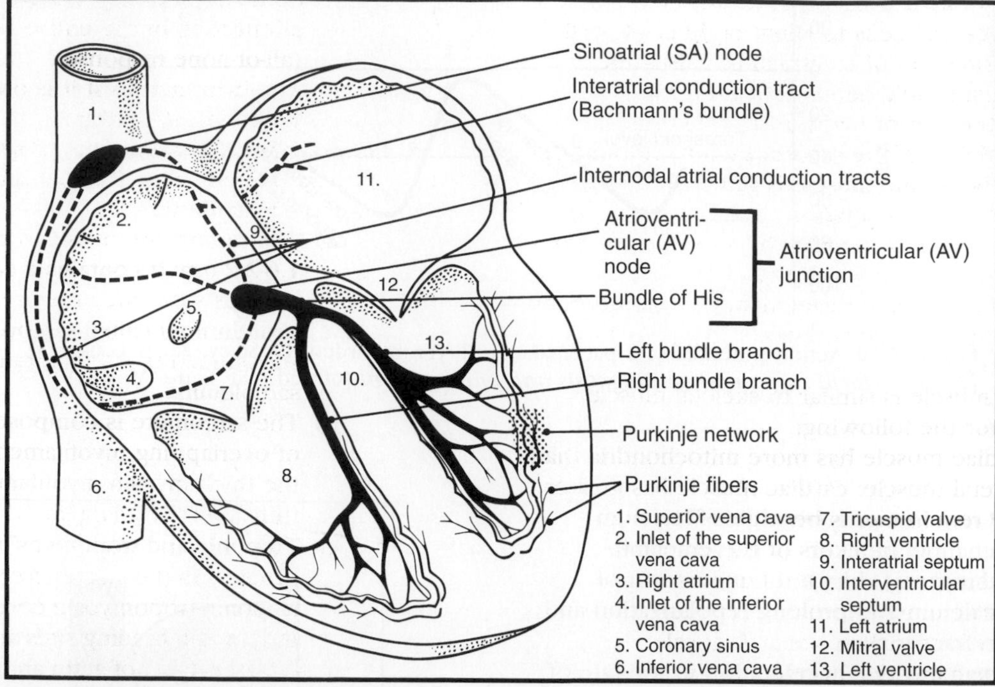

Figure 2-12 The conduction system. (From Huszar, R. J. [1994]. *Basic dysrhythmias: Interpretation and management.* [2nd ed.]. St Louis: Mosby.)

b) Located in the right atrial wall near opening of superior vena cava

2) Internodal pathways
   a) Three pathways between SA node and AV node
      i) Anterior tract (Bachmann's)
      ii) Middle tract (Wenckebach's)
      iii) Posterior tract (Thorel's)
3) Bachmann's bundle (interatrial pathway): pathway that takes the impulse from right atrium to left atrium
4) Atrioventricular (AV) node
   a) Located at the base of right atrium at top of interventricular septum
   b) Accounts for the physiologic delay of 0.08-0.12 seconds to allow the atria to depolarize completely, contract, and finish filling the ventricles before the ventricles are stimulated
   c) Contains no pacemaker cells; primary function is to slow the impulse down
5) Atrioventricular (AV) junction
   a) Tissue surrounding AV node and bundle of His that contains pacemaker cells
   b) Functions as a secondary pacemaker with intrinsic rate of 40-60 times per minute
6) Bundle of His
   a) First portion of intraventricular conduction system
7) Bundle branches
   a) Right bundle branch (RBB) takes the impulse to the right ventricular myocardium
   b) Left bundle branch (LBB) divides into three hemibundles
      i) Septal hemibundle depolarizes the interventricular septum in a left-to-right direction.
      ii) Left anterior hemibundle (LAH) depolarizes the anterior and superior left ventricle.
      iii) Left posterior hemibundle (LPH) depolarizes the posterior and inferior left ventricle.
      iv) Hemiblocks
         (a) Block of the septal hemibundle does not cause a clinically identifiable situation.
         (b) The posterior hemibundle is thicker than the anterior hemibundle and has a dual blood supply so less susceptible to block than the anterior hemibundle
   c) These three major branches (RBB, LAH, LPH) are referred to as *fascicles* as in *unifascicular, bifascicular,* and *trifascicular block.*
8) Purkinje fiber system
   a) The fascicles divide into the Purkinje fibers which continue to divide and take the impulse through the ventricular walls to terminate in the subendocardial surface of the ventricles.
   b) Acts as a final tertiary pacemaker if upper pacemakers fail at the inherent rate of 20-40 times per minute

9) Intercalated disks separate adjacent myocardial cells to allow rapid cell-to-cell transmission of electrical impulses and almost simultaneous activation and contraction of myocardial cells; this capability of the myocardium to respond as if it were one muscle is referred to as a *functional syncytium*.

g. Depolarization of cardiac chambers occurs from endocardium to epicardium.

h. Repolarization of cardiac chambers occurs from epicardium to endocardium.

12. Muscle mechanics

a. Cardiac muscle is similar to skeletal muscle except for the following:

1) Cardiac muscle has more mitochondria than skeletal muscle; cardiac muscle has greater ATP requirements because of the high energy requirements of the repetitive muscular action of the heart.

2) Cardiac muscle remains contracted 150-300 times longer than skeletal muscle.

3) Cardiac muscle forms a functional syncytium.

a) Intercalated disks lie between myocardial cells; they offer low electrical impedance, allowing electrical stimuli to pass with ease from cell to cell.

b) Stimulation of any muscle fiber results in stimulation of the entire muscle mass (all-or-none response).

c) The heart acts as if it is one muscle (i.e., functional syncytium).

b. Cardiac muscle ultrastructure (Figure 2-13)

1) A sarcomere is the basic contractile unit of the myocardium.

a) The sarcomere measures between 1.6-2.2 μm; it contains a centrally placed nucleus surrounded by intracellular protein fluid called sarcoplasm, which is surrounded by a membrane called a sarcolemma.

b) The sarcomere is composed of two sets of overlapping myofilaments, including thc thick myosin myofilament and the thin actin myofilament.

c) Troponin and tropomyosin are regulatory proteins in the sarcomere that form a troponin-tropomyosin complex to cover the myosin binding sites and inhibit cross-bridging of actin and myosin when the muscle is in a resting state.

d) The sarcoplasmic reticulum, a continuation of the sarcolemma, penetrates the cell to form a complex tubular (T tubule) system surrounding each fibril.

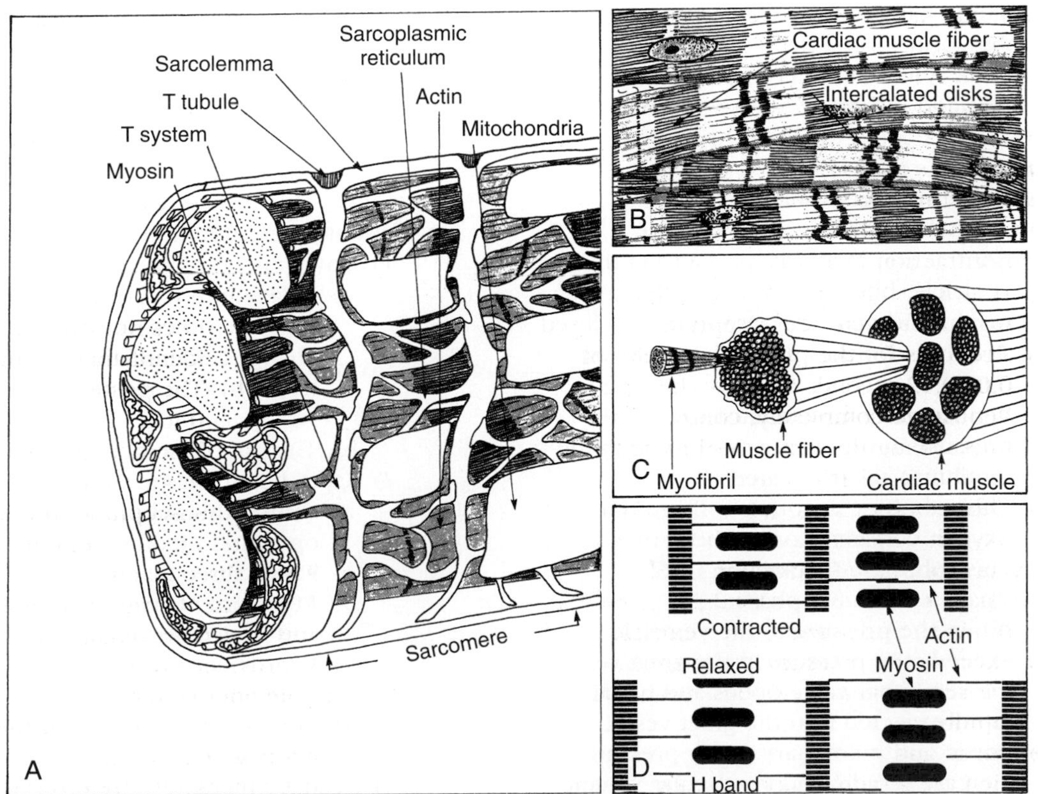

Figure 2-13 Cardiac muscle. **A,** The ultrastructure. **B,** Intercalated disks lie between muscle cells. **C,** Myofibrils form muscle fibers, which form cardiac muscle. **D,** Actin and myosin are myofilaments, which interlace in the presence of calcium to cause muscle contraction and shortening. (From Guzzetta C. E., & Dossey, B. M : [1992]. *Cardiovascular nursing: Holistic practice.* St Louis: Mosby.)

e) Calcium is stored in the sarcoplasmic reticulum and is necessary for the cross-bridging of actin and myosin.

c. Excitation-contraction process
   1) The wave of depolarization spreads through conduction system to myocardial muscle cell.
   2) The action potential reaches the sarcoplasmic reticulum, and the T tubules transmit the action potential from sarcolemma to interior of the cell.
   3) Calcium enters the cell during phase 2 of the action potential through calcium channels in the sarcolemma and the T tubules; more calcium is released from intracellular stores in the sarcoplasmic reticulum.
   4) Calcium binds with troponin to move the troponin and tropomyosin out of the way of the myosin binding sites.
   5) Actin and myosin myofilaments interact to form crossbridges that slide these overlapping myofilaments past one another.
   6) Shortening of the sarcomere occurs.
   7) Multiple sarcomere shortening, muscle contraction, and ejection of blood from the chamber occur.
   8) Calcium is pumped back into the sarcoplasmic reticulum which dissociates actin-myosin crossbridges; without the antagonist effect of calcium, troponin and tropomyosin form a troponin-tropomyosin complex which inhibits the cross-bridging of actin and myosin.
   9) Muscle relaxation occurs.

13. Cardiac cycle (Figure 2-14)
   a. Systole: the contraction phase
      1) Isovolumetric contraction: Subphase 1
         a) Contraction increases pressure in the ventricle, but there is no change in volume because the AV valves are closed and the semilunar valves have not yet opened.
         b) Ventricular pressure must exceed the pressure in the great vessel to open the semilunar valve.
         c) This subphase accounts for two thirds of oxygen consumption of the ventricle.
         d) This subphase follows the QRS.
      2) Maximal ejection: Subphase 2
         a) When the pressure in the ventricle exceeds the pressure in the great vessel, the semilunar valve opens and blood is rapidly ejected into the great vessel.
         b) Aortic and pulmonary artery pressures increase rapidly and ventricular volume decreases sharply.
         c) This subphase occurs during the ST segment.
      3) Reduced ejection (also referred to as *protodiastole*): Subphase 3

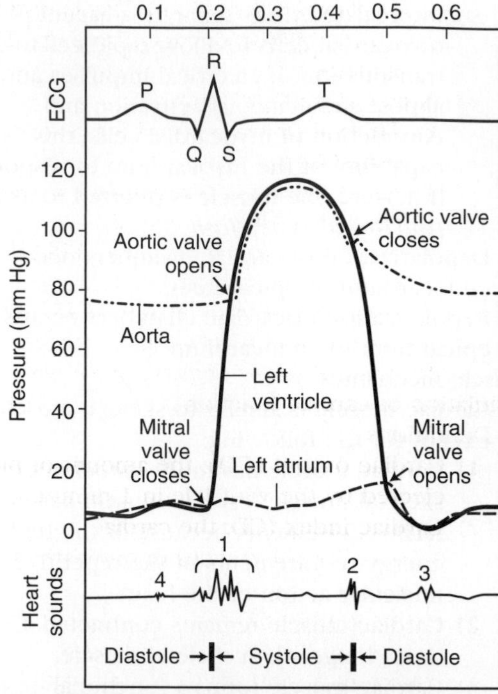

Figure 2-14 Wenger diagram: demonstrates the cardiac cycle showing ECG events, heart sounds, and pressure curves.

         a) Blood is slowly ejected from the ventricle to the great vessel.
         b) Ventricular pressure and volume decrease.
         c) When the pressure in the great vessel is greater than the pressure in the ventricle, the semilunar valve closes and systole ends.
         d) This subphase occurs during the T wave.
   b. Diastole: the relaxation phase
      1) Isovolumetric relaxation: Subphase 1
         a) Relaxation occurs and ventricular pressure decreases, but volume does not change because the semilunar valves have closed and the AV valves have not yet opened.
         b) This subphase occurs after the T wave.
      2) Rapid filling: Subphase 2
         a) During this subphase, the AV valves open and blood rushes into the ventricles.
         b) Atrial and ventricular pressures decrease and ventricular volume increases.
         c) Ventricular pressure is less than atrial pressure.
         d) This subphase occurs during the TP interval.
      3) Reduced filling (also referred to as *diastasis*): Subphase 3
         a) Atrial and ventricular pressures slowly increase and ventricular volumes increase with slow filling of ventricles.

b) Coronary artery blood flow is optimal.
c) This subphase occurs during the TP interval.

4) Atrial contraction: Subphase 4
a) This subphase is also referred to as the *atrial kick*.
b) Atrial contraction accounts for 15-30% of diastolic filling volume; may be up to 50% when left ventricular filling is impeded (e.g., mitral stenosis)
c) Atrial pressure decreases and ventricular volume and pressure increase.
d) This subphase occurs after P wave.

14. Regulation of cardiac function
a. Definitions
1) Cardiac output (CO): the amount of blood ejected by the ventricle in 1 minute
2) Cardiac index (CI): the cardiac output indexed for differences in body size by dividing by body surface area
3) Stroke volume (SV): the amount of blood ejected by the ventricle with each contraction; also defined as the difference between the end-diastolic volume and the end-systolic volume
4) Stroke index (SI): the stroke volume indexed for differences in body size by dividing by body surface area
5) Ejection fraction: percentage of blood in the ventricle that is ejected during systole; normal 55-75%
6) Afterload: the pressure against which the ventricle must pump; the pressure required to open the semilunar valve
7) Preload: the volume of blood in the ventricle at the end of diastole (end-diastolic pressure); determines the stretch on the myofibrils and the subsequent force of the next contraction (according to Starling's law of the heart)
8) Contractility: the force and velocity of the ejection of blood from the ventricle independent of preload and afterload

b. Intrinsic control of the heart
1) Determinants of cardiac output (Figure 2-15 and Table 2-1)
a) Heart rate
i) Definition: number of times per minute that the ventricles contract
ii) Evaluation
(a) Count the number of pulses palpable in 1 minute; the radial, brachial, femoral, or carotid pulses are most often used.
(b) If the apical rate is auscultated with a stethoscope or the HR on electrocardiogram (ECG) monitor is used to evaluate the HR, a palpable pulse with each audible heart sound or QRS must be confirmed.
iii) Effect of heart rate on cardiac output
(a) If heart rate is less than 50 or greater than 150 beats/min, cardiac output often falls and

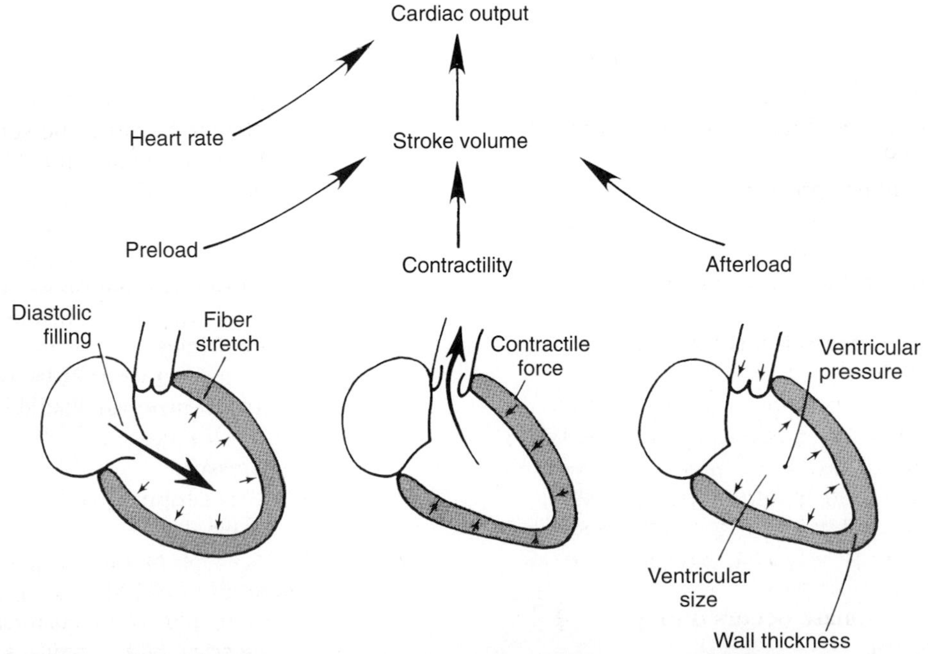

Figure 2-15 Determinants of cardiac output. (From Price, S. & Wilson, L. [2003]. *Pathophysiology: Clinical concepts of disease processes.* [6th ed.]. St. Louis: Mosby.)

Table 2-1 Determinants of Cardiac Output

	Conditions		Treatments	
Parameter	**Increased**	**Decreased**	**To increase**	**To decrease**

Heart rate: evaluated by palpation of pulse	• SNS stimulation (e.g., exercise, fever, infection, pain, anxiety, hypovolemia or hypervolemia, most physiologic or psychological stressors)
	• Drug effects (e.g., epinephrine, dopamine)
		• PNS (vagal) stimulation (e.g., Valsalva maneuver, coughing, suctioning, vomiting, carotid stimulation)
		• Conduction abnormalities (e.g., sinus arrest or block, second- or third-degree AV blocks) caused by ischemia, infarction, or inflammation
		• Drug effects (e.g., beta-blockers, digoxin)
			• Treatment of cause (e.g., reperfusion therapies for myocardial infarction, antiemetics for vomiting)
			• Parasympatholytic drugs (e.g., atropine)
			• Sympathomimetic drugs (e.g., epinephrine)
			• Pacemaker
				• Treatment of cause (e.g., antipyretics for fever, analgesics for pain, anxiolytics for anxiety)
				• Dependent upon rhythm:
				• Cardiac glycosides (e.g., digoxin)
				• Beta-blockers (e.g., propranolol, esmolol)
				• Calcium channel blockers (e.g., verapamil, diltiazem)
				• Other antidysrhythmic drugs dependent on rhythm
				• Vagal maneuvers
				  • Overdrive pacemaker
				  • Ablation
				• Cardioversion or defibrillation

Preload: evaluated by PAOP (LV) and RAP (RV) or RVEDV if a right ejection fraction (REF) catheter used	• Heart failure • Hypervolemia • Brady-dysrhythmias	• Hypovolemia • Excessive vasodilation (e.g., vasogenic shock) • Increased intrathoracic pressure (e.g., positive pressure mechanical ventilation) • Cardiac tamponade • Right ventricular failure or infarction (LV) • Tachydysrhythmias • Loss of atrial contraction (e.g., atrial fibrillation)	• Fluids • Isotonic crystalloids (e.g., normal (0.9%) saline, lactated Ringer's) • Colloids (e.g., albumin, plasma protein fraction [PPF], dextran, hetastarch) • Blood and/or blood products • Adjustment of vasodilator dosage	• Diuretics (e.g., furosemide) • Venous vasodilators (e.g., nitroglycerin, morphine sulfate, nitroprusside, calcium channel blockers [e.g., nifedipine]) • ACE inhibitors (e.g., captopril, enalapril) or angiotensin receptor blockers (ARBs) (e.g., losartan, valsartan) • Nesiritide (Natrecor)
Afterload: evaluated by calculation of SVR and SVRI (LV) and PVR and PVRI (RV)	• Vasoconstriction as from sympathetic nervous system (SNS) stimulation or vasopressors • Hypertension • Aortic stenosis • Hypercoagulability • Pulmonary hypertension (RV)	• Hypotension • Vasodilation (e.g., vasogenic shock such as septic shock, neurogenic shock, or anaphylactic shock)	• Adjustment of vasodilator dosage • Vasopressors (e.g., phenylephrine, norepinephrine, epinephrine, dopamine, vasopressin)	• Arterial vasodilators (e.g., nitroprusside, nitroglycerin greater than 1 mcg/kg/min, hydralazine, calcium channel blockers [e.g., nifedipine], alpha blockers [e.g., phentolamine, labetalol]) • ACE inhibitors (e.g., captopril, enalapril) or angiotensin receptor blockers (ARB) (e.g., losartan, valsartan), phosphodiesterase (PDE) inhibitors (e.g., milrinone, inamrinone) • Intraaortic balloon pump • Right ventricle specifically: oxygen, pulmonary vasodilators (e.g., aminophylline, nitric oxide, epoprostenol [Flolan], bosentan [Tracleer])

Table 2-1 Determinants of Cardiac Output—cont'd

	Conditions		Treatments	
Parameter	**Increased**	**Decreased**	**To increase**	**To decrease**
Contractility: evaluated by calculation of stroke volume and LVSWI (LV) and RVSWI (RV)	• SNS stimulation (see heart rate for selected factors that stimulate SNS) • Sympathomimetic drugs (e.g., epinephrine)	• Myocardial ischemia or infarction • Cardiomyopathy • Hypoxemia • Acidosis • Shock (i.e., myocardial depressant factor) • Drug adverse effects (e.g., barbiturates, anesthetics, beta-blockers, calcium channel blockers, most antidysrhythmics)	• Cardiac glycosides (e.g., digoxin) • Sympathomimetics (e.g., dobutamine, dopamine at medium [~5 mcg/kg/min] dose) • PDE inhibitors (e.g., milrinone, inamrinone) • Glucagon	• Beta-blockers (e.g., propranolol, metoprolol, esmolol) • Calcium channel blockers (e.g., diltiazem, verapamil)

LVSWI, Left ventricular stroke work index; *PVR,* pulmonary vascular resistance; *PVRI,* pulmonary vascular resistance index; *RVEDV,* right ventricular end-diastolic volume; *RVSWI,* right ventricular stroke work index; *SVR,* systemic vascular resistance; *SVRI,* systemic vascular resistance index.

the tendency to dysrhythmias increases.

iv) Effect of heart rate on myocardial oxygen consumption
   (a) Although an increase in heart rate may increase cardiac output, an increase in heart rate greater than 120 beats/min tends to increase myocardial oxygen demand more than the increase in coronary blood flow potentially causing ischemia, especially in patients with coronary artery disease.

v) Table 2-1 describes factors affecting heart rate.

b) Preload
   i) Definition: the stretch on the myofibrils at the end of diastole
      (a) The degree of myofibril stretch is affected by the ventricular volume.
      (b) While preload is a volume concept, it has traditionally been evaluated by the pressure in the ventricle at the end of diastole.
         (i) The relationship between volume and pressure is affected by the compliance of the ventricle.
         (ii) In a normally compliant ventricle, there is a linear relationship between volume and pressure.
         (iii) In a noncompliant ventricle, there is a disproportionate increase in pressure with changes in volume; this is referred to as *diastolic dysfunction.*
         (iv) Some causes of noncompliance of the ventricle include myocardial ischemia or infarction, ventricular hypertrophy, hypertrophic cardiomyopathy, restrictive pericarditis, and cardiac tamponade.
      (c) RV volumetric monitoring allows more accurate evaluation of preload through the evaluation of RV volumes rather than pressure and evaluation of RV ejection fraction.
   iii) Evaluation
      (a) Invasive: atrial pressure correlates to end-diastolic pressure for the respective ventricle
         (i) RV preload correlates to central venous pressure (CVP) or right atrial pressure (RAP) if no tricuspid valve disease
         (ii) LV preload correlates to pulmonary artery occlusive pressure (PAOP) or left atrial

Table 2-2 Clinical Indications of Hypoperfusion

Normal	Subclinical Hypoperfusion	Clinical Hypoperfusion	Shock
CI 2.5-4 L/min/m^2	CI 2.2-2.5 L/min/m^2	CI 2-2.2 L/min/m^2	CI less than 2 L/min/m^2
Normal	• No clinical indications of hypoperfusion though an expert nurse may detect subtle changes in the patient • Hypoperfusion at this stage is detected by hemodynamic monitoring	• Tachycardia • Narrowed pulse pressure • Tachypnea • Cool skin • Oliguria • Diminished bowel sounds • Restlessness → confusion	• Dysrhythmias • Hypotension • Tachypnea • Cold, clammy skin • Anuria • Absent bowel sounds • Lethargy → coma

pressure (LAP) if no mitral valve disease

(iii) RV volumetric monitoring (requires REF [right ejection fraction] catheter) allows measurement of right ventricular systolic volume, right ventricular end-diastolic volume, and right ventricular ejection fraction which are more accurate reflections of preload, especially in patients with decreased ventricular compliance.

(b) Noninvasive evaluation

(i) RV: jugular venous distention (JVD), hepatomegaly, and peripheral edema indicate high RV preload; flat neck veins when the patient is flat and oliguria indicate low RV preload

(ii) LV: S_3, crackles, and dyspnea indicate high LV preload; clinical indications of hypoperfusion (Table 2-2) indicate low LV preload.

iii) Effect of preload on stroke volume and cardiac output

(a) Starling's law of the heart and the Frank-Starling mechanism: Within physiologic limits, the greater the stretch on the myofibrils, the greater the force of the subsequent contraction (Figure 2-16).

(i) Both understretching and overstretching of the myofibrils result in a less than optimal contraction.

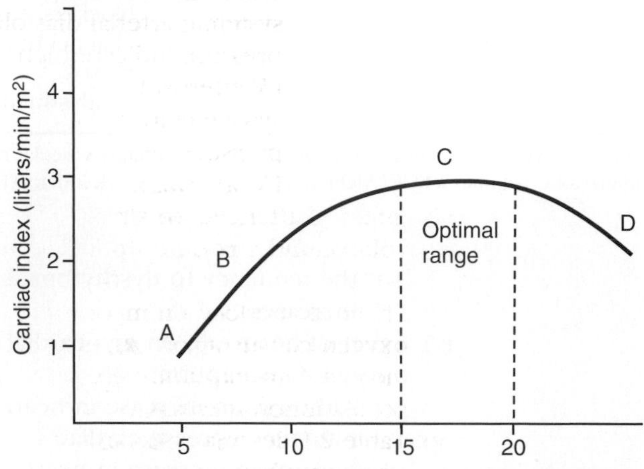

Figure 2-16 Relationship between PAOP and cardiac index. **A,** Understretched myofibrils resulting in decreased contractility and cardiac index. **B,** Normal stretched myofibrils resulting in normal (but suboptimal) cardiac index. **C,** Optimally stretched myofibrils resulting in optimal cardiac index. **D,** Overstretched myofibrils resulting in decreased contractility and cardiac index.

iv) Effect of preload on myocardial oxygen consumption: As preload increases, myocardial oxygen consumption increases.

v) Table 2-1 describes factors affecting preload

c) Afterload

i) Definition: the pressure against which the ventricle must pump to open the semilunar valve; affected by vascular resistance, ventricular diameter, and the mass and viscosity of blood

ii) Evaluation

(a) Invasive: calculated parameter

(i) RV afterload correlates to pulmonary vascular resistance (PVR) and pulmonary vascular resistance index (PVRI)

(ii) LV afterload correlates to systemic vascular resistance (SVR) and systemic vascular resistance index (SVRI)

(b) Noninvasive

(i) RV: Loud P_2 and high PA diastolic pressure indicate high RV afterload; low PA diastolic pressure indicates low RV afterload.

(ii) LV: Loud A_2, cool, pale extremities, and high systemic arterial diastolic pressure indicate high LV afterload; low systemic arterial diastolic pressure indicates low LV afterload.

iii) Effect of afterload on stroke volume and cardiac output (Figure 2-17)

iv) Effect of afterload on myocardial oxygen consumption: As afterload increases, myocardial oxygen consumption increases.

v) Table 2-1 describes factors affecting afterload.

d) Contractility

i) Definition: the force and velocity of the ejection of blood from the ventricle independent of preload and afterload

(a) Laplace's law states that the amount of contractile force generated within a chamber depends on the radius of the chamber and the thickness of its walls; therefore, the smaller the radius and the thicker the wall, the greater the force of contraction.

(b) Contractility is also significantly affected by endogenous catecholamines (e.g., epinephrine).

ii) Evaluation

(a) Invasive: calculated parameters

(i) RV contractility correlates to right ventricular stroke work index (RVSWI).

(ii) LV contractility correlates to left ventricular stroke work index (LVSWI).

(iii) Ejection fraction by REF catheter

(b) Noninvasive

(i) Clinical indicators of hypoperfusion (Table 2-2)

(ii) Diminished heart sounds

(iii) Ejection fraction by multiple gated acquisition (MUGA) scan or Doppler echocardiogram

iii) Effect of contractility on stroke volume and cardiac output (Figure 2-18)

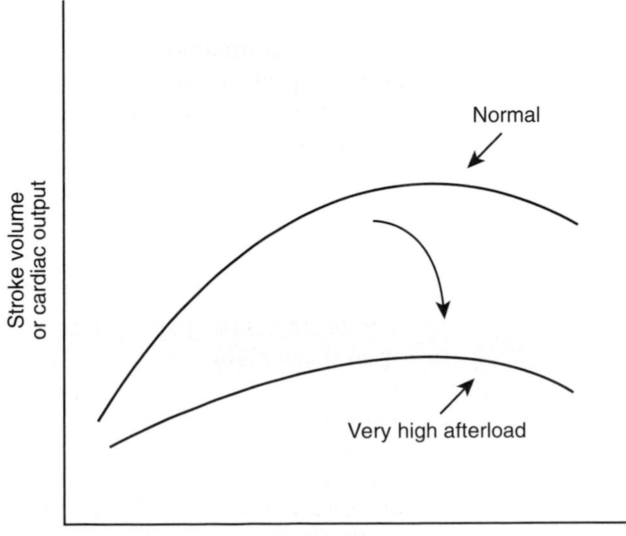

Figure 2-17 Relationship between afterload and stroke volume. (From Hicks, G. H. [2000]. *Cardiopulmonary anatomy and physiology*. Philadelphia: Saunders.)

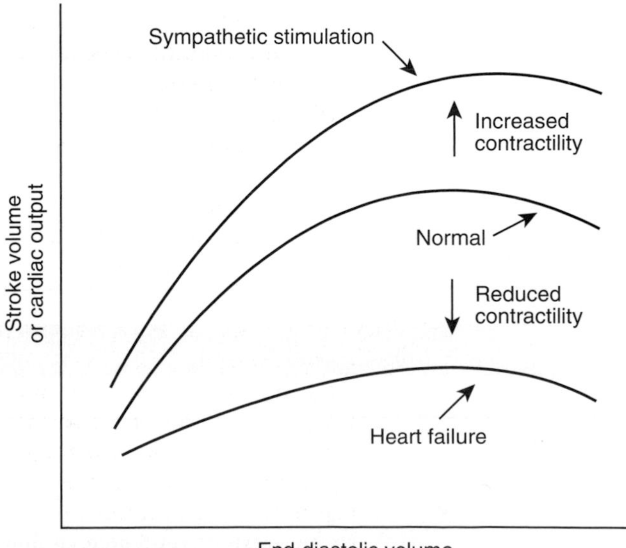

Figure 2-18 Relationship between contractility and stroke volume. (From Hicks, G. H. [2000]. *Cardiopulmonary anatomy and physiology*. Philadelphia: Saunders.)

iv) Effect of contractility on myocardial oxygen consumption: As contractility increases, myocardial oxygen consumption increases.
v) Table 2-1 describes factors affecting contractility.

c. Extrinsic control of the heart
1) Neurologic control of the heart
a) Autonomic nervous system
i) Terms used to describe cardiac effects
(a) Chronotropic: effect on heart rate
(b) Inotropic: effect on contractility
(c) Dromotropic: effect on conductivity
ii) Sympathetic nervous system (SNS)
(a) This branch is referred to as *fight or flight.*
(b) SNS is innervated by physiologic or psychological stress.
(c) It causes positive chronotropic, inotropic, and dromotropic effects.
(d) SNS receptors and effects are listed in Table 2-3.
(e) Sympathomimetic drugs are frequently used in critical care to augment these effects, especially after the patient's endogenous supplies are depleted; these drugs vary in their receptor stimulation and the potency of the stimulation (Table 2-4).

b) Parasympathetic (vagal) nervous system (PNS)
i) This branch maintains steady state.
ii) PNS causes negative chronotropic, inotropic, and dromotropic effects.
iii) Though the cardiovascular effects of the PNS are generally undesirable in critical care, they may decrease myocardial oxygen consumption by up to 50%.
iv) Parasympatholytic (or vagolytic) agents (e.g., atropine) block these effects.

c) Chemoreceptors
i) Chemoreceptors are located in carotid and aortic bodies.
ii) They are sensitive to changes in PaO_2, $PaCO_2$, and pH.
iii) Hypoxia, hypercapnia, and acidosis cause changes in heart rate and ventilatory rate.

d) Baroreceptor (or aortic) reflex
i) Baroreceptors are located in the carotid sinus and aortic arch.
ii) They are sensitive to increased arterial pressure.
iii) Medullary discharge causes vagal stimulation.
iv) Vagal stimulation results in a decrease in heart rate and contractility, which decreases cardiac output and arterial pressure.

e) Bainbridge reflex
i) Baroreceptors are located in the right atrium.

Table 2-3 Sympathetic Nervous System (Adrenergic) Receptors and Effects

Receptor	Location of Receptors	Effects
$Alpha_1$	Vessels	Vasoconstriction of most vessels, especially the arterioles
$Beta_1$	Heart	Increase in heart rate (chronotropic effect), contractility (inotropic effect), and conductivity (dromotropic effect)
$Beta_2$	Bronchial and vascular smooth muscle	Bronchodilation, vasodilation
Dopaminergic	Renal and mesenteric artery bed	Dilation of renal and mesenteric arteries

Table 2-4 Sympathomimetic Agents and Receptor Stimulation

Drug	$Alpha_1$	$Beta_1$	$Beta_2$
Phenylephrine	++++	0	0
Norepinephrine	++++	++	0
Epinephrine	++++	++++	++
Dopamine	++ greater than 5 mcg/kg/min; +++ greater than 10 mcg/kg/min	++++ less than 10 mcg/kg/min	+
Dobutamine	+	++++	++
Isoproterenol	0	++++	++++

ii) They are sensitive to increased venous pressure and right atrial pressure.
iii) Medullary discharge decreases vagal stimulation.
iv) Decreased parasympathetic tone causes an increase in heart rate and cardiac output which decreases venous pressure and right atrial pressure.

f) Respiratory reflex
i) Inspiration decreases intrathoracic pressure, which increases venous return to the right side of the heart, which causes the Bainbridge reflex; when the increased venous return reaches the left side of the heart, left ventricular cardiac output increases, which increases arterial blood pressure and decreases the heart rate through stimulation of baroreceptors.
ii) This process is at least partly responsible for sinus dysrhythmia; an interaction between the respiratory and cardiac centers in the medulla also contributes.

d. The endocrine function of the heart
1) Atrial natriuretic peptide (ANP)
a) Produced and stored by specialized atrial muscle cells
b) Triggers for ANP release
i) Primary cause of ANP release is increased atrial stretch.
ii) Other causes of ANP release include acute increase in intravascular volume, exercise, and endogenous or exogenous vasopressors.
c) Actions and effects: important regulator of blood volume and BP
i) Inhibits sodium transport in the collecting ducts of the kidney resulting in increased urine output
ii) Acts as an antagonist to angiotensin II, epinephrine, and endothelin, resulting in decrease in heart rate and vasodilation
iii) Diminishes the renin-angiotensin-aldosterone system, resulting in sodium and water excretion
iv) Decreases proliferation of cardiac fibroblasts and smooth muscle cells, resulting in the prevention of ventricular remodeling
2) Brain natriuretic peptide (BNP)
a) First discovered in animal brain tissue (hence the name) but it is produced by ventricular muscle tissue
b) Triggers for BNF release: increased intravascular volume
c) Actions and effects: similar to ANP with dilation of both arteries and veins
d) Measurement of BNP is being used both as a diagnostic study for diagnosis of heart failure as well as a therapeutic pharmacologic agent (i.e., nesiritide [Natrecor]) for heart failure
3) C-type natriuretic peptide
a) Lowest concentration of circulating plasma natriuretic peptides; distributed predominantly in the CNS, kidneys, and endothelial cells
b) Actions and effects: marked vasodilatory effects but no natriuretic effect
4) Endothelin
a) Potent vasoconstrictive peptides produced by endothelial cells
b) Causes an increase in renin, aldosterone, antidiuretic hormone, and SNS effects to increase systemic vascular resistance

Vascular System

1. Function: supply blood, nutrients, and hormones to the tissues and remove metabolic wastes from the tissues
2. Resistance to flow
a. Poiseuille's formula states that resistance depends on:
1) The length of the vessel
2) The radius of the vessel
3) The viscosity of the blood
b. Blood flow through the body is also influenced by neurologic stimulation affecting vascular tone and features that cause turbulence within the vascular lumen such as bifurcations or protrusions from the vessel wall into the vessel lumen (e.g., atherosclerosis).
3. Components of the vascular system (Figure 2-19)
a. Arteries
1) The arteries are the delivery system that distributes and regulates the amount of oxygenated blood flow to various tissue beds.
2) Arteries are able to stretch during systole and recoil during diastole.
3) The arterial system is a high-pressure circuit.
4) The layers of the arterial wall consist of the following: (Figure 2-20)
a) Intima: thin lining of endothelium and a small amount of elastic tissue; decreases resistance to flow and minimizes the chance of platelet aggregation
b) Media: smooth muscle and elastic tissue; changes the lumen diameter as needed
c) Adventitia: connective tissue; strengthens and shapes the vessels
b. Arterioles
1) Arterioles are vital to the maintenance of blood pressure and systemic vascular resistance
2) Arterioles may lead to any of the following:

a) Capillaries
b) Metarterioles
c) Precapillary sphincters which control blood flow into capillary bed

c. Capillaries
1) The capillary bed is the nutrient bed where exchange of gases, nutrients, and metabolites takes place by the process of diffusion.
2) Capillaries contain no smooth muscle.
3) The diameter of the capillary depends on changes in precapillary and postcapillary tone.
4) Capillary dynamics are influenced by four pressures (Figure 2-21).
a) Hydrostatic pressures push
i) Capillary hydrostatic pressure pushes fluid out of capillary and into interstitium.
ii) Interstitial hydrostatic pressure pushes fluid out of interstitium and into the capillary.

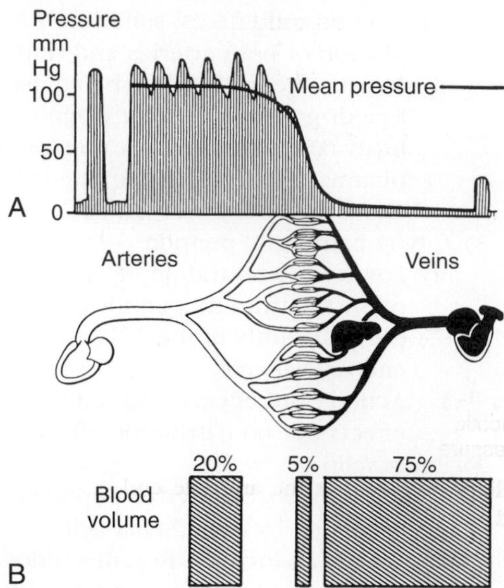

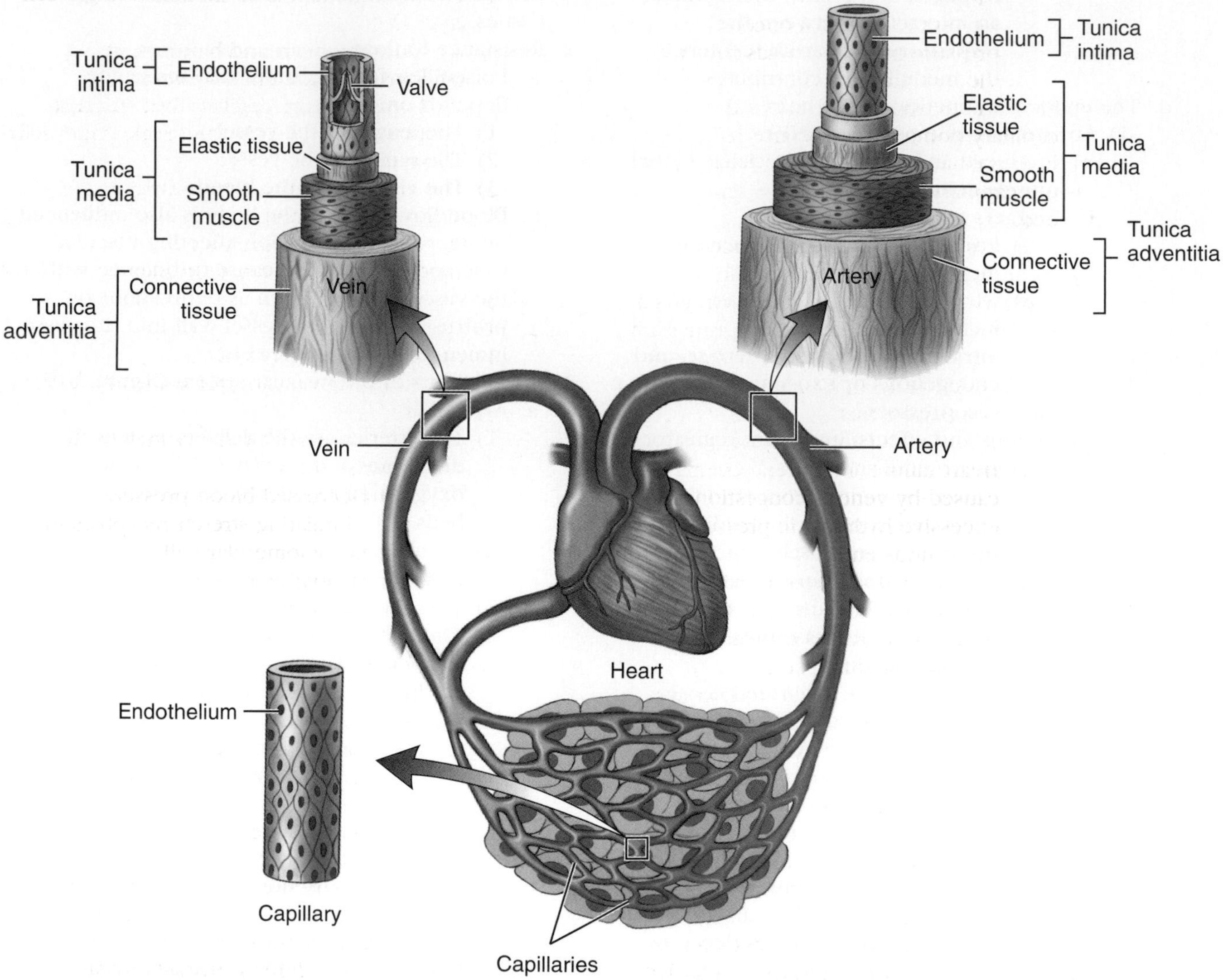

Figure 2-19 Components of the vascular system. **A,** Mean pressure in components of vascular system. **B,** Volume in components of vascular system. (From Rushmer, R: [1976]. *Cardiovascular dynamics* [4th ed.]. Philadelphia: Saunders.)

Figure 2-20 Blood vessel wall layers. (From Herlihy, B. [2011]. *The human body in health and illness.* [4th ed.]. St. Louis: Saunders.)

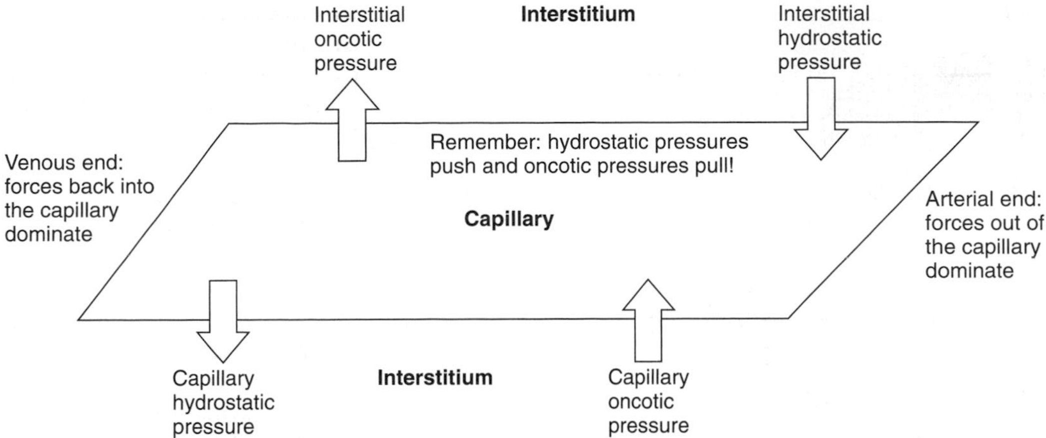

Figure 2-21 Capillary dynamics. Forces out of the capillary dominate at the arteriole end; forces back into the capillary dominate at the venule end.

b) Colloidal oncotic pressures pull
   i) Capillary colloidal oncotic pressure pulls and holds fluid in the capillary.
   ii) Interstitial colloidal oncotic pressure pulls and holds fluid in the interstitium.
c) Pressures pushing fluid out of the capillary dominate at the arterial end; pressures pushing fluid back into the capillary dominate at the venous end.
d) Edema is caused by an imbalance in these pressures or an increase in capillary permeability; *third spacing* is a term used to describe fluid accumulation in any space that is not intravascular or intracellular (e.g., interstitial edema, ascites, pleural effusion, pericardial effusion, lumen of the intestine).
   i) Heart failure: Peripheral edema is caused by venous congestion and excessive hydrostatic pressure at the venous end.
   ii) Protein malnutrition or liver disease: Decrease in plasma proteins decreases capillary colloidal oncotic pressure and allows excessive fluid to leak out of the capillary.

d. Veins
   1) The venous system is the return system that brings deoxygenated blood back to the heart and lungs.
   2) Veins act as a reservoir (i.e., capacitance vessels); the venous system holds 65-75% of total blood volume.
   3) The venous pump sends blood back to the right side of the heart; the skeletal muscles contract, compress veins, and propel blood toward the heart.
   4) Valves in the veins prevent retrograde blood flow.

e. Endothelium
   1) The endothelium is an immense single cell layer that:
      a) Lines the heart and blood vessels
      b) Surrounds the endocardium
      c) Comprises the capillary bed because capillaries are only this single endothelial layer
   2) The endothelium is instrumental in the following functions:
      a) Regulates vascular tone
      b) Prevents thrombus formation

4. Blood pressure
   a. Regulation
      1) Autonomic nervous system
      2) Renin-angiotensin-aldosterone (RAA) system (Figure 2-22)
         a) Renin secreted by the kidney in response to:
            i) Decreased blood pressure stimulating stretch receptors in juxtaglomerular cells
            ii) Sympathetic nervous system stimulation
            iii) Hyponatremia
         b) Renin stimulates the conversion of angiotensinogen to angiotensin I.
         c) Angiotensin I is converted to angiotensin II by angiotensin-converting enzyme (ACE) as the blood travels through the lung.
         d) Angiotensin II causes vasoconstriction and secretion of aldosterone.
         e) Vasoconstriction and sodium and water retention increases blood pressure and decreases renin secretion.
      3) Capillary fluid shifts: especially from interstitial to intravascular
      4) Local control mechanisms

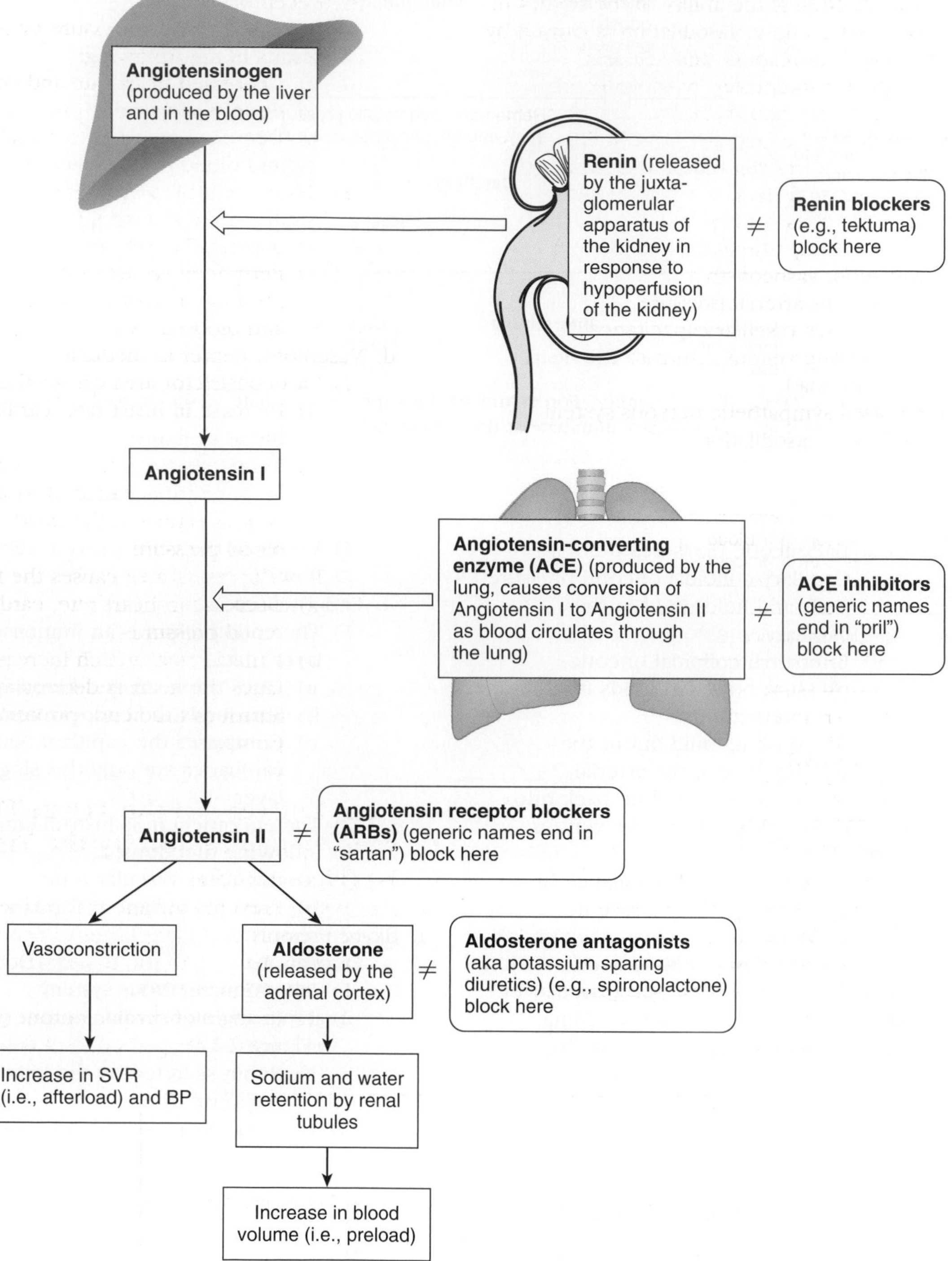

Figure 2-22 The renin-angiotensin-aldosterone system (RAAS) and drugs that block aspects of the RAAS.

b. Factors affecting arterial blood pressure (Figure 2-23)
c. Pulse pressure (Figure 2-24)
    1) The difference between systolic and diastolic pressures
    2) Affected by stroke volume and arterial elastance
d. Mean arterial pressure (Figure 2-24)
    1) The average pressure in the aorta and its major branches during cardiac cycle
    2) Calculated by either of the following formulae:
        a) [BP systolic + (BP diastolic × 2)] ÷ 3
        b) BP diastolic + 1/3 pulse pressure
    3) Normal: 70-105 mm Hg
    4) Affected by cardiac output and systemic vascular resistance

5. Control and regulation of peripheral blood flow
    a. Local control mechanisms

1) Autoregulation is the ability of the tissues to control blood flow; vasodilation is caused by hypoxia, hypercapnia, and acidosis.
2) Precapillary sphincters, which precede every capillary bed, relax and permit more blood flow when oxygen tension falls; they constrict and restrict blood flow when oxygen tension rises.

b. Autonomic nervous system
   1) Increased sympathetic nervous system stimulation: vasoconstriction
      a) Maintains arterial pressure
      b) Decreases vascular capacitance, increasing venous return to the heart and preload
   2) Decreased sympathetic nervous system stimulation: vasodilation

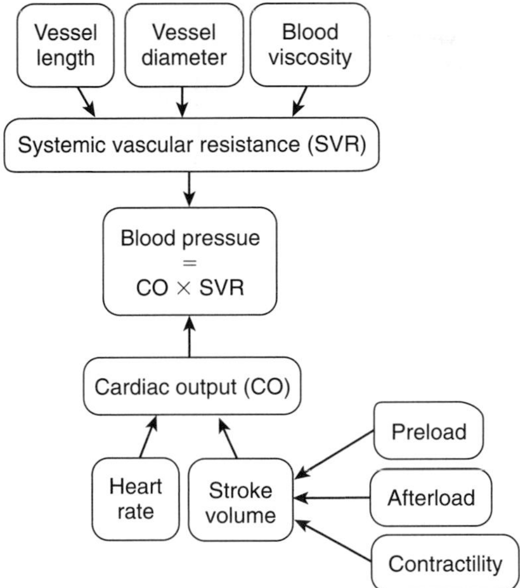

Figure 2-23 Determinants of blood pressure.

c. Baroreceptors
   1) Increase in blood pressure or blood volume results in the following:
      a) Decreased heart rate and contractility
      b) Peripheral vasodilation
      c) Decrease in systemic vascular resistance and blood pressure
   2) Decrease in blood pressure or blood volume results in the following:
      a) Increased heart rate and contractility
      b) Peripheral vasoconstriction
      c) Increase in systemic vascular resistance and blood pressure

d. Vasomotor center in medulla
   1) Vasoconstrictor area causes the following:
      a) Increase in heart rate, cardiac output, blood pressure
      b) Venoconstriction, which decreases vascular capacitance, thus increasing venous return to the heart, preload, and blood pressure
   2) Vasodepressor area causes the following:
      a) Decrease in heart rate, cardiac output, blood pressure
      b) Venodilation, which increases vascular capacitance, thus decreasing venous return to the heart, preload, and blood pressure

Oxygen Delivery to the Tissue (DO_2)/ Oxygen Consumption by the Tissues (VO_2) (Figure 2-25)

1. Parameters used to evaluate the balance between oxygen supply and oxygen consumption
   a. Oxygen delivery to the tissues (DO_2/DO_2I)
      1) DO_2 (Figure 2-26)
         a) Product of cardiac output (CO) and arterial oxygen content (CaO_2)

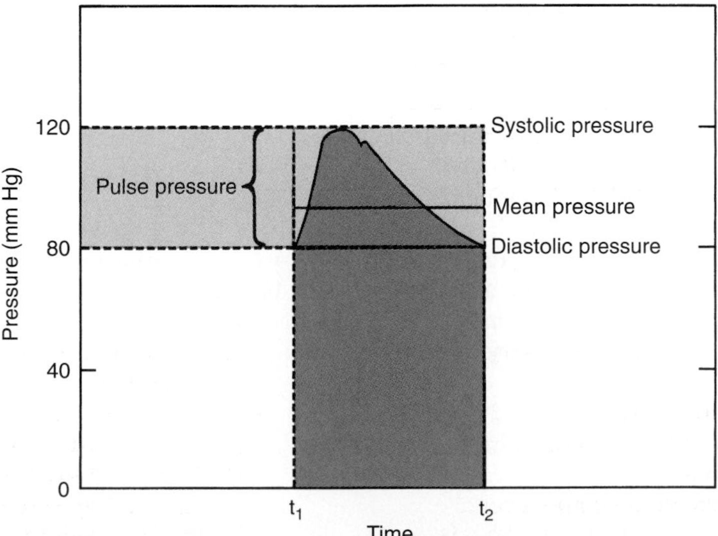

Figure 2-24 Blood pressure, pulse pressure (difference between systolic and diastolic pressures), and mean arterial pressure (calculated or measured average pressure). (Modified from Berne, R. M., & Levy, M. N. [1997]. *Cardiovascular physiology* [7th ed.]. St Louis: Mosby.)

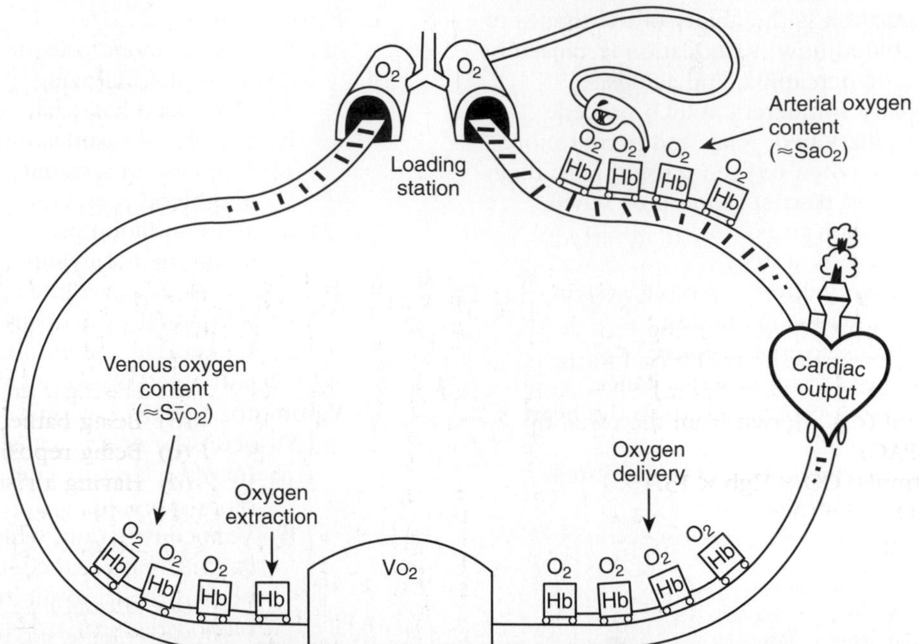

Figure 2-25 Schematic illustrating oxygen delivery/oxygen consumption (DO_2/VO_2). (From *Understanding continuous mixed venous oxygen saturation monitoring with the Swan-Ganz TD System*. Baxter Healthcare Corporation, Edwards Critical Care.)

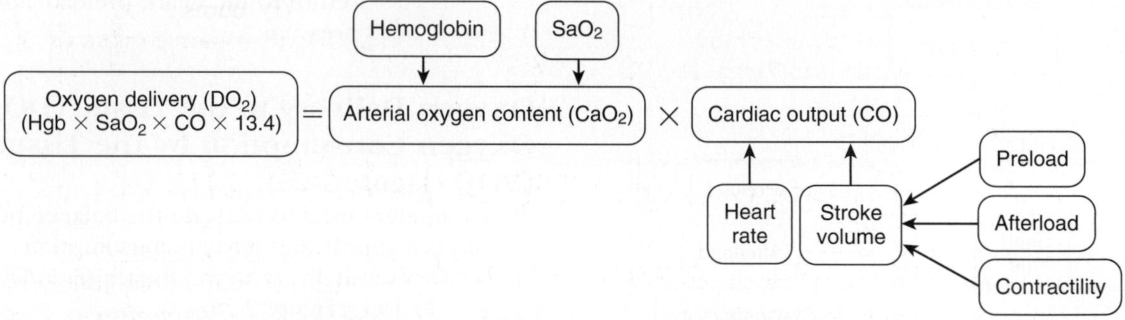

Figure 2-26 Determinants of oxygen delivery.

i) CO is a product of heart rate and stroke volume; stroke volume is affected by preload, afterload, and contractility.
  (a) Cardiac index (CI) is the CO ÷ body surface area (BSA).
ii) CaO_2 is a product of hemoglobin and arterial saturation.
  (a) CaO_2 is Hgb × SaO_2 (as a decimal) × 1.34 (the amount of oxygen that 1 gram of hemoglobin can carry if it is 100% saturated).
  (b) CaO_2 is normally 18-20 mL/dL.

b) Formula: CO × Hgb × SaO_2 × 13.4
  i) CO in liters/min
  ii) Hgb in g/dL
  iii) SaO_2 as a decimal (e.g., 95% is 0.95)

c) Normal DO_2: 900-1100 mL/min (~1000 mL/min)

2) DO_2I: DO_2 divided by body surface area so considers body size
  a) Formula: CI × Hgb × SaO_2 × 13.4
    i) CI in liters/min/m^2
    ii) Hgb in g/dL
    iii) SaO_2 as a decimal (e.g., 95% is 0.95)
  b) Normal: 550-650 mL/min/m^2 (~600 mL/min/m^2)

b. Oxygen consumption by the tissues (VO_2/VO_2I)
  1) Oxygen reserve in venous blood
    a) Saturation of venous blood (SvO_2)
      i) Determined by measuring the oxygen saturation in mixed venous blood in the pulmonary artery with an oximetric pulmonary artery catheter (PAC) or by blood gas analysis of a blood sample from the distal port of a PAC
      ii) Normal: 60-80%

b) Venous oxygen content (CvO_2) is a product of hemoglobin and arterial saturation.
  i) CvO_2 is Hgb × SvO_2 (as a decimal) × 1.34 (the amount of oxygen that 1 gram of hemoglobin can carry if it is 100% saturated).
  ii) CaO_2 is normally 18-20 mL/dL.

2) VO_2: volume of oxygen consumed by the tissues each minute
  a) Determined by comparing the oxygen content in the arterial blood to the oxygen content in the mixed venous blood (e.g., drawn from the distal tip of PAC)
  b) Formula: CO × Hgb × 13.4 × (SaO_2 − SvO_2)
  c) Normal VO_2: 200-300 mL/min (~250 mL/min)

3) VO_2I: VO_2 divided by body surface area so considers body size
  a) Formula: CI × Hgb × 13.4 × (SaO_2 − SvO_2)
  b) Normal: 110-160 mL/min/m^2 (~150 mL/min/m^2)

4) Oxygen extraction ratio (O_2ER)
  a) Evaluation of the amount of oxygen that is extracted from the arterial blood as it passes through the capillaries; ratio of the difference between the content of oxygen in the arterial blood and the content of oxygen in venous blood to the content of oxygen in the arterial blood
  b) Formula: (CaO_2 − CvO_2) ÷ CaO_2
  c) Normal: 22-30% (~25%)

5) Oxygen extraction index (O_2EI)
  a) Estimation of O_2ER calculated using only saturations
  b) Formula: (SaO_2 − SvO_2) ÷ SaO_2
  c) Normal: 20 to 27% (~25%)

c. Balance between supply and demand

1) Key point: The tissues normally use approximately 25% of the oxygen delivered and there is a 75% reserve.
  a) SaO_2 is normally ~100% and SvO_2 is normally ~75% *so the tissues used 25% and there is a 75% reserve.*
  b) CaO_2 is normally ~20 mL/dL and CvO_2 is normally ~15 mL/dL *so the tissues used 25% and there is a 75% reserve.*
  c) DO_2 is normally ~ 1000 mL/min and VO_2 is normally ~250 mL/min *so the tissues used 25% and there is a 75% reserve.*
  d) DO_2I is normally ~600 mL/min/m^2 and VO_2I is normally ~150 mL/min/m^2 *so the tissues used 25% and there is a 75% reserve.*

2) Oxygen reserve is reduced if DO_2 is decreased or VO_2 is increased
  a) Factors that decrease DO_2/DO_2I
    i) Decrease in SaO_2 (e.g., acute respiratory failure, decrease in the inspired oxygen level such as smoke inhalation, decrease in barometric pressure such as high altitudes)
    ii) Decrease in Hgb (e.g., anemia, hemorrhage)
    iii) Decrease in CO (e.g., heart failure, hypovolemia)
  b) Factors that increase VO_2/VO_2I
    i) Patient care activities
      (a) Having a dressing change
      (b) Being bathed
      (c) Being repositioned
      (d) Having a visitor
      (e) Being suctioned
      (f) Being weighed on a sling scale
      (g) Having a physical examination
    ii) Physiologic states
      (a) Agitation
      (b) Shivering
      (c) Fever
      (d) Increased work of breathing
      (e) Severe infection or sepsis
      (f) Burns
      (g) Multiple organ dysfunction syndrome (MODS)
      (h) Trauma
    iii) Anything that causes stimulation of SNS

3) Physiologic compensation for increased demand for oxygen at the cellular level
  a) Increase in cardiac output
  b) Redistribution of blood flow by recruiting underperfused capillary beds
  c) Increased oxygen extraction by the cells

4) Critical DO_2 point (Figure 2-27)
  a) A critical level of oxygen delivery exists where oxygen delivery and consumption are independent.
  b) When the critical oxygen delivery point is exceeded, oxygen consumption is dependent on oxygen delivery, and oxygen deficit, anaerobic metabolism, and lactic acidosis will occur.
    i) If SvO_2 improves with increase in DO_2, oxygen delivery and consumption are independent.
    ii) If SvO_2 does not improve with increase in DO_2, oxygen consumption is dependent on oxygen delivery.
  c) Lactic acidosis is the result of anaerobic metabolism, and elevated serum arterial lactate level indicates a tissue oxygen deficit.
    i) Normal serum arterial lactate level is less than 1 mmol/L.

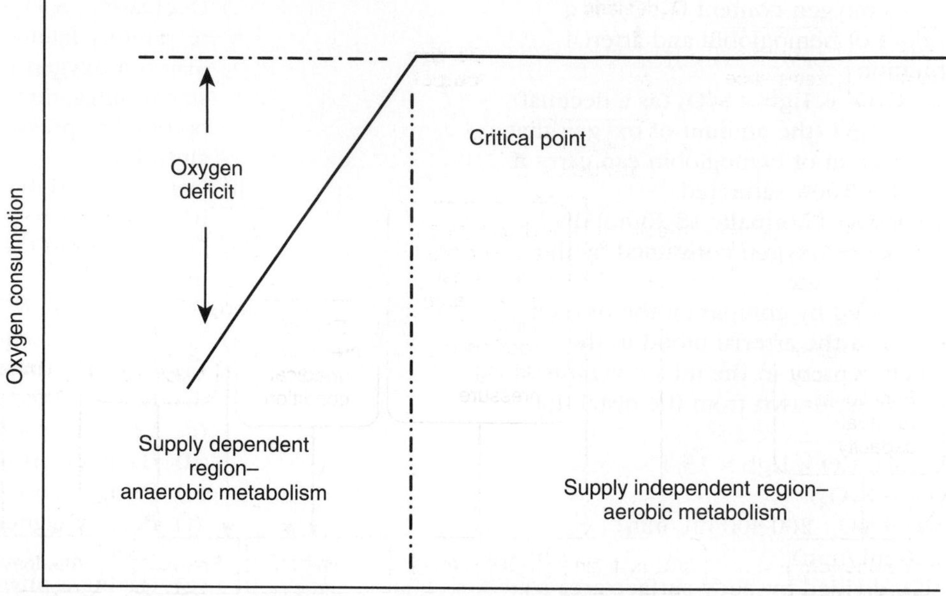

Figure 2-27 Critical oxygen delivery point. A critical level of oxygen delivery exists whereby oxygen delivery and consumption are interdependent of each other. Once this critical oxygen delivery point is exceeded, oxygen consumption becomes dependent on oxygen delivery. (From Dantzker, D. R., & Scharf, S. M. [1998]: *Cardiopulmonary critical care*. Philadelphia: Saunders.)

ii) Serum lactate levels greater than 2 mmol/L are associated with increased mortality.

d) Therapeutic efforts to decrease VO_2 and increase DO_2 may be utilized though the effects of optimization of DO_2 on mortality, morbidity, length of hospital stay, and hospital costs are still unclear.
   i) Increase DO_2.
      (a) Increase SaO_2 by using supplemental oxygen.
      (b) Increase Hgb by administering packed red cells.
      (c) Increase cardiac output by using inotropic agents.
   ii) Decrease VO_2.
      (a) Sedation
      (b) Muscle paralytics
      (c) Hypothermia

2. Oxygen supply and demand framework (Shackell & Gillespie, 2009) (Figure 2-28)
   a. Used to "guide patient assessment, link patient assessment data to physiologic concepts, draw conclusions about physiologic function, and select and understand rationale for patient care interventions" (Shackell & Gillespie, 2009).
   b. Serves as knowledge map to guide thinking in identifying problems and providing care

Cardiovascular Assessment

Interview

1. Chief complaint: identifies why the patient is seeking help and the duration of the problem
2. Symptoms related to cardiac disorders
   a. Chest pain: may also be identified as indigestion, burning, discomfort, tightness, pressure in midchest, epigastrium, or left arm (Table 2-5 describes differentiation of chest pain)
      1) PQRST format for describing complaint
         a) P
            i) Provocation: What provokes or worsens the pain?
            ii) Palliation: What relieves the pain? (Also include what was used but did not relieve pain.)
         b) Q
            i) Quality: What does the pain feel like?
         c) R
            i) Region: Where is the pain?
            ii) Radiation: If the pain radiates, to what area does the pain radiate?
         d) S
            i) Severity: How severe is the pain?
               (a) Pain scale: The most frequently used scale in adults is the 1-10 scale with 1 being negligible and 10 being the worst imaginable.
         e) T
            i) Timing: Is the pain intermittent or continuous? What is the relationship to other events or activities?
   b. Dyspnea
      1) Shortness of breath or "breathlessness"
      2) Exertional dyspnea

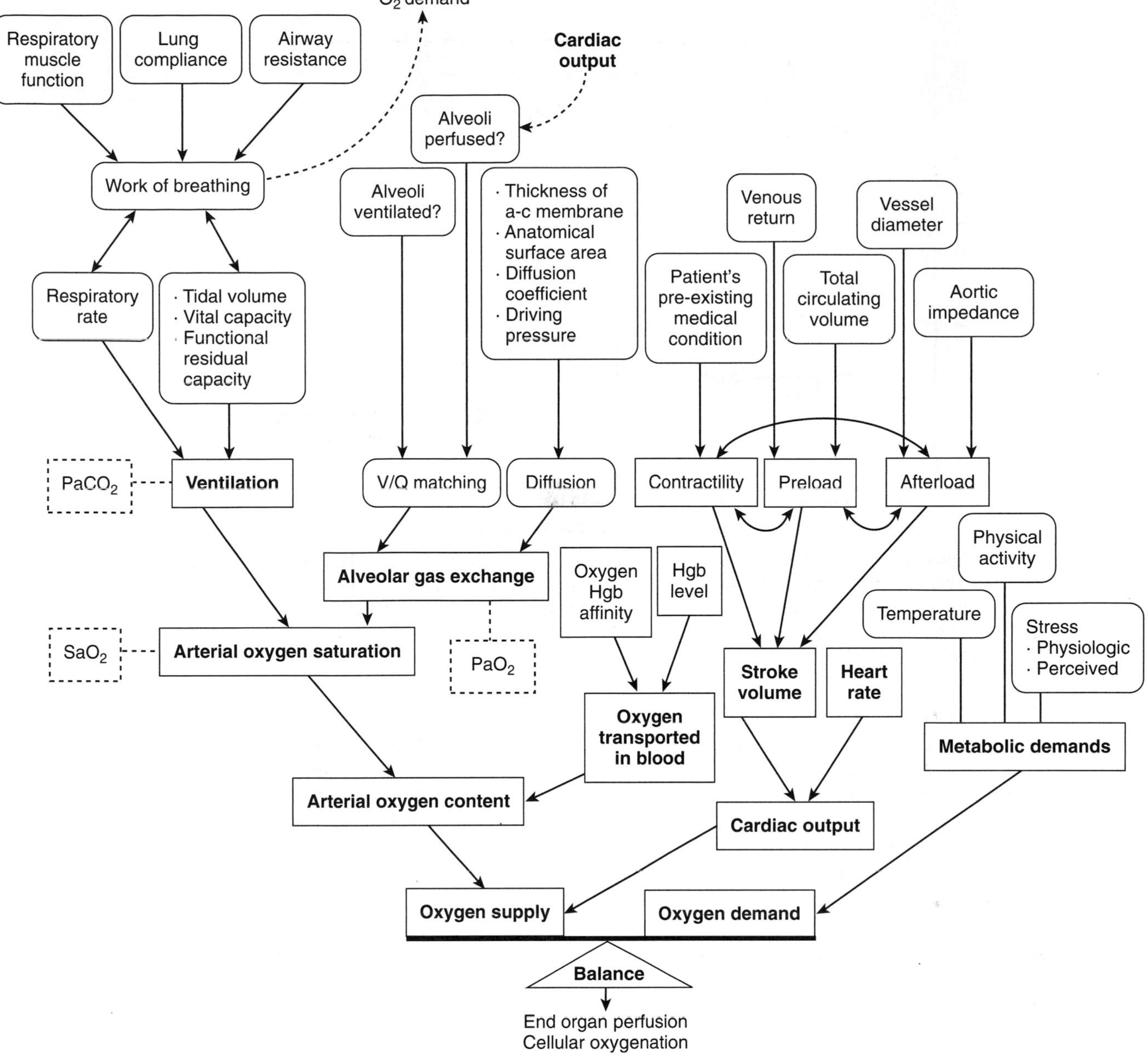

Figure 2-28 Oxygen supply and demand framework. (From Shackell, E., & Gillespie, M. [2009]. The oxygen supply and demand framework: A tool to support integrative learning. *Dynamics*, 20[4], 15-19.)

3) Orthopnea: Patient is unable to lie flat because of dyspnea.
4) Paroxysmal nocturnal dyspnea: patient awakens with a feeling of suffocation 1-2 hours after going to sleep; if accompanied by wheezing, may be called *cardiac asthma*

c. Cough
1) Quality: wet or dry
2) Productivity: appearance of expectorant
3) Frequency
4) Precipitating factors
5) Cardiac cough usually occurs at night and is precipitated by supine position, exertion, or by turning to one side.
6) Cough may be a side effect of ACE inhibitors or caused by heart failure, mitral stenosis, or pulmonary embolism.

d. Hemoptysis: may be related to pulmonary edema or pulmonary embolism

e. Palpitations
1) Unpleasant awareness of the heartbeat when at rest
2) May be described as skipping, pounding, thumping sensation
3) Associated with premature beats or other dysrhythmia
4) May be accompanied by syncope or chest pain

f. Syncope

Table 2-5 Differentiation of Chest Pain

Cause	Provocation	Palliation	Quality	Region/Radiation	Severity	Timing	Associated Signs/ Symptoms
Angina pectoris	• Exercise • Exertion • Exposure to cold • Emotional stress • Eating • Smoking	• Rest • Oxygen • Nitroglycerin • Calcium channel blocker (e.g., nifedipine)	• Heaviness or pressure • Tightness • Squeezing • Dull ache • Burning • Not always described as pain but as discomfort	• Substernal • May be diffuse and vague • May radiate to arms, neck, jaw, back, upper abdomen	• Mild to severe	• Gradual or sudden onset • Duration: usually 1-4 minutes but may be 5-15 minutes	• Tachycardia, tachypnea • Dyspnea • Nausea, vomiting • Diaphoresis • Weakness • Anxiety • May have ST-T wave changes with pain
Acute myocardial infarction	• No specific precipitator • Lifestyle change and stress • Usually occurs within 3 hours of awakening	• Narcotics • Reperfusion by fibrinolytic or percutaneous coronary intervention (e.g., angioplasty, atherectomy) • No relief with rest and/or nitroglycerin	• As for angina • Heaviness or pressure • May show Levine's sign (clenched fist over sternum)	• As for angina	• No symptoms to severe • Absence of pain is common in patients with diabetes mellitus and in older adults	• Sudden onset • Duration: longer than 30 minutes; usually 1-2 hours	• As for angina • Tachycardia, tachypnea • Dyspnea • Feeling of impending doom • S_4 • ECG changes: T wave inversion, ST segment elevation, eventually Q waves
Dissecting aortic aneurysm	• Peripheral vascular disease • Marfan's syndrome • Aortitis • Hypertension and/or hypertensive crisis • Chest trauma	• Narcotics • Surgery • No relief with rest and/or nitroglycerin	• Tearing • Ripping	• Anterior chest • Radiation to shoulders, neck, back, abdomen	• Severe	• Sudden onset • Worse at onset • Duration: hours to days	• Tachycardia, tachypnea • Dysphagia • Confusion • Diaphoresis • Syncope • Dyspnea • Anxiety • Unilateral absence of pulse; BP differences between sides • Motor/sensory changes • Murmur of aortic regurgitation

Pericarditis	• Myocardial infarction • Cardiac surgery • Trauma • Infections • Uremia • Lupus erythematosus	• Nonsteroidal antiinflammatory agents (e.g., ibuprofen; indomethacin) • Sitting up and leaning forward	• Sharp • Stabbing • Knifelike • Worsened by inspiration, coughing, movement, recumbent position	• Precordial • Substernal • Radiation to neck, shoulders, arms, back	• Mild to severe	• Sudden onset • Duration: days	• Tachycardia, tachypnea • Fever • Dyspnea • Pericardial friction rub • Leukocytosis • Diffuse concave • ST segment
Pulmonary embolism	• Venous stasis (e.g., immobility, pelvic surgery, atrial fibrillation) • Hypercoagulability (e.g., oral contraceptives, malignancy, polycythemia) • Injury to vessel wall (e.g., IVs, vascular surgery)	• Narcotics • High Fowler's position • Splinting of chest	• Sharp • Knifelike • Shooting • Deep ache • Pressure • Worsened by deep inspiration or coughing	• Substernal or lateral chest • Radiation to shoulder or neck	• Mild to severe	• Sudden onset • Duration: minutes to hours	• Tachycardia, tachypnea • Dyspnea • Pallor or cyanosis • Cough • Anxiety, feeling of impending doom • Sinus tachycardia or atrial dysrhythmias • Accentuated P_2 • Right-sided S_4, possible right-sided S_3 • If RVF: JVD • If pulmonary infarction: pleural friction rub, hemoptysis, fever
Pneumothorax	• Congenital bleb • Emphysematous bullous • Large tidal volumes or PEEP on mechanical ventilator • Chest trauma • Exacerbated by coughing, exertion, or Valsalva maneuver	• Narcotics • Insertion of chest tube	• Tearing • Sharp • Worsened by breathing	• Lateral chest • May radiate to shoulder, back, arms	• Mild to severe	• Sudden onset • Duration: hours to days	• Tachypnea • Tachycardia • Dyspnea • Anxiety • JVD • Hyperresonance to percussion of affected side • Diminished breath sounds on affected side • Subcutaneous emphysema may be seen • Tracheal deviation may be seen, especially with tension pneumothorax

Continued

Table 2-5 Differentiation of Chest Pain—cont'd

Cause	Provocation	Palliation	Quality	Region/Radiation	Severity	Timing	Associated Signs/ Symptoms
Pleuropulmonary (e.g., pleurisy)	• Respiratory infection • Aspiration	• Narcotics • Relief with sitting up	• Sharp • Worsened by coughing, inspiration, or movement	• Lateral chest • May radiate to shoulder, neck	• Moderate	• Gradual onset • Duration: days to weeks	• Tachypnea • Tachycardia • Dyspnea • Fever • Productive cough • Pleural friction rub
Gastrointestinal chest pain	• Cold liquids • Food intake, especially spicy foods, acidic foods or foods high in fat • Alcohol • Caffeine • Stress • Smoking • Exercise	• Sitting up • Antacids • Esophageal spasm (may be relieved by nitroglycerin)	• "Heartburn" • Dull, burning • Squeezing • Worsened by eating or supine position	• Retrosternal or lower substernal • Upper abdomen • Midline • May radiate to left arm, neck, jaw, upper abdomen, back, shoulder	• Mild to moderate	• Gradual or sudden onset • Duration: minutes to days	• Dyspnea • Diaphoresis • Anxiety • Dysphagia • Eructation • Vomiting
Musculoskeletal chest pain	• Neck or arm strain • Movement • Coughing • Deep breathing • CPR	• Rest • Heat • Nonsteroidal antiinflammatory agents (e.g., aspirin, ibuprofen)	• Soreness • Stabbing or sticking sensation • Tenderness • Worsened with inspiration and movement	• Localized to one side of chest	• Mild to moderate	• Gradual or sudden onset • Duration: weeks	• Tachypnea • Splinting respirations • Localized tenderness over site of pain
Psychosomatic chest pain	• Stress • Fatigue	• Rest • Anxiolytics	• Dull ache • Sharp • Stabbing • Superficial	• Precordium • Localized; frequently on left side • No radiation	• Mild to moderate	• Gradual or sudden onset • Duration: minutes to days	• Hyperpnea • Dyspnea • Palpitations • Dry mouth • Dizziness • Tingling of hands, mouth • Fatigue • Frequent sighing

BP, Blood pressure; *CPR*, cardiopulmonary resuscitation: *ECG*, electrocardiagram; *NTG*, nitroglycerin; S_4, fourth heart sound; *JVD*, jugular vein distention; P_2, pulmonic component of second sound; *PEEP*, positive end-expiratory pressure; *RVF*, right ventricular failure.

1) Effort syncope: transient loss of consciousness that occurs shortly after heavy activity is started; may be associated with aortic or subaortic stenosis
2) Stokes-Adams attack: dramatic loss of consciousness; related to heart block or dysrhythmia
3) Pacemaker syncope: syncope caused by malfunction or failure of an artificial pacemaker
4) Hypersensitive carotid sinus syncope: syncope caused by pressure applied on a carotid sinus body of a patient with atherosclerotic and hypersensitive carotid arteries

g. Headache: may be related to hypertension
h. Ascites: may be related to right ventricular failure (RVF)
i. Abdominal pain: may be related to RVF
j. Edema or weight gain: frequently related to RVF; also described as bloated feeling, swelling, tightening of clothing, tightening of shoes, marks left from constricting garments
k. Fatigue or weakness: may be related to RVF
l. Nocturia: may be related to HF or diuretic use
m. Diaphoresis: may be related to sympathetic nervous system stimulation or infection
n. Unexplained joint pain: may be related to rheumatic fever
o. Intermittent claudication: hip, thigh, or calf pain that occurs with exercise and ceases with rest; indicative of peripheral arterial disease
p. Peripheral skin changes: Decrease in hair distribution, skin color changes, skin ulcerations that will not heal, or a thin, shiny appearance to the skin may indicate peripheral vascular disease.
q. Calf tenderness: may be related to thrombophlebitis; may be accompanied by red, warm skin over vein
r. Varicose veins: dilated, sometimes painful, veins

3. History of present illness: use PQRST format
   a. Provocation, palliation
   b. Quality, quantity
   c. Region, radiation
   d. Severity
   e. Timing
   f. Associated symptoms
4. Past medical history
   a. Past illnesses
      1) Coronary artery disease
         a) Angina
         b) Myocardial infarction
      2) Cerebrovascular disease: transient ischemic attacks or stroke
      3) Dysrhythmias
      4) Hypertension
      5) Hyperlipidemia
      6) Peripheral vascular disease
      7) Rheumatic fever or rheumatic heart disease
      8) Murmur or known valvular heart disease
      9) Pulmonary disease (e.g., asthma, chronic obstructive pulmonary disease [COPD])
      10) Pulmonary embolism
      11) Connective tissue disorders
      12) Endocrine disorders, especially diabetes mellitus
      13) Kidney disease
      14) Alcoholism
      15) Anemia
      16) Bleeding disorders
   b. Past chest trauma: History of recent trauma is important to differentiate myocardial infarction from myocardial contusion; recent chest trauma would serve as a contraindication for fibrinolytics.
   c. Past surgical procedures
      1) Cardiac surgery: identify whether coronary artery bypass grafting, valve replacement, or other type of cardiac surgery
      2) Percutaneous coronary intervention (PCI) procedures: angioplasty; atherectomy; stent placement; valvuloplasty
      3) Pacemaker insertion
   d. Allergies and type of reaction
   e. Past diagnostic studies (e.g., stress ECG, cardiac catheterization, echocardiogram)
5. Family history
   a. Coronary artery disease (CAD)
   b. Cerebrovascular disease, including stroke
   c. Congenital heart defects
   d. Sudden cardiac death
   e. Peripheral vascular disease
   f. Hypertension
   g. Diabetes mellitus
   h. Hyperlipidemia
   i. Kidney disease
   j. Bleeding disorders
6. Social history
   a. Relationship with spouse or significant other; family structure
   b. Occupation
   c. Educational level
   d. Usual activity level and ability to perform activities of daily living
   e. Stress level and usual coping mechanisms
   f. Personality type
      1) Type A: sense of time urgency; hostility; aggression; ambition; competitiveness; impatience; frustration
      2) Type B: none of the above qualities
   g. Recreational habits
   h. Exercise habits
   i. Dietary habits
   j. Caffeine intake
   k. Tobacco use: recorded as pack-years (number of packs per day times the number of years he or she has been smoking)
   l. Alcohol use: recorded as alcoholic beverages consumed per month, week, or day
   m. Toxin exposure
   n. Travel

7. Medication history
   a. Prescribed drug, dose, frequency, time of last dose
   b. Nonprescribed drugs
      1) Over-the-counter drugs, including herbal supplements
      2) Substance abuse (e.g., cocaine, amphetamines)
   c. Patient's understanding of drug actions, side effects
   d. Drugs causing potential problems for patients with cardiovascular disease
      1) Sinus or cold remedies: may contain ephedrine and increase BP
      2) Over-the-counter weight reduction agents: may contain ephedrine
      3) Aspirin: prolongs blood clotting
      4) Tricyclic antidepressants: may cause dysrhythmias (e.g., torsades de pointes)
      5) Phenytoin: may cause dysrhythmias
      6) Phenothiazines: may cause dysrhythmias, hypotension
      7) Oral contraceptives: may predispose to embolus, thrombosis
      8) Doxorubicin (Adriamycin): may cause cardiomyopathy
      9) Lithium: may cause dysrhythmias
      10) Corticosteroids: cause sodium and fluid retention and exacerbate heart failure
      11) Theophylline preparations: cause tachycardia and may cause dysrhythmias
      12) Cardiac stimulants (e.g., cocaine): cause tachycardia and may cause dysrhythmias and coronary artery spasm
   e. Herbal supplements causing potential problems for patients with cardiovascular disease (Tachjian, Maria, and Jahangir, 2010)
      1) Alfalfa: may increase risk of bleeding with warfarin
      2) Black cohosh: may cause hypotension
      3) Ephedra: may increase heart rate and/or blood pressure; may cause fatal interactions with many cardiac drugs
      4) Garlic: may increase risk of bleeding with anticoagulants
      5) Ginger: may potentiate warfarin
      6) Ginkgo: may increase risk of bleeding with warfarin, aspirin, or COX-2 inhibitors
      7) Ginseng: may cause hypertension
      8) Goldenseal: may potentiate warfarin; may cause hypertension, hallucinations, or delirium
      9) Grapefruit juice: increases effects of statins, calcium-channel blockers
      10) Green tea: may decrease effect of warfarin
      11) Hawthorn: potentiates effects of cardiac glycosides and nitrates
      12) Kelp: increases effect of antihypertensives and anticoagulants
      13) Licorice root: may cause hypertension, hypokalemia, digoxin toxicity
      14) Oleander: may cause heart block, hyperkalemia, dysrhythmias, death
      15) St. John's wort: may increase heart rate and/or blood pressure; may decrease digoxin blood level

Landmarks (Figure 2-29)

1. Anatomical
   a. Clavicle
   b. Sternum
   c. Ribs
   d. Intercostal spaces
   e. Angle of Louis
   f. Xiphoid process
   g. Costal margin
   h. Costal angle
2. Imaginary
   a. Midsternal line (MSL)
   b. Midclavicular line (MCL)
   c. Anterior axillary line (AAL)
   d. Midaxillary line (MAL)
   e. Posterior axillary line (PAL)
   f. Scapular line
   g. Midspinal line
3. Location of heart
   a. Between the sternum and spinal column
   b. Lies between second ICS and fifth ICS
   c. Apex normally at fifth LICS at MCL

Inspection and Palpation

1. Vital signs
   a. Blood pressure (BP): sitting; lying; standing
      1) Reduction of up to 15 mm Hg in systolic and 5 mm Hg in diastolic BP when standing is normal; greater reduction indicates orthostatic changes.
         a) To assess for orthostatic changes, assist the patient to a standing position, wait 2-3 minutes, then repeat measurement of BP and heart rate.
      2) Variation of up to 15 mm Hg between arms is normal.
      3) BP in lower extremities is expected to be 10 mm Hg higher than in upper extremities.
      4) Narrowed pulse pressure frequently indicates vasoconstriction as occurs with innervation of sympathetic nervous system (SNS) (e.g., hypovolemic shock); widened pulse pressure frequently indicates excessive vasodilation as occurs with excessive vasodilatory mediator release (e.g., septic shock).
   b. Heart rate
      1) Rhythm if ECG monitor available
      2) Tachycardia frequently indicates innervation of SNS.
   c. Respiratory (ventilatory) rate: Tachypnea frequently indicates innervation of sympathetic nervous system (SNS).
   d. Temperature: Fever may indicate inflammatory or infectious process (e.g., myocardial infarction, pericarditis, endocarditis).

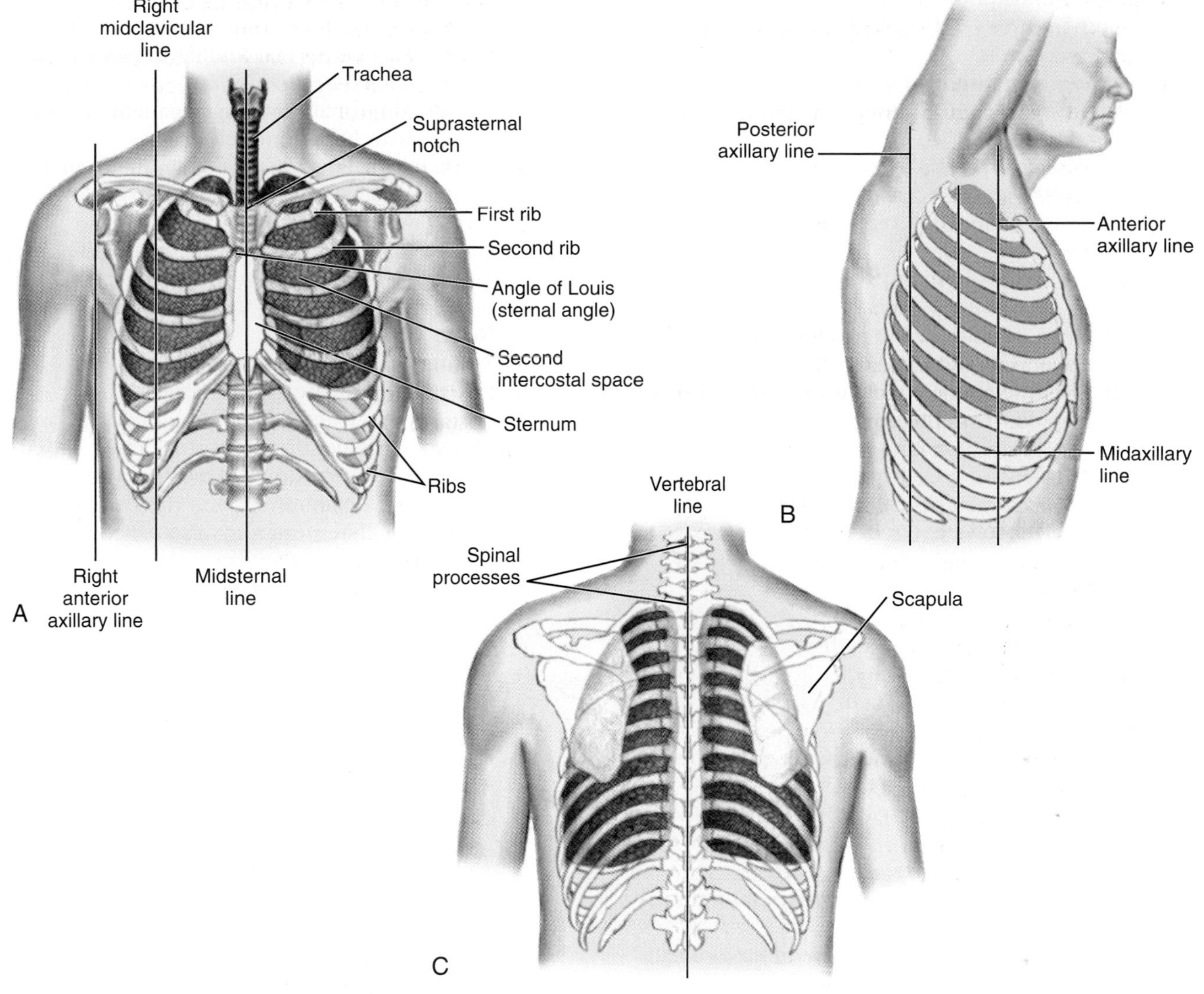

Figure 2-29 Landmarks of the thorax. **A,** Anterior. **B,** Right lateral. **C,** Posterior. (From Urden, L., Stacy, K., & Lough, M. [2010]. *Critical care nursing: Diagnosis and management* [6th ed.]. St. Louis: Mosby.)

e. Height
f. Weight: important indicator of fluid gain or loss

2. General survey
   a. Apparent health status: consistency of apparent age and chronological age
   b. Level of consciousness
   c. Gross deformity
   d. Nutritional status
   e. Stature/posture
   f. Gait
3. Skin and appendages
   a. Color
      1) Pallor: may be indication of anemia, sympathetic nervous system innervation, or sympathomimetic agents (e.g., phenylephrine [Neo-Synephrine], norepinephrine [Levophed], dopamine [Intropin])
      2) Cyanosis
         a) Peripheral (or cold) cyanosis is seen on fingertips, toes; associated with peripheral hypoperfusion or vasoconstriction
         b) Central (or warm) cyanosis is seen on lips, tongue, mucous membranes; associated with 5 grams of deoxygenated hemoglobin
            i) Central cyanosis may be a late or even impossible sign of hypoxemia in severely anemic patients.
            ii) Central cyanosis may be a relatively early sign of hypoxemia in polycythemic patients; patients with chronic bronchitis are nicknamed *blue bloaters - blue* because of chronic hypoxemia and *bloaters* because of chronic RVF.
         c) In dark-skinned patients, cyanosis appears as an ashen color.
      3) Ruddiness: related to polycythemia or hypercapnia

b. Moisture: diaphoresis; dryness
c. Temperature: Cold skin may be related to hypoperfusion.
d. Turgor: decrease in skin turgor, also referred to as *tenting*, related to interstitial dehydration
e. Edema
   1) Edema indicates increase in interstitial fluid of 30% above normal.
   2) Note the location of the edema.
      a) Facial
         i) Allergies: profound facial edema in anaphylaxis
         ii) Steroids: exogenous (e.g., prednisone) or endogenous (e.g., Cushing's syndrome)
         iii) Renal disease (e.g., nephrotic syndrome)
      b) Dependent edema: RVF
      c) Generalized edema (anasarca): end-stage HF; end-stage renal failure; severe hypoproteinemia
   3) Degree of pitting
      a) Grade 1+ = 0-¼ inch
      b) Grade 2+ = ¼-½ inch
      c) Grade 3+ = ½-1 inch
      d) Grade 4+ = >1 inch
f. Lesions
   1) Arterial disease may cause ulcers at toes or points of trauma.
   2) Venous disease may cause ulcers at sides of ankles.

4. Fingertips and nailbeds
   a. Color: bluish nailbeds with peripheral cyanosis
   b. Clubbing
      1) Loss of normal angle between base of nail and skin; clubbing present if angle is greater than 180 degrees
      2) Indicative of chronic hypoxia
   c. Splinter hemorrhages
      1) Red to black linear streaks under nailbed that run from base to tip of nail
      2) May indicate bacterial endocarditis
   d. Osler's nodes:
      1) Painful red subcutaneous nodules on fingertips
      2) May indicate embolization in infective endocarditis
5. Head and neck
   a. Face
      1) Facial expression
      2) Facial flushing: episodic facial flushing may indicate pheochromocytoma
   b. Head bobbing up and down with each heartbeat
      1) Referred to as *de Musset's sign*
      2) Indicates aortic aneurysm or regurgitation
   c. Eyes
      1) Xanthoma palpebrarum (also called *xanthelasma*)
         a) Benign, fatty, fibrous, yellowish plaque, nodule, or tumor on the eyelids
         b) Associated with hyperlipidemia
      2) Corneal arcus
         a) Light-colored ring surrounding the iris
         b) May be normal finding in elderly patient (called *arcus senilis*)
         c) Abnormal in younger patient; associated with hyperlipidemia
      3) Exophthalmos: may be seen in advanced HF with pulmonary hypertension
   d. Ears
      1) Diagonal bilateral earlobe creases (referred to as *McCarty's sign*): may indicate CAD if seen in individuals under 45 years of age
   e. Neck
      1) Jugular vein distention (JVD)
         a) To evaluate JVD (Figure 2-30)
            i) Place patient at a 45-degree angle
            ii) Identify the sternal angle: raised notch that is created where the manubrium and the body of the sternum join; also called *manubriosternal junction* or *angle of Louis*
            iii) Measure height of neck vein distention above the level of the sternal angle.
            iv) Normal height of neck vein distention is 1-3 cm above the sternal angle.
         b) Neck vein distention of greater than 3 cm above the sternal angle is indicative of any of the following:
            i) Right ventricular failure
            ii) Hypervolemia
            iii) Tension pneumothorax
            iv) Cardiac tamponade

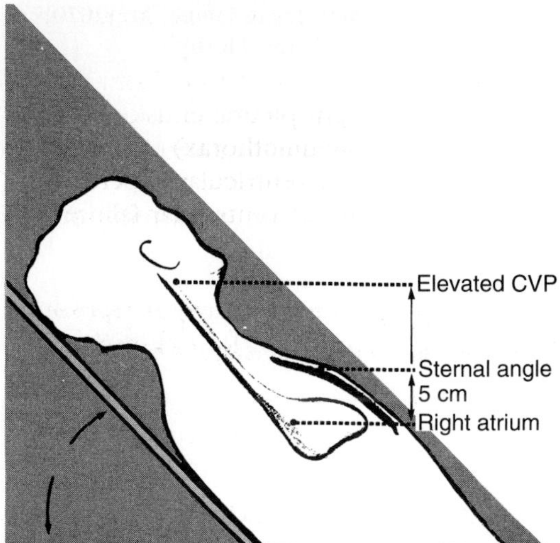

Figure 2-30 Jugular venous distention and estimation of central venous pressure: assess jugular venous distention with patient in 45-degree angle; determine height of jugular venous distention above the sternal angle; add 5 cm to this measurement to estimate central venous pressure in cm of water pressure. (From Guzzetta, C. E., & Dossey, B. M. [1992]. *Cardiovascular nursing: Holistic practice*. St Louis: Mosby.)

c) To estimate central venous pressure (CVP)
   i) The angle of Louis is assumed to be approximately 5 cm above the right atrium so 5 is added to the height of neck vein distention above the angle of Louis to estimate CVP.
   ii) Normal CVP is approximately 3-8 cm of H_2O pressure.

d) To evaluate hepatojugular (or abdominojugular) reflux
   i) The test is performed by applying pressure over right upper quadrant for 30-60 seconds while evaluating an increase in neck vein distention.
   ii) A positive result is a sustained increase in neck vein distention of 4 cm or more or a fall of 4 cm or more after release of pressure.
   iii) A positive result is an indication of heart failure

6. Precordium: Inspect and palpate entire precordium.
   a. Point of maximal impulse (PMI) or apical impulse
      1) Frequently visible and usually palpable; may not be palpable in patients with obesity, muscular chest wall, or an increased anterior-posterior diameter
      2) Location
         a) Normal location of the PMI is at the fifth LICS at the MCL.
         b) Lateral displacement is associated with any of the following:
            i) Left ventricular dilation (e.g., aortic or mitral insufficiency)
            ii) Upward displacement of the diaphragm (e.g., pregnancy, ascites)
            iii) Right to left mediastinal shift (e.g., right pleural effusion or tension pneumothorax)
            iv) Left ventricular hypertrophy (LVH) or left ventricular failure (LVF)
         c) Medial displacement may occur with any of the following:
            i) Downward displacement of the diaphragm (e.g., COPD)
            ii) Left to right mediastinal shift (e.g., left pleural effusion or tension pneumothorax)
      3) Intensity
         a) Normal intensity is only a light tap.
         b) Failure may increase the intensity and cause a heave.
      4) Size
         a) Normal size is approximately 1-2 cm.
         b) The size is more diffuse with ventricular aneurysm.
   b. Heave
      1) Lifting of the chest wall indicative of failure
      2) Left ventricular heave felt at or near the apex
      3) Right ventricular heave (or lift) felt at or near the sternum
   c. Thrill
      1) Palpable vibration associated with murmur or bruit
      2) Felt where the murmur is heard the loudest or at location of bruit

7. Abdomen
   a. Aortic pulsation
      1) Normally visible, especially during expiration
      2) Normally palpable at midline or slightly to left of midline; feel for lateral expansion which might be indicative of aneurysm

8. Extremities
   a. Arterial versus venous disease (Table 2-6)
   b. Temperature
      1) Coolness or coldness may indicate decreased blood flow due to hypoperfusion or vasoconstriction.
      2) Excessive warmth may indicate hyperthyroidism or fever.
   c. Peripheral pulses
      1) Location (Figure 2-31)

Table 2-6 Comparison of Clinical Indications of Arterial and Venous Peripheral Vascular Disease

	Arterial	Venous
Pain	• Excruciating in acute occlusion • Intermittent claudication in chronic occlusion	• Crampy pain • Homans' sign in thrombophlebitis
Pulses	• Diminished or absent	• Normal (but may be difficult to palpate due to edema)
Color	• Pale	• Normal or ruddy
Temperature	• Cool or cold	• Warm
Edema	• Absent	• Present; may be severe
Skin changes	• Thin, shiny, atrophic skin • Loss of hair • Thickened toenails	• Brown pigmentation at ankles
Ulcerations	• At toes or points of trauma	• At sides of ankles

a) Carotid: Palpate only lower half and never palpate both carotids simultaneously.
b) Brachial
c) Radial
d) Ulnar
e) Femoral
f) Popliteal
g) Posterior tibialis
h) Dorsalis pedis

2) Rate and rhythm
3) Amplitude
a) 0 = not palpable
b) 1+ = weak and thready, easily obliterated
c) 2+ = normal, not easily obliterated
d) 3+ = full and bounding, cannot obliterate

4) Capillary refill rate
a) Color should return to blanched area within 3 seconds; delay beyond 3 seconds indicates hypoperfusion.

5) Apical-radial pulse deficit
a) Performed by two nurses using one watch
b) Deficit (radial pulse rate less than apical rate) indicative of dysrhythmia (e.g., atrial fibrillation, ventricular ectopy)

6) Pulse contour (Figure 2-32)
a) Pulsus magnus
i) Strong, bounding pulses with rapid upstroke and downstroke
ii) Characteristic of any of the following:
(a) Hypertension
(b) Thyrotoxicosis
(c) Aortic insufficiency
(d) Patent ductus arteriosus
(e) Arteriovenous fistula

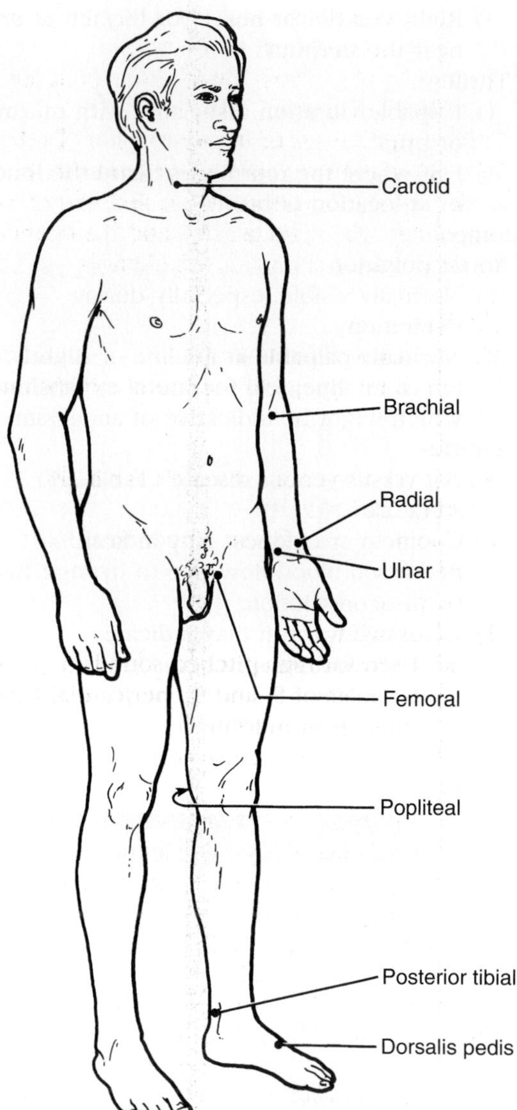

Figure 2-31 Locations of peripheral pulses. (From Lewis, S. M., & Collier, I. C. [1992]. *Medical-surgical nursing: Assessment and management of clinical problems* [3rd ed.]. St Louis: Mosby.)

ARTERIAL PULSE ABNORMALITIES

Type	Description
Pulsus magnus	Pulse is readily palpable, not easily obliterated by fingers, and does not fade Pulse is felt as a brisk impact; can occur with or without increased pulse pressure
Pulsus parvus	Pulse is difficult to feel, easily obliterated by the fingers, and may fade out Pulse is slow to rise, has a sustained summit, and falls slowly If both weak and variable in amplitude, pulse is termed "thready"
Pulsus alterans	Pulses have large amplitude beats followed by pulses of small amplitude Rhythm remains normal
Pulsus paradoxus	Pattern is exaggerated (greater than 10 mm Hg) during inspiration, and amplitude is increased during expiration Heart rate and rhythm are unchanged Inspiration Expiration Inspiration
Pulsus bisferiens (double-peaked)	Best felt by palpating carotid artery Two systolic peaks occur in disorders that cause rapid left ventricular ejection of large stroke volume with wide pulse pressure
Water-hammer, collapsing	Pulse has greater amplitude than normal pulse Pulse marked by rapid rise to a narrow summit followed by a sudden descent

Figure 2-32 Pulse contour. (Modified from Cannobio, M. M. [1990]. *Cardiovascular disorders*. St Louis: Mosby.)

b) Pulsus parvus
  i) Small, weak pulse
  ii) Characteristic of any of the following:
    (a) Aortic stenosis: also tardus (late)
    (b) Mitral stenosis
    (c) Constrictive pericarditis
    (d) Cardiac tamponade

c) Pulsus alternans
  i) Alternating pulse waves, every other beat being weaker than the preceding one
  ii) Characteristic of left ventricular failure

d) Pulsus paradoxus
  i) Pulsus paradoxus is an exaggeration of normal physiologic response to inspiration
    (a) The normal decrease in BP during inspiration is 10 mm Hg or less
    (b) BP drop of more than 10 mm Hg during inspiration is pulsus paradoxus
  ii) Pulsus paradoxus may be characteristic of any of the following conditions:
    (a) Pericardial effusion
    (b) Constrictive pericarditis
    (c) Cardiac tamponade
    (d) Severe lung disease
    (e) Advanced HF
    (f) Hemorrhagic shock

e) Pulsus bisferiens
  i) Two pulses palpated during systole with second slightly weaker than the first
  ii) Characteristic of any of the following:
    (a) Hypertrophic cardiomyopathy
    (b) Constrictive cardiomyopathy
    (c) Aortic stenosis or regurgitation

f) Water-hammer (or *Corrigan's*) pulse
  i) Increased pulse pressure with a rapid upstroke and downstroke and shortened peak
  ii) Characteristic of aortic regurgitation or patent ductus arteriosus (PDA)

d. Homan's sign
  1) Identified by dorsiflexing the foot with the knee slightly bent
  2) Homan's sign is present if the patient has pain in the calf with this action.
  3) Suggestive of thrombophlebitis but not definitive

e. Petechiae or ecchymosis

f. Varicose veins

g. Neurovascular assessment

Box 2-1 Clinical Manifestations of Acute Arterial Occlusion

Pain	Paresthesia
Pallor	Paralysis
Pulselessness	Polar (cold)

NOTE: These 6 Ps are your format for neurovascular assessment.

  1) Assess neurovascular status in all of the following situations:
    a) After cardiac catheterization
    b) After percutaneous coronary interventional (PCI) procedure (e.g., angioplasty, atherectomy, valvuloplasty)
    c) When the patient has intraaortic balloon pump catheter in place
    d) When the patient has a fracture of an extremity (to monitor for compartment syndrome)
    e) When the patient has a circumferential burn of an extremity
  2) Monitor for clinical indications of acute arterial occlusion: 6 Ps (Box 2-1)

h. Clinical indications of hypoperfusion (Table 2-2); Because hypoperfusion is progressive, the earlier these changes are identified, the more appropriate the management and the chances for successfully reversing the changes.

Auscultation

1. Qualities of a good stethoscope
  a. Snug-fitting earplugs to eliminate extraneous sounds
  b. Tubing
    1) Two tubings are preferable for high-frequency sounds.
    2) Tubing should be no longer than 12-15 inches.
  c. Chest piece
    1) Diaphragm
      a) Used for high-pitched sounds (e.g., S_1, S_2, splits of S_1 and S_2, pericardial friction rubs, most murmurs)
      b) Held firmly against skin
    2) Bell
      a) Used for low-pitched sounds (e.g., S_3, S_4, murmurs of AV valve stenosis)
      b) Held only tightly enough against skin to create a seal
2. Auscultatory areas (Figure 2-33)
  a. Mitral: fifth LICS at MCL
  b. Tricuspid: fifth LICS at LSB
  c. Erb's point: third LICS at LSB
  d. Pulmonic: second LICS at LSB
  e. Aortic: second RICS at RSB
3. Method of cardiac auscultation
  a. Ensure a quiet room by turning off television and radio and asking others to be quiet.
  b. Listen to all four auscultatory areas with both bell and diaphragm.

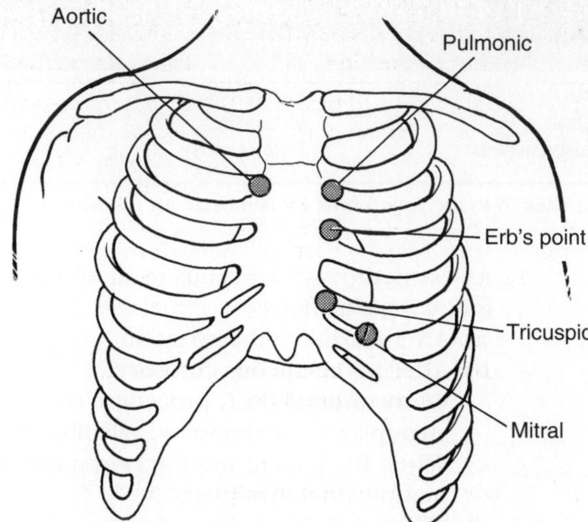

Figure 2-33 Cardiac auscultatory areas. (From Price, S. & Wilson, L. [2003]. *Pathophysiology: Clinical concepts of disease processes* [6th ed.]. St Louis: Mosby.)

c. Concentrate on one cardiac event at a time: S_1; S_2; systole; diastole

4. Heart sounds
   a. Rules to consider
      1) Left-sided heart events precede right-sided heart events (i.e., the mitral component [M_1] precedes the tricuspid component [T_1] of S_1, and the aortic component [A_2] precedes the pulmonic component [P_2] of S_2).
      2) Left-sided heart events are normally louder than right-sided heart events (i.e., M_1 is the loudest component of S_1, and A_2 is the loudest component of S_2).
      3) Left-sided heart events are normally loudest during expiration, and right-sided heart events are normally loudest during inspiration.
   b. S_1
      1) Caused by closure of the AV valves: mitral and tricuspid
      2) Marks the end of diastole and the beginning of systole
      3) Loudest at the apex
      4) Note if a single sound or split.
      5) Note any increase in intensity (closing snap).
   c. S_2
      1) Caused by closure of the semilunar valves: aortic and pulmonic
      2) Marks the end of systole and the beginning of diastole.
      3) Loudest at the base
      4) Note if a single sound or split.
      5) Note any increase in intensity.
   d. Splits
      1) Split S_1
         a) Both components (M_1 and T_1) of S_1 can be heard.
         b) A split S_1 is heard best at the tricuspid area.
         c) A narrowly split S_1 may be normal.
         d) A split S_1 is more often abnormal than normal and associated with any of the following:
            i) Right bundle branch block
            ii) Left ventricular (epicardial) pacemaker
            iii) Left ventricular ectopy
      2) Split S_2
         a) Both components (A_2 and P_2) of S_2 can be heard.
         b) A split S_2 is heard best at the pulmonic area.
         c) Inspiratory only split of S_2 is normal
            i) Called a physiologic split of S_2
            ii) Normal and frequently heard in individuals under 50 years of age
            iii) Split only during inspiration
            iv) Caused by changes in intrathoracic pressure related to ventilation; increased venous return to right ventricle and decreased venous return to left ventricle delay pulmonic valve closure (P_2).
         d) Expiratory split of S_2 is abnormal.
            i) Increased splitting during inspiration (split on expiration but split more during inspiration); associated with any of the following:
               (a) Right bundle branch block
               (b) Left ventricular ectopy
               (c) Left ventricular (epicardial) pacemaker
               (d) Severe mitral regurgitation
               (e) Pulmonary stenosis
               (f) Pulmonary hypertension
               (g) Ventricular septal defect
            ii) Fixed splitting (split the same on inspiration and expiration); associated with atrial septal defect
            iii) Paradoxical split (split on expiration but not on inspiration); associated with any of the following:
               (a) Left bundle branch block
               (b) Right ventricular (endocardial) pacemaker
               (c) Right ventricular ectopy
               (d) Severe aortic stenosis or regurgitation
               (e) Patent ductus arteriosus
   e. Extra heart sounds (Table 2-7 is a summary of extra heart sounds)
      1) S_3
         a) Also called a ventricular gallop
         b) Dull, low-pitched sound occurring early in diastole after S_2; may sound like "Ken-tuc-ky" with the "ky" being the S_3

Table 2-7 Extra Sounds

Sound	Cause	Timing	Location	Pitch	Position	Respiratory Effect
S_3 (also called ventricular gallop)	Rapid ventricular filling into dilated ventricle	Early diastole (rapid filling subphase of diastole)	Mitral if LV; tricuspid if RV	Low	Heard best in left lateral position	LV S_3 increases with expiration; RV S_3 increases with inspiration
S_4 (also called atrial with gallop)	Atrial contraction into noncompliant ventricle	Late diastole (atrial contraction subphase of diastole)	Mitral area if LV; tricuspid area if RV	Low	Heard best in left lateral position	LV S_4 increases with expiration; RV S_4 increases with inspiration
Quadruple rhythm	All four heart sounds are heard	S_3 heard in early diastole, and S_4 heard in late diastole	Apex	Low	Heard best in left lateral position	As for S_3, S_4
Summation gallop	S_1, S_2 heard along with merged S_3 and S_4; occurs with tachycardia	Mid-diastole	Apex	Low	Heard best in left lateral position	As for S_3, S_4
Pericardial friction rub	Inflammation of the pericardium	Systolic, early diastolic, and late diastolic components	Lower left sternal border	High	Heard best with patient leaning forward	Heard best if patient holds breath after expiration
Pericardial knock	Constriction of the pericardium	Early diastole	Lower left sternal border	Low	Heard best with patient leaning forward or in left lateral position	Heard best if patient holds breath after expiration
Ejection click	Opening of defective semilunar valve	Early systole	Aortic or pulmonic	High	Heard best with patient leaning forward	Aortic: not affected by respiratory phase Pulmonic: increased with expiration
Midsystolic click	Prolapse of mitral valve leaflet	Midsystole	Mitral	High	Heard best in left lateral position	Increased with expiration
Opening snap	Abrupt recoil of stenotic atrioventricular valve	Early diastole	Mitral	High	Heard best in left lateral position	Mitral: increased with expiration Tricuspid: increased with inspiration
Mediastinal crunch	Pneumomediastinum; heart movements displacing air that is present in the mediastinum	Random	Apex or lower left sternal border	High	Heard best in left lateral position	Increased with inspiration

LV, Left ventricle; *RV,* right ventricle; S_1, first heart sound; S_2, second heart sound; S_3, third heart sound; S_4, fourth heart sound.

c) Caused by rapid rush of blood into a dilated ventricle; considered abnormal in patients over 30 years of age
d) Heard best with bell, with the patient lying on the left side
   i) Left-sided S_3
      (a) Heard best at apex
      (b) Heard best during expiration
   ii) Right-sided S_3
      (a) Heard best at sternum
      (b) Heard best during inspiration
e) Associated primarily with failure
f) May also be associated with any of the following:
   i) Fluid overload
   ii) Cardiomyopathy
   iii) Ventricular septal defect or patent ductus arteriosus
   iv) Mitral or tricuspid regurgitation

2) S_4
   a) Also called an *atrial gallop*
   b) Dull, low-pitched sound occurring late in diastole before S_1; may sound like "Ten-nes-see" with the "Ten" being the S_4
   c) Due to atrial contraction of blood into a noncompliant ventricle; abnormal in adults

- d) Heard best with bell with patient lying on the left side
  - i) Left-sided S_4: heard best at apex
  - ii) Right-sided S_4: heard best at sternum
- e) Associated with any of the following:
  - i) Myocardial ischemia or infarction
  - ii) Hypertension
    - (a) Systemic: left-sided S_4
    - (b) Pulmonary: right-sided S_4
  - iii) Ventricular hypertrophy
  - iv) AV blocks
  - v) Severe aortic or pulmonic stenosis

3) Quadruple rhythm: all four heart sounds heard
4) Summation gallop
   - a) All four heart sounds with tachycardia
   - b) Merging of S_3 and S_4 causes a louder mid-diastolic sound
5) Pericardial friction rub
   - a) High-pitched "to-and-fro" scratchy sound; usually triphasic including systolic, early diastolic, and late diastolic components
   - b) Heard best at the fourth-fifth intercostal space at lower (LSB) with patient leaning forward
   - c) Differentiate between pericardial and pleural friction rubs: Ask the patient to hold breath; if the rub persists, it is a pericardial friction rub.
   - d) Caused by inflammation of the pericardium; commonly heard after MI or cardiac surgery
6) Pericardial knock
   - a) Loud, early-diastolic sound heard best at lower LSB
   - b) Caused by constrictive pericarditis
7) Snaps
   - a) Opening snap
     - i) Short, high-pitched sound heard early in diastole at third-fourth LICS at LSB; earlier, sharper, higher pitched than S_3
     - ii) Caused by either of the following:
       - (a) Opening of stenotic AV valve; usually precedes a diastolic murmur
       - (b) Increased flow (e.g., ventricular septal defect, patent ductus arteriosus)
   - b) Closing snap
     - i) Really a loud S_1
     - ii) Caused by closure of AV valve
8) Clicks: high-pitched sounds heard during systole
   - a) Aortic ejection click
     - i) High-pitched sound heard early in systole over aortic area to apex; may precede systolic ejection murmur
     - ii) Caused by aortic valve disease or dilated aorta (e.g., aortic aneurysm or coarctation)
   - b) Pulmonic ejection click
     - i) High-pitched sound heard early in systole over pulmonic area
     - ii) Caused by pulmonic valve disease, pulmonary embolism, pulmonary hypertension, hyperthyroidism
   - c) Midsystolic click
     - i) High-pitched sound heard best at apex or lower left sternal border
     - ii) May occur alone or prior to a late systolic murmur
     - iii) Due to mitral valve prolapse or mitral regurgitation
   - d) Prosthetic valve click: metallic click caused by opening and closing of prosthetic valve
9) Mediastinal crunch
   - a) Crunching sound heard best at apex or along LSB in left lateral position
   - b) Caused by air in mediastinum

f. Murmurs

1) Causes of turbulence (referred to as a *murmur* if intracardiac or referred to as a *bruit* if extracardiac) (Figure 2-34)
   - a) Increased flow across a normal valve (e.g., flow murmur)
     - i) May also be called *functional* (as opposed to structural); always soft (not louder than grade II/VI) and systolic (but never holosystolic)
     - ii) Caused by any of the following:
       - (a) Hyperthermia
       - (b) Anemia
       - (c) Pregnancy
       - (d) Hyperthyroidism
   - b) Forward flow through a stenotic valve
   - c) Backward flow through a regurgitant (also called *insufficient* or *incompetent*) valve
   - d) Flow through an AV fistula or septal defect
   - e) Flow into a dilated chamber or a portion of a vessel
2) Description
   - a) Timing
     - i) Systolic
       - (a) Holosystolic: AV regurgitation or ventricular septal defect
       - (b) Ejection (midsystolic): semilunar stenosis
       - (c) Late: papillary muscle dysfunction, mitral valve prolapse, hypertrophic cardiomyopathy (previously called *idiopathic hypertrophic subaortic stenosis*)
     - ii) Diastolic
       - (a) Early diastolic: semilunar regurgitation

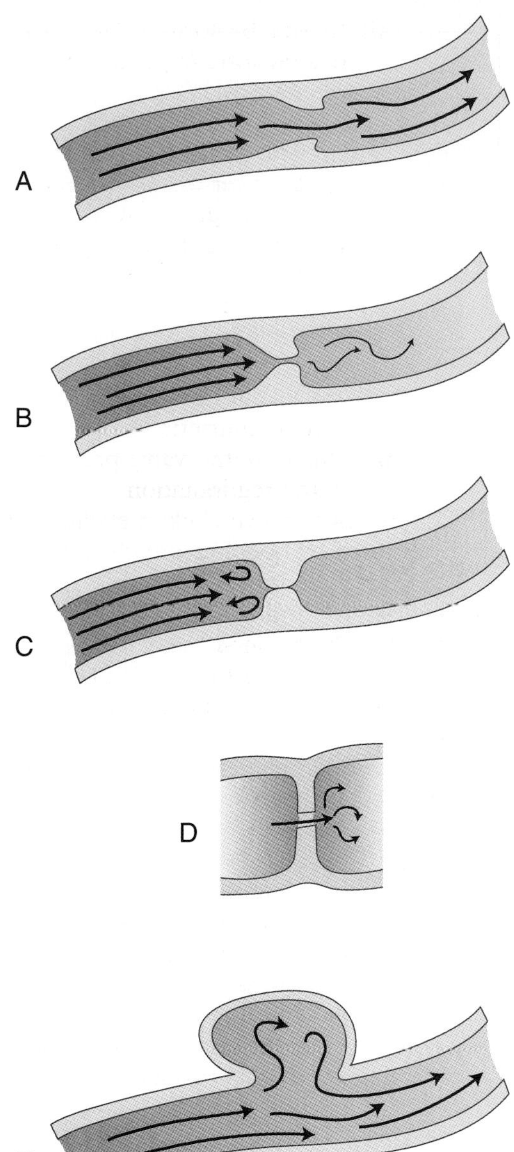

Figure 2-34 Causes of turbulence. **A,** Increased flow across a normal valve. **B,** Forward flow through a stenotic valve. **C,** Backward flow through an incompetent valve. **D,** Flow through a septal defect or an AV fistula. **E,** Flow into a dilated chamber or a portion of a vessel.

(b) Mid-diastolic or late diastolic: AV stenosis

b) Location: place at which the murmur is loudest

c) Radiation: direction in which the murmur radiates

d) Intensity: Levine scale

i) Grade I/VI: barely audible, difficult to detect

ii) Grade II/VI: clearly audible but quiet

iii) Grade III/VI: moderately loud, without a thrill

iv) Grade IV/VI: loud; with or without a thrill

v) Grade V/VI: very loud, thrill present, audible with stethoscope partially off the chest

vi) Grade VI/VI: loudest possible, thrill present, audible with stethoscope off the chest

e) Configuration

i) Crescendo: gets louder

ii) Decrescendo: gets softer

iii) Crescendo-decrescendo: louder then softer

iv) Plateau: even intensity throughout

f) Pitch

i) High pitched (heard best with diaphragm)

(a) Mitral and tricuspid regurgitation

(b) Aortic and pulmonic stenosis

(c) Aortic and pulmonic regurgitation

ii) Low pitched (heard best with bell): mitral and tricuspid stenosis

g) Quality

i) Soft

ii) Harsh

iii) Blowing

iv) Musical

v) Rumbling

vi) Rough

3) Differentiation of murmurs (Figure 2-35)

5. Vascular sound

a. Bruit

1) Turbulent sound

2) May be heard over carotids, aorta, renals, iliacs, femorals

3) Associated with plaque or aneurysm

b. Doppler pulse

1) A Doppler stethoscope is used to identify presence of pulse if the pulse is not palpable and may be used to confirm that the pulse palpated is the patient's and not the nurse's.

c. Doppler pressure

1) A Doppler stethoscope is used to measure the blood pressure distal to vascular lesions or surgery.

2) Apply sphygmomanometer on the calf or below the graft site and inflate to a pressure above the patient's systolic brachial pressure; allow pressure to decrease and note pressure when pulse is audible again; note posterior tibial pressure and dorsalis pedis pressures.

3) Use the best pressure (posterior tibial or dorsalis pedis) to calculate the ankle-brachial index (ABI).

a) Divide the systolic pressure from the leg by the brachial systolic pressure (ankle/brachial) to calculate the ABI.

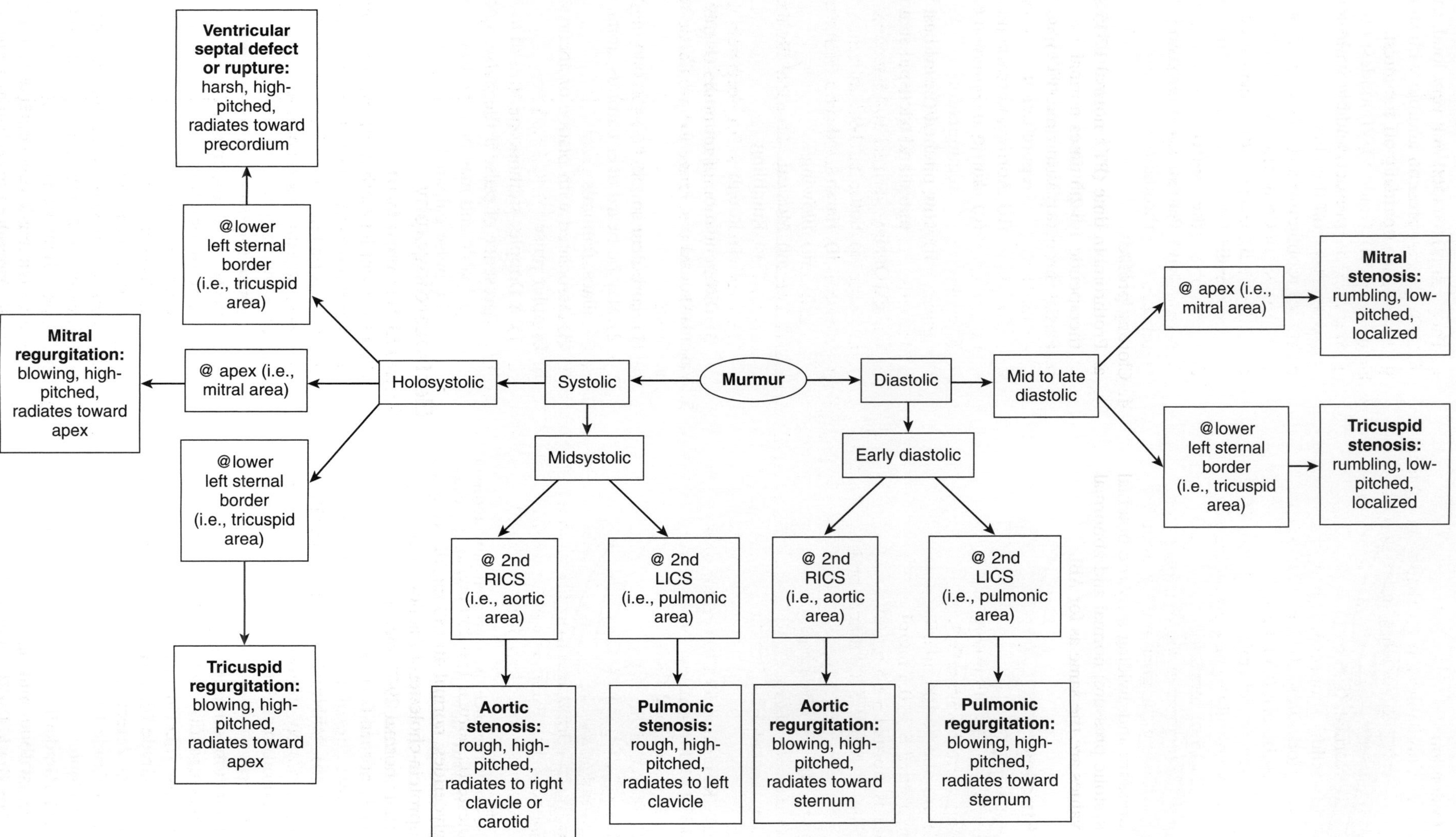

Figure 2-35 Murmurs. *LICS,* left intercostal space; *RICS,* right intercostal space.

b) Evaluation
   i) Unreliable: greater than 1; consider using toe/brachial index described later
   ii) Normal: 0.95 to 1
   iii) Mildly abnormal: 0.95-0.75
   iv) Moderately abnormal: 0.75-0.5
   v) Ischemia: 0.50-0.25
   vi) Severe ischemia: less than 0.25
   vii) Clinically significant: decrease of 0.15 or more
c) Some recommend toe/brachial index (TBI) using the great toe's systolic pressure and dividing it by the brachial systolic pressure; normal and abnormal values are the same as for ABI.

Diagnostic Studies

1. Serum chemistries
   a. Sodium: normal 136-145 mEq/L
   b. Potassium: normal 3.5-5 mEq/L
   c. Chloride: normal 96-106 mEq/L
   d. Calcium: normal 8.5-10.5 mg/dL
   e. Phosphorus: normal 3-4.5 mg/dL
   f. Magnesium: normal 1.5-2.2 mEq/L or 1.8-2.4 mg/dL
   g. Glucose: normal 70-110 mEq/L
   h. BUN: normal 5-20 mg/dL
   i. Creatinine: normal 0.7-1.5 mg/dL
   j. Enzymes
      1) Total CK: normal 55-170 U/L for males; 30-135 U/L for females
      2) CK-MB: 0% of total CK
      3) LDH: 90-200 IU/L
      4) LDH-1: 17-25% of total LDH
   k. Muscle proteins
      1) Myoglobin: normal less than 110 ng/mL
      2) Troponin I: normal less than 1.5 ng/mL
      3) Troponin T: normal less than 0.1 ng/mL
   l. Lipid profile
      1) Cholesterol: normal 150-200 mg/dL
      2) Triglycerides: normal 40-150 mg/dL
      3) Lipoprotein-cholesterol fractionation
         a) HDL: normal 29-77 mg/dL
         b) LDL: normal 62-130 mg/dL
   m. Homocysteine: normal less than 15 μmol/L
   n. C-reactive protein: normal less than 1 mg/dL
   o. Brain-type natriuretic peptide (BNP): normal less than 100 picograms/mL
      1) Heart failure
         a) Mild: 100-300 pg/mL
         b) Moderate: 300-700 pg/mL
         c) Severe: more than 700 pg/mL
      2) May also be earlier indicator of acute myocardial infarction than either CK-MB or troponin I
2. Arterial blood gases
   a. pH: normal 7.35-7.45
   b. $PaCO_2$: normal 35-45 mm Hg
   c. HCO_3 : normal 22-26 mM
   d. Base excess: −2 - +2
   e. PaO_2: normal 80-100 mm Hg
   f. SaO_2: greater than 95%
   g. Arterial lactate: less than 1 mmol/L
3. Hematology
   a. Hematocrit: normal 40-52% for males; 35-47% for females
   b. Hemoglobin: normal 13-18 g/dL for males; 12-16 g/dL for females
   c. White blood cells (WBC): normal 3500-11,000/mm^3
   d. Erythrocyte sedimentation rate: normal up to 15 mm/hr for males; up to 20 mm/hr for females
4. Clotting profile
   a. Prothrombin time (PT): normal 12-15 seconds; therapeutic 1.5-2.5 times normal
   b. Partial thromboplastin time (PTT): normal 60-90 seconds; therapeutic 1.5-2.5 times normal
   c. Activated partial thromboplastin time (aPTT): normal 25-38 seconds; therapeutic 1.5-2.5 times normal
   d. Activated clotting time (ACT): normal 70-120 seconds; therapeutic 150-190 seconds
   e. Thrombin time: normal 10-15 seconds
   f. Bleeding time: normal 1-9.5 minutes
   g. International normalized ratio (INR): normal less than 2
      1) Therapeutic range for atrial fibrillation: 1.5-2.5
      2) Therapeutic range for deep vein thrombosis (DVT) or pulmonary embolus (PE): 2-3
      3) Therapeutic range for prosthetic valves: 2.5-3.5
   h. Platelets: normal 150,000-400,000/mm^3
5. Urine
   a. Glucose: normal negative
   b. Ketones: normal negative
   c. Specific gravity: 1.005-1.03
   d. Osmolality: 50-1200 mOsm/liter
6. Other diagnostic studies (Table 2-8)

Electrocardiography

General Information

1. The electrocardiograph measures and records the electrical activity of the heart by measuring electrical potential at the skin surface; the electrocardiogram is a recording of that activity.
2. An electrocardiogram is used to detect or demonstrate any of the following:
   a. Rhythm disturbances
   b. Conduction defects
   c. Electrolyte imbalances
   d. Drug effects and toxicity
   e. Chamber enlargement or hypertrophy
   f. Myocardial ischemia, injury, or infarction
3. ECG paper (Figure 2-36)
   a. Horizontal axis measures time
      1) Each small (1 mm) box is equal to 0.04 seconds

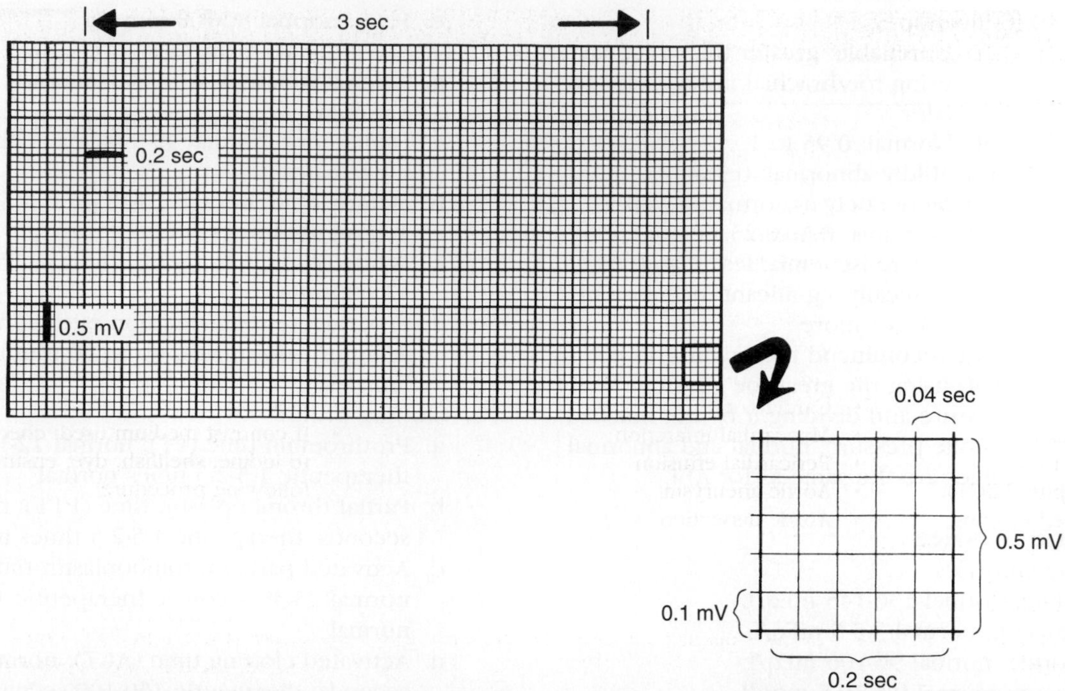

Figure 2-36 ECG paper: Horizontal axis represents time with each small block equal to 0.04 second and each large block equal to 0.2 second with 3-second intervals marked off at top of paper; vertical axis represents voltage when standardized with each small block equal to 0.1 mV and each large block equal to 0.5 mV. (From Kinney, M. R., et al. [1998]. *AACN's clinical reference for critical-care nursing* [4th ed.]. St Louis: Mosby.)

Table 2-8 Cardiovascular Diagnostic Studies

Study	Evaluates	Comments
Aortography	• Aortic valve insufficiency • Aneurysms or dissection of ascending aorta • Coarctation of the aorta • Injuries to the aorta and major branches	• Contrast medium used: check for allergy to iodine, shellfish, dye; ensure hydration following procedure • Monitor for clinical indications of anaphylaxis (e.g., flushing, urticaria, stridor) • Monitor puncture site
Cardiac biopsy	• Effect of cardiotoxic drugs • Evidence of cardiac transplant rejection • Inflammatory heart disease • Tumors • Cardiomyopathy	• Observe closely for signs of cardiac perforation and/or cardiac tamponade

Cardiac catheterization and coronary angiography	• Severity of coronary artery stenosis
	• Cardiac muscle function
	• Pressures within the heart
	• Cardiac output and ejection fraction
	• Blood gas analysis within chambers
	• Allows angioplasty, atherectomy, intracoronary stents, or lasers to reduce coronary artery obstruction
		• Prior to test:
		  • Check for allergy to iodine, shellfish, dye (contrast medium used)
		• After the test:
		  • Ensure hydration following procedure (contrast medium used)
		  • Keep extremity in which catheter was placed immobilized in a straight position for 6-12 hours
		  • Monitor arterial puncture point for hemorrhage or hematoma; collagen (e.g., AngioSeal) or stitch device (e.g., Perclose) may be used
		  • Monitor neurovascular status of affected limb
		  • Note complaints of back pain and vital sign changes (may indicate retroperitoneal hemorrhage)

Table 2-8 Cardiovascular Diagnostic Studies—cont'd		
Study	**Evaluates**	**Comments**
Chest x-ray	• Cardiac size and shape and chamber size • Abnormalities of the lungs, ribs, pleura, pulmonary vasculature • Presence of pleural effusions • Presence of thoracic aneurysm or calcification of the aorta • Presence and location of catheters, pacemaker and automatic implantable cardiac defibrillator (AICD) leads	• Inquire about possibility of pregnancy
Computed tomography (CT) Electron beam computerized tomography (EBCT): high speed imaging provides improved view of vascular structures including calcification	• Left ventricular wall motion • Cardiac tumors • Myocardial infarction • Pericardial effusion • Aortic aneurysm • Aortic dissection	• May be done with or without contrast medium • If contrast medium used: check for allergy to iodine, shellfish, dye; ensure hydration following procedure
Digital subtraction angiography	• Vascular disease and degree of occlusion	• Contrast medium used: check for allergy to iodine, shellfish, dye; ensure hydration following procedure • Monitor for clinical indications of anaphylaxis (e.g., flushing, urticaria, stridor) • Monitor puncture site
Doppler ultrasonography Duplex ultrasonography	• Vascular disease and degree of occlusion	

Echocardiography
• M-mode: single ultrasound beam
• 2-D: planar ultrasound beam; wider view of heart and structures
• Doppler: addition of Doppler to demonstrate flow of blood through the heart
• Color flow: Doppler blood flow superimposed on 2-D echocardiogram
• Stress echocardiography: images before, during, and after exercise or pharmacologic stress
• Transesophageal echocardiography (TEE): transducer placed in esophagus
	• Chamber size and wall thickness
	• Valve functioning
	  • Papillary muscle functioning
	  • Prosthetic valve functioning
	• Ventricular wall motion abnormalities
	• Intracardiac masses
	• Presence of pericardial fluid
	• Intracardiac pressures (Doppler)
	• Ejection fraction and cardiac output (Doppler)
	• Valve gradients (Doppler)
	• Intracardiac shunts (Doppler)
	• Thoracic aneurysm (transesophageal)
		• Transesophageal echocardiography is particularly better if patient is obese, has COPD, chest wall deformity, chest trauma, or thick chest dressings
		• Monitor for methemoglobinemia if local anesthetic (e.g., Cetacaine) is used
		• If TEE, monitor for clinical indications of esophageal perforation (i.e., sore throat, dysphagia, epigastric or substernal pain)

Electrocardiography (ECG)	• Dysrhythmias • Conduction defects including intraventricular blocks • Electrolyte imbalance • Drug toxicity • Myocardial ischemia, injury, infarction • Chamber hypertrophy	• List what drugs the patient is receiving on ECG request • Be alert to electrical safety hazards

Continued

Table 2-8 Cardiovascular Diagnostic Studies—cont'd

Study	Evaluates	Comments
Electrophysiologic studies (EPS)	• Dysrhythmias under controlled circumstances • Best therapy for control of dysrhythmia: drug, required dosage of therapy; pacemaker; catheter ablation	• Patients may have near-death experience during EPS; encourage expression of fears, concerns, anxieties • Monitor puncture site
Holter monitor	• Suspected dysrhythmias over 24-48 hour period • Pacemaker function • Silent ischemia	• Instruct patient regarding importance of diary-keeping
Intravascular ultrasound (IVUS)	• Coronary artery size and patency • Structure of vessel wall • Coronary artery stent position and patency • Aorta and presence of aneurysm, aneurysm dissections	• As for cardiac catheterization
Magnetic resonance imaging (MRI)	• Three-dimensional view of the heart • Anatomy and structure of the heart and great vessels including: cardiomyopathy; congenital defect; masses; aneurysm • Changes in chemistry of tissues before structural changes occur	• Does not involve radiation or dyes • Cannot be used in patients with any implanted metallic device, including pacemakers, implantable defibrillators, metallic heart valves, intracranial aneurysm clips
Multiple-gated acquisition (MUGA) scan (radionuclide angiography)	• Ventricular size and ventricular wall motion • Cardiac output, cardiac index, end-systolic volume, end-diastolic volume, and ejection fraction • Intracardiac shunts	• Assure patient that amount of radioactive material is minimal
Pericardiocentesis and pericardial fluid analysis	• Presence of blood, pus, pathogens, or malignancy • Also used for emergency relief of cardiac tamponade	• Observe closely for signs of cardiac tamponade

Peripheral angiography	• Atherosclerotic plaques, occlusion, aneurysms, or traumatic injury	• Prior to test:
		  • Contrast medium used: check for allergy to iodine, shellfish, dye
		• After the test:
		  • Contrast medium used, ensure hydration postprocedure
		  • Keep extremity in which catheter was placed immobilized in a straight position for 6-12 hours
		  • Monitor arterial puncture point for hemorrhage or hematoma
		  • Monitor neurovascular status of affected limb
		  • Monitor for indications of systemic emboli

Plethysmography: arterial or venous	*Arterial* • Patency of peripheral arteries and presence of occlusive vascular disease *Venous* • Patency of peripheral venous system and presence of deep vein thrombosis	• Requires one normal extremity since one extremity is compared to the other
Positron emission tomography (cardiac PET scan)	• Severity of coronary artery stenosis • Collateral circulation • Patency of bypass grafts • Size and location of infarcted tissue	• Assure patient that amount of radioactive material is minimal
Sestamibi exercise testing and scan Sestamibi-dipyridamole stress test (for patients with physical limitation preventing exercise)	• Myocardial ischemia during exercise (ischemic areas show increased uptake of radioactivity [hot spots])	• Monitor for myocardial ischemia

Table 2-8 Cardiovascular Diagnostic Studies—cont'd

Study	Evaluates	Comments
Signal-averaged ECG	• Presence of late electrical potentials which may be responsible for malignant ventricular dysrhythmias; may be performed before and after ablation	• Patient must lie still for 10 minutes
Stress electrocardiography (also referred to as *Exercise Tolerance Test* [ETT])	• Persons with high risk for CAD, patients with known CAD, or post-CABG patients for ischemia with exercise or pharmacologic agents (e.g., adenosine, dipyridamole, dobutamine) if patient cannot tolerate exercise • Exercise-induced dysrhythmias	• One millimeter or greater transient ST segment depression 80 msec after the J point is suggestive of CAD • Monitor closely for exercise-induced hypotension or ventricular dysrhythmias • Adenosine is the preferred agent for pharmacologic stress test because it has a short half-life and does not require reversal agent
Technetium-99 pyrophosphate scan	• Size, location of acute MI (infarcted areas show increased uptake of radioactivity ["hot spots"] 1-7 days after MI)	• Assure patient that amount of radioactive material is minimal • Peak accuracy at 12-48 hours after initial symptoms
Thallium stress electrocardiography	• Myocardial ischemia during exercise (ischemic areas show decreased uptake of radioactivity [cold spots])	• Assure patient that amount of radioactive material is minimal
Thallium-201 scan	• Myocardial ischemia (ischemic areas show decreased uptake of radioactivity [cold spots])	• Assure patient that amount of radioactive material is minimal
Vectorcardiography	• Chamber hypertrophy • Bundle branch blocks and hemiblocks • Myocardial ischemia or infarction	
Venography (ascending contrast phlebography)	• Deep leg veins • Presence of deep vein thrombosis (DVT) • Competence of deep vein valves • May be used to locate suitable vein for arterial bypass graft	• Contrast medium used: check for allergy to iodine, shellfish, dye; ensure hydration postprocedure • Monitor for clinical indications of anaphylaxis (e.g., flushing, urticaria, stridor) • Monitor puncture site
Ventriculography	• Ventricular wall motion • Wall thickness • Ventricular aneurysm • Mitral valve motion • LV end-diastolic volume, end-systolic volume, stroke volume, ejection fraction • Intracardiac shunt	• Contrast medium used: check for allergy to iodine, shellfish, dye; ensure hydration postprocedure • Monitor for clinical indications of anaphylaxis (e.g., flushing, urticaria, stridor) • Monitor puncture site

2) Each large (5 mm) box is equal to 0.2 seconds
3) Small marks at the top of the paper identify 3-second intervals

b. Vertical axis measures voltage
1) Useful only if standardized, as on multiple-lead ECG; rhythm strips are not generally standardized because the size (i.e., gain) can be changed
2) If standardized
a) Each small (1 mm) box is equal to 0.1 mV
b) Each large (5 mm) box is equal to 0.5 mV

4. Rule of electrical flow
a. Impulses traveling toward the positive pole of a lead cause a positive deflection.
b. Impulses traveling toward the negative (or away from the positive) pole of a lead cause a negative deflection.

Rhythm Strip Analysis

1. Monitoring leads
a. Standard electrode placement with 5-lead system (Figure 2-37)
1) White (right arm): just below right clavicle
2) Black (left arm): just below left clavicle
3) Brown

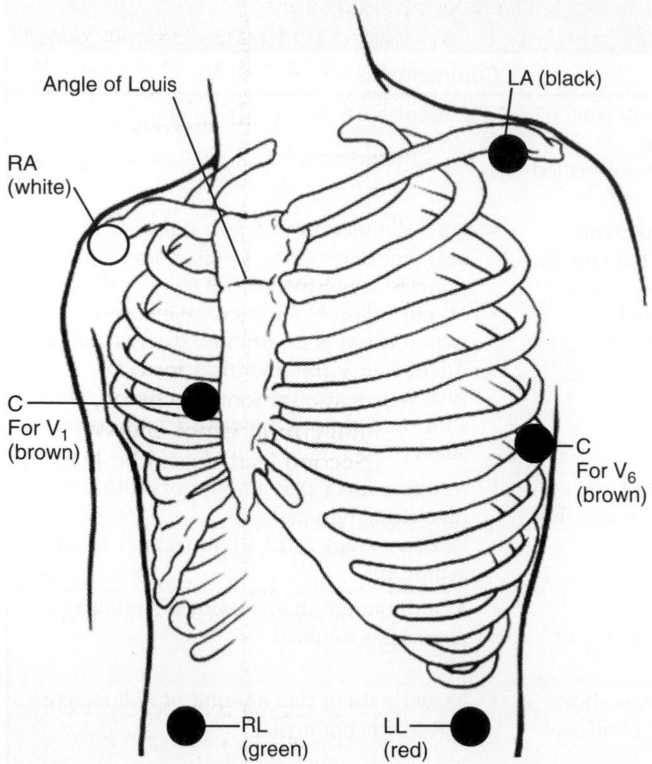

Figure 2-37 Standard electrode placement for monitoring with 5-lead system. (From Drew, B [2002]. *Philips—AACN cardiac monitoring pocket reference*. Philips PN #5990-0487. Aliso Viejo, CA: American Association of Critical-Care Nurses.)

a) For V_1: fourth ICS at right sternal border
b) For V_6: fifth ICS at left midaxillary line

4) Green (right leg): lower chest, above and to right of umbilicus
5) Red (left leg): lower chest, above and to left of umbilicus
6) NOTE: Remember White on the right, Snow over grass, Smoke over fire, Brown on the ground (Barill, 2003)
7) Available leads: I, II, III, aVR, aVL, aVF, or V (which V lead depends on placement of the brown lead)

b. Typical leads monitored in three-lead system (Figure 2-38)
   1) Lead II: positive (red) at lower left torso; negative (white) under right clavicle; ground (black) under left clavicle (NOTE: remember White to the right. Smoke over fire [Barill, 2003])
   2) Modified chest leads (MCLs):
      a) MCL_1
         i) Monitor: set at lead I
         ii) Lead placement: positive (black) at fourth ICS at RSB; negative (white) under left clavicle; ground (red) under right clavicle
      b) MCL_6
         i) Monitor: set at lead II
         ii) Lead placement: positive at fifth ICS at left midaxillary line (MAL)

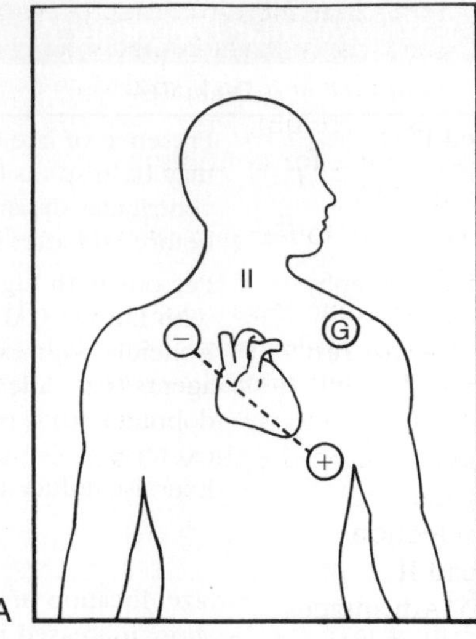

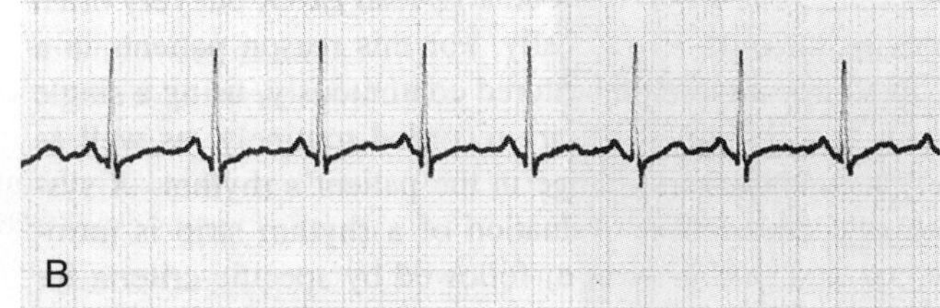

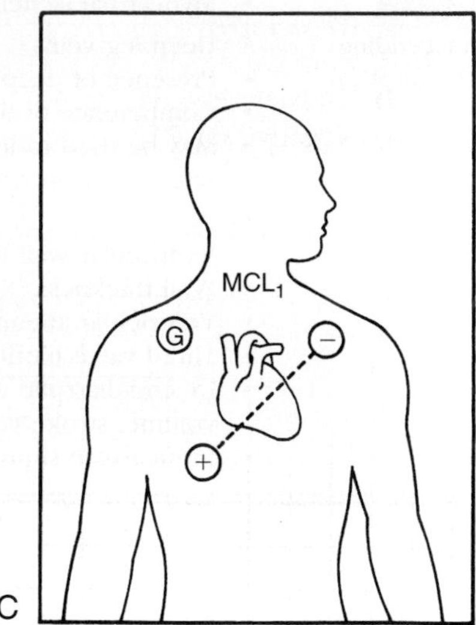

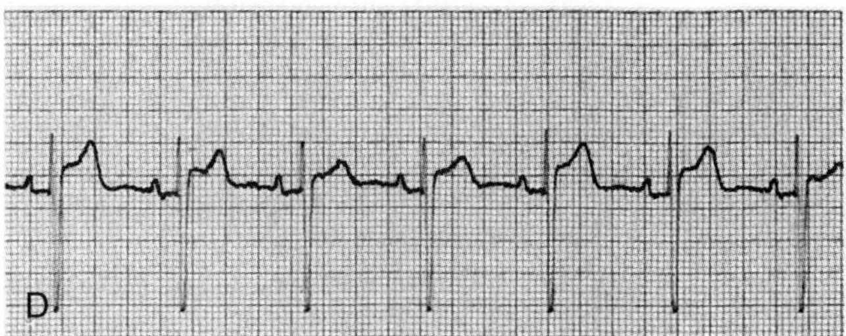

Figure 2-38 Monitoring leads. **A,** Electrode placement for lead II. **B,** Representation of appearance of ECG in lead II. **C,** Electrode placement for MCL_1. **D,** Representation of appearance of ECG in MCL_1. (From Urden L. D., Lough M. E., & Stacy K. M. [1995]. *Priorities in critical care nursing*. St Louis: Mosby.)

c) Note that the difference between MCLs and true V leads is that V leads are unipolar and preferred if available and MCLs are bipolar

c. Lead placement for continuous derived 12-lead ECG (EASI™)
   1) E (brown): lower part of the sternum at the fifth ICS
   2) A (red): right midaxillary line at fifth ICS
   3) S (black): upper part of the sternum
   4) I (white): left midaxillary line at fifth ICS
   5) Fifth electrode (green) can be placed anywhere on the torso; it serves as a ground.

d. Lead selection
   1) Lead II
      a) Advantages
         i) Upright P and QRS waves
         ii) Normal appearance
      b) Disadvantage: ectopy and aberrancy look-alike
      c) Clinical indication: atrial dysrhythmias
   2) V_1 or MCL_1
      a) Advantages
         i) Better differentiation of ectopy from aberrancy
         ii) Differentiation of LBBB from RBBB
         iii) Differentiation of LV ectopy from RV ectopy
      b) Disadvantages
         i) Diphasic P wave
         ii) Negative QRS
      c) Clinical indications
         i) Diagnosis of wide QRS complexes (e.g., differentiation of ventricular ectopy from supraventricular tachycardia with aberrancy, differentiation of RBBB or LBBB): V_1 and/or V_6
         ii) Ischemia, injury, infarction: however, two leads are best
            (a) Second lead is determined by lead with significant ST segment elevation (patient's ischemic fingerprint).
            (b) If the patient's ischemic fingerprint is not known: Second lead should be lead III or V_3.
         iii) Pacemaker: V_1
         iv) Heart failure and/or cardiomyopathy to monitor for the development of bundle branch block: V_1
   3) V_6 or MCL_6
      a) Advantages as for V_1; may be especially helpful if incision/dressing prevents placement of lead at sternum

2. Components of a single cardiac cycle (Figure 2-39)
   a. P wave
      1) Represents atrial depolarization
      2) First deflection from the isoelectric line
      3) Normal P wave: no more than 2.5 mm tall and no more than 0.11 seconds wide

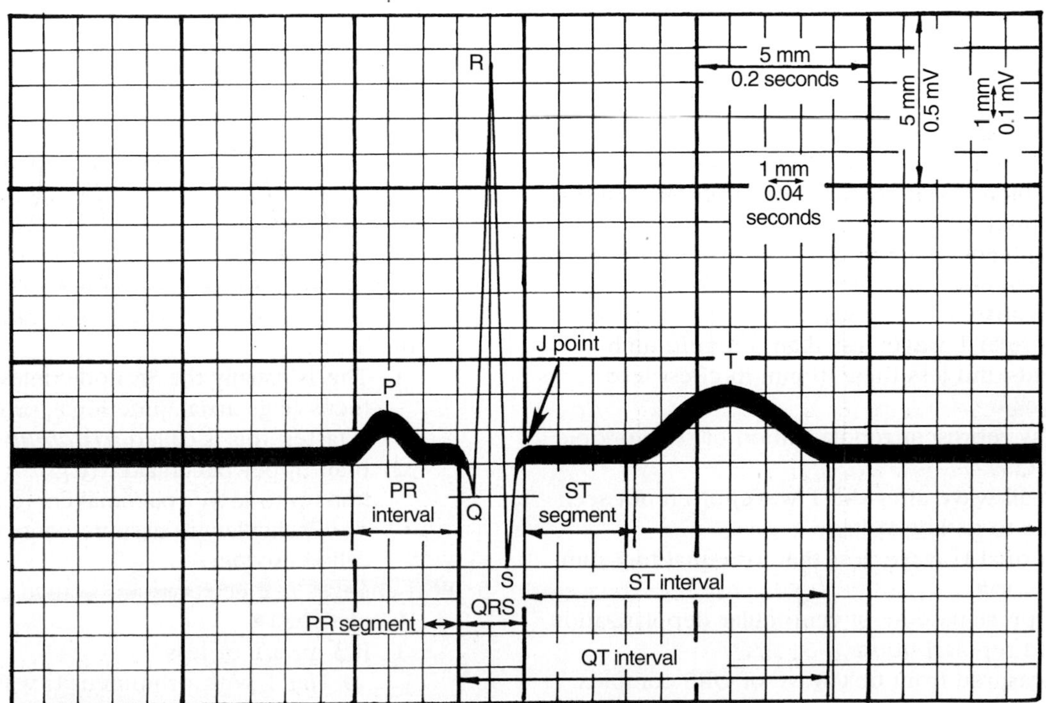

Figure 2-39 Components of a single cardiac cycle. (From Seidel, J. C. [1986]. *The Methodist Hospital: Basic electrocardiography: a modular approach.* St Louis: Mosby.)

b. PR segment
   1) Represents the delay in AV node
   2) Isoelectric line between P wave and QRS complex
c. PR interval
   1) Represents atrial depolarization + delay in AV node
   2) Measured from beginning of P wave to beginning of QRS complex
   3) Normal PR interval: 0.12 to 0.2 seconds
d. Q wave: the first negative wave after the P wave but before the R wave
e. R wave: the first positive wave after the P wave
f. S wave: the negative wave after the R wave
g. QRS complex
   1) Represents ventricular depolarization
   2) May have one, two, or all three: Q, R, S
      a) Case indicates size; for example qRS indicates a small q and large R and S
      b) An apostrophe after an R indicates that it is a second R (i.e., R prime) as in bundle branch blocks; so, for example, rSR' indicates small R, large S, large second R
   3) Measured from beginning of the first wave of complex to the end of last wave of complex
   4) Normal QRS interval: 0.06 to 0.11
   5) Normal QRS amplitude: less than 30 mm in chest leads
h. ST segment
   1) Represents the time during which the ventricles have completely depolarized and the beginning of repolarization
   2) Located between the QRS complex and the beginning of the T wave
   3) Normally isoelectric at baseline
i. J point
   1) The angle at which the QRS complex ends and the ST segment begins
   2) The J point deviates from the isoelectric line if the ST segment is elevated or depressed.
j. T wave
   1) Represents ventricular repolarization
   2) Wave after the QRS; may be positive or negative
   3) Normal T wave: less than 5 mm in limb leads and less than 10 mm in chest lead
k. U wave
   1) May represent repolarization of the Purkinje fibers
   2) Small wave after the T wave; often not seen due to its low voltage
   3) Normal U wave: less than or equal to 1 mm
l. QT interval
   1) Represents time of ventricular depolarization and repolarization
   2) Measured from first wave of QRS complex to the end of the T wave
   3) Normal QT interval based on heart rate; the slower the heart rate, the longer the normal QT; the faster the heart rate, the shorter the normal QT
      a) For heart rates 60-100/min, the normal QT interval is less than half of the RR interval.
   4) To correct for changes in heart rate (especially for heart rates not 60-100/min), calculate the QTc.
      a) Formula: QT ÷ square root of the R-R interval
      b) Normal QTc: 0.32-0.44
   5) Indications for monitoring of QT interval
      a) Congenital long QT syndrome
      b) Significant bradycardia (less than 50 beats per minute)
      c) Antidysrhythmics that are known to prolong the QT interval
         i) IA: quinidine, procainamide, disopyramide (Norpace)
         ii) IC: flecainide (Tambocor), propafenone (Rythmol)
         iii) II/III: sotalol (Betapace)
         iv) III: ibutilide (Corvert), dofetilide (Tikosyn)
      d) Electrolyte imbalances
         i) Hypokalemia
         ii) Hypomagnesemia
         iii) Hypocalcemia
      e) Tricyclic antidepressants (e.g., amitriptyline [Elavil], nortriptyline [Pamelor])
      f) Antibiotics: fluoroquinolones (e.g., gemifloxacin, moxifloxacin), macrolides (e.g., azithromycin), erythromycin
      g) Cerebrovascular disease (e.g., intracranial or subarachnoid hemorrhage, stroke, intracranial trauma)
      h) Hypothermia
      i) Hypothyroidism
      j) Hypoglycemia
      k) Myocardial ischemia or infarction
      l) Heart failure or cardiomyopathy

3. Steps in analysis of a rhythm strip (Table 2-9)
4. Criteria for basic dysrhythmias and blocks (Table 2-10)
   a. The pacemaker rule: The fastest rate will control the heart.
      1) This is usually the SA node unless an irritable focus (e.g., atrial, junctional, or ventricular) is faster; this is called *irritability*.
      2) If an upper pacemaker (e.g., SA node) fails, it is up to lower pacemakers (e.g., junctional or ventricular) to assume control: this is called *escape*.
5. ECG changes in electrolyte imbalance
   a. Hypokalemia
      1) If 3 mEq/L or less
         a) Flat T with prominent U wave
         b) T wave and U wave of approximately the same amplitude
         c) ST segment flattening and/or depression

Table 2-9 Rhythm Strip Analysis

Component	Assessment
Regularity (rhythm)	• Is it regular? • Is it irregular? • Are there any patterns to the irregularity? • Are there any ectopic beats; if so, are they early (premature) or are they late (escape)? • Is regularity of P waves and QRS complexes the same? (If there is only one P wave for each QRS, only one regularity needs to be recorded)

Rate	• *Methods*
	  • Count dark lines between P waves or QRS complexes as 300, 150, 100, 75, 60, 50, 43, 38, 33, 30
	  • Count number of QRS complexes in a 6-second strip and multiply by 10
	  • Use a rate ruler
	• Are atrial and ventricular rates the same? (If there is only one P wave for each QRS, only one rate needs to be recorded)

P waves	• Are the P waves regular? • Is there one P wave for every QRS? • Is there a P wave in front of the QRS or behind it? • Is the P wave normal and upright in lead II? • Are there more P waves than QRS complexes? • Do all P waves look alike? • Are irregular P waves associated with ectopic beats? If so, are they early (premature) or late (escape)?
PR intervals	• Is PRI measurement within normal range? • (Normal interval: 0.12-0.2 seconds) • Are all PRIs constant? • If PRI varies, is there a pattern to the changing measurements?
QRS complexes	• Is QRS measurement within normal limits? (normal interval: 0.06-0.11 seconds) • Are all QRS complexes of equal duration? • Do all QRS complexes look alike? • Are unusual QRS complexes associated with ectopic beats? If so, are they early (premature) or late (escape)?
QT interval	• Is the QT measurement within normal limits? (measured QT less than half of previous R-R interval or QTc of 0.32-0.44)
Patient presentation	• Is the patient symptomatic? • Are there clinical indications of hypoperfusion such as hypotension, syncope, or chest pain?

2) If 2 mEq/L or less
   a) U wave taller than T wave
   b) Prolongation of QT interval
   c) ST segment depression
3) If 1 mEq/L or less
   a) U wave fuses with T wave.

b. Hyperkalemia
1) If greater than 6 mEq/L
   a) ST segment disappears and T waves become tall, narrow, and peaked.
   b) QRS complex widens.
2) If 6.5 mEq/L or greater
   a) QRS complex widens more.
   b) P wave widens and flattens.
3) If 7.5 mEq/L or greater
   a) Sinus arrest with disappearance of P waves
4) If 10-12 mEq/L or greater
   a) Wide QRS merged with T wave
   b) Ventricular fibrillation or asystole

c. Hypocalcemia
1) Prolonged QT
2) Prolonged ST segment

d. Hypercalcemia
1) Shortened QT
2) Shortened ST segment

e. Hypomagnesemia
1) Prolonged QT
2) Broad, flattened T wave

f. Hypermagnesemia
1) PR, QT prolonged
2) Prolonged QRS

6. Drug effects on the ECG

a. Digitalis
1) Scooping of ST-T wave (known as *digitalis effect*)
2) Shortened QT
3) PR interval may be prolonged

b. Type IA antidysrhythmics (e.g., procainamide, quinidine, disopyramide)
1) QT prolongation
2) T wave flattening

Table 2-10 Criteria For Basic Dysrhythmias and Blocks

Rhythm	Rate	Regularity	P Waves	PR Interval	QRS Duration
Normal sinus rhythm	60-100/min	Atrial and ventricular rhythms regular	Normal	0.12-0.2 second and constant	Less than 0.12 second
Sinus bradycardia	Less than 60/min	Atrial and ventricular rhythms regular	Normal	0.12-0.2 second and constant	Less than 0.12 second
Sinus tachycardia	Greater than 100/min (usually 100-160/min)	Atrial and ventricular rhythms regular	Normal	0.12-0.2 second and constant	Less than 0.12 second
Sinus dysrhythmia	Usually 60-100/min but may be slower or faster	Atrial and ventricular rhythms regularly irregular; rate increases with inspiration (so R-R interval shortens) and decreases with expiration (so R-R interval lengthens); difference between shortest and longest R-R less than 0.12 second	Normal	0.12-0.2 second and usually constant; may vary slightly with rate variation	Less than 0.12 second
Sinus block (sinus exit block)	Dependent on underlying rhythm	Atrial and ventricular rhythms regular with an irregularity; R-R interval at block measures an exact multiple of the normal R-R interval	One or more entire cardiac cycle is absent; P wave absent during block	None during block	QRS absent during block
Sinus arrest	Dependent on underlying rhythm	Atrial and ventricular rhythms regular with an irregularity (a pause); R-R interval at pause measures more or less than an exact multiple of the normal R-R interval	Indefinite period of time without an entire cardiac cycle; P wave absent during arrest	None during arrest	QRS absent during arrest
Premature atrial contractions	Dependent on underlying rhythm	Dependent on underlying rhythm; PAC interrupts underlying rhythm	P wave of this early beat differs from sinus P; the ectopic P wave is early and may be flattened, notched, or lost in preceding T wave	Usually 0.12-0.2 second but may be greater than 0.2	Less than 0.12 second
Wandering atrial pacemaker	Usually 60-100/min	Atrial and ventricular rhythms usually slightly irregular	P waves look different beat to beat; at least 3 different-looking P waves	0.12-0.2 second and may vary	Less than 0.12 second
Supraventricular tachycardia*	Greater than 100/min; usually 150-250/min	Atrial and ventricular rhythms regular	P waves are impossible to distinguish; may be lost in QRS or preceding T wave	Cannot measure	Less than 0.12 second
Atrial tachycardia	150-250/min	Atrial and ventricular rhythms regular	P wave differs from sinus P; may merge with preceding T wave	0.12-0.2 second	Less than 0.12 second
Multifocal atrial tachycardia (also called chaotic atrial rhythm)	Usually 100-150/min	Atrial and ventricular rhythms usually slightly irregular	P waves look different beat to beat; at least 3 different-looking P waves	0.12-0.2 second and may vary	Less than 0.12 second

*Supraventricular tachycardia refers to any narrow QRS tachycardia with a focus that cannot be definitely identified; the term should be used only when a more definitive diagnosis cannot be made.

Table 2-10 Criteria For Basic Dysrhythmias and Blocks—cont'd

Rhythm	Rate	Regularity	P Waves	PR Interval	QRS Duration
Atrial flutter	Atrial rate approximately 300/min; ventricular rate varies with conduction through the AV node; 2:1 atrial flutter has a ventricular rate of approximately 150/min, 4:1 atrial flutter has a ventricular rate of approximately 75/min	Atrial flutter waves regular; ventricular rhythm (response) usually regular	No true P waves; flutter waves have characteristic sawtooth appearance	No true P waves	Less than 0.12 second
Atrial fibrillation	Atrial rate greater than 350/min; ventricular rate varies greatly depending on conduction through AV node	Atrial fibrillatory waves irregular; ventricular rhythm irregularly irregular	No true P waves; fibrillatory waves manifested by quivering baseline	No true P waves	Less than 0.12 second
Premature junctional contraction	Dependent on underlying rhythm	Dependent on underlying rhythm; PJC interrupts underlying rhythm	P wave if visible will be inverted; may be in front of, in, or after the QRS complex	Can be measured only if P wave is in front of QRS; PR will be less than 0.12 second if measurable	Less than 0.12 second
Junctional escape rhythm	40-60/min	Atrial and ventricular rhythms regular	If visible, P wave inverted; may be in front of, in, or after the QRS complex	Can be measured only if P wave is in front of QRS; PR will be less than 0.12 second if measurable	Less than 0.12 second
Accelerated junctional rhythm	60-100/min	Atrial and ventricular rhythms regular	If visible, P wave inverted; may be in front of, in, or after the QRS complex	Can be measured only if P wave is in front of QRS; PR will be less than 0.12 second if measurable	Less than 0.12 second
Junctional tachycardia	Greater than 100/min; usually 100-180/min	Atrial and ventricular rhythms regular	If visible, P wave inverted; may be in front of, in, or after the QRS complex	Can be measured only if P wave is in front of QRS; PR will be less than 0.12 second if measurable	Less than 0.12 second
First-degree AV nodal block	Dependent on underlying rhythm	Dependent on underlying rhythm	P wave normal	Greater than 0.2 second	Less than 0.12 second

Continued

Table 2-10 Criteria For Basic Dysrhythmias and Blocks—cont'd

Rhythm	Rate	Regularity	P Waves	PR Interval	QRS Duration
Second-degree AV nodal block Type I* (Wenckebach)	Atrial rate dependent on underlying rhythm; ventricular rate dependent on conduction ratio; atrial rate greater than ventricular rate	Atrial rhythm regular, ventricular rhythm irregular (P-P is regular but R-R is irregular); groupings identifiable between P waves that were not conducted	P waves normal, but some P waves not followed by a QRS	Normal PR interval progressively lengthens until a P wave is not followed by a QRS; entire cycle begins again with normal PR interval	Less than 0.12 second
Second-degree AV nodal block Type II*	Atrial rate dependent on underlying rhythm; ventricular rate dependent on conduction ratio but usually less than 60/min; atrial rate greater than ventricular rate	Atrial rhythm regular, ventricular rhythm regular or irregular depending on whether conduction ratio varies or is constant; P-P regular, but some R-Rs may be twice normal	P waves normal, but there are P waves not followed by a QRS without preceding progressive lengthening	Usually 0.12-0.2 second of conducted P waves but may be longer; constant for each conducted QRS	0.12 second or longer
Third-degree (or complete) AV block	Atrial rate dependent on underlying rhythm; ventricular rate dependent on focus of escape rhythm (40-60/min if escape focus is junctional, 20-40/min if escape focus is ventricular)	Atrial rhythm regular, ventricular rhythm usually regular; P-P regular; R-R usually regular	Normal but P waves not followed by (associated with) QRS	No consistent PR interval; no relationship between the P waves and the QRS complexes	Less than 0.12 second if escape focus is junctional; 0.12 second or longer if escape focus is ventricular
Left bundle branch block (LBBB)	Dependent on underlying rhythm	Dependent on underlying rhythm	P wave normal	0.12-0.2 second as long as no coexisting AV nodal block	0.12 second or longer; QRS is negative in V_1
Right bundle branch block (RBBB)	Dependent on underlying rhythm	Dependent on underlying rhythm	P wave normal	0.12-0.2 second as long as no coexisting AV nodal block	0.12 second or longer; QRS is positive in V_1
Premature ventricular contraction	Dependent on underlying rhythm	Dependent on underlying rhythm; PVC interrupts underlying rhythm	No associated P wave	No associated P wave; cannot measure PR	0.12 second or longer; QRS of PVC looks different than normal QRSs
Monomorphic ventricular tachycardia	100-250/min *VT is usually ~150/min; VT at 200-250/min may be called ventricular flutter	Ventricular rhythm usually regular; if dissociated P waves are identifiable, atrial rhythm regular	No associated P waves but may have dissociated P waves scattered through the rhythm	No associated P waves; cannot measure PR	0.12 second or longer; QRS of VT looks different than normal QRSs

*2:1 block is a second-degree block but may be either Type I or Type II; the QRS width may be helpful in differentiating between the two; if the QRS is of normal width, it is probably Type I, if the QRS is 0.12 or greater, it is probably Type II.

Table 2-10 Criteria For Basic Dysrhythmias and Blocks—cont'd

Rhythm	Rate	Regularity	P Waves	PR Interval	QRS Duration
Polymorphic ventricular tachycardia (torsades de pointes)	150-250/min	Ventricular rhythm may be regular	None	None	0.12 second or longer with QRS that seems to twist around a center line; gradual alteration in the amplitude and direction of the QRS
Ventricular fibrillation	None	Irregular; chaotic baseline	None	None	None
Idioventricular rhythm	20-40/min	Ventricular rhythm usually regular; no atrial activity	None	None	0.12 second or longer
Accelerated idioventricular rhythm	40-100/min	Ventricular rhythm usually regular; no atrial activity	None	None	0.12 second or longer
Asystole	None	No atrial or ventricular activity	None	None	None

Multiple-Lead ECG Analysis

1. ECG leads (Figure 2-40)
   a. Limb leads: frontal plane
      1) Lead I: + at LA (left arm); - at RA (right arm)
      2) Lead II: + at F (foot); - at RA
      3) Lead III: + at F (foot); - at LA
      4) Lead aVR: unipolar RA
      5) Lead aVL: unipolar LA
      6) Lead aVF: unipolar F
   b. Chest leads: horizontal plane
      1) Lead V_1: 4ICS at right sternal border (RSB)
      2) Lead V_2: 4ICS at left sternal border (LSB)
      3) Lead V_3: halfway between V_2 and V_4
      4) Lead V_4: 5ICS at left midclavicular line (LMCL)
      5) Lead V_5: 5ICS at left anterior axillary line (LAAL)
      6) Lead V_6: 5ICS at left midaxillary line (LMAL)
      7) R wave gets taller across the precordium from V_1 to V_6 (referred to as *normal progression of the R wave across the precordium*); the S wave gets smaller across the precordium (V_1 to V_6).
      8) Conditions associated with poor R wave progression across the precordium include the following:
         a) Anterior myocardial infarction
         b) Left bundle branch block
         c) Emphysema
      9) Conditions associated with low voltage across the precordium include the following:
         a) Emphysema
         b) Pericardial effusion
         c) Myocardial infarction
         d) Obesity
   c. Specialty leads
      1) Posterior leads
         a) Lead V_7: 5ICS at left posterior axillary line (LPAL)
         b) Lead V_8: halfway between V_7 and V_8
         c) Lead V_9: 5ICS next to vertebral column
      2) Right ventricular leads
         a) Lead V_{4R}: 5ICS at RMCL
         b) Lead V_{5R}: 5ICS at RAAL
         c) Lead V_{6R}: 5ICS at RMAL
         d) The standard 12 leads plus V_{4R}-V_{6R} and $V_{7\text{-}9}$ make the 18 leads of an 18-lead ECG
         e) Right ventricular leads routinely performed on patients with ECG indicators of inferior MI (33-50% of patients with inferior MI have concurrent right ventricular infarction)
2. Mean QRS axis
   a. Represents the average direction of ventricular depolarization
   b. Described on a 360-degree circle
      1) Normal axis
         a) Downward and to the left (0-90 degrees)
         b) Caused by the normal direction of depolarization from superior to inferior and the larger muscle mass of the left ventricle
      2) Left axis deviation (LAD)
         a) Upward and to the left (0 to -90 degrees)
         b) May be caused by any of the following:

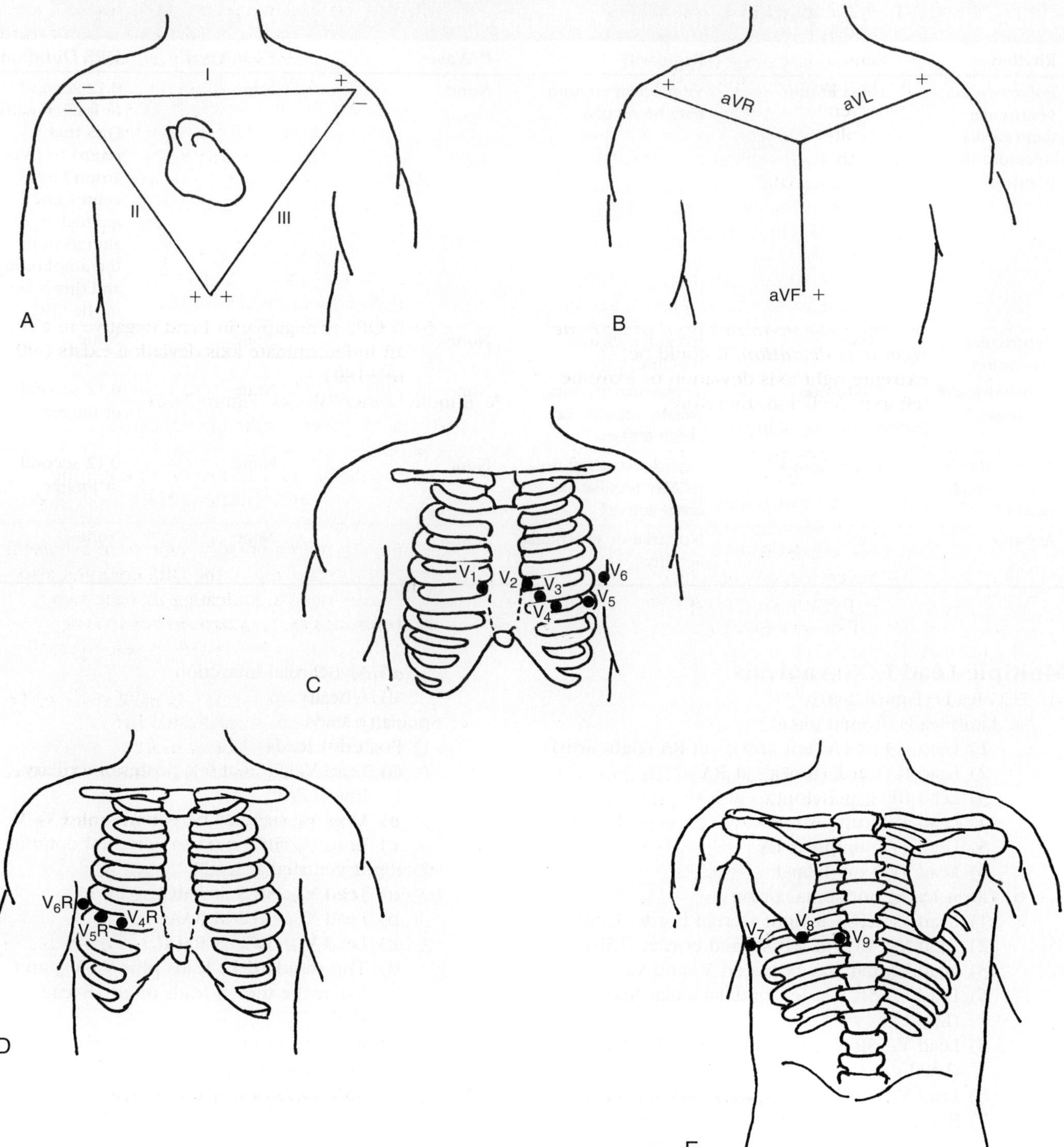

Figure 2-40 ECG leads. **A,** Bipolar limb leads: I, II, III. **B,** Unipolar limb leads: aVR, aVL, aVF. **C,** Standard chest leads: V_1-V_6. **D,** Right ventricular leads: V_{4R}-V_{6R}. **E,** Posterior leads: V_7-V_9.

i) Normal variant: only considered abnormal if more negative than -30 degrees
ii) Left ventricular hypertrophy
iii) Left anterior hemiblock
iv) Inferior myocardial infarction
v) Wolff-Parkinson-White syndrome with a right accessory pathway
vi) Ventricular pacemaker
vii) Mechanical shift of heart to more horizontal: ascites; pregnancy; abdominal tumor

3) Right axis deviation (RAD)
   a) Downward and to the right (+90 to ±180 degrees)
   b) May be caused by any of the following:
      i) Normal variant: only considered abnormal if more positive than +110 degrees

ii) Right ventricular hypertrophy (RVH)
iii) Pulmonary embolism
iv) Left posterior hemiblock
v) Lateral myocardial infarction
vi) Wolff-Parkinson-White syndrome with a left accessory pathway
vii) Dextrocardia
viii) Mechanical shift of heart to more vertical: emphysema

4) Indeterminate axis
   a) Upward and to the right (-90 to ±180)
   b) Though this axis deviation is frequently referred to as *no-man's land* or *extreme right axis deviation,* it could be extreme right axis deviation or extreme left axis deviation; therefore, indeterminate is more appropriate.
   c) May be caused by any of the following:
      i) Ventricular tachycardia
      ii) Ventricular pacemaker
      iii) Multiple infarctions
      iv) Hyperkalemia
      v) Severe right ventricular hypertrophy (e.g., severe pulmonary disease)

c. Quadrant method (Figure 2-41)
   1) Determine which quadrant where the mean QRS axis is located by using the direction of the QRS in leads II and aVF.
      a) Lead I
         i) Positive pole is at the left arm, and negative pole is at the right arm.
         ii) If the mean QRS axis is to the left, there will be a predominantly positive QRS in lead I.
         iii) If the mean QRS axis is to the right, there will be a predominantly negative QRS in lead I.
      b) Lead aVF
         i) Positive pole is at the foot.
         ii) If the mean QRS axis is downward, there will be a predominantly positive QRS in lead aVF.
         iii) If the mean QRS axis is upward, there will be a predominantly negative QRS in lead aVF.
   2) If QRS is positive in I and positive in aVF, mean QRS axis is normal (0 to +90).
   3) If QRS is positive in I and negative in aVF, a left axis deviation exists (0 to -90).
   4) If QRS is negative in I and positive in aVF, a right axis deviation exists (+90 to ±180).
   5) If QRS is negative in I and negative in aVF, an indeterminate axis deviation exists (-90 to ±180)

3. Bundle branch blocks (Figure 2-42)
   a. Block of either bundle branch causes the following:
      1) A delay in the conduction through the ventricles and a prolongation of the QRS interval
      2) Branching (commonly referred to as *rabbit ears*) or slurring of the QRS complex also usually occurs, indicating that the two ventricles are depolarized out of sync.
      3) T wave deflection in the opposite direction of the QRS
   b. LBBB is a bifascicular block (loss of both major hemibundles) and is manifested by:
      1) QRS of 0.12 seconds or more
      2) QRS which is positive in V_6 and negative in V_1
         a) Monophasic QRS or rsR' complex in V_6
         b) rS or QS in V_1
   c. Right bundle branch block (RBBB) is a unifascicular block and is manifested by:
      1) QRS of 0.12 seconds or more
      2) QRS which is positive in V_1 and negative in V_6

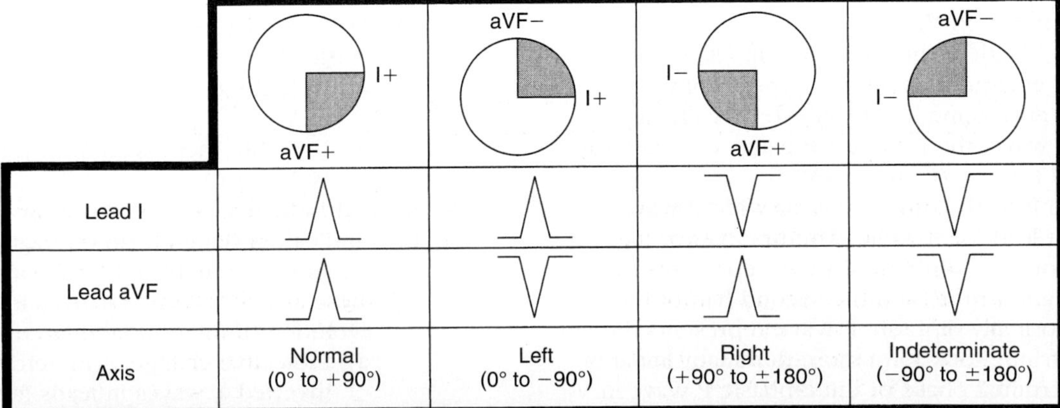

Figure 2-41 Quadrant method of axis determination. (Modified from Kinney, M. R., et al. [1998]. *AACN's clinical reference for critical-care nursing* [4th ed.]. St Louis: Mosby.)

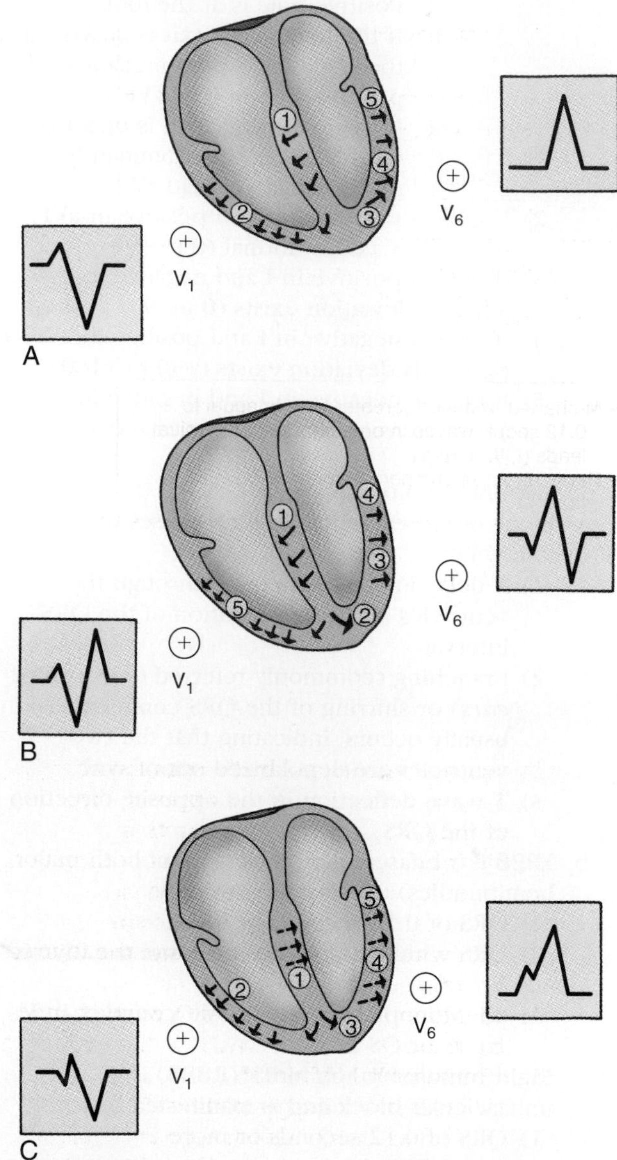

Figure 2-42 A, Normal ventricular depolarization. **B,** Right bundle branch block. **C,** Left bundle branch block. (From Urden, L., Stacy, K., & Lough, M. [2010]. *Critical care nursing: Diagnosis and management* [6th ed.]. St. Louis: Mosby.)

a) rSR' in V_1
b) Wide terminal S wave in leads I and V_6

4. Chamber enlargement and/or hypertrophy
   a. Atrial enlargement is manifested by changes in the P wave; the two best P wave leads are lead II and lead V_1. (Figure 2-43)
      1) In lead II: Look for tall or wide P waves.
      2) In lead V_1 or MCL_1: The first half of the normally diphasic P wave represents the right atrium, and the second half of the normally diphasic P wave represents the left atrium; look for a more dominant initial or terminal phase of the diphasic P wave in V_1 or MCL_1.
      3) Right atrial enlargement is manifested by the following ECG changes:
         a) Tall (greater than 2.5 mm), peaked P wave in II (sometimes referred to as *P-pulmonale*)
         b) Larger initial phase of the diphasic P wave normally seen in V_1
      4) Left atrial enlargement is manifested by the following ECG changes:
         a) Wide (greater than or equal to 0.12 second), notched P wave in II (sometimes referred to as *P-mitrale*)
         b) Larger terminal phase of the biphasic P wave normally seen in V_1
   b. Ventricular hypertrophy is manifested by changes in the QRS; look at changes in the precordial leads for ventricular hypertrophy.
      1) Right ventricular hypertrophy causes a change in the usual left ventricular dominance across the precordial leads. (Figure 2-44)
         a) QRS amplitude: R wave larger than S wave in V_1, V_2; S wave larger than R wave in V_5, V_6 (indicative of change from the normal dominance of the left ventricle to dominance of right ventricle)
         b) Right axis deviation: QRS negative in I; QRS positive in aVF
         c) May have right atrial enlargement
         d) ST-T wave changes in V_1, V_2 indicative of right ventricular strain
      2) Left ventricular hypertrophy causes an exaggeration of the usual left ventricular dominance across the precordial leads (Figure 2-45)
         a) QRS amplitude
            i) Deepest S in V_1 or V_2 plus tallest R in V_5 or V_6 greater than or equal to 35 mm
            ii) R in lead aVL greater than or equal to 12 mm
         b) Left axis deviation: QRS is positive in I; QRS negative in aVF
         c) May have left atrial enlargement
         d) ST-T wave changes in V_5, V_6 indicative of left ventricular strain
      3) NOTE: Remember WiLLiaM MaRRoW (Right bundle branch block, 2010)
         a) In LBBB, there is a W in V1 and an M in V_6
         b) In RBBB, there is an M in lead V1 and a W in lead V_6
5. Myocardial ischemia, injury, infarction
   a. ECG indicators (Figure 2-46 on page 71.)
      1) Ischemia is manifested by T wave changes; these are the earliest changes in the evolution of myocardial infarction.
         a) Indicative change: symmetrically inverted T waves in leads facing the ischemic area
         b) Reciprocal change: tall T waves in leads opposite the ischemic area

Condition	P wave appearance		Mnemonic features
	Lead II	Lead V_1	
Normal sinus rhythm (NSR)		or	• The P should be upright in lead II if there is sinus rhythm • The P may be upright, negative or biphasic in lead V_1 with sinus rhythm
RAE (=**P** **P**ulmonale)	2.50		• **P**rominent (greater than or equal to 2.5 mm tall) **p**eaked P waves in the **p**ulmonary leads (II, III, and aVF)
LAE (=**P** **M**itrale)	0.12	or	• **M**-shaped, widened (greater than or equal to 0.12 sec) P waves in one or more of the **m**itral leads (I, II, or aVL) • Deep, negative component to the P wave in lead V_1

Figure 2-43 Atrial enlargement. *RAE,* Right atrial enlargement; *LAE,* left atrial enlargement. (From Grauer, K. [1998]. *A practical guide to ECG interpretation* [2nd ed.]. St. Louis: Mosby.)

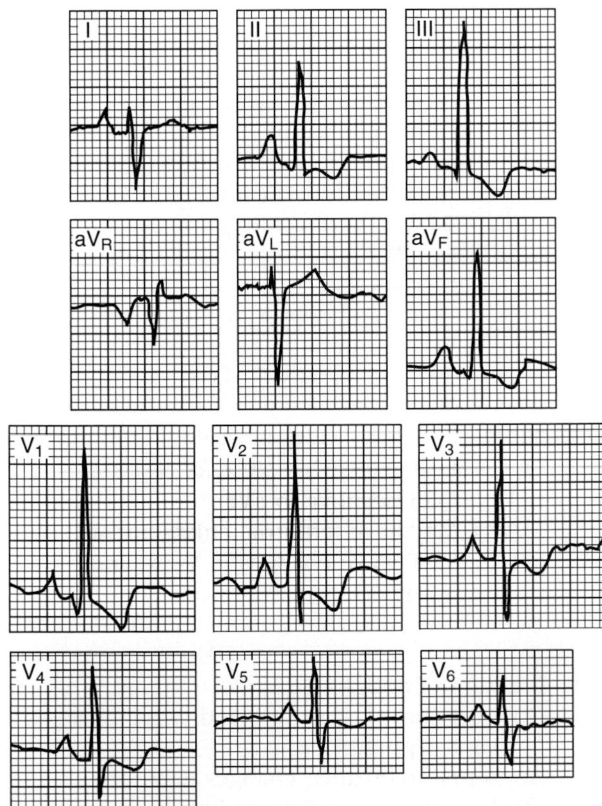

Figure 2-44 Right ventricular hypertrophy with right atrial enlargement. Note tall, peaked P waves in lead II with dominant initial component of the P wave in V_1 as evidence of right atrial enlargement. Note dominant R wave in V_1 and reverse progression of the R wave across the precordium along with right axis deviation and right ventricular strain (ST segment depression and asymmetrical T wave inversion in V_1, V_2) as evidence of right ventricular hypertrophy. (From Conover, M. B. [2003]. *Understanding electrocardiography.* [8th ed.]. St. Louis: Mosby.)

2) Injury is manifested by ST segment changes; these are intermediate changes in the evolution of myocardial infarction.
   a) Indicative change: ST segment elevation in leads facing the injured area
   b) Reciprocal change: ST segment depression in leads opposite the injured area
3) Infarction is manifested by Q wave changes; these are the latest changes in the evolution of myocardial infarction.
   a) Indicative change: pathologic Q wave (0.04 second wide and/or 25% height of R wave) in leads facing the necrotic area
   b) Reciprocal change: tall R waves in leads opposite the necrotic area
   c) Q waves
      i) Are normal in many leads; to be pathologic (i.e., indicative of infarction) must be 0.4 second wide and 25% of the height of the R wave
      ii) Take up to 24 hours to develop
      iii) Relate to mass loss of myocardium
      iv) Prevented by successful reperfusion therapies (e.g., fibrinolytics, PCI)
4) Some conditions may make ECG diagnosis of MI difficult by changing the morphology of the QRS, the ST segment, and/or the T waves; some examples include the following:
   a) Unstable angina (e.g., Wellens syndrome)

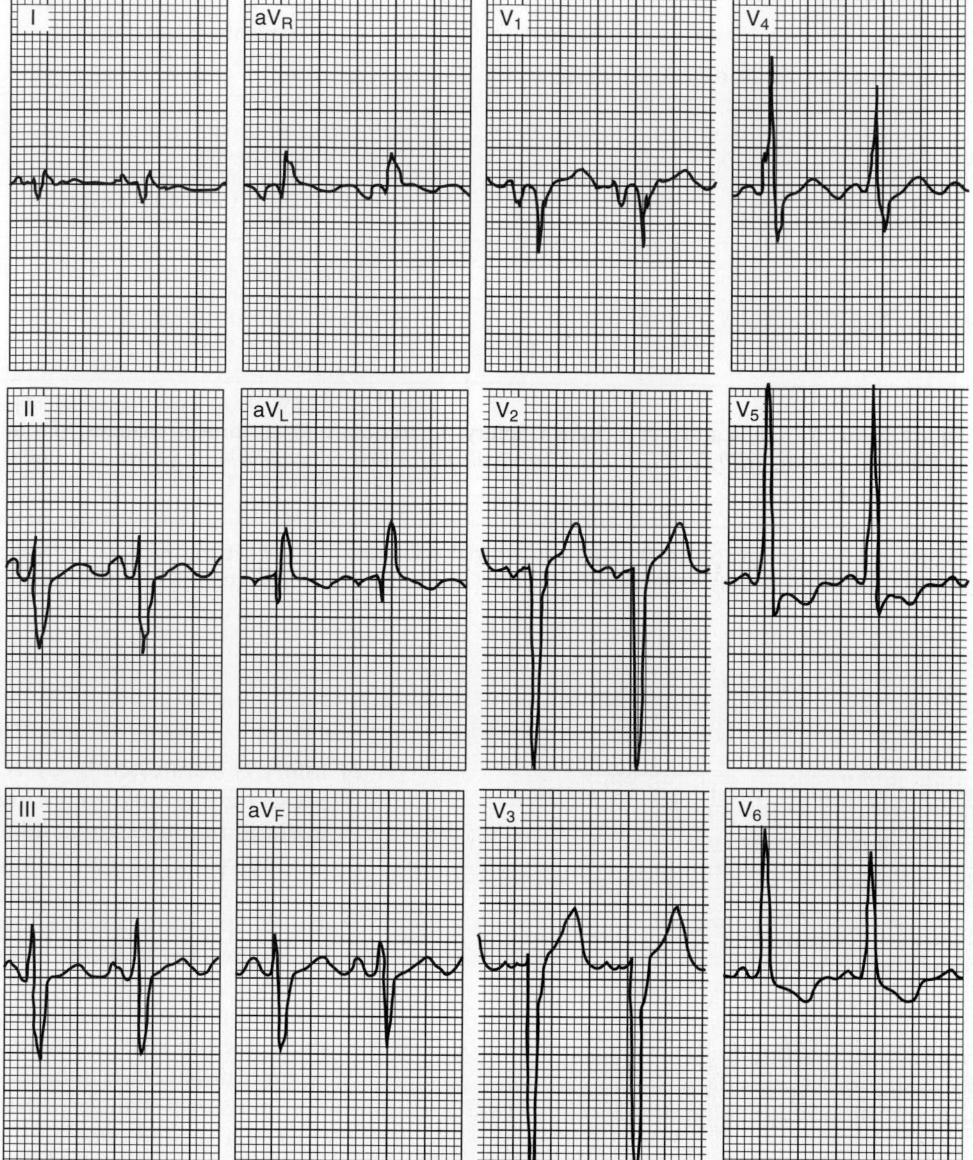

Figure 2-45 Left ventricular hypertrophy with left atrial enlargement. Note wide, notched P waves in lead II with dominant terminal component of the P wave in V_1 as evidence of left atrial enlargement. Note deep S wave in V_2 and tall R wave in V_5 with left axis deviation and left ventricular strain (ST segment depression and asymmetrical T wave inversion in V_5, V_6) as evidence of left ventricular hypertrophy. (From Conover, M. B. [2003]. *Understanding electrocardiography* [8th ed.]. St. Louis: Mosby.)

b) Ventricular pacemakers
c) LBBB: Chance of acute MI is more likely if the following are present:
  i) New onset
  ii) ST segment depression of 1 mm in leads V_1, V_2
  iii) ST segment elevation of more than 5 mm
d) Ventricular hypertrophy
e) Wolff-Parkinson-White syndrome
f) Pericarditis
g) Hypothermia
h) Hemorrhagic stroke
i) Electrolyte imbalances

b. Location (Table 2-11)
  1) Anterior left ventricle: indicative changes in V_3, V_4 (possibly V_2)
  2) Septal: indicative changes in V_1, V_2
  3) Lateral left ventricle: indicative changes in I, aVL and/or V_5, V_6
    a) I, aVL are considered high lateral leads
    b) V_5, V_6 are considered low lateral leads
  4) Inferior left ventricle: indicative changes in II, III, aVF
  5) Posterior left ventricle
    a) Reciprocal changes in V_1, V_2
    b) Indicative changes in V_7, V_8, or V_9
      i) V_8 and V_9 are the most significant.

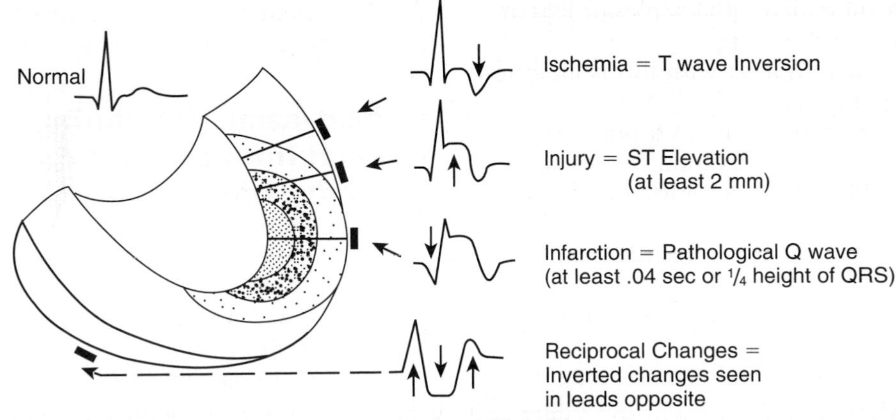

Figure 2-46 ECG indicators of ischemia, injury, infarction, and reciprocal changes. (From Harvey, M. [2000]. *Study guide to core curriculum for critical care nursing* [3rd ed.]. Philadelphia: Saunders.)

Table 2-11 ECG Lead Correlation with Myocardial Infarction Locations

Location	Coronary Artery Affected	Indicative Leads	Reciprocal Leads
Anterior	LAD	(V_2), V_3, V_4	V_7, V_8, V_9
Septal	LAD	V_1, V_2	V5, V_6
Anteroseptal	LAD	V_1, V_2, V_3, (V_4)	I, aVL
Lateral	LCA	I, aVL (high lateral), V_5, V_6 (low lateral)	II, III, aVF
Anterolateral	LCA	V_3, V_4, V_5, V_6, (I, aVL)	II, III, aVF
Inferior	RCA	II, III, aVF	I, aVL
RV	RCA	V_{4R}, V_{5R}, V_{6R} may be transient	I, aVL
Posterior	RCA and/or LCA	V_7, V_8, V_9 or reciprocal in V_1, V_2, V_3	V_1, V_2, V_3

NOTE: Changes may also be seen in leads in parentheses.

Table 2-12 Determination of Age of Myocardial Infarction

Description	ECG Characteristics	Time from Onset of Pain
Hyperacute	• ST segment elevation • Tombstone-shaped T waves or T wave inversion	Minutes to hours
Acute	• ST segment elevation • T wave inversion • Pathologic Q waves	Hours to days
Recent	• T wave inversion • Pathologic Q waves	Weeks to months
Old	• Pathologic Q waves	After several months

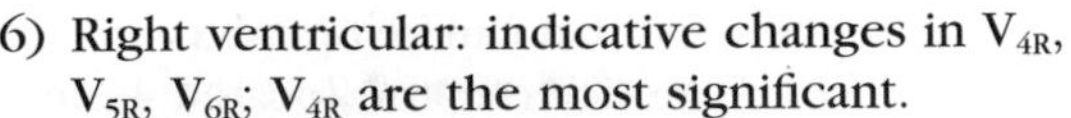

6) Right ventricular: indicative changes in V_{4R}, V_{5R}, V_{6R}; V_{4R} are the most significant.

c. Determination of age of MI (Table 2-12)

6. ECG changes in angina
   a. Variant (also referred to as *Prinzmetal's* or *vasospastic*) angina
      1) Angina at rest caused by spasm of the coronary artery or arteries

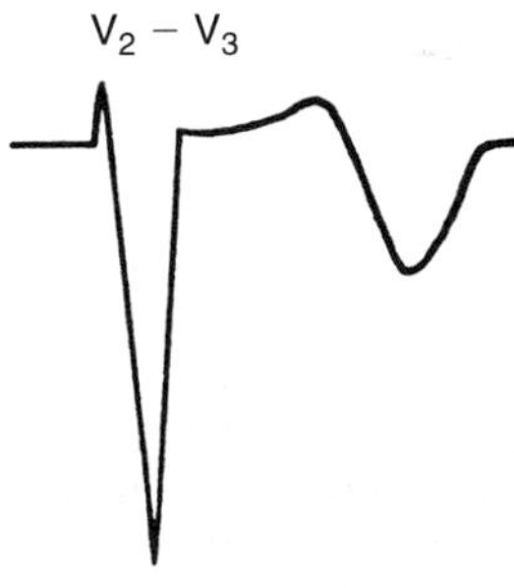

Figure 2-47 Wellens syndrome. (From Conover, M. [2003]. *Understanding electrocardiography* [8th ed.] St. Louis: Mosby.)

      2) Manifested by ST segment elevation with pain
   b. Wellens syndrome (Figure 2-47)
      1) Group of signs that are associated with occlusion of proximal left anterior descending artery and high risk of sudden cardiac death in a patient with unstable angina
         a) Symmetrical, deeply inverted T waves in V_2 and V_3 that persist even when the patient is pain free
         b) Little or no ST segment elevation
         c) Little or no enzyme elevation

d) No development of Q waves or loss of precordial R waves
2) Cardiac catheterization with PCI is indicated
7. ECG changes in pericarditis
   a. ST segment normal in V_1 and aVR but all other leads show ST segment elevation
   b. Depression of PR interval in limb leads and left chest leads (V_5, V_6)
   c. Decrease in QRS voltage if pericardial effusion present
8. ECG changes in myocardial trauma (e.g., myocardial contusion)
   a. Nonspecific ST and T wave changes; infarction pattern if necrosis
   b. High risk of dysrhythmias and AV nodal blocks
9. ECG changes in hypothermia (seen when temperature less than 30° C)
   a. J wave (also referred to as an *Osborne wave*): rounded waves above the isoelectric line between the QRS complex and the early part of the ST segment; usually seen best in lead II and V leads
   b. ST segment elevation
   c. Prolonged intervals
10. ECG changes in hypothyroidism
   a. ST segment depression
   b. Prominent T waves with T wave inversion
   c. May have LVH

ST Segment Monitoring

1. Continuous monitoring of ST segment for changes associated with ischemia because the ischemia may not cause chest pain (referred to as *silent* ischemia)
2. Indications
   a. Acute coronary syndrome
   b. Myocardial infarction
   c. Following PCI: optional depending on clinical indications such as chest pain, dysrhythmias
   d. During and following cardiac surgery
   e. During and following noncardiac surgery in patients at risk of myocardial ischemia
3. Lead choice
   a. Choose a lead that best demonstrates ST changes during ischemia, evolving MI, or at the time of balloon occlusion at the time of PCI (referred to as the patient's *ischemic fingerprint*).
   b. If information regarding the ischemic fingerprint is not available, use lead III and V_3.
4. Note significant changes in the ST segment: ST segment elevation or depression of at least 1 mm for at least 60 seconds is considered significant.
   a. ST segment elevation represents more severe, usually transmural, ischemia.
   b. ST segment depression represents less severe, usually subendocardial, ischemia or reciprocal changes of ischemia.
   c. Other causes of ST segment deviation include electrolyte imbalances, pericarditis, hypothermia, ventricular aneurysm, hypothyroidism, hyperventilation, pulmonary infarction, and drugs such as digoxin.

Hemodynamic Monitoring

General Information Regarding Hemodynamic Monitoring

1. Definition: monitoring of blood flow generally through the use of invasive catheters
2. Uses
   a. Measure hemodynamic pressures and record waveforms
      1) Arterial catheter: systemic arterial blood pressure including systolic, diastolic, and mean
      2) Central venous pressure catheter: central venous pressure measured as a mean
      3) Pulmonary artery catheter (PAC)
         a) Allows measurement of the following:
            i) Right atrial pressure measured as a mean
            ii) Pulmonary artery pressure (PAP) including systolic, diastolic, and mean
            iii) Pulmonary artery occlusive pressure (PAOP) measured as a mean as an indirect reflection of left atrial pressure
            iv) Cardiac output usually measured by thermodilution technique
         b) Lumens of a typical PAC (Figure 2-48)
            i) Proximal lumen opens in the right atrium and allows measurement of right atrial pressure and administration of infusions; this port is also used for bolus injections for the thermodilution measurement of cardiac output.
            ii) Proximal infusion lumen: many catheters have another right atrial port to be used for central infusions.
            iii) Distal lumen: opens at the distal tip of the catheter; PAP is measured at this port with the balloon deflated, and PAOP is measured at this port with the balloon inflated
            iv) Balloon lumen: allows inflation of the balloon at the distal tip of the catheter for measurement of PAOP; a 1.5 mL capacity balloon is attached to the port and there is a gate-valve that can be opened and closed
            v) Thermistor: located 4 cm proximal to the balloon, the thermistor measures core body temperature and temperature changes that occur with injectates during thermodilution cardiac output measurements

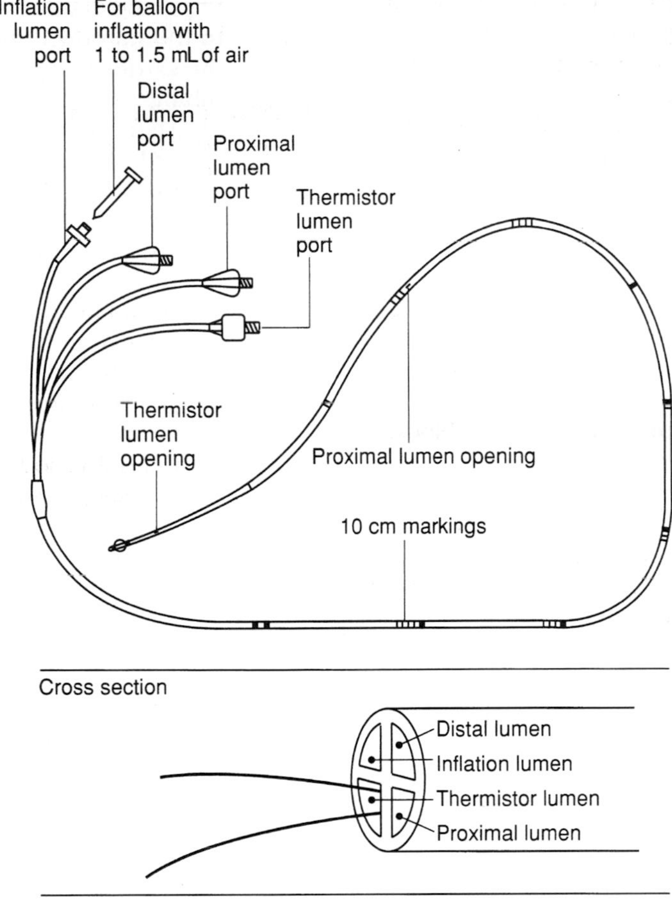

Figure 2-48 Pulmonary artery catheter. (From Visalli, F., & Evans, P. [1981]. The Swan-Ganz catheter: A program for teaching safe effective use. *Nursing* 81[11],1.)

vi) There are black lines on the catheter every 10 cm; each thin line indicates 10 cm; a thick line indicates 50 cm.

c) Specialized catheters also allow the evaluation of the following:
   i) Continuous cardiac output (CCO)
   ii) SvO_2: oxygen saturation of mixed venous blood
   iii) $ScvO_2$: oxygen saturation of venous blood in the superior vena cava
   iv) REF: right ventricular end-systolic volume, right ventricular end-diastolic volume, right ventricular stroke volume, and right ventricular ejection fraction

b. Obtain blood samples.
   1) Arterial catheter
      a) Intermittent arterial samples for arterial blood gases and serum arterial lactate
      b) Continuous intraarterial blood gas monitoring allows measurement of pH, PaO_2, $PaCO_2$ through the use of fiberoptic and electrochemical sensors in an intraarterial catheter.
   2) Central venous catheter: venous
   3) Pulmonary artery catheter
      a) Right atrial (proximal port): venous
      b) Pulmonary artery (distal port): mixed venous

c. Provide central venous access for administration of fluids or drugs.
   1) Central venous catheter: usually triple-lumen
   2) Pulmonary artery catheter (PAC)
      a) Right atrial (proximal) port
      b) Pulmonary artery (distal) port: saline flush solution to ensure patency; heparin may be added to flush solution (though still controversial), but this port should not be used for fluid or drug administration
      c) VIP (i.e., venous infusion port) catheters: provide an extra right atrial port

d. Perform intracardiac pacing via specialized PAC

3. Common indications for hemodynamic monitoring
   a. Shock of any etiology
   b. Myocardial infarction especially with:
      1) Acute left or right ventricular failure
      2) Refractory pain
      3) Significant hypotension or hypertension
      4) Right ventricular infarction
      5) Mechanical complications (e.g., papillary muscle rupture, rupture of interventricular septum)

c. High-risk surgical patient
d. Acute right ventricular failure (e.g., after pulmonary embolism)
e. Severe valvular disease
f. Cardiac tamponade
g. Pulmonary edema of uncertain etiology: used to differentiate between cardiac and noncardiac pulmonary edema
h. Pulmonary hypertension
i. Acute respiratory failure (e.g., acute respiratory distress syndrome)
j. Need for evaluation of fluid status and guide fluid resuscitation (e.g., burns, multiple trauma, complex surgical procedures especially in patients with preexisting cardiopulmonary disease)
k. Need for evaluation of hemodynamic response to potent pharmacologic agents (e.g., hypertensive crisis treated with nitroprusside)

4. Relative contraindications of invasive hemodynamic monitoring
   a. Severe coagulopathy
   b. Severe pulmonary hypertension
   c. Presence of a prosthetic tricuspid or pulmonic valve
   d. Presence of an endocardial pacemaker
   e. Lack of trained physicians and nurses
5. Controversies regarding invasive hemodynamic monitoring
   a. It is unclear which patients actually benefit from invasive hemodynamic monitoring (i.e., benefits outweigh risks) though research efforts to link hemodynamic monitoring with improvement in outcomes continue.
   b. A retrospective observation study (i.e., no controls of confounding variables) showed an association between invasive monitoring and an increase in mortality. (Connors et al., 1996)
      1) There was a 65% reduction in the use of PACs between 1993 and 2004 with a significant drop after this 1996 publication. (Wiener & Welch, 2007)
   c. Some significant issues to consider include the following:
      1) There is an institutional and human tendency to "routinize" technology (Benner, 2003) such as invasive monitoring.
      2) Studies suggest that nurses' and physicians' knowledge regarding hemodynamic waveforms and data interpretation is limited.
      3) Interrater variability and lack of reproducibility continue to be problematic in evaluating values.
   d. Vincent et al. (2008) recommend that rather than abandoning invasive hemodynamic monitoring, the following should be ensured:
      1) Correct measurement
      2) Correct interpretation
      3) Correct application
6. Components of a pressure monitoring system (Figure 2-49)
   a. Physiologic signal: intravascular pressure carried to the transducer by a catheter (inserted into the cardiovascular circuit) and fluid-filled tubing
      1) Static pressure is produced by the volume of blood in the vascular system at zero flow
      2) Dynamic pressure is produced by the heart; equal to flow × resistance
      3) Hydrostatic pressure is related to the density of the fluid, gravity, and the height of the column of blood between the heart and the vessels
         a) "Zeroing" the pressure monitoring system by leveling the air-fluid interface of the transducer at the phlebostatic axis (which correlates to the atrial level), turning the stopcock to open the system to air, and ensuring that the digital display and the graphic representation both indicate zero corrects for the hydrostatic gradient.
   b. Transducer: converts the mechanical signal to an electrical signal
   c. Monitor
      1) Amplifier: device that increases the magnitude of the electrical signal and filters out electrical interference
      2) Oscilloscope: device that displays the resultant signal as a pressure waveform and as a numerical value
      3) Recorder: device that records the pressure waveform on paper for analysis

Hemodynamic Parameters (Table 2-13)

1. Arterial and ventricular pressures measured as systolic/diastolic while atrial pressures measured as a mean
2. Systemic arterial blood pressure
   a. Pressure in a systemic artery; reflects systemic arterial blood pressure
   b. Blood pressure = CO × SVR; changes in blood pressure are due to either a change in cardiac output or systemic vascular resistance.
   c. Measured by a catheter in a peripheral artery or the second lumen of an intraaortic balloon catheter (central aortic arterial line)
      1) Radial artery site is the preferred peripheral site due to collateral circulation provided by the ulnar artery.
         a) Allen's test must be performed prior to any radial artery puncture to assess patency of radial-ulnar arch; this test is performed by compressing both the radial and ulnar artery to blanch the hand; when the ulnar artery is released, evaluate the time until return of color; if longer than 7 seconds, this radial artery should not be punctured (for arterial blood gases or for radial artery cannulation).

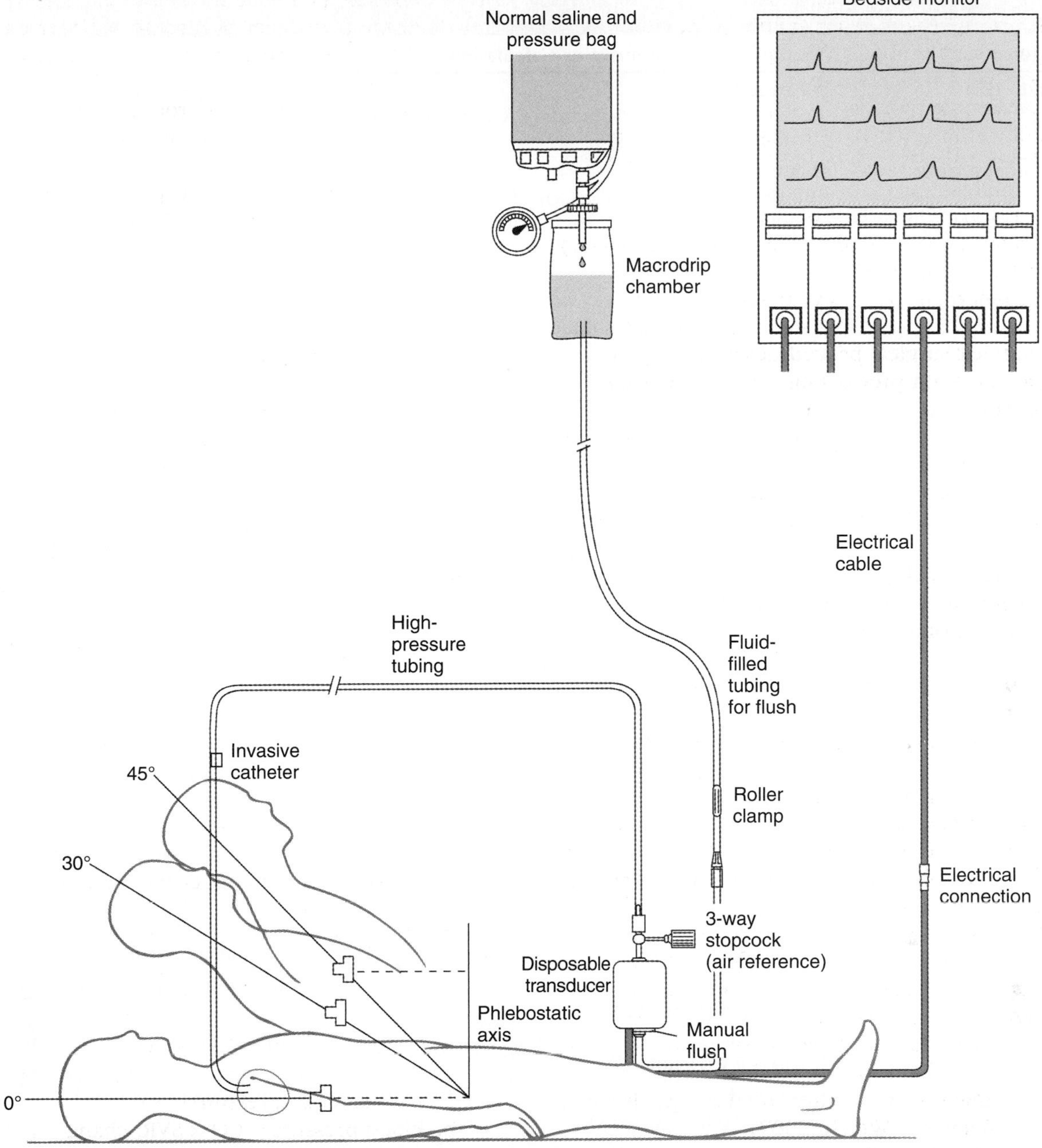

Figure 2-49 Components of a pressure monitoring system. (From Urden, L., Stacy, K., & Lough, M. [2010]. *Critical care nursing: Diagnosis and management* [6th ed.]. St. Louis: Mosby.)

2) Neurovascular assessment of the limb distal to any arterial line is essential; thrombosis or embolization may cause acute arterial occlusion and loss of limb.

d. Systolic arterial pressure: maximal pressure with which the blood is ejected from the left ventricle

e. Diastolic arterial pressure: reflects the rapidity of flow of the ejected blood through the arterial system and the vessel's elasticity

1) Diastolic pressure is expected to be higher (and pulse pressure to be narrowed) if there is endogenous catecholamine release or the patient is receiving sympathomimetic agents (e.g., epinephrine, dopamine [Intropin], or norepinephrine [Levophed]).

2) Diastolic pressure is expected to be lower (and pulse pressure to be widened) if there are excessive vasodilatory mediators (e.g., septic shock, anaphylactic shock).

f. Mean arterial pressure: average pressure occurring in the aorta and its major branches during the cardiac cycle; mean arterial pressure of at least 60 mm Hg is necessary to perfuse the vital organs

g. Normal pressure values

Table 2-13 Hemodynamic Parameters, Methods of Measurement or Calculation, and Normals

Parameter	Method of Measurement or Calculation	Normal
Heart rate (HR)	Measured: Count rate at apex or number of R waves by ECG monitor	60-100 beats/min
Mean arterial pressure (MAP)	Calculated: [BP systolic + (BP diastolic × 2)] ÷ 3 Systolic and diastolic pressures can be obtained by direct (arterial line) or indirect (auscultated using a sphygmomanometer)	70-105 mm Hg (Normal systolic BP is 90-140 mm Hg; normal diastolic BP is 60-90 mm Hg)
Cardiac output (CO)	Measured: Usually by thermodilution technique	4-8 L/min
Cardiac index (CI)	Calculated: CO ÷ by body surface area (BSA)	2.5-4 L/min/m^2
Stroke volume (SV)	Calculated: CO ÷ HR	60-120 mL/beat
Stroke index (SI)	Calculated: SV ÷ BSA	30-65 mL/m^2/beat
Central venous pressure (CVP)	Measured: At the tip of a catheter (frequently multilumen) in the superior vena cava; may be measured with a transducer or a water manometer	2-6 mm Hg (transducer) 3-8 cm H_2O (water manometer)
Right atrial pressure (RAP)	Measured: At the proximal port of the PAC; this port is located in the right atrium	2-6 mm Hg 3-8 cm H_2O
Pulmonary artery pressure (PAP)	Measured: At the distal port of the PAC with the balloon deflated; the tip is located in a pulmonary arteriole	Systolic (PAs): 15-30 mm Hg Diastolic (PAd): 5-15 mm Hg Mean (PAm): 10-20 mm Hg
Pulmonary artery occlusive pressure (PAOP)	Measured: At the distal port of the PAC with the balloon inflated; because right heart pressures are blocked by the inflated balloon, PAOP indirectly reflects left atrial pressure, left ventricular end-diastolic pressure (LVEDP), and left ventricular preload	8-12 mm Hg (NOTE: Though 8-12 mm Hg is "normal," many patients require a higher pressure [as high as 15-20 mm Hg] to achieve optimal stretch on the myofibrils and optimal preload)
Systemic vascular resistance (SVR)	Calculated: [(MAP − RAP) × 80] ÷ CO	800-1400 dynes/sec/cm^{-5}
Systemic vascular resistance index (SVRI)	Calculated: [(MAP − RAP) × 80] ÷ CI	2000-2400 dynes/sec/cm^{-5}/m^2
Pulmonary vascular resistance (PVR)	Calculated: [(PAm − PAOP) × 80] ÷ CO	100-250 dynes/sec/cm^{-5}
Pulmonary vascular resistance index (PVRI)	Calculated: [(PAm − PAOP) × 80] ÷ CI	225-315 dynes/sec/cm^{-5}/m^2
Left ventricular stroke work index (LVSWI)	Calculated: [SI × (MAP − PAOP)] × 0.0136	45-65 g•m/m^2
Right ventricular stroke work index (RVSWI)	Calculated: [SI × (PAm − RAP)] × 0.0136	5-12 g•m/m^2
Coronary artery perfusion pressure (CAPP)	Calculated: Diastolic BP − PAOP	60-80 mm Hg
Right ventricular end-diastolic volume (RVEDV)	Measured: By thermodilution method with REF PAC	100-160 mL
Right ventricular end-diastolic volume index (RVEDVI)	Calculated: RVEDV ÷ BSA	60-100 mL/m^2
Right ventricular end-systolic volume (RVESV)	Measured: By thermodilution method with REF PAC	50-100 mL

Table 2-13 Hemodynamic Parameters, Methods of Measurement or Calculation, and Normals—cont'd

Parameter	Method of Measurement or Calculation	Normal
Right ventricular end-systolic volume index (RVESVI)	Calculated: RVESV ÷ BSA	30-60 mL/m^2
Right ventricular ejection fraction (REF)	Measured: By thermodilution method with REF PAC	40-60%
Arterial oxygen saturation (SaO_2)	Measured: By pulse oximetry or by arterial blood gas analysis	95-100%
Mixed venous oxygen saturation (SvO_2)	Measured: By SvO_2 port of a fiberoptic oximetric PAC or by mixed venous blood gas analysis	60-80%
Central venous oxygen saturation ($ScvO_2$)	Measured: By fiberoptic oximetric central venous catheter or by venous blood gas analysis	65-85%
Arterial oxygen content (CaO_2)	Calculated: $1.34 \times Hgb \times SaO_2$	18-20 mL/dL
Venous oxygen content (CvO_2)	Calculated: $1.34 \times Hgb \times SvO_2$	12-16 mL/dL
Oxygen delivery (DO_2)	Calculated: $CO \times CaO_2 \times 10$	900-1100 mL/min
Oxygen delivery index (DO_2I)	Calculated: $CI \times CaO_2 \times 10$	550-650 mL/min/m^2
Oxygen consumption (VO_2)	Calculated: $CO \times Hgb \times 13.4 \times (SaO_2 - SvO_2)$	200-300 mL/min
Oxygen consumption index (VO_2I)	Calculated: $CI \times Hgb \times 13.4 \times (SaO_2 - SvO_2)$	110-160 mL/min/m^2
Oxygen extraction ratio (O_2ER)	Calculated: $CaO_2 - CvO_2/CaO_2$	22-30%
Oxygen extraction index (O_2EI)	Calculated: $SaO_2 - SvO_2/SaO_2$	20-27%

1) Systolic: 90-140 mm Hg
2) Diastolic: 60-90 mm Hg
3) Mean: 70-105 mm Hg

h. Causes of abnormal pressures (Table 2-14)
   1) Arterial catheter versus cuff pressures
      a) Arterial catheters are a direct measurement and therefore more accurate (assuming proper zeroing, leveling, and dynamic response) especially in shock states, severe hypertension, vasoconstriction, and obesity.
         i) Indirect blood pressure measurements including auscultation and oscillometric methods tend to underestimate systolic pressure and overestimate diastolic pressure.
         ii) Mean arterial pressures tend to be the same even in these situations and is a more consistent evaluation of perfusion pressure.
      b) Expect radial artery catheters to show a pressure slightly higher (~10 mm Hg) than brachial cuff measurement because the radial artery is smaller than the brachial artery.
      c) If there is a significant variation between pressure measured by arterial catheter and pressure auscultated using a sphygmomanometer other than in the situations listed earlier, do the following:
         i) Check the pressure monitoring system for air bubbles, occlusions, and positioning of catheter against wall of artery.
         ii) Ensure that the air-fluid interface of the transducer is level with the phlebostatic axis.
         iii) Ensure adequate damping of the pressure monitoring system.

i. Normal waveform (Figure 2-24)

3. Right atrial pressure (RAP)
   a. Pressure in the right atrium
   b. Reflects venous return to right heart; also, reflects right ventricular end-diastolic pressure and preload as long as right ventricular compliance and tricuspid valve function are normal

Table 2-14 Causes of Abnormal Hemodynamic Pressures

Parameter	Increased	Decreased
Systemic arterial blood pressure *Normals:* • *Systolic: 90-140 mm Hg* • *Diastolic: 60-90 mm Hg* • *Mean: 70-105 mm Hg*	• Increase in systemic vascular resistance (e.g., hypertension, sympathetic nervous system innervation) • Increase in cardiac output (e.g., hyperthyroidism)	• Decrease in systemic vascular resistance (e.g., sepsis, anaphylaxis) • Decrease in cardiac output (e.g., myocardial infarction, tachydysrhythmias)

Right atrial pressure (RAP)
Normals:
• *2-6 mm Hg mean*
• *3-8 cm H_2O*
	• Hypervolemia
	• Tricuspid valve dysfunction: stenosis or regurgitation
	• Right ventricular failure or infarction
	• Ventricular septal defect (VSD) with left-to-right shunt
	• Pulmonic stenosis
	• Pulmonary hypertension
	  • Active: hypoxemic pulmonary vasoconstriction (PaO_2 less than 60 mm Hg)
	    – Pulmonary embolism (PE)
	    – Chronic obstructive pulmonary disease (COPD)
	    – Acute respiratory distress syndrome (ARDS)
	  • Passive: mitral valve dysfunction (stenosis or regurgitation)
	• Positive-pressure ventilation
	• Constrictive pericarditis
	• Cardiac tamponade
	• Mitral valve dysfunction: stenosis or regurgitation
	• Chronic left ventricular failure (RAP would be a late indication of LVF)
		• Hypovolemia
		• Vasodilation
		  • Venous vasodilators (e.g., nitroglycerin, morphine)
		  • Endogenous systemic vasodilation (e.g., septic shock, anaphylactic shock, neurogenic shock)

Right ventricular pressure *Normals:* • *Systolic: 15-30 mm Hg* • *End-diastolic: 0 to 8 mm Hg*	• Right ventricular failure or infarction • Ventricular septal defect (VSD) with left → right shunt • Pulmonary hypertension • Mitral valve dysfunction: stenosis or regurgitation • Constrictive pericarditis • Cardiac tamponade • Chronic left ventricular failure	• Hypovolemia • Excessive vasodilation (e.g., vasodilators, septic shock, anaphylactic shock, neurogenic shock)
Pulmonary artery pressure (PAP) *Normals:* • *Systolic: 15 to 30 mm Hg* • *Diastolic: 5 to 15 mm Hg* • *Mean: 10 to 20 mm Hg*	• Hypervolemia • Ventricular septal defect with left → right shunt • Pulmonary hypertension • Positive-pressure ventilation • Mitral valve dysfunction: stenosis or regurgitation • Constrictive pericarditis • Cardiac tamponade • Left ventricular failure	• Hypovolemia • Excessive vasodilation (e.g., vasodilators, septic shock, anaphylactic shock, neurogenic shock)
Pulmonary artery occlusive pressure (PAOP) *Normal:* • *8 to 12 mm Hg*	• Positive-pressure ventilation especially with positive end-expiratory pressure (PEEP) • Hypervolemia • Mitral valve dysfunction: stenosis or regurgitation • Constrictive pericarditis • Cardiac tamponade • Left ventricular failure • Severe aortic stenosis	• Hypovolemia • Excessive vasodilation (e.g., vasodilators, septic shock, anaphylactic shock, neurogenic shock)

Table 2-14 Causes of Abnormal Hemodynamic Pressures—cont'd

Parameter	Increased	Decreased
Cardiac output and cardiac index *Normal:* • *CO 4-8 L/min* • *CI 2.5-4 L/min*	• Sympathetic nervous system (SNS) innervation (endogenous catecholamines) (e.g., stress, exercise) • Exogenous catecholamines (e.g., epinephrine, isoproterenol, dobutamine, dopamine) • Other positive inotropes (e.g., digitalis, amrinone) • Infection, early sepsis • Hyperthyroidism • Anemia	• Decreased contractility (e.g., myocardial infarction [MI], cardiomyopathy, beta-blockers) • Increased afterload (e.g., systemic or pulmonary hypertension, aortic or pulmonic stenosis, polycythemia) • Alteration in preload: excessively increased (e.g., hypervolemia, HF) or decreased (e.g., hypovolemia, cardiac tamponade, mitral or tricuspid valve disease) • Significantly increased or decreased heart rate (e.g., bradydysrhythmias, tachydysrhythmias)

SvO_2
Normal: 60-80%
$ScvO_2$
Normal: 70-80%
	• Increased oxygen supply and delivery
	  • Increased SaO_2 (e.g., increased FiO_2, CPAP, or PEEP)
	  • Increase in cardiac output/cardiac index (inotropes, IABP, ventricular assist device, decrease in excessive afterload, hyperdynamic [i.e., early] stage of septic shock)
	  • Increased hemoglobin (e.g., blood administration)
	• Decreased oxygen demand
	  • Anesthesia and/or analgesics
	  • Muscle paralysis or sedation
	  • Hypothermia
	  • Sleep
	  • Hypothyroidism
	  • Beta-blockers
	• Decreased oxygen extraction at tissue level
	  • Early sepsis
	  • Cyanide toxicity
	• Shift of oxyhemoglobin dissociation curve to the left (e.g., alkalosis, hypothermia, decreased levels of 2, 3-DPG)
	• Technical problems
	  • PAC in occluded position
	  • Deposits of fibrin on the tip of the catheter
		• Decreased oxygen supply and delivery
		  • Decrease in SaO_2 (e.g., decreased FiO_2, CPAP, or PEEP, suctioning, acute respiratory failure, pulmonary edema)
		  • Decrease in cardiac output/ cardiac index (e.g., shock, heart failure, hypovolemia, dysrhythmias, excessive CPAP or PEEP, negative inotropes, excessive afterload)
		  • Decrease in Hgb (e.g., anemia, hemorrhage) or abnormal hemoglobin (e.g., methemoglobinemia, sickle cell anemia)
		• Increased metabolic needs (e.g., seizures, shivering, restlessness, pain, hyperthermia, increased work of breathing, increased metabolic rate, exertion [e.g., turning, bathing, active range of motion])
		• Increased oxygen extraction at tissue level (e.g., early sepsis)
		• Shift of oxyhemoglobin dissociation curve to the right (e.g., acidosis, hyperthermia)

c. Measured through catheter in superior vena cava (central venous catheter [i.e., CVP]) or at the proximal port of PAC (i.e., RAP)
   1) Insertion of a CVP catheter or PAC
      a) Preceded by insertion of a venous introducer into the internal jugular, subclavian, or femoral vein; the right internal jugular vein is the preferred site because the risk of pneumothorax is reduced by the use of the internal jugular vein
      b) The catheter is then threaded through the introducer into place with the CVP catheter tip in the superior vena cava and the PAC tip in a pulmonary arteriole in the dependent area (West zone 3) though the RAP is measured from the proximal port, which is in the right atrium.
   2) Though these parameters (CVP and RAP) are not actually the same, they are the same in practicality and are frequently used interchangeably.
   3) Central venous pressure may be measured by a water manometer in cm H_2O pressure or by a transducer in mm Hg pressure.
   4) RAP from the proximal port of the PAC is generally measured by a transducer in mm Hg.
   5) To convert values, remember that 1 mm Hg is equal to 1.36 cm H_2O.

   d. Normal pressure value: 2-6 mm Hg mean (or 3-8 cm H_2O)
   e. Causes of abnormal pressures (see Table 2-14)
   f. Normal waveform (Figure 2-50)
4. Right ventricular pressure
   a. Pressure in the right ventricle
   b. Measured only during insertion of the PAC as the distal tip of the PAC is floated through the right ventricle
   c. Normal pressure values
      1) Systolic: 15-30 mm Hg
      2) End-diastolic: 0-8 mm Hg
   d. Causes of abnormal pressures (see Table 2-14)
   e. Normal waveform (Figure 2-51)
5. Pulmonary artery pressure (PAP) (Box 2-2)
   a. Pressure in the pulmonary artery with the balloon **deflated**
   b. Measured from the distal tip of the PAC with balloon **deflated**
      1) PA systolic pressure (PAs): pressure in the pulmonary artery during RV systole
      2) PA end-diastolic pressure (PAd): pressure in the pulmonary artery at the end of RV diastole; reflects left atrial pressure in the absence of pulmonary disease and LVEDP in the absence of pulmonary disease and mitral valve dysfunction
   c. Normal pressure values
      1) Systolic: 15-30 mm Hg
      2) Diastolic: 5-15 mm Hg
      3) Mean: 10-20 mm Hg
   d. Causes of abnormal pressures (see Table 2-14)
   e. Correlation between PAd and PAOP
      1) PAd is normally 2-4 mm Hg greater than PAOP
      2) PAd 5 mm Hg or more greater than PAOP can be caused by any of the following:
         a) Tachycardias greater than 125 beats/min
         b) Pulmonary hypertension
            i) Active: hypoxemic pulmonary vasoconstriction with PaO_2 less

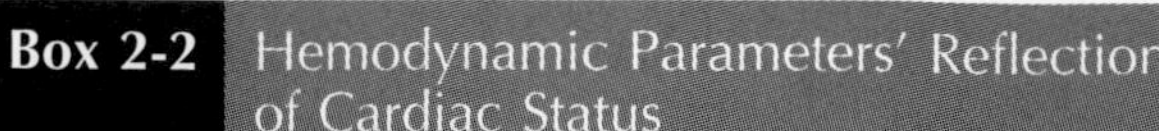

RAP = Right heart
PAd = Pulmonary vascular bed
PAOP = Left heart

NOTE: One of the ways to remember causes of abnormal pressures is to consider that pressure behind the problem will be increased while pressure in front of the problem will be decreased. For example, in massive pulmonary embolism and acute cor pulmonary, the PAOP would be decreased (in front of the problem) and the PAd and RAP will be increased (behind the problem).

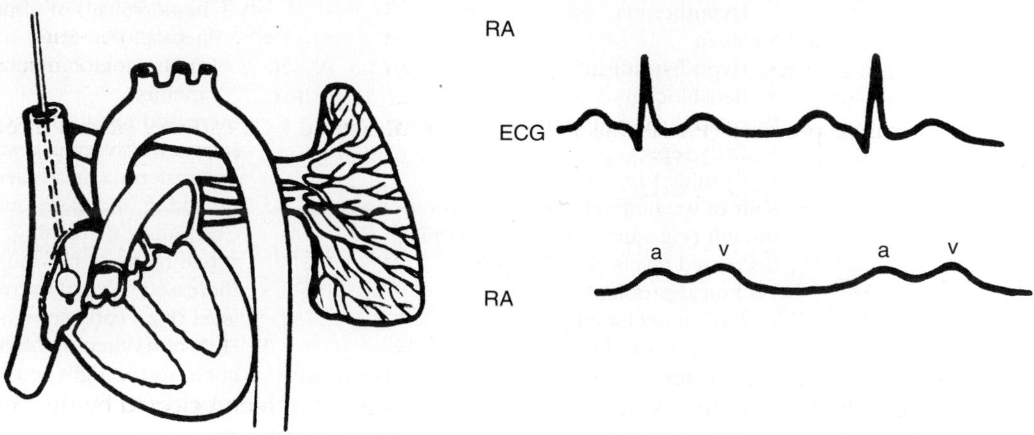

Figure 2-50 Right atrial waveform. (Courtesy Baxter Healthcare, Irvine, CA.)

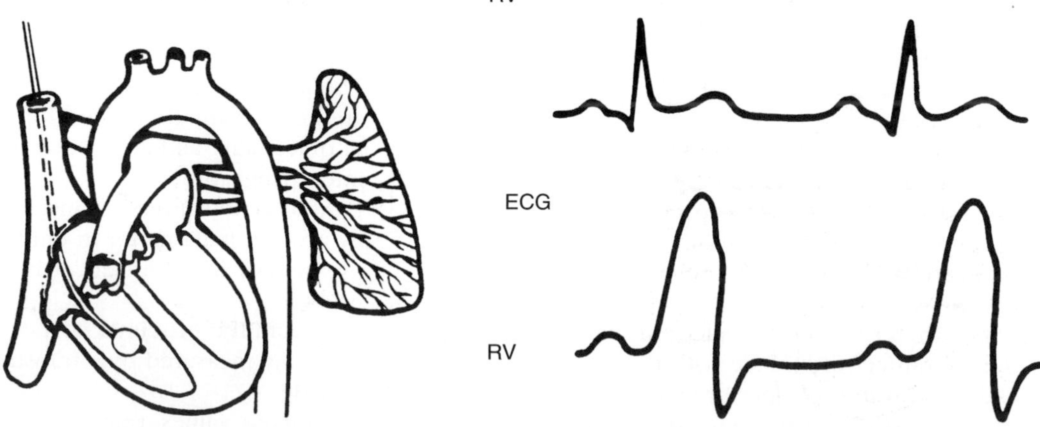

Figure 2-51 Right ventricular waveform. (Courtesy Baxter Healthcare, Irvine, CA.)

than 60 mm Hg (e.g., acute respiratory distress syndrome [ARDS], chronic obstructive pulmonary disease [COPD], pulmonary embolism [PE])
ii) Passive: mitral valve dysfunction (stenosis or regurgitation)

3) The difference between the PAd and the PAOP is sometimes referred to as the R to L gradient and is most helpful in differentiating cardiac from noncardiac (e.g., ARDS) pulmonary edema.
   a) If the PAd is elevated but the PAOP is normal (R to L gradient of greater than 5 mm Hg): This is an indication of pulmonary hypertension, and pulmonary edema is noncardiac pulmonary edema caused by an increase in alveolocapillary membrane permeability with leaking of fluid into the pulmonary interstitium and alveolus.
   b) If the PAd and the PAOP are both elevated (R to L gradient 5 mm Hg or less): This is an indication of cardiac pulmonary edema caused by an increase in the pulmonary capillary hypostatic pressure pushing fluid into the pulmonary interstitium and alveolus.

f. Normal waveform (Figure 2-52)
g. Changes in waveform (Table 2-15)
   1) Fling (also referred to as *whip*) (Figure 2-53)
   2) Damped (Figure 2-54)

6. Pulmonary artery occlusive pressure (PAOP) (also referred to as *pulmonary capillary wedge pressure* [PCWP] or *pulmonary artery wedge pressure* [PAWP])
   a. Pressure in the pulmonary artery with the balloon inflated; reflects pressure from the left atrium in the absence of pulmonary hypertension
   b. Measured from the distal tip of the PAC with the balloon inflated; the balloon blocks right heart pressures from the distal tip; left atrial pressure reflects left ventricular end-diastolic pressure and LV preload in the absence of mitral valve disease or left atrial tumor
   c. Normal pressure value: 8-12 mm Hg (measured as a mean); remember that some patients require a PAOP as high as 15-20 mm Hg for optimal preload
   d. Causes of abnormal pressures (see Table 2-14)
   e. Normal waveform (Figure 2-55)
      1) The *a* wave correlates with atrial contraction: It is the first wave seen after the QRS using dual channel recording.
      2) The *v* wave correlates with ventricular contraction: It is the first wave after the T wave using dual channel recording.
   f. Changes in waveform (Table 2-15)
      1) Large *a* waves
      2) Large *v* waves
      3) Large *a* waves and large *v* waves
   g. PAOP greater than PAd caused by any of the following:
      1) PAd artificially low or PAOP artificially high
      2) Mitral regurgitation with mean of PAOP used rather than the *a* wave amplitude (since mitral regurgitation causes large *v* waves on the PAOP waveform, it increases the PAOP if the mean is used; use the mean of the *a* wave measurement when there are large *v* waves) (Figure 2-56)
      3) Forceful atrial contraction

7. Left atrial pressure (LAP)
   a. Pressure in the left atrium; reflects left ventricular end-diastolic pressure and LV preload in the absence of mitral valve disease or left atrial tumor
   b. Measured by a catheter placed directly in the left atrium, usually placed during cardiac surgery
   c. A PAC usually used to measure PAOP as an indirect reflection of LAP because of the risk of complications related to direct LA catheter (e.g., air embolism, cardiac tamponade)
   d. Normals, waveforms, etc., as for PAOP

8. Cardiac output
   a. Amount of blood ejected by the ventricle each minute
   b. Invasive method utilizing a PAC and thermodilution technique
      1) Intermittent: method

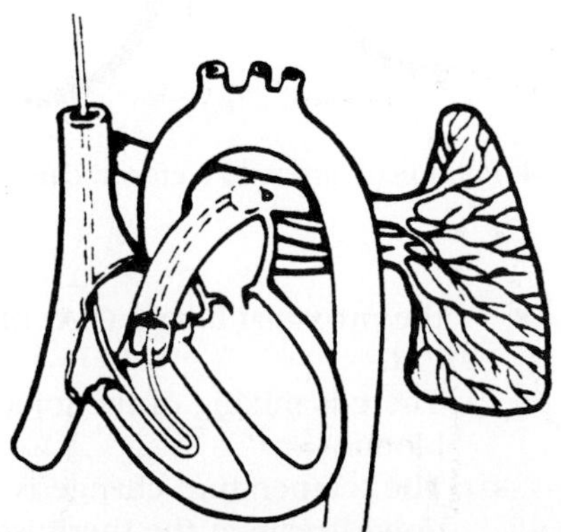

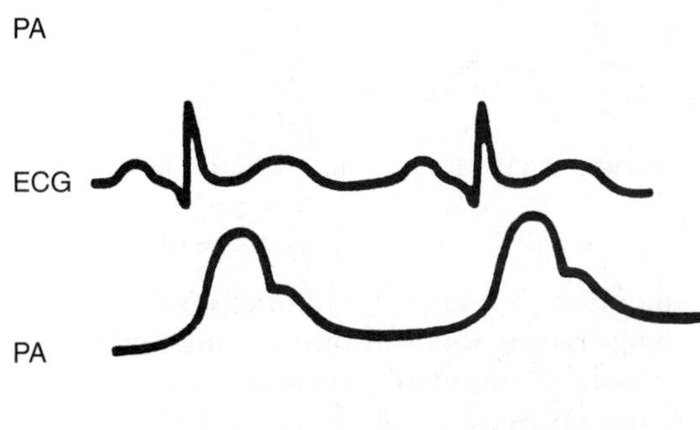

Figure 2-52 Pulmonary artery waveform. (Courtesy Baxter Healthcare, Irvine, CA.)

Table 2-15 Hemodynamic Waveform Abnormalities

Abnormality	Cause	Implications/Treatment
Pulmonary Artery		

Fling (or whip) (Figure 2-53)	• Excessive catheter length in RA or RV
	• Catheter tip is located near the pulmonic valve
		• Turn patient to left side to see if catheter will float out into PA
		• Monitor closely for indications that the catheter has flipped back into RV
		  • Loss of dicrotic notch characteristic of an arterial waveform
		  • Decrease in diastolic pressure to close to 0 mm Hg
		  • Ventricular ectopy: PVCs, possible ventricular tachycardia
		• Inflate balloon to increase the chance that it will float distally back into position
		• Catheter needs to be repositioned distally for fling or if catheter is in RV

Damped (Figure 2-54)	• Air bubbles within the pressure monitoring system • Catheter occlusion (e.g., fibrin at the tip of the catheter or catheter tip against the wall of the vessel) • Spontaneous occluded position	• Check the system for bubbles or blood; check that stopcocks are all positioned correctly and that stopcocks are covered with dead-end stopcock port covers (no holes) • Try to aspirate the catheter; DO NOT FLUSH because catheter may be in wedge position; if a clot is aspirated, discard and flush catheter • If still damped, ask patient to take deep breaths, cough, and turn to side; if still in spontaneous occluded position, catheter needs to be repositioned proximally
Pulmonary Artery Occlusive Pressure (PAOP) Waveform		
Large *a* waves	• Mitral stenosis • Severe aortic stenosis • Hypertension • AV block with AV asynchrony	

Large *v* waves	• Mitral regurgitation
	• Ventricular septal defect
		• Note: **In patients with large V waves:**
		  • The mean PAOP may be higher than PAd; do not use mean as the pressure value for PAOP
		  • Use the measurement of the *a* wave for the pressure value for PAOP because the mitral valve is open during the *a* wave (atrial contraction) and this value has better correlation with LVEDP

Large *a* and *v* waves (looks like M)	• Cardiac tamponade • Constrictive pericarditis • Hypervolemia • Left ventricular failure	

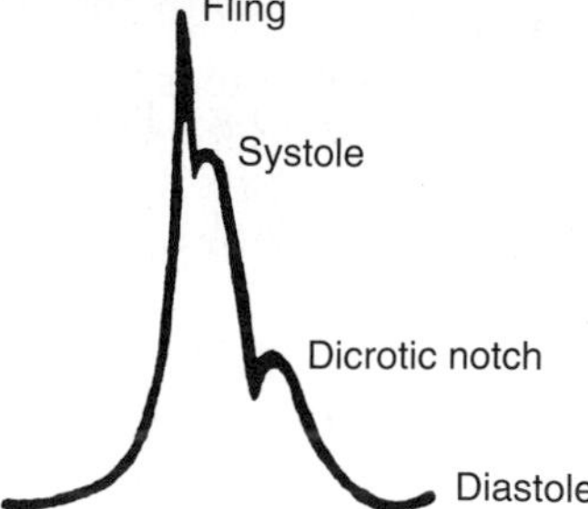

Figure 2-53 Pulmonary artery waveform: catheter fling (or whip).

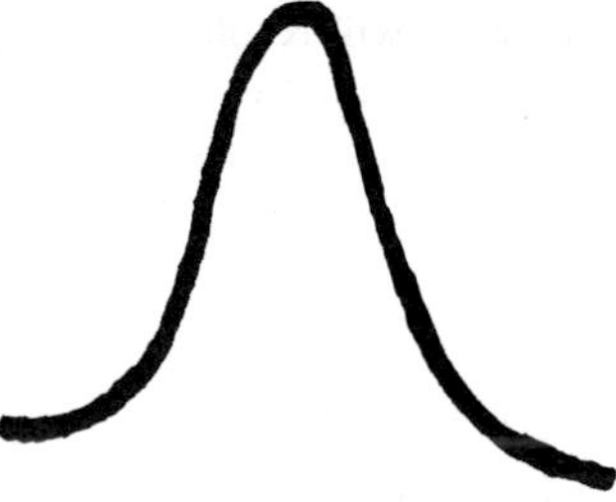

Figure 2-54 Pulmonary artery waveform: damped waveform.

a) Injection of a known volume of a known temperature solution into an unknown volume of blood at a known temperature
b) The injectate solution (usually normal saline) is injected into the proximal lumen (RA) of the PAC.
c) There is mixing of the injectate with the blood.
d) The temperature change is sensed downstream at the thermistor located 4 cm from the distal tip of the PAC.

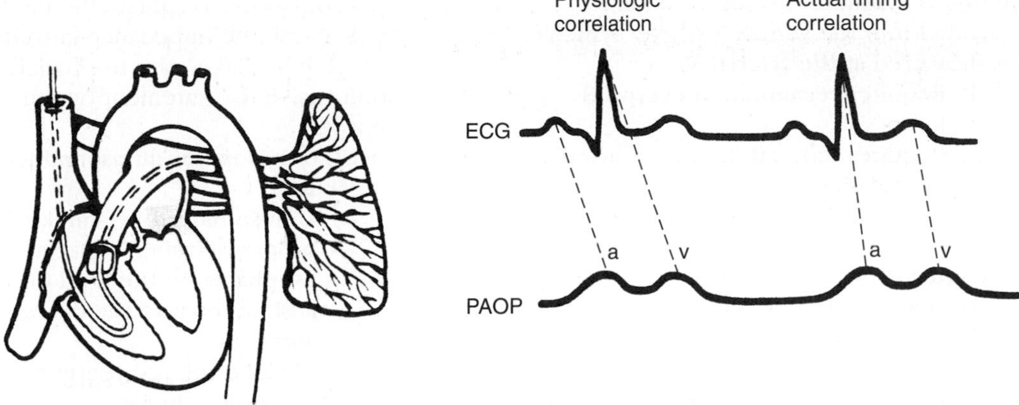

Figure 2-55 Pulmonary artery occlusive pressure waveform. Though the *a* wave correlates physiologically to atrial depolarization and the P wave and the *v* wave correlate physiologically with the QRS and ventricular depolarization, tubing and catheter cause a time delay. In actuality, the first wave seen after the QRS is the *a* wave, and the first wave seen after the T wave is the *v* wave. (Adapted from and courtesy Baxter Healthcare, Irvine, CA.)

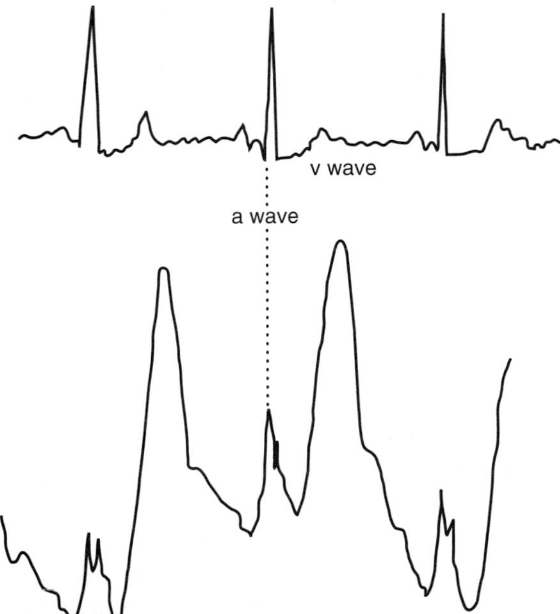

Figure 2-56 PAOP waveform of a patient with mitral regurgitation. Note the very large *v* waves. Use of the mean of the PAOP waveform or the *v* wave will result in an exaggerated PAOP. Since the mitral valve is open during the *a* wave, the mean of the *a* wave is a better reflection of the left ventricular end-diastolic pressure. (From Druding, M. C. [2000]. Integrating hemodynamic monitoring and physical assessment. *Dimens Crit Care Nurs, 19*[4], 25-30.)

e) The amount of the unknown volume of blood is deduced from the amount of change in temperature.
f) Calculate the average of three measurements that are within 10% of a median value.

2) Continuous (referred to as *continuous cardiac output* [CCO])
   a) Method
      i) A thermal filament in the right ventricle creates a signal by warming the blood as it flows by
      ii) The thermistor at the distal tip measures the temperature of the blood downstream.
      iii) The computer produces a thermodilution curve and calculates the cardiac output.
      iv) The cardiac output is updated approximately every 5 minutes.
   b) Advantages over intermittent method
      i) More accurate especially in patients with low output states
      ii) Continuously updated
      iii) Decreases required nursing time
      iv) Eliminates interrater reliability caused by variability in injectate volume, rate of injection, and selection or elimination of values for averaging
      v) Reduces risks of contamination and fluid overload
   c) Disadvantage: catheter approximately three times the cost of conventional catheter

c. Minimally invasive methods
   1) Pulse contour waveform analysis method allows derivation of CO, SV, and stroke volume variability (SVV) from analysis of the arterial waveform.
   2) Method: requires a venous catheter and an arterial catheter
      a) Lithium dilution cardiac output (PulseCO by LiDCO): requires calibration using a subtherapeutic dose of lithium to be injected into the venous catheter which is measured at the arterial sensor
         i) Requires recalibration every 4-8 hours
         ii) Cannot be used in patients on therapeutic lithium
      b) Pulse contour cardiac output system (PiCCO by Pulsion Medical Systems)

requires calibration using cold saline injected into the venous catheter which is measured at the arterial sensor
   i) Requires recalibration every 4-8 hours
   ii) Requires femoral or axillary arterial cannulation
c) Vigileo (Edwards Lifesciences) uses a specialized (i.e., Flotrac) sensor added to the arterial pressure monitoring system
   i) Does not require calibration
   ii) Provides CO, SV, SVV, and SVR

d. Noninvasive measurement by bioimpedance
   1) Utilizes thoracic electrical bioimpedance technology
      a) Impedance (Z): resistance to flow of electrical current
   2) Method
      a) Four dual sensors are placed on each side of the neck and thorax.
      b) A low-amplitude, high-frequency electrical signal is emitted from the outer sensors through the thorax.
      c) Blood is an excellent conductive medium, and electricity follows the path of least resistance; the aorta is the largest, most distensible, blood-filled vessel in the thoracic cavity.
      d) Aortic blood flow is readily tracked by this method.
   3) Allows continuous measurement of the following parameters
      a) Composite parameters
         i) Cardiac output
         ii) Cardiac index
         iii) Stroke volume
      b) Thoracic fluid status: base thoracic impedance (Zo): normal 20-30 ohms for males and 25-35 for females
      c) Afterload: SVR: normal 800-1200 dynes/sec/cm^{-5}
      d) Contractility
         i) Change in impedance over time (dZ/dt): normal 0.8-2.5 ohms/second
         ii) Acceleration contractility index (ACI): normal 2-5 ohms/second
         iii) Left cardiac work index (LCWI): normal 3-5 kg/min/m^2
         iv) Preejection period: normal 0.05-0.12 second
         v) Ventricular ejection time: normal 0.25-0.35 second
      e) Change in impedance/change in time (dZ/dt)
   4) Causes no risk or discomfort to the patient but the patient must be supine, recumbent, and quiet
   5) Contraindicated in patients with impedance-driven pacemakers that calculate minute ventilation to regulate the pacemaker rate because the impedance current may cause the pacemaker rate to accelerate

e. Noninvasive measurement by transesophageal Doppler
   1) Utilizes Doppler ultrasound technology
   2) Method
      a) Ultrasound probe, similar to an orogastric tube, is placed in the esophagus to the level of the third ICS and oriented to the descending thoracic aorta.
      b) Image displayed represents changes in blood flow in the descending thoracic aorta with each systolic cycle.
   3) Allows measurement or calculation of cardiac output and index, stroke volume and index, SVR and SVRI, flow time corrected for heart rate, peak velocity of blood during systole, stroke distance, minute distance, and mean acceleration
      a) Preload: Flow Time Corrected (FTc)
      b) Contractility: Peak velocity (PV)
      c) Afterload: Velocity and Flow Time

f. Normal value: CO 4-8 L/min; CI 2.5-4 L/min

g. Causes of abnormal parameter (see Table 2-14)

9. Mixed venous oxygen saturation (SvO_2)
   a. Oxygen saturation of the blood as it returns to the lung for reoxygenation
      1) Represents the average of the venous oxygen saturations of all organs and tissues
      2) Provides a global perspective of how well the body's demand for oxygen is met by the amount of oxygen supplied
   b. Measurement
      1) Blood gas analysis of blood drawn from the distal lumen of the PAC
      2) Fiberoptic oximetric PAC
         a) Perform calibration as indicated.
            i) In vitro before the catheter is inserted
            ii) In vivo every 24 hours
         b) Monitor the signal quality indicator to ensure reliability.
         c) Note that accuracy may be affected by hematocrit, catheter position, blood temperature or pH.
   c. Normal SvO_2: 60-80%
      1) Affected by changes in DO_2 and/or VO_2
   d. Causes of abnormal parameter (see Table 2-14)

10. Central venous oxygen saturation ($ScvO_2$)
   a. Oxygen saturation of the blood in the superior vena cava
      1) Serves as a surrogate for SvO_2 before PAC inserted or when PAC placement is not possible such as when admission to a critical care unit is not possible or not yet necessary
      2) Though the $ScvO_2$ consistently overestimates the SvO_2 (by around 5-15%) under shock

conditions, there is a close correlation between the two parameters.

b. Measurement
   1) Blood gas analysis of blood drawn from a catheter in the superior vena cava or right atrium
   2) Fiberoptic oximetric central venous catheter (e.g., Edwards PreSep) inserted into the jugular or subclavian vein with the tip in the superior vena cava or right atrium
      a) Femoral vein placement is not recommended; Davison et al (2010) found that more than 50% of values from a fcmoral catheter diverged more than 5% from $ScvO_2$ values.
c. Normal $ScvO_2$: greater than 70%
   1) Affected by changes in DO_2 and/or VO_2
d. Causes of abnormal parameter as for SvO_2

11. Right ventricular parameters
   a. Measured with special REF PAC
   b. Normal values for right ventricular parameters (see Table 2-14)
12. Oxygenation parameters
   a. Calculated parameters
   b. Normal values for oxygenation parameters (see Table 2-14)
13. Gastric tonometry
   a. Detects regional alterations in tissue perfusion based on the concept that the splanchnic circulation is the first body system to be affected by inadequate perfusion
   b. Method
      1) A vented nasogastric tube with a tonometer balloon located a few inches from the catheter's distal tip is placed into the stomach; a three-way stopcock is at the proximal end of the tonometer port.
      2) The tonometer balloon is filled with saline and is permeable to carbon dioxide.
      3) After a period of equilibration, saline samples taken from the balloon are analyzed for CO_2 to reflect the $PiCO_2$ (intramucosal carbon dioxide) at the same time that arterial blood is drawn for bicarbonate level.
      4) The pHi is then calculated; a low pHi (less than 7.2) indicates perfusion abnormality.
   c. Trends are monitored and interventions evaluated by changes in pHi.
14. Sublingual capnography
   a. Detects regional alterations in tissue perfusion; developed to overcome limitations and difficulties of gastric tonometry
   b. Method: A sensor is placed under the patient's tongue and held in place for 60-90 seconds.
   c. Increases in $P_{sl}CO_2$ correlate with decreases in arterial BP and CI and an increase in serum lactate.

Use of Hemodynamic Monitoring for Clinical Decision-Making

1. Maximize accuracy, reproducibility, and reliability of measured parameters.
   a. The transducer must be leveled and balanced to zero (i.e., *zeroed*) with each head-of-bed position change and/or at least every 12 hours.
      1) Level the air-fluid interface of the transducer to the phlebostatic axis at the time of setup, anytime the head of bed is changed, anytime that the transducer and monitoring cable are disconnected, or at any time the accuracy of the pressure readings are questionable.
         a) The air-fluid interface (also referred to as the *air reference port*) of the transducer needs to be leveled using either a laser or carpenter's level with the phlebostatic axis to ensure accuracy of measurement; the phlebostatic axis correlates with the right atrium and is at the fourth intercostal space and midway between the sternum anterior and the spine posterior (Figure 2-57); this reference point is used if the patient is supine.
            i) Mark the phlebostatic axis on the patient's chest so that clinicians are consistent.
            ii) Be aware of the clinical importance of having the air-fluid interface level with the phlebostatic axis (Frazier, 2008).
               (a) If transducer too high, readings will be too low (2 mm Hg lower for every 1 inch above the phlebostatic axis).
               (b) If transducer too low, readings will be too high (2 mm Hg higher for every 1 inch below the phlebostatic axis).
         b) If the patient is supine, there is no need to put the head of bed flat to take pressure measurements as long as the head of bed is elevated no more than 60 degrees and the air-fluid interface is at the level of the phlebostatic axis (Figure 2-57).
         c) Patients may also be lateral 20, 30, or 90 degrees or prone for pressure readings (Bridges, 2009).
            i) Reference point for 30 degrees: half the distance from surface of the bed to the left sternal border
            ii) Reference point for 90 degrees right: fourth ICS at midsternum
            iii) Reference point for 90 degrees left: fourth ICS at left sternal border

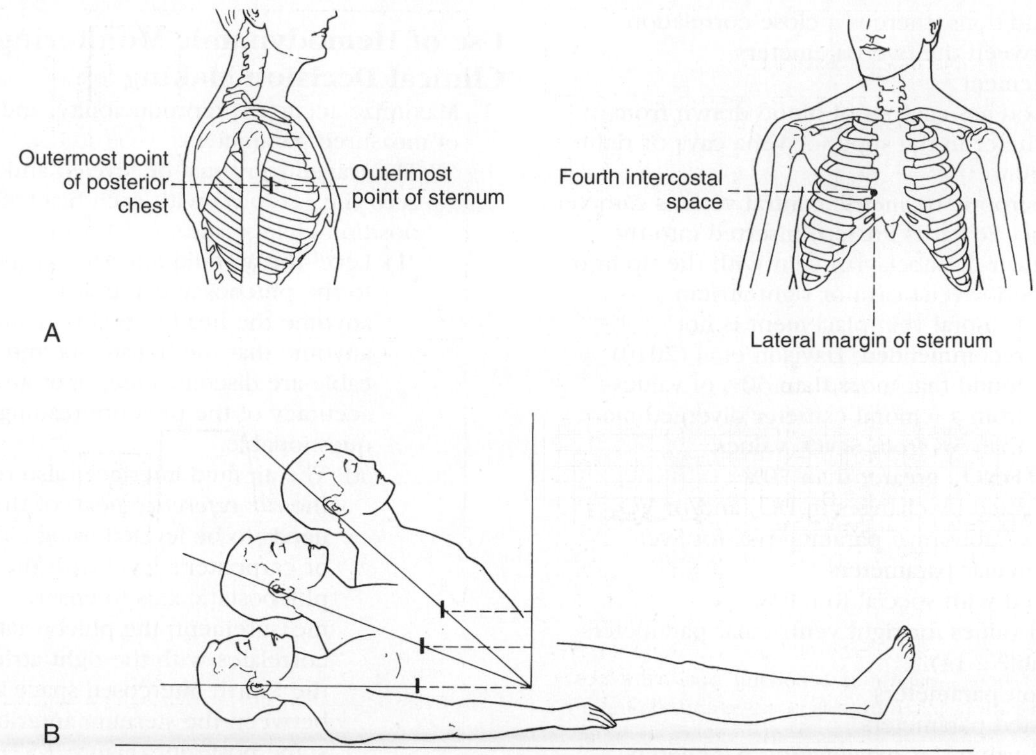

Figure 2-57 Phlebostatic axis. **A,** Location of phlebostatic axis. **B,** Note that the measurements are accurate with head of bed elevated up to 45 degrees as long as the air-fluid interface is level with the phlebostatic axis. (From Flynn, J. B. M., & Bruce, N.P. [1993]. *Introduction to critical care skills.* St Louis: Mosby.)

d) Wait 5-15 minutes after any position change before obtaining pressure measurements (Bridges, 2009).

2) Zero referencing at the time of setup, anytime the head of bed is changed, anytime that the transducer and monitoring cable are disconnected, or at any time the accuracy of the pressure readings is questionable
   a) Zero referencing the transducer requires closing the transducer to the patient, opening of the stopcock closest to the transducer to air, and ensuring that the monitor and the recorder read O ± 1 mm Hg.
   b) This negates the force exerted by the atmosphere so that only cardiovascular pressures are sensed, measured, and recorded.

b. Ensure accurate calibration.
   1) Calibration ensures the accuracy of a quantitative measuring instrument
   2) Transducer calibration
      a) To calibrate, a known pressure (e.g., using a sphygmomanometer) is exerted on the transducer to see that the monitor measures and displays it correctly.
      b) Reusable transducers require calibration before use; disposable transducers are precalibrated and only require calibration if the accuracy of the measurements is questionable
   3) Monitor calibration
      a) Some monitors require calibration.
      b) Consult the operating manual for specific instructions for the monitor in use.
   4) Oximetry calibration
      a) SvO_2 oximeters require calibration with the oxygen saturation measured from blood drawn from the distal port of the PAC (frequently referred to as *mixed venous oxygen saturation*).
      b) This calibration is done in vitro prior to catheter insertion and in vivo daily and anytime that the fiberoptics may have been damaged, the oximeter module is disconnected from the fiberoptic PAC, or the SvO_2 values are questionable.

c. Analyze the graphic recording with simultaneous ECG as the most reliable means of measuring hemodynamic pressure at end-expiration (Figure 2-58).
   1) Graphic method is more reliable than digital or cursor methods.
   2) Pressure readings obtained at end-expiration minimize the effects of intrathoracic pressure changes because intrathoracic

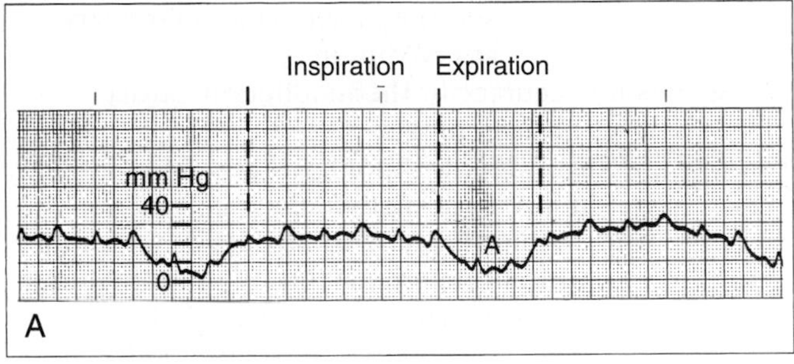

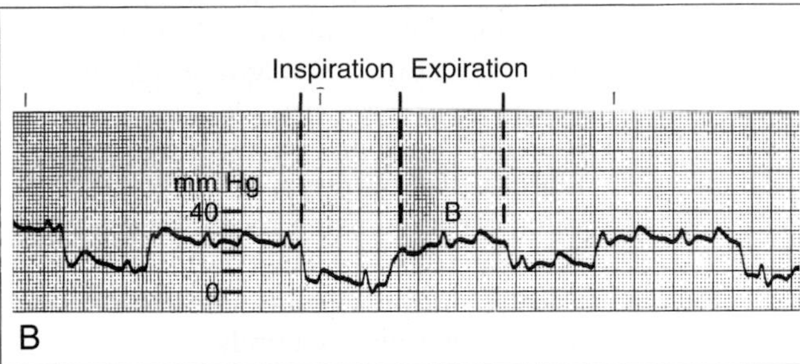

Figure 2-58 Hemodynamic measurements are done at end-expiration. **A,** When a patient is receiving positive pressure mechanical ventilation, inspiration is positive and expiration is neutral. Readings should be done at the valley. Remember: volume ventilator - valley. **B,** When a patient is spontaneously breathing or on pressure-cycled ventilator, inspiration is negative and expiration is positive. Readings should be done at the peak. Remember: patient or pressure ventilator - peak. (Reprinted with permission from Schermer, L. [1998]. Physiologic and technical variables affecting hemodynamic measurements. *Crit Care Nurse*, 8[2], 33-40.)

pressure is closest to atmospheric pressure at the end of expiration.

a) Spontaneously breathing patient: expiration is positive (high point of fluctuation)
b) Mechanically ventilated patient: expiration is neutral (low point of fluctuation)
c) Remember: ventilator valley, patient peak

d. Ensure proper PAC position in West's lung zone III.
   1) PAOP pressure measurements are most accurate when the PAC tip is located in West's lung zone III because pulmonary venous pressure is higher than the surrounding alveolar pressure and all capillaries are open.
   2) The PAC tip is below the level of the left atrium when the catheter is in this position.
   3) Indications that the PAC tip is in zone III (Martin, 2006; Bridges, 2006)
      a) Confirmed by chest x-ray: Tip is below the left atrium on frontal chest x-ray.
      b) PAd greater than PAOP
      c) Normal PAOP waveform with clearly identifiable *a* and *v* waves
      d) Respiratory variation in PAd greater than respiratory variation in PAOP

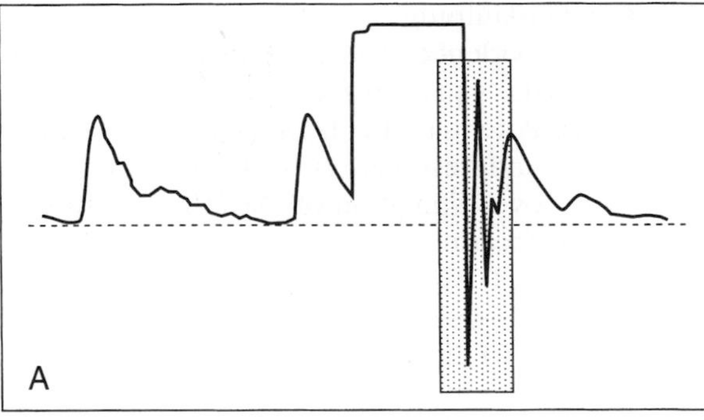

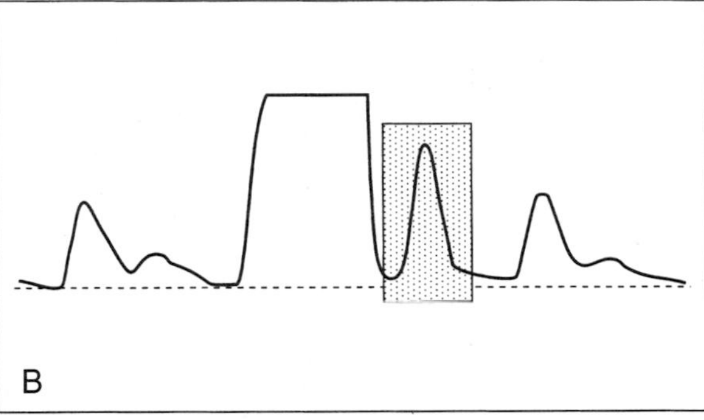

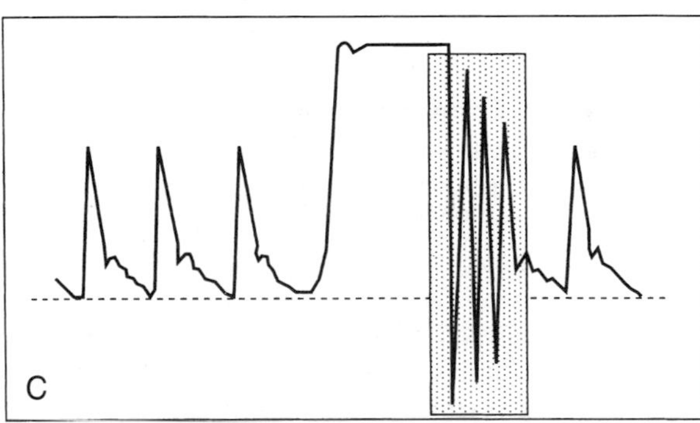

Figure 2-59 Square wave test using the fast-flush valve. **A,** Normal test and accurate waveform. **B,** Overdamped. **C,** Underdamped.

      e) Change in PEEP results in a change in PAOP of less than one half of the change in PEEP.

e. Ensure adequate damping using the square wave test (also referred to as *dynamic response test* or *frequency response test*) (Figure 2-59) on initial pressure monitoring setup, at least every 12 hours, when the system has been opened (e.g., zeroing, drawing blood, tubing change), whenever the waveform appears distorted or damped, or at any time the accuracy of the pressure readings is questionable.
   1) Fast-flush the system causing the waveform to square off at the top of the screen.
   2) Analyze the waveform after the flush.
      a) One or two oscillations indicate an optimally damped system.
      b) No peaks should be more than 1 mm apart, and the second peak should be less than one third of the height of the first peak.

3) Overdamping
   a) Evidence: There are no oscillations after the square wave.
   b) Potential effects on pressure readings: underestimation of systolic and overestimation of diastolic pressures
   c) Treatment
      i) Check for occlusion (e.g., kinks, clots) or air in system.
      ii) Ensure that noncompliant tubing is in place between the catheter and the transducer.
      iii) Ensure tight-fitting connections.
4) Underdamping
   a) Evidence: more than two oscillations after square wave or more than one to two blocks between bounces
   b) Potential effects on pressure readings: overestimation of systolic and underestimation of diastolic pressures
   c) Treatment
      i) Restrict catheter and tubing length to 4 feet maximum.
      ii) Add a damping device to absorb unwanted frequency vibration or turn a stopcock slightly.

f. Obtain chest x-ray after insertion of CVP or PAC to ensure proper positioning of the catheter.
   1) The tip of a CVP catheter is positioned in the proximal superior vena cava.
   2) The tip of a PAC is positioned in a pulmonary arteriole in lung zone 3.
      a) When the catheter tip of the PAC is inserted in lung regions in which alveolar pressure exceeds venous pressure (zones 1 and 2), PAOP will not accurately represent left atrial pressure; also PEEP in a patient who is hypovolemic or has noncompliant lungs can convert a zone 3 into a zone 1 or 2, causing discrepancies between PAOP and left atrial pressure.
      b) An ideally positioned PAC will occlude the pulmonary arteriole and show a PAOP waveform when between 1.25-1.5 mL of air has been used to inflate the 1.5-mL capacity balloon.
         i) When a PAOP waveform is seen when less than 1.25 mL has been injected into the 1.5 mL capacity balloon, the catheter is too distal and prone to cause arteriolar occlusion without balloon inflation (referred to as *spontaneous wedge*).
         ii) When the balloon is inflated to obtain a PAOP measurement, the nurse must observe the monitor and stop injecting air into the balloon as soon as the PA waveform converts to a PAOP waveform to avoid overwedging and potentially fatal pulmonary artery rupture.

g. Ensure accuracy of thermodilution cardiac output measurements.
   1) Utilize CCO technology if possible.
   2) If intermittent methodology is used
      a) Room temperature injectates for cardiac output determination by thermodilution are adequate as long as a 12° F difference exists between blood temperature and injectate temperature; keep injectate solution and tubing away from direct sunlight and heat lamps.
      b) Iced injectates may be used in low or high cardiac output states or if the CO value obtained using room temperature is suspected to be inaccurate.
      c) Cardiac output injectate must be injected within 4 seconds.
   3) Enter the appropriate computation constant into the cardiac output computer, or monitor for calculation of cardiac output; catheter size and type and injectate volume and temperature determine the computation constant.

2. Ensure patency of the catheter by maintaining a saline flush system.
   a. Heparin may be added, though currently controversial; usual heparin concentration is 1 unit of heparin/1 mL of flush solution.
      1) Heparin is contraindicated in patients with a history of heparin-induced thrombocytopenia (HIT) (also referred to as *heparin-associated thrombosis and thrombocytopenia* [HATT] or *white clot syndrome*).
   b. Intermittent flush devices deliver 3-5 mL/hr as long as the pressure bag is maintained at 300 mm Hg

3. Correlate numerical value of parameter with the patient's clinical presentation.
   a. Hemodynamic parameter changes may precede clinical presentation changes (e.g., subclinical hypoperfusion).
   b. Hemodynamic parameter changes may reflect inaccurate measurements; care must be taken to be consistent in measuring techniques.
   c. Note trends of change of measured parameters over time and in response to therapeutic interventions.
   d. Notify the physician of significant changes from patient's normal.
      1) PA systolic more than 4-7 mm Hg
      2) PA diastolic more than 4-7 mm Hg
      3) PAOP more than 4 mm Hg

4. Utilize hemodynamic parameters in clinical decision making
   a. Determination of best PEEP: PEEP that will give the best PaO_2 and SaO_2 without causing a drop in CO and CI

b. Determination of best PAOP or optimal point on Starling's curve
   1) PAOP that will give the best stroke volume and cardiac output without producing pulmonary edema
   2) Right ventricular end-diastolic volume may be a more valid parameter to monitor in evaluation of best stretch and filling volumes
      a) The main issue is whether pressure truly reflects volume.
      b) Pressure is not a reflection of volume in patients with poor ventricular compliance.
      c) These measurements require a special REF PAC.
c. Determination of true PAOP with patients on PEEP (especially important if patient is on high levels of PEEP)
   1) Convert cm H_2O measurement of PEEP to mm Hg by dividing by 1.36
   2) Subtract one half of the PEEP (in mm Hg) from the measured PAOP to get a "true" PAOP when evaluating fluid status and filling volumes.
   3) This is of questionable clinical value because trends, rather than absolute pressure measurements, are of the most clinical significance.
d. Utilization of the patient's clinical presentation and hemodynamic parameters to detect physiologic alterations and responses to therapy (Table 2-16)
   1) Use indexes to evaluate parameters (e.g., cardiac index versus cardiac output).
   2) Utilize therapeutic manipulations (e.g., drug administration and titration, fluid therapy, IABP) to optimize cardiac output and vital organ perfusion while minimizing myocardial oxygen consumption (Figure 2-60).

5. Prevent, detect, and assist in management of complications of hemodynamic monitoring (Table 2-17).

Table 2-16 Hemodynamic Profiles for Selected Critical Care Conditions

Condition	Clinical Presentation	Hemodynamic Presentation
Cardiogenic shock	• Tachycardia, hypotension, tachypnea • S_3 • Crackles • Dyspnea • JVD • Hepatomegaly • Peripheral edema • Oliguria	• CO/CI decreased • RAP, PAP, PAOP increased • SVR, SVRI increased • LVSWI decreased • SaO_2, SvO_2 decreased • DO_2 decreased
Hypovolemic shock	• Flat neck veins • Tachycardia, hypotension, tachypnea • Oliguria	• CO/CI decreased • RAP, PAP, PAOP decreased • SVR, SVRI increased • SvO_2 decreased • DO_2 decreased
Anaphylactic shock	• Hypotension, tachypnea • Tachycardia • Angioedema • Warmth, erythema, pruritus, hives • Wheezing, stridor	• CO/CI decreased • RAP, PAP, PAOP decreased • SVR, SVRI decreased • SvO_2 decreased • DO_2 decreased
Neurogenic shock	• Hypotension, tachypnea • Bradycardia • Warm, dry, flushed skin • Hypothermia • Neurologic deficit	• CO/CI decreased • RAP, PAP, PAOP decreased • SVR, SVRI decreased • SvO_2 decreased • DO_2 decreased
Septic shock (early) (late as in hypovolemic shock)	• Tachycardia, hypotension, tachypnea • Hyperthermia • Irritability, confusion • Warm, moist, flushed skin	• CO/CI increased • RAP, PAP, PAOP decreased • SVR, SVRI decreased • SvO_2 increased • DO_2 increased; VO_2 decreased
Pulmonary hypertension (chronic obstructive pulmonary disease, pulmonary embolism, mitral valve disease, hypoxemia)	• Tachycardia • JVD may occur • Dyspnea	• RAP may be increased • PVR greater than 250 dynes/sec/cm^{-5} • PAm greater than 20 mm Hg • PAd more than 5 mm Hg greater than PAOP • SaO_2, SvO_2 decreased

Continued

Table 2-16 Hemodynamic Profiles for Selected Critical Care Conditions—cont'd

Condition	Clinical Presentation	Hemodynamic Presentation
Cardiac pulmonary edema	• Tachycardia • Dyspnea • Crackles • S_3	• CO/CI decreased • RAP, PAP, PAOP increased • SVR, SVRI increased • PVR, PVRI increased • SaO_2, SvO_2 decreased • DO_2 decreased
Noncardiac pulmonary edema (e.g., ARDS)	• Dyspnea • Crackles • Evidence of decreased lung compliance (e.g., increased work of breathing if patient spontaneously breathing, increased peak and plateau pressures if patient is being mechanically ventilated)	• PAP elevated, PAOP normal • PVR, PVRI increased • SaO_2, SvO_2 decreased • DO_2 decreased
Cardiac tamponade	• "Fullness" in chest • Tachycardia, hypotension, tachypnea • Muffled heart sounds • JVD • Electrical alternans	• CO/CI decreased • RAP, PAP, PAOP increased • Equalization of intracardiac pressures; RAP, PAd, PAOP will all be increased within a 5 mm Hg variation • Large *a* and *v* waves (M) on PAOP waveform • Pulsus paradoxus (drop in BP more than 10 mm Hg during inspiration) • SvO_2 decreased • DO_2 decreased
Papillary muscle rupture (acute mitral regurgitation)	• Tachycardia, hypotension, tachypnea • Dyspnea • Crackles • S_3 • New holosystolic murmur at apex	• CO/CI decreased • RAP, PAP, PAOP increased • Large *v* waves on PAOP waveform • SaO_2, SvO_2 decreased • DO_2 decreased
Rupture of ventricular septum	• Tachycardia, hypotension, tachypnea • New holosystolic murmur at lower left sternal border	• Inaccurate cardiac output measurement: because cardiac output measurement by thermodilution is actually a right ventricular cardiac output, measured cardiac output will be high but the cardiac output from the left ventricle is actually low • RAP, PAP increased • Large *v* waves on PAOP waveform may be seen • SvO_2 (or mixed venous oxygen saturation) increased • Increased oxygen gradient (oxygen step-up) between blood drawn from proximal port (RA) and distal port (PA) • DO_2 decreased
Left ventricular infarction	• Chest pain • S_4 at apex • ECG changes of LVMI	• Significance of hemodynamic compromise determined by amount of ventricular ischemia/injury/infarction and the wall(s) affected • CO/CI may be decreased • RAP, PAP, PAOP may be increased • LVSWI may be decreased
Right ventricular infarction	• Chest pain • S_4 at sternum • Distended jugular neck veins • Clear lungs • ECG changes of RVMI	• Significance of hemodynamic compromise determined by amount of ventricular ischemia/injury/infarction • CO/CI may be decreased • RAP may be increased • PAP, PAOP may be decreased • RVSWI may be decreased

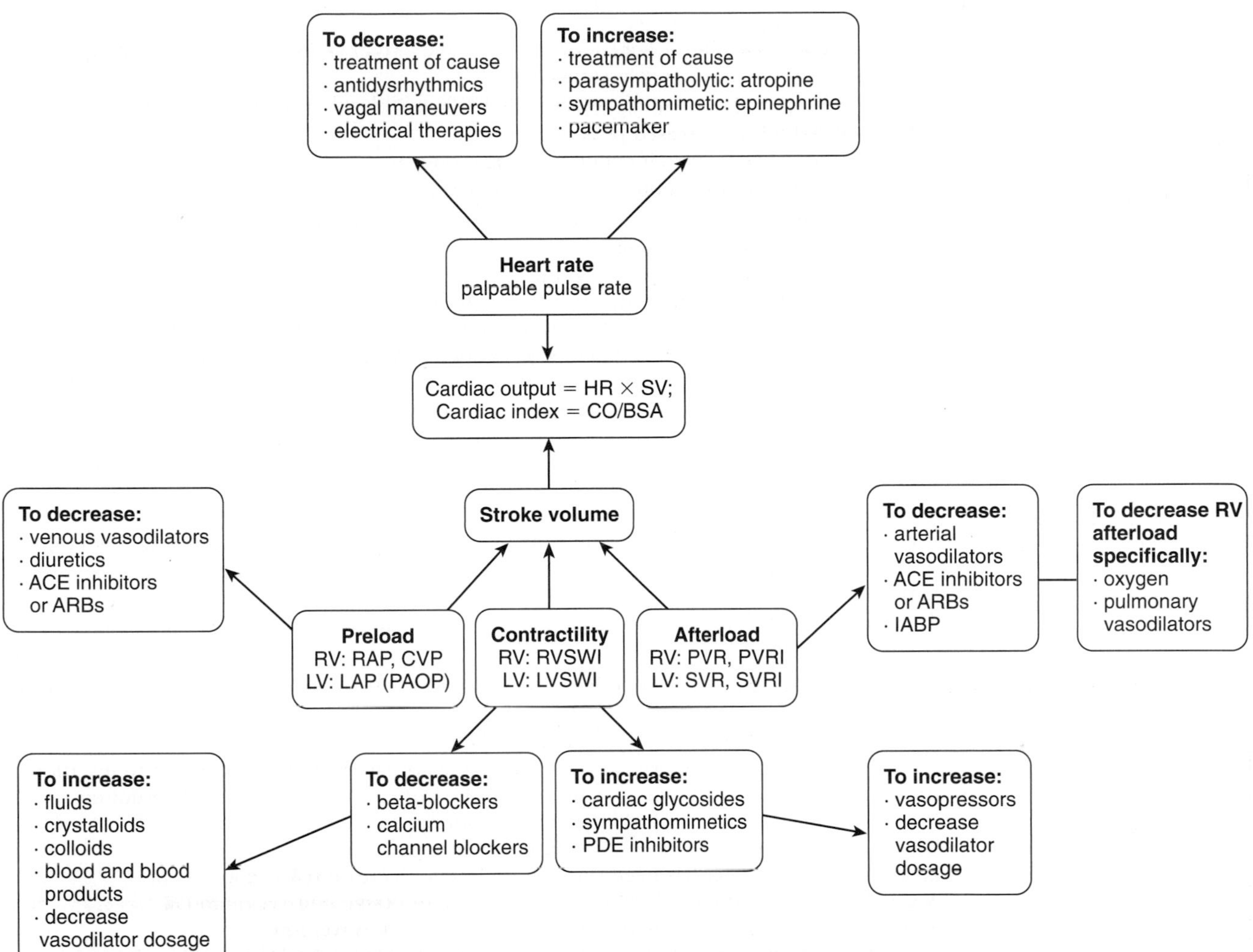

Figure 2-60 Therapeutic manipulations to optimize cardiac output and vital organ perfusion and/or minimize myocardial oxygen consumption. *ACE,* Angiotensin converting enzyme; *ARB,* angiotensin receptor blocker; *BSA,* body surface area; *CO,* cardiac output; *CVP,* central venous pressure; *HR,* heart rate; *IABP,* intraaortic balloon pump; *LAP,* left atrial pressure; *LV,* left ventricle; *LVSWI,* left ventricular stroke work index; *PAOP,* pulmonary artery occlusive pressure; *PDE,* phosphodiesterase; *PVR,* pulmonary vascular resistance; *PVRI,* pulmonary vascular resistance index; *RAP,* right atrial pressure; *RV,* right ventricle; *RVSWI,* right ventricular stroke work index; *SV,* stroke volume; *SVR,* systemic vascular resistance; *SVRI,* systemic vascular resistance index.

Table 2-17 Complications of Hemodynamic Monitoring

Complications	Prevention/Detection/Treatment
Air emboli	• Utilize Trendelenburg position for insertion of deep vein catheters • Place sterile gloved finger over needle hub with any disconnection during insertion to prevent air emboli • Aspirate air from flush solution bag to avoid air embolus with inadvertent emptying of flush solution bag • Flush all lumens with saline prior to insertion of catheters • Monitor the pressure monitoring system for air bubbles • Use only Luer-Lok connections • Have the patient hold his or her breath during catheter-tubing disconnects (e.g., tubing changes or removal of deep vein catheters) • If air embolus is suspected, turn patient to left side with head down (i.e., Durant's maneuver) and administer oxygen
Arterial puncture (during venous cannulation)	• Hold pressure for at least 5-10 minutes; a longer time may be required for patients on anticoagulants or patients who have received fibrinolytics
Balloon rupture	• Test the balloon before insertion by inflating the balloon and holding it in a basin of sterile saline and watching for bubbling • Store catheters away from sunlight and heat • Limit the length of time that catheter is left in (ideally less than 72 hours) • Limit the number of times the balloon is inflated to only when indicated (balloons are expected to last about 72 inflations); use PAd as a reflection of LVEDP in patients without pulmonary hypertension • Do not overinflate balloon; stop injecting air as soon as the PAOP waveform is seen • Do not aspirate air from the balloon; allow passive deflation and reattach the empty syringe to the balloon port • Indications that the balloon has ruptured include inability to obtain PAOP waveform and absence of resistance during inflation • If balloon rupture has occurred, label balloon lumen accordingly so that others do not continue to try to inflate balloon; use PAd as a reflection of LVEDP in patients without pulmonary hypertension; if a PAOP is required, a new PAC must be inserted • This complication is particularly dangerous in right-to-left shunt (e.g., neonates); adults typically shunt left-to-right
Clotting and catheter occlusion	• Maintain saline drip with an intermittent flush device; heparin may be added but is currently controversial • Monitor for any change in waveform (e.g., damping)

Dysrhythmias: usually ventricular dysrhythmias or RBBB	• Have emergency equipment (including transcutaneous pacemaker) available during insertion
	• Inflate balloon to capacity (e.g., 1.5 mL) when the catheter is in the right atrium during insertion so that the balloon cushions the catheter tip
	• Observe the ECG monitor closely during insertion
	• Ensure that the catheter has been sutured in place to decrease risk of movement
	• Assess PAP waveform for indications that the catheter has flipped back into RV
	  • Request catheter repositioning for catheter fling or RV waveform
	  • If RV waveform is noted, inflate balloon to capacity (e.g., 1.5 mL) to cushion the catheter tip
	  • Turn patient to left side to encourage distal migration of catheter back into pulmonary artery
	  • Deflate balloon after successful repositioning back into the pulmonary artery
	• Observe the ECG monitor closely during removal of the PAC; the catheter should be removed in a smooth continuous movement with balloon deflated

Emboli	• Aspirate if you suspect a small clot rather than flush
Exsanguination	• Use only Luer-Lok connections • Maintain alarms in ON position; pressure alarms are usually set 10-20 mm Hg above and below the patient's normal
Fluid overload	• Limit the number of fast flushes • Use 5 mL instead of 10 mL for cardiac outputs when indicated or use continuous cardiac output which requires no fluid boluses for determination of cardiac output • Limit the frequency of cardiac outputs to every 4 hours unless required more often
Hematoma	• Maintain pressure for 5-10 minutes with single-thickness pressure dressing after catheter removal; a longer time may be required for patients on anticoagulants or patients who have received fibrinolytics
Hypothermia	• Use room temperature injectate • Apply blankets, radiant heaters as needed

Table 2-17 Complications of Hemodynamic Monitoring—cont'd

Complications	Prevention/Detection/Treatment
Infection	• Encourage percutaneous catheter insertion (results in a much lower incidence of infection than does cutdown) • Change the flush solution bag whenever it is empty or every 72-96 hours or according to your hospital protocol • Change the tubing every 72-96 hours or according to your hospital protocol • Dress and inspect the site using sterile technique every 72-96 hours or according to your hospital protocol • Avoid clear semipermeable dressings in patients with oily skin • Use normal saline rather than D_5W for the flush solution • Flush well after drawing blood samples; do not allow dried blood to stay in stopcock ports or tubing • Limit the number of stopcocks in the pressure monitoring system • Replace all vented stopcock covers with nonvented "deadend" caps • Utilize strict sterile technique with blood sampling and cardiac outputs • Encourage use of catheter sleeve through which the PAC is threaded; allows for sterile catheter manipulation • Limit the length of time that catheter is left in place (ideally less than 72-96 hours) • Monitor for clinical indications of infection at catheter insertion site: redness, warmth, induration, purulent drainage, and pain at insertion site • Monitor for clinical indications of catheter sepsis: fever, chills, leukocytosis, positive blood culture and/or catheter culture
Microshock	• Recognize that this risk is due to elimination of the skin as a protection from microshock in patients with intracardiac catheters • Ensure that all electrical equipment is properly functioning and grounded • Do not touch the patient and a piece of electrical equipment at the same time
Nerve palsy	• Maintain limbs in functional position (e.g., do not keep the wrist hyperextended to prevent ulnar nerve palsy)
Pneumothorax, hemothorax, chylothorax during insertion	• Have chest x-ray taken after central vein catheter cannulation • Assist with insertion of chest tube if pneumothorax (air in pleural space), hemothorax (blood in pleural space), or chylothorax (lymph fluid in pleural space) occurs
Pulmonary artery rupture	• Recognize patients at high risk: elderly patients, patients with pulmonary hypertension, patients receiving anticoagulant, fibrinolytic, or platelet aggregation inhibitor therapy, hypothermic patients, postcardiac surgery patients • Inflate balloon with only enough air to cause PAOP waveform; do not overinflate and limit inflation time to a maximum of 15 seconds because both prolonged inflation and excessive balloon volume put too much tension on the vessel wall • Monitor patient for sudden onset of hemoptysis especially after inflation of balloon, dyspnea, and hypotension as indications of pulmonary artery rupture • If rupture of the pulmonary artery does occur: increase the FiO_2, suction the airway, position the patient with the affected lung down, assist with intubation with double-lumen endotracheal tube, use PEEP or PAC balloon inflation for tamponade effect as prescribed, monitor vital signs and oxygenation levels closely for changes, and prepare the patient for surgery if requested
Pulmonary infarction	• Inflate balloon only long enough for graphic recording • Continuously monitor PAP so that if catheter advances into PAOP position, it will be noted and the catheter repositioned • Request proximal repositioning if it takes less than 1.25 mL to achieve occluded position because this indicates that the catheter is positioned too distal and may spontaneously occlude the pulmonary arteriole (commonly referred to as *spontaneous wedge*) and cause ischemia and infarction • Monitor for chest pain, dyspnea, and decreased SaO_2 as an indication of pulmonary infarction

Thrombosis	• Maintain saline drip with intermittent flush device (IFD); keep pressure bag at 300 mm Hg so that IFD is functional
	  • Heparin may be added to flush solution with usual concentration of 1 unit/mL; while this practice has been shown to improve patency, it increases the risk of heparin-induced thrombocytopenia (HIT)
	• Limit the length of time that catheter is left in (ideally less than 72 hours)
	• Prevent trauma to the intima by skillful catheter insertion
	• To prevent/detect arterial thrombosis with arterial catheters
	  • Select the site with collateral flow (e.g., radial artery)
	  • Utilize the smallest catheter feasible (e.g., 20 gauge for radial artery cannulation)
	  • Perform neurovascular assessment hourly to promptly detect acute arterial occlusion
	• If arterial occlusion occurs, assist with intraarterial fibrinolytic or embolectomy

LEARNING ACTIVITIES

CHAPTER 2

NOTE: Remember that you won't see questions like these on the CCRN examination, but these activities allow you to approach the content from a different perspective to remember it better. Multiple-choice questions (like on the CCRN examination) are available on the Elsevier website.

1. Complete the following crossword puzzle dealing with cardiovascular anatomy and physiology.

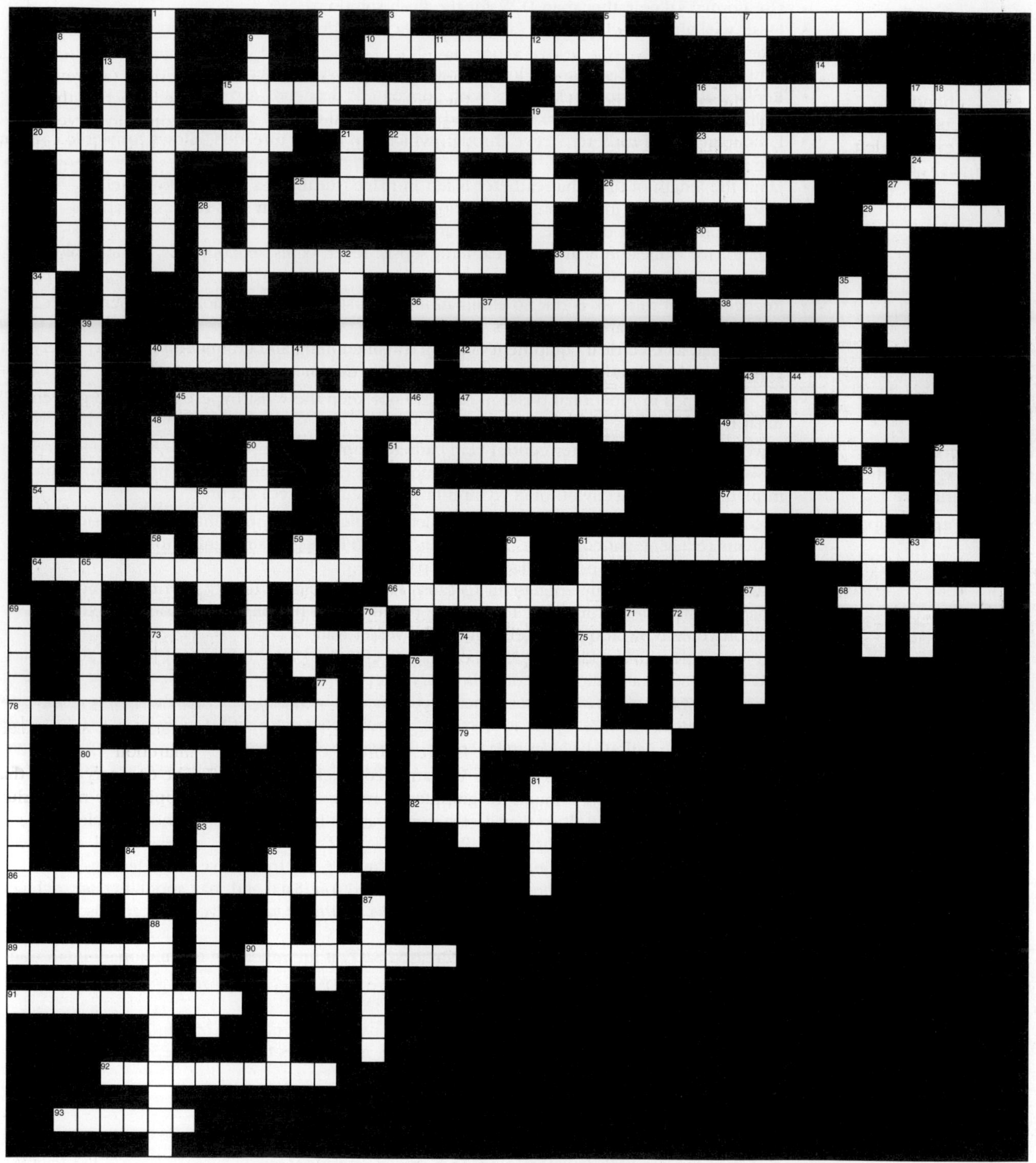

ACROSS

6. The term used to describe the effect on contractility
10. These receptors are located in the renal and mesenteric artery bed, and stimulation causes vasodilation of those vascular beds
15. The type of disks that lie between myocardial cells to allow rapid transmission of the cardiac impulse
16. The interatrial pathway is frequently referred to as _____'s bundle
17. The calculated parameter used to evaluate left ventricular contractility (abbrev.)
20. This innermost layer of the heart which lines the heart chamber and the heart valves
22. The left bundle branch is divided into left anterior and left posterior _____
23. During this refractory period, the cardiac muscle cell cannot respond no matter how strong the impulse is
24. This calculated parameter is used to evaluate left ventricular afterload (abbrev.)
25. The term used to describe the effect on heart rate
26. Rapid depolarization that allows cardiac muscle to contract in concert as if it were one muscle; this is referred to as a functional ____
29. Crossbridging of actin and ____ causes muscle shortening
31. Calcium is necessary for _____ which causes muscle shortening
33. The muscles which contract to close the atrioventricular valves
36. The type of pressure that pushes (such as out of the capillary and into the interstitium)
38. This layer of the serous pericardium is synonymous with the epicardium
40. The ability of the cardiac cells to respond to a stimulus
42. Another term for antidiuretic hormone
43. The valve that lies between the right ventricle and the pulmonary artery
45. A mineralocorticoid secreted by the adrenal cortex which causes sodium and water retention
47. These receptors are located in the right atrium and are sensitive to increased venous pressure
49. This refractory period is frequently referred to as the vulnerable period
51. The relaxation phase of the cardiac cycle
54. A neurotransmitter for the sympathetic nervous system that causes an increase in heart rate and contractility along with vasoconstriction
56. The pressure against which the ventricle must pump in order to open the semilunar valve
57. These fibers penetrate the ventricle to transmit the electrical impulse through to the endocardium
61. Pulse ____ is the difference between systolic and diastolic blood pressure
62. Elevation of this level in the blood is an indication of hypoxia and anaerobic metabolism
64. Occurs when sodium rushes into the cell causing it to become less negative
66. The fluid in the pericardial space acts as a ____
68. This layer of the pericardium acts as a barrier against infection and neoplastic invasion
73. This reflex causes an increase in heart rate with inspiration and a decrease in heart rate with expiration
75. The relationship between filling volume and contractility is frequently referred to as ____'s law of the heart
78. The type of receptors that are located in the carotid and aortic bodies which are sensitive to PaO_2, $PaCO_2$, and pH
79. The basic contractile unit of the myocardium
80. The valve between the left atrium and the aorta
82. DO_2 is a calculated parameter representing the ____ of oxygen to the tissues
86. A precursor of angiotensin
89. An increase in epicardial fat is associated with _____
90. The type of vessel that forms the nutrient bed for the tissues
91. High pressure lower cardiac chambers
92. Vasoconstrictive peptide produced by endothelial cells
93. Phase 1 of the action potential may be referred to as the ____ channel

DOWN

1. The portion of the cardiac wall which includes fibrous and serous layers
2. Fluid accumulation in spaces outside the intracellular and intravascular spaces is referred to as _____ spacing
3. The amount of blood that is ejected by the left ventricle per minute (abbrev.)
4. This peptide is associated with increased intravascular volume and is increased in heart failure (abbrev.)
5. The atrial contraction is frequently referred to as the atrial ____
7. The valve that lies between the right atrium and the right ventricle
8. The outermost layer of the artery
9. VO_2 is a calculated parameter representing the ____ of oxygen by the tissues
11. The ability of the cardiac cells to initiate electrical impulses regularly and spontaneously
12. Parameter used to evaluate right ventricular preload (abbrev.)
13. Cell layer that lines heart and blood vessels
14. The natural pacemaker of the heart is this node (abbrev.)
18. The function of these structures is to maintain unidirectional blood flow through the heart
19. A rupture of this innermost layer of the artery caused by plaque triggers the intrinsic pathway of clotting in atherosclerosis
21. Parameter used to evaluate right ventricular afterload (abbrev.)
26. The branch of the autonomic nervous system that is frequently referred to as the "fight or flight" system
27. The contraction phase of the cardiac cycle
28. The type of pressure that pulls (such as into the capillary from the interstitium)
30. The coronary artery that supplies the anterior left ventricle and the anterior two thirds of the septum (abbrev.)
32. Recovery; return to predominance on intracellular potassium and extracellular sodium
34. Vascular resistance is dependent upon the length and radius of the vessel and the viscosity of the blood is referred to as _____'s formula
35. A cardiac contractile protein used in the diagnosis of myocardial infarction
37. The coronary artery that supplies the right atrium, right ventricle, and inferior wall of the left ventricle
39. A cardiac muscle fiber
41. These receptors are located in the heart and stimulation increases heart rate, contractility, and conductivity
43. The two important factors in coronary artery perfusion are time and _____
44. The coronary artery that supplies blood to the left atrium and the lateral left ventricle (abbrev.)
46. The outmost layer of the cardiac wall

48. Diastolic BP - PAOP (abbrev.)
50. Term for the contractile state of the heart, irrespective of preload
52. Jugular venous distention is an indication of increased preload of the _____ ventricle
53. The _____ fraction is the percentage of blood that was in the ventricle at the end of diastole that was pumped out during systole
55. The substance secreted by the kidney in response to hypoperfusion of the kidney
58. Pressure receptors
59. The valve that lies between the left atrium and the left ventricle
60. This type of cardiac cell has automaticity
61. Phase 3 of the action potential may be referred to as the ___ channel
63. Low pressure upper cardiac chambers
65. The branch of the autonomic nervous system that maintains a steady state
67. Parasympathetic stimulation is frequently referred to as _____ stimulation
69. The "powerhouse" of the cell which uses nutrients and oxygen to make ATP
70. The effect on conductivity
71. The measured parameter used to evaluate left ventricular preload
72. These receptors are located in the vessels, and stimulation causes vasoconstriction
74. The _____ potential must be met for depolarization to occur
76. The effect of venous return on the heart which stretches the myofibrils and, therefore, determines the force of the next contraction
77. During this subphase of diastole and systole, no blood is moving
81. This middle layer of the artery becomes calcified in arteriosclerosis limiting the ability of the artery to dilate
83. The branches of the intraventricular conduction system are referred to as ____
84. Cellular energy (abbrev.)
85. This circulation consists of interarterial vessels that anastomose with each other as the result of gradual coronary artery occlusion
87. Phase 2 of the action potential is referred to as the ____ channel
88. Inflammation or infarction of this layer of the heart is associated with contractility problems

2. Identify the coronary artery that usually supplies the following structures. Identify the coronary artery as LAD (left anterior descending artery), LCA (left circumflex artery), or RCA (right coronary artery).

Structure	Coronary Artery
Anterior left ventricle	
AV node	
Bundle branches	
Inferior left ventricle	
Lateral left ventricle	
Left atrium	
Posterior left ventricle	
Right atrium	
Right ventricle	
SA node	
Septum	

3. Identify the determinants of myocardial oxygen supply and myocardial oxygen demand.

Myocardial Oxygen Supply	Myocardial Oxygen Demand

4. Identify the *primary* factor or factors affected in each condition and the primary effect or effects of each treatment; indicate increase or decrease of heart rate, preload, afterload, or contractility by appropriate arrows (↑ or ↓). (NOTE: Sympathetic nervous system responses may be seen in any of these conditions but they are secondary, not primary.)

Conditions				
Aortic stenosis	___Heart Rate	___Preload	___Afterload	___Contractility
Bradydysrhythmias	___Heart Rate	___Preload	___Afterload	___Contractility
Cardiac tamponade	___Heart Rate	___Preload	___Afterload	___Contractility
Cardiogenic shock	___Heart Rate	___Preload	___Afterload	___Contractility
Cardiomyopathy	___Heart Rate	___Preload	___Afterload	___Contractility
Heart failure	___Heart Rate	___Preload	___Afterload	___Contractility
Hypertension	___Heart Rate	___Preload	___Afterload	___Contractility
Hypovolemia	___Heart Rate	___Preload	___Afterload	___Contractility
Left ventricular myocardial infarction	___Heart Rate	___Preload	___Afterload	___Contractility
Neurogenic shock	___Heart Rate	___Preload	___Afterload	___Contractility
Pulmonary hypertension	___Heart Rate	___Preload	___Afterload	___Contractility
Right ventricular myocardial infarction	___Heart Rate	___Preload	___Afterload	___Contractility
Septic shock—early	___Heart Rate	___Preload	___Afterload	___Contractility
Septic shock—late	___Heart Rate	___Preload	___Afterload	___Contractility
Tachydysrhythmias	___Heart Rate	___Preload	___Afterload	___Contractility
Treatments				
Aminophylline	___Heart Rate	___Preload	___Afterload	___Contractility
Digoxin (Lanoxin)	___Heart Rate	___Preload	___Afterload	___Contractility
Dobutamine (Dobutrex)	___Heart Rate	___Preload	___Afterload	___Contractility
Dopamine (3-5 mcg/kg/min)	___Heart Rate	___Preload	___Afterload	___Contractility
Dopamine (5-10 mcg/kg/min)	___Heart Rate	___Preload	___Afterload	___Contractility
Dopamine (greater than 10 mcg/kg/min)	___Heart Rate	___Preload	___Afterload	___Contractility
Fluid challenge	___Heart Rate	___Preload	___Afterload	___Contractility
Furosemide (Lasix)	___Heart Rate	___Preload	___Afterload	___Contractility
Intraaortic balloon pump	___Heart Rate	___Preload	___Afterload	___Contractility
Isoproterenol (Isuprel)	___Heart Rate	___Preload	___Afterload	___Contractility
Milrinone (Primacor)	___Heart Rate	___Preload	___Afterload	___Contractility
Nesiritide (Natrecor)	___Heart Rate	___Preload	___Afterload	___Contractility
Nitroglycerin	___Heart Rate	___Preload	___Afterload	___Contractility
Nitroprusside (Nipride)	___Heart Rate	___Preload	___Afterload	___Contractility
Phenylephrine (Neo-Synephrine)	___Heart Rate	___Preload	___Afterload	___Contractility
Propranolol (Inderal)	___Heart Rate	___Preload	___Afterload	___Contractility
Vasopressin (Pitressin)	___Heart Rate	___Preload	___Afterload	___Contractility

5. Match the receptor of the sympathetic nervous system with its physiologic effect.

___ 1. Increase in heart rate, contractility, conductivity
___ 2. Dilation of the renal and mesenteric arteries
___ 3. Vasoconstriction
___ 4. Vasodilation and bronchodilation

a. Alpha$_1$
b. Beta$_1$
c. Beta$_2$
d. Dopaminergic

6. Identify which of these sympathomimetic (adrenergic) drugs cause the most powerful stimulation of each of these receptors.

___ 1. Alpha$_1$
___ 2. Beta$_1$
___ 3. Beta$_2$
___ 4. Dopaminergic

a. Albuterol (Proventil)
b. Fenoldopam (Corlopam)
c. Phenylephrine (Neo-Synephrine)
d. Dobutamine (Dobutrex)

7. Identify the formula for each of these parameters.

Parameter	Formula
a. Cardiac output (CO)	
b. Stroke index (SI)	
c. Blood pressure (BP)	
d. Coronary artery perfusion pressure (CAPP)	
e. Mean arterial pressure (MAP)	
f. Systemic vascular resistance (SVR)	
g. Delivery of oxygen to the tissues (DO_2)	

8. Match the heart sound to possible cause.

HEART SOUND

___ 1. S_1
___ 2. S_2
___ 3. Physiologic split of S_2
___ 4. Paradoxical split of S_2
___ 5. Fixed, wide split of S_2
___ 6. S_3
___ 7. S_4
___ 8. Pericardial friction rub
___ 9. Midsystolic click
___ 10. Holosystolic murmur
___ 11. Systolic ejection murmur
___ 12. Early diastolic murmur
___ 13. Mid- to late-diastolic murmur

POSSIBLE CAUSES

a. Changes in intrathoracic pressure created by ventilation
b. Atrial septal defect; acute pulmonary hypertension; pulmonic stenosis
c. Pericarditis
d. Aortic stenosis; pulmonic stenosis
e. Mitral stenosis; tricuspid stenosis
f. LBBB; right ventricular pacemaker or ectopy; severe aortic valve disease; patent ductus arteriosus
g. Mitral regurgitation; tricuspid *regurgitation;* ventricular septal defect
h. HF; fluid overload; cardiomyopathy; ventricular septal defect; patent ductus arteriosus
i. Closure of aortic and pulmonic valves
j. Mitral valve prolapse; mitral regurgitation
k. Closure of mitral and tricuspid valves
l. Aortic regurgitation; pulmonic regurgitation
m. Myocardial ischemia or infarction; hypertension; ventricular hypertrophy; AV block; severe aortic or pulmonic stenosis

9. Complete the following table describing common murmurs.

Condition	Timing	Location	Pitch
Mitral regurgitation			
Mitral stenosis			
Aortic regurgitation			
Aortic stenosis			
Mitral valve prolapse			
Papillary muscle dysfunction or rupture			
Ventricular septal defect or rupture			

10. Match the dysrhythmia to the appropriate characteristic.

___ 1. Normal sinus rhythm
___ 2. Sinus bradycardia
___ 3. Sinus tachycardia
___ 4. Premature atrial contraction
___ 5. Atrial fibrillation
___ 6. Atrial flutter
___ 7. Supraventricular tachycardia
___ 8. Premature junctional contraction
___ 9. Junctional escape rhythm
___ 10. Accelerated junctional rhythm
___ 11. Junctional tachycardia
___ 12. Premature ventricular complex
___ 13. Accelerated idioventricular rhythm
___ 14. Ventricular tachycardia
___ 15. Ventricular fibrillation
___ 16. Asystole
___ 17. First-degree AV block
___ 18. Second-degree AV block, type I
___ 19. Second-degree AV block, type II
___ 20. Third-degree AV block

a. PR interval greater than 0.2 second
b. Early P wave which looks different from other P waves followed by normal QRS
c. Sawtooth waves on baseline, no clearly identifiable P waves, normal QRS
d. QRS is early, greater than 0.12 second, with T wave in opposite direction of QRS
e. Regular rhythm, normal P waves, normal QRS complexes, rate less than 60/min
f. Quivering baseline, irregularly irregular occurring QRSs.
g. QRS complex is early with inverted P wave immediately (less than 0.12 second) prior to the QRS, in the QRS or immediately after the QRS
h. Regular rhythm with rate of 40-60/min with narrow QRS with inverted P wave immediately (less than 0.12 second) prior to the QRS, in the QRS or immediately after the QRS
i. Flat line, no QRS complexes
j. Regular rhythm, normal P waves, normal QRS complexes, rate greater than 100/min
k. Regular rhythm, normal P waves, normal QRS complexes, rate 60-100/min
l. Progressive PR lengthening until a P wave is not followed by a QRS
m. Regular rhythm with rate of 60-100/min with narrow QRS with inverted P wave immediately (less than 0.12 second) prior to the QRS, in the QRS or immediately after the QRS
n. Wide QRS (greater than 0.12 second) rhythm with rate of 40-100/min
o. Regular rhythm with rate of greater than 100/min with narrow QRS with inverted P wave immediately (less than 0.12 second) prior to the QRS, in the QRS or immediately after the QRS
p. Regular rhythm with rate 150-250/min without clearly discernible P waves with narrow QRS
q. P wave not followed by QRS without preceding progression of PR interval
r. No relationship between P waves and QRS complexes; escape rhythm established by AV junction or ventricle
s. Irregular baseline, absence of QRS complexes
t. Wide QRS (greater than 0.12 second) rhythm with rate greater than 100/min

11. Analyze the following ECG rhythm strips. All strips are 6 seconds.

a.

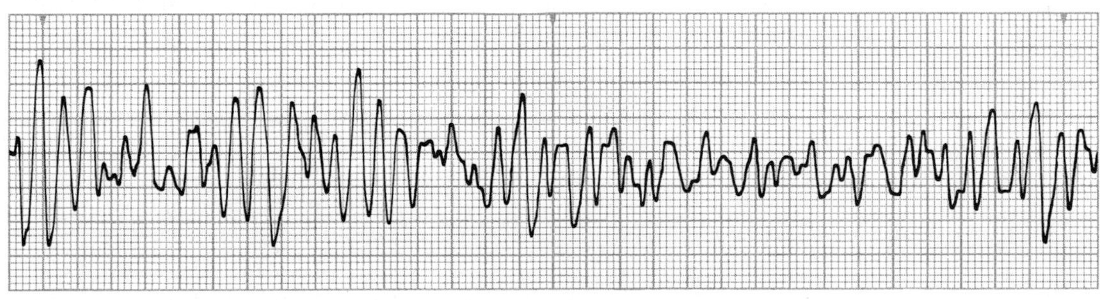

Interpretation ____

b.

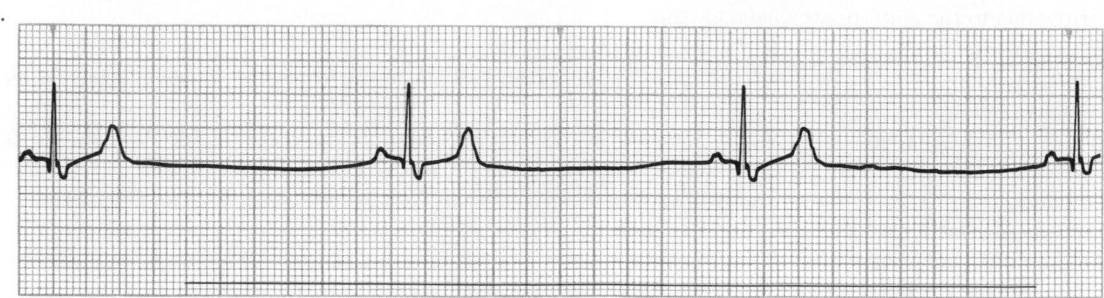

Interpretation ____________________

c.

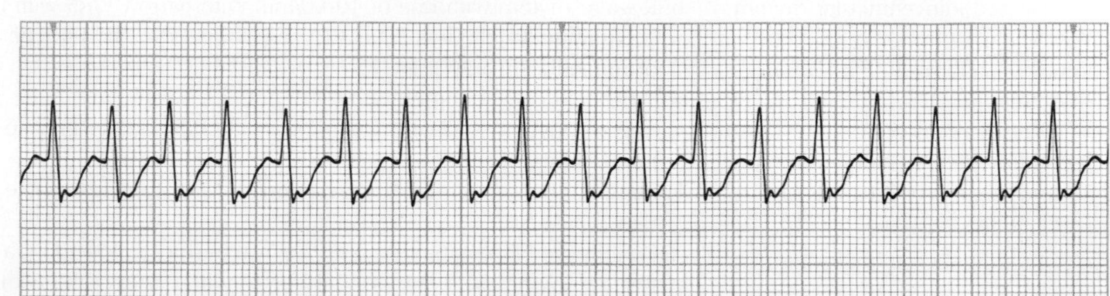

Interpretation ____________________

d.

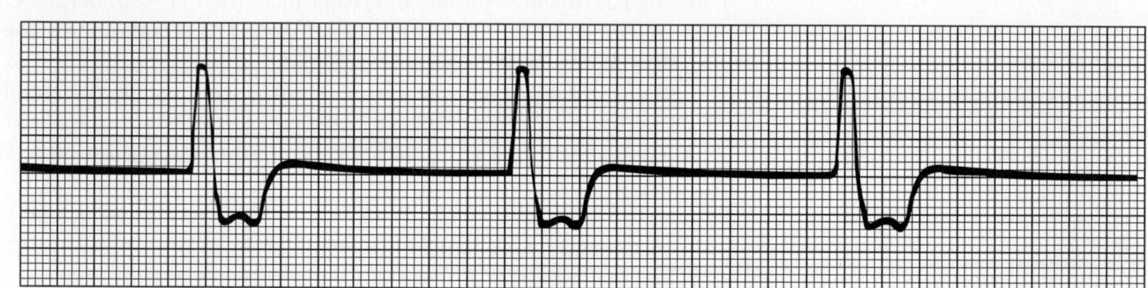

Interpretation ____________________

e.

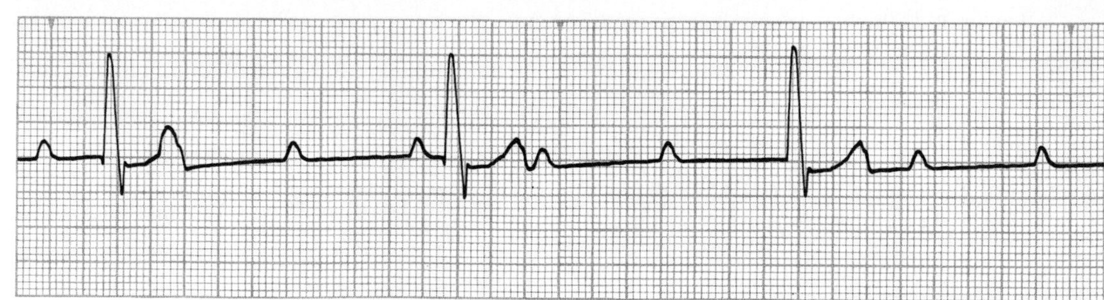

Interpretation ____________________

f.

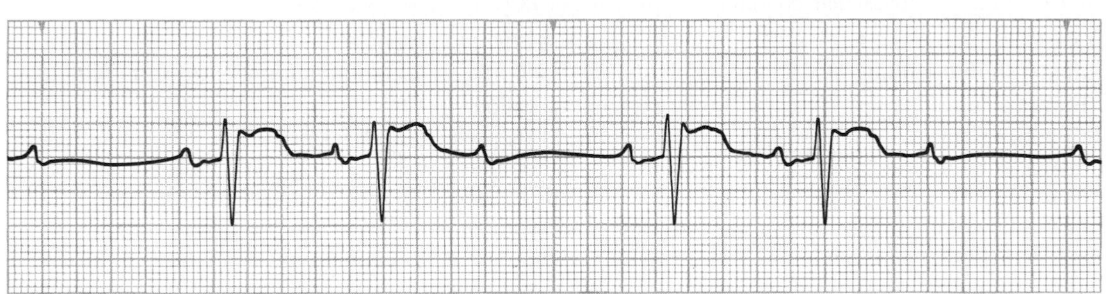

Interpretation ____________________

g.

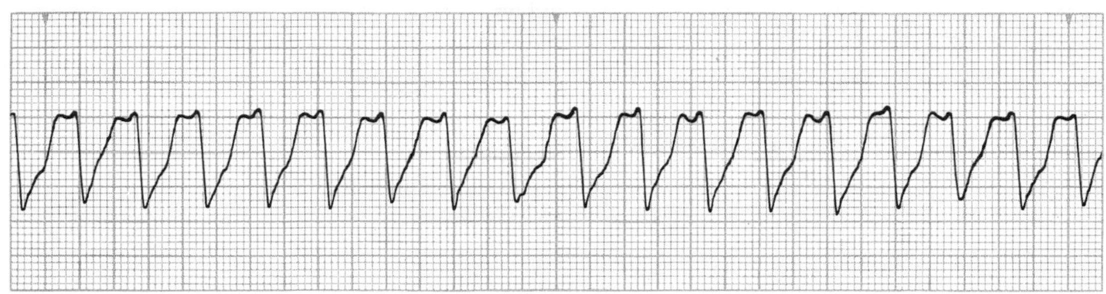

Interpretation ____________________

h.

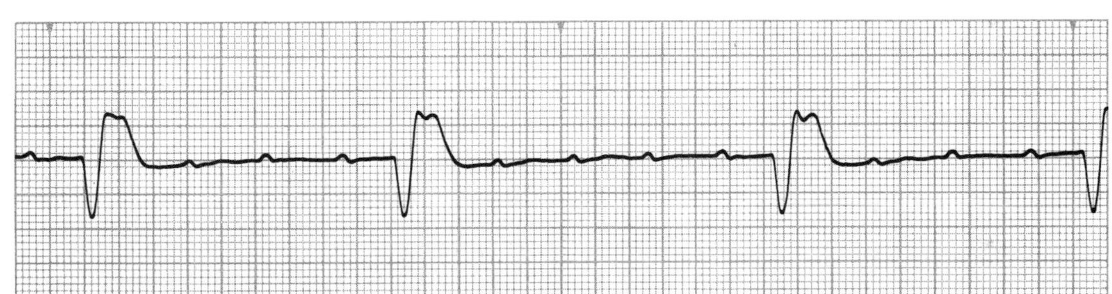

Interpretation ____________________

i.

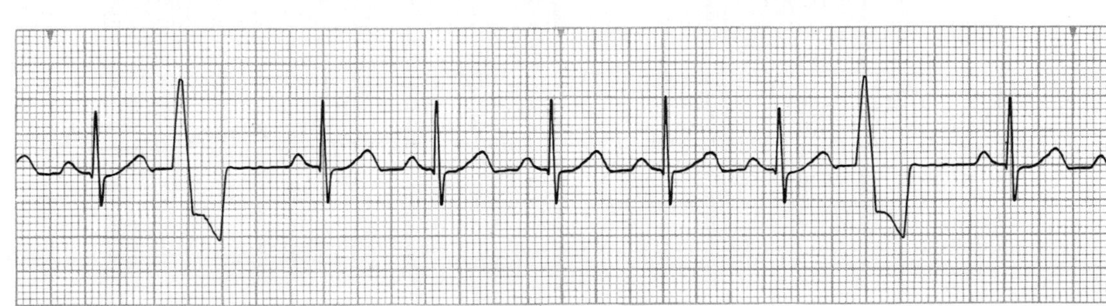

Interpretation ____________________

12. Match the following cardiovascular conditions to their major ECG diagnostic features.

CONDITION

___ 1. Acute myocardial infarction
___ 2. Hypercalcemia
___ 3. Hyperkalemia
___ 4. Hypocalcemia
___ 5. Hypokalemia
___ 6. Left atrial enlargement
___ 7. Left bundle branch block
___ 8. Left ventricular hypertrophy
___ 9. Pericarditis
___ 10. Variant angina
___ 11. Right atrial enlargement
___ 12. Right bundle branch block
___ 13. Right ventricular hypertrophy
___ 14. Wellens syndrome

ECG DIAGNOSTIC FEATURES

a. Symmetrically, deeply inverted T waves in V_2, V_3 with little or no ST segment elevation
b. Prolonged QT, prolonged ST segment
c. R wave larger than S wave in V_1, V_2, S wave larger than R wave in V_5, V_6, right axis deviation, ST-T wave changes in V_1, V_2
d. Diffuse ST segment elevation across the precordium
e. Wide (greater than 0.11 second), notched P wave in lead II, dominant terminal component of P wave in V_1
f. Wide (0.12 second or greater than) QRS below the baseline in V_1
g. Q waves at least 0.04 second wide and/or $\frac{1}{4}$ height of R wave along with ST segment elevation and symmetrically inverted T waves
h. Increased QRS amplitude, left axis deviation, ST-T wave changes in V_5, V_6
i. Wide (0.12 second or greater than) QRS above the baseline in V_1
j. Tall (greater than 2.5 mm) peaked P wave in lead II, dominant initial component of P wave in V_1
k. Shortened QT, shortened ST segment
l. Flat T waves, prominent U wave, ST segment depression
m. ST segment elevation with pain
n. Tall peaked T waves, widening of QRS complex, atrial asystole

13. Match the cardiac wall to the lead grouping that is used to evaluate that wall.

LEAD GROUPINGS

___ 1. II, III, aVF
___ 2. V_{4R}
___ 3. I, aVL
___ 4. V_1, V_2
___ 5. V_3, V_4
___ 6. V_5, V_6
___ 7. V_8, V_9

CARDIAC WALL

a. Anterior
b. Lateral (high)
c. Lateral (low)
d. Posterior
e. Right ventricular
f. Septal
g. Inferior

14. Analyze the following 12-lead ECGs for bundle branch block. Identify if left or right bundle branch block.

a.

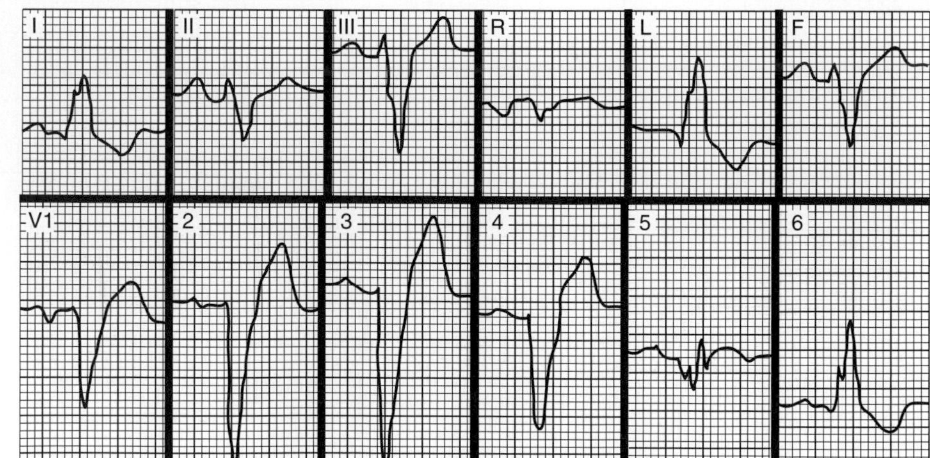

Interpretation: ______________________________

b.

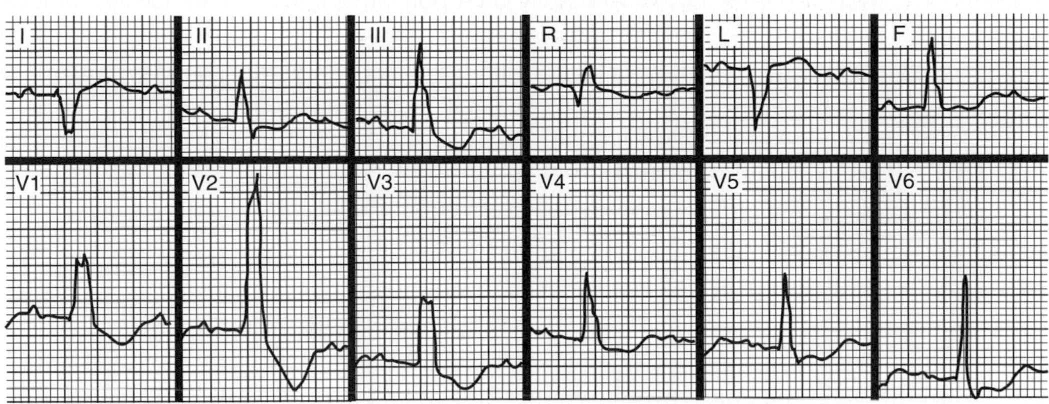

Interpretation ____________________

15. Analyze the following 12-lead ECGs for atrial enlargement or ventricular hypertrophy.

a.

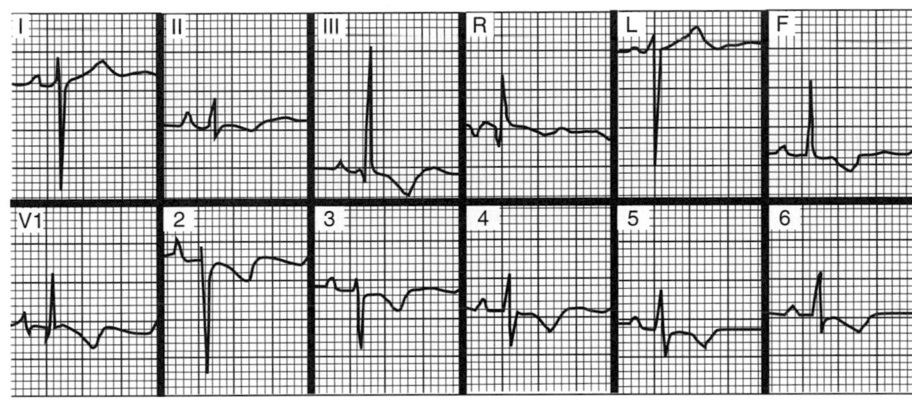

Interpretation ____________________

b.

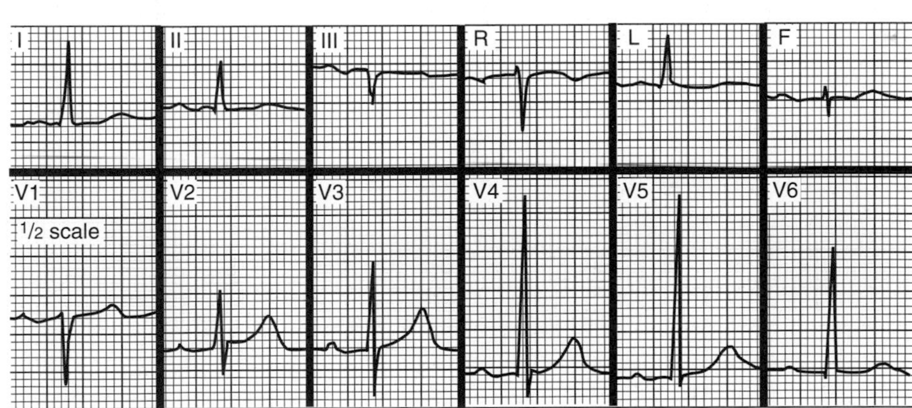

Interpretation ____________________

16. Analyze the following 12-lead ECGs from patients with acute chest pain for indications of MI. Identify location and age of MI if present.

a.

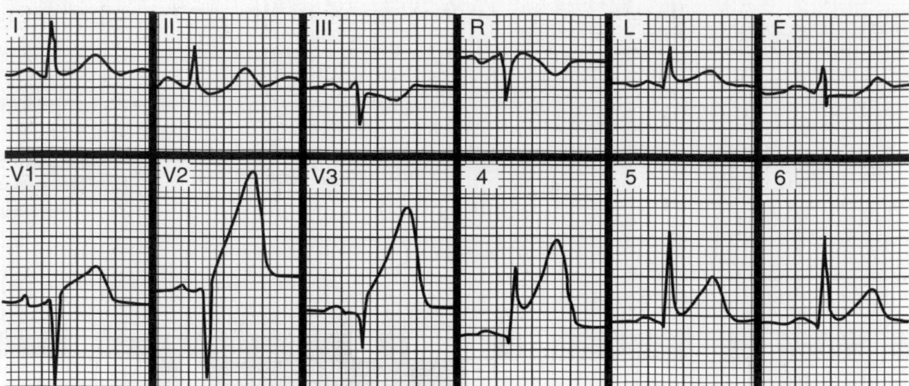

Interpretation: ______________________________

b.

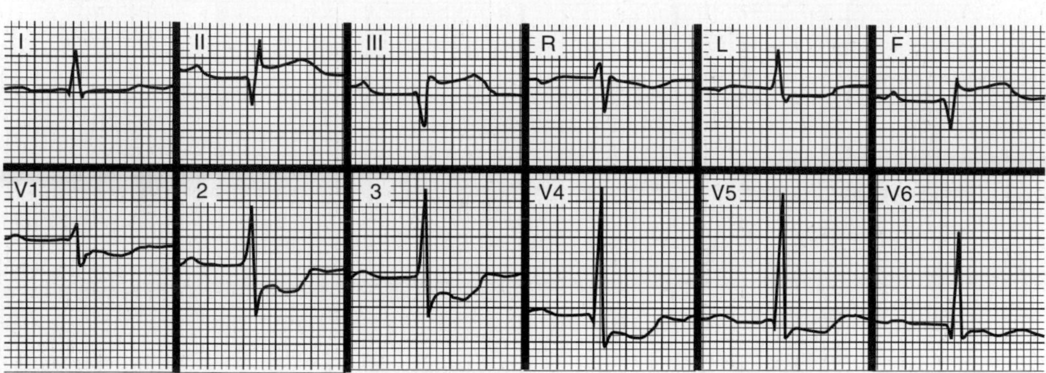

Interpretation ______________________________

17. Complete the following crossword puzzle dealing with hemodynamic monitoring.

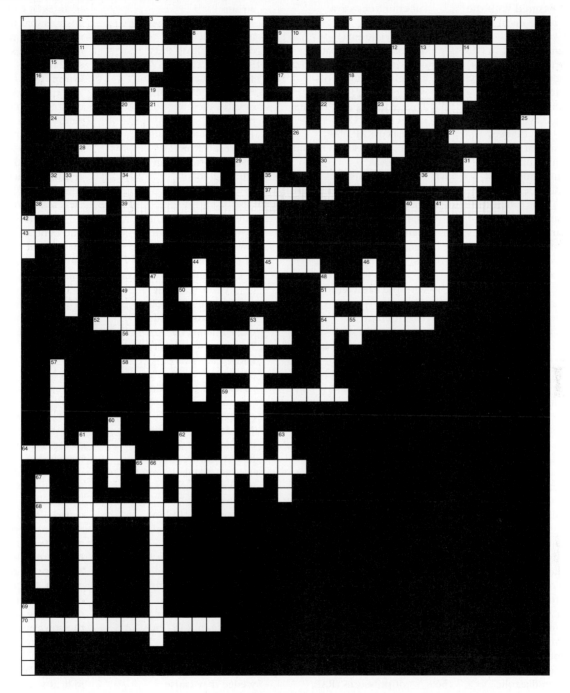

ACROSS

1. PAP is measured with the balloon at the distal end of the PAC _____
7. Right ventricular volumetric monitoring is performed using this type of catheter (abbrev.)
9. The relaxation phase of the cardiac cycle
11. Gastric _____ detects regional alterations in tissue perfusion using gastric intramucosal carbon dioxide
13. Oxygen ___ is when the O_2 saturation in the pulmonary artery is higher than in the right atrium; indication of ventricular septal rupture
16. The ___ notch of the PA waveform represents closure of the pulmonic valve
17. Diastolic BP minus PAOP (abbrev.)
21. This type of monitoring is the monitoring of blood flow generally through the use of invasive catheters
23. The most common site for arterial catheters for monitoring of blood pressure
24. DO_2 is an abbreviation for oxygen ___
25. The amount of blood ejected from the heart each beat (abbrev.)
26. Rupture of the ventricular septum results in an _____ in SvO_2
27. Indications of PAC migration back into the right ventricle include loss of dicrotic notch, decrease in diastolic pressure, and ___
28. This type of shock results in decreased CO, decreased RAP, PAP, PAOP, increased SVR and tachycardia
30. The *a* wave of the PAOP waveform represents contraction of the ___
32. Air in the pleural space; a potential complication of central venous catheter insertion
36. ___ nerve palsy occurs when the wrist is maintained in hyperextended position
37. The pressure in the superior vena cava (abbrev.)
38. An intermittent ___ device maintains patency of a catheter by delivering a minimal amount of solution each hour
39. This type of shock results in decreased CO, increased RAP, PAP, PAOP, increased SVR, and tachycardia
41. Using more air than required to cause a PAOP waveform may cause pulmonary artery ___ manifested by massive hemoptysis
43. In-___ calibration of a SvO_2 catheter is done with the catheter inside the body
45. This therapy is particularly useful when a patient with significantly elevated SVR is too hypotensive to safely use arterial vasodilators (abbrev.)
49. This type of cardiac output monitoring allows for less risk of contamination and frequently updated values (abbrev.)
50. This drug may be added to flush solution to prevent catheter occlusion
51. The *v* wave of the PAOP waveform represents contraction of the ___
52. The average blood pressure over time (abbrev.)
54. This device records the pressure waveform on paper for analysis
56. ___ of pressures (RAP, PAd, PAOP) is an indication of cardiac tamponade
58. Pulmonary ___ is evidenced by PVR greater than 250 dynes/sec/cm^{-5}, PA mean greater than 20 mm Hg, and difference between PAd and PAOP is 5 mm Hg or greater
59. This device increases the magnitude of an electrical signal and filters out electrical interference
64. The phlebostatic axis is at the fourth ICS and ___; correlates with the location of the right atrium
65. This type of shock results in decreased CO, decreased RAP, PAP, PAOP, decreased SVR, and tachycardia
68. Zeroing the transducer negates the effect of ___ pressure
70. This fatal complication can result from disconnection of an arterial line

DOWN

2. This type of monitoring is indicated for patients with hypertensive crisis or on vasoactive drugs
3. The determination of best ____ is the ___ that results in the best SaO_2 without dropping the CO/CI (abbrev.)
4. To ___ a transducer, a known amount of pressure is exerted on the transducer to see that the pressure is measured correctly
5. The derived parameter calculated by using height and weight; used in calculation of indexed parameters (abbrev.)
6. The amount of blood ejected by the heart in 1 minute (abbrev.)
7. The parameter that is measured from the proximal port of the PAC (abbrev.)
8. The major cause of a decrease in RAP, PAP, and PAOP
10. Leaving the PAC balloon inflated or a spontaneous wedge may cause pulmonary ___
12. PAOP is measured with the balloon at the distal end of the PAC _____
13. $ScvO_2$ is advocated to be used in this type of shock to evaluate the optimization of oxygen delivery
14. The parameter measured from the distal tip of the PAC with the balloon inflated; indirectly measures LAP (abbrev.)
15. SvO_2 may be evaluated by drawing a ___ venous blood gas
18. This type of calibration of an SvO_2 catheter ensures that the oximeter values are consistent with mixed venous oxygen saturation
19. Lymph fluid in the pleural space; a potential complication of central venous catheter insertion
20. To ___ the transducer, it is opened to air and the baseline on the monitor and the numeric value is adjusted
22. Elevated blood levels of _____ indicate hypoxia
25. The contraction phase of the cardiac cycle
29. The device that converts a mechanical signal to an electrical signal
31. When the dicrotic notch on the PA waveform is lost and the amplitude is lessened
33. This type of shock results in decreased CO, decreased RAP, PAP, PAOP, decreased SVR, and bradycardia
34. This device displays the electrical signal as a pressure waveform and a numerical value
35. Inflation of the balloon at the distal tip of the PAC causes ___ and blocks right heart pressures to allow measurement of left heart pressure
40. This type of response test ensures adequate damping of a pressure monitoring system using the square wave test
41. SvO_2 is a reflection of oxygen ___
42. The calculated parameter indicative of left ventricular afterload (abbrev.)
44. The lumen of the PAC that measures the temperature of the blood in the pulmonary artery
46. In-___ calibration of an SvO_2 catheter is done with the catheter outside the body
47. VO_2 is an abbreviation for oxygen ___
48. To ___ a PAC is to use more air than is required to cause a PAOP waveform

53. This type of technology allows for the noninvasive measurement of cardiac output through cutaneous sensors
55. The amount of blood ejected by the heart in 1 minute and indexed to body size (abbrev.)
57. The stretch on the myofibrils that determines the force of the next contraction
59. Represents the pressure required to open the semilunar valve
60. The calculated parameter indicative of left ventricular contractility and indexed to body size (abbrev.)
61. Technique for measuring cardiac output
62. This early stage of this type of shock results in increased CO, decreased RAP, PAP, PAOP, decreased SVR, and tachycardia
63. Excessive artifact on the PA waveform caused by excessive movement of the catheter
66. _____ assessment of the limb with an arterial line is important in the detection of acute arterial occlusion
67. The original brand name of PAC (2 words)
69. The air-fluid interface of the transducer must be ___ with the phlebostatic axis

18. Match the pathologic condition with its hemodynamic profile.

___ 1. Cardiac tamponade
___ 2. Noncardiac pulmonary edema
___ 3. Cardiac pulmonary edema
___ 4. Rupture of interventricular septum
___ 5. Pulmonary hypertension
___ 6. Papillary muscle rupture
___ 7. Right ventricular MI
___ 8. Cardiogenic shock
___ 9. Hypovolemic shock

a. ↑ RAP, ↓ PAOP, ↓ CO/CI, SvO_2, DO_2
b. ↑ PAP and PAOP, ↑ SvO_2, large v waves on PAOP waveform, falsely ↑ CO/CI, new systolic murmur at lower left sternal border
c. ↑ PAP and PAOP, large *v* waves on PAOP waveform, new systolic murmur at apex
d. PAd, PVR, PAm are all ↑ and the difference between PAd and PAOP is greater than 5 mm Hg
e. ↓ RAP, PAP, PAOP, ↑ SVR, ↓ CO/CI, SvO_2, DO_2
f. ↑ RAP, PAP, PAOP, ↑ SVR, ↓ SaO_2, SvO_2, DO_2
g. ↑ PAP and PAOP, crackles, ↓ SaO_2, SvO_2, DO_2
h. ↑ PAP, normal or decreased PAOP, crackles, ↓ SaO_2, SvO_2, DO_2
i. RAP, PAd, and PAOP are all ↑ and within 5 mm Hg of one another, large *a* and large *v* waves on PAOP waveform, ↓ CO/CI, SvO_2, DO_2

19. Identify whether the parameters in these case studies are decreased, normal, or increased. Discuss implications and treatment goals.

a. Patient A is a 44-year-old male who was transported to the Emergency Department after having chest pain for 6 hours. He had ST segment elevation from V_2-V_6. He also has a history of two previous MIs, and the ECG shows a previous inferior MI. The next day, Q waves are noted from V_2-V_6 despite fibrinolytic therapy administered in the Emergency Department. He is now hypotensive with an S_3 audible at his cardiac apex and crackles audible in his lung bases. Urine output has been marginal for the last 2 hours. The physician inserts a PAC to allow better evaluation of current status as well as response to therapy. The patient's BSA is 1.7 m^2

Parameter	↑, ↓, or Normal	Parameter	↑, ↓, or Normal
BP: 88/70 mm Hg		SV: 23 mL/beat	
MAP: 76 mm Hg		SI: 14 mL/m^2/beat	
HR: 128 beats/min		SVR: 1813 dynes/sec/cm^{-5}	
RAP: 8 mm Hg		SVRI: 3022 dynes/sec/cm^{-5}	
PAP: 42/26 mm Hg		PVR: 240 dynes/sec/cm^{-5}	
PAm: 31 mm Hg		PVRI: 400 dynes/sec/cm^{-5}	
PAOP: 22 mm Hg		LVSWI: 10.3 g • m/m^2	
CO: 3 L/min		RVSWI: 2.7 g • m/m^2	
CI: 1.8 L/min/m^2		SvO_2: 51%	
SaO_2: 88% on 5 L/min via nasal cannula		DO_2I: 318 mL/min/m^2	

Implications and treatment goals: ____

____

b. Patient B is a 52-year-old being admitted to the critical care unit after surgery for repair of hemothorax after a gunshot wound. The Post Anesthesia Care Unit (PACU) nurse gives you a report of massive blood loss before surgery; estimated blood loss in the OR was 1 L. He has had 5 L of lactated Ringer's and 2 units of packed red blood cells. Past medical history includes MI 5 years ago and angioplasty 2 years ago for intractable angina. A PAC was inserted prior to surgery to evaluate fluid status and cardiac function and to aid in fluid resuscitation. The patient's BSA is 1.9 m^2.

Parameter	↑, ↓, or Normal	Parameter	↑, ↓, or Normal
BP: 92/70 mm Hg		SV: 24 mL/beat	
MAP: 77 mm Hg		SI: 13 mL/m^2/beat	
HR: 122 beats/min		SVR: 2097 dynes/sec/cm^{-5}	
RAP: 1 mm Hg		SVRI: 4053 dynes/sec/cm^{-5}	
PAP: 20/6 mm Hg		PVR: 221 dynes/sec/cm^{-5}	
PAm: 11 mm Hg		PVRI: 427 dynes/sec/cm^{-5}	
PAOP: 3 mm Hg		LVSWI: 13.1 g • m/m^2	
CO: 2.9 L/min		RVSWI: 1.8 g • m/m^2	
CI: 1.5 L/min/m^2		SvO_2: 50%	
SaO_2: 98% on 5 L/min via nasal cannula		DO_2I: 138 mL/min/m^2	
Hgb: 7 g/dL			

Implications and treatment goals:____

The Cardiovascular System: Pathologic Conditions

CHAPTER 3

Cardiopulmonary Arrest

Definition

A sudden cessation of the cardiac output and effective circulation; cardiac arrest is followed by ventilatory cessation

Etiology

1. Dysrhythmias
2. Electrical shock
3. Drowning
4. Asphyxiation
5. Trauma
6. Hypothermia
7. Terminal phases of a chronic illness (CPR may not be attempted on this patient according to advanced directives and "do not resuscitate" [DNR] orders)

Pathophysiology

1. Cardiac arrest ceases delivery of oxygen and removal of carbon dioxide, causing tissue hypoxia and metabolic (i.e., lactic) acidosis.
2. Ventilatory arrest causes hypercapnia, respiratory acidosis, and hypoxemia.
3. Cerebral cortex is irreversibly damaged within 4-6 minutes at normal body temperature and severe neurologic deficit or biological death occurs

Clinical Presentation

1. Loss of consciousness
2. Absence of breathing; agonal breathing may be a precursor to cardiopulmonary arrest
3. Absence of central pulses
4. Absence of auscultated or palpated blood pressure
5. Anoxic seizures may occur
6. Urinary and bowel incontinence may occur
7. ECG
   a. Most commonly ventricular fibrillation
   b. Less commonly ventricular tachycardia
   c. Rarely asystole
   d. Cardiopulmonary arrest with a stable electrical rhythm (referred to as *pulseless electrical activity [PEA]*)

Collaborative Management

1. Recognize the factors that are crucial in survival; these are referred to as the *chain of survival* by the American Heart Association (AHA) (Hazinski et al., 2010).
   a. Immediate recognition of cardiac arrest and activation of the emergency response system
   b. Early cardiopulmonary resuscitation (CPR) with emphasis on chest compressions; reasons for recent change from ABC to CAB (Field et al., 2010)
      1) Most cardiac arrests occur as a result of ventricular fibrillation or pulseless ventricular tachycardia in adults, and chest compressions and defibrillation are most crucial to survival.
      2) ABC sequence delayed chest compressions due to the time required to look, listen, feel for airflow, open the airway, and start mouth-to-mouth ventilation or retrieve a barrier or other ventilation equipment; in the new sequence, ventilation is only delayed until after a cycle of 30 compressions.
      3) Because lay persons are reluctant to give mouth-to-mouth ventilation to a stranger, compressions are more promptly initiated with the new Hands-Only™ CPR for those lay rescuers.
   c. Rapid defibrillation
   d. Effective advanced life support
   e. Integrated postcardiac arrest care
2. Recognize cardiac arrest and activate the emergency response system
   a. Complete assessment: if the person is unresponsive and either not breathing or only gasping
   b. Call for help: Call 911 for out-of-hospital cardiac arrest, or follow specific protocol (e.g., Code Blue) for in-hospital cardiac arrest.
   c. Retrieve defibrillator
3. Provide basic life support (BLS) as recommended by current AHA guidelines

a. Circulation
   1) Assess a carotid pulse for no more than 10 seconds.
   2) Deliver compressions.
      a) Place heel of one hand over the lower half of sternum; place the other hand over the first hand.
      b) Compress the sternum at a depth of at least 2 inches at a rate of at least 100/min.
         i) New guidelines emphasize that the provider push hard and fast, allowing the chest to completely recoil after each compression.
         ii) Compression ratio is 30 : 2 for CPR to adults.
         iii) All rescue efforts, including defibrillation, insertion of advanced airways, intravenous access, and administration of medications, should be performed with minimal interruption of compressions.
         iv) Compressions should be maintained without pauses for ventilation.

b. Airway and ventilation
   1) After the initial 30 compressions, open the airway using head tilt–chin lift maneuver; jaw thrust maneuver is no longer recommended in initial establishment of airway.
   2) If the patient is adequately breathing, position him or her on the left side in recovery position.
   3) If the patient is not breathing or breathing inadequately, health care providers should deliver two breaths using any of the following methods:
      a) Mouth to mask ventilation
      b) Manual resuscitation bag-valve-mask secured over nose and mouth
      c) Manual resuscitation bag to endotracheal (ET) tube or tracheostomy tube if already in place
   4) Note that each rescue breath does make the chest rise.
   5) Continue rescue breathing every 6 to 8 seconds (8-10 breaths/min); note that hyperventilation is associated with poor survival rates.

c. Coordination of compressions and ventilation: Maintain a ratio of 30 compressions to 2 ventilations for one or two rescuers.

d. Considerations
   1) CPR performed expertly provides only 25-30% of normal cardiac output, but most of this goes to the upper body, including the heart and brain.
   2) Mortality rates increase despite prompt CPR if advanced cardiac life support (ACLS) is delayed beyond 12 minutes.
   3) Resistance of ventricular dysrhythmias to defibrillation occurs over time; prompt defibrillation is critical to survival.

4. Initiate rapid defibrillation.
   a. Principle: By delivering a shock of sufficient strength, a critical mass of myocardium is depolarized simultaneously, allowing emergence of a dominant normal rhythm.
   b. Uses
      1) Pulseless ventricular tachycardia and ventricular fibrillation
      2) Unstable or refractory ventricular tachycardia with a pulse
      3) May also be used in asystole where the rhythm is unclear and could be fine VF
   c. Timing: should be performed for ventricular fibrillation or pulseless ventricular tachycardia as soon as defibrillator is available
      1) Ideally within 3 minutes
      2) Minimal delay between cessation of CPR and defibrillation and defibrillation and resumption of CPR
   d. Method for manual defibrillation
      1) Check pulse: Make sure that ventricular fibrillation pattern is not merely artifact caused by loose ECG electrode
      2) Remove any foil-lined patches from the patient's chest (e.g., nitroglycerin patches) because they may cause arcing and patient burns; patient must be dry and not in contact with any metallic objects.
      3) Turn defibrillator on and make sure that the synchronizer switch is off so that charge is delivered as soon as buttons are pushed; most defibrillators automatically reset to nonsynchronized mode so you can immediately defibrillate if ventricular fibrillation occurs after cardioversion.
      4) Apply defibrillation pads to chest for paddle placement or apply conductive jelly to paddles.
         a) Four pad/paddle positions are equally effective (Link et al., 2010).
            i) Anterolateral (considered the default position)
            ii) Anteroposterior: This paddle placement may be better for obese patients, patients with hyperinflated lungs (e.g., COPD), and for patients with an implantable cardioverter-defibrillator (ICD).
            iii) Anterior-left infrascapular
            iv) Anterior-right infrascapular
         b) Pacemakers
            i) In patients with permanent pacemakers, the paddles should not be placed within 8 cm of the pulse generator (Link et al., 2010).
            ii) Turn temporary pacemaker pulse generator off during defibrillation.

5) Charge to appropriate voltage for defibrillation
   a) Biphasic: 150-200 joules for a biphasic truncated exponential waveform or 120 joules for a rectilinear biphasic waveform; if unknown, use maximum available
      i) Advantages of biphasic defibrillation is that it offers equal or better efficacy at lower energies than traditional monophasic waveform defibrillators (less than or equal to 200 joules are safe and have equal or greater efficiency for terminating VF when compared with higher energy monophasic shock), less risk of myocardial injury, and skin burns.
      ii) In the first phase, the current moves from one paddle to the other (as in monophasic defibrillation) and in the second phase, the current reverses direction.
   b) Monophasic: 360 joules
6) Apply paddles to defibrillation pads or jellied paddles to chest using firm (~25 pounds) pressure.
7) Say the word *clear* and ensure that no one is touching the patient or the bed.
8) Press both discharge buttons simultaneously.
9) Resume CPR, beginning with chest compressions; note that current guidelines recommend only one shock before resuming CPR.
10) Recheck rhythm after 5 cycles (~2 minutes).
   a) If rhythm and pulse are restored, administer antidysrhythmic drug therapy.
   b) If rhythm and pulse are not restored, continue with appropriate algorithm.

e. Method for using an automatic external defibrillator (AED)
   1) Attach the device to the patient: Put one pad to the right of the sternum below the right clavicle and the other pad lateral to the apex in the left midaxillary line.
   2) Turn the device on.
   3) Ensure that the patient is completely still and no one is touching the patient.
   4) Press the analyze button. The device will signal "stand clear" and perform a 3-second analysis.
   5) If ventricular tachycardia or ventricular fibrillation is detected, the AED will charge to 200 joules (biphasic) and display a "shock indicated" message.
   6) Call "clear" and ensure that no one is touching the patient.
   7) Press the shock button to deliver the shock if it was indicated.
   8) If rhythm and pulse are restored, antidysrhythmic drug therapy will be administered.
   9) If rhythm and pulse are not restored, continuance of CPR and appropriate algorithm

f. Successful defibrillation is less likely if any of the following is present:
   1) Hypoxia
   2) Severe acidosis
   3) Alkalosis
   4) Local ionic imbalance
   5) Ischemia
   6) Long VF duration

g. Complications
   1) Dysrhythmias: asystole, bradycardia, AV blocks, ventricular fibrillation
   2) Hypotension
   3) Myocardial damage
   4) Pulmonary edema
   5) Emboli
   6) Muscle pain
   7) Skin burns

5. Provide effective advanced cardiac life support (ACLS) as recommended by current American Heart Association (AHA) guidelines.
   a. Utilization of ACLS algorithms to provide assistance with decision-making in a cardiopulmonary arrest (Figures 3-1 to 3-3)
   b. Identification and treatment of the cause of cardiac arrest, especially important in treatment of PEA
      1) 5 Hs: hypovolemia, hypoxia, hydrogen ion (acidosis), hyper/hypokalemia, and hypothermia
      2) 5 Ts: tension pneumothorax, tamponade (cardiac), toxins, thrombosis (coronary), and thrombosis (pulmonary)
   c. Oxygen therapy
      1) Administer 100% oxygen during cardiopulmonary arrest with a bag-valve-mask; a reservoir bag or tubing attached to the bag-valve-mask is required to achieve as high a concentration of oxygen as possible.
      2) Remember that there is no contraindication to 100% oxygen during cardiopulmonary arrest.
   d. Vascular access
      1) Determination of patency of existing central or peripheral IV or heparin lock; if a central vein catheter is in place when the arrest occurs, it should be used to administer drugs during the resuscitation
      2) Antecubital or external jugular veins are preferred if a venous catheter or additional venous catheters must be established.
         a) Peak drug concentrations are lower and circulation times are longer when drugs are administered by peripheral sites compared with central sites.

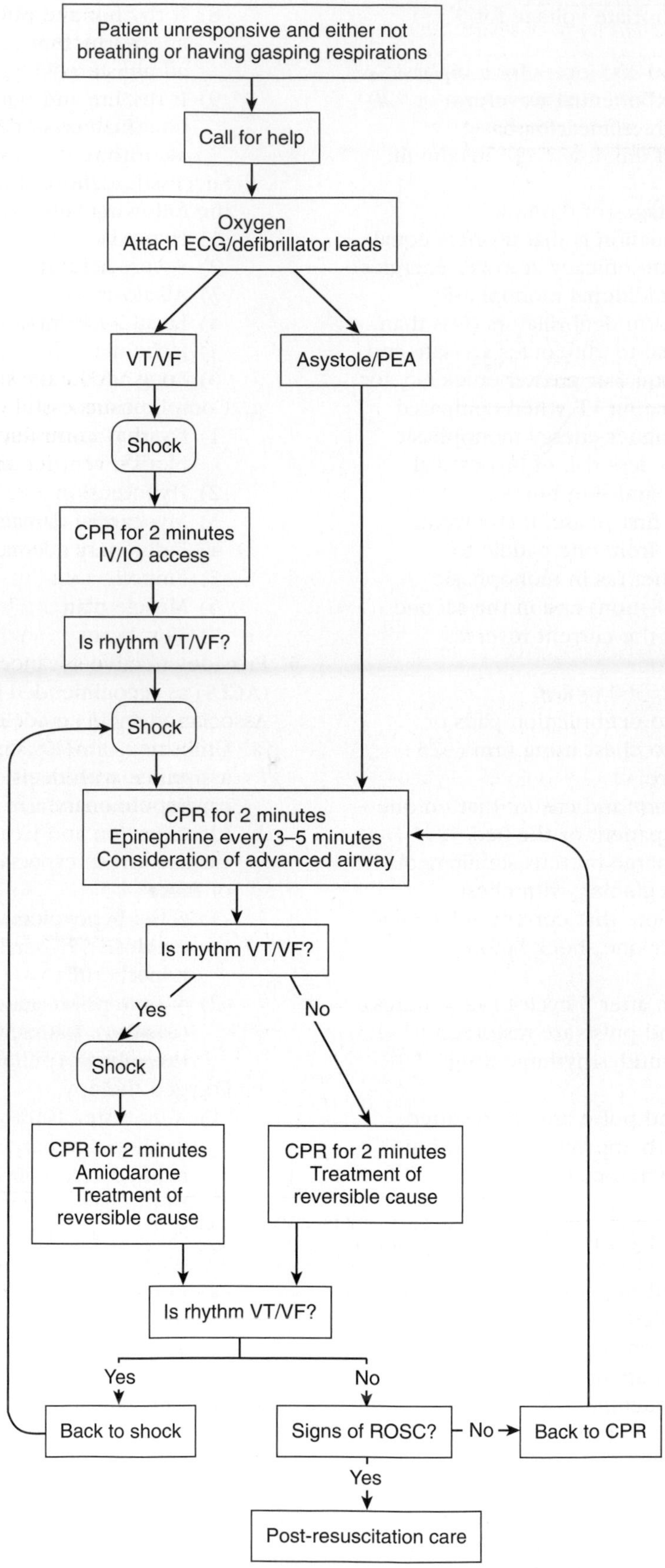

Figure 3-1 ACLS cardiac arrest algorithm. *CPR,* cardiopulmonary resuscitation; *ECG,* electrocardiogram; *PEA,* pulseless electrical activity; *ROSC,* return of spontaneous circulation; *VF,* ventricular fibrillation; *VT,* ventricular tachycardia. (Data from Neumar, R. W., Otto, C. W., Link, M. S., Kronick, S. L., Shuster, M., Callaway CW, et al. [2010]. Part 8: Adult advanced cardiovascular life support: 2010 American Heart Association guidelines for cardiopulmonary resuscitation and emergency cardiovascular care. *Circulation, 122*[18 Suppl 3], S729-767.)

b) If peripheral venous access is used for resuscitation drugs, administer bolus drugs rapidly, follow with a 20-mL saline, and elevate the extremity for 10-20 seconds.

3) Central vein cannulation may be performed.
   a) The major disadvantage of central vein cannulation during cardiopulmonary arrest is the need to stop CPR.
      i) Internal jugular and subclavian sites require cessation of CPR.
      ii) Femoral vein cannulation does not require cessation of CPR.
   b) Another consideration is that unsuccessful central vein cannulation may contraindicate the use of fibrinolytics and increase the risk of bleeding with the use of glycoprotein IIb/IIIa agents (e.g., abciximab [ReoPro], eptifibatide [Integrilin], tirofiban [Aggrastat]) and anticoagulants.
4) Distal wrist and hand veins and distal saphenous veins in the legs are the least favorable sites for drug administration during CPR.
5) Intraosseous access may be used if intravenous access is not available; drugs administered by IO route take approximately 2 minutes to reach the heart.

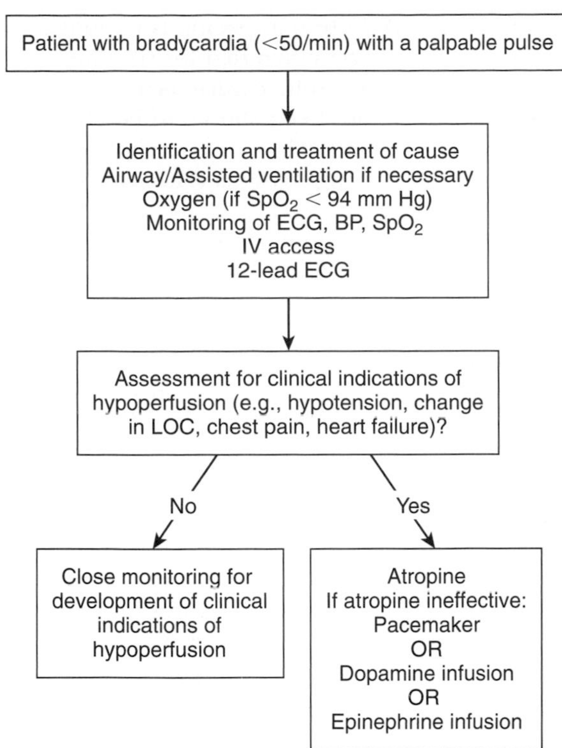

Figure 3-2 Bradycardia algorithm. *BP,* blood pressure; *ECG,* electrocardiogram; *LOC,* level of consciousness; *SpO_2,* oxygen saturation by pulse oximetry. (Data from Neumar, et al. [2010]. Part 8: Adult advanced cardiovascular life support: 2010 American Heart Association Guidelines for Cardiopulmonary Resuscitation and Emergency Cardiovascular Care. *Circulation*, 122[18 Suppl 3], S729-767.)

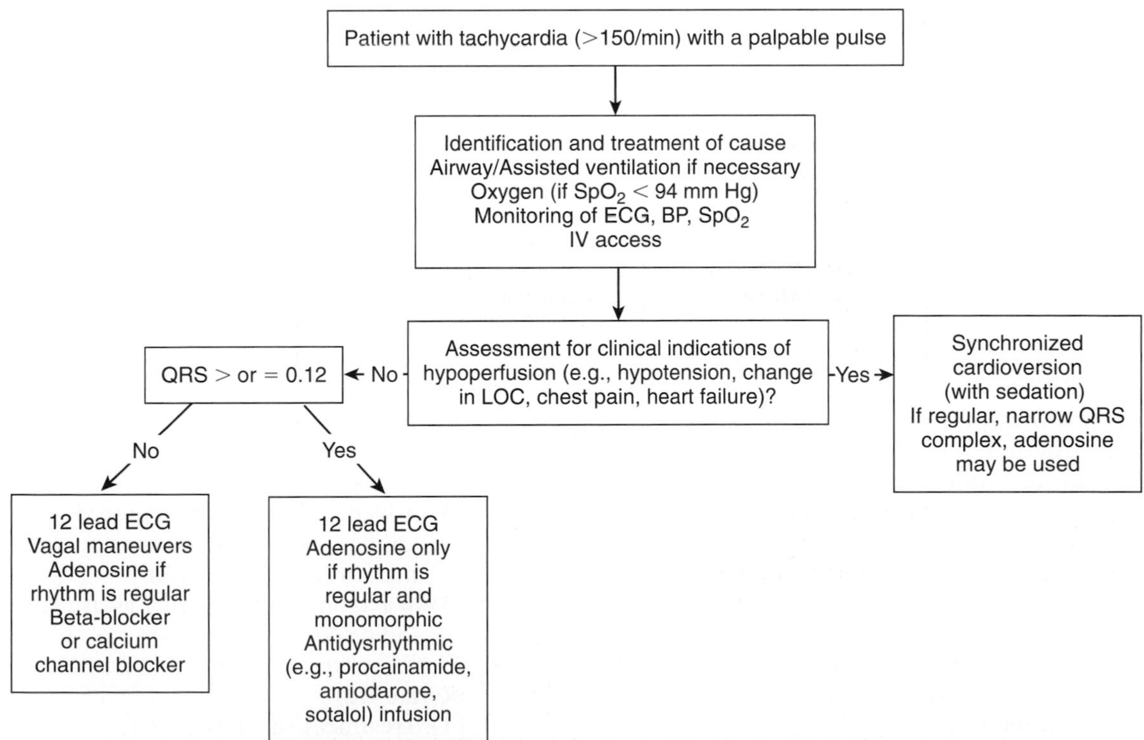

Figure 3-3 Tachycardia algorithm. *BP,* blood pressure; *ECG,* electrocardiogram; *IV,* intravenous; *LOC,* level of consciousness; *SpO_2,* oxygen saturation by pulse oximetry. (Data from Neumar, et al. [2010]. Part 8: Adult advanced cardiovascular life support: 2010 American Heart Association Guidelines for Cardiopulmonary Resuscitation and Emergency Cardiovascular Care. *Circulation*, 122[18 Suppl 3], S729-767.)

e. Endotracheal intubation
   1) Attempt as soon as feasible, but defibrillation and administration of epinephrine are first and second priorities.
   2) Hyperventilation with 100% oxygen should precede any intubation attempt.
   3) Confirm endotracheal tube placement by listening for equal bilateral breath sounds along with esophageal detector device, end-tidal carbon dioxide indicator, or capnography; chest x-ray is obtained after the patient is stabilized.
      a) Capnography is recommended for confirmation and monitoring of ET tube placement and the quality of CPR (Hazinski, 2010).
   4) Advantages of endotracheal intubation include reduction of the risk of vomiting and aspiration and provision of a relative airway seal.
   5) If IV route cannot be established but endotracheal tube placement has been achieved, some emergency drugs can be given via the ET tube; however, intravenous route is preferred.
      a) Epinephrine, lidocaine, atropine, and naloxone may be administered via the ET tube.
      b) ET administration requires adjusting the dose to 2-2.5 times the usual dose and diluting the drug with isotonic saline to make a total volume of at least 10 mL; follow with several quick insufflations with the manual resuscitation bag.
   6) Two alternative airway techniques are placed orally and are inserted past the hypopharynx but not into the trachea.
      a) Laryngeal mask airway (LMA)
      b) Esophageal-tracheal Combitube (ETC)

f. Intravenous fluids: Normal saline is used to maintain adequate preload and to mix intravenous drug infusions.

g. Pharmacologic agents as indicated in algorithms (Figures 3-1 to 3-3)

h. Electrical therapies to change an abnormal cardiac rhythm to a normal one
   1) Defibrillation for ventricular fibrillation or pulseless ventricular tachycardia as previously described
   2) Cardioversion for unstable supraventricular tachycardia or ventricular tachycardia with a pulse
   3) Temporary pacemaker: for patients who have problem with impulse formation and/or conduction
      a) Indications
         i) Symptomatic bradycardia nonresponsive to drug therapy (e.g., atropine)
         ii) Symptomatic AV blocks
         iii) Note that pacing is no longer recommended for patients with asystolic cardiac arrest; it has not been shown to be effective and delays or interrupts chest compressions (Link et al., 2010).
      b) Types
         i) Transcutaneous pacemaker
            (a) Large surface skin electrodes applied anterior and posterior
               (i) Posterior: positive electrode applied between spine and left scapula at level of heart
               (ii) Anterior: negative electrode applied at left fourth ICS at midclavicular line
            (b) May be painful for patient and should be replaced by transvenous lead as soon as possible
         ii) Transvenous pacemaker for patients who do not respond to drugs or transcutaneous pacing
            (a) Lead is threaded into the apex of the right ventricle via subclavian or internal jugular vein.

6. Provide quality postcardiac arrest care (Peberdy et al., 2010).
   a. Recognize that care after return of spontaneous circulation (ROSC) significantly impacts patient survival with optimal quality of life.
   b. Identify and treat reversible causes of cardiac arrest.
   c. Optimize ventilation and oxygenation.
      1) Avoidance of hyperventilation; keep $PaCO_2$ within between 40-45 mm Hg
      2) Oxygen to maintain SaO_2 at greater than or equal to 94%
         a) Close monitoring of ABGs and decrease of oxygen when possible to prevent oxygen toxicity
         b) Use of hyperoxygenation with 100% oxygen during suctioning to avoid hypoxemia
      3) Advanced airways as required
      4) Limitation of tidal volume to 6-8 mL/kg to prevent acute lung injury
      5) Waveform capnography as available and indicated
   d. Treat hypotension (i.e., systolic BP less than 90 mm Hg)
      1) Treatment of causes
      2) Intravenous or intraosseous boluses
      3) Inotropic or vasopressor agents as indicated
      4) Antidysrhythmics as indicated
   e. Utilize therapeutic hypothermia if the patient is unresponsive but with an adequate BP following

resuscitation; shown to improve neurologic recovery and reduce mortality rate

1) Indications
   a) Out-of-hospital cardiac arrest as the result of ventricular fibrillation or pulseless ventricular tachycardia; may also be used for in-hospital cardiac arrest
   b) Persistent change in neurologic function after ROSC
   c) Able to maintain BP with or without vasopressors after ROSC
2) Contraindications (Pyle et al., 2007)
   a) Less than 18 years of age
   b) Coma of other etiology prior to cardiac arrest
   c) Pregnancy
   d) Terminal illness (e.g., late-stage cancer)
   e) Intracerebral hemorrhage
   f) Surgery within 14 days
   g) Systemic infection or sepsis
   h) Known bleeding or coagulopathy
3) Method
   a) Prepare patient for initiation of cooling.
      i) Intubation and mechanical ventilation
      ii) Foley catheter
      iii) Temperature monitoring via use of internal temperature monitor: urinary bladder, rectal, or pulmonary artery
   b) Initiate cooling within 2-6 hours of cardiac arrest and maintain body temperature between 32-34°C for 24 hours along with drugs to sedate and prevent shivering.
      i) Cooling methods: At least one study (Tomte et al., 2011) has found no difference in outcomes between surface and core cooling methods.
         (a) Surface
            (i) Ice packs applied to armpits, neck, torso, groin
            (ii) Air circulating cooling system
            (iii) Fans
            (iv) Cold water or alcohol sponge baths or sprays
            (v) Cooling blanket under and over the patient with a sheet between the blanket and the patient (i.e., cooling blanket, sheet, patient, sheet, cooling blanket)
         (b) Core
            (i) Cold intravenous infusions: 1-2 L of 4°C normal saline or lactated Ringer's solution by peripheral or femoral vein access; 30 mL/kg over 30 minutes is a common protocol
            (ii) Gastric lavage may be used.
            (iii) Endovascular cooling catheters may be used.
            (iv) Extracorporeal circulation may be used.
      ii) Close monitoring of vital signs, CBC, PT, aPTT, INR, serum chemistries, ABGs every 12 hours
      iii) Control of discomfort and shivering
         (a) Shivering causes increase in oxygen consumption.
         (b) Sedation with benzodiazepines such as midazolam (Versed) is indicated; muscle paralytics such as vecuronium or pancuronium may be required.
            (i) Drug clearance is decreased during hypothermia.
   c) Rewarm gradually (0.25-0.5°C/hr) over 24 hours to avoid hypotension and cerebral edema.
4) Complications
   a) Infection: decrease in number and function of neutrophils and decreased antibody production
   b) Impaired tissue oxygenation: shift in oxyhemoglobin dissociation curve to the left impairs drop off of oxygen at tissue level
   c) Coagulopathy
   d) Dysrhythmias
      i) Atrial fibrillation with temperature less than 32°C
      ii) Ventricular fibrillation with temperature less than 30°C
   e) Hyperglycemia
   f) Electrolyte imbalance: Hypokalemia, hypophosphatemia, and hypomagnesemia due to cold-induced diuresis

f. Facilitate coronary reperfusion as indicated for STEMI or high suspicion of acute MI.
   1) Percutaneous coronary intervention (e.g., angioplasty, atherectomy, stent placement)

g. Provide advanced critical care management as required.
   1) Prevention, close monitoring, and/or correction of electrolyte imbalance
   2) Prevention, close monitoring, and/or correction of hypoglycemia or hyperglycemia
   3) Prevention, close monitoring, and/or correction of myocardial stunning with

inotropic agents, fluid management, and/or intraaortic balloon pump (IABP)
  4) Prevention, close monitoring, and/or correction of acute renal injury with fluid management and renal replacement therapy
  5) Prevention, close monitoring, and/or correction of acute brain injury
    a) Avoidance of calcium, which has been shown to cause cerebral vessel spasm
    b) Avoidance of dextrose in water: use isotonic normal saline rather than D_5W; the dextrose in D_5W is quickly metabolized to leave only hypotonic water; this contributes to hypoosmolality and potentially cerebral edema
    c) Positioning: Elevate head of bed 30 degrees; avoid neck flexion or rotation; avoid hip flexion
    d) Increased cerebral perfusion pressure: Increase MAP and decrease intracranial pressure (ICP) as indicated; the following pharmacologic agents may be used:
      i) Analgesics to reduce pain
      ii) Anticonvulsants (e.g., phenytoin [Dilantin]) to prevent seizures
      iii) Isotonic or hypertonic solutions
      iv) Sedatives and muscle paralytics (e.g., pancuronium [Pavulon]) to decrease cerebral oxygen requirements
      v) Osmotic agents (e.g., mannitol [Osmitrol]) to increase cortical circulation and reduce cerebral edema
      vi) Calcium channel blockers (e.g., nimodipine [Nimotop]) to prevent cerebral vasospasm
      vii) Steroid (e.g., methylprednisolone [Solu-Medrol]) to reduce cerebral edema

7. Monitor for complications of CPR
  a. Fracture of sternum, ribs
  b. Hemothorax
  c. Pneumothorax
  d. Laceration of abdominal viscera especially the liver
  e. Myocardial contusion
  f. Cardiac rupture
8. Special circumstance: cardiac arrest with hypothermia
  a. If body temperature is less than 95°F (35°C)
    1) Initial treatment
      a) Perform CPR.
      b) Defibrillate for the initial series of three shocks for ventricular fibrillation or pulseless ventricular tachycardia.
      c) Intubate and ventilate with warm, humidified oxygen.
      d) Obtain IV access and administer warmed IV saline.
  b. If core temperature is less than 86°F (30°C)
    1) Continue CPR but withhold IV medications.
    2) Continue with warm inspired oxygen and warm IV fluids.
    3) Also peritoneal lavage with warm saline, extracorporeal rewarming, and esophageal rewarming tubes may be used.
  c. If core temperature is greater than 86°F (30°C)
    1) Continue CPR and administer IV medications but space longer than usual ACLS intervals.
    2) Repeat defibrillation for pulseless VT or VF as core temperature rise above 95°F.

Psychosocial Considerations

1. The patient
  a. During the resuscitation
    1) Touch the patient's hand and talk to them during the resuscitation efforts.
    2) Maintain the patient's modesty and dignity during the resuscitation efforts with drapes, curtains, and doors; ensure that all team members are respectful of the patient.
  b. After the resuscitation
    1) Patients frequently (~40%) have near-death experience during cardiac arrest but are frequently reluctant to discuss it.
      a) As the patient regains consciousness, assure them that they are not alone; reorient the patient to person, place, and time.
      b) Consider asking the patient if he or she remembers anything that occurred during the time their heart was stopped.
  c. If the resuscitation efforts are unsuccessful: Provide respectful and culturally sensitive care of the body.
2. The family
  a. Need for information
    1) If the patient's condition has been worsening, the family should be informed of the worsening condition.
    2) If the cardiopulmonary arrest was sudden, they should be informed about what has happened, what is being done, and an estimate of how long it may be before more information will be available.
      a) If information must be conveyed by telephone, they should be told that the situation is serious but not told of a death by telephone.
  b. Need for privacy
    1) Escort the family to a family conference room where they can grieve apart from other visitors but do not leave them alone.
    2) Ask if someone, such as a religious leader or a family member or friend, can be telephoned; offer to call someone from

pastoral services or have a social worker or a volunteer to be there with them.
    3) Allow the family to "tell their story" but do not give inappropriate reassurance.
    4) Be honest; do not give inappropriate reassurance but be hopeful, warm, and caring.
  c. Family presence during cardiopulmonary arrest is being advocated today as part of holistic care.
    1) The family's wishes should be adhered to if they do not conflict with the wishes of the patient.
    2) Consideration must be given to the family members' coping abilities.
    3) If a family member (generally limited to one member) desires to be present during resuscitation efforts:
      a) Prepare the family members for what to expect.
      b) Drape the patient appropriately.
      c) Set limits prior to entering the room; explain where they may stand and if they may touch the patient, such as hold the patient's hand.
      d) If the patient is not responding to resuscitation efforts and death is imminent, allow the family member time to talk to the patient.
      e) If the code team asks the family member to leave, escort him or her out, and make sure that someone stays with the family member.
  d. If resuscitation efforts are successful, allow family visitation as soon as possible.
  e. If the resuscitation efforts are unsuccessful:
    1) The family is usually informed of the patient's death by the physician.
    2) Express your sympathy.
    3) Answer whatever questions the family asks.
    4) Ask the family members if they desire to see the body and prepare them for what they will see.
    5) Prepare the body for visitation by discarding trash and removing clutter; remove the endotracheal tube if legally acceptable (i.e., not a coroner's case) and remove any blood from the face and hands.
    6) Place a couple of chairs close to the body and escort the family to the bedside; stay with them.
    7) Contact the organ transplant coordinator.
3. Other patients
  a. Screen the patient being resuscitated from other patients.
  b. Make sure that other patients are being cared for during resuscitation efforts on a patient.
4. The staff
  a. Ensure constructively critical multidisciplinary debriefing of the resuscitation efforts aids in quality improvement, team building, and stress reduction.
    1) Performance of the team as a team; critique of the poor performance of an individual member should not occur in a group setting
    2) Adequacy of supplies and equipment
  b. Counseling services should be available for staff.

Evaluation

1. Patient airway, adequate oxygenation (i.e., normal PaO_2, SpO_2, SaO_2) and ventilation (i.e., normal $PaCO_2$)
2. Absence of clinical indications of respiratory distress
3. Stable cardiac rate and rhythm
4. Stable hemodynamic status
5. Alert and oriented with no neurologic deficit
6. Control of chest pain, discomfort, or dyspnea

Dysrhythmias and Blocks

Definitions

1. Dysrhythmia: any cardiac rhythm other than sinus rhythm at a normal rate
  a. Sinus
  b. Atrial
  c. Junctional
  d. Ventricular
2. Block: failure of an intrinsic impulse to be conducted through the conduction system
  a. AV blocks: differentiation of degrees and types of blocks (Figure 3-4)
  b. Bundle branch blocks
    1) Left bundle branch block
      a) Hemiblocks: blockage of one of the two major branches of the LBB; these are diagnosed by axis deviation and exclusion of other causes
        i) Left anterior hemiblock
        ii) Left posterior hemiblock
    2) Right bundle branch block

Etiology

1. General
  a. Congenital
    1) Long QT syndrome
      a) Two types with separate gene affected
        i) Romano-Ward syndrome
        ii) Lange-Nielsen syndrome: associated with deafness
      b) Manifestations
        i) ECG characteristics: prolonged QT interval; sustained or nonsustained torsades de pointes
        ii) Loss of consciousness, seizures, or cardiac arrest
    2) Brugada syndrome
      a) Autosomal dominant pattern in 50% of cases; more common in Southeast Asians and Japanese
      b) Manifestations
        i) ECG characteristics

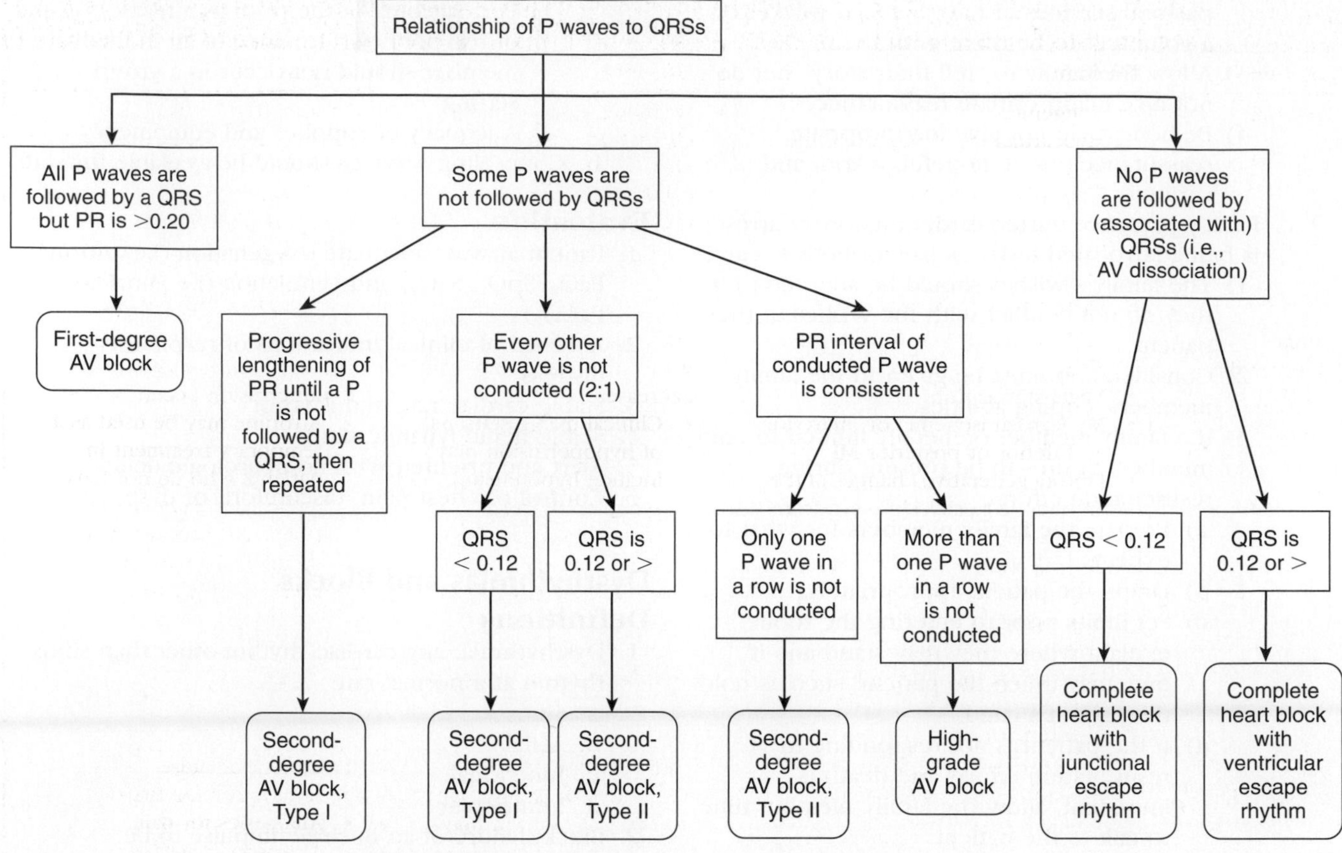

Figure 3-4 Differentiation of degrees and types of AV block.

(a) ST segment elevation and negative T wave in leads V_1 and V_2

(b) RBBB

(c) Prolonged PR interval

ii) Sudden cardiac arrest may occur as a result of polymorphic ventricular tachycardia and ventricular fibrillation; dysrhythmias may be triggered by: Antidysrhythmics (IA, IC, or III) which prolong the QT interval; antimalarials; antidepressants (e.g., tricyclics such as amitriptyline [Elavil]); fever; hyperglycemia; cocaine; or lithium

3) Accessory pathways
   a) Wolff-Parkinson-White (WPW) syndrome
   b) Long-Ganong-Levine syndrome
   c) Mahaim fibers

b. Myocardial ischemia or infarction

c. Hypoxemia/hypoxia

d. Electrolyte imbalance

e. Acid-base imbalance

f. Sympathetic nervous system stimulation via endogenous catecholamines or sympathomimetic drugs (e.g., epinephrine, dopamine)

g. Parasympathetic (i.e., vagal) stimulation

h. Drug effects or toxicity

1) "Holiday heart" syndrome caused by excessive alcohol consumption; this binge drinking may cause acute dysrhythmias, usually a supraventricular tachycardia

2. Etiology specific to each dysrhythmia (Table 3-1)

Pathophysiology: Arrhythmogenic Mechanisms

1. Problems with impulse formation
   a. Altered automaticity
      1) Enhanced automaticity
         a) Abnormal condition of latent pacemaker cells in which their firing rate is increased beyond their inherent rate (even nonpacemaker cells may depolarize spontaneously)
         b) Resting membrane potential is less negative or threshold potential is lower, increasing the chance of depolarization.
         c) Caused by:
            i) Hypoxia
            ii) Hypercapnia
            iii) Ischemia, infarction
            iv) Hypokalemia, hypocalcemia
            v) Catecholamines
            vi) Hyperthermia
            vii) Digitalis toxicity
            viii) Stretching of the heart muscle

Text continued on p. 126

Table 3-1 Basic Dysrhythmia and Block Management

Rhythm	Etiology	Significance	Treatment

General	• Congenital
	• Myocardial ischemia, infarction
	• Hypoxia
	• Electrolyte imbalance
	• Acid-base imbalance
	• Sympathetic or parasympathetic stimulation
	• Drug effect or toxicity
		• Dependent on patient's clinical presentation
		• Monitor for clinical manifestations of hypoperfusion
			• Treatment of cause
			• General emergency management for any symptomatic patient
			  • Oxygen
			  • Intravenous access
			  • Multiple-lead ECG if rhythm interpretation requires or if ischemia is suspected

Sinus bradycardia	• Athletic heart
	• Sleep
	• Vagal stimulation
	• Myocardial ischemia or infarction
	  • Inferior or posterior MI
	• Fibrodegenerative changes of the SA node (e.g., sick sinus syndrome)
	• Increased ICP
	• Hypothermia
	• Hypothyroidism
	• Neurogenic shock
	• Cervical or mediastinal tumor
	• Drug effect: digitalis; beta-blockers; calcium channel blockers; opiates
		• Depends on rate
		• If too slow, cardiac output decreases
		  • Clinical manifestations of hypoperfusion may include hypotension, syncope, dyspnea, change in level of consciousness, chest pain, HF, anxiety
		  • Escape beats (atrial, junctional, or ventricular) may occur
			• None if asymptomatic
			• If clinical manifestations of hypoperfusion occur:
			  • Atropine may be used as a temporary treatment in patients who do not have myocardial ischemia
			  • Pacemaker; dopamine or epinephrine may also be used in some cases

Sinus tachycardia	• SNS stimulation caused by psychological or physiologic stressors (e.g., stress, fear, anxiety, pain, anger, infection, exercise, dehydration)
	• Hypoxia
	• Anemia
	• Myocardial ischemia or infarction
	  • Anterior MI
	• Hypovolemia or hypervolemia
	• Shock
	• Hyperthyroidism
	• Heart failure
	• Inflammatory heart disease
	• Pulmonary embolism
	• Fibrodegenerative changes (e.g., sick sinus syndrome with tachy-brady manifestation)
	• Drug effect: epinephrine, isoproterenol; dopamine; atropine; caffeine; nicotine; amphetamines; cocaine; alcohol; aminophylline
		• Usually not significant except in patients with heart disease—then may cause angina, MI, HF, or shock	• Treatment of cause
			  • Anxiolytics for anxiety
			  • Analgesics for pain
			  • Antipyretics for fever
			  • Fluids for hypovolemia
			  • Treatment of HF
			  • Avoidance of stimulants
			  • Beta-blockers for hyperthyroidism
			• Usually does not require other treatment but the following may also be used:
			  • Oxygen
			  • Sedation and/or beta-blocker may be used to decrease or block the effects of catecholamines

Sinus dysrhythmia	• Normal; variation in sympathetic and parasympathetic stimulation during ventilation • In older patient, may indicate sick sinus syndrome • Digitalis toxicity	• Normal variation • May be seen in digitalis toxicity	• None • Discontinuance of digitalis if toxicity is cause
Sinus block (sinus exit block)	• Fibrodegenerative changes of the sinus node (e.g., sick sinus syndrome) • Ischemia of SA node (e.g., MI) • Vagal stimulation • Carotid sinus hypersensitivity • Inflammatory heart disease (e.g., myocarditis) • Drug toxicity: digitalis, quinidine, procainamide	• Depends on frequency and duration of pauses • If patient loses consciousness (Stokes-Adams attacks) very significant and requires treatment	• Discontinuance of digitalis if toxicity is cause • Atropine • Pacemaker if frequent pauses, long pauses, or if patient having syncope (i.e., Stokes-Adams attacks)

Continued

Table 3-1 Basic Dysrhythmia and Block Management—cont'd

Rhythm	Etiology	Significance	Treatment
Sinus arrest	• Fibrodegenerative changes (e.g., sick sinus syndrome) • Ischemia of SA node (e.g., MI) • Vagal stimulation • Carotid sinus hypersensitivity • Electrolyte imbalance • Drug toxicity: digitalis, beta-blockers	• Depends on frequency and duration of pauses • If patient loses consciousness (i.e., Stokes-Adams attacks) considered significant and requires treatment	• Discontinuance of digitalis if toxicity is cause • Atropine • Pacemaker if frequent pauses, long (greater than 3 seconds) pauses, or if patient having Stokes-Adams attacks
Premature atrial contractions	• SNS stimulation caused by psychological or physiologic stressors (e.g., stress, fear, anxiety, pain, anger, infection, exercise, dehydration) • Hypoxia • Myocardial ischemia or infarction • Valvular heart disease (e.g., mitral stenosis; mitral valve prolapse) • Heart failure • Inflammatory heart disease (e.g., myocarditis) • Electrolyte imbalance • Drug effect: caffeine; nicotine; alcohol • Drug toxicity: digitalis	• Usually benign but may precede atrial tachycardia, flutter, or fibrillation • Considered significant if greater than 6/min	• Treatment of cause • Usually no treatment necessary; but if frequent, treatment may include digitalis, quinidine, propranolol, beta-blockers, calcium channel blockers, or anxiolytics
Wandering atrial pacemaker	• Vagal stimulation • Sinus bradycardia • Digitalis toxicity	• May represent multiple atrial escape beats	• Usually none needed • Discontinuance of digitalis if toxicity is suspected • Atropine may be used to increase slow sinus rate

Atrial tachycardia (Paroxysmal atrial tachycardia [PAT] refers to the sudden interruption of sinus rhythm by a rapid ectopic focus—starts and ends abruptly)	• SNS stimulation caused by psychological or physiologic stressors (e.g., stress, fear, anxiety, pain, anger, infection, exercise, dehydration)
	• Hypoxia
	• Myocardial ischemia or infarction
	• Valvular heart disease (e.g., mitral valve prolapse)
	• Chronic obstructive pulmonary disease
	• Hyperthyroidism
	• Inflammatory heart disease (e.g., myocarditis)
	• Wolff-Parkinson-White syndrome
	• Drug effect: caffeine; nicotine; alcohol
	• Drug toxicity: digitalis (frequently PAT with block)
		• Patient may experience palpitations and clinical manifestations of hypoperfusion (e.g., hypotension, syncope, chest pain, HF) because diastolic filling time and preload is greatly reduced
		• Myocardial oxygen consumption is increased and myocardial oxygen supply is decreased so myocardial ischemia may occur or worsen
			• Depends on patient's tolerance, cause, and history of previous attacks
			• Discontinuance of digitalis if toxicity is suspected
			• Initial treatment: vagal stimulation; adenosine; if the rhythm persists, continue with the following:
			  • Calcium channel blockers (e.g., diltiazem [Cardizem], verapamil [Calan])
			  • Beta-blockers
			  • Digoxin if not the cause
			  • Synchronized cardioversion
			• Other considerations
			  • Right atrial pacing
			  • Ablation may be indicated for recurrent AV nodal reentrant tachycardia
			• NOTE: if QRS is wide (e.g., associated with WPW): do NOT use adenosine, beta-blockers, calcium channel blockers, or digoxin; preferred agent is amiodarone; if WPW, ablation is preferred long-term treatment

Multifocal atrial tachycardia (may also be called chaotic atrial rhythm)	• Pulmonary hypertension (e.g., COPD, pulmonary embolism) • Valvular heart disease • Heart failure • Electrolyte imbalance • Drug toxicity: digitalis	• Demonstrates atrial irritability which may lead to atrial tachycardia, flutter, fibrillation	• Treatment of cause: electrolyte replacement, treatment of heart failure, etc. • Discontinuance of digitalis if toxicity is suspected • If normal LV function: verapamil, beta-blocker, amiodarone, digoxin, flecainide, propafenone • If abnormal LV function: amiodarone, diltiazem, digoxin

Table 3-1 Basic Dysrhythmia and Block Management—cont'd

Rhythm	Etiology	Significance	Treatment

Atrial fibrillation	• Myocardial ischemia or infarction
	  • Especially anterior MI
	• Valvular heart disease (e.g., mitral or tricuspid stenosis or regurgitation)
	• Heart failure
	• Cardiomyopathy
	• Hyperthyroidism
	• Inflammatory heart disease (e.g., pericarditis)
	• Hypertension
	• Postcardiotomy
	• Pulmonary hypertension (e.g., COPD, pulmonary embolism)
	• Wolff-Parkinson-White syndrome
	• Drug effect: alcohol
		• No effective atrial contraction, so loss of atrial kick
		• Mural thrombi formation predisposes to emboli
		• Significance varies greatly on rate: may cause clinical manifestations of hypoperfusion (e.g., hypotension, syncope, chest pain, HF)
			• Rate control
			  • Normal LV function: beta-blocker or calcium channel blocker for rate control at rest and during exercise; digoxin as a second-line drug (only controls rate at rest)
			  • Abnormal LV function: digoxin, diltiazem, or amiodarone
			• Though no additional treatment is required acutely if rate is controlled (between 60-100/min), it is desirable to actually convert the AF to NSR if possible to reduce the risk of stroke and increase ventricular diastolic filling volume and cardiac output (considered rhythm control and maintenance)
			  • Normal LV function with duration less than 48 hours: cardioversion or amiodarone, ibutilide, dofetilide, procainamide, disopyramide, flecainide, propafenone, sotalol
			  • Abnormal LV function of less than 48-hour duration: cardioversion or amiodarone
			  • Duration greater than 48 hours or unknown duration: anticoagulation with INR 2-3 for 3 weeks followed by cardioversion
			• If slow ventricular response rate: atropine or pacemaker may be needed
			  • Digitalis should be considered as cause of slow ventricular response rate; withhold if digitalis is cause
			• NOTE: If associated with WPW, do NOT use adenosine, calcium channel blockers, or digoxin; preferred agent is amiodarone
			• Other nonacute considerations
			  • Overdrive pacing
			  • Implantable atrial defibrillator
			  • Ablation or maze procedure may be performed
			• Long-term anticoagulation is needed for chronic AF to prevent mural thrombi and risk for embolic stroke; desirable INR 2-3

Continued

Table 3-1 Basic Dysrhythmia and Block Management—cont'd

Rhythm	Etiology	Significance	Treatment
Atrial flutter	• Myocardial ischemia or infarction • Valvular heart disease • Heart failure • Cardiomyopathy • Hyperthyroidism • Inflammatory heart disease (e.g., pericarditis) • Hypertension • Postcardiotomy • Pulmonary hypertension (e.g., COPD, pulmonary embolus) • Drug effect: alcohol • Drug toxicity: digitalis	• No effectiveness of atrial contraction • Significance varies greatly depending on rate • If rate is very rapid may cause clinical manifestations of hypoperfusion (e.g., hypotension, syncope, chest pain, HF) because diastolic filling time and preload is greatly reduced	• As for atrial fibrillation • Though adenosine is not indicated for treatment of atrial flutter, it may slow the rhythm enough to recognize the flutter waves • Anticoagulation may be prescribed for atrial flutter, but the risk of mural thrombi and stroke is considered lower than for atrial fibrillation
Premature junctional contraction	• SNS stimulation caused by psychological or physiologic stressors (e.g., stress, fear, anxiety, pain, anger, infection, exercise, dehydration) • Hypoxia • Myocardial ischemia or infarction • Especially inferior MI • Valvular heart disease • Heart failure • Electrolyte imbalance • Drug effect: nicotine; caffeine; alcohol • Drug toxicity: digitalis • Also etiology as for PACs	• Usually benign but may predispose to junctional tachycardia if frequent	• Usually none necessary but sedation or beta-blockers may be used • Discontinuance of digitalis if toxicity is cause • Sedation • Beta-blockers
Junctional escape rhythm	• Vagal stimulation • SA block • Complete AV block • Myocardial ischemia or infarction • Valvular heart disease • Hypoxia • Postcardiotomy • Drug toxicity: digitalis	• Protects patient from asystole • Do not suppress	• Note that this is *not* irritability; it is escape, so it is treated by accelerating the sinus node • Atropine • Pacemaker may be needed • Discontinuance of digitalis if digitalis toxicity is cause; it is a frequent cause of this rhythm
Accelerated junctional rhythm	• Vagal stimulation • SA block • Complete AV block • Myocardial ischemia or infarction • Reperfusion of myocardium • Hypoxia • Inflammatory heart disease (e.g., myocarditis) • Postcardiotomy • Drug toxicity: digitalis	• Protects patient from asystole • Do not suppress	• Treat failure of sinus node • Discontinuance of digitalis if digitalis toxicity is cause; it is a frequent cause of this rhythm
Junctional tachycardia	• Myocardial ischemia or infarction • Reperfusion of myocardium • Inflammatory heart disease • Postcardiotomy • Drug toxicity: digitalis, theophylline	• Usually stops spontaneously and is usually tolerated well	• Treat cause • Discontinuance of digitalis if digitalis toxicity is cause • Vagal stimulation • Adenosine • Amiodarone • Beta-blockers or calcium channel blockers if normal LV function

Table 3-1 Basic Dysrhythmia and Block Management—cont'd

Rhythm	Etiology	Significance	Treatment
First degree AV block	• Normal variation • Congenital • Fibrodegenerative changes of the conduction system • Vagal stimulation • Myocardial ischemia or infarction • Myocardial contusion • Cardiomyopathy • Postcardiotomy • Inflammatory heart disease (e.g., myocarditis) • Electrolyte imbalance • Drug toxicity: digitalis; beta-blockers; calcium channel blockers	• Relatively benign but may progress to second or third degree block	• Close observation for progression of block • Discontinuance of digitalis if digitalis toxicity is cause • Drugs or pacemaker not needed unless there is also a sinus bradycardia with hypoperfusion
Second degree AV block type I (previously referred to as Mobitz I; also known as Wenckebach)	• Fibrodegenerative changes of the conduction system • Myocardial ischemia or infarction • Inferior or posterior MI • Postcardiotomy • Inflammatory heart disease • Myocardial contusion • Drug toxicity: digitalis; beta-blockers; calcium channel blockers	• Block is at AV node • Occurs more often in inferior MIs (RCA lesion) • Relatively benign: usually transient, and does not usually progress to complete heart block	• Does not usually require treatment • Close monitoring for progression of block • Discontinuance of digitalis if digitalis toxicity is cause • Transvenous pacemaker or atropine may be used if rate slow and patient symptomatic
Second degree AV block type II (previously referred to as Mobitz II)	• Myocardial ischemia or infarction • Anterior MI • Hypertension • Valvular heart disease • Conduction system fibrosis • Inflammatory heart disease (e.g., myocarditis) • Postcardiotomy • Myocardial contusion	• Block is at bundle of His which accounts for the slight widening of the QRS complex • Occurs more often in anterior MIs (LAD lesion) • Ominous as it often progresses to CHB	• Atropine may be used but is not usually helpful • Transcutaneous or transvenous pacemaker

Third degree (or complete) AV block	• Myocardial ischemia or infarction
	• Conduction system fibrosis
	• Inflammatory heart disease
	• Postcardiotomy
	• Myocardial contusion
	• Hypoxia
	• Electrolyte imbalance
	• Drug toxicity: digitalis
		• If no escape rhythm is established, the patient has ventricular asystole	• Close observation for clinical manifestations of hypoperfusion if inferior MI with junctional escape rhythm
			• Atropine may be used but is not usually helpful
			• Pacemaker especially if:
			  • Anterior MI
			  • Inferior MI with ventricular escape rhythm

Left bundle branch block (LBBB)	• Myocardial ischemia or infarction • Anterior MI • Fibrodegenerative changes of the conduction system • Postcardiotomy	• Bifascicular block considered more serious than RBBB especially in presence of acute MI • Monitor this patient closely during pulmonary artery catheter insertion because RBBB may occur causing trifascicular block	• New LBBB in acute MI may be treated with prophylactic pacemaker especially if an AV block is also present
Right bundle branch block (RBBB)	• Myocardial ischemia or infarction • Anterior or inferior MI • Fibrodegenerative changes of the conduction system • Postcardiotomy • Pulmonary artery catheter insertion • Acute pulmonary embolus	• None; cardiac output is not affected by delayed ventricular depolarization (wide QRS)	• Close monitoring for development of LBBB

Continued

Table 3-1 Basic Dysrhythmia and Block Management—cont'd

Rhythm	Etiology	Significance	Treatment

Premature ventricular contraction	• SNS stimulation caused by psychological or physiologic stressors (e.g., stress, fear, anxiety, pain, anger, infection, exercise, dehydration or adrenergic drugs [e.g., epinephrine, dopamine])
	• Hypoxia
	• Acidosis
	• Myocardial ischemia or infarction
	• Reperfusion of myocardium
	• Heart failure
	• Cardiomyopathy
	• Myocardial contusion
	• Ventricular aneurysm
	• Valvular heart disease
	• Electrolyte imbalance
	• Drugs: caffeine, nicotine, alcohol, cocaine
	• Drug toxicity: digitalis; aminophylline
		• PVCs of most significance: may predispose to VT or VF
		  • Frequent (greater than 6/min)
		  • Bigeminal
		  • Multifocal
		  • R on T phenomenon
		  • Couplets
		  • Runs of ventricular tachycardia (3 or more PVCs in a row)
		• Pulse amplitude of PVC is reduced due to decreased filling time
			• Treatment of cause (e.g., oxygen, electrolyte replacement, discontinue digitalis)
			• No treatment required if only occasional, unifocal, and does not occur on previous T wave (R on T)
			• If frequent, multifocal, R on T, couplets, or runs of VT or symptomatic: amiodarone, lidocaine, beta-blockers

Monomorphic ventricular tachycardia	• SNS stimulation caused by psychological or physiologic stressors (e.g., stress, fear, anxiety, pain, anger, infection, exercise, dehydration or adrenergic drugs [e.g., epinephrine, dopamine]) • Hypoxia • Acidosis • Myocardial ischemia or infarction • Reperfusion of myocardium • Cardiomyopathy • Myocardial contusion • Ventricular aneurysm • Valvular heart disease • Postcardiotomy • R on T PVC • Electrolyte imbalance • Drugs: caffeine, nicotine, alcohol, cocaine • Drug toxicity: digitalis	• Ominous as may progress to ventricular fibrillation • Symptoms depend on underlying heart disease, rate, and duration of VT • May cause angina, HF, shock	• Treatment of cause • If normal LV function: procainamide, amiodarone, lidocaine, sotalol • If impaired LV function: amiodarone, lidocaine, cardioversion • If having hypotension, chest pain, or pulmonary edema: immediate sedation and cardioversion • If pulseless: treat as VF (e.g., CPR, defibrillation, vasopressin or epinephrine, amiodarone, etc.)

Table 3-1 Basic Dysrhythmia and Block Management—cont'd

Rhythm	Etiology	Significance	Treatment

Polymorphic ventricular tachycardia (torsades de pointes if preceded by prolonged QT)	• Class IA antidysrhythmics (e.g., procainamide, quinidine, disopyramide) or class IC antidysrhythmics (e.g., flecainide, propafenone)
	• Class III antidysrhythmics (e.g., sotalol, amiodarone)
	• Tricyclic antidepressants (e.g., amitriptyline [Elavil])
	• Phenothiazines (e.g., chlorpromazine [Thorazine])
	• Organic insecticides
	• Electrolyte imbalance (especially hypomagnesemia, hypocalcemia, hypokalemia)
	• Congenital long QT syndrome or Brugada syndrome
	• Marked bradycardia
	• Hypothermia
	• Subarachnoid hemorrhage
		• No effective perfusion
		• May go into and out of this rhythm
			• Treatment of cause
			• Prevention of torsades de pointes: close monitoring of QT interval and discontinuance of any offending drug when QT prolongs to greater than half of the RR interval
			• Discontinuance of any offending drug if characteristic torsades pattern seen
			• If QRS normal:
			  • Electrolyte replacement
			  • Amiodarone, beta-blocker, lidocaine, procainamide, sotalol
			• If QRS prolonged (suggests torsades)
			  • Electrolyte replacement especially magnesium
			  • Overdrive pacing
			  • Isoproterenol
			  • Phenytoin
			  • Lidocaine
			• If impaired LV function: amiodarone, lidocaine, cardioversion

Ventricular fibrillation	• SNS stimulation caused by psychological or physiologic stressors (e.g., stress, fear, anxiety, pain, anger, infection, exercise, dehydration) or adrenergic drugs [e.g., epinephrine, dopamine]) • Hypoxia • Myocardial ischemia or infarction • R on T PVC • Electrical shock including microshock • Brugada syndrome (familial) • Drowning • Hypothermia • Drug toxicity: digitalis • Dying heart	• Lethal within 4-6 minutes • No cardiac output • Symptoms include: loss of consciousness, pulse, heart sounds, ventilation; BP; anoxic seizures	• CPR until defibrillator available and ready, then after defibrillation, and between successive defibrillation attempts • Immediate defibrillation (150-200 joules [biphasic energy], 360 joules [monophasic energy]) • Vasopressin or epinephrine • Intubation • Antidysrhythmics: amiodarone or lidocaine • Postresuscitation care

Idioventricular rhythm	• Vagal stimulation
	• Failure of higher pacemakers (e.g., ischemia or fibrosis of conduction system)
	• Myocardial ischemia or infarction
	• Third-degree AV block
	• Drug toxicity: digitalis
		• Protects the patient from asystole but very unreliable
		• Do not suppress
			• Acceleration of higher pacemakers with atropine
			• Pacemaker
			• If pulseless:
			  • CPR
			  • Epinephrine
			  • Pacemaker
			  • Consideration and treatment of causes

Accelerated idioventricular rhythm	• Failure of higher pacemakers (e.g., ischemia or fibrosis of conduction system) • Myocardial ischemia or infarction • Reperfusion of myocardium • Drug toxicity: digitalis	• Protects the patient from asystole but very unreliable • Do not suppress	• Acceleration of higher pacemakers with atropine • Pacemaker

Continued

Table 3-1 Basic Dysrhythmia and Block Management—cont'd

Rhythm	Etiology	Significance	Treatment

Asystole	• Vagal stimulation
	• Hypoxia
	• Acidosis
	• Shock
	• Myocardial ischemia or infarction
	• Third-degree AV block
	• Anaphylaxis
	• Hypothermia
	• Drug overdose
	• Dying heart
		• Lethal within 4-6 minutes
		• No cardiac output
		• Symptoms include: loss of consciousness, pulse, heart sounds, ventilation; BP; anoxic seizures
			• CPR
			• Epinephrine
			• Confirmation of rhythm in second lead to rule out ventricular fibrillation
			• Consideration of causes and treatment accordingly
			  • 5 Hs: hypovolemia, hypoxia, hydrogen ion (acidosis), hyper/hypokalemia, and hypothermia
			  • 5 Ts: tension pneumothorax, tamponade (cardiac), toxins, thrombosis (coronary), and thrombosis (pulmonary)

d) Cause of most atrial, junctional, and ventricular ectopic beats, accelerated junctional rhythm, accelerated idioventricular rhythm, and some ventricular tachycardia

2) Depressed automaticity
   a) Resting membrane potential is more negative or threshold potential is higher, decreasing the chance of depolarization.
   b) Caused by any of the following:
      i) Vagal stimulation
      ii) Hyperkalemia, hypercalcemia
      iii) Decreased catecholamines
      iv) Hypothermia
      v) Beta-blockers
   c) Cause of bradycardia or blocks

b. Triggered activity
   1) Repetitive ectopic firing caused by afterdepolarizations; an afterdepolarization is an abnormal electrical impulse that occurs during or after repolarization of an action potential
   2) If an afterdepolarization is strong enough to reach threshold, a triggered beat or rhythm occurs.
   3) This activity is not self-gencrating but is dependent on the preceding beat.
   4) They may be early or late.
      a) Early: occur when the QT is prolonged
         i) Caused by: prolongation of repolarization and effective refractory period
         ii) Example: torsades de pointes
      b) Delayed: the result of elevated intracellular calcium
         i) Caused by
            (a) Electrolyte imbalances
            (b) Catecholamines
         ii) Cause of tachycardias of digitalis toxicity

2. Problems with impulse conduction
   a. Reentry (Figure 3-5): the most common mechanism for tachydysrhythmias
      1) An impulse travels through an area of the myocardium and depolarizes it, but then reenters the same area to depolarize it again.
      2) Requirements
         a) An available circuit: Reentry can occur in areas of the heart where conduction velocity is abnormally slow.
         b) Unequal responsiveness of two segments of the circuit (i.e., delay in one limb of the circuit)
         c) An area of slowed conduction or unidirectional block
            i) Conduction must be slow enough to allow time for the previously stimulated area to recover the ability to conduct.
            ii) The area of unidirectional block provides a return pathway for the original stimulus to reenter a previously stimulated area and time to repolarize.
      3) Caused by:
         a) Myocardial ischemia or infarction
         b) Electrolyte imbalance
         c) Antidysrhythmic drugs
      4) Cause of any of the following:
         a) Some ectopy
         b) Some ventricular tachycardias
         c) Most supraventricular tachycardias
         d) Tachycardias seen with accessory pathways
   b. Accessory pathways (Figure 3-6)
      1) Lown-Ganong-Levine syndrome
         a) Caused by:
            i) AV nodal bypass tract
            ii) AV node smaller than normal

iii) Fibers running through AV node that do not have the built-in delay feature that nodal fibers have

b) Cause of:

i) History of palpitations

ii) Tachydysrhythmias with short PR, normal QRS

2) WPW syndrome

a) Caused by Kent bundle which bypasses the AV node

i) Type A: Kent bundle on left; R wave in V_1 with inverted T wave and depressed ST

ii) Type B: Kent bundle on right; QS in V_1 with upright T wave and elevated ST

b) Cause of:

i) Tachydysrhythmias

(a) History of palpitations

(b) Short PR, wide QRS with slurring of first portion of QRS (referred to as a *delta wave*) (Figure 3-7)

(c) QRS morphology during tachycardia

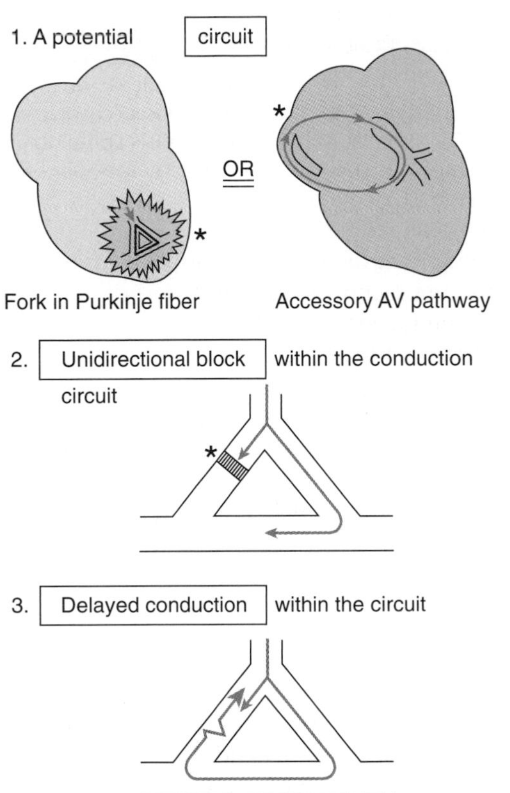

Figure 3-5 Reentry. Requirements for reentry include 1) a potential conduction circuit or circular conduction pathway, 2) a block or delay within part of the circuit, and 3) delayed conduction within the remainder of the circuit. *AV,* atrioventricular. (From Aehlert, B. [2011]. *ECGs made easy* [4th ed.]. St. Louis: Mosby.)

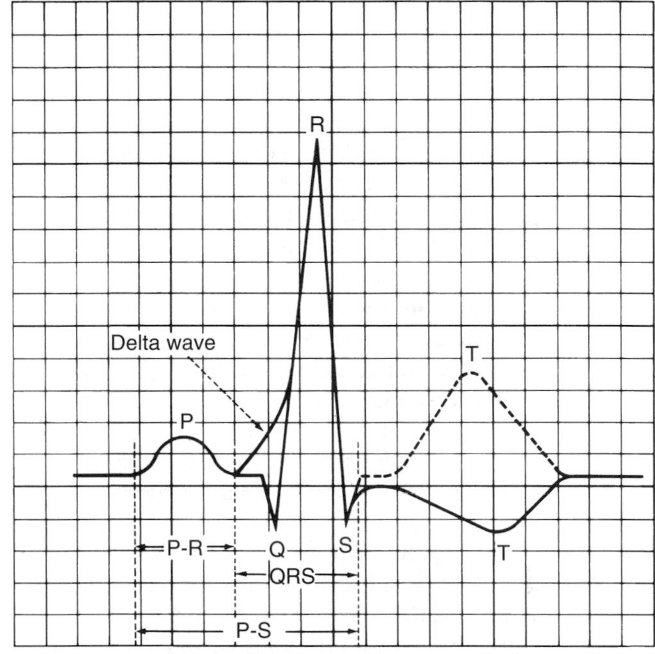

Figure 3-7 Wolff-Parkinson-White syndrome. Note the short PR interval, the delta wave, widened QRS complex, and T wave inversion characteristic of preexcitation. (From Kinney, M. R., et al. [1998]. *AACN's clinical reference for critical-care nursing* [4th ed.]. St. Louis: Mosby.)

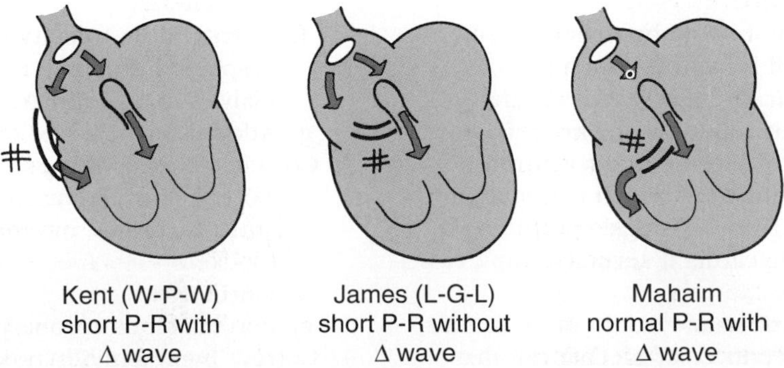

Figure 3-6 Accessory pathways. Location of accessory pathways and corresponding ECG characteristics. *L-G-L,* Lown-Ganong-Levine; *W-P-W,* Wolff-Parkinson-White. (From Aehlert, B. [2009]. *ECGs made easy* [3rd ed.]. St. Louis: Mosby.)

(i) Wide QRS: Sinus impulse may take accessory pathway around the mandatory delay in the AV node (referred to as *preexcitation*) causing severe supraventricular tachycardias with a wide QRS
(ii) Narrow QRS: Impulse may also take AV node but reenter via accessory pathway; narrow QRS

(d) Treatment
(i) Antidysrhythmics: amiodarone, flecainide, procainamide, propafenone, or sotalol
(ii) Cardioversion if drugs fail to convert
(iii) Avoid adenosine, calcium channel blockers, and digoxin.
(iv) Long-term treatment: ablation via catheter or surgically

3) Mahaim fibers
a) Caused by nodoventricular or fasciculoventricular fibers
b) Cause of:
i) Tachydysrhythmias
(a) History of palpitations
(b) Normal PR interval with LBBB pattern
ii) Normal PR, narrow QRS with rS in lead III when in sinus rhythm

c. Aberrant conduction
1) Aberrant conduction occurs most often when:
a) Rate is rapid.
b) Very premature atrial contractions
c) There are changes in cycle length (e.g., atrial fibrillation [QRS which ends a short cycle length after a long cycle length is likely to be conducted aberrantly is referred to as *Ashman's phenomenon*]).
2) Since one of the bundle branches (usually the right) is still refractory when a supraventricular impulse reaches it, the impulse must travel down the nonrefractory bundle and across to the other ventricle; this causes a wide QRS which is frequently mistaken for a PVC if a single complex or ventricular tachycardia if several complexes in a row
3) Unlike ectopy, aberrancy is no more serious than the supraventricular mechanism that caused it (e.g., atrial fibrillation with aberrancy is no more clinically significant than atrial fibrillation).
4) QRS morphology is the most important criterion in the differentiation between ectopy and aberrancy, but other criteria may also be helpful (Table 3-2); multiple-lead ECG is often helpful to identify P waves and in looking at the morphology of the QRS.
5) Ectopy is more common than aberrancy; if in doubt, always assume ectopy and treat accordingly.

Clinical Presentation

1. Anxiety, restlessness
2. Vertigo, syncope
3. Weakness, fatigue, activity intolerance
4. Palpitations
5. Chest pain
6. Clinical indications of LVF: dyspnea; S_3; crackles
7. Clinical indications of hypoperfusion (see Table 2-2 on page 26)
8. Diagnostic studies
   a. Electrocardiography: multiple-lead ECG
   b. Serum electrolyte levels
   c. Drug levels
   d. Arterial blood gases

Collaborative Management

1. Assess for clinical manifestations of hypoperfusion (see Table 2-2 on page 26): follow ACLS algorithms for lethal dysrhythmias (see Cardiopulmonary Arrest section of this chapter).
2. Treat etiology of the dysrhythmia; some examples include the following:
   a. Decrease psychological and physical stress.
   b. Correct ischemia/infarction if possible with reperfusion therapies such as percutaneous coronary intervention (PCI) or fibrinolytics.
   c. Correct hypoxemia and hypoxia with oxygen.
   d. Correct electrolyte imbalance with electrolyte replacement or restriction/dialysis.
   e. Correct acid-base imbalance by treating the cause.
      1) Improve oxygen delivery to the tissues if lactic acidosis
      2) Insulin and fluid administration for diabetic ketoacidosis
      3) Dialysis for renal failure with metabolic acidosis
   f. Correct drug toxicity by withholding the suspected drug and antidote (e.g., Digibind) or dialysis if appropriate.
   g. Administer beta-blockers for hyperthyroidism.
3. Correct ischemia if possible.
   a. Coronary artery vasodilators and/or antispasmodics: nitrates; calcium channel blockers
   b. Fibrinolytics
   c. Percutaneous coronary intervention
4. Correct hypoxemia/hypoxia
   a. Improve SaO_2 (e.g., oxygen, endotracheal intubation, mechanical ventilation, positive end-expiratory pressure [PEEP]).

Table 3-2 Differentiation between Ventricular Ectopy and Aberrancy

Features	Favoring Ventricular Ectopy	Favoring Supraventricular Origin with Aberrancy
Rate	• 130-150/min	• Greater than 150/min
Regularity	• Regular	• Irregular (because most likely to be atrial fibrillation)
P wave	• None or dissociated (AV dissociation) • Inverted P wave after QRS (retrograde conduction to atria)	• Premature
QRS width	• Greater than 0.14 seconds	• 0.12-0.14 seconds
QRS morphology	• Initial vector opposite normal beats • Precordial concordance (all QRSs V_1-V_6 positive or all QRSs V_1-V_6 negative) • QRS morphology similar to previously seen PVCs	• Initial vector same as normal beats
QRS morphology in V_1 NOTE: Upper case letters indicate large waves, lower case letters indicate small waves	• Monophasic R • Rr' with left peak taller • Biphasic qR • Biphasic Rs or rS	• Monophasic QS • Biphasic rS • Triphasic rSR' or rR'
QRS morphology in V_6 NOTE: Upper case letters indicate large waves, lower case letters indicate small waves	• Monophasic QS • Biphasic qR • Biphasic rS	• Monophasic R • Triphasic qRs
Fusion beats	• Yes	• No
Compensatory pause after single beat or at end of run	• Yes	• No
Axis	• Indeterminate or LAD of −30 or greater	• Normal or RAD
Patient history	• History of PVCs • History of heart disease	• History of PACs, atrial fibrillation • History of preexisting bundle branch block
Response to carotid massage	• No effect on ventricular rate	• Often causes at least temporary slowing of ventricular rate
BP	• Usually very low or absent (but may be normal)	• Moderately low or normal
Consciousness	• Frequently unconscious (but may be conscious)	• May complain of lightheadedness
Seizures	• Frequently present (but may be absent)	• Absent

   b. Improve cardiac output (e.g., inotropes, vasodilators, intraaortic balloon pump).
   c. Improve hemoglobin (e.g., blood).
5. Correct electrolyte imbalances.
   a. Replace deficient electrolytes.
   b. Decrease excessive electrolyte levels (e.g., electrolyte restriction, diuretics, ion exchange resins, dialysis).
6. Correct acidosis.
   a. Improve perfusion to correct metabolic acidosis caused by lactic acid.
   b. Initiate dialysis for patients with renal failure.
   c. Provide hydration and insulin therapy for patients in diabetic ketoacidosis.
   d. Improve ventilation to correct respiratory acidosis.
7. Eliminate cause of catecholamine release or block effects.
   a. Treat pain.
   b. Decrease anxiety with relaxation techniques and anxiolytics.
   c. Administer beta-blockers for cardioprotection as prescribed.
8. Initiate standing orders (e.g., IV, oxygen, multiple-lead ECG)
9. Initiate antidysrhythmic therapy as indicated by standing orders or as prescribed.
   a. Vaughan-Williams classification system (Table 3-3)
   b. Drugs and treatments of choice for each dysrhythmia (see Table 3-1)
      1) Information regarding indications, actions, dosage, contraindications, and adverse effects of selected antidysrhythmic agents (Table 3-4)
   c. Monitor closely for adverse effects of antidysrhythmic agents.

Table 3-3 Vaughan-Williams Antidysrhythmic Classification System

Class	Effect	Examples
IA	• Blocks sodium influx which depresses the rate of depolarization • Delays repolarization and prolongs action potential duration • Decreases contractility (negative inotrope) • Prolongs QT (torsades de pointes potential) and QRS duration	• Quinidine • Procainamide (Pronestyl) • Disopyramide (Norpace)
IB	• Blocks sodium influx during phase 0 which depresses the rate of depolarization • Accelerates repolarization and shortens action potential duration • Suppresses ventricular automaticity in ischemic tissue	• Lidocaine (Xylocaine) • Mexiletine (Mexitil) • Phenytoin (Dilantin)
IC	• Blocks sodium influx which depresses the rate of depolarization • Does not change repolarization and action potential duration • Has pronounced proarrhythmogenic potential	• Flecainide (Tambocor) • Propafenone (Rythmol)

II	• Depresses SA node automaticity
	• Increases refractory period of atrial and AV junctional tissue to slow conduction velocity
	• Shortens action potential duration
	• Inhibits sympathetic activity (i.e., blocks beta receptors)
	• Reduces atrial and ventricular contractility
		• Beta-blockers
		  • Propranolol (Inderal)
		  • Esmolol (Brevibloc)
		  • Acebutolol (Sectral)
		  • Sotalol (Betapace) (both II and III)

III	• Blocks potassium movement during phase III • Delays repolarization and increases action potential duration • Prolongs effective refractory period	• Amiodarone (Cordarone) • Sotalol (Betapace) (both II and III) • Ibutilide (Corvert) • Dofetilide (Tikosyn)

IV	• Blocks calcium movement during phase II
	• Depresses automaticity in the SA and AV nodes
	• Prolongs the conduction time in the AV junction and increases the refractory period at the AV junction
	• Decreases contractility
		• Calcium channel blockers
		  • Verapamil (Calan)
		  • Diltiazem (Cardizem)

Misc.	• Blocks reentry mechanism • Shortens action potential of atrial tissue with little or no effect on action potential of ventricle • Prolongs AV nodal refractory period • Decreases SA node automaticity and slows sinus rate	• Adenosine (Adenocard)
Misc.	• Blocks parasympathetic nervous system effects to increase SA node firing rate and improve AV nodal conduction	• Atropine
Misc.	• Slows conduction through AV node • Prolongs AV nodal refractory period • Decreases SA node automaticity and slows sinus rate	• Digoxin

10. Utilize electrical therapies as indicated.
    a. Cardioversion
        1) Uses
            a) Urgent cardioversion is used for tachydysrhythmias (other than sinus) that is rapid enough to cause hemodynamic compromise or that has not responded to antidysrhythmic drug therapy.
            b) Elective cardioversion is performed for tachydysrhythmias that are reasonably well-tolerated hemodynamically but have not responded to antidysrhythmic drug therapy.
        2) Contraindications
            a) Tachydysrhythmias that result from digitalis toxicity
            b) Nonsustained tachydysrhythmias
            c) Long-standing atrial fibrillation
            d) Atrial fibrillation with normal or slow ventricular rate in the absence of AV nodal blocking drugs
            e) Multifocal atrial tachycardia
        3) Method: as for defibrillation except:
            a) Conscious patients should be sedated with diazepam (Valium), lorazepam (Ativan), or midazolam (Versed).
            b) Elective procedures should be preceded by at least a 6-hour fast.
            c) Anterior-posterior electrode placement is preferable for cardioversion of atrial fibrillation.
            d) Emergency equipment and drugs must be available.
            e) Synchronizer switch is on so that charge is delivered only during QRS, avoiding the descending limb of the T wave.
            f) Voltage is from 50-200 joules (Neumar et al., 2010).
                i) Narrow and regular: 50-100 J
                ii) Narrow and irregular: 120-200 J biphasic or 200 J monophasic
                iii) Wide and regular: 100 J
                iv) Wide and irregular: Defibrillate with 120-200 J biphasic or 360 J

Text continued on p. 142

Table 3-4 Selected Antidysrhythmic Agents

Drug	Classification/ Actions	Indications	Administration	Adverse Effects	Nursing Implications
Procainamide hydrochloride (Pronestyl)	**Class IA Antidysrhythmic** • Increases atrial refractoriness • Decreases automaticity, conductivity, contractility • Causes peripheral vasodilation	• Supraventricular dysrhythmias • Ventricular dysrhythmias	• PO 0.5-1 g every 4-6 hours • IM 250-500 mg every 4-6 hours • IV injection: 50-100 mg every 5 minutes • Stop injections and start maintenance infusion when suppression of dysrhythmia; widening of QRS by 50%; hypotension; or a total of 17 mg/kg occur • IV infusion: mix 2 g in 500 mL (4 mg/mL) and infuse at 1-4 mg/min • Therapeutic blood level 3-10 mcg/mL	• Bradycardia • Hypotension with IV administration • AV block • Dysrhythmias including torsades de pointes • Anorexia, nausea, vomiting, abdominal pain, diarrhea • Hepatic dysfunction • Bitter taste • Rash, urticaria • Fever • Mental depression • Hallucinations • Seizures • Bone marrow depression, thrombocytopenia • Worsening HF • Lupus-like syndrome	• Monitor BP, HR, ECG • ECG effects include increased PR interval, QRS width, and QT interval • Note contraindications: known hypersensitivity, myasthenia gravis, AV block • Use cautiously in renal disease, liver disease, HF, respiratory depression, patient receiving digitalis • Administer PO drug with food • Instruct patient to report fever, rash, muscle pain, bruising or bleeding, diarrhea, chest pain
Lidocaine hydrochloride (Xylocaine)	**Class IB Antidysrhythmic** • Decreases ventricular automaticity and excitability • Increases ventricular fibrillation threshold	• Ventricular dysrhythmias	• IV injection: • VF: 1.5 mg/kg repeated every 3-5 minutes • VT: 1 mg/kg repeated every 5-10 minutes • Maximum: 3 mg/kg • IV infusion: mix 2 g in 500 mL (4 mg/mL) and infuse at 1-4 mg/min • Therapeutic blood level: 2-5 mcg/mL	• Hypotension • SA arrest • AV block • Nausea, vomiting • Tremors • Restlessness • Lightheadedness • Anaphylaxis *Clinical indications of toxicity (in relative order of occurrence)* • Perioral paresthesias • Feelings of dissociation • Dizziness • Drowsiness • Euphoria • Mild agitation • Dysarthria • Hearing impairment • Disorientation • Confusion • Muscle twitching • Seizures • Respiratory arrest	• Monitor BP, HR, ECG • Note contraindications: known hypersensitivity, AV block, supraventricular dysrhythmias, sick sinus syndrome • Use cautiously in liver disease, HF, respiratory depression, malignant hyperthermia, and in older adults • Note that toxicity incidence is increased if patient has HF or liver disease, has low lean body mass or is elderly, or is concurrently taking cimetidine (Tagamet) or beta-blocker • Note that the administration of prophylactic lidocaine after MI is no longer recommended; while the incidence of ventricular fibrillation is decreased, the incidence of asystole is increased

Continued

Table 3-4 Selected Antidysrhythmic Agents—cont'd

Drug	Classification/ Actions	Indications	Administration	Adverse Effects	Nursing Implications
Mexiletine (Mexitil)	**Class IB Antidysrhythmic** • Decreases ventricular automaticity and excitability • Increases ventricular fibrillation threshold	• Life-threatening ventricular dysrhythmias	• PO: initial dose of 200-400 mg followed by 200-400 bid, tid, or qid; maximum 1200 mg/day	• Proarrhythmia including PVCs, ventricular tachycardia, torsades de pointes, PACs, supraventricular tachycardia, bradycardia, AV block, bundle branch block • Hypotension • Nausea, vomiting • Diarrhea or constipation • Elevated liver enzymes • Palpitations • Chest pain • Dyspnea • Headache • Paresthesia, tremors, nystagmus, ataxia, dysarthria • Tinnitus • Blurred vision • Dizziness • Drowsiness, insomnia • Confusion • Seizures	• Monitor HR, BP, ECG • Note contraindications: second- or third-degree block or sick sinus syndrome without pacemaker, cardiogenic shock • Administer with meals to decrease GI adverse effects • Note that risk of toxicity is greater if patient is concurrently receiving cimetidine (Tagamet) or beta-blocker; dosage is adjusted in heart failure and liver disease • Monitor closely for clinical indications of toxicity: tremor; dizziness; ataxia; nystagmus
Flecainide (Tambocor)	**Class IC Antidysrhythmic** • Blocks sodium influx during phase 0 which depresses the rate of depolarization • Does not change repolarization and action potential duration	• Life-threatening or refractory ventricular dysrhythmias • Atrial or ventricular dysrhythmias that do not respond to other drugs	• PO: 50-200 mg twice daily; maximum dose 400 mg/day	• Proarrhythmia including PVCs, ventricular tachycardia, torsades de pointes, PACs, supraventricular tachycardia, bradycardia, SA block or arrest, AV block, bundle branch block • Nausea, vomiting, abdominal pain, constipation • Dyspnea • Chest pain • Headache • Drowsiness • Dizziness • Blurred vision • Tremor • Dry mouth	• Monitor HR, BP, ECG • Report widening of QRS of greater than 25% • Monitor closely for heart failure • Note contraindications: known hypersensitivity, second- or third-degree AV block, cardiogenic shock • Use cautiously in heart failure, SA or bifascicular blocks or sick sinus syndrome without a pacemaker, renal disease, liver disease, myasthenia gravis • Use cautiously in patient also receiving another negative inotropic agent (e.g., verapamil, procainamide, beta-blocker) • Correct electrolyte imbalance prior to therapy if possible

Propafenone (Rythmol)	**Class IC Antidysrhythmic** • Blocks sodium influx during phase 0 which depresses the rate of depolarization • Does not change repolarization and action potential duration	• Life-threatening or refractory ventricular dysrhythmias • Atrial fibrillation	• PO: 150-300 mg tid; maximum 900 mg/day	• Proarrhythmia including PVCs, ventricular tachycardia, torsades de pointes, PACs, supraventricular tachycardia, bradycardia, SA block or arrest, AV block, bundle branch block • AV block • Nausea, vomiting, constipation • Heart failure • Dyspnea, bronchospasm • Dizziness • Diplopia • Paresthesia • Headache • Bitter or metallic taste • Leukopenia, agranulocytosis, thrombocytopenia, anemia • Bruising	• Monitor HR, BP, ECG • Report widening of QRS of greater than 25% • Monitor closely for clinical indications of heart failure • Note contraindications: heart failure, cardiogenic shock, SA, AV, bifascicular blocks or sick sinus syndrome without a pacemaker, myasthenia gravis, COPD, hypotension • Use cautiously in patients with renal or liver disease; dosage may be adjusted • Use cautiously if the patient is also receiving another negative inotropic agent (e.g., verapamil, procainamide, beta-blocker) • Use cautiously in patients receiving digitalis because this drug can increase plasma concentration • Use cautiously in patients receiving oral anticoagulants because propafenone can increase plasma concentration • Administer with food to diminish GI adverse effects • Correct electrolytes prior to therapy • Instruct patient to report recurrent or persistent infection

Continued

Table 3-4 Selected Antidysrhythmic Agents—cont'd

Drug	Classification/ Actions	Indications	Administration	Adverse Effects	Nursing Implications
Propranolol (Inderal)	**Noncardioselective Beta-Blocker Class II Antidysrhythmic** • Decreases heart rate, contractility, automaticity, excitability, conductivity • Depresses sinus node automaticity • Increases AV nodal refractoriness and decreases conduction velocity • Decreases myocardial oxygen consumption	• Supraventricular and ventricular dysrhythmias • Hypertension • Angina • Pheochromocytoma • Hyperthyroid crisis • Myocardial infarction (primary prevention and secondary prevention of extension and reinfarction) • Hypertrophic cardiomyopathy	• PO: 10-80 mg tid or qid • IV injection: 0.1 mg/kg in 3 divided doses at rate not to exceed 1 mg/min • IV infusion: mix 20 mg in 250 mL (0.08 mg/mL); usual dose 3-8 mg/hr • Therapeutic blood level 0.04-0.90 mcg/mL	• Bradycardia • AV block • Hypotension • Nausea, vomiting, diarrhea • Fatigue, lethargy • Rash • Syncope • HF • Bronchospasm, especially in patients with asthma • Mental depression • Hyperglycemia in type 2 DM • Asymptomatic hypoglycemia in type 1 DM • Impotence • Emotional lability • Insomnia • Agranulocytosis, thrombocytopenia	• Monitor HR, BP, ECG • Monitor for clinical indications of heart failure • Note contraindications: known hypersensitivity, sinus bradycardia, AV block greater than first degree, HF, shock, asthma, Raynaud's syndrome • Use cautiously in diabetes mellitus, renal disease, hyperthyroidism, COPD, liver disease, myasthenia gravis, peripheral vascular disease, hypotension • May potentiate the hypoglycemic effects of insulin and prevents sympathetic symptoms of hypoglycemia • Note that this drug limits cardiac reserve and exercise capacity because heart rate cannot increase • Note that this drug masks sympathetic clinical indications of shock because receptors are blocked
Esmolol (Brevibloc)	**Cardioselective Beta-Blocker Class II Antidysrhythmic** • Decreases heart rate, contractility, automaticity, excitability, conductivity • Depresses sinus node automaticity • Increases AV nodal refractoriness and decreases conduction velocity • Decreases myocardial oxygen consumption	• Supraventricular tachycardia • Intraoperative or postoperative tachycardia and/or hypertension	• IV injection: loading dose of 500 mcg/kg over 1 minute followed by maintenance dose of 50 mcg/kg/min for 4 minutes • If desired effect does not occur, repeat the loading dose of 500 mcg/kg over 1 minute and follow with a dose increased by 50 mcg/kg/min for 4 minutes (e.g., 500 + 100, 500 + 150, 500 + 200) • IV infusion: when desired effect is achieved, no additional loading doses are needed and the maintenance dose is increased by 50 mcg/kg/min and maintained	• Bradycardia • Hypotension • AV block • Nausea, vomiting • Fatigue, lethargy • HF • Bronchospasm, especially in patients with asthma • Urinary retention • Inflammation and induration at injection site	• Monitor HR, BP, ECG • Monitor for clinical indications of heart failure • Note contraindications: known hypersensitivity, bradycardia, AV block greater than first degree, HF, shock, asthma • Use cautiously in diabetes mellitus, renal disease, hyperthyroidism, COPD, liver disease, myasthenia gravis, peripheral vascular disease, hypotension • May potentiate the hypoglycemic effects of insulin and prevents sympathetic symptoms of hypoglycemia; masks sympathetic clinical indications of shock because receptors are blocked

Metoprolol (Lopressor)	**Cardioselective Beta-Blocker Class II Antidysrhythmic** • Decreases heart rate, contractility, automaticity, excitability, conductivity • Depresses sinus node automaticity • Increases AV nodal refractoriness and decreases conduction velocity • Decreases myocardial oxygen consumption	• Hypertension • Angina • Myocardial infarction (primary prevention and secondary prevention of extension and reinfarction)	• PO: 100-450 mg daily in one or two doses • IV injection: 5 mg IV slowly at 5-minute intervals to a total of 15 mg	• Bradycardia • AV block • Hypotension • Nausea, vomiting, diarrhea, constipation • Fatigue, lethargy • Rash • Syncope • HF • Dyspnea, wheezing • Mental depression • Hyperglycemia in type 2 DM • Asymptomatic hypoglycemia in type 1 DM • Impotence • Emotional lability • Agranulocytosis, thrombocytopenia	• Monitor HR, BP, ECG • Monitor for clinical indications of heart failure • Note contraindications: known hypersensitivity, sinus bradycardia, AV block greater than first degree, HF, shock, asthma, Raynaud's syndrome • Use cautiously in diabetes mellitus, renal disease, hyperthyroidism, COPD, liver disease, myasthenia gravis, peripheral vascular disease, hypotension • May potentiate the hypoglycemic effects of insulin and prevents sympathetic symptoms of hypoglycemia • Note that this drug limits cardiac reserve and exercise capacity because heart rate cannot increase • Note that this drug masks sympathetic clinical indications of shock because receptors are blocked
Sotalol (Betapace) (NOTE: Class II and III)	**Class II and III Antidysrhythmic** • Depresses SA node automaticity • Increases refractory period of atrial and AV junctional tissue to slow conduction • Shortens action potential duration • Inhibits sympathetic activity • Blocks potassium movement during phase III • Increases action potential duration • Prolongs effective refractory period	• Life-threatening or refractory ventricular dysrhythmias	• PO: initial 80 mg bid followed by 160-320 mg/ daily divided into two to three doses • IV injection: 100 mg (1.5 mg/kg) over 5 minutes	• Proarrhythmia including torsades de pointes, sinus bradycardia; second- or third-degree AV block • Heart failure • Hypotension • Dyspnea • Bronchospasm (especially in patients with history of asthma) • Headache	• Monitor HR, BP, ECG • Report prolongation of QT interval to more than half of RR interval or hypotension • Monitor serum glucose in patients with DM • Monitor closely for clinical indications of heart failure • Note contraindications: second- or third-degree AV block, SA block without pacemaker, QT prolongation • Do not administer concurrently or within 4 hours of class IA antiarrhythmics or other class III antiarrhythmics; do not administer with other drugs that prolong the QT interval such as phenothiazines, tricyclic antidepressants • Correct electrolytes prior to therapy • Warn patient not to discontinue abruptly

Continued

Table 3-4 Selected Antidysrhythmic Agents—cont'd

Drug	Classification/ Actions	Indications	Administration	Adverse Effects	Nursing Implications
Amiodarone hydrochloride (Cordarone)	**Class III Antidysrhythmic** • Prolongs the action potential and effective refractory period	• Life-threatening or refractory ventricular dysrhythmias • Refractory supraventricular dysrhythmias especially those caused by WPW	• PO: loading dose of 800-1600 mg/day for 1-3 weeks; then 600-800 mg/day for 1 month; then 200-800 mg daily • IV injection (loading dose): 150 mg over 10 minutes followed by: • IV infusion: mix 900 mg in 500 mL (1.8 mg/mL); usual dose is 1 mg/min for the next 6 hours followed by 0.5 mg/min • Use central venous catheter if more concentrated solution is used • Use solutions diluted in PVC containers within 2 hours; solutions diluted in glass or polyolefin containers within 24 hours • Administer through PVC tubing because dosing has taken into account adsorption to tubing • Therapeutic blood level 1.5-2.5 mcg/mL	• Hypotension • Proarrhythmia including PVCs, ventricular tachycardia, torsades de pointes, PACs, supraventricular tachycardia, bradycardia, SA block or arrest, AV block, bundle branch block • HF • Nausea, vomiting • Dizziness • Headache • Fatigue, malaise, muscle weakness • Corneal microdeposits • Rash, photosensitivity • Altered liver enzymes, hepatotoxicity • Hyperthyroidism, hypothyroidism • Blue-gray skin discoloration • Tremors, peripheral neuropathies, extrapyramidal symptoms • Cough, progressive dyspnea, pulmonary fibrosis	• Monitor HR, BP, ECG, breath sounds, electrolytes, liver function studies, thyroid function studies, pulmonary function studies, chest x-ray, neurologic symptoms • Monitor for clinical indications of heart failure, pulmonary fibrosis • Note contraindications: known hypersensitivity, marked sinus bradycardia, second- or third-degree AV block unless functioning pacemaker, cardiogenic shock • Use cautiously in patients with sinus node disease, conduction disturbances, severely depressed ventricular function, and marked cardiomegaly • Do not confuse amiodarone (an antidysrhythmic agent) with amrinone (an inotropic agent) • Advise methylcellulose ophthalmic solution and annual eye examinations for patients on long-term therapy • Advise use of sun protection factor (SPF) 15 sunscreen and sunglasses for patients on long-term therapy • Monitor for drug interactions: interacts with digitalis, anticoagulants, beta-blockers, calcium channel blockers, phenytoin, and class I antidysrhythmics • If used concurrently with digitalis, monitor closely for indications of digitalis toxicity • Administer PO drug with food to decrease GI adverse effects

Ibutilide (Corvert)	**Class III Antidysrhythmic** • Blocks potassium movement during phase III • Increases action potential duration • Prolongs effective refractory period	• Recent onset atrial fibrillation or atrial flutter	• IV infusion: mix 1 mg in 50 mL and infuse over 10 minutes for patients weighing over 60 kg (0.01 mg/kg in patients weighing less than 60 kg); may be repeated after 10 minutes if needed • Discontinue if atrial fibrillation or flutter terminates, a new dysrhythmia occurs, or if prolongation of the QT occurs	• Proarrhythmia including PVCs, ventricular tachycardia, torsades de pointes, PACs, supraventricular tachycardia, bradycardia, AV block, bundle branch block • Hypotension	• Monitor HR, BP, ECG • Report widening of QRS by greater than 25% or prolongation of QT interval to more than half of RR interval or hypotension • Correct electrolyte imbalances (especially hypokalemia) before initiating ibutilide • Administer anticoagulants for 2-3 weeks as prescribed for patients with atrial fibrillation of more than 2-3 days duration • Note contraindications: patients with second- or third-degree AV block, SA block without pacemaker, hypersensitivity to ibutilide, congenital or acquired long QT syndrome, in patient receiving verapamil or drugs that prolong the QT interval • Use cautiously in patients receiving digitalis because this drug may mask the cardiotoxicity associated with excessive digoxin levels • Do not administer concurrently or within 4 hours of class IA antiarrhythmics or other class III antiarrhythmics; do not administer with other drugs that prolong the QT interval such as phenothiazines, tricyclic antidepressants

Continued

Table 3-4 Selected Antidysrhythmic Agents—cont'd

Drug	Classification/ Actions	Indications	Administration	Adverse Effects	Nursing Implications
Dofetilide (Tikosyn)	**Class III Antidysrhythmic** • Blocks potassium movement during phase III • Increases action potential duration • Prolongs effective refractory period	• Recent onset atrial fibrillation or atrial flutter • Maintenance of sinus rhythm in patients with highly symptomatic atrial flutter or atrial fibrillation of greater than 1 week duration	• PO: 500 mcg twice daily • Initiation of this oral therapy requires hospitalization for monitoring of QT interval while dosage is adjusted • Dosage is also adjusted according to creatinine clearance	• Proarrhythmia including PVCs, ventricular tachycardia, torsades de pointes, PACs, supraventricular tachycardia, bradycardia, AV block, bundle branch block • Hypotension • Nausea • Syncope • Chest pain	• Monitor HR, BP, ECG • Report widening of QRS by greater than 25% or prolongation of QT interval to more than half of RR interval or hypotension • Correct electrolyte imbalances (especially hypokalemia or hypomagnesemia) before initiating dofetilide • Note contraindications: patients with second- or third-degree AV block, SA block without pacemaker, hypersensitivity to dofetilide, in patient receiving verapamil or drugs that prolong the QT interval • Do not administer concurrently or within 4 hours of class IA antiarrhythmics or other class III antiarrhythmics; do not administer with other drugs that prolong the QT interval such as phenothiazines, tricyclic antidepressants
Verapamil (Calan)	**Calcium Channel Blocker** **Class IV Antidysrhythmic** • Depresses rate of SA node • Increases refractoriness of AV node • Relaxes vascular smooth muscle decreasing SVR, BP	• Supraventricular dysrhythmias • Angina • Hypertension • Hypertrophic cardiomyopathy	• PO: 40-120 mg every 6 hours • IV injection: 0.075-0.15 mg/kg (5-10 mg); may be repeated in 15-30 minutes at 5-10 mg • Maximum: 20 mg • IV infusion: mix 50 mg in 250 mL (200 mcg/mL); usual dose is 1-5 mcg/kg/min • Therapeutic blood level 0.1-0.15 mcg/mL	• Bradycardia • AV block • Hypotension • Nausea • Constipation or diarrhea • Elevated liver enzymes • Headache • Dizziness • Heart failure	• Monitor HR, BP, ECG, liver function studies, breath sounds, heart sounds • Note contraindications: known hypersensitivity, AV block, sick sinus syndrome, WPW, advanced HF, cardiogenic shock • Use cautiously in HF, hypotension, liver disease, renal disease, patients receiving digitalis or beta-blockers • Do not give concurrently with IV beta-blockers • Administer calcium (500 mg-1 g IV over 10 minutes) as prescribed prior to IV verapamil to prevent hypotension

Diltiazem (Cardizem)	**Calcium Channel Blocker** • Relaxes vascular smooth muscle decreasing preload and afterload • Relieves coronary artery spasm • Slows SA and AV nodal conduction times	• Angina • Coronary artery spasm • Mild HF • Hypertension • Hypertrophic cardiomyopathy • Supraventricular tachycardia	• PO: 30-60 mg every 6 hours • IV injection: 0.15-0.25 mg/kg (20 mg average) over 2 minutes, may be repeated in 15 minutes at 0.35 mg/kg (25 mg average) over 2 minutes • IV infusion: mix 125 mg in 100 mL for a total volume of 125 mL (1 mg/mL) and infuse at 5-15 mg/hr	• Bradycardia • Dysrhythmias • AV block • Hypotension • Nausea • Headache • Flushing • Fatigue • Drowsiness • Edema • Rash • Renal failure • Transient elevation in liver enzymes	• Monitor HR, BP, ECG • Note contraindications: known hypersensitivity, severe hypotension, second- or third-degree AV block, SSS, WPW, acute MI, pulmonary edema • Use cautiously in HF, hypotension, liver disease, renal disease, older adult
Digitalis (Digoxin, Lanoxin, Digitoxin, lanatoside C)	**Cardiac Glycoside** • Increases cardiac contractility to increase CO • Increases the refractory period of the AV node • Decreases sinus node firing rate • Decreases atrial automaticity • Increases ventricular automaticity • Increases GFR and urine output	• HF • Supraventricular tachycardias, especially in patients with HF	• IV, PO • Digitalizing dose: 0.75-1.5 mg dose over 24 hours, usually in 4 doses of 0.25 mg • Administer IV dose over 5 minutes • Maintenance dose: 0.125-0.5 mg qd • Therapeutic blood level 0.5-2 ng/mL	*Toxic effects* • Anorexia, nausea, vomiting, diarrhea • Fatigue, muscle weakness • Agitation • Hallucinations • Visual disturbances • SA and AV blocks • Junctional and ventricular dysrhythmias, *Treatment of toxicity* • Discontinue drug • Correct hypoxemia, ischemia, acid-base or electrolyte imbalance • Treat tachydysrhythmias as prescribed: usually lidocaine • Treat bradydysrhythmias as prescribed: usually atropine or pacemaker • Administer Digibind as prescribed for life-threatening dysrhythmias or blocks • Correction of hypokalemia is recommended before Digibind • Average dose is 400-800 mg over 30 minutes or IV bolus if cardiac arrest • Administered through inline filter • Reversal of digitalis toxicity occurs within 30-60 minutes, but digoxin levels remain elevated	• Monitor apical HR, ECG, serum electrolytes, especially potassium, calcium, magnesium • Note contraindications: known hypersensitivity, sick sinus syndrome, SA or AV block, ventricular tachycardia, hypertrophic cardiomyopathy, WPW • Use cautiously in patients with acute MI, hypothyroidism, liver disease, renal disease, hypothyroidism, older adult • Assess patient for clinical indications of digitalis toxicity • Withhold for 1-2 days before elective electrical cardioversion

Continued

Table 3-4 Selected Antidysrhythmic Agents—cont'd

Drug	Classification/ Actions	Indications	Administration	Adverse Effects	Nursing Implications
Adenosine (Adenocard)	**Endogenous Nucleoside Unclassified Antidysrhythmic** • Slows conduction through the AV node • Interrupts the reentry pathways through the AV node to restore normal sinus rhythm	• Supraventricular tachycardias including those associated with WPW • Not effective in atrial fibrillation or atrial flutter but may slow rate so that fibrillatory or flutter waves can be identified	• IV injection: 6 mg IV; must be given within 6 seconds; repeat at 12 mg IV if conversion is not achieved within 1-2 minutes; 12 mg dose may be repeated once • Must be administered as quickly as possible (referred to as IV "slam") due to very short half-life (10 seconds); administer as quickly as possible into NS flush or insert Y connector into line to push NS flush as quickly as possible after pushing adenosine as quickly as possible	• Transient dysrhythmias at the time of conversion (including short asystolic pause) • Pause may be prolonged especially in patients with sick sinus syndrome • Hypotension if large doses are used • Nausea • Facial flushing • Headache • Dyspnea • Bronchospasm • Chest pressure • Recurrence of dysrhythmias	• Monitor HR, BP, ECG, BP and depth, breath sounds • Note contraindications: known hypersensitivity, second- or third-degree AV block, sick sinus syndrome, ventricular dysrhythmias • Use cautiously in patients with asthma or older adults • Decrease initial dosage as prescribed in patients receiving dipyridamole (Persantine), diazepam (Valium), phenobarbital, or carbamazepine (Tegretol); initial dose may be prescribed as 3 mg • Increase initial dosage as prescribed in patients receiving aminophylline or another xanthine; initial dose may be prescribed as 12 mg • Store at room temperature; solution must be clear at time of use

Atropine sulfate Ipratropium (Atrovent)	**Anticholinergic (also called parasympatholytic)** • Decreases vagal tone • Increases sinus rate • Slightly increases conduction through the AV node • Relaxes smooth muscle; prevents bronchospasm • Decreases GI, tracheobronchial secretions	• Symptomatic sinus bradycardia • Asystole • Preoperative preparation for surgery • Anticholinesterase insecticide (organophosphate) poisoning • Bronchospasm; asthma	• IV injection: 0.5-2 mg (0.5 mg given as initial dose in sinus bradycardia, 1 mg given as initial dose in asystole, 2 mg given as initial dose in organophosphate poisoning); repeated as needed at 3-5 minute intervals • Maximum: 0.04 mg/kg (usually approximately 3 mg) • Nebulizer: 0.025 mg/kg diluted with 3-5 mL of normal saline every 6-8 hours • Hand-held inhaler: 2 puffs every 6-8 hours	• Tachycardia, palpitations • Bradycardia if given slowly or in dose of less than 0.5 mg • Hypotension • Dry mouth • Blurred vision, dilated pupils • Urinary retention • Constipation, paralytic ileus • Headache • Dizziness • Restlessness • Increased myocardial oxygen consumption and chest pain in patients with CAD • NOTE: Ipratropium (by inhalation) causes virtually no systemic adverse effects	• Monitor HR, BP, ECG, urine output, bowel sounds • Note contraindications: known hypersensitivity to belladonna, glaucoma, GI obstruction, myasthenia gravis, thyrotoxicosis, ulcerative colitis, prostatic hypertrophy, tachydysrhythmias • Use cautiously in renal disease, HF, hyperthyroidism, hepatic disease, hypertension • Use cautiously in acute MI: do not administer atropine for bradycardia unless the patient is symptomatic; increasing heart rate increases myocardial oxygen consumption and can increase infarction size • Do not use pupils as a reflection of brain status after atropine: pupils will be dilated and nonreactive • Use hard candy to help alleviate side effect of dry mouth unless contraindicated
Isoproterenol (Isuprel)	**Unclassified Antidysrhythmic; Beta-Selective Adrenergic Agent** • Increases heart rate, contractility, conductivity • Shortens repolarization and QT interval • Causes bronchodilation	• Bradycardia refractory to other drugs • Torsades de pointes	• Mix 1 mg in 250 mL (4 mcg/mL); infuse at 2-20 mcg/min	• Tachycardia, palpitations • Hypotension • Ventricular dysrhythmias • Chest pain • Flushing • Headache • Nausea, vomiting • Anxiety, tremor • Hyperglycemia	• Monitor BP, HR, ECG • Note contraindications: tachydysrhythmias, digitalis toxicity, angina, narrow angle glaucoma • Use cautiously in older adults and those with hyperthyroidism, chest pain, hypertension, psychoneurosis, diabetes mellitus

monophasic rather than synchronized cardioversion.
g) Antidysrhythmic drug therapy is used after sinus rhythm is restored.
4) Complications: as for defibrillation
b. Defibrillation: See Cardiopulmonary Arrest.

11. Utilize pacemaker therapies for patients who have problem with impulse formation and/or conduction.
a. Definition: an electronic device that delivers an electrical stimulus to the heart to cause depolarization of the myocardium and increase or decrease the heart rate
1) Terminology used to discuss pacemakers (Table 3-5)
b. Indications for pacemaker
1) Sick sinus syndrome with syncope
a) Symptomatic bradydysrhythmias
b) Sinus block or sinus arrest with ventricular asystole
c) Alternating tachycardia and bradycardia (called *tachy-brady syndrome*)
2) Hypersensitive carotid sinus syndrome
3) AV blocks
a) Second degree AV block type I with symptomatic bradycardia
b) Second degree AV block type II
c) Third degree AV block
4) Bundle branch block with AV block
5) Bifascicular block (i.e., LBBB or RBBB with hemiblock) with acute MI
6) Trifascicular block (e.g., bilateral bundle branch block)
7) Refractory tachydysrhythmias unresponsive to drug therapy or cardioversion (referred to as *tachycardia overdrive*); an important treatment modality for torsades de pointes
8) Hypertrophic cardiomyopathy or heart failure are indications for biventricular pacing.
9) Prophylactic use during cardiac surgery in patients with acute coronary syndrome or cardiac dysrhythmias
10) Note that pacemakers are not currently recommended for cardiac arrest with ventricular asystole.
c. Components
1) Pulse generator
a) Components
i) Battery
(a) Lithium-iodide batteries in permanent pacemakers last approximately 7-10 years
ii) Microprocessor that controls pacing (voltage) and sensing
b) Types
i) Single chamber atrial
ii) Single chamber ventricular
iii) Dual chamber atrioventricular
iv) Dual chamber biventricular
2) Lead(s)
a) Atrial
b) Ventricular
3) Electrode(s)
a) Unipolar
i) Negative only
ii) Metal of pulse generator acts as positive
b) Bipolar
i) Positive: proximal; sensing
ii) Negative: distal; pacing
d. Types of pacemakers
1) Temporary or permanent
a) Temporary (external pulse generator): hours to weeks
i) Transthoracic epicardial
(a) Electrodes attached to epicardium of atrium, ventricle, or both during cardiac surgery and brought through the chest wall
ii) Transvenous endocardial
(a) Pacing lead(s) inserted percutaneously via internal jugular or subclavian vein and advanced into RA or RV or both
iii) Transcutaneous
(a) Percutaneous leads applied to chest and back; used during cardiac arrests until transvenous pacer can be inserted
b) Permanent (internal pulse generator): months to years
i) Transvenous endocardial: lead inserted into cephalic vein and advanced into RA or RV; pulse generator implanted in subcutaneous fat under clavicle
ii) Epicardial: electrodes sewn onto epicardium (thoracotomy required); pulse generator implanted in subcutaneous fat of abdomen
2) Asynchronous vs synchronous
a) Asynchronous
i) Also called *fixed rate*
ii) The pacemaker delivers a pacing stimulus at a fixed rate regardless of the heart's intrinsic activity.
iii) Will cause competition with the heart's intrinsic activity and the pacing stimulus may land during the descending limb of the T wave
iv) Rarely seen today
b) Synchronous
i) Also called *demand*
ii) The pacemaker delivers a pacing stimulus only when the heart's

Table 3-5	Pacemaker Terminology
Artifact	The spike recorded on the ECG depicting the electrical energy discharge from the pulse generator
A-V interval	In a dual-chamber pacemaker, the period of time between an atrial event (sensed or paced) and a paced ventricular event
Blanking period	The interval of time during which the pacemaker cannot sense any events
Burst pacing	The delivery of rapid, multiple electrical stimuli; typically used to interrupt a fast heart rate
Capture	Depolarization of the atria and/or ventricle by an electrical stimulus delivered by an artificial pacemaker; one-to-one capture occurs when each electrical stimulus causes a corresponding depolarization
Committed (DVI) operation	A characteristic of some DVI pacemakers whereby a ventricular stimulus always follows an atrial stimulus regardless of intrinsic ventricular activity
Cross talk	The phenomenon that can occur in dual-chamber pacemakers in which a stimulus from the atrial lead is sensed by the ventricular lead, or vice versa, resulting in an inappropriate pacemaker response such as inhibiting or resetting of the refractory period.
Demand pacemaker	A pacemaker that only discharges when the patient's heart rate drops below the pacemaker's preset rate
Dual-chamber pacing (i.e., AV sequential)	The pacing in both the atria and the ventricles to artificially restore the natural contraction sequence of the heart; also called *physiologic pacing*
Electrode	The uninsulated conductive portion of a pacing lead which makes electrical contact with tissue
Electromagnetic interference (EMI)	Radiated or conducted energy—either electrical or magnetic—which can interfere with or disrupt the function of a pulse generator
End-of-life	The point at which a pacemaker signals that it should be replaced because its battery is nearing depletion
Escape interval	The time between a paced or sensed cardiac event and the subsequent pacing stimulus of a pulse generator
Fusion beat	A spontaneous cardiac depolarization which occurs coincidentally with a paced depolarization; the paced and natural depolarization waveforms fuse
Hysteresis	A pacing parameter which allows a longer escape interval after a sensed event, allowing perpetuation of the patient's intrinsic rhythm
Inhibited	A common type of pacemaker that does not pace when its output is suppressed by sensed spontaneous cardiac events occurring at a rate more rapid than the pacing rate
Intrinsic	Inherent; belonging to or originating from the heart itself
Lead	The insulated wire or wires that carry electrical signals to and from the heart, a connector pin, and stimulating, sensing electrode(s)
Milliamperage (mA)	The unit of measurement used for electrical stimulus (i.e., output) generated by a pacemaker
Multisite pacing	The ability of a pacemaker to stimulate more than one site, such as biventricular pacing
Myopotentials	Electrical signals that originate in body muscles; these signals may be sensed by the pacemaker and falsely interpreted as depolarization
Output	An electric stimulus delivered by the pulse generator; measured in milliamperage (mA)
Pacemaker syndrome	A collection of signs and symptoms related to the adverse hemodynamic effects of ventricular pacing, usually attributed to the absence of synchrony between the atrial and ventricular contractions
Pacing mode	The manner in which a pacemaker provides artificial rate and rhythm support in the presence of dysrhythmia; identified by a three- or five-letter code.
Programmable	A pulse generator with a pacing mode and/or parameters that can be changed noninvasively at any time by means of an external programmer
Pulse generator	The portion of the pacing system that produces electrical pulses and contains the power supply and electronic circuit
Pulse width	The duration of the pacing pulse expressed in millisecond; also called *pulse duration*
Rate responsive or rate modulated pacing	The ability of a pacemaker to increase or decrease its rate in response to the heart's intrinsic rate or detected changes in the body (i.e., body activity, atrial activity, respiratory rate)
Refractory period	The time during which the pacemaker's sensing mechanism becomes nonresponsive to cardiac activity

Continued

Table 3-5 Pacemaker Terminology—cont'd

Safety pacing	In some DVI and DDD pacemakers, following atrial pacing, the pacemaker is designed to trigger a ventricular pacing output if ventricular sensing occurs during the first portion of the programmed A-V interval; this ensures a ventricular depolarization if the event sensed was electrical interference
Sensing	The ability of the pacemaker to detect the patient's intrinsic activity and respond appropriately by either triggering or inhibiting output
Sensing threshold	The minimum atrial or ventricular intracardiac signal amplitude required to inhibit or trigger a demand pacemaker
Sensitivity	The degree to which a pacemaker is responsive to levels of electrical activity in the heart
Stimulation threshold	The minimum electrical stimulus needed to obtain consistent capture
Telemetry	The ability of the pacemaker to send information (i.e., programmed status, measurements, signals to the programmer)
Tracking	When ventricular pacing is synchronized to sensed atrial activity
Triggered	To deliver an electrical stimulus upon detecting a spontaneous depolarization
V-A interval	With dual-chamber pacemakers, the period of time elapsing from a ventricular event (sensed or paced) to the next scheduled atrial pace

From Medtronic. (2005). *Pacing Glossary*. Retrieved September 8, 2012, from https://wwwp.medtronic.com/medtronicconnect/resources/presentationtools//1332879501392/MedtronicPacingGlossary2007.pdf.

Table 3-6 The NASPE/BPEG Generic (NBG) Pacemaker Code

Position I	Position II	Position III	Position IV	Position V
Chamber(s) paced O = None A= Atrium V = Ventricle D = Dual (A+V)	Chamber(s) sensed O = None A= Atrium V = Ventricle D = Dual (A+V)	Response to sensing O = None T = Triggered I = Inhibited D = Dual (T + I)	Rate modulation R = Rate modulation	Multisite pacing O = None A= Atrium V = Ventricle D = Dual (A+V)

From Bernstein, A. D., Daubert, J. C., Fletcher, R. D., Hayes, D. L., Luderitz, B., Reynolds D.W., et al. (2002). The revised NASPE/BPEG generic code for antibradycardia, adaptive-rate, and multisite pacing. North American Society of Pacing and Electrophysiology/British Pacing and Electrophysiology Group. *PACE, 25*(2), 260-264.

intrinsic pacemaker fails to function at a predetermined rate.

iii) The pacing stimulus will be either inhibited or triggered when the intrinsic activity is seen.

e. North American Society of Pacing and Electrophysiology (NASPE) generic code (Table 3-6)

f. Pacemaker modes (Table 3-7)

1) Atrial: AOO, AAI
   a) Pacing stimulus occurs before the P wave
   b) Requires an intact AV nodal conduction
2) Ventricular: VOO, VAT, VVI, VVT, VDD
   a) Pacing stimulus occurs before the QRS complex
3) Atrioventricular (AV) sequential: DOO, DVI, DDD
   a) Maintains AV synchrony and the hemodynamic benefit of the atrial kick
   b) Pacing stimulus before both or either P wave or QRS complex
   c) Sufficient AV delay set to allow atrial depolarization and contraction to complete ventricular filling
4) Multisite: atriobiventricular (also referred to as *cardiac resynchronization therapy*)
   a) Used in severe heart failure in patients with ventricular depolarization asynchrony
   b) Placement of a left ventricular lead (either placed directly on the left ventricle [epicardial] by thoracotomy approach or endocardially via the coronary sinus) along with right ventricular and right atrial leads
   c) An atrioventricular delay adequate to allow atrial contraction to contribute optimally to ventricular filling
   d) Optimal timing of stimulation of both ventricles; this may be with one ventricle stimulated slightly before the other rather than simultaneous,
   e) May or may not include an implantable cardioverter-defibrillator
5) Rate-responsive: the heart rate is adjusted according to demands for cardiac output
   a) Heart rate changes are stimulated by changes in muscle activity, minute

Table 3-7 Pacemaker Modes

Code	Description	Indications	Advantages	Disadvantages
AOO	Fixed rate atrial pacer	• Consistently slow sinus rate with intact AV nodal conduction	• Single lead • Maintains AV synchrony	• Atrial competition • No protection in case of AV nodal block
AAI	Demand atrial pacer	• Sick sinus syndrome • Sinus arrest • Sinus bradycardia • Must have intact AV nodal conduction	• Single lead • Maintains AV synchrony	• No protection in case of AV nodal block
VOO	Fixed rate ventricular pacer	• Complete heart block with slow idioventricular rhythm • Rarely used today	• Single lead • Protection from ventricular asystole	• Ventricular competition with possible stimulation of ventricular dysrhythmias
VAT	Atrial triggered ventricular pacer	• Complete heart block with intact sinus node	• Synchronized AV conduction with atrial "kick" optimizes cardiac output • Ventricular rate increases with atrial rate so more exercise responsive	• Two leads • May cause pacemaker-mediated tachycardia: rapid ventricular response in sinus or atrial dysrhythmias • May cause pacemaker-mediated tachycardia
VVI	Demand ventricular pacer	• Sick sinus syndrome • Sinus bradycardia • Sinus arrest • Complete heart block	• Single lead • Simple and reliable • Inexpensive • Protection from ventricular asystole • Little chance of competitive rhythms	• Loss of synchronized AV conduction and atrial "kick" may reduce cardiac output • Not rate responsive • (NOTE: VVIR is a VVI with rate responsiveness
VVT	Pacing stimulus delivered if needed or not; stimulus depolarizes ventricle if no intrinsic depolarization; stimulus lands harmlessly in QRS if intrinsic depolarization	• Sick sinus syndrome • Sinus bradycardia • Sinus arrest • Complete heart block	• Single lead • Can evaluate pacer function even if intrinsic activity faster than pacer rate	• Loss of synchronized AV conduction and atrial "kick" may reduce cardiac output • Not rate responsive • Difficult to evaluate QRS morphology
VDD	Ventricular pacer that can be atrial triggered or inhibited by intrinsic ventricular depolarization	• Sick sinus syndrome • Sinus bradycardia • Sinus arrest • Complete heart block	• Maintains AV synchrony • If atrial activity is present as pacer functions in atrial triggered mode; if no atrial activity, paces the ventricle in demand mode with inhibition to intrinsic ventricular depolarization	• Two leads • May cause pacemaker-mediated tachycardia • Does not pace the atria, so loss of atrial contraction if no intrinsic atrial activity
DOO	Fixed rate AV sequential pacer	• Consistently slow atrial and ventricular rate	• Synchronized AV conduction with atrial "kick" optimizes cardiac output	• Two leads • Not rate responsive • Atrial and ventricular competition
DVI	Fixed rate atrial pacer with demand ventricular pacer	• Sick sinus syndrome • Sinus bradycardia • Sinus arrest • Complete heart block	• Synchronized AV conduction with atrial "kick" optimizes cardiac output	• Two leads • Not rate responsive • Blind to intrinsic atrial activity so atrial competition and even atrial fibrillation may occur
DDD	Demand atrial and ventricular pacer; ventricular pacing may be atrial triggered or ventricular inhibited	• Sick sinus syndrome • Sinus bradycardia • Sinus arrest • Complete heart block	• Synchronized AV conduction with atrial "kick" optimizes cardiac output • Near normal physiologic function	• Two leads • Most expensive • May cause pacemaker-mediated tachycardia • Difficult troubleshooting • Is not used in atrial fibrillation

ventilation, or blood changes in temperature or pH
b) Rate-responsive modes: AAIR, VVIR, DDDR

g. Collaborative management
1) Assess for proper functioning
a) Determination of the type of pacemaker
b) ECG evidence of pacing (Figure 3-8 and Figure 3-9)
i) Spike before paced event
ii) Wide QRS if ventricular pacer
iii) Presence of T wave confirms ventricular depolarization
iv) Presence of fusion beats
c) Determination of settings
i) Rate: usually set at 70-90/min but higher than the intrinsic rate for tachycardia overdrive
ii) Mode (see Table 3-7)
iii) Output: usually set at 1.5-2 times the pacing threshold
(a) The pacing threshold is determined by decreasing the mA until capture is lost and then increased until capture is once again obtained; typical pacing threshold is 1-1.5 mA so the mA is usually set at 1.5-3.
iv) Sensitivity: usually set at approximately 2-5 mV
v) AV interval: like a PR interval for AV sequential pacemakers
d) Systematic assessment of rhythm strip in patient with pacemaker (Aehlert, 2011)
i) Identify the patient's intrinsic rate and rhythm.
ii) Determine if there is evidence of paced activity (i.e., pacing artifact).
(a) If there is evidence of atrial pacing, evaluate the paced interval to determine rate and regularity.
(b) If there is evidence of ventricular pacing, evaluate the paced interval to determine rate and regularity.
iii) Evaluate the escape interval.
(a) Compare the escape interval to the paced interval; these should be the same unless there is hysteresis.
iv) Analyze the rhythm strip for electrical complications of failure to fire, failure to capture, failure to sense, or oversensing (Table 3-8)

2) Specific to temporary pacemaker
a) Maintain electrical safety.
i) Ensure proper grounding of equipment.
ii) Touch side rails before touching patient to discharge static electricity.
iii) Wear rubber gloves when making adjustments.
iv) Keep patient and linens dry.
v) Avoid sources of electromagnetic interference (EMI) (e.g., electrocautery, defibrillation, MRI, transcutaneous electrical nerve stimulation (TENS) units, radiation therapy, lithotripsy).
b) Prevent complications.
i) Cover dial to prevent accidental changes in settings.
ii) Limit mobility of affected extremity to prevent accidental catheter dislodgement.

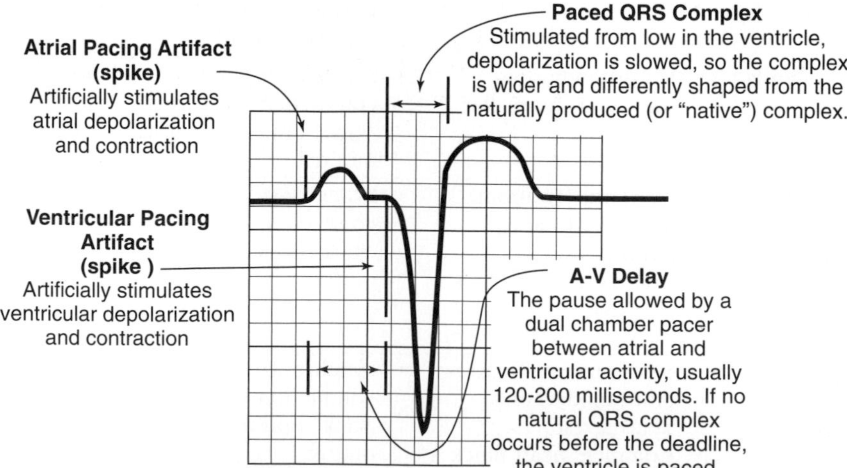

Figure 3-8 ECG evidence of pacing. (From Witherall, C. [1990]. Questions nurses ask about pacemakers. *Am J Nurs*, 90 [12], 20.)

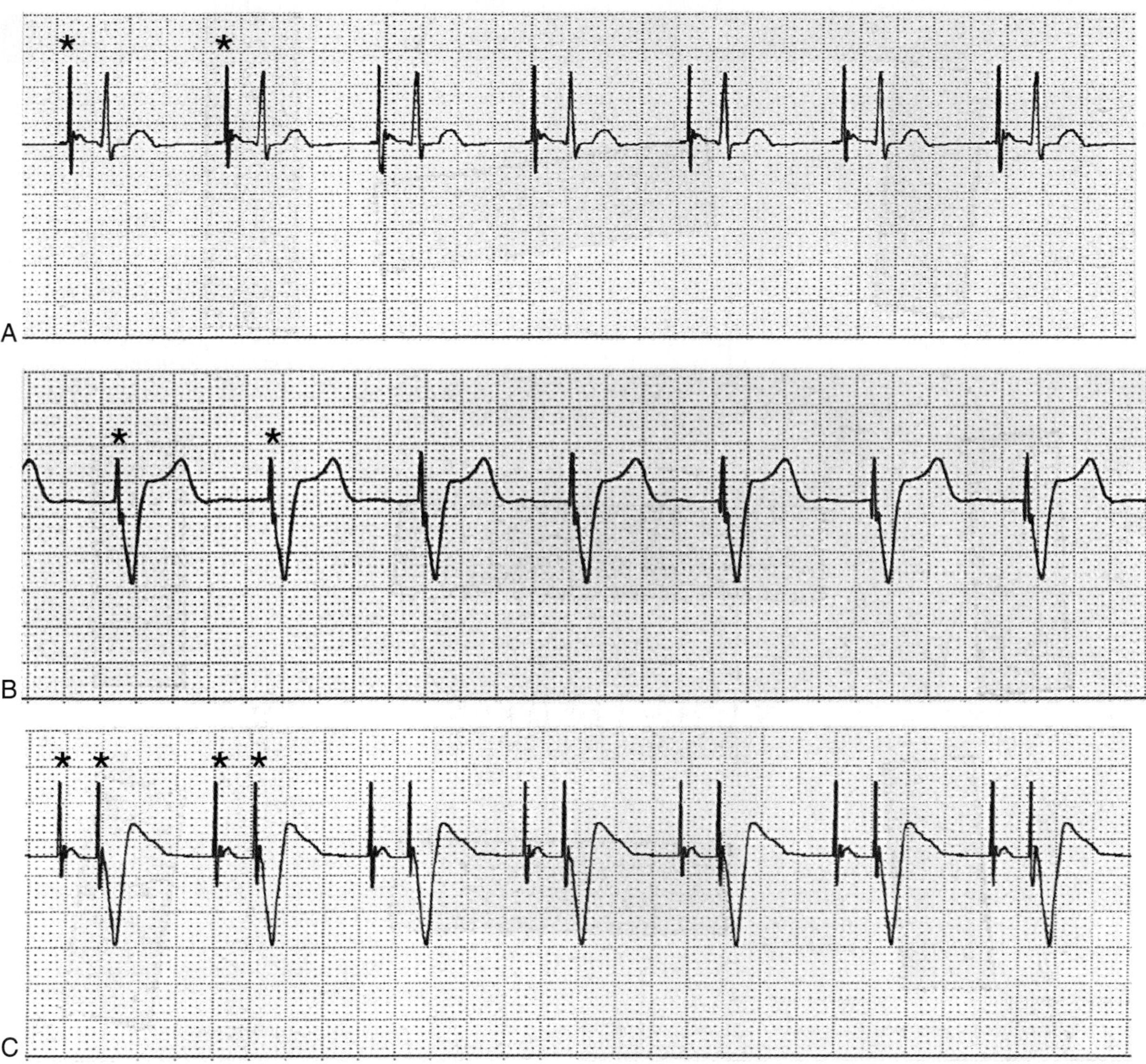

Figure 3-9 Pacing examples. **A,** Atrial pacing. **B,** Ventricular pacing. **C,** Dual-chamber pacing. Each asterisk represents a pacemaker artifact (i.e., spike). (From Urden, L., Stacy, K., & Lough, M. [2010]. *Critical care nursing: Diagnosis and management* [6th ed.]. St. Louis: Mosby.)

iii) Observe catheter site for signs of infection.
iv) Assist with establishment of pacing threshold and set mA slightly above this; usually initially set at between 3-5 mA depending on pacing threshold.
v) Observe cardiac monitor for pacemaker malfunction.

3) Specific to permanent
  a) Prevent complications.
    i) Limit mobility of affected upper extremity for 48 hours to prevent lead dislodgement.
    ii) Encourage arm exercise after 48 hours to prevent frozen shoulder (ankylosis).
    iii) Observe incision for signs of infection.
    iv) Observe cardiac monitor for pacemaker malfunction.
  b) Provide patient and family instruction.
    i) How to take pulse, symptoms to report
    ii) Sources of electromagnetic interference (EMI) to avoid (e.g., MRI, metal detectors, radio transmitters, electrical generating plants)
    iii) Avoidance of lifting anything over 5 pounds with the arm closest to the pacemaker for 1-2 months
    iv) Avoidance of lifting arm closest to the pacemaker above the head for 1-2 months
    v) Clinical indications of pacemaker malfunction (e.g., dyspnea, syncope, chest pain, fatigue,

Table 3-8 Pacemaker Electrical Malfunctions

Malfunction	Causes	Interventions
Failure to fire (pace): pacemaker does not fire when it is physiologically indicated for it to fire • Recognized by pauses longer than the automatic interval and absence of pacer spike at end of escape interval	• Loose connections • Battery depletion • Lead displacement • Lead fracture • Sensing malfunction (e.g., electromagnetic interference [EMI])	• Tighten connections if temporary • Replace battery or pulse generator • Lead repositioning or replacement may be needed • Evaluate patient's own rhythm and patient's response; if inadequate, administer atropine and/or apply external transcutaneous pacemaker; CPR may be required • May be caused by sensing malfunction; to identify a sensing malfunction, convert pacemaker to asynchronous by placing a magnet over an implanted pacemaker or switching to asynchronous on an external pacemaker; if pacer spikes seen in asynchronous mode, sensing malfunction exists • Remove source of EMI
Failure to capture: pacemaker fires but depolarization does not occur • Recognized by spike not followed by depolarization (e.g., P wave if atrial pacer or QRS if ventricular pacer)	• Displacement of lead • Lead fracture • Increased pacing thresholds (e.g., electrolyte imbalance, drug toxicity, acid-base imbalance, ischemia) • Fibrosis or scar tissue at thc lead tip • Battery failure • Chamber perforation • Complexes not visible	• Position patient on left side or to whatever position patient was in when capture was last seen • Increase mA • May require lead repositioning, lead replacement • Replace battery or pulse generator • Check chest x-ray for lead fracture and lead placement • Correct metabolic or electrolyte imbalance • Consider drug levels and toxicity • Check for diaphragmatic pacing and monitor or cardiac tamponade if catheter perforation is suspected • May require external transcutaneous pacing or CPR
Undersensing or failure to sense: pacemaker fails to recognize intrinsic activity (e.g., P wave or QRS) • Recognized by pacer spikes falling closer to the intrinsic beats than the escape interval; spikes land indiscriminately throughout the cardiac cycle including potentially on the descending limb of the T wave	• Displacement of lead • Lead fracture • Sensitivity set too low or set on asynchronous • Disconnection of sensing circuit • Inadequate signal (e.g., low P or QRS voltage) • Battery failure • Increased sensing threshold (e.g., edema or fibrosis at lead tip) • Chamber perforation	• Position patient on left side or to whatever position sensing was last seen • Lead repositioning or replacement may be necessary • Make sure that pacer is not set on asynchronous • Increase sensitivity (i.e., turn down the mV) • Check connections on temporary pacemaker • Administer lidocaine if the QRSs that are not sensed are PVCs • Check chest x-ray for lead placement or lead fracture • Replace battery or pulse generator • If patient's own rhythm adequate, turn pacer off or heart rate down to minimum • If patient's own rhythm inadequate, increase pacer rate to override patient's own rhythm
Oversensing pacemaker recognizes extraneous electrical activity or the wrong intrinsic electrical activity as the inhibiting event • Recognized by absence of pacer spikes and failure to fire	• Sensitivity set too high • Electromagnetic interference (EMI) • Oversensing of P waves or T waves • Myopotentials • Crosstalk (no ventricular pacing)	• Decrease sensitivity (i.e., turn up the mV) • Remove from EMI; ensure that all equipment is properly grounded • Decrease atrial output, decrease ventricular sensitivity, increase ventricular blanking period • May require external transcutaneous pacing or CPR

peripheral edema, persistent hiccups)
vi) Wound care (e.g., keeping clean and dry until healed)
vii) Importance of carrying pacemaker identification card and informing healthcare providers of presence of pacemaker

4) Monitor for complications
   a) Frozen shoulder
   b) Infection
   c) Pneumothorax
   d) Myocardial perforation
   e) Catheter or lead displacement
   f) Hematoma
   g) Dysrhythmias
      i) Pacemaker-mediated tachycardia: a rapid paced rhythm which can occur with atrial tracking pacemakers; it begins with and is sustained by ventricular events which are conducted retrogradely to the atria; the pacemaker senses this retrograde atrial depolarization and then delivers a stimulus to the ventricle, causing a ventricular depolarization, which again is conducted retrogradely to the atria; the cycle repeats itself to produce a tachycardia.
   h) Electrical malfunction (Table 3-8)

12. Prepare and care for the patient with an implantable cardioverter-defibrillator (ICD).
   a. Definition: implantable device to provide for immediate termination of VT or VF in patients in whom these dysrhythmias cannot be pharmacologically or surgically controlled
   b. Tiered therapy (also called *third-generation*) devices have all of the following (Morton & Fontaine, 2009):
      1) Bradycardia pacing: VVI/DDD/VDD
      2) Antitachycardia pacing: burst
      3) Low-energy cardioversion: 1-8 J
      4) High-energy cardioversion: 15-36 J
      5) Defibrillation: 30-36 J
   c. Indications
      1) One or more episodes of spontaneous VT or VF in a patient in whom EPS and/or spontaneous ventricular dysrhythmias cannot be used to accurately predict the efficacy of other treatment
      2) Recurrent episodes of sustained VT or VF in a patient in whom antidysrhythmic therapy is suboptimal due to intolerance or noncompliance
      3) Persistent inducibility of sustained VT or VF during EPS despite antidysrhythmic therapy and/or ablation
      4) VF in a patient with no evidence of structural heart disease and no detectable suppressing triggering factors
   d. Contraindications
      1) Frequent episodes of VT or VF (greater than 2 events/month)
      2) Uncontrolled HF
      3) Less than 6-12 months of productive life expectancy
      4) History of noncompliance
      5) Extreme psychological barriers to use of the device
   e. Components
      1) Generator
         a) Processes information from the lead system and delivers the electrical impulses
         b) Stores information about the patient's heart rhythm and therapy delivered
         c) Placed in the left upper quadrant of abdomen or under the clavicle
         d) Usually lasts about 3-5 years before replacement required
      2) Leads record heart rhythm and carry pulses and shocks from the generator to the heart
         a) Atrial lead
         b) Ventricular lead
   f. Method
      1) System evaluates heart rate and probability density function (PDF).
         a) PDF diagnoses the amount of time the QRS spends away from the isoelectric baseline
      2) System is turned on and off by using a donut-shaped magnet.
         a) Device is usually not turned on during early postoperative period due to frequent occurrence of sinus tachycardia during this period.
      3) When VT is sensed, the ICD will first initiate antitachycardia pacing.
      4) If the VT is not successfully pace-terminated, the ICD will cardiovert the rhythm with low-energy synchronized shocks.
      5) If the rhythm deteriorates to VF or if VF is the initial rhythm, the ICD will defibrillate at a higher energy level.
      6) Once a shock is delivered, the device senses the rhythm.
      7) If sinus rhythm is not restored, up to five shocks of 25-35 joules are delivered.
      8) If the electrical rhythm deteriorates to bradycardia or asystole, the bradycardia back-up pacing function is activated.
   g. Collaborative management
      1) Provide postprocedure management as for pacemaker insertion
      2) Monitor for dysrhythmias and evaluate effectiveness of ICD if firing occurs; administer antidysrhythmic agents as prescribed

3) If cardiopulmonary arrest occurs, do the following:
   a) Obtain emergency equipment and prepare to cardiovert or defibrillate
   b) Treat this patient as you would any patient in cardiopulmonary arrest; do not wait for the device.
   c) Do not place defibrillator paddles within 8 cm of the generator.
   d) Anterior-posterior paddle placement may be more effective.
4) Deactivate the ICD using a magnet as requested by the physician.
5) Monitor for complications.
   a) Observe incision for signs of infection.
   b) Observe for clinical indications of cardiac tamponade.
6) Encourage the patient to express fears and concerns about being shocked; consider referral to support group.
7) Monitor for complications.
   a) Atelectasis
   b) Pneumonia
   c) Pneumothorax
   d) Lead migration
   e) Lead fracture

13. Prepare and care for the patient having ablation therapy.
   a. Use: to eradicate dysrhythmia in patients who experience frequent, disabling, or life-threatening dysrhythmias that are not suppressed with pharmacologic therapy or in whom pharmacologic therapy is not well-tolerated
   b. Types
      1) Radiofrequency catheter ablation
         a) A catheter is placed in the heart via cardiac catheterization.
         b) Radiofrequency energy is applied to the area in which the dysrhythmia originates or an accessory pathway (e.g., WPW).
         c) Controlled, localized necrosis occurs
         d) Postprocedure care is as for cardiac catheterization or angioplasty; monitor closely for dysrhythmias.
      2) Surgical ablation: the area in which the dysrhythmia originates is either excised or eliminated by cryosurgery or laser.
14. Prepare for and care for the patient having maze procedure for atrial fibrillation.
   a. Performed either by cardiothoracic surgery or PCI
   b. A maze of carefully planned sutures or laser-created cuts create an electrical conduction route through atrial myocardium, corralling and herding chaotic atrial impulses from the SA node to the AV node.
   c. Provide postoperative management as for cardiothoracic surgery or PCI, depending on procedure performed.

Acute Coronary Syndrome

Definitions

1. Arteriosclerosis: a group of diseases characterized by thickening and loss of elasticity (calcification) of arterial walls
   a. Atherosclerosis: the most common form of arteriosclerosis; a chronic disease process characterized by the build-up of fatty plaque along the subintimal layer of arteries leading to a decrease in arterial lumen
   b. Progression (Figure 3-10)
2. Coronary artery disease: a progressive disease of the coronary arteries that results in narrowing and obstruction of the vessels and eventually myocardial ischemia; may also be referred to as *ischemic heart disease, coronary heart disease,* or *atherosclerotic heart disease*
3. Acute coronary syndrome: the group of clinical symptoms compatible with myocardial ischemia and differentiated by ECG findings; includes the following (Figure 3-11):
   a. Unstable angina: patient presenting with chest pain, no ST segment elevation, and normal cardiac biomarkers
      1) De novo angina: new onset angina
      2) Crescendo angina: angina that has increased in frequency, intensity, or duration
      3) Preinfarction: angina of prolonged duration that occurs even at rest
      4) Wellens syndrome: angina with deep T wave inversion in V_2, V_3 indicative of critical proximal LAD stenosis
      5) Variant (also called *Prinzmetal's* or *vasospastic*): angina with ST segment elevation related to coronary artery spasm
   b. Myocardial infarction: electrical and mechanical death of a portion of the myocardium
      1) ST elevation
         a) ST segment elevation MI: patient presenting with chest pain, elevated cardiac biomarkers, and ST segment elevation
         b) Non-ST segment elevation MI: patient presenting with chest pain and elevated cardiac biomarkers but no ST segment elevation
      2) Location: Table 3-9 describes wall of MI along with coronary artery affected, indicative ECG leads, and anticipated complications
         a) Left ventricular myocardial infarction (LVMI): most MIs are LV
            i) Anterior LV: 42%
            ii) Septal LV: 10%
            iii) Lateral LV: 10%
            iv) Inferior LV: 33%
            v) Posterior LV: 5%
         b) Right ventricular myocardial infarction (RVMI)

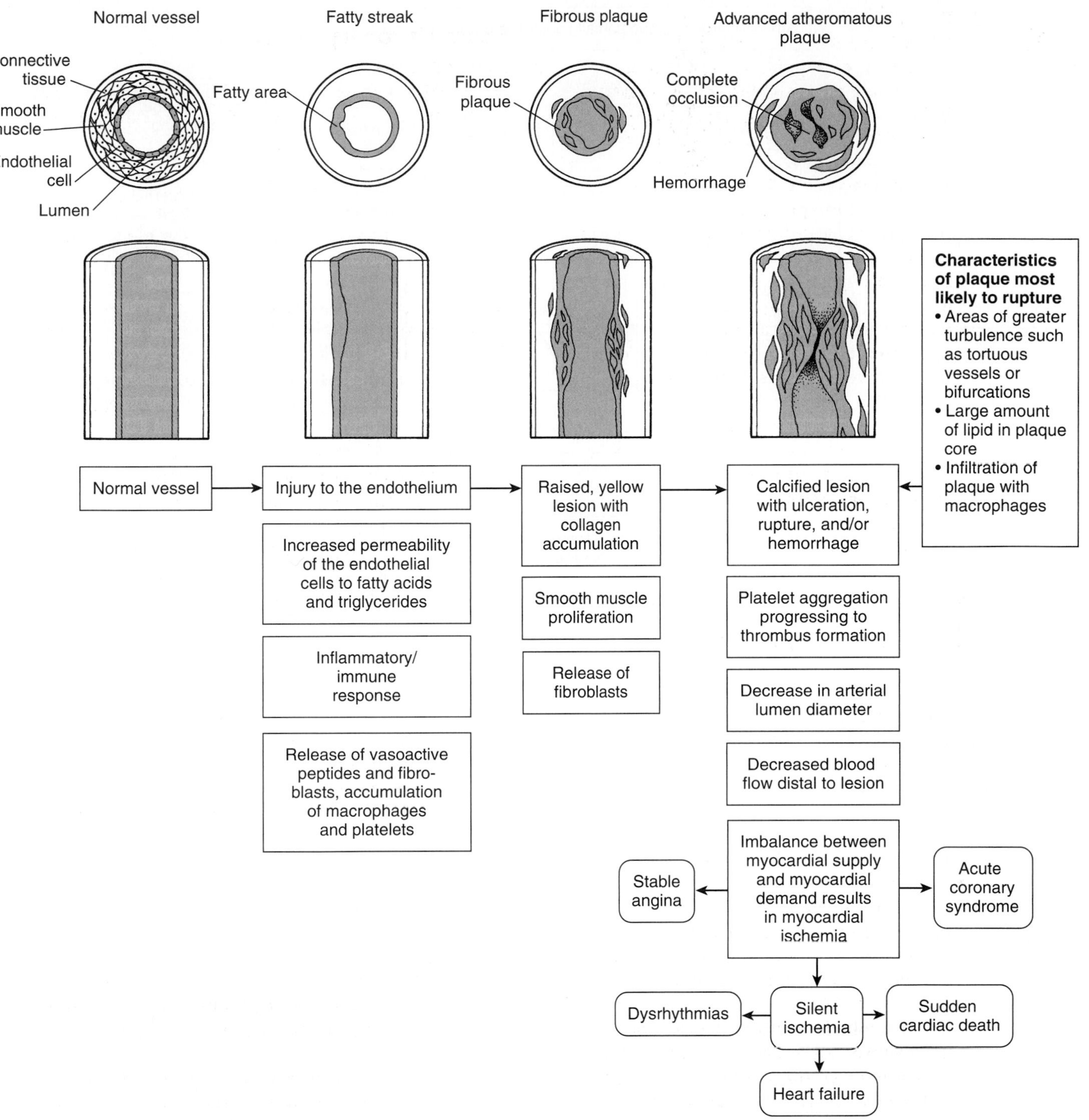

Figure 3-10 Progression of atherosclerosis. (Modified from Thelan, L. A., Urden, L. D., Lough, M. E., & Stacy, K. M. [1998]. *Critical care nursing: Diagnosis and management* [3rd ed.]. St. Louis: Mosby.)

i) Concurrent with inferior LVMI; one third of all inferior MIs have concurrent RV infarction
ii) Rarely isolated: isolated RVMI more common in patients with right ventricular hypertrophy (e.g., COPD)
iii) Smaller infarct due to decreased oxygen requirements of right ventricle
iv) Almost always transmural

Etiology

1. Etiology of arteriosclerosis/atherosclerosis
   a. Nonmodifiable risk factors
      1) Heredity: when siblings or parents develop CAD before 55 years of age
         a) Maternal history of CAD before 65 years conveys greater risk than paternal history in women.
         b) Several risk factors have genetic predisposition (e.g., hypertension, hyperlipidemia, diabetes mellitus).

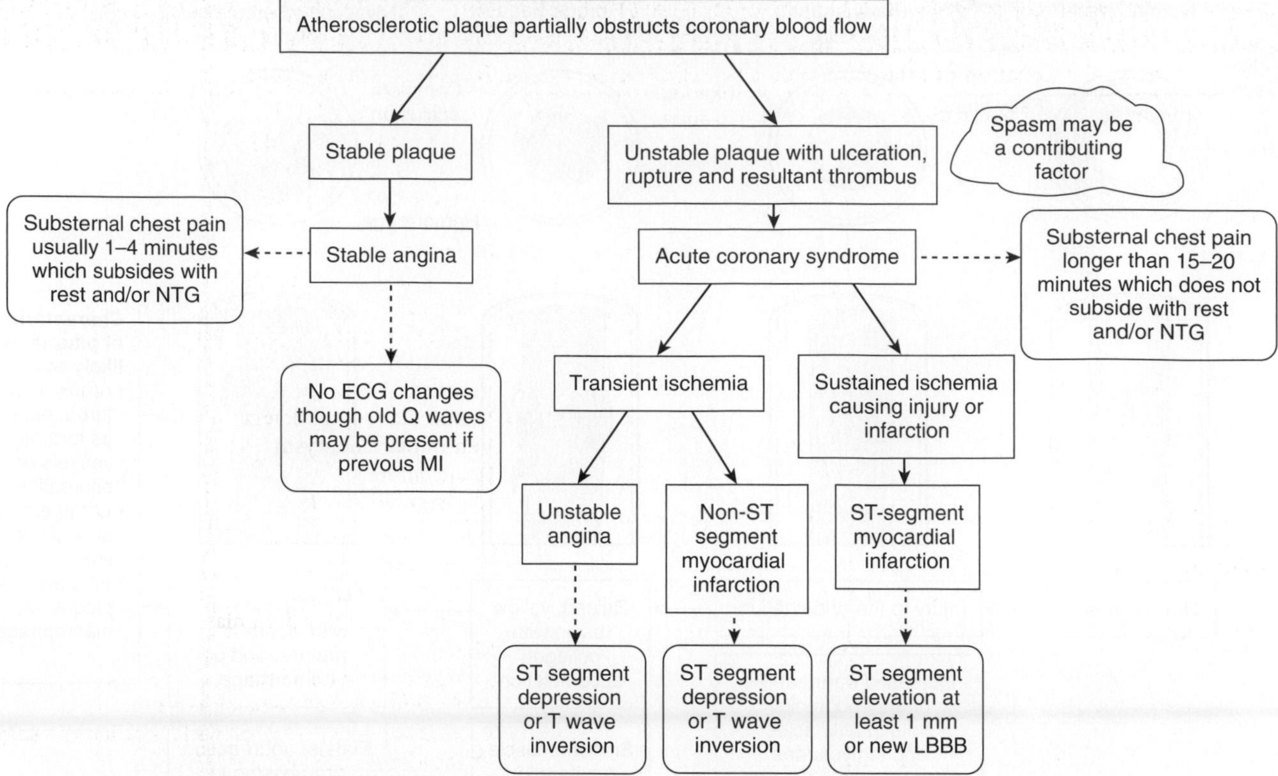

Figure 3-11 Differentiation of stable angina from acute coronary syndrome. Dotted lines connect pathology to the clinical presentation. *LBBB,* left bundle branch block; *NTG,* nitroglycerin; *MI,* myocardial infarction.

2) Advancing age: older than 45 years for males and older than 55 years for females
3) Gender: Males have twice the risk of premenopausal females; risk increases in women after menopause.

b. Modifiable risk factors
1) Hypertension: BP greater than 140/90 mm Hg or requiring antihypertensive agents to achieve BP less than 140/90 mm Hg
2) Hyperlipidemia: elevated levels of cholesterol, triglycerides, or low-density lipoproteins (LDL) and/or decreased levels of high density lipoproteins (HDL); desirable levels of lipids are the following:
   a) Cholesterol level less than 200 mg/dL
   b) LDL level less than 100 mg/dL for patients with heart disease or diabetes mellitus; less than 130 for patients with two or more risk factors; less than 160 for patients with only one risk factor
   c) HDL level greater than 40 mg/dL
   d) Triglyceride level less than 150 mg/dL
3) Smoking: increases LDL level, platelet aggregation, and fibrinogen level, and may cause vasospasm; elevated carbon monoxide levels decrease the oxygen-carrying capacity of hemoglobin; complete smoking cessation is desired
4) Diabetes mellitus or glucose intolerance
   a) Control of blood glucose in patients with diabetes mellitus is advocated to control risk of sequelae including CAD; desirable fasting glucose level is less than 150 mg/dL.
   b) Diabetes is also associated with increased levels of LDL and triglycerides and obesity.
5) Hyperhomocysteinemia: homocysteine level greater than 14 µmol/L
   a) Homocysteine is an essential sulfur-containing amino acid formed during the processing of dietary protein; elevated levels are toxic to the vascular endothelium and increase coagulability.
   b) Deficiencies of folate, vitamin B_{12}, and vitamin B_6 have all been implicated in elevated levels of homocysteine; elevated levels of homocysteine may be successfully reduced by folate, vitamin B_{12}, and/or pyridoxine therapy.
6) Sedentary lifestyle: Exercise is inversely related to cardiovascular mortality; sedentary people are also more likely to be obese, hypertensive, and diabetic.
7) Stress
   a) Chronic stress promotes the long-term development of CAD.

Table 3-9 Myocardial Infarction Summary

Coronary Artery	Location of Infarct	Indicative ECG Leads	Anticipated Complications

Left main coronary artery	Extensive anterior	V_1-V_6	• Sudden cardiac death
			• Dysrhythmias especially:
			  • Sinus tachycardia
			  • Atrial dysrhythmias
			  • Ventricular dysrhythmias
			• Blocks
			  • First-degree AV block
			  • Second-degree AV block type II
			  • Third-degree AV block with ventricular escape
			  • Bundle branch block
			• Ventricular rupture
			• Ventricular septal defect
			• Ventricular aneurysm
			• Heart failure
			• Cardiogenic shock

Left anterior descending artery	Septal	V_1, V_2	• Dysrhythmias especially:
			  • Sinus tachycardia
			  • Atrial fibrillation
			  • Ventricular dysrhythmias
			• Blocks
			  • First-degree AV block
			  • Second-degree AV block type II
			  • Third-degree AV block with ventricular escape
			  • Bundle branch block
			• Ventricular septal rupture

	Anterior	V_3, V_4	• Dysrhythmias especially:
			  • Sinus tachycardia
			  • Atrial fibrillation
			  • Ventricular dysrhythmias
			• Blocks
			  • First-degree AV block
			  • Second-degree AV block type II
			  • Third-degree AV block with ventricular escape
			  • Bundle branch block
			• Ventricular aneurysm
			• Heart failure
			• Cardiogenic shock

Left circumflex artery	Lateral	High: I, aVL Low: V_5, V_6	• Dysrhythmias • Heart failure

Right coronary artery	Inferior	II, III, aVF	• Dysrhythmias especially:
			  • Sinus bradycardia
			  • Sinus arrest
			  • Junctional rhythms
			  • Ventricular dysrhythmias
			• Blocks
			  • SA blocks
			  • First-degree AV block
			  • Second-degree AV block type I
			  • Third-degree AV block usually with AV junctional escape
			  • Bundle branch block
			• Papillary muscle rupture
			• Heart failure

Continued

Table 3-9 Myocardial Infarction Summary—cont'd

Coronary Artery	Location of Infarct	Indicative ECG Leads	Anticipated Complications

	Posterior	Reciprocal changes in V_1, V_2
		Indicative changes in V_7-V_9 (especially V_8, V_9)
			• Dysrhythmias especially:
			  • Sinus bradycardia
			  • Sinus arrest
			  • Junctional rhythms
			  • Ventricular dysrhythmias
			• Blocks
			  • First-degree AV block
			  • Second-degree AV block type I
			  • Third-degree AV block usually with AV junctional escape
			• Papillary muscle rupture with acute mitral regurgitation

	Right ventricular	V_{4R}-V_{6R} (especially V_{4R})	• Dysrhythmias especially:
			  • Sinus bradycardia
			  • Sinus arrest
			  • Junctional rhythms
			  • Ventricular dysrhythmias
			• Blocks
			  • First-degree AV block
			  • Second-degree AV block type I
			  • Third-degree AV block usually with AV junctional escape
			  • Bundle branch block
			• Papillary muscle rupture with acute tricuspid regurgitation
			• Right ventricular failure

b) Acute stress increases catecholamine levels, myocardial oxygen consumption, and dysrhythmia potential.
c) Personality type A with aggression may also contribute.

8) Obesity: body weight greater than 120% of ideal body weight; ideal body weight is desirable
   a) Obesity also contributes to hypertension, hyperlipidemia, glucose intolerance, and sedentary lifestyle.
   b) Midline fat is of greater risk than hip and thigh fat (apple versus pear).
   c) BMI greater than 30 is considered obese and increases cardiac risk.
   d) Metabolic syndrome (i.e., combination of BMI >30 kg/m2, elevated triglycerides and reduced HDL, hypertension, and fasting serum glucose >110 mg/dl or type 2 DM) increases the risk of CAD.
9) Oral contraceptives: increase risk of MI especially in smokers; increases BP; smoking cessation is desirable for all people but especially in women who use oral contraceptives

c. Protective factors
   1) Exercise: elevates HDL, decreases BP and resting HR, decreases body fat, and increases endogenous tissue plasminogen activator (tPA) levels
      a) Intensity: sufficient to increase heart rate to 50-80% of predicted maximal heart rate
      b) Duration: 20-30 minutes
      c) Frequency: at least three times per week
      d) Type of exercise: Recommendation is to vary the type of exercise to prevent boredom, but walking is an excellent form of exercise for almost all patients.
   2) Stress management: reduces catecholamine levels, decreases blood pressure, reduces muscle tension
      a) Methods include daily stretching, breathing exercises, meditation, prayer, and yoga.
   3) High-fiber, low fat diet: reduces total cholesterol
   4) Alcohol (1-2 beverages per day): increases HDL and may decrease platelet aggregation; overall health benefit diminishes after 1-2 alcoholic beverages per day
   5) ASA (81-325 mg daily): prevents platelet aggregation and decreases inflammation (one postulated contributor to CAD)
   6) Omega-3 fatty acids: decrease platelet aggregation, increase HDL levels, decrease triglyceride levels
      a) Alpha linolenic acid found in canola oil, walnuts, flaxseeds
      b) Eicosapentaenoic acid (EPA) and docosahexaenoic acid (DHA) found in salmon, trout, sardines
   7) Flavonoids: antioxidant effect, induce nitric oxide formation, may inhibit platelet aggregation; found in tea and cocoa

8) Loving relationships
   a) Decrease the overall incidence of CAD, though mechanisms are unclear; loneliness and depression have been identified as contributing factors to CAD
   b) Pets also have a beneficial effect by decreasing stress and depression.

2. Etiology of MI
   a. Arteriosclerosis/atherosclerosis
   b. Coronary artery thrombosis
   c. Coronary artery spasm
   d. Cocaine-induced: Excessive sympathetic stimulation causes tachycardia, hypertension, arterial vasoconstriction and spasm; coronary artery spasm may cause MI especially non-Q wave infarction.
   e. Combination of these factors: Most MIs are caused by atherosclerosis and thrombosis.
   f. Other less commonly seen causes
      1) Severe prolonged hypotension
      2) Sudden, severe anemia
      3) Chest trauma (e.g., myocardial contusion)
      4) Trauma to coronary artery or arteries
      5) Aortic stenosis or insufficiency
      6) Thyrotoxicosis
      7) Blood dyscrasias
      8) Aortic dissection
      9) Arteritis
      10) Carbon monoxide poisoning

Clinical Presentation

1. Subjective
   a. Pain: 75-85% of all patients with MI have pain
      1) Provocation: emotional or physical stress; may occur at rest
      2) Palliation: not relieved by oxygen, rest, and/or nitrates; relieved by narcotics and/or reperfusion (e.g., fibrinolytics or PCI)
      3) Quality
         a) Frequently described as pressure on the chest
         b) May also be described as knifelike, stabbing, burning, or indigestion
         c) May feel like usual anginal pain but more severe
         d) Atypical pain common in women
         e) If described as tearing or ripping, consider dissecting aortic aneurysm
      4) Region/radiation
         a) Primary location is usually chest but may be epigastric (especially with inferior MI).
         b) Radiation is usually to the left arm, left elbow, left shoulder, both arms, or jaw.
         c) If radiating to back, consider dissecting aortic aneurysm.
      5) Severity: from vague, slight discomfort to severe pain; more intense than the patient's typical anginal pain
      6) Timing
         a) Most MIs occur within 3 hours of awakening.
         b) The pain is continuous from onset with a duration of 20 minutes or more.
         c) Pain that comes and goes for as long as several days before the actual MI is referred to as a *stuttering MI pattern*: intermittent pain before continuous pain is preinfarction angina.
   b. Silent MI: As many as 25% of all patients with MI have no pain.
      1) More likely in the elderly or diabetic patient
      2) Clues suggesting possible silent MI: new onset heart failure or acute change in mental status, unexplained abdominal pain, unexplained dyspnea or fatigue
   c. Associated symptoms
      1) Nausea and vomiting: seen more often in inferior or posterior MI
      2) Dyspnea or orthopnea: seen more often in anterior MI
      3) Diaphoresis
      4) Palpitations
      5) Apprehension
2. Objective
   a. Heart rate and rhythm
      1) Tachycardia: seen more often in anterior MI
      2) Bradycardia: seen more often in inferior MI
   b. Normotension, hypotension, hypertension
      1) Hypertension: seen more often in anterior MI
      2) Hypotension: seen more often in inferior MI
      3) Equality in arms: Inequality in arms indicates possible dissecting thoracic aortic aneurysm.
   c. Tachypnea
   d. Elevated temperature: may occur 48-72 hours after MI
   e. Levine's sign: clenched fist held over sternum
   f. May have JVD: indicative of RVF; commonly seen in RV infarction
   g. May have abnormal PMI: downward and lateral displacement
   h. Heart sound changes
      1) May have diminished heart sounds: related to decreased contractility
      2) May have S_4: indicative of left ventricular noncompliance; common for first 24 hours
      3) May have S_3: early sign of LVF
      4) May have pericardial friction rub: indicative of pericarditis
      5) May have systolic murmur of mitral regurgitation (high-pitched, blowing, holosystolic murmur loudest at apex which radiates to the axilla); may indicate LVF or papillary muscle dysfunction or rupture
      6) May have murmur of ventricular septal rupture (high-pitched, harsh, holosystolic murmur loudest at lower left sternal border)
   i. May have carotid, aortic, or femoral bruits
   j. May have clinical indications of hypoperfusion (see Table 2-2 on page 26)
   k. May have clinical indications of heart failure

1) LVF (e.g., S_3, crackles, dyspnea) in left ventricular infarction
2) RVF (e.g., JVD, hepatomegaly, peripheral edema) in right ventricular infarction

3. Serum
   a. Leukocyte count: increased (usually 12,000-15,000/mm^3) at 48-72 hours in acute MI
   b. Erythrocyte sedimentation rate (ESR): increased at 48-72 hours in acute MI
   c. CRP: increased in acute MI
   d. IL-6: increased in acute MI; marker of increased mortality in acute MI
   e. Cardiac biomarkers (Table 3-10)
      1) Positive serum isoenzymes
         a) CK: positive CK-MB (greater than 3%) is indicative of MI; highly specific test for MI
         b) LDH: normally LDH_2 is greater than LDH_1; LDH_1 greater than LDH_2 (referred to as *flipped LDH*) is indicative of MI; does not occur until 48-72 hours after the onset of pain
      2) Increased serum muscle proteins
         a) Myoglobin: muscle protein; high sensitivity but low specificity; excellent early negative predictive value
         b) Troponin: contractile protein
            i) Cardiac troponin I (cTnI): found only in cardiac muscle; more specific but later rise and peak
            ii) Cardiac troponin T (cTnT): found in cardiac muscle as well as skeletal muscle; less specific than I, especially in patients with renal failure but earlier rise and peak

4. ECG
   a. ST segment depression in unstable angina
   b. ST segment elevation in variant angina
   c. As a diagnostic tool for acute MI: most helpful when clearly abnormal
      1) If initial ECG nondiagnostic, repeat ECGs should be done every 30 minutes until pain cessation or the ECG is clearly diagnostic and definitive therapy can be initiated
      2) The typical criteria for prompt reperfusion therapies (e.g., PCI, fibrinolytics) in acute MI include either of the following:
         a) ST segment elevation of greater than or equal to 1 mm in at least 2 continuous leads
         b) New left bundle branch block
      3) There are multiple problems with ECG diagnosis of MI
         a) Lag time of hours (or even days) may exist before diagnostic ECG changes become evident; first ECG diagnostic only 50% of the time.
         b) Changes may be subtle.
         c) Previous ECG may not be available for comparison.
         d) Changes may be obscured by a competitive condition.
            i) LBBB or ventricular pacemaker obscures anterior MI.
            ii) WPW obscures anterior MI.
            iii) Left anterior hemiblock obscures inferior MI.
            iv) Left posterior hemiblock obscures lateral MI.
            v) Ventricular hypertrophy may obscure anterior or lateral MI.
         e) 15 or 18 leads are used to prevent missing an infarction in a traditionally "electrically silent" area of the heart; sensitivity and inclusion for reperfusion therapy is increased through the use of right ventricular and posterior lead
            i) 18-lead ECG: 12 standard, 3 right ventricular leads, 3 posterior leads
            ii) 15-lead ECG: 12 standard + V_{4R} + V_8 + V_9
   d. ECG indicators (see Electrocardiography section of Chapter 2 and Figure 2-46)
   e. Locations, indicative leads, coronary artery affected (see Electrocardiography section of Chapter 2 and Table 2-11)
   f. Determination of the age of the MI (see Electrocardiography section of Chapter 2 and Table 2-12)

Table 3-10 Cardiac Biomarkers for Acute MI

Test	Normal Values	Abnormal Values Consistent with MI	Time to Rise (after Injury)	Peak (after Injury)	Return to Normal (after Injury)
CK-MB	0% of total CK	Greater than 3%	6-10 hours	12-24 hours	2-3 days
LDH_1	17-25% of total LDH	Greater than 40%	8-24 hours	72 hours	8-14 days
Myoglobin	Men: 20-90 ng/mL Women: 10-75 ng/mL	Men: greater than 90 ng/ml Women: greater than 75 ng/mL	1-4 hours	6-12 hours	1-2 days
Cardiac troponin I (cTnI)	Less than 1.5 ng/mL	Greater than 4 ng/mL	4-6 hours	18 hours	1-2 weeks
Cardiac troponin T (cTnT)	Less than 0.1 ng/mL	Greater than 0.2 ng/mL	3-4 hours	24 hours	2-3 weeks

5. Echocardiography
   a. Normal wall motion: strong predictor of nonischemic pain
   b. Reduced wall motion: strong predictor of ischemia/infarction
   c. May show mechanical complications (e.g., ventricular septal defect, papillary muscle rupture)
6. Chest x-ray: may show cardiomegaly, indications of heart failure
7. Cardiac catheterization: will likely show coronary artery occlusion; percutaneous coronary intervention (PCI) may be performed after diagnosis
8. Radionuclide studies
   a. Technetium-99 pyrophosphate scan: infarcted areas show up as "hot spots"
   b. Thallium-201 scan: ischemic or infarcted areas show up as "cold spots"

Pathophysiology

1. LVMI (Figure 3-12)
2. RVMI (Figure 3-13)

3. Factors affecting mortality
   a. Age
   b. Left ventricular ejection fraction
   c. Number of occluded vessels
   d. Previous history of MI
   e. Presence of cardiogenic shock: associated with loss of 40% of LV muscle mass; may be from one MI or several cumulative MIs
   f. NOTE: Females have twice the mortality of males; probably related to the fact that they tend to be older and have more significant risk factors (e.g., diabetes mellitus, hypertension) when they develop their MI.

Collaborative Management

1. Provide care according to national guidelines (Figure 3-14).
2. Manage cardiopulmonary arrest if required.
   a. Ventricular fibrillation frequently occurs within 1 hour: early identification of clinical indications of MI and hospitalization is very important.

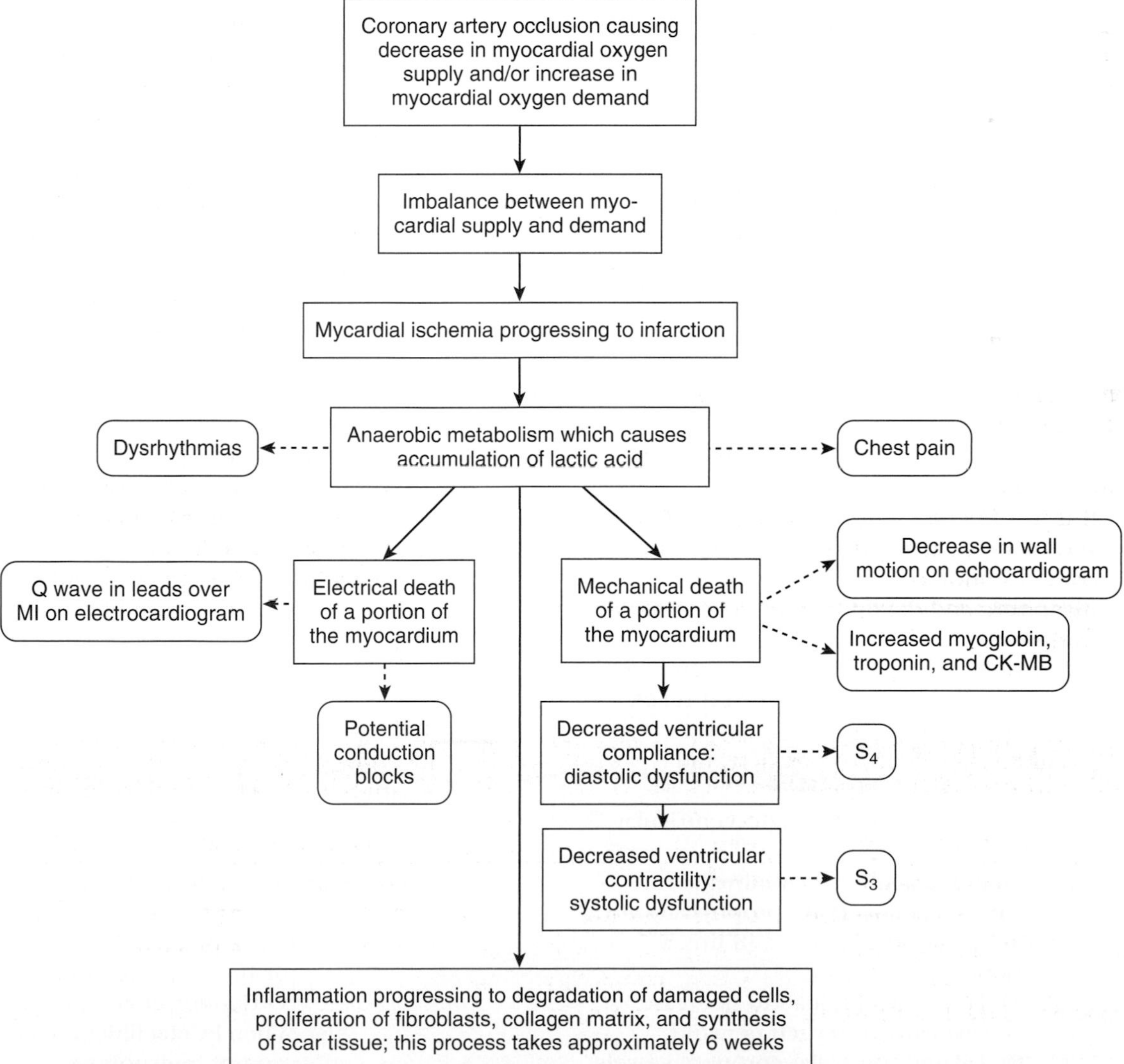

Figure 3-12 Pathophysiology of myocardial infarction. Dotted lines connect pathology to the clinical presentation.

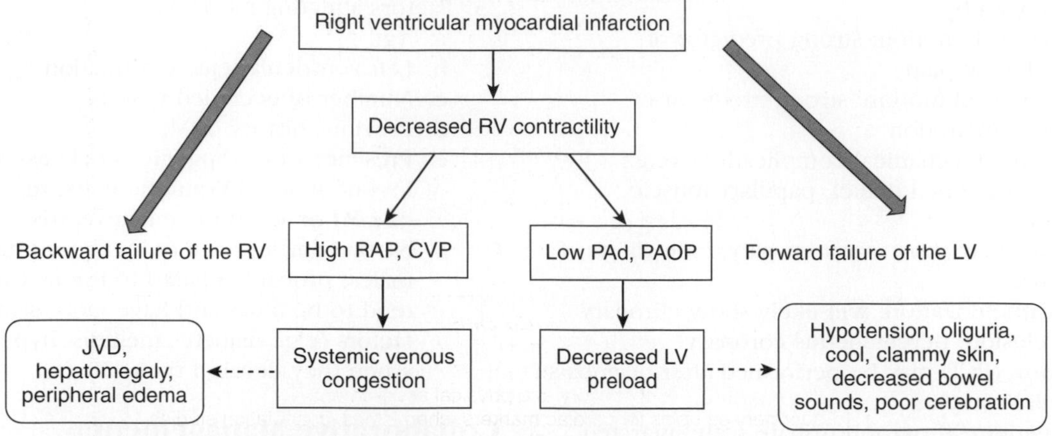

Figure 3-13 Pathophysiology of right ventricular MI. Dotted lines connect pathology to the clinical presentation. *CVP,* central venous pressure; *JVD,* jugular venous distention; *LV,* left ventricular; *PAd,* pulmonary artery diastolic pressure; *PAOP,* pulmonary artery occlusive pressure; *RAP,* right atrial pressure; *RV,* right ventricular.

b. Manage airway, oxygenation, and circulation using BLS, and ACLS.

3. Monitor ECG, vital signs, physical examination, and hemodynamic parameters for changes.
   a. Safely and accurately monitor the patient's hemodynamic parameters as indicated; hemodynamic monitoring is likely to be useful in the following situations in acute MI.
      1) Persistent chest pain
      2) Persistent tachycardia
      3) Significant hypertension or hypotension
      4) Significant left ventricular or right ventricular failure
      5) Intravenous inotropic or vasoactive agents
      6) New systolic murmur
   b. Utilize hemodynamic parameters in evaluating clinical status for changes and responses to prescribed therapies.
4. Reduce size of myocardial infarction: myocardial salvaging techniques
   a. Treat pain promptly and adequately: decreases catecholamine release and myocardial oxygen demand
      1) Morphine sulfate: 2-4 mg IV every 5 minutes pain relief
         a) Actions: decreases preload; decreases catecholamine release via pain relief (which decreases heart rate and afterload); decreases anxiety and restlessness
         b) Cautions: inferior MI; right ventricular MI
      2) Nitroglycerin: usually given initially sublingually; may be given prophylactically at 25-100 mcg/min IV for 24-48 hours
         a) Actions
            i) Decreases preload to decrease myocardial oxygen demand
            ii) Dilates epicardial coronary vessels to increase myocardial oxygen supply
            iii) Augments the analgesic effect of morphine
         b) Caution: may cause reflex tachycardia; beta-blockers may be needed
      3) Calcium channel blockers (e.g., nifedipine [Procardia]); especially for variant angina
      4) Reperfusion therapies (e.g., fibrinolytics, PCI): relieve pain by reestablishing blood flow and aerobic metabolism
      5) IABP: may be used for intractable pain as it increases coronary artery perfusion pressure (Figures 3-15 through 3-17 and Table 3-11)
   b. Increase myocardial oxygen supply
      1) Administer oxygen at 2-6 L/min per nasal cannula for 24-48 hours
         a) Probably has little effect on the myocardial arterial oxygen content of otherwise normal individuals but may significantly improve oxygenation of an ischemic myocardium especially in patients with hypoxemia from pulmonary edema
         b) Even in the absence of pulmonary edema or other complications, it seems that some patients develop modest hypoxemia early during the course of acute MI.
      2) Provide either emergent PCI or fibrinolytics to reestablish patency of the infarct-related artery (IRA) within the benchmark time frame
         a) Assist with decision making regarding reperfusion therapies.
            i) When PCI facilities are available, PCI is preferred over fibrinolytics for the majority of patients (O'Connor et al., 2010).
            ii) When PCI facilities are not available, prompt transport to a facility with PCI capability is preferred over fibrinolytics if

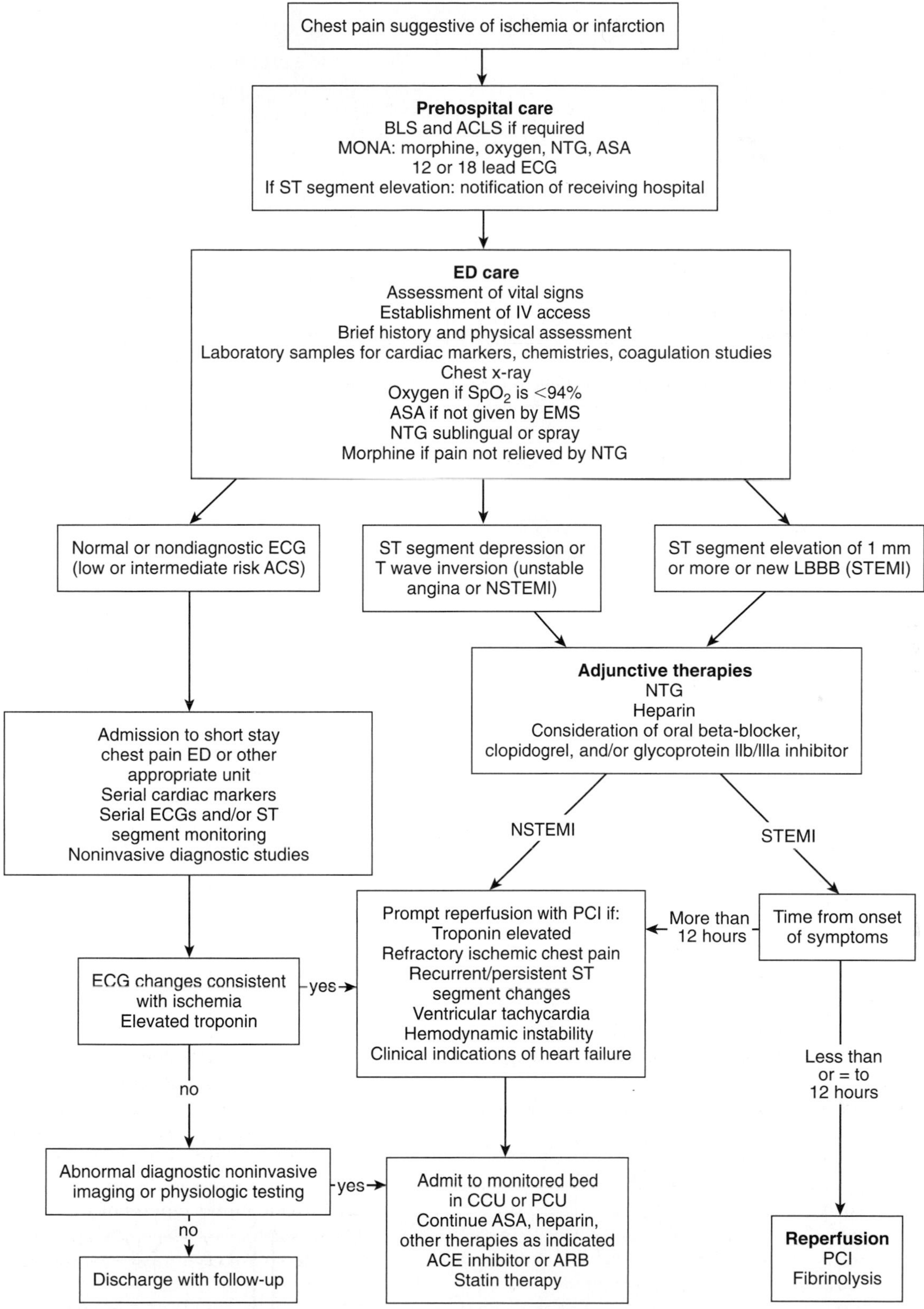

Figure 3-14 ACS management algorithm. *ACLS,* advanced cardiac life support; *ACS,* acute coronary syndrome; *ARB;* angiotensin receptor blocker; *ASA,* aspirin; *BLS,* basic life support; *CCU,* critical care unit; *ECG,* electrocardiogram; *EMS,* emergency medical services; *IV,* intravenous; *LBBB,* left bundle branch block; *MONA,* morphine, oxygen, nitroglycerin, aspirin; *NSTEMI,* Non-ST segment elevation myocardial infarction; *NTG,* nitroglycerin; *PCI,* percutaneous coronary intervention; *PCU,* progressive care unit; *SpO_2,* oxygen saturation by pulse oximetry; *STEMI,* ST segment elevation myocardial infarction. (Data from O'Connor, R. E., Brady, W., Brooks, S. C., Diercks, D., Egan, J., Ghaemmaghami, C., et al. [2010]. Part 10: Acute coronary syndromes: 2010 American Heart Association guidelines for cardiopulmonary resuscitation and emergency cardiovascular care. *Circulation*, 122[18 Suppl 3], S787-817.)

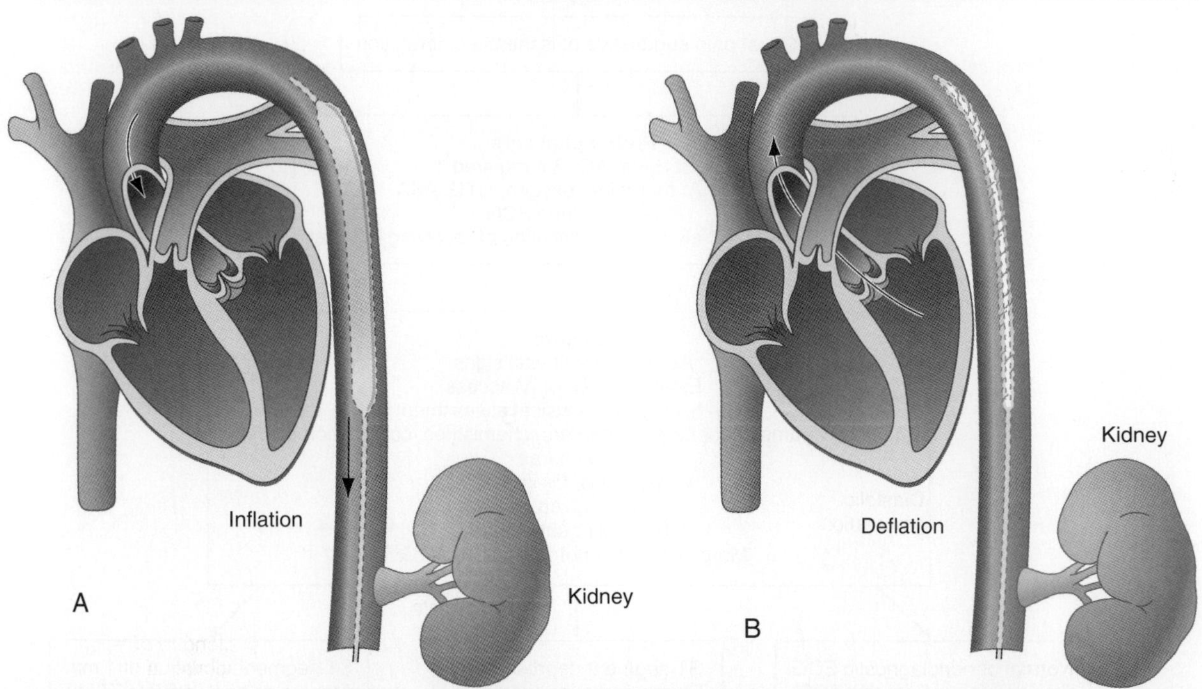

Figure 3-15 Intraaortic balloon pump movement. **A,** Inflation during diastole moves blood toward the heart to increase coronary artery perfusion pressure. **B,** Deflation during systole moves blood away from the heart to decrease afterload. (From Carlson, K. K. [Ed.]. [2009]. *AACN Advanced critical care nursing.* St. Louis: Saunders.)

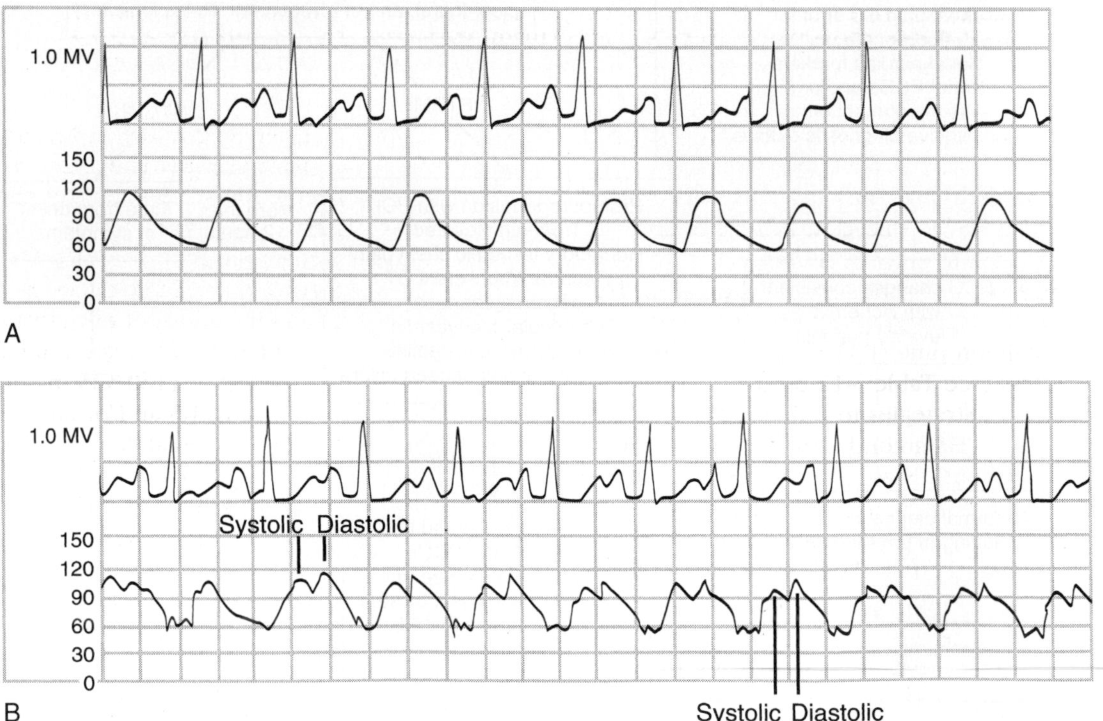

Figure 3-16 Simultaneous electrocardiographic and arterial blood pressure recordings before *(panel A)* and during *(panel B)* intraaortic balloon counterpulsation. The peak diastolic (coronary perfusion) pressure is increased and the peak systolic pressure is decreased during counterpulsation. (From Darovic, G. O. [2002]. *Hemodynamic monitoring: Invasive and noninvasive clinical application* [3rd ed.]. Philadelphia: Saunders.)

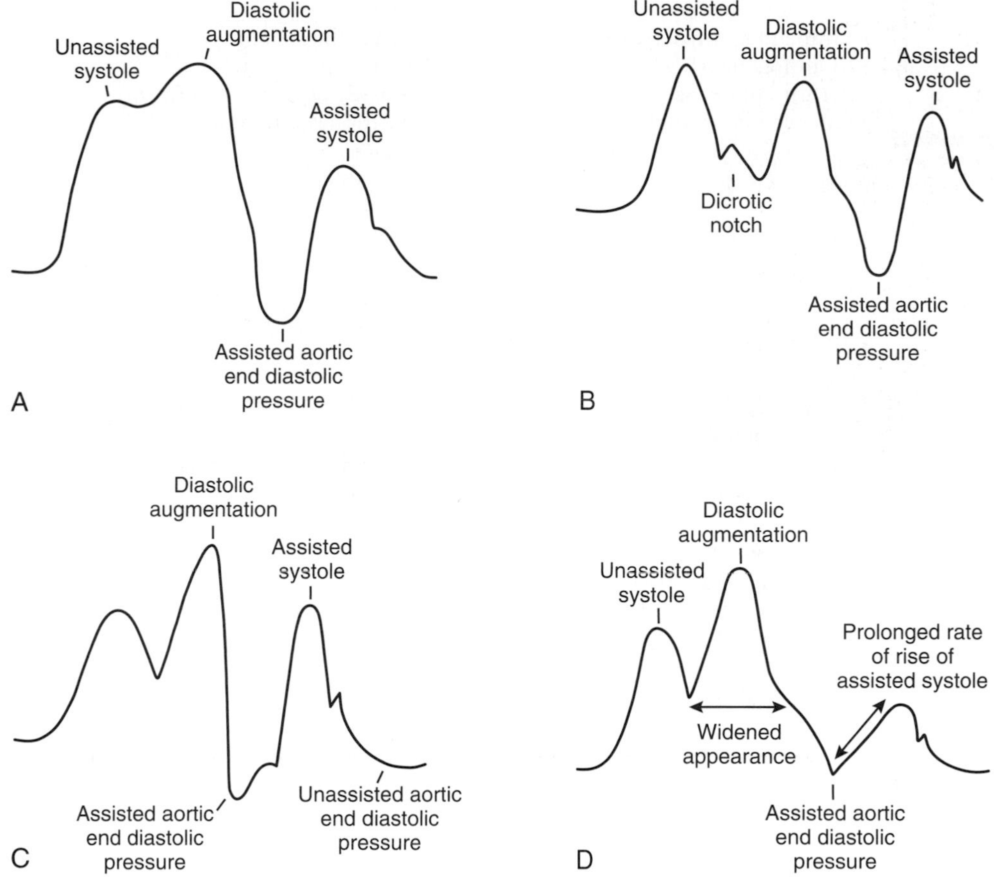

Figure 3-17 Inaccurate IABP timing. **A,** Early inflation. **B,** Late inflation. **C,** Early deflation. **D,** Late deflation. (From Datascope Corporation [1989]. *Mechanics of intraaortic balloon counterpulsation*. Montvale, NJ: Datascope.)

transfer to PCI time is less than 120 minutes (O'Connor et al., 2010).

b) Assist in prompt preparation of the patient for emergent PCI if PCI is determined to be the appropriate method of reperfusion for this specific patient; the goal is to achieve a door-to-balloon time (DTBT) of 90 minutes or less (see Table 3-12 on page 164)
   i) Strategies to reduce STEMI DTBT (Hammond, 2010; Farwell, 2010)
      (a) Establish protocols that define the process and facilitate crucial assessment studies (e.g., ECG, troponin) and interventions (IV, ASA).
      (b) Empower EMS and/or ED physician to activate the STEMI team; eliminate unnecessary consults.
      (c) Facilitate sharing of information through computerization.
      (d) Provide feedback to participants so that improvements can continue.

c) Administer fibrinolytics if they are determined to be the appropriate method of reperfusion for this specific patient; the goal is to achieve door-to-needle time of 60 minutes or less (see Table 3-13 on page 166)

d) Either primary PCI or fibrinolytics are preceded by platelet aggregation inhibitors and/or anticoagulants.
   i) Platelet aggregation inhibitors
      (a) ASA (160-325 mg initially and daily) and/or another antiplatelet drug (e.g., clopidogrel [Plavix], prasugrel [Effient]) to decrease platelet aggregation and clot extension
      (b) GP IIb/IIIa platelet receptor blockers (e.g., abciximab [ReoPro], eptifibatide [Integrilin], tirofiban HCl [Aggrastat]) (see Table 3-14 on page 168)
   ii) Anticoagulants (Table 3-14)
      (a) Unfractionated heparin may be prescribed for 24-48 hours to maintain aPTT 45-60 seconds
         (i) Indirect thrombin inhibitor

Text continued on p. 178

Table 3-11 Intraaortic Balloon Pump

Indications	• Unstable angina refractory to medical therapy • Impending myocardial infarction or myocardial infarction • Cardiogenic shock or severe left ventricular failure • Heart failure, as a bridge to left ventricular assist device or transplant • Mechanical complications of acute MI (e.g., ruptured papillary muscle with acute mitral regurgitation, acute ventricular septal rupture) • Ischemia-related intractable ventricular dysrhythmias • High-risk patient undergoing coronary percutaneous intervention • Preoperative, perioperative, and/or postoperative support prior to coronary artery bypass graft or other major surgery • Difficulty weaning from cardiopulmonary bypass • Myocardial contusion • Septic shock
Contraindications	Absolute • Aortic valve regurgitation • Aortic dissection • Patients with chronic end-stage heart disease who are not awaiting a cardiac transplant • Patients with irreversible brain damage or terminal condition Relative • Aortic aneurysm • Uncontrolled sepsis • Severe bilateral peripheral vascular disease (e.g., absent femoral pulse); if patient has had bilateral femoropopliteal bypass grafts, the balloon may be placed via the left axillary artery into the ascending aorta • Coagulopathy • Tachydysrhythmias

Actions (Figure 3-15)	• Balloon is inflated during diastole to increase myocardial oxygen supply
	  • Increases coronary artery blood flow by displacing blood retrograde toward the aortic arch and increasing diastolic blood pressure
	  • Increases blood flow to the renal arteries and lower extremities by displacing blood antegrade toward the renal and lower extremities arteries
	  • Increases MAP to improve tissue perfusion
	• Balloon is deflated immediately prior to systole to decrease myocardial oxygen demand
	  • Decreases left ventricular afterload by decreasing systolic BP

Insertion and mechanics	• Catheter with balloon is inserted via femoral artery (NOTE: The catheter may be inserted via iliac, subclavian, or axillary artery if the femoral artery is not an option)
	• Balloon is positioned in descending thoracic aorta between left subclavian and renal arteries
	  • The tip of the catheter should be at the 2nd-3rd ICS, 1-2 cm from the left subclavian artery and above the renal arteries by chest x-ray
	  • The balloon occludes 80% of the aortic diameter when inflated
	• Helium to inflate the balloon is shuttled into and out of the balloon by a pump which is housed in a console at the bedside

Timing (Figure 3-16)	• By ECG
	  • Inflated after the T wave
	  • Deflated prior to QRS
	• By arterial waveform (NOTE: Newly IABP catheters have fiberoptic pressure sensors in the tip that provide real-time pressure signals because the signal travels at the speed of light rather than assuming a delay with fluid-filled transducer systems)
	  • Inflated at the dicrotic notch
	  • Deflated at the end-diastolic dip immediately prior to systole
	• Inflation and deflation are usually triggered by ECG but fine timing is done by the nurse using the arterial waveform
	• Frequency may be 1:1, 1:2, or 1:3 but timing is always adjusted in 1:2 setting

Assessment	• HR: a normalization of heart rate is desirable • BP: a decrease in systolic BP, an increase in diastolic BP, and an increase in MAP is desirable • CO/CI: an increase in cardiac output/index is desirable • PAP/PAOP: a decrease in PAP and PAOP is desirable • A decrease in the amplitude of *v* wave on the PAOP waveform is desirable in patients with mitral regurgitation or ventricular septal rupture • SaO_2: an increase in SaO_2 is desirable • SvO_2: an increase in SvO_2 is desirable • Urine output: an increase in urine output is desirable • Complaints of chest pain: a decrease in chest pain is desirable • ECG: a decrease in the presence or frequency of dysrhythmias is desirable • Neurovascular status of affected limb: the presence of palpable pulses and a warm limb with normal capillary refill is desirable

Table 3-11 Intraaortic Balloon Pump—cont'd	
Brief summary of nursing management	• Assess the parameters described earlier • Ensure optimal timing of balloon inflation and deflation • Titrate pharmacologic therapies to augment the mechanical therapy of the IABP • Ensure positioning of the patient with head of bed elevation greater than 30 degrees and avoidance of hip flexion • Observe for complications and provide appropriate management for the prevention of complications

Complications: prevention and treatment	• Thrombosis causing lower extremity ischemia
	  • Insertion precautions
	    — Use the smallest sheath that will allow the catheter to be advanced through it;
	    — Select the limb with the best pulse
	  • Dextran 40 as prescribed as an antiplatelet aggregation agent
	  • Restraint of affected leg to prevent displacement of the balloon and trauma to intima of artery
	  • Neurovascular assessment of the affected limb every hour
	  • If limb ischemia is noted: treatment may include any of the following:
	    — Removal of catheter with placement of the sheath and catheter in the other femoral artery if the IABP is still needed
	    — Catheter thrombectomy
	    — Femorofemoral graft
	    — Lidocaine or papaverine: to decrease arterial spasm
	• Catheter displacement causing renal or left upper extremity ischemia
	  • Elevation of head of bed no more than 20-30 degrees to prevent displacement of the balloon
	  • Restraint of affected limb to prevent displacement of the balloon
	  • Close monitoring of urine output
	  • Notification of physician of significant changes in urine output
	  • Neurovascular assessment of left arm every hour
	• Emboli
	  • Dextran 40 as prescribed as an antiplatelet aggregation agent
	  • Heparin may be prescribed
	  • Avoidance of allowing the balloon to remain static (noninflating) for more than 30 minutes; clots may form in the folds of the balloon and be embolized when the balloon is then reinflated
	• Infection
	  • Sterile dressing changes daily or every other day
	  • Close monitoring of the site for erythema, edema, induration, warmth
	• Aortic dissection
	  • Attention to complaints of back pain, vital sign changes
	  • Removal of catheter and repair of aorta if dissection occurs
	• Anemia
	  • Attention to presence of petechiae or ecchymosis, platelet counts
	  • Discontinuance of heparin
	  • Blood and/or blood products may be prescribed
	• Balloon complications
	  • Leak
	    — Attention to increase in volume or frequency of refilling
	    — Replacement of catheter if leak occurs to prevent gas embolism
	  • Rupture
	    — Attention to blood in catheter
	    — Replacement of catheter if rupture occurs to prevent entrapment
	• Inaccurate timing (Fig. 3-17)
	  • Inflation is too early: aortic valve closes too early and stroke volume is decreased
	  • Inflation is too late: diastolic augmentation is decreased
	  • Deflation is too early: less increase in coronary artery perfusion pressure and less of a decrease in afterload
	  • Deflation is too late: increase in afterload
	• Inadequate pumping: usually due to dysrhythmias
	  • Timing method changed from ECG to arterial line

Continued

Table 3-11 Intraaortic Balloon Pump—cont'd

Weaning	• Indications • Cardiac index greater than 2.0 L/min • PAOP less than 18 mm Hg • MAP greater than 70 mm Hg • SVR less than 1400 dynes/sec/cm^{-5} • SpO_2 greater than 94% • Absence of anginal pain • Urine output at least 0.5 mL/kg/hr • Absence of clinical indicators of hypoperfusion • Methods • May be done by decreasing the frequency (e.g., from every cardiac cycle to every other cardiac cycle to every third cardiac cycle) • May be done by decreasing the volume in the balloon with each inflation (e.g., decreased by 25% with each weaning step)
Balloon removal	• Gown, mask, eye protection must be used • Pump is turned off, sutures are removed, catheter is removed and inspected to ensure that the entire catheter has been removed • Firm pressure is applied to the insertion site for at least 15 minutes but may be required for more than 30 minutes if the patient has been receiving anticoagulants; a vascular hemostasis device may be used • Pressure dressing to insertion site for 2-4 hours • Monitor site frequently for the next 4-8 hours for bleeding or hematoma formation

Table 3-12 Percutaneous Coronary Interventions

Procedures	• Percutaneous transluminal coronary angioplasty (PTCA): inflation of a balloon-tipped catheter in an area of coronary artery stenosis from plaque; plaque is pushed back against the wall of the vessel and fractured (controlled trauma) • Cutting balloon microsurgical dilation catheter system: microsurgical blades mounted longitudinally on an angioplasty balloon to open narrowed artery; as the balloon expands radially, the blades are exposed and incise plaque in the arteries; claimed to facilitate maximum dilatation of the target lesion with more precision and less trauma than conventional angioplasty • Coronary artery stent: use of a metal mesh tube that acts as a scaffolding device to support a coronary artery and maintain patency after PTCA; previously used only in case of acute closure, most PTCA procedures include planned stent placements • Stents are usually stainless steel but may be nitinol, tantalum, or another metal • Stents have usually been thought of as a coil but they may be a mesh, slotted tube, ring, or another design • Stents are either deployed by balloon expansion or they may be self-expanding • Stents may be drug-eluting (i.e., drug-eluting stent [DES]) to reduce the risk of neointimal hyperplasia and restenosis rates — Sirolimus, an immunosuppressive agent, to prevent proliferation of normal tissue and inflammation — Paclitaxel, an antineoplastic agent, to inhibit cell proliferation and migration • Brachytherapy: use of intracoronary irradiation to reduce risk of restenosis; combined with PTCA or stent placement • Coronary atherectomy: removal of plaque from a coronary artery by a high-speed diamond-tipped (rotational) or shaving (directional) device • Directional coronary atherectomy (DCA): a directional device shaves pieces of the atheroma into the catheter tip • Coronary rotational ablation (Rotablator): a diamond-coated burr drills through the atheroma and pulverizes the plaque • Transluminal extraction catheter (TEC): a motorized cutting head shaves the atheroma from the arterial wall and suctions out the pieces • Excimer laser coronary atherectomy (ELCA): use of a laser to vaporize the atheroma • AngioJet: high speed saline jet; most effective for thrombus

Table 3-12 Percutaneous Coronary Interventions—cont'd

Indications	• Unstable or chronic angina • Acute or postacute MI • Postcoronary artery bypass graft with postoperative angina • Patient must be surgical candidate (in case of coronary artery dissection)
Contraindications	• Left main CAD (unless there is a patent bypass around it, referred to as *protected*) • Stenosis of coronary artery at orifice • Variant angina • Critical valvular disease
Action	• The goal of percutaneous coronary interventions is to reduce the degree of coronary artery stenosis; the intervention is considered successful if the degree of stenosis is reduced to 20-30% stenosis without serious complications
Assessment	• Vital signs: BP, HR, RR, T • ECG: monitor closely for ST segment elevation • Sheath insertion site: usually femoral but may be radial • Neurovascular status of affected limb • Any complaints of chest pain • Any complaints of back pain

Brief summary of specific nursing management	• Monitor for myocardial ischemia: note any new chest pain, ST segment elevation especially if PCI performed for acute ischemia or infarction
	• Assess puncture site frequently to detect bleeding and/or hematoma formation
	  • Control systolic BP to less than 150 mm Hg and diastolic BP less than 90 mm Hg with antihypertensives as prescribed
	  • Monitor platelet count and aPTT (patient will receive platelet aggregation inhibitors and either unfractionated or low-molecular-weight heparin to prevent reocclusion)
	  • Immobilize groin by restraining with sheet stretched over knee on affected side and tucked on each side of bed rather than restraining ankle
	  • Perform neurovascular checks to detect peripheral ischemia related to femoral artery thrombosis
	• Monitor for clinical indications of retroperitoneal hemorrhage: postural tachycardia and/or hypotension; back and/or flank pain; Grey-Turner's sign; decrease in hemoglobin and hematocrit (unfortunately there are no early indications)
	• Keep affected limb straight and immobile; head of bed should be elevated no more than 30 degrees as long as the sheath is in place and for 4-8 hours after removal
	• Assist with removal or remove sheath (depending on hospital protocol) if not completed in the cardiac catheterization laboratory; Perclose, VasoSeal, or Angio-Seal may be used when the sheath was removed in the cardiac catheterization laboratory
	  • If IV heparin has been infusing, it will be discontinued and the ACT needs to be less than 150 seconds; if unfractionated heparin is to be restarted, it will be restarted several hours after sheath removal; low-molecular-weight heparin subcutaneously may be used
	  • Pain control and sedation (e.g., local infiltration with lidocaine or IV morphine and/or midazolam [Versed] or lorazepam [Ativan])
	  • Apply pressure to where the sheath entered the artery which is about 1 inch above the skin entry site
	  • Manual pressure or mechanical pressure devices (e.g., C-clamp, FemoStop) may be used
	  • Pressure is held for at least 30 minutes or until hemostasis achieved
	  • Control of bleeding must be maintained while peripheral pulses are still palpated

Continued

Table 3-12 Percutaneous Coronary Interventions—cont'd

Complications: prevention and treatment	• Acute reocclusion or closure due to:
	  • Trauma to intima initiating clotting cascade
	    — ASA and heparin are used to prevent thrombosis
	    — GP IIb/IIIa platelet receptor blockers (e.g., abciximab [ReoPro], eptifibatide [Integrilin], or tirofiban HCl [Aggrastat]) are used for PCI in ACS patients who have not been receiving clopidogrel
	    — ASA and clopidogrel (Plavix) are maintained after the procedure
	      • Prasugrel (Effient) is another platelet receptor blocker that may be used but should not be used for ACS patients with stroke or transient ischemic attack
	    — Monitor aPTT; usually maintained at 50-70 seconds
	    — Proton pump inhibitor is recommended with dual antiplatelet therapy
	  • Coronary artery spasm
	    — Nitroglycerin infusion and/or calcium channel blockers are frequently used
	    — Note: new onset chest pain or ST segment changes should be reported immediately
	• Coronary artery dissection: due to catheter trauma; necessitates placement of stent or, in severe cases, emergent coronary artery bypass graft
	• Cardiac tamponade: due to cardiac perforation
	• Dysrhythmias: due to ischemia or reperfusion
	• Pseudoaneurysm: due to catheter dissection of artery
	• Hemorrhage or hematoma: due to anticoagulated state
	  • Retroperitoneal hemorrhage or hematoma
	  • Femoral artery puncture site hemorrhage or hematoma
	• Embolic complications (e.g., myocardial infarction, cerebral infarction, peripheral emboli)
	• Chronic restenosis: due to intimal hyperplasia
	• Hypotension, bradycardia (vagal reaction): due to increased parasympathetic nervous system during sheath removal; atropine is effective

Postprocedure education	• Information about devices placed: give the patient a stent identification card with date, facility, type, and site of implant • Care of site used for catheter insertion (femoral or radial) • Need for drugs to maintain stent patency: usually aspirin and clopidogrel • Avoid magnetic resonance imaging (MRI) scans within 8 weeks of stent placement • Symptoms to report: site pain, chest pain, bleeding

Table 3-13 Fibrinolytic Therapy

Actions	• Activate plasminogen to plasmin, the active agent which breaks down clots (speeds up the normal fibrinolytic process to allow early reperfusion)
	• Limit cellular necrosis and decrease infarction size
	• Decrease mortality, morbidity
	  • Short-term: reestablishing arterial patency
	  • Long-term: maintaining ejection fraction

Fibrinolytic agents (Table 3-14)	• Streptokinase (SK) (rarely used today)
	• Recombinant tissue plasminogen activator (rt-PA)
	  • Alteplase (Activase): short-half life so administered as a bolus followed by infusion
	  • Tenecteplase (TNKase): longest half-life so administered as a one-time bolus
	• Recombinant plasminogen activator (r-PA)
	  • Reteplase (Retavase): intermediate half-life so administered as two boluses 10 minutes apart
	• Urokinase (rarely used in acute MI but may be used in peripheral arterial occlusion)

Indications	• History strongly suggestive of MI • ST segment elevation of more than 1 mm in at least two contiguous leads or new LBBB • Pain of less than 6 hours or still having pain (Note: as long as the patient is having pain, salvageable myocardium is assumed because dead myocardium does not metabolize aerobically or anaerobically, and neither lactic acid or pain would be produced)
Absolute contraindications	• Active internal bleeding • History of hemorrhagic stroke, intracranial neoplasm, AV malformation, or aneurysm • Intracranial or intraspinal surgery or trauma within 2 months • Known bleeding disorder (e.g., thrombocytopenia, hemophilia) • Suspected aortic aneurysm or acute pericarditis • Systolic BP greater than or equal to 200 mm Hg and/or diastolic BP greater than or equal to 120 mm Hg • Prolonged (more than 10 minutes) or traumatic CPR • Pregnancy • Streptokinase is contraindicated if the patient has received streptokinase or had a streptococcal infection within the last 6-9 months but tPA can still be used

Table 3-13 Fibrinolytic Therapy—cont'd	
Relative contraindications	• Major surgery or trauma within 10 days • Recent gastrointestinal or genitourinary bleeding • Cerebrovascular disease • Oral anticoagulant therapy • Systolic BP greater than or equal to 180 mm Hg and/or diastolic BP greater than or equal to 110 mm Hg • Significant liver dysfunction • Septic thrombophlebitis • Subacute bacterial endocarditis • High likelihood of left heart thrombus (e.g., mitral stenosis with atrial fibrillation, ventricular aneurysm, left atrial myxoma) • Diabetic hemorrhagic retinopathy • Advanced age (greater than 70-75 years) with consideration of physiologic age, severity of concomitant diseases, mental status • Any condition when bleeding would be a significant hazard or would be difficult to manage (e.g., recent femoral artery puncture or sheath)

Clinical indications of reperfusion	• Pain cessation
	• ST segment return to baseline
	• Reperfusion dysrhythmias
	  • Sinus bradycardia
	  • Idioventricular rhythm, accelerated idioventricular rhythm
	  • AV blocks
	  • Ventricular irritability: PVCs, ventricular tachycardia, ventricular fibrillation
	• CK washout: early or markedly elevated CK peak

Assessment	• Heart rate • Blood pressure • ECG rhythm; note reperfusion dysrhythmias • Clinical indications of reperfusion • Bleeding (e.g., puncture points, gums, saliva, sputum, gastric secretions, stools, urine) • Complaints of chest pain, back pain, or headache

Brief summary of nursing management	• Administer adjuvant therapy: tPA is followed by ASA, heparin (SK causes significant fibrinogen depletion, and heparin is not indicated due to increased bleeding risk)
	• Monitor for clinical indications of reperfusion; notify physician if these are not seen so that emergent PCI can be scheduled
	• Avoid punctures: arterial; IV, IM, subcutaneous
	  • Apply pressure until hemostasis is achieved if punctures are required after fibrinolytics initiated
	  • Insert multiple (usually 2-3) IV catheters prior to initiation of fibrinolytic therapy; one of these catheters may be used for venous sampling
	• Monitor stools, urine, emesis, sputum, saliva for blood
	• Monitor for complications

Complications	• Hemorrhage
	  • At site of vascular puncture: 80% incidence
	  • GI or GU bleeding: 15-20% incidence
	  • Intracranial bleed: 1% incidence
	• Reocclusion: monitor for new pain and/or ST segment changes
	• Allergic reactions to streptokinase
	  • Monitor for urticaria, fever, bronchospasm, dyspnea, stridor, or dysrhythmias
	  • Administer diphenhydramine (Benadryl) and/or hydrocortisone (Solu-Cortef) as prescribed in attempt to prevent allergic reaction
	• Reperfusion dysrhythmias: usually transient
	  • Administer antidysrhythmics or perform cardioversion or defibrillation as indicated for sustained ventricular tachycardia or ventricular fibrillation (prophylactic antidysrhythmics are no longer recommended with fibrinolytic therapy)
	  • Administer atropine or apply transcutaneous pacemaker for symptomatic bradycardia or block

Table 3-14 Drugs that Affect Clotting Used for Patients with Myocardial Infarction

Drug	Classification/ Actions	Indications	Administration	Adverse Effects	Nursing Implications

Abciximab (ReoPro)	Platelet aggregation inhibitor (GP IIb/IIIa platelet receptor blocker)
	• Inhibits platelet aggregation and platelet-mediated thrombosis
		• Acute coronary syndrome with or without percutaneous coronary intervention (PCI)
		• PCI when risk for thrombosis is high
			• IV injection: 0.25 mg/kg administered between 10 minutes and 1 hour before the start of the PTCA or atherectomy followed by infusion
			• IV infusion: 0.125 mcg/kg/min (10 mcg/min maximum) for 12 hours
				• Bleeding
				  • Intracranial hemorrhage
				  • Hematuria
				  • Hematemesis
				  • Bleeding at sheath site or other puncture point
				• Thrombocytopenia
				• Hypotension
				• Bradycardia
				• Nausea, vomiting, abdominal pain
				• Chest pain
				• Back pain
				• Headache
				• Pain at injection site
				• Allergic reaction, anaphylaxis (especially with repeat administration)
					• Monitor PT, aPTT, or ACT, platelet count
					• Administer with aspirin and heparin therapy as prescribed
					• Note contraindications: patients with active internal bleeding, clinically significant bleeding in the GI or GU tract within the last 6 weeks, bleeding diathesis, history of CVA within the last 2 years or CVA with significant residual neurologic deficit, intracranial neoplasm, aneurysm, or AV malformation, severe uncontrolled hypertension, oral anticoagulants within 7 days unless prothrombin time is less than 1.2 × control, thrombocytopenia, presumed or documented history of vasculitis, major surgery or trauma within the last 6 weeks, pericarditis, known hypersensitivity to abciximab or murine proteins
					• Use cautiously in patients who weigh less than 75 kg, patients older than 65 years of age, patients with a history of GI disease, patients receiving fibrinolytics
					• Do not administer with dextran
					• Monitor oral secretions, sputum, vomitus, NG aspirate, stool, urine for blood
					• Limit venipuncture and urinary catheterization as possible; use IV catheter with saline lock for blood sampling; avoid noncompressible IV sites
					• Avoid nasotracheal and nasogastric tubes if possible
					• Avoid automatic BP cuffs
					• Administer platelets as prescribed for thrombocytopenia
					• Store refrigerated, do not shake (should be clear), administer through filter

Eptifibatide (Integrilin)	**Platelet aggregation inhibitor** (GP IIb/IIIa platelet receptor blocker)
	• Inhibits platelet aggregation and platelet-mediated thrombosis
		• Acute coronary syndrome with or without percutaneous coronary intervention (PCI)
		• PCI when risk for thrombosis is high
			For acute coronary syndrome
			• IV injection: 180 mcg/kg over 1-2 minutes followed by:
			• IV infusion: 2 mcg/kg/min for up to 72 hours; decreased to 0.5 mcg/kg/min during PCI and continued for 24 hours after PCI
			For PCI without acute coronary syndrome
			• IV injection: 135 mcg/kg over 1-2 minutes before procedure followed by:
			• IV infusion: 0.5 mcg/kg/min for 24 hours
				• Bleeding
				  • Intracranial hemorrhage
				  • Hematuria
				  • Hematemesis
				  • Bleeding at sheath site
				• Hypotension
					• Monitor PT, aPTT, or ACT, platelet count
					• Note contraindications: active internal bleeding, clinically significant bleeding in the GI or GU tract within the last 6 weeks, bleeding diathesis, history of CVA within the last 2 years or CVA with significant residual neurologic deficit, intracranial neoplasm, aneurysm, or AV malformation, severe uncontrolled hypertension, oral anticoagulants within 7 days unless prothrombin time is less than 1.2 × control, thrombocytopenia, presumed or documented history of vasculitis, major surgery or trauma within the last 6 weeks, pericarditis, known hypersensitivity to eptifibatide, renal failure, thrombocytopenia
					• Administer with aspirin and heparin therapy as prescribed
					• Monitor oral secretions, sputum, vomitus, NG aspirate, stool, urine for blood
					• Limit venipuncture and urinary catheterization as possible; use IV catheter with saline lock for blood sampling; avoid noncompressible IV sites
					• Avoid nasotracheal and nasogastric tubes if possible
					• Avoid automatic BP cuffs
					• Administer platelets as prescribed for thrombocytopenia
					• Store refrigerated

Continued

Table 3-14 Drugs that Affect Clotting Used for Patients with Myocardial Infarction—cont'd

Drug	Classification/ Actions	Indications	Administration	Adverse Effects	Nursing Implications

Tirofiban HCl (Aggrastat)	**Platelet aggregation inhibitor** (GP IIb/IIIa platelet receptor blocker)
	• Inhibits platelet aggregation and platelet-mediated thrombosis
		• Acute coronary syndrome with or without PCI	• IV infusion: premixed as 25 mg in 500 mL; usual dose is 0.4 mcg/kg/min for 30 minutes and then continued at 0.1 mcg/kg/min (dosage is decreased in renal failure)	• Bleeding
				  • Intracranial hemorrhage
				  • Hematuria
				  • Hematemesis
				  • Bleeding at sheath site
				• Hypotension
				• Bradycardia
				• Pelvic pain
					• Monitor PT, aPTT, or ACT, platelet count
					• Note contraindications: active internal bleeding, clinically significant bleeding in the GI or GU tract within the last 6 weeks, bleeding diathesis, history of CVA within the last 2 years or CVA with significant residual neurologic deficit, intracranial neoplasm, aneurysm, or AV malformation, severe uncontrolled hypertension, oral anticoagulants within 7 days unless prothrombin time is less than 1.2 × control, thrombocytopenia, presumed or documented history of vasculitis, major surgery or trauma within the last month, pericarditis, known hypersensitivity to tirofiban
					• Use cautiously in patients who weigh less than 75 kg, patients older than 65 years of age, patients with a history of GI disease, patients receiving fibrinolytics, patients with thrombocytopenia
					• Administer with aspirin and heparin therapy as prescribed
					• Limit venipuncture and urinary catheterization as possible; use IV catheter with saline lock for blood sampling; avoid noncompressible IV sites
					• Monitor oral secretions, sputum, vomitus, NG aspirate, stool, urine for blood

Recombinant tissue plasminogen activator (rt-PA) alteplase (Activase)	**Fibrinolytic**
	• Converts plasminogen to plasmin at fibrin surface
	• Causes clot-specific lysis
		• Acute myocardial infarction (chest pain strongly suggestive of acute MI; ST segment of at least 1 mm in at least two leads)
		• Massive pulmonary embolism (with RVF or refractory hypoxemia)
		• Thrombotic stroke
			For acute MI
			• IV injection: 15 mg followed by:
			• IV infusion: 0.75 mg/kg (not to exceed 50 mg) over next 30 minutes, followed by 0.5 mg/kg (not to exceed 35 mg) over the next 60 minutes
			• Heparin started within 1 hour of initial dose
			For ischemic stroke
			• Total dose: 0.9 mg/kg with maximum dose of less than or equal to 90 mg
			• IV injection: 10% of this total dose over 1 minute followed by:
			• IV infusion: remaining 90% of this total dose administered over 60 minutes
			• Anticoagulants and platelet aggregation inhibitors are not used for at least 24 hours
			For acute pulm nary embolism
			• IV infusion: 100 mg at 50 mg/hr for 2 hours
			For acute arterial occlusion
			• 0.05-0.1 mg/kg/hr by local intraarterial infusion
			• Reconstitution in sterile water only
				• Severe, spontaneous bleeding including potential cerebral, retroperitoneal, GU, GI bleeding, surface bleeding
				• Reperfusion dysrhythmias
					• Monitor aPTT, PT, thrombin time, fibrinogen, neurologic status, and for signs of hemorrhage
					• Note contraindications: active bleeding; history of cerebral hemorrhage, intracranial neoplasm, AV malformation or aneurysm; recent (within 2 months) intracranial or intraspinal surgery or trauma; known bleeding disorder; severe uncontrolled hypertension; prolonged CPR
					• Use cautiously in recent (within 10 days) major surgery, GI, GU bleeding, or trauma; hypertension with SBP greater than 180 mm/Hg or DBP greater than 110 mm/Hg; high likelihood of left heart thrombus; acute pericarditis; significant liver dysfunction; pregnancy; retinopathy; septic thrombophlebitis; advanced age (greater than 70-75 years); patients receiving oral anticoagulants; any condition in which bleeding constitutes a significant hazard or would be particularly difficult to manage because of its location
					• Monitor for indications of reperfusion in MI
					  • Cessation of pain
					  • ST segments descending back to baseline
					  • Reperfusion dysrhythmias (ventricular ectopy including PVCs, VT or VF, accelerated idioventricular rhythm, junctional escape rhythms, bradycardia)
					  • Early CK peak
					• Note that signs of reperfusion are much more subtle in PE and thrombotic stroke
					• Limit venipuncture and urinary catheterization as possible; use IV catheter with saline lock for blood sampling; avoid noncompressible IV sites
					• Administer all drugs through existing IVs started before initiation of fibrinolytic therapy or by mouth
					• Avoid nasotracheal and nasogastric tubes if possible
					• Avoid automatic BP cuffs
					• Monitor oral secretions, sputum, vomitus, NG aspirate, stool, urine for blood
					• Bleeding precautions are maintained for 12-24 hours

Continued

Table 3-14 Drugs that Affect Clotting Used for Patients with Myocardial Infarction—cont'd

Drug	Classification/ Actions	Indications	Administration	Adverse Effects	Nursing Implications
Recombinant tissue plasminogen activator (rt-PA) tenecteplase (TNKase)	**Fibrinolytic** • Converts plasminogen to plasmin at fibrin surface • Causes clot-specific lysis	• Acute myocardial infarction (chest pain strongly suggestive of acute MI; ST segment of at least 1 mm in at least 2 leads)	• IV injection over 5 seconds • Less than 60 kg: 30 mg • Less than or equal to 60-less than 70 kg: 35 mg • Greater than or equal to 70-less than 80 kg: 40 mg • Greater than or equal to 80-less than 90 kg: 45 mg • Greater than or equal to 90 kg: 50 mg • Heparin administered concurrently	• Severe, spontaneous bleeding including potential cerebral, retroperitoneal, GU, GI bleeding, surface bleeding • Reperfusion dysrhythmias	• Monitor aPTT, PT, thrombin time, neurologic status, and for signs of hemorrhage • Note contraindications: active bleeding; history of cerebral hemorrhage, intracranial neoplasm, AV malformation or aneurysm; recent (within 2 months) intracranial or intraspinal surgery or trauma; known bleeding disorder; severe uncontrolled hypertension; prolonged CPR • Use cautiously in recent (within 10 days) major surgery, GI, GU bleeding, or trauma; hypertension with SBP greater than 180 mm/Hg or DBP greater than 110 mm/Hg; high likelihood of left heart thrombus; acute pericarditis; significant liver dysfunction; pregnancy; retinopathy; septic thrombophlebitis; advanced age (greater than 70-75 years); patients receiving oral anticoagulants; any condition in which bleeding constitutes a significant hazard or would be particularly difficult to manage because of its location

- Identify indications of reperfusion in MI:
  - Cessation of pain
  - ST segments descending back to baseline
  - Reperfusion dysrhythmias (ventricular ectopy including PVCs, VT or VF, accelerated idioventricular rhythm, junctional escape rhythms, bradycardia)
  - Early CK peak
- Limit venipuncture and urinary catheterization as possible; use IV catheter with saline lock for blood sampling; avoid noncompressible IV sites
- Avoid nasotracheal and nasogastric tubes if possible
- Avoid automatic BP cuffs
- Administer all drugs through existing IVs started before initiation of fibrinolytic therapy or by mouth
- Monitor oral secretions, sputum, vomitus, NG aspirate, stool, urine for blood
- Bleeding precautions are maintained for 12-24 hours

Continued

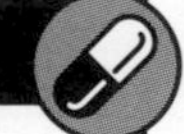

Table 3-14 Drugs that Affect Clotting Used for Patients with Myocardial Infarction—cont'd

Drug	Classification/ Actions	Indications	Administration	Adverse Effects	Nursing Implications

Recombinant plasminogen activator (r-PA) reteplase (Retavase)	**Fibrinolytic**
	• Converts plasminogen to plasmin at fibrin surface
	• Causes clot-specific lysis
		Acute myocardial infarction (chest pain strongly suggestive of acute MI; ST segment of at least 1 mm in at least two leads)	• IV injection of 10 units over 2 minutes initially followed by 10 units over 2 minutes after 30 minutes
			• Heparin administered concurrently
				• Severe, spontaneous bleeding including potential cerebral, retroperitoneal, GU, GI bleeding, surface bleeding
				• Reperfusion dysrhythmias
					• Monitor aPTT, PT, thrombin time, neurologic status, and for signs of hemorrhage
					• Note contraindications: active bleeding; history of cerebral hemorrhage, intracranial neoplasm, AV malformation or aneurysm; recent (within 2 months) intracranial or intraspinal surgery or trauma; known bleeding disorder; severe uncontrolled hypertension; prolonged CPR
					• Use cautiously in recent (within 10 days) major surgery, GI, GU bleeding, or trauma; hypertension with SBP greater than 180 mm/Hg or DBP greater than 110 mm/Hg; high likelihood of left heart thrombus; acute pericarditis; significant liver dysfunction; pregnancy; retinopathy; septic thrombophlebitis; advanced age (greater than 70-75 years); patients receiving oral anticoagulants; any condition in which bleeding constitutes a significant hazard or would be particularly difficult to manage because of its location
					• Identify indications of reperfusion in MI
					  • Cessation of pain
					  • ST segments descending back to baseline
					  • Reperfusion dysrhythmias (ventricular ectopy including PVCs, VT or VF, accelerated idioventricular rhythm, junctional escape rhythms, bradycardia)
					  • Early CK peak
					• Limit venipuncture and urinary catheterization as possible; use IV catheter with saline lock for blood sampling; avoid noncompressible IV sites
					• Avoid nasotracheal and nasogastric tubes if possible
					• Avoid automatic BP cuffs
					• Administer all drugs through existing IVs started before initiation of fibrinolytic therapy or by mouth
					• Monitor oral secretions, sputum, vomitus, NG aspirate, stool, urine for blood
					• Bleeding precautions are maintained for 12-24 hours

Heparin sodium	**Anticoagulant** • Prevents conversion of prothrombin to thrombin • Prevents conversion of fibrinogen to fibrin • Prevents extension of existing clots • Decreases platelet aggregation	• Unstable angina or myocardial infarction • Maintenance of arterial patency after PCI or fibrinolytic therapy • Prevention of thrombus formation during periods of inactivity • Deep vein thrombosis • Pulmonary emboli • Peripheral arterial emboli • Transient ischemic attacks or reversible ischemic neurologic deficit • Disseminated intravascular coagulation (controversial) • Maintenance of arterial line patency	• Subcutaneous: usually prophylactic, dose is 5000 units every 12 hours (also called mini-heparin) • IV injection: usually 80 units/kg (maximum 10,000 units) followed by infusion (only 60 units/kg recommended if patient is receiving fibrinolytics or GP IIb/IIIa inhibitors) • IV infusion: mix 25,000 units in 500 mL (50 units/mL)and infuse at 18 units/kg/hr (maximum 1000 units/hr) (only 12 units/kg recommended if patient is receiving fibrinolytics or GP IIb/IIIa inhibitors); dose is adjusted to achieve aPTT of 1.5-2.5 times the laboratory control • NOTE: the trend in IV weight-dosed heparin is to decrease the amount of heparin (60 units/kg for injection followed by 12 units/kg/hr for infusion) and desirable aPTT (45-60 seconds) Maximum: 40,000 units/day	• Hemorrhage with excessive aPTT • Hypertension or hypotension • Hypersensitivity reaction including bronchospasm • Fever • Hepatitis • Hyperkalemia especially in patients with renal failure • Thrombocytopenia (caused by immune response referred to as heparin induced thrombocytopenia (HIT)	• Monitor aPTT and platelet count and for signs of hemorrhage • Note petechiae and request platelet count if petechiae noted; heparin usually discontinued if platelet count is less than 100,000/mm^3 • Administer lepirudin (Refludan) or argatroban as prescribed for heparin-induced thrombocytopenia (HIT) • Note contraindications: known hypersensitivity, active bleeding, blood dyscrasias (except DIC), suspected intracranial hemorrhage, severe hypertension, peptic ulcer disease, open wounds, recent surgery, endocarditis, shock, threatened abortion • Use cautiously in alcoholism, liver disease, renal disease, older adults • Monitor oral secretions, sputum, vomitus, NG aspirate, stool, urine for blood • Ensure that protamine sulfate (antidote) is available • Avoid IM, arterial, or venous punctures if at all possible • Hold pressure for longer than usual if punctures necessary • Do not discontinue suddenly: warfarin will usually have already been started and the PT within therapeutic range before heparin is discontinued • Do not aspirate before subcutaneous administration and do not massage after administration • Note that NTG interacts with heparin, causing more heparin to be required to achieve therapeutic aPTT; monitor aPTT closely with significant NTG dosage changes or discontinuance

Continued

Table 3-14 Drugs that Affect Clotting Used for Patients with Myocardial Infarction—cont'd

Drug	Classification/ Actions	Indications	Administration	Adverse Effects	Nursing Implications
Heparin: low-molecular-weight enoxaparin (Lovenox) dalteparin sodium (Fragmin)	**Anticoagulant** • Inhibits thrombin activity • Prevents DVT • Does not prevent platelet aggregation	• High risk for DVT • Acute coronary syndrome	Enoxaparin (Lovenox) • SC: 30 mg bid Dalteparin sodium (Fragmin) • SC: 2500 international units daily starting 1-2 hours before surgery and repeated qd for 5-10 days postoperatively Ardeparin (Normiflo) • SC: 50 antifactor Xa IU/kg every 12 hours beginning the evening before surgery and continued until the patient is ambulatory Tinzaparin sodium (Innohep) • SC: 175 factor antifactor Xa IU/kg daily for approximately 6 days or until adequate anticoagulation with warfarin	• Bleeding • Epidural or spinal hematoma (especially when used with patients with epidural or spinal anesthesia) • Fever • Elevation of liver enzymes • Thrombocytopenia • Chest pain	• Note that LMW heparin does not require routine laboratory monitoring because it does not usually alter PT or aPTT • Note that contraindications and cautions are as for heparin • Obtain baseline platelet count; monitor for petechiae • Monitor oral secretions, sputum, vomitus, NG aspirate, stool, urine for blood • Ensure that protamine sulfate (antidote) is available • Avoid IM, arterial, or venous punctures if at all possible • Hold pressure for longer than usual if punctures necessary • Administer deep subcutaneously but avoid IM injection
Bivalirudin (Angiomax)	**Anticoagulant: Direct Thrombin Inhibitor** • Prevents conversion of prothrombin to thrombin including both free and clot-bound thrombin	• Unstable angina in patients undergoing PCI	• IV injection: 0.75-1 mg/kg followed by IV infusion • IV infusion: mix 250 mg in 250 mL of normal saline (1 mg/mL) and infuse at 1.75-2.5 mg/kg/hr for 4 hours then decrease infusion to 0.2 mg/kg/hr for an additional 14-20 hours if needed	• Bleeding • Back pain • Generalized pain • Headache • Nausea • Hypotension	• Monitor PT, aPTT, CBC, and for signs of bleeding • Note that contraindications and cautions are as for heparin • Obtain baseline platelet count and aPTT; monitor aPTT every 4 hours; ACT may also be used • Anticoagulant effects are increased in patients receiving platelet aggregation inhibitors, fibrinolytics, or other anticoagulants • Monitor oral secretions, sputum, vomitus, NG aspirate, stool, urine for blood • Avoid IM, arterial, or venous punctures if at all possible • Hold pressure for longer than usual if punctures necessary • Protect infusion from direct sunlight

Warfarin (Coumadin, Panwarfin)	**Anticoagulant** • Depresses synthesis of prothrombin by the liver • Prevents extension of clot and secondary thromboembolic complications	• Deep vein thrombosis • Valvular heart disease • Atrial dysrhythmias • Postvalve replacement	• PO: 2-10 mg daily depending on PT and international normalized ratio (INR) • INR 2-3 — MI — DVT prophylaxis or treatment — Pulmonary embolus — Valvular heart disease — Atrial fibrillation — Tissue heart valve • INR 2.5- 3.5 — Mechanical heart valve	• Hemorrhage with excessive PT • Agranulocytosis, leukopenia • Hepatitis • Diarrhea • Fever • Rash • Skin necrosis: occurs during the first several days of warfarin therapy; lesions occur on extremities, breasts, trunk, penis • Cholesterol microemboli causing purple toe syndrome	• Monitor PT and for signs of hemorrhage • Note contraindications: known hypersensitivity, bleeding disorders, leukemia, peptic ulcer disease, liver disease, severe hypertension, endocarditis, acute nephritis, blood dyscrasias, eclampsia, suspected intracranial hemorrhage, open wounds, recent surgery, threatened abortion • Use cautiously in alcoholism, pregnancy, lactation, during menses, during use of any drainage tube, older adult, or in any patient in whom slight bleeding is dangerous • Ensure that vitamin K (AquaMephyton) is available • Avoid IM, arterial, or venous punctures if at all possible • Hold pressure for longer than usual if punctures necessary • Monitor oral secretions, sputum, vomitus, NG aspirate, stool, urine for blood • Do not discontinue suddenly • Teach patient to avoid trauma and increase amounts of vitamin K (green leafy vegetables), and how to monitor for bleeding • Teach the patient to report fever or rash; usually necessitates discontinuance

(ii) Initial dosing should be weight-based, then infusion is adjusted by aPTT results
(iii) Usual dose of unfractionated heparin: bolus of 60 units/kg, then infusion of 12 units/kg/hr

(b) Low-molecular-weight heparin subcutaneous
(i) Indirect thrombin inhibitor
(ii) Lower incidence of heparin induced thrombocytopenia (HIT) than unfractionated heparin

(c) Bivalirudin (Angiomax) (Table 3-14)
(i) Direct thrombin inhibitor
(ii) Most frequently used after PCI

(d) Warfarin (Table 3-14) is usually prescribed for at least 3 months in patients with any of the following:
(i) Anterior Q wave MI
(ii) Heart failure
(iii) Severe left ventricular dysfunction
(iv) Atrial fibrillation
(v) Previous embolic event

3) Prepare patient for coronary bypass grafting as indicated; coronary artery bypass graft (Table 3-15) is utilized to provide arterial or venous conduits to redirect coronary blood flow around occluded coronary arteries
4) Treat anemia if present: maintain Hgb greater than 12 g/dL if possible.
5) Maintain coronary artery perfusion pressure.
   a) Use caution in administration of NTG and other vasoactive agents because they may decrease CAPP by decreasing the aortic root pressure.
   b) NTP is contraindicated during ischemic pain because it may cause coronary artery steal and decrease coronary artery perfusion pressure.
6) Control dysrhythmias.
   a) Tachydysrhythmias decrease the time for coronary artery filling and may decrease cardiac output.

Table 3-15 Coronary Artery Bypass Grafting (CABG)

Procedures	• Types of bypasses
	  • Arterial bypass (preferred because of better long-term patency rates)
	    — Internal thoracic (also called internal mammary) arteries
	    — Gastroepiploic artery
	    — Inferior epigastric arteries
	    — Radial arteries
	  • Vein grafts
	    — Saphenous veins
	    — Brachial veins
	• Surgical approaches
	  • Median sternotomy with cardiopulmonary bypass (CPB)
	    — CPB provides a motionless heart and a bloodless field
	    — Complications of CPB include systemic inflammatory response syndrome (SIRS), coagulopathy, atelectasis, acute respiratory distress syndrome, cerebral microemboli, thrombotic stroke, post-CPB encephalopathy, renal insufficiency, dysrhythmias
	  • Off-pump coronary artery bypass graft (OPCABG)
	    — May be performed through small median sternotomy or anterior thoracotomy
	    — Bypass is performed on a beating heart
	    — Avoids complications related to cardiopulmonary bypass
	  • Minimally invasive direct (MIDCABG)
	    — Performed through anterior thoracotomy
	    — May be used for proximal LAD and select lesions of RCA or circumflex
	    — Bypass is performed on a beating heart
	    — Avoids complications related to cardiopulmonary bypass
	    — Thoracoscopy may be used

Indications	• Left main artery disease or three vessel disease • Double vessel disease if one of vessels is proximal LAD • Single or double vessel disease with angina unresponsive to medical therapy • CAD with ejection fraction less than 35% • Emergent conditions such as unstable angina, acute MI with persistent pain or shock, or coronary artery dissection during interventional cardiology procedures

Table 3-15 Coronary Artery Bypass Grafting (CABG)—cont'd

Action	• The goal of coronary artery bypass graft is to provide arterial or venous conduits to redirect coronary blood flow around occluded coronary arteries
Assessment	• Vital signs: HR, BP, RR, T • Hemodynamic parameters: RAP, PAP, PAOP, CO, CI, SVR, PVR, LVSWI, RVSWI • Oxygenation parameters: SaO_2, SvO_2; arterial blood gases • Serum electrolytes • Mediastinal and pleural tube drainage • Complaints of incisional pain, chest pain, dyspnea • Incision for bleeding, separation, or redness and induration

Brief summary of specific nursing management	• Relieve pain
	  • Administer narcotics and sedatives for relief of incisional pain
	  • Provide instruction regarding splinting during coughing and turning
	  • Report ischemic pain; titrate NTG for relief of ischemic pain
	• Monitor closely for hemodynamic changes: titrate drug therapy to optimize cardiac output and minimize myocardial oxygen consumption
	  • Pharmacologic support of this patient may include dobutamine, dopamine, nitroglycerin, nitroprusside
	  • Vasopressors may be used to increase coronary artery perfusion pressure and maintain patency of grafts; monitor for excessive afterload and myocardial oxygen consumption as well as excessive vasoconstriction and peripheral hypoperfusion
	  • Nitroglycerin at low dose is frequently used to reduce spasm
	• Monitor closely for hemorrhage: mediastinal tube, pleural tubes, incision
	  • Administer intravenous fluids, blood and/or blood products, and albumin as prescribed
	  • Maintain patency of mediastinal and pleural tubes
	  • Be alert for sudden reduction of drainage via mediastinal tube because occlusion may cause cardiac tamponade
	• Monitor closely for changes in perfusion
	  • Note any complaints of chest pain, ST segment elevation, dysrhythmias
	  • Note any changes in appearance or volume of urine
	  • Note any changes in level of consciousness or neurologic function
	  • Note any changes in SaO_2, PAP, PVR
	  • Note any changes in bowel sounds, abdominal distention, abdominal pain
	• Monitor the ECG for dysrhythmias or blocks
	  • Replace electrolytes as prescribed; potassium and magnesium imbalances predispose to dysrhythmias
	  • Administer antidysrhythmics as prescribed; prophylactic antidysrhythmics (e.g., amiodarone) may be given to prevent atrial fibrillation
	  • Utilize epicardial pacing wires for symptomatic bradycardias or blocks
	• Prevent/monitor for complications

Complications: prevention and treatment	• Potential complications during surgery
	  • Cerebral or myocardial infarction
	  • Hemorrhage: greater risk with internal thoracic artery implant
	  • Inability to wean from cardiopulmonary bypass: intraaortic balloon pump and/or VAD used
	• Potential complications during postoperative period
	  • Immediate
	    — Heart failure with hypotension and/or pulmonary edema
	    — Hemorrhage
	    — Cardiac tamponade
	    — Dysrhythmias
	    — MI
	    — Hypertension
	    — Cerebral embolism
	    — Acute respiratory failure (e.g., atelectasis, ARDS)
	    — Renal failure
	    — Electrolyte imbalance (e.g., hypokalemia, hypocalcemia, hypomagnesemia)
	    — Graft closure
	    — Coagulopathy
	  • Intermediate
	    — Donor site infection
	    — Sternal wound infection: especially if patient is diabetic and/or internal thoracic (i.e., mammary) artery used for bypass

b) Bradydysrhythmias increase the time for coronary artery filling but may decrease cardiac output.

7) Administer calcium channel blockers or NTG for coronary artery spasm.
   a) Especially important in cocaine-induced MI

8) Utilize intraaortic balloon pump as prescribed (see Table 3-11).

c. Decrease myocardial oxygen consumption.

1) Administer beta-blockers as prescribed to decrease heart rate and contractility to decrease myocardial oxygen consumption.
   a) Actions
      i) Decrease incidence of dysrhythmias and increase ventricular fibrillation threshold.
      ii) Block the effects of catecholamines (cardioprotection).
      iii) Reduce infarct size and severity of HF.
   b) Agents: Metoprolol (Lopressor) 5 mg IV every 2 minutes × 3 is usually given, but atenolol (Tenormin) or esmolol (Brevibloc) may be used.
   c) Contraindications
      i) Heart rate less than 50 beats/min
      ii) Second- or third-degree AV block
      iii) Systolic BP less than 100 mm Hg
      iv) Heart failure
      v) Bronchospasm
         (a) No beta-blockers should be given to a patient with active bronchospasm.
         (b) Cardioselective beta-blockers (e.g., metoprolol or esmolol) may be given to a patient with a history of bronchospastic lung disease (e.g., asthma), but noncardioselective beta-blockers (e.g., propranolol) should not be given.
      vi) Cocaine-induced MI: Blocking beta receptors allows unopposed alpha receptors to increase vasoconstriction and vasospasm; nitroglycerin and/or a calcium channel blocker (e.g., diltiazem [Cardizem]) is more likely to be prescribed along with a benzodiazepine (e.g., diazepam [Valium]) to reduce agitation and seizure potential.

2) Administer ACE inhibitors (e.g., captopril [Capoten], enalapril [Vasotec]) or angiotensin-blockers (e.g., losartan [Cozaar], valsartan [Diovan]) as prescribed to attenuate ventricular remodeling.
   a) Action: Block the vasoconstriction and sodium and water retention associated with activation of the renin-angiotensin-aldosterone system.
   b) Indications in acute MI: anterior or large inferior MI or evidence of HF
   c) ACE inhibitors block the conversion of angiotensin I to angiotensin II; angiotensin-blockers block angiotensin II and do not block the breakdown of bradykinin, so are less likely to cause cough.
   d) Caution: hypotension

3) Administer vasodilators as prescribed.
   a) Venous vasodilators (usually nitroglycerin) to decrease preload
   b) Arterial vasodilators (usually nitroprusside) to decrease afterload
   c) Caution: hypotension; careful titration necessary to decrease myocardial oxygen consumption but to prevent hypoperfusion

4) Monitor serum glucose and administer insulin as required to maintain serum glucose below 150 mg/dL.

5) Provide physical and emotional rest.
   a) Maintain bed rest for 24 hours, then gradually increase in activity as long as patient is hemodynamically stable; allow rest after meals, personal hygiene, toileting, and physical therapy.
   b) Prevent Valsalva maneuver.
      i) Teach patient to exhale when turning in bed.
      ii) Administer stool softeners as prescribed.
      iii) Provide bedside commode for elimination.
   c) Explain procedures thoroughly: monitor alarms; equipment; visiting hours; reasons for procedures
   d) Keep family informed regarding patient's progress and status.
   e) Provide for patient's comfort.
      i) Provide prompt pain control: analgesics
      ii) Provide nausea control: antiemetics, mouth care
      iii) Provide for physical comfort: temperature control; lighting; noise control
   f) Instruct patient regarding relaxation techniques; encourage utilization of these techniques; utilize calming music, white noise, or nature sounds to aid in relaxation.
   g) Provide appropriate nutrition: clear liquid to soft diet; usually low sodium
      i) Caffeine: may have up to 4-5 caffeinated beverages/24 hr as long as dysrhythmias do not occur
      ii) Iced water: no restriction

h) Administer anxiolytics as prescribed: usually diazepam (Valium), lorazepam (Ativan), or alprazolam (Xanax)
   i) Note common emotional responses seen in acute MI and treat appropriately. (Table 3-16)

d. Collaborative management specific to RV infarctions
   1) Assess for clinical indications of RVMI, especially in the patient with acute inferior MI.
      a) ECG changes in V_{4R}, V_{5R}, V_{6R}
      b) Increased RAP, decreased PAOP
      c) Decreased CO, CI, MAP, increased SVR
      d) Right-sided S_4
      e) Clinical indications of RVF: jugular venous distention (JVD), hepatojugular reflux, right-sided S_3, murmur of tricuspid insufficiency
      f) Minimal to absent pulmonary congestion
   2) Administer therapy specific to right ventricular infarction.
      a) Maintain adequate filling volumes.
         i) Measure RAP and PAOP; patients with significant right ventricular infarction usually require hemodynamic monitoring.
         ii) Administer volume: usually in the form of colloids (e.g., dextran, plasma protein fraction, albumin); fluids administered until PAOP is increased by greater than 5 mm Hg but PAOP and RAP should not exceed 20 mm Hg
         iii) Avoid use of diuretics and/or venous vasodilators; if dilators are needed, selective arterial dilators

Table 3-16 Emotional Responses Seen in Acute Myocardial Infarction

Response	Indications	Collaborative Management
Anxiety	• Increased verbalization • Inability to concentrate • Restlessness, apprehension • Sleep disturbances • Tremors • Tachycardia, mild hypertension	• Be consistent with patient assignment • Provide orientation to unit, procedures, equipment, etc. • Assess usual coping mechanisms • Invite patient to ask questions • Keep family informed about patient condition • Encourage participation in rehabilitation program
Denial	• Avoidance of discussion of heart attack • Discussions kept on a social, humorous level • Minimization of severity (e.g., "little heart attack") • Noncompliance with activity and diet restrictions; smoking • Overly cheerful demeanor • Repetition of same questions to different staff members	• Listen but do not reinforce denial • Assess consequences of denial: denial decreases in-hospital mortality but increases incidence of sudden cardiac death after discharge • Assess the threat causing the need for denial • Provide counseling if patient still in denial at time of discharge • Encourage participation in rehabilitation program
Depression	• Listlessness, disinterest • Expressions of hopelessness, pessimism • Abbreviated verbal responses (e.g., monosyllable answers) • Slowness in movement and speech • Withdrawn behavior • Anorexia • Sad look, crying	• Voice your observations (e.g., "you look sad") • Let patient know that it is normal to feel this way • Encourage verbalization of feelings • Allow and encourage crying • Encourage participation in rehabilitation program
Anger	• Open opposition to treatment regimen • Expressions of disappointment or frustration • Passive-aggressive behavior • Sarcasm • Voices anger, screaming, cursing	• Acknowledge angry or hostile feelings • Explore cause of anger • Let patient know that these feelings are normal • Let spouse and family know that anger is normal • Be matter-of-fact about expressions of anger • Encourage participation in rehabilitation program
Aggressive sexual behavior	• Frequent seductive comments • Frequent initiation of sexually related conversion • Frequent boasts about past sexual interests and prowess • Flirtatious compliments • Attempts to hold, fondle, or kiss parts of nurse's body • Deliberate exposure of genitals	• Be honest and simply tell the patient that such behavior makes you uncomfortable if it does • Accept compliments with a simple "thank you" • Arrange sexual counseling for patient and spouse • Encourage participation in rehabilitation program

should be used (e.g., hydralazine [Apresoline]) so that preload is not decreased.

b) Maintain contractility: Inotropes (e.g., dobutamine) are frequently required.

e. Monitor for, prevent, and treat complications. (Table 3-17)

f. Provide instruction and counseling regarding lifestyle modification and need for pharmacologic therapy.

1) Nonpharmacologic therapies

a) Well-balanced diet to maintain normal weight maintenance

i) Low in saturated fat and transfatty acids while including monounsaturated fats (e.g., olive oil, canola oil)

ii) High in fiber

(a) Fresh fruit and vegetables

(b) Whole grains

iii) Adequate low-fat proteins

iv) Low (2-3 g/day) sodium may be recommended.

v) ADA diet for control of blood glucose for patient with DM

b) Cessation of tobacco use

c) Limitation of alcohol consumption to 1-2 alcoholic beverages daily

d) Regular aerobic exercise in moderation

e) Adequate rest and relaxation

f) Stress reduction: relaxation; imagery, biofeedback

g) Differentiation between symptoms of angina and MI

h) Changes in sexual activity that may be helpful

Table 3-17 Complications of Myocardial Infarction

Complication	Clinical Indications	Prevention/Treatment
Dysrhythmias and conduction system defects	• Change in rhythm or conduction on rhythm strip or multiple-lead ECG • Indications of hypoperfusion may be evident	• Close monitoring for changes in rhythm or conduction • Beta-blocker as a cardioprotective agent as prescribed • Magnesium, potassium, or calcium to correct electrolyte imbalance as prescribed • Antidysrhythmic agents as indicated and prescribed • Application of external pacemaker or insertion of transvenous pacemaker as indicated • Cardioversion or defibrillation as indicated

Heart failure	• Tachycardia, tachypnea
	• Clinical indications of LVF
	  • Dyspnea, orthopnea, cough
	  • S_3
	  • Crackles in lung bases
	• Clinical indications of RVF
	  • Jugular venous distention
	  • Hepatomegaly, splenomegaly
	  • Peripheral edema
	• Chest x-ray shows pulmonary venous congestion, cardiomegaly
	• Increased RAP, PAP, PAOP (PAOP usually greater than 20 mm Hg)
		• Oxygen
		• Sodium and fluid restriction
		• ACE inhibitors (e.g., captopril, enalapril)
		• Beta-blockers (e.g., metoprolol, carvedilol)
		• Diuretics (e.g., furosemide, bumetanide)
		• Vasodilators (e.g., nitroglycerin)
		• Inotropic agents (e.g., dobutamine, milrinone, digoxin)

Cardiogenic shock	• Tachycardia, tachypnea, hypotension • Clinical indications of LVF • Clinical indications of RVF • Clinical indications of hypoperfusion (see Table 2-2 on page 26) • Urine output less than 0.5 mL/kg/hr • Cool to cold skin • Diminished to absent bowel sounds • Lethargy to confusion to coma • Chest x-ray shows pulmonary venous congestion, cardiomegaly • Decreased CO/CI (usually less than 2 L/min/m^2) • Increased PAOP (usually greater than 18 mm Hg) • Increased SVR (usually greater than 2000 dynes/sec/cm^{-5})	• Oxygen • Sodium and fluid restrictions • ACE inhibitors (e.g., captopril, enalapril) • Inotropic agents (e.g., digoxin, dobutamine, inamrinone or milrinone) • Diuretics (e.g., furosemide, bumetanide) • Vasodilators (e.g., nitroglycerin, nitroprusside) • IABP • Ventricular assist devices • Emergent revascularization: fibrinolytics, PCI; CABG

Table 3-17 Complications of Myocardial Infarction—cont'd

Complication	Clinical Indications	Prevention/Treatment
Papillary muscle dysfunction/rupture	• New holosystolic murmur loudest at apex • Clinical indications of LVF • Clinical indications of hypoperfusion • Increased PAP, PAOP • Large V waves on PAOP waveform • Echocardiography shows mitral regurgitation	• Vasodilators (e.g., nitroprusside, nitroglycerin) • IABP • Surgical replacement of mitral valve with concurrent CABG
Ventricular septal rupture	• New holosystolic murmur loudest at lower left sternal border (LLSB) • Chest pain, dyspnea • Syncope • Increased PAP, PAOP • Increased SvO_2 • Increased CO/CI by thermodilution method of measurement (inaccurate) • Clinical evidence of hypoperfusion • Hypotension	• Vasodilators (e.g., nitroglycerin, nitroprusside) • IABP • Surgical correction of ventricular septal defect with concurrent CABG unless rupture is small

Cardiac wall rupture	• Clinical indications of hypoperfusion
	• Clinical indications of cardiac tamponade
	  • Jugular venous distention
	  • Muffled heart sounds
	  • Hypotension
	  • Increased RAP, PAP, PAOP with equalization within 5 mm Hg
	• Sinus tachycardia or pulseless electrical activity
	• Eventual cardiopulmonary arrest with PEA
		• Pericardiocentesis
		• CPR; internal cardiac massage may be necessary
		• Surgical repair may be attempted (survival is rare)

Ventricular aneurysm	• Diffuse PMI, left ventricular heave • Atrial fibrillation or ventricular dysrhythmias • Persistent ST segment elevation • Chest x-ray shows left ventricular dilation • Echocardiography shows dyskinesis, left ventricular dilation • Clinical indications of LVF may be present • Clinical indications of systemic emboli may be present: cerebral emboli; peripheral emboli with acute arterial occlusion	• Antidysrhythmics (e.g., amiodarone) • Anticoagulants (e.g., heparin followed by warfarin) • Treatment of HF: ACE inhibitors, beta-blockers, diuretics, vasodilators, inotropes • Surgical resection may be performed • Ablative procedures may be necessary for recurrent ventricular dysrhythmias
Pericarditis	• Fever • Chest pain which worsens with deep breath and lessens sitting up and with leaning forward • Pericardial friction rub • Elevated WBC, sedimentation rate • Diffuse ST segment elevation across the precordial leads • Chest x-ray may show pericardial effusion	• Aspirin or nonsteroidal antiinflammatory drugs (e.g., ibuprofen, naproxen); colchicine may also be used • Discontinuance of anticoagulants • Pericardiocentesis may be required for pericardial effusion • Close monitoring for clinical indications of cardiac tamponade
Dressler's syndrome (also referred to as *postmyocardial infarction syndrome*): late pericarditis which is thought to be autoimmune	• Fever • Chest pain which worsens with deep breath and lessens sitting up and with leaning forward • Pericardial friction rub • Elevated WBC, sedimentation rate • Diffuse ST segment elevation across the precordial leads • Chest x-ray may show pericardial effusion	• Aspirin or colchicine • Corticosteroids (e.g., prednisone) may be prescribed • Pericardiocentesis may be required for pericardial effusion • Close monitoring for clinical indications of cardiac tamponade

Sudden cardiac death	• Cardiopulmonary arrest	• Preventive measures include:
		  • Risk factor modification
		  • Antiplatelet aggregation therapy (e.g., ASA)
		  • Beta-blockers
		  • Encouragement of family members to learn CPR
		• Treatment: BLS and ACLS

2) Pharmacologic agents
   a) Prescribed medication regimen for secondary prevention of MI: aspirin, beta-blocker, ACE inhibitor (if indicated)
   b) Control of cardiac risk factors
      i) Antihypertensives for hypertension
      ii) Lipid-reducing therapy (e.g., statin) for hyperlipidemia
      iii) Oral hypoglycemics and/or insulin for diabetes mellitus
      iv) Thyroid hormone replacement or suppressive agents for thyroid disorders

Heart Failure

Definitions

1. Heart failure: a clinical syndrome characterized by dyspnea, activity intolerance, and fluid overload which adversely affects the patient's functional status and quality of life (Hunt et al., 2001)
   a. Clinical indications of intravascular and interstitial volume overload (e.g., dyspnea, crackles, edema)
   b. Clinical indications of tissue hypoperfusion (e.g., fatigue, exercise intolerance)
2. Acute decompensated heart failure: the sudden or gradual onset of the signs or symptoms of heart failure which necessitate unplanned office visits, emergency departments visits, or hospitalization; a nearly universal finding is pulmonary and systemic congestion due to increased left- and right-heart filling pressures (Gheorghiade et al., 2005)
3. Pulmonary edema
   a. Fluid in the alveolus
   b. Impairs gas exchange and causes hypoxemia by impairing the diffusion between alveolus and capillary
   c. May be cardiac versus noncardiac; frequently differentiated using PAOP and the difference between PA diastolic pressure and PAOP
      1) Cardiac pulmonary edema
         a) Caused by acute left ventricular failure
         b) Elevated PAP, elevated PAOP; difference between PA diastolic and PAOP less than 5 mm Hg
         c) Fluid is *pushed* from the pulmonary capillary into the interstitium and finally into the alveolus due to increased pulmonary capillary hydrostatic pressure
      2) Noncardiac pulmonary edema
         a) Most common cause is acute respiratory distress syndrome (ARDS); may also be caused by drowning
         b) Elevated PAP, normal PAOP; difference between PA diastolic and PAOP greater than 5 mm Hg
         c) Fluid *leaks* from the pulmonary capillary into the interstitium and alveolus due to increased permeability of the damaged alveolocapillary membrane

Etiology

1. Risk factors
   a. **#1** CAD, especially with history of MI
   b. Congenital heart disease
   c. Valvular heart disease
   d. Hypertension
   e. Diabetes
   f. Obesity
   g. Alcoholism
   h. Smoking
   i. High or low hematocrit
   j. Sedentary life style
   k. High-fat/high-salt diet
2. Etiologic factors (Table 3-18)
3. Causes of decompensation in a patient with heart failure
   a. Progression of left ventricular dysfunction
   b. New or worsening ischemia
   c. Hypoxemia
   d. Worsening of anemia
   e. Drugs such as nonsteroidal antiinflammatory drugs (NSAIDs), initiation of beta-blocker dosage at too high dosages
   f. Hypertension
   g. New dysrhythmia, particularly atrial fibrillation
   h. Missed or suboptimal medication
   i. Dietary indiscretion, such as high-salt foods
   j. Alcohol

Table 3-18 Etiologic Factors of Heart Failure

Left Ventricular Failure	Right Ventricular Failure
• CAD/LV infarction	• LVF
• Cardiomyopathy	• CAD/RV infarction
• Hypertension	• Pulmonary hypertension
• Dysrhythmias	• Passive: mitral valve disease
• Volume overload	• Active: hypoxemia; pulmonary embolism
• Valvular disease: mitral or aortic	• Dysrhythmias
• Ventricular septal defect	• Volume overload
• Coarctation of aorta	• Valvular disease: mitral or pulmonic
• Myocarditis	• Ventricular septal defect
• Cardiac tamponade	• Cardiomyopathy
	• Myocardial contusion
	• LVF
	• CAD/RV infarction
Biventricular Failure	
Increased demand	Electrolyte imbalance
• Thyrotoxicosis	• Hyponatremia
• Anemia	• Hypokalemia
• Pregnancy	• Hypocalcemia
• Systemic infection	• Hypomagnesemia
• Beriberi	• Hypophosphatemia
• Paget's disease	

4. Common comorbidities in a patient with heart failure
   a. Coronary artery disease
   b. Myocardial infarction
   c. Hypertension with systolic BP greater than 140 mm Hg
   d. Renal insufficiency
   e. Hyperlipidemia
   f. Diabetes mellitus
   g. Atrial fibrillation
   h. COPD and/or asthma

Pathophysiology

1. Adaptive compensatory processes progress to maladaptive process: In the short-term, mechanisms compensate for the failing heart, but in the long term, all of these factors trigger a process of pathologic growth and remodeling. (Figure 3-18)
   a. Signal-modulating inhibitors: Primary therapies are directed toward blocking dysfunctional compensatory mechanisms.
      1) SNS: beta-blockers, alpha- and beta-blockers
      2) Renin-angiotensin-aldosterone system: ACE inhibitors and angiotensin II receptor blockers (ARBs)
      3) Aldosterone: aldosterone antagonists
2. Interrelationship between LVF and RVF (Figure 3-19)

Classifications of Heart Failure

1. Location: left or right; note that the most common cause of right ventricular failure is left ventricular failure
2. Onset: acute or chronic
3. Output state: low-output (e.g., myocardial infarction, cardiomyopathy) or high-output (e.g., thyrotoxicosis, anemia)
4. Type of pumping defect: backward (i.e., high volume and engorgement behind the failing ventricle) versus forward (i.e., low filling volume for the ventricle in front of the failing ventricle)
5. Relationship to the cardiac cycle: systolic (60-70%) or diastolic (30-40%)
   a. Systolic dysfunction (pump problem): inability of the ventricle to shorten against a load; the

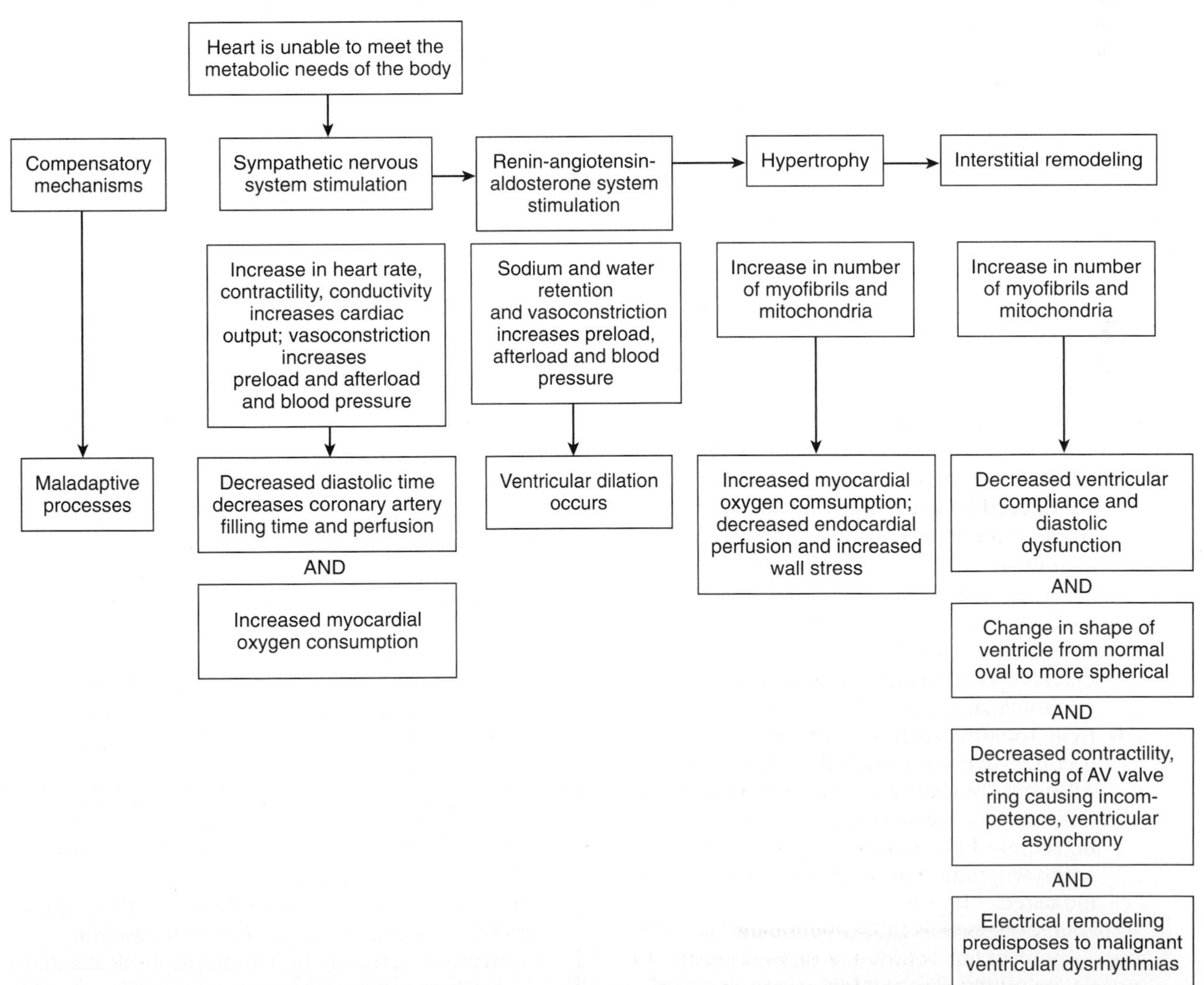

Figure 3-18 Progression of adaptive compensatory mechanisms to maladaptive processes.

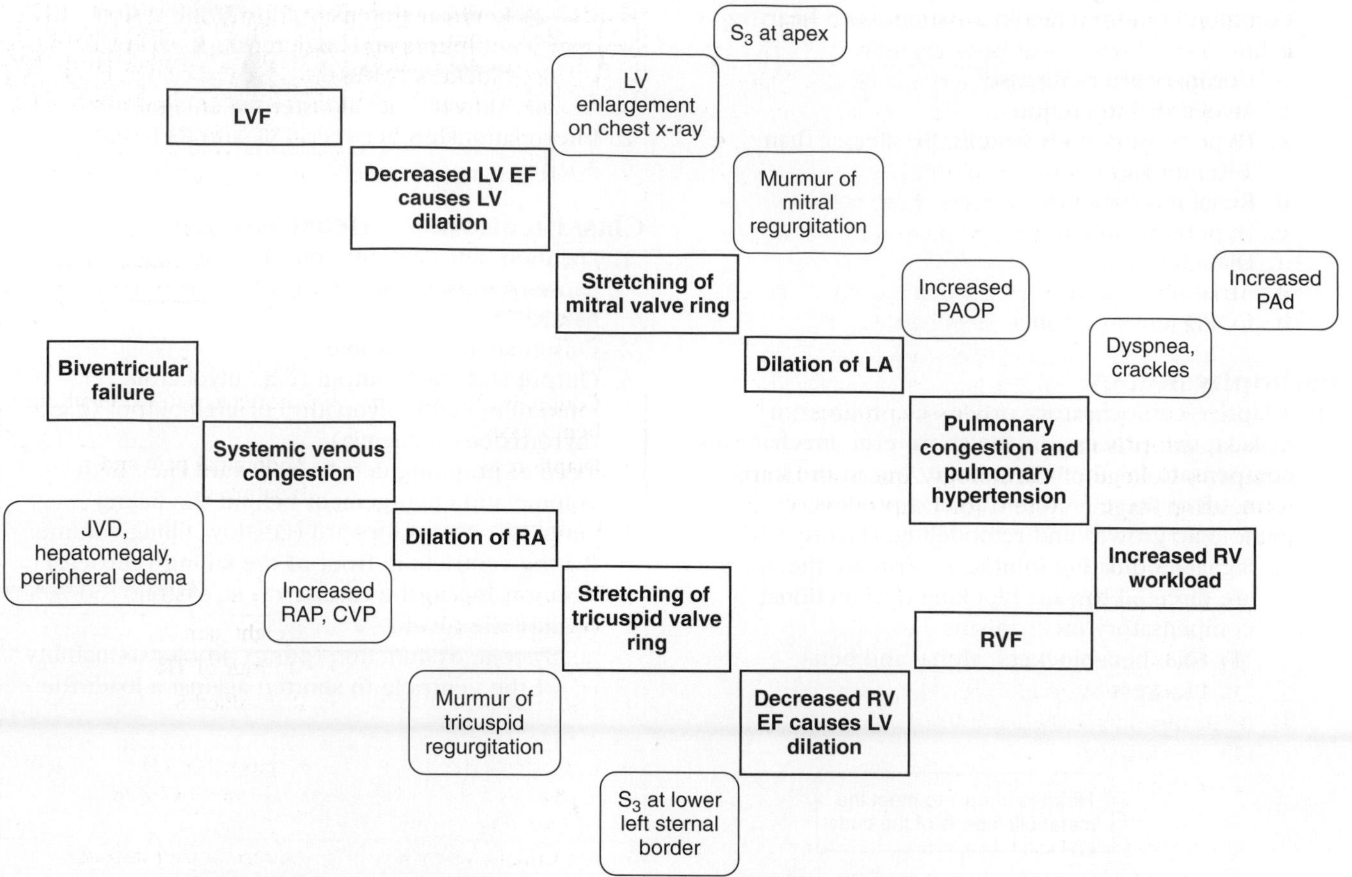

Figure 3-19 Left ventricular failure progressing to biventricular failure. *CVP,* central venous pressure; *EF,* ejection fraction; *JVD,* jugular venous distention; *LA,* left atrium; *LV,* left ventricular; *LVF,* left ventricular failure; *PAd,* pulmonary artery diastolic pressure; *PAOP,* pulmonary artery occlusive pressure; *RA,* right atrium; *RAP,* right atrial pressure; *RV,* right ventricle; *RVF,* right ventricular failure.

left ventricle loses its ability to contract normally against progressive increases in afterload

1) Possible causes: myocardial infarction; myocardial contusion; myocarditis; dilated cardiomyopathy; hypertension; valvular heart disease; electrolyte imbalance; dysrhythmias
2) Hemodynamics: decreased contractility; EF less than 40%; increased cardiac volumes and pressures
3) Clinical indications: displaced PMI; JVD; S_3; crackles; dyspnea; peripheral edema; cardiomegaly
4) Drug therapy: treatment of cause, diuretics if congestive symptoms; ACE inhibitor or ARB; beta-blocker or alpha- and beta-blocker but not pure alpha-blocker; inotropes may be required for diuretic-resistant congestion; antidysrhythmics and anticoagulants may be indicated

b. Diastolic dysfunction (filling problem): an impairment in left ventricular filling at near normal or mildly elevated left atrial and ventricular pressures; due to decrease in ventricular compliance; small changes in volume are associated with a disproportionate increase in pressure

1) Possible causes: myocardial ischemia; hypertrophic cardiomyopathy; ventricular hypertrophy; constrictive pericarditis or cardiac tamponade; valvular heart disease; aging
2) Hemodynamics: increased contractility; normal EF; increased cardiac pressures with normal or slightly increased cardiac volumes
3) Clinical indications: S_4; crackles; dyspnea; peripheral edema; precordial heave; normal heart sound
4) Drug therapy: treatment of cause, diuretics if congestive symptoms, ACE inhibitor or ARB, beta-blocker or alpha- and beta-blocker, calcium channel blocker, control of tachydysrhythmias

6. New York Heart Association functional classification
   a. Class I: patients with cardiac disease but without resulting limitation of physical activity; ordinary physical activity does not cause undue fatigue, palpitation, dyspnea, or angina

b. Class II: patients with cardiac disease resulting in slight limitation of physical activity; they are comfortable at rest; ordinary physical activity results in fatigue, palpitation, dyspnea, or angina
c. Class III: patients with cardiac disease resulting in marked limitation of physical activity; they are comfortable at rest; less than ordinary activity causes fatigue, palpitation, dyspnea, or angina
d. Class IV: patients with cardiac disease resulting in inability to carry on any physical activity without discomfort; symptoms of cardiac insufficiency or angina may be present even at rest; if any physical activity is attempted, discomfort is increased

7. American College of Cardiology/American Heart Association staging system for heart failure (Hunt et al., 2001)
   a. A: high risk for developing heart failure
      1) Hypertension
      2) CAD
      3) Diabetes mellitus
      4) Family history of cardiomyopathy
   b. B: asymptomatic heart failure
      1) Previous MI
      2) Left ventricular systolic dysfunction
      3) Asymptomatic valvular disease
   c. C: symptomatic heart failure
      1) Known structural heart disease
      2) Shortness of breath and fatigue
      3) Reduced exercise tolerance
   d. D: Refractory end-stage heart failure
      1) Marked symptoms at rest despite maximal medical therapy

Clinical Presentation (Table 3-19)

1. First symptoms frequently cough, exertional dyspnea, edema, or fatigue
2. Proportional pulse pressure
   a. Calculation: (systolic BP – diastolic BP)/systolic BP
   b. Proportional pulse pressure of less than 25% is associated with a cardiac index of less than 2.2 L/min/m^2
3. Serum
   a. Electrolyte levels: may reveal and/or confirm imbalances especially hypokalemia, hypocalcemia, and hypomagnesemia
   b. Albumin levels: may show hypoproteinemia, which can contribute to edema
   c. Arterial blood gases: may show hypoxemia (especially if pulmonary edema present) and acid-base imbalances (including lactic acidosis in severe hypoperfusion states)
   d. Drug levels: may reveal abnormal levels of digoxin, antidysrhythmic agents
   e. Thyroid profile: may reveal abnormal thyroid function
   f. CBC: may show anemia or leukocytosis
   g. BUN, creatinine: may be elevated to detect renal impairment

Table 3-19 Clinical Indications of Left Ventricular, Right Ventricular, and Biventricular Failure

Left Ventricular Failure	Right Ventricular Failure
• Tachypnea, dyspnea, orthopnea, PND	• Jugular venous distention
• Tachycardia	• Hepatojugular reflux
• Left-sided S_3	• Dependent pitting edema
• Displaced PMI, heave at apex	• Heave at sternum
• Crackles, wheezes	• Hepatomegaly/splenomegaly
• Cough, frothy sputum, hemoptysis	• Anorexia, nausea, vomiting
• Diaphoresis	• Abdominal pain and bloating
• Pulsus alternans	• Ascites
• Oliguria	• Nocturia
• Weakness, fatigue	• Weakness, fatigue
• Mental confusion	• Weight gain
• Murmur of MR	• Murmur of TR
• ABGs: decreased PaO_2, SaO_2	• Right-sided S_3
• Hemodynamics • Elevated PA, PAOP • Decreased CO/CI	• Hemodynamics • Elevated CVP, RAP
• Abnormal chest x-ray • Cardiomegaly • Engorged pulmonary vasculature • Kerley B lines • Pleural effusion	• Abnormal liver function studies • ALT • AST • LDH
• ECG • Left atrial enlargement • Left ventricular hypertrophy • Atrial dysrhythmias	• ECG • Right atrial enlargement • Right ventricular hypertrophy • Atrial dysrhythmias

   h. Brain-type natriuretic peptide (BNP)
      1) Normal: less than 100 g/mL; levels greater than 100 g/mL indicate HF
      2) Elevated BNP level correlates with an increased left ventricular end-diastolic pressure and volume and PAOP.
         a) Other conditions associated with increased BNP levels
            i) Left ventricular failure
            ii) Cardiac inflammation
            iii) Primary pulmonary hypertension
            iv) Renal failure
            v) Ascitic cirrhosis
            vi) Endocrine disorders (e.g., primary hyperaldosteronism, Cushing's syndrome)
            vii) May be elevated in elderly patients

b) May replace chest x-ray as the test of choice in differential diagnosis of dyspnea in acute care setting
i. Urine: may show proteinuria and/or presence of RBCs or casts
4. Diagnostic studies
a. Chest x-ray: shows cardiac enlargement and dilation; may show pulmonary congestion
b. Cardiac catheterization and coronary angiography
1) May show coronary artery disease or valve abnormalities
2) Cardiac pressures increased and ejection fraction decreased in systolic dysfunction
3) Cardiac pressures increased and ejection fraction normal in diastolic dysfunction
c. Computed tomography (CT): may be used to evaluate left ventricular wall motion and detect cardiac tumors, MI, aortic aneurysm
d. Echocardiography: shows changes in chamber size, wall thickness, and valve motion
e. Electrocardiography (ECG)
1) May show myocardial ischemia/infarction
2) May show atrial enlargement and/or ventricular hypertrophy
f. Multiple-gated acquisition (MUGA) scan: may be used to evaluate cardiac function, determine ejection fraction, and detect wall motion abnormalities
5. Hemodynamic parameters
a. Increase in volume indicators: RAP, PAP, PAOP
b. Decrease in cardiac output/index
c. Increase in systemic vascular resistance: SVR
d. Increase in pulmonary vascular resistance: PVR
e. Hemodynamic subtypes of heart failure (Figure 3-20)

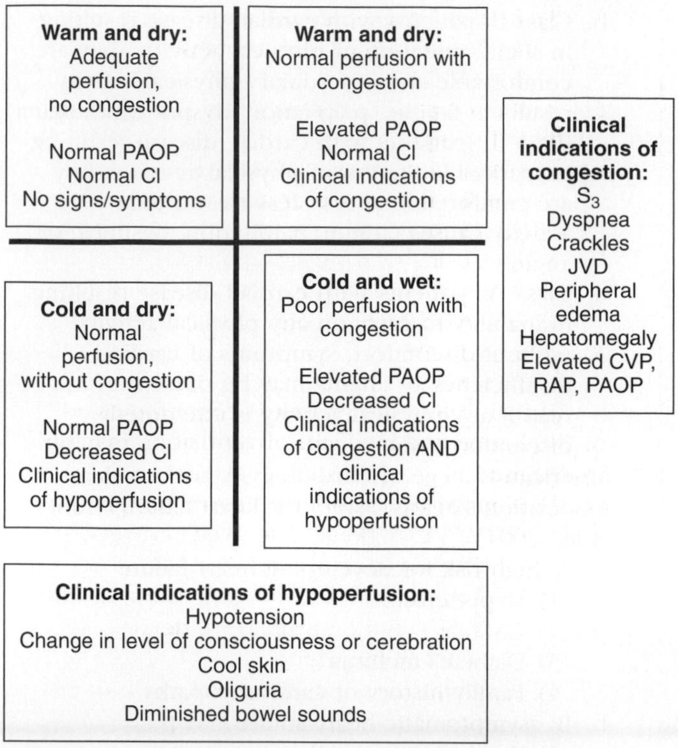

Figure 3-20 Hemodynamic subtypes of heart failure. *CI,* cardiac index; *CVP,* central venous pressure; *JVD,* jugular venous distention; *PAOP,* pulmonary artery occlusive pressure; *RAP,* right atrial pressure. (Adapted from Stevenson, L. W., & Perloff, J. K. [1989]. The limited reliability of physical signs for estimating hemodynamics in chronic heart failure. *JAMA,* 261[6], 884-888.)

Collaborative Management

1. Treat the cause and/or contributing factors if possible
a. Reperfusion in acute MI along with neurohormonal antagonism with beta-blocker (or alpha-/beta-blocker [e.g., carvedilol]) and ACE inhibitor
b. Revascularization of patients with coronary artery disease
c. Valve replacement if required, especially for acute valvular disorder such as ruptured papillary muscle with acute mitral regurgitation
d. Treatment of symptomatic or life-threatening dysrhythmias with antidysrhythmic agents, electrical therapies (e.g., cardioversion, defibrillation, pacemaker, automatic implantable cardiac defibrillator), or surgical procedures (e.g., ablation)
e. Continuous positive airway pressure (CPAP) for obstructive sleep apnea, which is common in patients with HF
f. Avoidance of certain pharmacologic agents
1) Antidysrhythmics being used to suppress asymptomatic dysrhythmias
2) Most calcium channel blockers
3) NSAIDs (increase resistance to diuretics)
2. Be aware of recommended medical treatment by ACC/AHA heart failure stage (Jessup et al., 2009).
a. A: treatment of hypertension and diabetes, control of metabolic syndrome, avoidance of alcohol and illicit drugs, smoking cessation, exercise, lipid control
b. B: all interventions for stage A plus the following:
1) ACE inhibitor and ARB in appropriate patients
2) Beta-block or alpha- and beta-blocker in appropriate patients
3) Consideration of ICD
c. C: all interventions for stages A and B plus the following:
1) Drugs for routine use
a) ACE inhibitor
b) Beta-blocker or alpha- and beta-blocker
c) Diuretics for fluid retention
2) Drugs for selected patients
a) Aldosterone antagonists (e.g., spironolactone)
b) ARB
c) Digitalis
d) Hydralazine/nitrates

3) Devices in selected patients
   a) Resynchronization therapy
   b) AICD

d. D: all interventions for stages A, B, and C plus the following:
   1) Discussion of end of life care
   2) Consideration of extraordinary measures
      a) Chronic inotropes
      b) Permanent mechanical support
      c) Cardiac transplantation
      d) Experimental surgeries or drugs

3. Improve oxygenation
   a. Oxygen by nasal cannula at 2-6 L/min to maintain SaO_2 of 95% unless contraindicated
   b. Intubation and mechanical ventilation may be required
      1) Noninvasive positive-pressure ventilation (BiPAP) may be used to avert intubation.
         a) Positive-pressure ventilation during inspiration (pressure support ventilation [PSV]) during inspiration decreases the work of breathing
         b) Continuous positive-pressure airway pressure (CPAP) during expiration: increases the driving pressure of oxygen to improve oxygenation; decreases intrapulmonary shunt by opening collapsed alveoli; decreases surface tension and work of breathing
      2) Positive end-expiratory pressure (PEEP) may be required if patient is on mechanical ventilation
         a) Increases the driving pressure of oxygen
         b) Decreases shunt by opening alveoli that are collapsed (alveolar recruitment) and keeps alveoli open at low distending pressure if they are still open
         c) Decreases surface tension and work of breathing
         d) Positive alveolar pressure prevents the transudation of fluid into the alveoli
   c. Elimination of accumulated fluid: diuretics
   d. Treatment of anemia: more than half of patients with HF are anemic with hemoglobin less than 12 g/dL and treatment of anemia improves cardiac function
      1) Packed red blood cells may be required acutely if anemia is significant.
      2) Erythropoietin (Epogen)
      3) Iron

4. Decrease myocardial oxygen consumption.
   a. Physical and emotional rest
      1) Allow rest after meals, personal hygiene, toileting, physical therapy, etc.
      2) Prevent Valsalva maneuver.
         a) Teach patient to exhale when turning in bed.
         b) Administer stool softeners as prescribed.
         c) Provide bedside commode for elimination.
      3) Explain procedures thoroughly: monitor alarms; equipment; visiting hours; reasons for procedures
      4) Keep family informed regarding patient's progress and status.
      5) Provide for physical comfort: temperature control; lighting; noise control
      6) Instruct patient regarding relaxation techniques; encourage utilization.
      7) Provide appropriate nutrition: soft low-sodium (2-3 g/day) diet
      8) Administer anxiolytics as prescribed: usually diazepam (Valium), lorazepam (Ativan), or alprazolam (Xanax).
   b. Beta-blocker (or alpha- and beta-blocker) as prescribed
      1) Indications: heart failure as the result of systolic and diastolic dysfunction; usually used for Class II, III HF
      2) Actions
         a) Acts as a cardioprotective agent to protect the heart from excessive catecholamines
         b) Decreases left ventricular mass and volume
         c) Changes the shape of the ventricle from spherical to elliptical
         d) Increases exercise capacity
      3) Agents
         a) Carvedilol (Coreg): alpha- and noncardioselective beta-blocker
         b) Bisoprolol (Zebeta): cardioselective beta-blocker
         c) Sustained release metoprolol (Lopressor, Toprol): cardioselective beta-blocker
         d) Dosages are started low and gradually increased while monitoring closely for decompensation because beta-blockers tend to decrease contractility
      4) Contraindications for the use of beta-blockers in heart failure
         a) Decompensated heart failure
         b) Cardiogenic shock
         c) Acute pulmonary edema
         d) Hemodynamic instability (requiring IV inotropic support)
         e) Bronchial asthma (cardioselective beta-blockers may be used cautiously)
         f) Second- or third-degree AV block
         g) Sick sinus syndrome
         h) Severe hepatic impairment

5. Decrease preload
   a. Positioning: low Fowler's position with legs dependent
   b. Sodium and fluid restrictions acutely
      1) Fluid restriction to less than 2000 mL/24 hr
      2) Sodium restriction to less than 2-3 g/24 hr
      3) Daily measurement of weight to detect early fluid retention

c. Diuretics
  1) Indication: heart failure with evidence of or a predisposition to fluid retention
  2) Action: Eliminate symptoms as well as physical signs of fluid retention, such as JVD and/or edema.
  3) Agents
    a) Usually loop diuretics (e.g., furosemide [Lasix], bumetanide [Bumex])
      i) Continuous infusion may be superior to intermittent boluses.
    b) Aldosterone antagonists (e.g., aldosterone [Aldactone], eplerenone [Inspra]) may be used with loop diuretics or alone.
      i) Relatively weak diuretic in patients with normal renin; however, it is much more effective in patients who have edema associated with either increased production or decreased elimination of renin
      ii) Benefits are synergistic to the benefits of ACE inhibitors
      iii) Close monitoring of potassium levels is necessary especially when patient is also on an ACE inhibitor or ARB.
      iv) Contraindicated in patients with renal insufficiency
    c) Two or more diuretics may be prescribed together
    d) Short-term use of a drug that increases renal blood flow, such as fenoldopam (Corlopam), may be prescribed.
  4) Cautions
    a) Overuse will decrease blood volume, decrease CO, and lead to organ hypoperfusion and prerenal azotemia.
    b) Diuretics may alter the efficacy and toxicity of other drugs used to treat heart failure (e.g., ACE inhibitors, beta-blockers).

d. ACE inhibitors and angiotensin II receptor blockers (ARBs)
  1) Indications: heart failure as the result of systolic and diastolic dysfunction
  2) Action:
    a) ACE inhibitors block conversion of angiotensin I to angiotensin II and the resultant vasoconstriction and aldosterone release.
    b) ARBs block angiotensin II and the resultant vasoconstriction and aldosterone release.
      i) ARBs are frequently used if a patient has angioedema or cough as a result of ACE inhibitors; they are also preferred with African-Americans.
  3) Agents
    a) ACE inhibitors: captopril (Capoten), enalapril (Vasotec), lisinopril (Zestril, Prinivil), ramipril (Altace), benazepril HCl (Lotensin), quinapril HCl (Accupril), fosinopril (Monopril), moexipril HCl (Univasc), trandolapril (Mavik), perindopril (Aceon)
    b) ARBs: losartan (Cozaar), valsartan (Diovan), telmisartan (Micardis), irbesartan (Avapro), candesartan (Atacand), eprosartan (Teveten), olmesartan (Benicar)
    c) If neither ACE inhibitors nor ARBs are tolerated, the combination of nitrates and hydralazine (Apresoline) may be prescribed
  4) Cautions
    a) Hypotension
    b) Angioedema, especially ACE inhibitors
    c) Hyperkalemia especially when in combination with an aldosterone antagonist such as spironolactone (Aldactone)
    d) Proteinuria and renal failure

e. Nesiritide (Natrecor): recombinant form of B-type natriuretic peptide (BNP)
  1) Indication: decompensated heart failure with dyspnea at rest or with minimal activities and clinical evidence of fluid overload
    a) Systolic and diastolic dysfunction
    b) Decompensation is defined as sustained deterioration in function of at least one NYHA class, usually associated with evidence of total body salt and water overload
  2) Action: binds to the alpha-type natriuretic peptide receptor on the surface of vascular smooth muscle and endothelial cells
    a) Dilates arteries and reduces SVR
    b) Dilates veins and reduces PAOP
    c) Decreases aldosterone and norepinephrine levels
    d) Inhibits RAA system and endothelin pathways prompting the release of fluid and sodium from the body
    e) Improves symptoms of decompensated HF more than NTG with less proarrhythmogenesis and tachycardia than dobutamine
  3) Contraindications
    a) Hypovolemia
    b) Profound hypotension (e.g., cardiogenic shock)
    c) Aortic stenosis
    d) Hypertrophic or restrictive cardiomyopathy
    e) Constrictive pericarditis or cardiac tamponade

4) Controversy: Recent studies indicate that nesiritide worsens renal function; its use has decreased significantly in the last five years.

f. Endothelin receptor antagonist: tezosentan (Veletri)
1) Action: vasodilation
2) Does not increase heart rate, but higher doses were associated with hypotension
3) Recent studies results have been mixed in terms of benefit.

g. Venous vasodilators (e.g., nitroglycerin [Tridil], morphine)
1) Not recommended in diastolic dysfunction
2) Be familiar with the effects of commonly used vasodilators (Table 3-20)

h. Dialysis: if the patient is in renal failure

i. Continuous renal replacement therapy (CRRT): may be used to manage the overhydration in heart failure refractory to traditional therapies such as fluid restriction and diuretics

6. Decrease afterload.
a. Nitroprusside: particularly helpful for hypertensive patients
b. Calcium channel blockers
1) Most calcium channel blockers should be avoided in the treatment of heart failure; amlodipine (Norvasc) and felodipine (Plendil) may be used in diastolic dysfunction.
c. ACE inhibitors or ARBs: prevent activation of angiotensin II with the resultant vasoconstriction and increase in afterload
d. Renal artery angioplasty, stents: indicated for patient with renal artery stenosis
e. Pulmonary vasodilators may be used to reduce pulmonary hypertension.
f. Intraaortic balloon pump: especially helpful in patients who have very high afterload that is refractory to arterial vasodilators or who are too hypotensive to utilize arterial dilators to reduce afterload

7. Increase contractility
a. Inotropic agents
1) Indications
a) Temporary treatment of diuretic-refractory decompensation
b) Stage D heart failure to improve quality of life
i) Note that inotropic agents do increase myocardial oxygen consumption; they have not been shown to improve survival and are generally not recommended
2) Hemodynamic effects (Table 3-21)
3) Agents (Table 3-22)
a) Cardiac glycosides (e.g., digoxin)
i) Recommended to improve symptoms in patients with heart failure due to left ventricular systolic dysfunction with dilated ventricle and should be used together with diuretics, ACE inhibitors, and beta-blockers
ii) Actions
(a) Improve cardiac contractility by inhibiting Na, K -ATPase; increases ejection fraction and exercise tolerance
(b) Inhibit SNS and reduces norepinephrine and renin activity
(c) Slow the heart rate in atrial fibrillation
iii) Major drawback: the narrow therapeutic/toxic ratio
b) Sympathetic stimulants (e.g., dobutamine)
i) Used primarily if HF in presence of acute MI
ii) Actions
(a) Increases contractility by stimulating beta receptors so may increase ectopy potential
(b) Dobutamine is preferred (unless patient is hypotensive) because it causes less tachycardia than dopamine

Table 3-20 Vasoactive Effects of Selected Drugs

Drug	Arteries	Veins
Clevidipine (Cleviprex)	Yes	No
Fenoldopam mesylate (Corlopam)	Yes	No
Hydralazine (Apresoline)	Yes	No
Milrinone (Primacor)	Yes	Yes
Minoxidil (Loniten)	Yes	No
Morphine sulfate	No	Yes
Nesiritide (Natrecor)	Yes	Yes
Nicardipine (Cardene)	Yes	Yes
Nifedipine (Procardia)	Yes	Yes
Nitroglycerin (Tridil)	Only if greater than 1 mcg/kg/min	Yes
Nitroprusside (Nipride)	Yes	Yes
Phentolamine (Regitine)	Yes	Yes
Prazosin (Minipress)	Yes	Yes

Table 3-21 Hemodynamic Effects of Inotropic Agents

Drug	CO/CI	MAP	PAOP	SVR	Heart Rate
Digoxin	↑	⇔	⇔	⇔	↓
Dobutamine	↑	↑	↓	↓	⇔ or ↑
Dopamine	↑	↑	↑	↑	↑
Inamrinone/ Milrinone	↑	⇔	↓	↓	⇔

Table 3-22 Inotropic Agents

Drug	Classification/ Actions	Indications	Administration	Adverse Effects	Nursing Implications
Dopamine hydrochloride (Intropin)	**Sympathomimetic** • Dosage determines action • 2-5 mcg/kg/min causes beta stimulation (increases contractility) • 5-10 mcg/kg/min causes alpha and beta stimulation (increases contractility and causes vasoconstriction) • Dosages greater than 10 mcg/kg/min cause predominant alpha stimulation (vasoconstriction)	• Low cardiac output states (2-10 mcg/kg/min) • Vasogenic forms of shock (10 or greater than mcg/kg/min)	• IV infusion: mix 400 mg in 250 mL (1600 mcg/mL) and infuse at 0.5-20 mcg/kg/min depending on desired effect • Maximum: 20 mcg/kg/min • Administer through central venous catheter if possible; if administered peripherally, use a large vein • Do not administer with alkaline solutions	• Tachycardia • Ventricular ectopy • Hypertension or hypotension • Nausea, vomiting • Dyspnea • Headache • Palpitations • Chest pain in patients with CAD • Tissue necrosis with high dosages or extravasation	• Monitor HR, BP, ECG, PA, PAOP, SVR, CI, urine output • Note contraindications: known hypersensitivity, uncorrected tachydysrhythmias, ventricular fibrillation, pheochromocytoma, hypertrophic cardiomyopathy, and in patients receiving MAO inhibitors • Use cautiously in peripheral vascular disease • Consider the cause of hypotension instead of automatically initiating dopamine to increase the blood pressure; *improve perfusion* by treating the cause of hypotension (e.g., volume replacement, inotropes, preload or afterload reduction) • Provide volume expansion during weaning; taper gradually to wean • Do not administer if discolored • Prevent extravasation because necrosis may occur; treat extravasation with phentolamine (Regitine)
Dobutamine hydrochloride (Dobutrex)	**Sympathomimetic** • Increases cardiac contractility and cardiac output • Decreases preload and possibly afterload	• Cardiogenic shock • Low cardiac output states	• IV infusion; mix 250 mg in 250 mL (1000 mcg/mL) and infuse at 2-40 mcg/kg/min • Maximum: 40 mcg/kg/min • Administer through central venous catheter if possible; if administered peripherally, use a large vein • Do not administer with alkaline solutions	• Tachycardia • Ventricular ectopy • Hypertension or hypotension • Nausea, vomiting • Dyspnea • Headache • Anxiety • Paresthesia • Palpitations • Chest pain	• Monitor BP, HR, ECG, PA, PAOP, SVR, CI • Note contraindications: known hypersensitivity, hypertrophic cardiomyopathy • Use cautiously in patients with hypertension or ventricular dysrhythmias • Note that the increase in heart rate is less than with dopamine • Use with nitroprusside as prescribed in cardiogenic shock; dobutamine increases contractility and decreases preload (and to a lesser degree afterload) and nitroprusside decreases afterload and preload

Inamrinone (Inocor) Note change in generic name to avoid confusion between previously named amrinone and amiodarone	**PDE Inhibitor Inotrope** • Increases cardiac contractility • Relaxes vascular smooth muscle to cause vasodilation of arteries and veins and decrease afterload and preload	• Heart failure: short-term (less than 5 days) management of patients with HF who have not responded to traditional therapy of digitalis, diuretics, and/or vasodilators	• IV injection: 0.75 mg/kg over 2-3 minutes; may repeat in 30 minutes • IV infusion: mix 500 mg in 500 mL (1000 mcg/mL) and infuse at 5-15 mcg/kg/min • Maximum: 10 mg/kg/day • Do not reconstitute with dextrose	• Ventricular dysrhythmias • Hypotension • Anorexia, nausea, vomiting, abdominal pain, diarrhea • Increased liver enzymes, hepatotoxicity • Hypokalemia • Tremor • Thrombocytopenia (inamrinone more than milrinone) • Chest pain • Hypersensitivity reactions • Headache • Burning at injection site • Fever • Blurred vision (milrinone)	• Monitor heart rate, BP, ECG, PA, PAOP, CI, SVR, platelet counts, liver function studies, electrolytes (especially potassium), BUN, creatinine • Platelet count below 150,000/mm^3 usually requires dosage reduction • Platelet count below 100,000/mm^3 usually requires discontinuance • Note contraindications: known hypersensitivity to this drug or bisulfites (preservative), severe aortic or pulmonic valvular disease, hypertrophic cardiomyopathy, ventricular dysrhythmias • Use cautiously in renal disease, liver disease, atrial dysrhythmias, older adult • Use cautiously in acute MI because myocardial oxygen consumption is increased • Correct hypokalemia and hypovolemia before or during inamrinone use • Note that milrinone is more frequently prescribed than inamrinone because of the greater incidence of thrombocytopenia with inamrinone
Milrinone (Primacor)			• IV injection: 50 mcg/kg over 10 minutes • IV infusion: mix 30 mg in 250 mL (120 mcg/mL); usual dose 0.375-0.75 mcg/kg/min (less if renal insufficiency)		

and decreases afterload rather than increases afterload such as dopamine does
iii) Parenteral only
c) PDE inhibitors (e.g., milrinone [Primacor], inamrinone [Inocor])
i) Used only if no response to digitalis, diuretics, vasodilators
ii) Actions
(a) Increases contractility by inhibiting phosphodiesterase
(b) Causes vasodilation to decrease preload and afterload
iii) Parenteral only

b. Mechanical cardiac support devices
1) The supply of acceptable donor hearts remains insufficient for the number of patients who require them; mechanical devices offer an alternative (at least temporary); devices continue to be developed and tested as a permanent alternative to cardiac transplantation.
2) Goal: to stabilize and improve the hemodynamic condition of the patient with loss of ventricular function
3) Complications: infection and thromboembolism are most significant; bleeding; hypertension
4) Ventricular assist device (VAD): used in severe cases especially if patient is a candidate for cardiac transplantation (Table 3-23)

c. Surgical approaches
1) Dynamic cardiomyoplasty
a) Latissimus dorsi muscle (LDM) wrapped around the heart and stimulated by electrical impulses to contract with each heartbeat
b) High perioperative mortality in NYHA class IV patients along with overall high long-term mortality and lack of

Table 3-23 Ventricular Assist Device

Indications	• Bridge to recovery: use of a device until the heart recovers and transplantation is not required • Persistent heart failure despite aggressive therapy but with potential for recovery if the heart is given time to rest • Inability to wean from cardiopulmonary bypass • Cardiogenic shock refractory to pharmacologic or IABP therapy • Stunned (may also be referred to as *hibernating*) myocardium • Bridge to bridge: use of a short-term device with replacement later with a long-term device • Bridge to transplant: use of a device to support the patient until a donor heart is available • End-stage heart disease awaiting suitable donor for cardiac transplant • Destination therapy: use of a permanent device as an alternative to transplantation • Class IV HF with ejection fraction less than 25%, on continuous inotropic therapy, but not a candidate for cardiac transplantation • Physiologic indications despite pharmacologic support or IABP therapy • MAP less than 60 mm Hg • Systolic less than 90 mm Hg • PAOP or RAP greater than 20-25 mm Hg • Urine output less than 20 mL/hr • Cardiac index less than 2 L/min/m^2 • Ejection fraction less than 25% • May be used with IABP
Contraindications	• Irreversible, extensive heart disease; no possibility of being weaned from VAD and patient not a candidate for cardiac transplant • Prolonged cardiac arrest with resultant neurologic damage • Multiple organ failure • Significant complications or disease (e.g., chronic renal failure, cancer with metastasis, severe hepatic disease, significant blood dyscrasias, severe COPD)
Actions	• Maintains systemic circulation and tissue perfusion with flow assistance • Decreases myocardial workload to promote ventricular recovery • Reversal of ventricular dilation, regression of left ventricular hypertrophy, reversal of ventricular remodeling
Devices	Total artificial heart: CardioWest, Abiomed Displacement pumps: Thoratec, ABIOMED BVS 5000, HeartMate XVE, Novacor LVAD Rotary/continuous flow/axial pumps: HeartMate II, MicroMed DeBakey, Jarvik 2000 FlowMaker, Impella, Berlin Heart Incor LVAD, TandemHeart Percutaneous VAD, VentrAssist LVAD, Bio-Medicus Magnetically levitated pumps: Levitronix CentriMag All devices have cannula, pump, and external power source

Table 3-23 Ventricular Assist Device—cont'd

Insertion and mechanics	Requires an extended median sternotomy Left ventricular assist device (LVAD) • Outflow circuit anastomosed to patient aorta or femoral artery • Inflow circuit anastomosed to left atrium or ventricle • Left atrium is usually used in the pending recovery patient • Left ventricle is usually used in the bridge to transplant patient Right ventricular assist device (RVAD) • Outflow circuit anastomosed to patient's pulmonary artery • Inflow circuit anastomosed to right atrium Biventricular assist device (Bi-VAD) • Both ventricles are supported; the main advantage here is that with either LVAD or RVAD the unassisted ventricle may fail Implanted Device • The pump unit may be implanted into the abdominal wall • Controller unit and power source are attached to the pump unit by a percutaneous lead
Assessment	• HR: a normalization of heart rate is desirable • BP: an increase in MAP is desirable • CO/CI: an increase in cardiac output/index is desirable • Thermodilution CO will not be accurate in patients with RVAD; use Fick formula (calculation of CO using mixed venous oxygen saturation and arterial oxygen saturation) • PAP/PAOP: a decrease in PAP and PAOP is desirable • SaO_2: an increase in SaO_2 is desirable • SvO_2: an increase in SvO_2 is desirable • Urine output: an increase in urine output is desirable • Complaints of chest pain: a decrease in chest pain is desirable • ECG: a decrease in the presence or frequency of dysrhythmias is desirable • Neurovascular status of affected limb: the presence of palpable pulses and a warm limb with normal capillary refill is desirable
Brief summary of nursing management	• Assess the parameters described earlier • Titrate pharmacologic therapies to augment the mechanical therapy of the VAD • Adjust fluid balance by administering colloids, crystalloids, or diuretics as prescribed • Prevent hazards of immobility: turn side to side when hemodynamics are stabilized; passive range of motion; utilize special mattresses and beds as indicated • Observe for complications and provide appropriate management for the prevention of complications • Provide emotional support to the patient and family; utilize social services, pastoral care, and support groups as indicated

Complications: prevention and treatment	• Thromboembolism: heparin may be prescribed
	• Hemolysis
	• Bleeding
	  • Monitor ACT while on heparin
	  • Monitor for bleeding, including cardiac tamponade
	  • Administer blood and blood products as indicated
	  • Prevent tubing disconnection; all connections should be clearly visible and securely connected
	• Infection
	  • Monitor CBC, body temperature, and heart rate
	  • Monitor for pain, tenderness, heat, redness at exit site and abdominal pump pocket
	  • Assess breath sounds and chest x-ray; pneumonia is common because of immobilization; ventilatory assistance is required with some VADs
	• Dysrhythmias
	• Cerebral emboli
	• Respiratory failure
	• Renal failure
	• Air embolism
	• Mechanical failure
	• Psychological complications (e.g., depression, anxiety)
	• Anxiety concerning device failure and infection

Weaning	• The following parameters with VAD off are required prior to weaning the patient from the VAD
	  • MAP greater than 60 mm Hg
	  • RAP (RVAD) or PAOP (LVAD) less than 25 mm Hg
	  • CI greater than 2 L/min/m^2
	• The VAD flow is decreased
	• Anticoagulation is recommended during weaning
	• VAD removal is done in the OR

demonstrated survival advantage over medical therapy; not recommended at this time

2) Partial left ventriculectomy (also referred to as the *Batista heart failure procedure*): most suited for dilated cardiomyopathy
   a) Resection of a wedge of left ventricular wall to restore the volume-mass-diameter relationship of the left ventricle; mitral and/or tricuspid valve may be replaced concurrently
   b) ACC/AHA guidelines conclude that procedure currently considered not useful/effective and in some cases can be harmful
3) Dor procedure (also referred to as *endoventricular circular patch plasty*)
   a) Areas of hypofunctioning myocardium are cut out and the opening in the wall is repaired with a synthetic or autologous tissue circular patch.
   b) Evidence is unclear and the current ACC/AHA guidelines do not address this procedure.
4) Left-ventricular splints and wraps: in clinical trials
   a) Goal: arrest and reverse remodeling of the failing heart
   b) Devices
      i) Myocor Myosplint: two epicardial pads and a transventricular tension member; the two pads are placed on the surface of the heart with the load-bearing tension member passing through the ventricle, connecting the pads and drawing the ventricular walls toward one another
      ii) Acorn Cardiac Support Device: wraps the heart in a mesh bag to prevent further dilation and failure; the Dacron wrap is pulled over the base of the heart and attached with sutures
      iii) Evidence is unclear and the current ACC/AHA guidelines do not address these procedures.
5) Cardiac transplantation
   a) Indications for cardiac transplantation in heart failure patient
      i) Class III or IV and a life expectancy of less than 24 hours
      ii) Under 65 years of age at the time of listing; if retransplantation or heart-kidney or heart-liver, the age of 55 years is generally used
      iii) Acute heart failure or cardiogenic shock as a result of acute MI that is refractory to medical therapy and requires mechanical support or patients who can not be weaned from cardiopulmonary bypass are candidates unless they have contraindications

8. Manage dysrhythmias
   a. Atrial
      1) Atrial dysrhythmias frequently resolve with treatment of HF because atrial stretch, and, therefore, atrial irritability is decreased
      2) Digoxin: decreases ventricular response rate by increasing refractoriness of AV node
      3) Anticoagulants: used to prevent mural thrombi and embolic events
   b. Ventricular
      1) Antidysrhythmics as prescribed
         a) Class I antidysrhythmics (e.g., procainamide, lidocaine) should not be used except for immediately life-threatening ventricular dysrhythmia.
         b) Some Class III antidysrhythmics, such as amiodarone, do not appear to increase the risk of death and are preferred over class I agents.
      2) Correction of electrolyte deficiencies that may cause dysrhythmias and alter the efficacy and safety of antidysrhythmic agents
   c. Dual-chamber pacemaker with rate modulation
      1) Beneficial for patients with severe heart failure with poor activity tolerance
      2) Increases heart rate in response to physical activity
   d. Cardiac resynchronization therapy (CRT): atriobiventricular pacing
      1) Indications in HF patients: 30-50% of patients with HF have ventricular asynchrony and the 80% of patients with advanced HF have LBBB with resultant ventricular asynchrony
         a) Ejection fraction of 35% or less
         b) QRS of at least 130 milliseconds (0.13 seconds)
         c) NYHA class III to IV
      2) Actions
         a) Restores synchronous ventricular contraction to optimize left ventricular filling and improve cardiac output
         b) Improved exercise tolerance
         c) Improved quality of life
         d) Reduction in mortality
      3) Collaborative management: as for newly implanted pacemakers and for HF
         a) Monitor for 100% ventricular capture as well as any lengthening of the QRS that might indicate loss of capture of one of the ventricles (usually the left ventricle)
         b) Restrict movement of the arm to prevent lead dislodgement or bleeding in the pacemaker pocket; give instructions regarding: avoidance of pushing, pulling, or lifting anything heavier than 5 pounds for 1-2 weeks after surgery; what

symptoms to report; and other instructions as for implanted pacemaker
c) Monitor for complications: infection

9. Provide collaborative management specific to RVF (cor pulmonale).
   a. Treat the cause
      1) Hypoxemia: oxygen to maintain SaO_2 of at least 90%
      2) Primary pulmonary hypertension: (nitric oxide, epoprostenol [Flolan]) may be indicated depending on etiology
      3) Pulmonary embolism
         a) Anticoagulants
         b) Fibrinolytics if RVF and/or refractory hypoxemia
      4) Dysrhythmias: cardioversion, antidysrhythmic agents, pacemaker, resynchronization therapy
   b. Ensure volume optimization.
      1) Treatment of fluid overload: sodium restriction, diuretics, CRRT
      2) Treatment of hypovolemia: fluid administration
   c. Administer inotropic agents as required; especially when poor right ventricular contractility (e.g., right ventricular MI)
10. Monitor for complications.
   a. Deep vein thrombosis/pulmonary embolism
   b. Progressive deterioration
   c. Dysrhythmias: common cause of sudden death
   d. Complications of therapy
      1) Fluid and electrolyte imbalance: hypokalemia; hypocalcemia; hypomagnesemia due to diuretic therapy
      2) Digitalis toxicity
   e. Depression
   f. Anxiety
   g. Sleep disturbances
11. Provide instruction and counseling regarding lifestyle modification and need for pharmacologic therapy.
   a. Nonpharmacologic therapies
      1) Weight normalization
      2) Dietary modifications
         a) Low saturated fat
         b) Low (2-3 g/day) sodium
         c) ADA diet for control of blood glucose for patient with DM
      3) Cessation of tobacco use
      4) Limitation of alcohol consumption to 1-2 alcoholic beverages daily
      5) Regular aerobic exercise in moderation
      6) Complementary therapies: relaxation; imagery, biofeedback
      7) Stress reduction
      8) Yearly flu and pneumococcal vaccine
      9) Recognition of symptoms of HF and when to call the physician
      10) Measurement of body weight is the best way to monitor when to initiate and titrate diuretic therapy.
         a) Teach the patient to notify the physician if he or she gains 2 lb/day for more than 2 days or a total of 5 lb in 1 week.
   b. Pharmacologic agents
      1) Prescribed medication regimen for HF
      2) Control of hypertension, hyperlipidemia, diabetes mellitus, and thyroid disorders
      3) Avoidance of drugs that may worsen HF: nonsteroidal antiinflammatory drugs

Cardiomyopathy

Definition

Disorder causing destruction of cardiac muscle fibers (i.e., myofibrils) leading to impaired contractility and cardiac output (Figure 3-21)

Dilated (Previously Called *Congestive*) Cardiomyopathy

1. Etiology
   a. Idiopathic
   b. Infection, especially viral (e.g., coxsackievirus B, arbovirus)

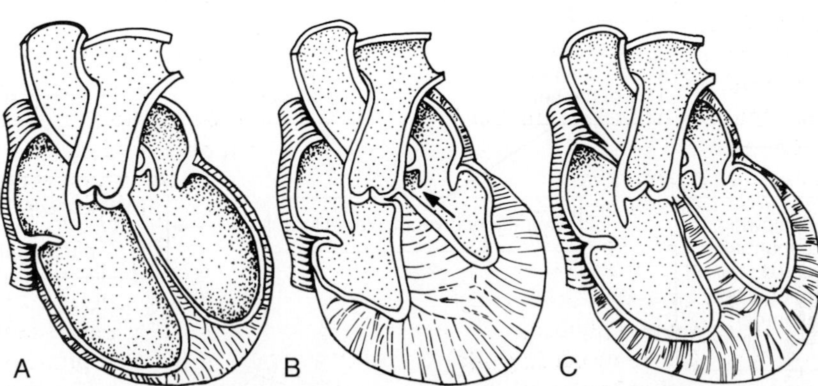

Figure 3-21 Cardiomyopathies. **A,** Dilated. **B,** Hypertrophic. **C,** Restrictive. (From Kinney, M. R., Packa, D. R., & Dunbar, S. B. [1993]. *AACN's clinical reference for critical-care nursing* [3rd ed.]. St. Louis: Mosby.)

c. Toxins (e.g., doxorubicin [Adriamycin], daunorubicin [Cerubidine], alcohol, lead, arsenic, cobalt)
d. Electrolyte, vitamin or nutrient deficiency
  1) Hypokalemia
  2) Hypocalcemia
  3) Hypophosphatemia
  4) Thiamine deficiency
e. Pregnancy
f. Neuromuscular disorders (e.g., myasthenia gravis, muscular dystrophy)
g. Connective tissue disorders (e.g., lupus, scleroderma, rheumatoid disease)
h. Infiltrative disorders (e.g., sarcoidosis, amyloidosis)
i. Hyperthyroidism

2. Pathophysiology (Figure 3-22)
3. Clinical presentation
  a. Subjective
    1) Fatigue, weakness, decreased exercise tolerance
    2) Chest pain
    3) Palpitations
    4) Syncope
    5) Symptoms of HF: dyspnea; edema
  b. Objective
    1) Orthostatic BP changes
    2) May have murmurs of tricuspid and/or mitral regurgitation
    3) Signs of biventricular failure
      a) LVF: S_3; crackles; PMI displaced laterally
      b) RVF: JVD; peripheral edema; hepatomegaly
  c. Diagnostic
    1) Chest x-ray
      a) Cardiomegaly
      b) Pulmonary congestion
      c) Possibly pleural effusion
    2) Electrocardiography
      a) Biventricular hypertrophy, biatrial enlargement
      b) Dysrhythmias: atrial fibrillation common
      c) Blocks: BBB may be seen

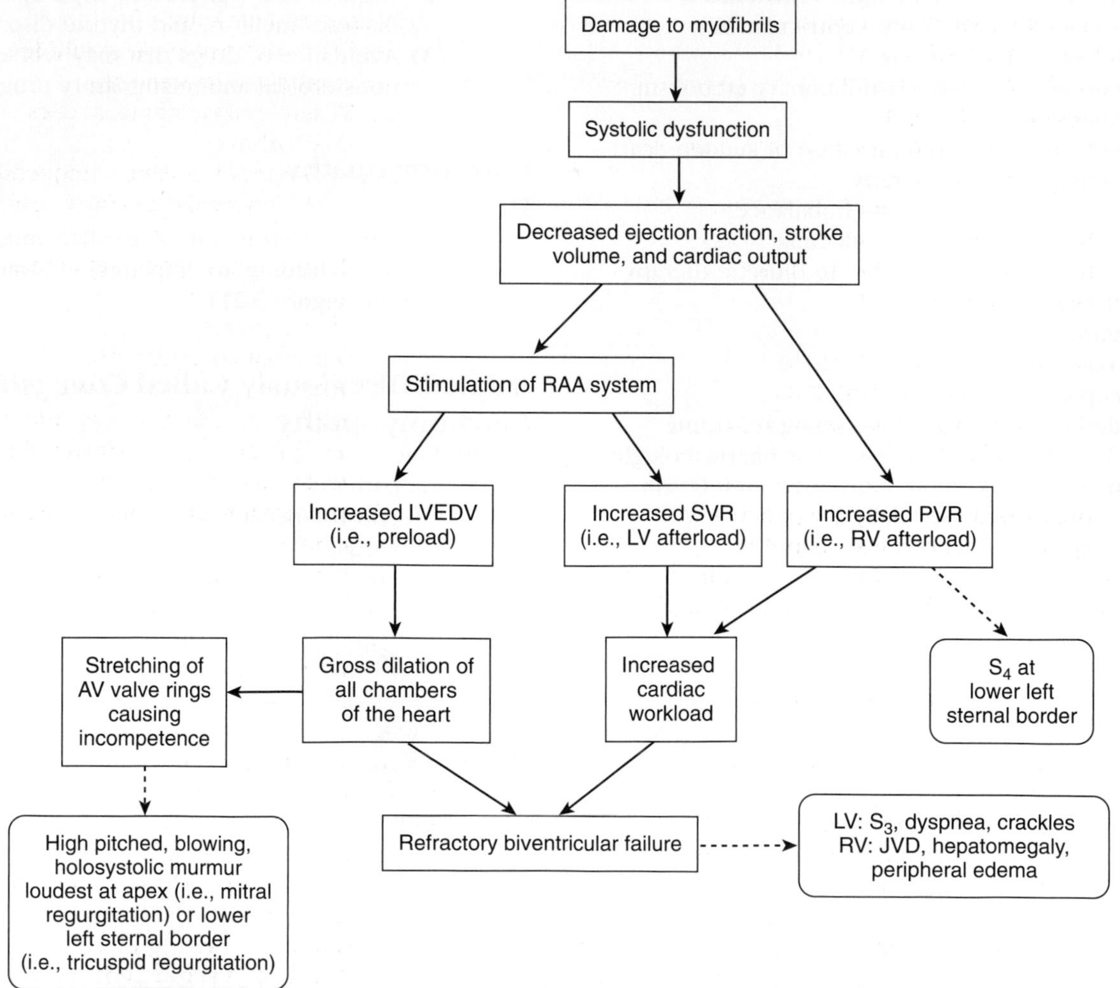

Figure 3-22 Pathophysiology of dilated cardiomyopathy. Dotted lines connect pathology to the clinical presentation. *AV,* atrioventricular; *JVD,* jugular venous distention; *LV,* left ventricular; *LVEDV,* left ventricular end-diastolic volume; *PVR,* pulmonary vascular resistance; *RAA,* renin-angiotensin-aldosterone; *RV,* right ventricular; *SVR,* systemic vascular resistance.

3) Echocardiography
   a) Decreased ventricular wall motion
   b) Decreased ejection fraction
   c) Enlarged chamber size
   d) Abnormal wall motion
4) Cardiac catheterization
   a) Elevated PAP, LAP, LVEDP
   b) Decreased cardiac output
   c) Decreased ejection fraction
   d) Mitral and/or tricuspid regurgitation
   e) RAP, RVEDP may be elevated if RVF present

4. Collaborative management
   a. Provide care as for HF.
      1) Oxygen by nasal cannula at 2-6 L/min to maintain SaO_2 of 95% unless contraindicated
      2) ACE inhibitor (e.g., captopril)
      3) Beta-blocker (e.g., metoprolol) or alpha- and beta-blocker (e.g., carvedilol) may be prescribed
      4) Vasodilators (e.g., nitrates)
      5) Diuretics (e.g., furosemide)
      6) Inotropes (e.g., digoxin) may be required
      7) Cardiac resynchronization therapy (CRT): atriobiventricular pacing
   b. Decrease myocardial oxygen consumption
      1) Activity restrictions
      2) Sodium restrictions
      3) Physical comfort: temperature; lighting; noise control
      4) Anxiolytics as prescribed and indicated: usually diazepam (Valium); lorazepam (Ativan); or alprazolam (Xanax)
   c. Monitor for complications
      1) Dysrhythmias
         a) Atrial fibrillation: digoxin
         b) Ventricular dysrhythmias: antidysrhythmic agents (e.g., amiodarone), ICD
      2) Systemic emboli: anticoagulation frequently prescribed especially for patients with ejection fractions less than 30%
   d. Assist in preparation of the patient for mitral valve replacement or cardiac transplantation as requested.

Hypertrophic Cardiomyopathy

1. Types
   a. Nonobstructive: ventricular free wall hypertrophied
   b. Obstructive: both ventricular free wall and interventricular septum are hypertrophied; genetically transmitted
2. Etiology
   a. Heredity: genetically transmitted autosomal dominant trait
   b. Idiopathic
   c. Neuromuscular disorders (e.g., Friedreich's ataxia)
   d. Hypoparathyroidism
3. Pathophysiology (Figure 3-23)
4. Clinical presentation
   a. Subjective
      1) Dyspnea, orthopnea, PND
      2) Chest pain
      3) Palpitations
      4) Syncope
   b. Objective
      1) PMI displaced laterally
      2) Crackles
      3) S_4
      4) Murmurs
         a) Subaortic stenosis: systolic ejection murmur loudest along left sternal border; increases with Valsalva maneuver, decreases with squatting position
         b) Mitral regurgitation: holosystolic blowing murmur loudest at apex radiates to axilla
   c. Diagnostic
      1) Chest x-ray
         a) Left atrial dilation
         b) Cardiomegaly
         c) Pulmonary congestion
      2) Electrocardiography
         a) Left atrial enlargement and left ventricular hypertrophy
         b) ST and T wave abnormalities
         c) Dysrhythmias
            i) Atrial fibrillation frequently seen
            ii) Ventricular dysrhythmias may be seen
         d) Blocks: left anterior hemiblock frequently seen
      3) Echocardiography
         a) Left atrial enlargement
         b) Increased thickness of the left ventricular free wall and interventricular septum causing narrowing of the left ventricular outflow tract
         c) Abnormal wall motion especially of septum
         d) Mitral regurgitation possible
      4) Cardiac catheterization
         a) Elevated LVEDP
         b) Mitral regurgitation may be evident
         c) Left ventricular outflow pressure gradient
5. Collaborative management
   a. Prevent obstruction of the left ventricular outflow tract
      1) Administer beta-blockers and/or calcium channel blockers as prescribed to decrease contractility and myocardial oxygen consumption; these agents also decrease the heart rate to improve ventricular filling.
      2) Avoid inotropic agents that would increase the outflow tract obstruction.
      3) Prepare patient for percutaneous or surgical procedures as requested.

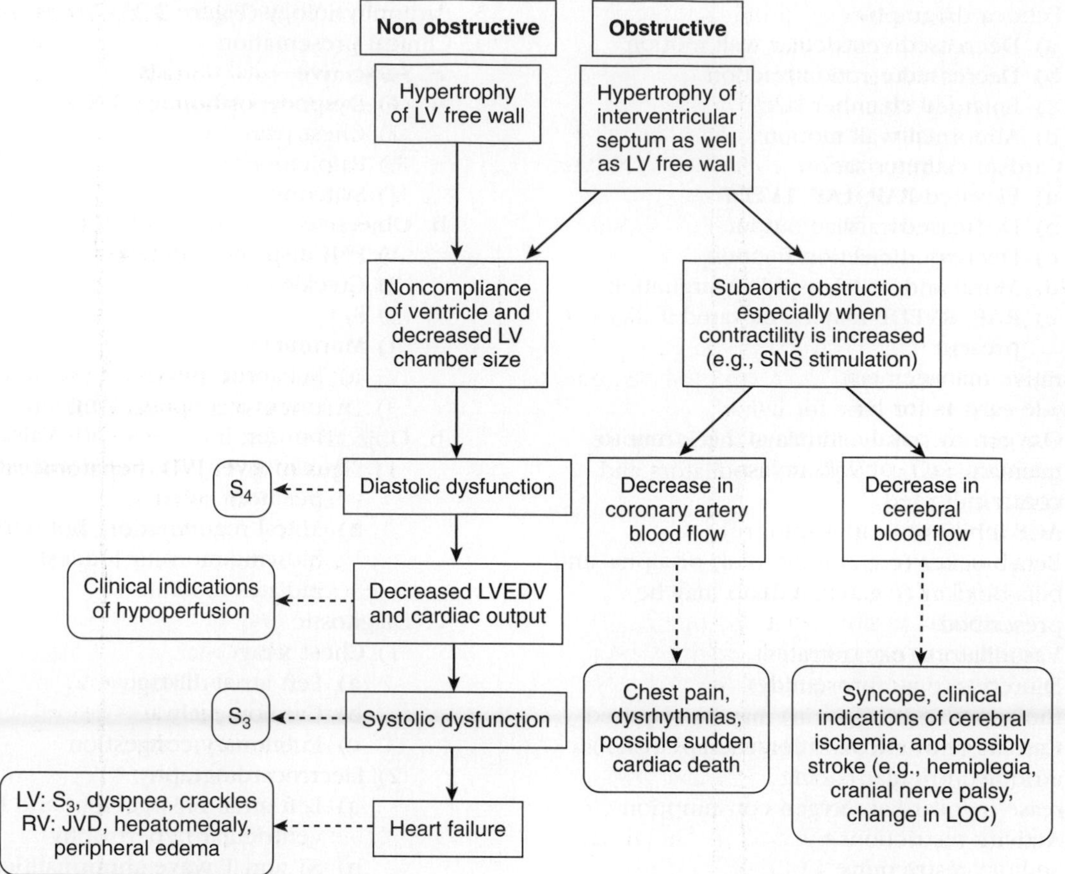

Figure 3-23 Pathophysiology of hypertrophic cardiomyopathy. Dotted lines connect pathology to the clinical presentation. *AV,* atrioventricular; *JVD,* jugular venous distention; *LV,* left ventricular; *LVEDV,* left ventricular end-diastolic volume; *PVR,* pulmonary vascular resistance; *RAA,* renin-angiotensin-aldosterone; *RV,* right ventricular; *SNS,* sympathetic nervous system; *SVR,* systemic vascular resistance.

a) Ventricular septal myectomy: recommended for left ventricular outflow obstruction if symptoms continue despite optimal medical therapy
   i) Surgical removal of a portion of the hypertrophied septum
   ii) Requires thoracotomy and cardiopulmonary bypass
   iii) Mitral valve usually replaced concurrently
   iv) Complications include septal perforation, blocks, and dysrhythmias along with the complications of cardiac surgery with cardiopulmonary bypass
b) Percutaneous transluminal septal myocardial ablation (PTSMA)
   i) Recommended for left ventricular outflow obstruction if symptoms continue despite optimal medical therapy and the patient is a suboptimal surgical candidate or the patient prefers it after a discussion of options
   ii) Percutaneous coronary intervention to isolate the septal perforator branch of the left anterior descending coronary artery and inject 98% ethanol to cause selective infarction of a portion of the septum to prevent movement of the septum toward the left ventricular free walls to keep the outflow tract open
      (a) Contraindications include inadequate septal thickness, right bundle branch block, mitral valve disease, and greater than 50% occlusion of RCA.
   iii) Temporary pacemaker is usually in place for 24-48 hours
   iv) CK-MB and troponin should peak 7 hours after ablation
   v) IV or oral analgesics may be required
   vi) Care as for any other PCI along with monitoring for dysrhythmias,

heart blocks, stroke, cardiac tamponade, and hypotension

c) Dual-chamber pacing
   i) Shortening of the AV interval minimizes contraction of the septum and decreases the outflow tract obstruction
   ii) Usually used in conjunction with pharmacologic agents

b. Maintain adequate filling volumes
   1) Administer intravenous fluids as prescribed.
   2) Administer beta-blockers and calcium channel blockers to decrease the heart rate allowing more time for filling.
   3) Use caution or avoid drugs that decrease preload such as venous vasodilators and diuretics.

c. Monitor for complications.
   1) Dysrhythmias
      a) Atrial: Digoxin is not used as it may increase outflow tract obstruction; diltiazem or verapamil may be used.
      b) Ventricular: antidysrhythmics (e.g., amiodarone)
   2) Systemic emboli: Anticoagulants frequently prescribed, especially for patients with ejection fractions less than 30%.

d. Assist in preparation of the patient for cardiac transplantation as requested.

Restrictive: Least Common

1. Etiology
   a. Idiopathic
   b. Infiltrative disorders (e.g., sarcoidosis, amyloidosis)
   c. Endomyocardial fibrosis
   d. Glycogen deposition
   e. Hemochromatosis
   f. Radiation
   g. Lymphoma
   h. Connective tissue disorders (e.g., scleroderma)
2. Pathophysiology (Figure 3-24)
3. Clinical presentation
   a. Subjective
      1) Chest pain
      2) Fatigue, weakness
      3) Dyspnea, orthopnea, PND
   b. Objective
      1) Signs of RVF: JVD, hepatomegaly, peripheral edema, right-sided S_3
      2) May also have signs of LVF: left-sided S_3, crackles
   c. Diagnostic
      1) Chest x-ray
         a) Cardiomegaly
         b) Pulmonary congestion
         c) Possibly pleural effusion
      2) Electrocardiography
         a) Low QRS voltage
         b) AV blocks are common
      3) Echocardiography
         a) Atrial enlargement
         b) Enlarged ventricular outside dimension but small ventricular chamber
         c) Pericardial effusion may be evident
      4) Cardiac catheterization: elevated RAP, RVEDP, PAP, LAP, LVEDP

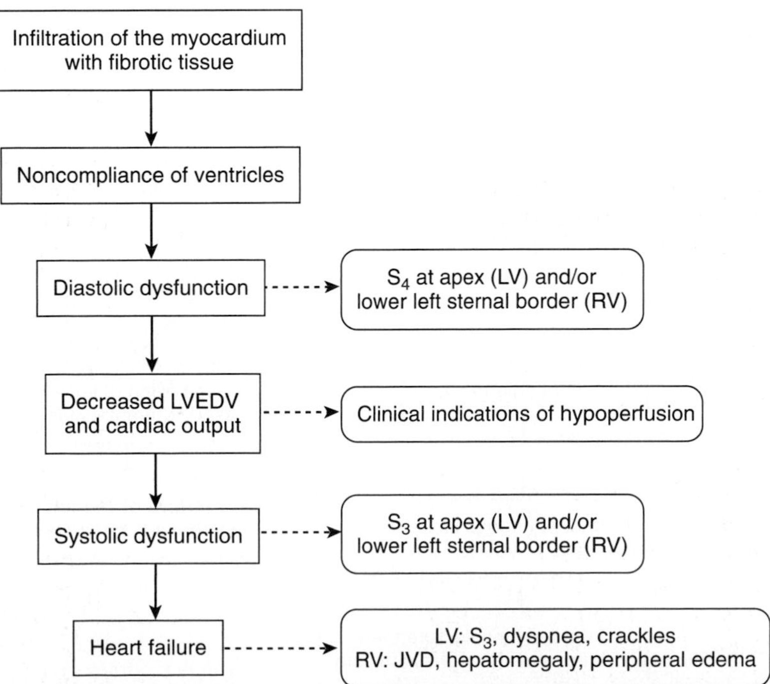

Figure 3-24 Pathophysiology of restrictive cardiomyopathy. Dotted lines connect pathology to the clinical presentation. *JVD,* jugular venous distention; *LV,* left ventricular; *LVEDV,* left ventricular end-diastolic volume; *RV,* right ventricular.

4. Collaborative management
    a. Treat the cause: may include steroids
    b. Provide care as for HF
        1) Oxygen by nasal cannula at 2-6 L/min to maintain SaO_2 of 95% unless contraindicated
        2) ACE inhibitors (e.g., captopril)
        3) Beta-blockers (e.g., metoprolol)
        4) Vasodilators (e.g., nitrates)
        5) Diuretics (e.g., furosemide)
        6) Inotropes (e.g., digoxin)
    c. Monitor for complications
        1) Dysrhythmias
            a) Atrial fibrillation: digoxin
            b) Ventricular dysrhythmias: antidysrhythmic agents (e.g., amiodarone)
        2) AV blocks: pacemaker may be needed
        3) Systemic emboli: anticoagulants frequently prescribed, especially for patients with ejection fractions less than 30%
    d. Assist in preparation of the patient for cardiac transplantation as requested.

Indications for Cardiac Transplantation

1. Heart disease
    a. Severe functional limitations
    b. Poor prognosis
    c. Not surgically correctable
    d. Unresponsive to medical therapy
    e. Pulmonary vascular resistance (PVR) normal or reversible with therapy (if pulmonary hypertension is severe and irreversible, the patient may be a candidate for a heart-lung transplant)
2. Age of 70 years or less
3. Lack of intrinsic disease in other organ systems that would limit long-term survival or be worsened by immunosuppressive therapy
4. Favorable psychosocial profile
5. Blood negative for HIV and HBV

Valvular Heart Disease

Definition

An acquired or congenital disorder of a cardiac valve; characterized by stenosis (obstruction) or regurgitation (backward flow) of blood

Mitral Regurgitation (Insufficiency, Incompetence)

1. Etiology
    a. Trauma
    b. Rheumatic heart disease (RHD) or other form of infective endocarditis
    c. Papillary muscle dysfunction or rupture, rupture of chordae tendineae
    d. Congenital malformation of mitral valve
    e. Mitral valve prolapse (MVP) (also referred to as *Barlow's syndrome* or *floppy mitral valve syndrome*)
    f. LV dilation from LVF
    g. Hypertrophic cardiomyopathy
    h. Marfan's syndrome
    i. Calcification of mitral valve leaflets
    j. Scleroderma
    k. Prosthetic valve dysfunction
2. Pathophysiology (Figure 3-25)

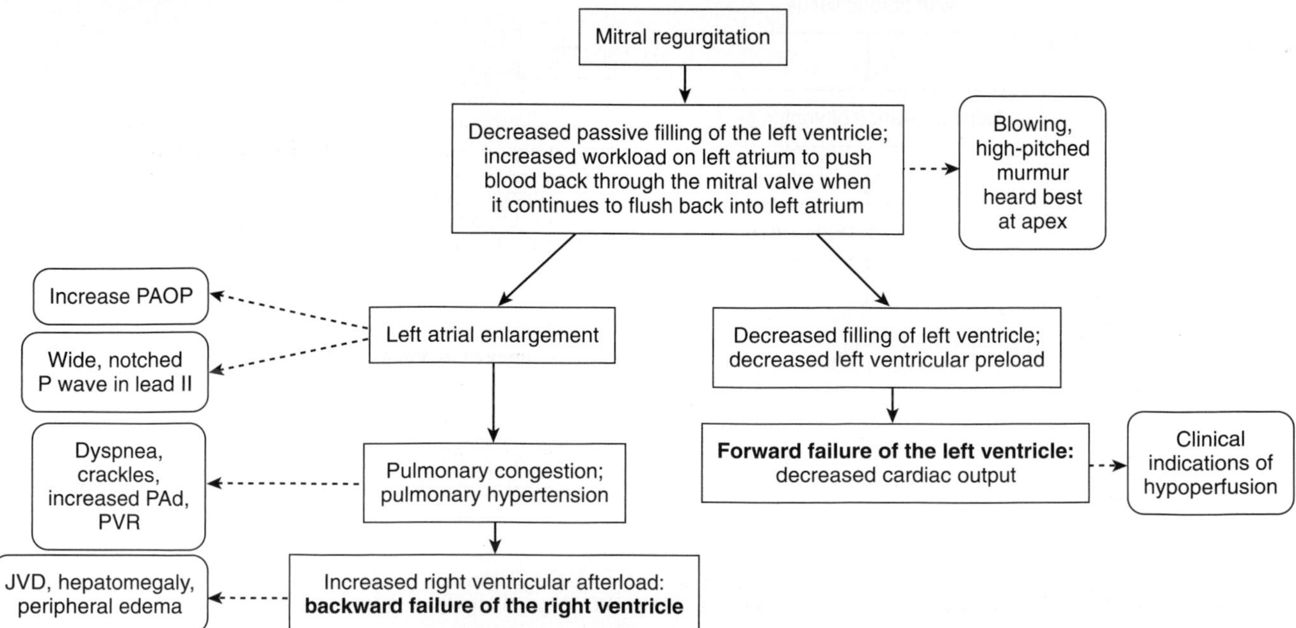

Figure 3-25 Pathophysiology of mitral regurgitation. Dotted lines connect pathology to the clinical presentation. *JVD,* jugular venous distention; *PAd,* pulmonary artery diastolic pressure; *PAOP,* pulmonary artery occlusive pressure; *PVR,* pulmonary vascular resistance.

3. Clinical presentation
    a. Subjective
        1) Dyspnea, orthopnea, paroxysmal nocturnal dyspnea (PND); may have cough
        2) Chest pain may occur but is not common
        3) Palpitations may occur
        4) Weakness, fatigue
        5) Anxiety
    b. Objective
        1) Tachycardia
        2) Diaphoresis
        3) Confusion
        4) PMI displaced laterally; may be more diffuse
        5) Crackles may be present
        6) Heart sound changes
            a) S_2 may be widely split
            b) Right-sided S_3, S_4 may be heard
            c) Holosystolic murmur: high-pitched, blowing, loudest at apex, and radiates to axilla
        7) Signs of RVF: JVD; hepatomegaly; peripheral edema
    c. Diagnostic
        1) Hemodynamic monitoring: PAOP waveform shows large *v* waves
        2) Chest x-ray
            a) Cardiomegaly
            b) Left atrial enlargement
            c) Left ventricular hypertrophy
            d) Pulmonary congestion may be present
        3) Electrocardiography
            a) Left atrial enlargement
            b) Left and/or right ventricular hypertrophy
            c) Dysrhythmias: most frequently atrial fibrillation
        4) Echocardiography
            a) Thickening, prolapse, and calcification of mitral valve
            b) Right ventricular, left atrial, and left ventricular enlargement
        5) Cardiac catheterization
            a) Increased left atrial and ventricular pressures
            b) Regurgitation of blood from the left ventricle to the left atrium

Mitral Stenosis

1. Etiology
    a. RHD
    b. Endocarditis
    c. Congenital
    d. Tumors of left atrium (e.g., atrial myxoma)
    e. Calcification of mitral annulus
2. Pathophysiology (Figure 3-26)
3. Clinical presentation
    a. Subjective
        1) Dyspnea, orthopnea, PND, crackles
        2) Cough, hemoptysis
        3) Fatigue, weakness
        4) Palpitations
        5) Dysphagia
        6) Hoarseness
        7) Syncope may occur.
        8) Chest pain may occur but is rare.
    b. Objective
        1) Ruddy face (mitral facies)
        2) RV heave palpable at sternum
        3) Heart sound changes
            a) Loud S_1: referred to as *closing snap*
            b) Loud P_2

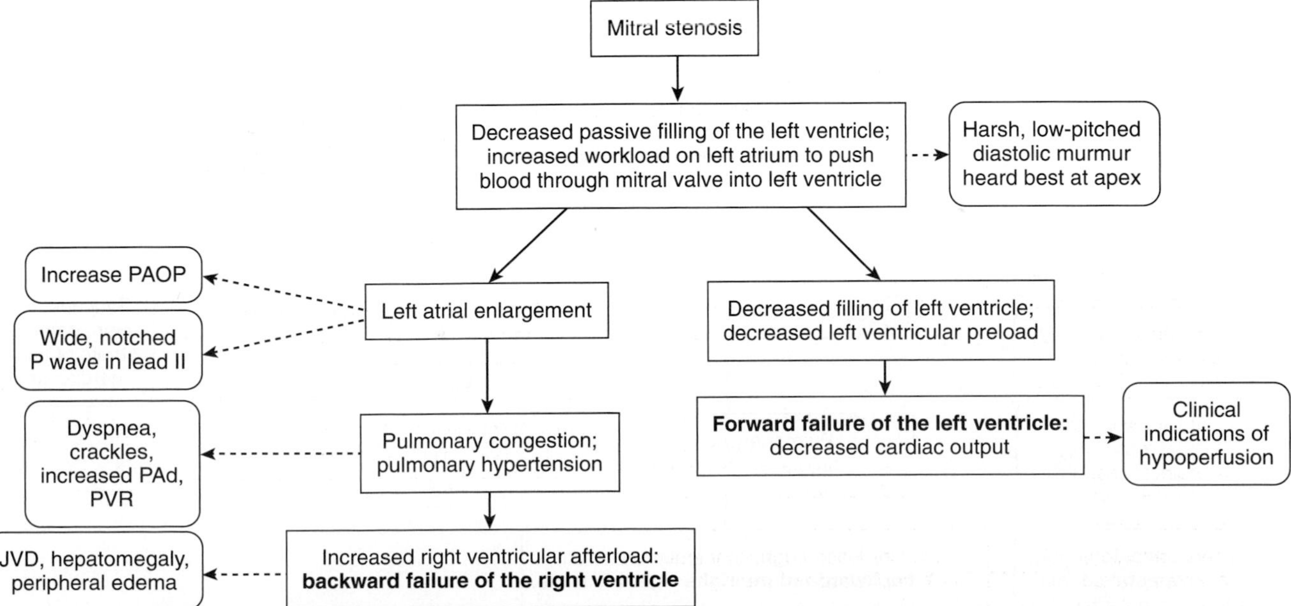

Figure 3-26 Pathophysiology of mitral stenosis. Dotted lines connect pathology to the clinical presentation. *JVD,* jugular venous distention; *PAd,* pulmonary artery diastolic pressure; *PAOP,* pulmonary artery occlusive pressure; *PVR,* pulmonary vascular resistance.

c) Right-sided S_3, S_4
d) Opening snap
e) Mid-diastolic murmur: harsh, rumbling, loudest at apex; may have associated thrill
4) Signs of RVF: JVD; hepatomegaly; peripheral edema
c. Hemodynamic parameters: PAOP waveform shows large *a* waves
d. Diagnostic
1) Chest x-ray
a) Left atrial enlargement
b) Pulmonary congestion
c) Right ventricular hypertrophy
d) Mitral valve calcification
2) Electrocardiography
a) Left atrial enlargement (frequently referred to as *P-mitrale*)
b) Right ventricular hypertrophy
c) Dysrhythmias: most frequently atrial fibrillation
3) Echocardiography
a) Abnormal movement and thickening of valve leaflets and narrowing of mitral valve orifice
b) Left atrial enlargement
c) Right ventricular hypertrophy
4) Cardiac catheterization
a) Elevated pressure gradient across mitral valve
b) Elevated RAP, PAP, LAP

Aortic Regurgitation (Insufficiency, Incompetence)

1. Etiology
a. RHD
b. Calcification
c. Congenital malformation (e.g., bicuspid aortic valve)
d. Endocarditis
e. Syphilis
f. Marfan's syndrome
g. Hypertension
h. Connective tissue disease (e.g., lupus erythematosus)
i. Aortic dissection
j. Trauma
2. Pathophysiology (Figure 3-27)
3. Clinical presentation

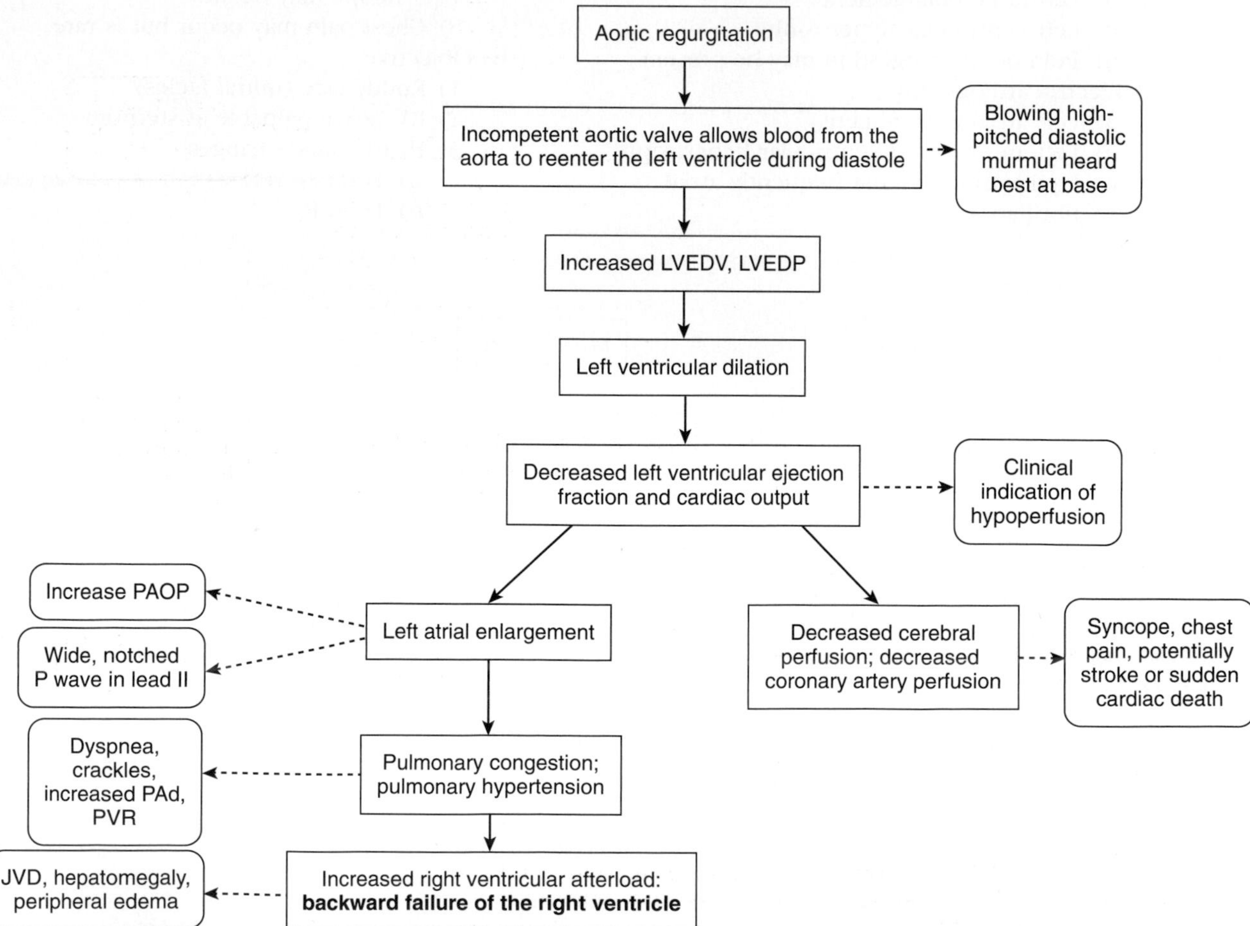

Figure 3-27 Pathophysiology of aortic regurgitation. Dotted lines connect pathology to the clinical presentation. *JVD,* jugular venous distention; *LVEDP,* left ventricular end-diastolic pressure; *LVEDV,* left ventricular end-diastolic volume; *PAd,* pulmonary artery diastolic pressure; *PAOP,* pulmonary artery occlusive pressure; *PVR,* pulmonary vascular resistance.

a. Subjective
   1) Fatigue
   2) Cough
   3) Symptoms of HF: dyspnea; orthopnea; PND
   4) Exertional chest pain
   5) Syncope
   6) Palpitations
b. Objective
   1) Musset's sign: nodding of the head with each systole
   2) Widened pulse pressure
   3) Water-hammer (also called *Corrigan's*) pulse: rapid rise that collapses suddenly
   4) PMI displaced laterally and downward
   5) Hill's sign: Popliteal is greater than brachial BP by 40 mm Hg or more.
   6) Quincke's sign: visible capillary pulsation of nailbeds when fingertip is pressed
   7) Signs of HF: S_3, crackles, JVD, hepatomegaly, peripheral edema
   8) Heart sound changes
      a) Diastolic murmur: high-pitched, blowing, decrescendo, loudest at base, may radiate to the apex; may have associated thrill
      b) May have aortic ejection click
      c) Systolic murmur: may have systolic ejection murmur
c. Diagnostic
   1) Chest x-ray
      a) Left atrial enlargement
      b) Left ventricular hypertrophy
      c) Pulmonary congestion
   2) Electrocardiography
      a) Sinus tachycardia
      b) Left ventricular hypertrophy
      c) Left atrial enlargement
   3) Echocardiography
      a) Poor aortic valve motion
      b) Thickening of aortic valve
      c) Left ventricular hypertrophy
      d) Left atrial enlargement
   4) Cardiac catheterization
      a) Elevated LAP, LVEDP
      b) Regurgitation from aorta to left ventricle

Aortic Stenosis

1. Etiology
   a. RHD
   b. Calcification
   c. Congenital bicuspid valve
   d. Aortic coarctation
2. Pathophysiology (Figure 3-28)

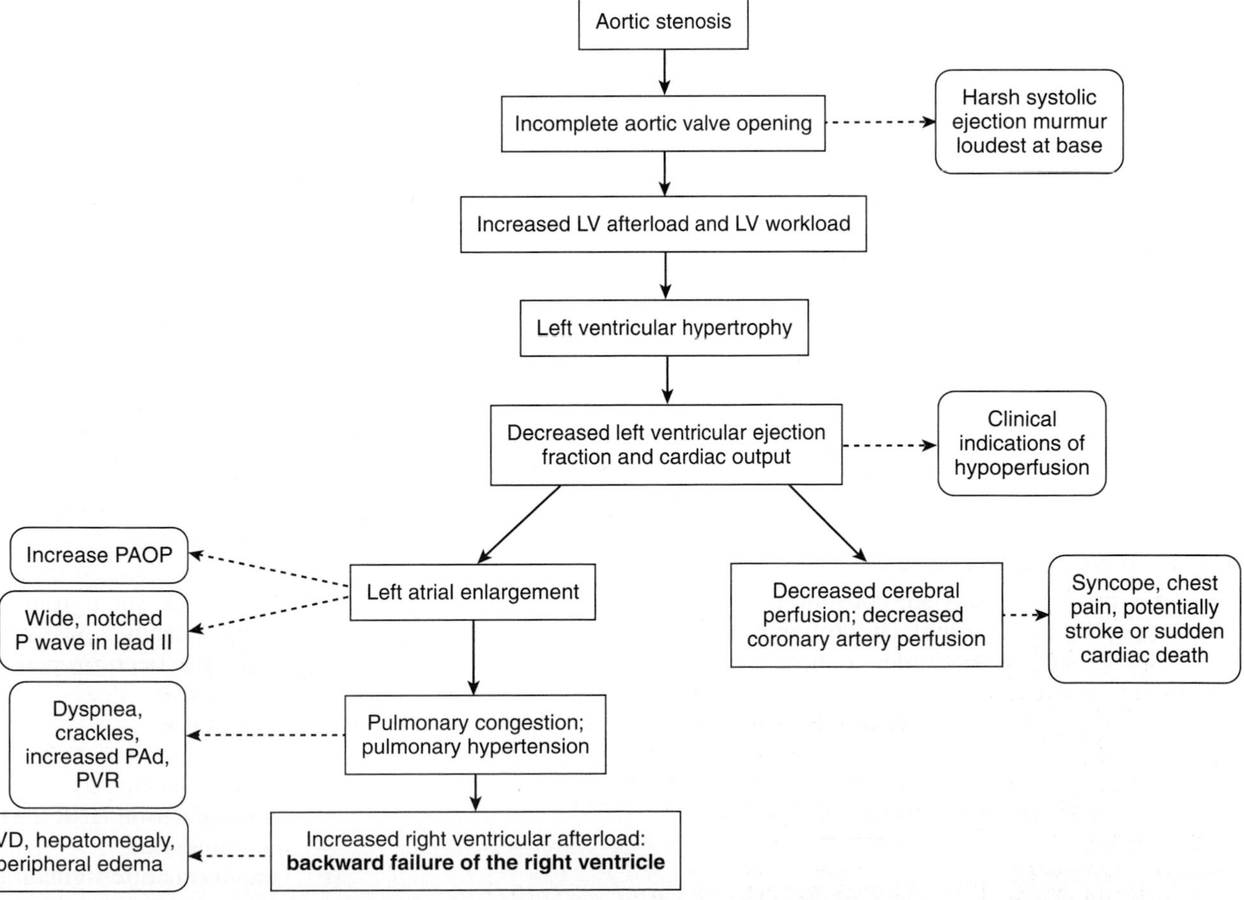

Figure 3-28 Pathophysiology of aortic stenosis. Dotted lines connect pathology to the clinical presentation. *JVD,* jugular venous distention; *LV,* left ventricular; *LVEDP,* left ventricular end-diastolic pressure; *LVEDV,* left ventricular end-diastolic volume; *PAd,* pulmonary artery diastolic pressure; *PAOP,* pulmonary artery occlusive pressure; *PVR,* pulmonary vascular resistance.

3. Clinical presentation
   a. Subjective
      1) Chest pain, especially on exertion
      2) Syncope, especially on exertion
      3) Symptoms of LVF: dyspnea; orthopnea; PND
      4) Fatigue, weakness
      5) Palpitations
   b. Objective
      1) Narrow pulse pressure
      2) PMI displaced laterally and/or downward
      3) Signs of LVF: S_3; crackles
      4) Heart sound changes
         a) May have split S_1
         b) Paradoxical split of S_2
         c) Systolic ejection murmur: harsh, crescendo/decrescendo, loudest at aortic area radiating to the neck
         d) May have aortic ejection click
   c. Diagnostic
      1) Chest x-ray
         a) Calcification of aortic valve may be seen
         b) Cardiomegaly
         c) Left atrial enlargement
         d) Left ventricular hypertrophy
         e) Pulmonary congestion
         f) Right ventricular hypertrophy
      2) Electrocardiography
         a) Left atrial enlargement (P-mitrale)
         b) Left ventricular hypertrophy
         c) Dysrhythmias: most frequently atrial fibrillation
         d) Blocks: AV blocks; left bundle branch block
      3) Echocardiography
         a) Aortic valve leaflet thickening and decreased movement of the leaflets
         b) Calcification of aortic valve
         c) High-pressure gradient between left ventricle and aorta
         d) Left ventricular hypertrophy
         e) Possibly right ventricular hypertrophy
      4) Cardiac catheterization
         a) Significant pressure gradient
         b) Elevated LAP, LVEDP

Collaborative Management

1. Decrease myocardial oxygen consumption
   a. Oxygen by nasal cannula at 2-6 L/min to maintain SaO_2 of 95% unless contraindicated
   b. Sodium restrictions
   c. Physical comfort: temperature, lighting, noise control
   d. Anxiolytics as prescribed: usually diazepam (Valium); lorazepam (Ativan); or alprazolam (Xanax)
2. Provide care for HF
   a. ACE inhibitors (e.g., captopril)
   b. Beta-blockers (e.g., metoprolol) may be prescribed.
   c. Vasodilators (e.g., nitrates) but should be avoided in severe AS
   d. Diuretics (e.g., furosemide) but should be used with caution in severe AS
   e. Inotropic agents: Digitalis may be used especially if supraventricular tachydysrhythmias are present.
3. Monitor for complications.
   a. Dysrhythmias: usually atrial fibrillation
   b. Blocks: Permanent pacemaker may be necessary.
   c. Emboli (mural thrombi): potential for pulmonary, cerebral, renal, splenic, mesenteric embolus; antiembolic measures including anticoagulation
   d. Endocarditis: prophylactic antibiotics prior to any invasive procedures, dental procedures for prevention
4. Prepare patient for surgical repair or replacement of the affected valve as requested.
   a. Valvuloplasty: percutaneous coronary intervention to repair a valve utilizing a balloon-tipped intracardiac catheter; considered palliative since restenosis rate is high
   b. Commissurotomy: surgical separation of the thickened adherent leaves of a stenosed valve (usually mitral)
   c. Valve repair
      1) Open commissurotomy: Fused commissures are incised to reestablish mobility.
      2) Valve leaflet reconstruction: Fibrous pericardium is frequently used for patches.
      3) Annuloplasty: insertion of a ring to correct the dilation of the valve annulus
      4) Repair of elongated chordae tendineae by suturing within or to the side of a papillary muscle
   d. Valve replacement: replacement of the native valve with a mechanical or biological prosthetic valve
      1) Types of valve replacement
         a) Bioprosthetic valves: last approximately 5-10 years
            i) Types
               (a) Homografts: human cadaver valves that have been specially treated for surgical use
               (b) Heterograft: valve from an animal, usually a pig or cow, which has been prepared for surgical use
            ii) Anticoagulation
               (a) Short-term (~3 months after valve replacement) anticoagulation (INR 2-3) is recommended
               (b) Long-term anticoagulation is recommended if atrial fibrillation or left atrial thrombus

b) Mechanical valves: last approximately 10-15 years
   i) Stainless steel, carbon, or other durable material
   ii) Anticoagulation: long-term anticoagulation is recommended (INR is 2-3.5 depending on type of valve)
c) Pulmonary autograft (also referred to as *Ross procedure*)
   i) The patient's own pulmonic valve is used to replace the diseased aortic valve with a homograft or heterograft implanted into the pulmonic position.
2) Postoperative management as for CABG with close monitoring for AV nodal blocks

Hypertensive Crises

Definitions

1. Hypertension: elevation in blood pressure above 140/90 mm Hg on at least three separate occasions
2. Hypertensive crisis: rapid rise in BP and occurs when BP elevation is severe enough to cause the threat of immediate vascular necrosis and end-organ damage; BP usually greater than 180/120 mm Hg or MAP greater than 150 mm Hg
   a. Hypertensive urgencies: an acute or chronic BP elevation not associated with any observable acute organ damage
      1) Do not usually require critical care unit admission
      2) Usually safely treated with oral antihypertensive agents to reduce BP to baseline over 24-48 hours
   b. Hypertensive emergencies: an acute elevation of BP that is associated with acute and ongoing organ damage to the kidneys, brain, heart, eyes, or vascular system
      1) No absolute BP level but BP is usually greater than 240/140 mm Hg
      2) BP must be lowered within minutes to a few hours to reduce potential complications of new or progressive end-organ damage
      3) Requires immediate hospitalization in a critical care unit and intravenous antihypertensive agents

Etiology

1. Primary
   a. Untreated or inadequately treated essential (idiopathic) hypertension
      1) Risk factors: family history; black race; obesity; hyperlipidemia; diabetes or glucose intolerance; tobacco use; excessive alcohol intake; high-fat and/or high-sodium diet; stress; sedentary lifestyle; aging; oral contraceptives
      2) Poor compliance frequently a factor in hypertensive crisis; factors closely related to poor compliance include lack of symptoms (i.e., the silent killer), side effects of pharmacologic agents, costs of pharmacologic agents
2. Secondary
   a. Cerebrovascular conditions (e.g., thrombotic or hemorrhagic stroke)
   b. CNS injuries
      1) Head injury
      2) Spinal cord injury: autonomic dysreflexia is hypertension with bradycardia that occurs in patients with spinal cord injury T6 or above in response to noxious stimuli
   c. Aortic dissection or coarctation
   d. Renal disease
      1) Increased renin-angiotensin levels
         a) Renin-secreting tumor
         b) Renovascular disease
      2) Acute glomerulonephritis
      3) Chronic pyelonephritis
      4) Postrenal transplant
   e. Pregnancy: preeclampsia, eclampsia, HELLP (hemolysis, elevated liver enzyme levels, and low platelet count) syndrome
   f. Burns
   g. Drug side effects: oral contraceptives; steroids; cocaine; amphetamines; methamphetamine, decongestants
   h. Drug interactions: MAO inhibitors and tyramine; disulfiram (Antabuse) and alcohol
   i. Drug withdrawal: clonidine, beta-blockers, ACE inhibitors, alcohol
   j. Endocrine disorders (e.g., pheochromocytoma, Cushing's syndrome, primary hyperaldosteronism)
   k. Vasculitis
   l. Scleroderma or other connective tissue disease
   m. Peri/postoperative hypertension, especially cardiac or vascular surgery

Pathophysiology

See Figure 3-29.

Clinical Presentation

1. General
   a. Significant elevation in BP above normal (see Table 3-24)
   b. Epistaxis may occur.
2. Cardiovascular involvement may be present.
   a. Chest pain
   b. Signs of left ventricular hypertrophy: PMI displaced to left, S_4, ECG indicators of left ventricular hypertrophy (i.e., deep S in V_1, V_2 and tall R in V_5, V_6)
   c. Signs of left ventricular failure/pulmonary edema: dyspnea; orthopnea; left ventricular heave; S_3; crackles
3. Renal involvement may be present.
   a. Nocturia
   b. Pressure-related diuresis

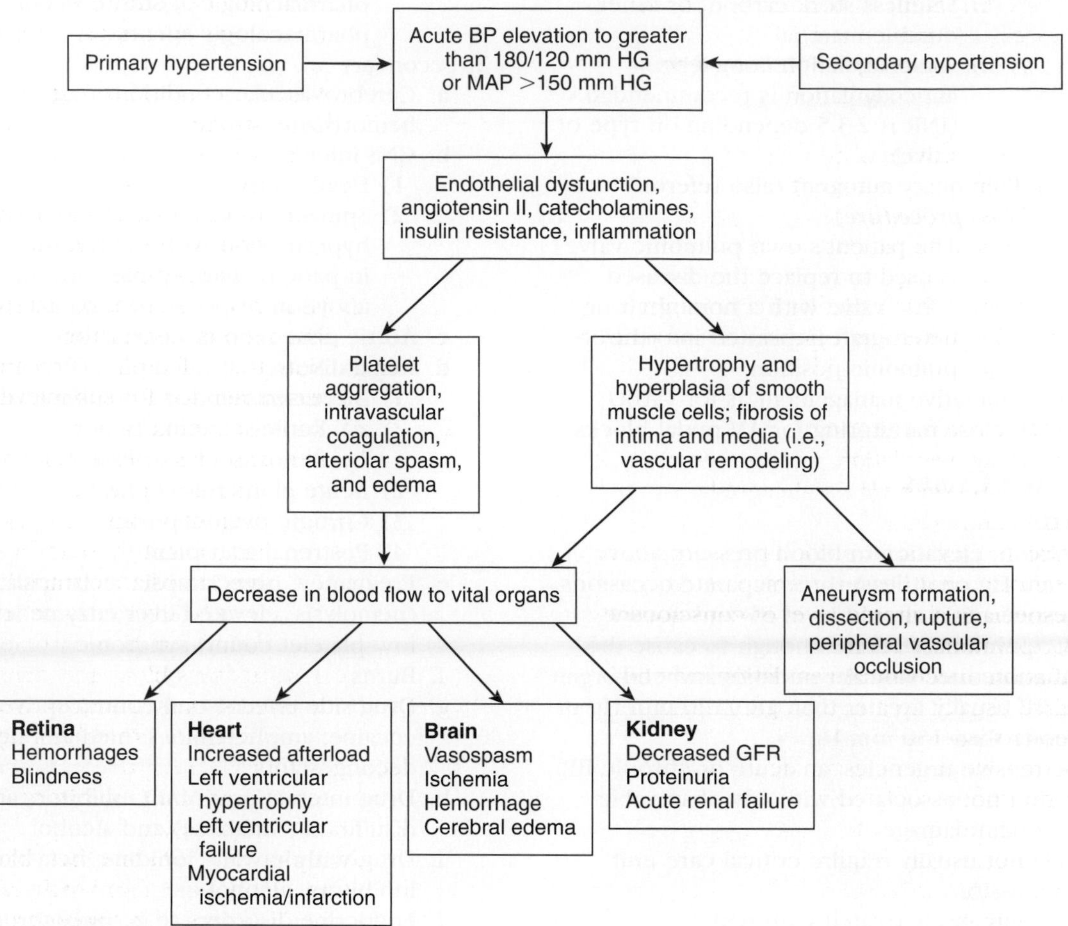

Figure 3-29 Pathophysiology of hypertensive crisis. *BP,* blood pressure; *GFR,* glomerular filtration rate; *MAP,* mean arterial pressure.

Table 3-24 Classification of BP Levels According to JNC7

BP Category	Systolic (mm Hg)	and/or	Diastolic (mm Hg)
Optimal	Less than 120	and	Less than 80
Normal	Less than 130	and	Less than 85
Hypertensive			
Stage 1	140 to 159	or	90 to 99
Stage 2	160 or greater	or	100 or greater

Adapted from Bakris, G. (2003). *The implications of JNC 7 for antihypertensive treatment protocols.* Retrieved May 9, 2010, from www.medscape.com/viewprogram/2513_pnt.

c. Hematuria

d. Elevated BUN and creatinine

4. Retinal involvement may be present.
   a. Visual disturbances (e.g., blurred vision, reduced visual acuity, photophobia, temporary loss of vision)
   b. Funduscopic changes (Keith-Wagener-Barker classification)
      1) Grade I: arteriolar narrowing
      2) Grade II: focal arteriolar spasm
      3) Grade III: hemorrhages and exudates
      4) Grade IV: papilledema
5. Neurologic involvement may be present especially in hypertensive encephalopathy.
   a. Occipital or anterior headache especially in the morning; may be severe
   b. Nausea, vomiting
   c. Seizures
   d. Altered mental status: irritability, confusion, agitation progressing to lethargy and coma
   e. Focal neurologic signs (e.g., cranial nerve palsy, sensory or motor deficits, aphasia; positive Babinski's reflex)
6. Diagnostic
   a. Serum
      1) Potassium: Hypokalemia occurs in primary hyperaldosteronism.
      2) BUN and creatinine may be elevated.
      3) Lipid profile to evaluate additional cardiac risk
      4) Aldosterone may be elevated.

b. Captopril challenge test: Plasma renin level is measured before and one hour after 25 mg of captopril (Capoten) to confirm or rule out renovascular hypertension.
c. Urine: hematuria or proteinuria may be present
d. Chest x-ray
    1) Cardiomegaly may be present.
    2) Pulmonary edema may be present.
    3) Widening of mediastinum suggests dissecting thoracic aortic aneurysm.
e. Electrocardiography: may show left atrial enlargement, left ventricular hypertrophy
f. CT of brain: may show cerebral edema and/or hemorrhage

Collaborative Management

1. Maintain airway, ventilation, and oxygenation.
    a. Oxygen: 2-6 L/min via nasal cannula
    b. Airway maintenance
        1) Oropharyngeal or nasopharyngeal airway or endotracheal intubation may be required especially if altered level of consciousness or pulmonary edema
    c. Ventilation: mechanical ventilation may be required especially if neurologic impairment or pulmonary edema
2. Decrease myocardial oxygen consumption.
    a. Activity restriction initially
    b. Sodium restriction to less than 2 g/24 hr
    c. Smoking cessation
    d. Physical comfort: temperature control; lighting; noise control
    e. Anxiolytics as prescribed: usually diazepam (Valium); lorazepam (Ativan); or alprazolam (Xanax)
3. Decrease blood pressure gradually.
    a. Reduction of MAP by no more than 20-25% within the first hour because blood pressure decreased too aggressively may cause neurologic damage by significantly decreasing cerebral perfusion pressure. (NOTE: If aortic dissection has occurred, BP is reduced more aggressively but reduction takes place within 5-10 minutes.)
        1) Monitor BP closely.
            a) An invasive arterial catheter is indicated in hypertensive emergency.
            b) If neurologic changes occur, BP reduction should be slowed or temporarily stopped.
    b. Antihypertensive agents (Table 3-25)
        1) Vasodilators
            a) Nitroprusside (Nipride)
                i) Mixed arterial and venous vasodilator but predominantly arterial
                ii) Usually first-line agent for hypertensive emergency
            b) Hydralazine (Apresoline): selectively arterial vasodilator
            c) Fenoldopam mesylate (Corlopam): selectively arterial vasodilator with dopaminergic stimulation
            d) Clevidipine (Cleviprex): selectively arterial vasodilator
            e) Nitroglycerin (NTG): Effects are dose-dependent.
                i) Venous vasodilator at doses of less than 1 mcg/kg/min
                ii) Mixed arterial and venous vasodilator when dose greater than 1 mcg/kg/min
            f) Nicardipine (Cardene): mixed arterial and venous vasodilator
            g) Note that nifedipine (Procardia) is not recommended for sublingual use.
        2) Sympathetic blockers
            a) Alpha-blockers block vasoconstriction
                i) Phentolamine (Regitine): especially helpful if hypertension due to autonomic dysreflexia since bradycardia contraindicates beta-blocker; also particularly helpful in pheochromocytoma
            b) Beta-blockers block the reflex tachycardia associated with vasodilators.
                i) Esmolol (Brevibloc): rapid acting, cardioselective beta-blocker
                ii) Contraindicated in heart failure, heart block
            c) Alpha- and beta-blockers: block both vasoconstriction and tachycardia
                i) Labetalol (Normodyne): alpha- and noncardioselective beta-blocker
                    (a) Particularly helpful in patients with intracranial hypertension because direct vasodilators would increase intracranial volume and pressure
        3) ACE inhibitor
            a) Enalaprilat (Vasotec) (only IV ACE inhibitor)
        4) Diuretics: usually loop diuretics (e.g., furosemide [Lasix], bumetanide [Bumex])
            a) Use of diuretics is controversial because these patients may have had significant diuresis related to excessive glomerular filtration rate
    c. Condition-specific management (Feldstein, 2007)
        1) Hypertensive encephalopathy: labetalol, nicardipine, nitroprusside
        2) Heart failure: nitroglycerin or nitroprusside
        3) Myocardial ischemia: nitroglycerin
        4) Aortic dissection: labetalol or nitroprusside and esmolol
        5) Adrenergic crisis: phentolamine or nitroprusside and esmolol
        6) Preeclampsia/eclampsia: hydralazine
        7) Perioperative/postoperative: clevidipine or nicardipine or esmolol or nitroprusside or nitroglycerin or fenoldopam

Text continued on page 215

Table 3-25 Selected Drugs Used for Hypertensive Emergency

Drug	Classification/ Actions	Indications	Administration	Adverse Effects	Nursing Implications
Vasodilators					
Clevidipine (Cleviprex)	**Calcium Channel Blocker** • Relaxes arteriolar smooth muscle decreasing SVR, afterload, and BP	• Hypertension	• IV infusion:1-2 mg/hr; may be doubled every 90 seconds until BP approaches target; then increased by less than double every 5-10 minutes • Maximum: 21 mg/hr for 24 hours	• Nausea and vomiting • Headache • Insomnia • Tachycardia • Rebound hypertension • Exacerbation of heart failure	• Monitor HR, BP, blood lipids • Metabolized by blood ester hydrolysis to form inactive metabolites; advantage in renal or hepatic insufficiency • Note contraindications: allergy to soybeans, soy products, eggs, or egg products, defective lipid metabolism, pancreatitis, hyperlipidemia, severe aortic stenosis • Use caution in patients with heart failure • Consider lipid calories in daily nutritional plan • Infusion must be changed every 12 hours • Use cautiously in the elderly
Enalaprilat (IV), enalapril (PO) (Vasotec)	**ACE (Angiotensin Converting Enzyme) Inhibitor** • Inhibits conversion of angiotensin I to angiotensin II • Prevents vasoconstriction and aldosterone secretion to decrease preload and afterload	• HF • Hypertension	• PO: 5-40 mg daily • IV injection: 1.25 mg over 5 minutes every 6 hours	• Tachycardia • Hypotension especially after first dose • Anorexia • Fatigue • Headache • Loss of taste • Diarrhea • Rash, angioedema • Dizziness • Photosensitivity • Proteinuria, nephrotic syndrome, renal failure • Pancytopenia • Hyperkalemia • Bronchospasm • Cough	• Monitor HR, BP, urine output, protein in urine, serum potassium, WBC • Monitor WBC and differential before treatment and periodically during treatment • Note contraindications: known hypersensitivity, AV block, hypotension • Use cautiously in renal disease, lupus, scleroderma, hypovolemia, leukemia, diabetes mellitus, thyroid disease, COPD, asthma, hyperkalemia and in patients on drugs that may affect WBC counts or immune response • Monitor for allergic reaction: rash, fever, pruritus, urticaria; antihistamines may be used; discontinuance may be necessary • Administer thiazide diuretics as prescribed; frequently given together • Angiotensin II blocker (e.g., losartan [Cozaar], valsartan [Diovan]) may be prescribed if cough develops • Indicated for hypertension with HF

Fenoldopam mesylate (Corlopam)	**Vasodilator Antihypertensive** • Relaxes vascular smooth muscle decreasing preload (PAOP) and afterload (SVR) • Stimulates dopaminergic receptors causing diuresis	• Severe hypertension (short-term treatment) • Need to improve renal flow such as after potentially nephrotoxic dyes and contrast media	• IV infusion: mix 10 mg in 250 mL (40 mcg/mL); usual dose is 0.1-0.3 mcg/kg/min; may be increased in increments 0.05-0.1 mcg/kg/min every 15 minutes until target BP is reached • Maximum: 1.7 mcg/kg/min	• Tachycardia, hypotension • Ventricular dysrhythmias • Dizziness • Anxiety • Headache • Flushing • Nausea, vomiting, abdominal pain • Hypokalemia • Increased intraocular pressure • Increased intracranial pressure	• Monitor HR, BP, urine output, serum potassium, neurologic status • Note contraindications: known hypersensitivity to fenoldopam or sulfite, intracranial hypertension • Use caution in patients with glaucoma or ocular hypertension and in patients on other drugs which may cause hypotension (e.g., beta-blockers) • Indicated especially for postoperative hypertension or hypertension with renal insufficiency
Hydralazine (Apresoline)	**Vasodilator Antihypertensive** • Relaxes arteriolar smooth muscle decreasing SVR, afterload, and BP	• Hypertension • Afterload reduction	• PO: 10-50 mg every 6-8 hours • IV injection: 5-20 mg over 3-5 minutes every 4-6 hours • Maximum: 400 mg/day	• Tachycardia • Orthostatic hypotension • Anorexia, nausea, vomiting, diarrhea • Sodium retention • Weight gain • Palpitations • Flushing • Headache • Tremors • Dizziness • Lupus-like syndrome • Exacerbation of HF or chest pain • Leukopenia, agranulocytosis	• Monitor HR, BP, ECG • Note contraindications: known hypersensitivity to hydralazine, coronary artery disease, mitral valve disease, severe aortic stenosis • Use cautiously in renal disease, cerebrovascular disease • Administer beta-blockers as prescribed for reflex tachycardia because it may cause myocardial ischemia • Indicated for pregnancy-related hypertension (i.e., eclampsia)
Nicardipine (Cardene)	**Calcium Channel Blocker** • Relaxes vascular smooth muscle decreasing preload and afterload	• Hypertension • Angina pectoris	• PO: 20 mg tid initially; may be increased to 20-40 mg tid after 3 days if tolerated well • IV infusion: mix 25 mg in 240 mL (0.1 mg/mL) and infuse at 5 mg/hr (50 mL/hr); may be increased by 2.5 mg/hr (25 mL/hr) every 5 minutes until desired BP reduction is achieved • Do not mix in lactated Ringer's solution • Maximum: 15 mg/hour	• Tachycardia • Hypotension • Nausea, vomiting, heartburn • Flushing • Headache • Chest pain • Heart failure • Hepatitis • Renal failure • Local irritation at injection site	• Monitor HR, BP • Note contraindications: known hypersensitivity, sick sinus syndrome, second- or third-degree AV block, systolic BP less than 90 mm Hg, severe aortic stenosis • Use caution in HF, hypotension, liver disease, renal insufficiency or failure, and in the elderly • Indicated for postoperative hypertension

Continued

Table 3-25 Selected Drugs Used for Hypertensive Emergency—cont'd

Drug	Classification/ Actions	Indications	Administration	Adverse Effects	Nursing Implications
Nitroglycerin (Tridil)	**Nitrates** • Relaxes smooth muscle to reduce preload (PAOP) (and afterload [SVR] if greater than 1 mcg/kg/min) • Dilates coronary collateral circulation • Relieves coronary artery spasm	• Acute angina • Prophylactic use before activities that may cause angina • Heart failure (preload reduction)	• Sublingual: 0.3-0.4 mg at 5 minute intervals to a maximum of three tablets or metered-dose sprays • PO (isosorbide): 5-40 mg every 6 hours • Transdermal: 1-4 inches every 8 hours • IV infusion: mix 50 mg in 250 mL (200 mcg/mL); initial dose 5-10 mcg/min, increase by 5-10 mcg/min every 5 minutes until desired results are achieved (e.g., control of chest pain, preload reduction) • Maximum: 400 mcg/min • Administer in glass bottle and via non-PVC tubing	• Tachycardia or bradycardia • Hypotension or hypertension • Palpitations • Weakness • Apprehension • Flushing • Dizziness • Syncope • Headache • Methemoglobinemia with resultant reduction in SaO_2, SpO_2, and tissue oxygen delivery	• Monitor HR, BP, urine output • Monitor RAP, PA, PAOP, SVR, CI if nitroglycerin is being administered IV and pulmonary artery catheter has been inserted • Note contraindications: known hypersensitivity, anemia, intracranial hypertension, cerebral hemorrhage, hypertrophic cardiomyopathy, right ventricular infarction, sildenafil (Viagra) or vardenafil (Levitra) within the last 24 hours • Use cautiously in hypotension; IV nitroglycerin is titratable and preferred in acute situations • Decrease nitrate tolerance by scheduling oral nitrates with nitrate-free period at night and by removing transdermal nitrates at night • Administer ASA or acetaminophen for headache; usually dose-related • Teach patient to protect tablets from light and moisture and replace every 3 months • Teach patient to limit NTG to three tablets every 5 minutes and if no relief is obtained, to go to the ED • Teach patient to apply nitroglycerin paste to any relatively hairless area between the knees and shoulders and to rotate sites to prevent maceration • Note that patients receiving IV NTG and heparin IV concurrently require more heparin to achieve therapeutic aPTT; monitor aPTT closely with NTG dosage changes or discontinuance • Indicated especially for hypertension with chest pain

Nitroprusside (Nipride)	**Vasodilator Antihypertensive**
	• Relaxes vascular smooth muscle decreasing preload (PAOP) and afterload (SVR)
		• Hypertensive crisis
		• HF (preload and afterload reduction)
		• Cardiogenic shock
		• BP control during and after vascular surgery
			• IV infusion: mix 50 mg in 250 mL (200 mcg/mL) and infuse at 0.25-10 mcg/kg/min
			• Maximum: 10 mcg/kg/min for 10 minutes only
			• Protect from light by wrapping aluminum foil around bag or bottle; it is not necessary to wrap foil around tubing but avoid exposure of tubing to direct sunlight
				• Nausea, vomiting, abdominal pain
				• Headache
				• Tinnitus
				• Dizziness
				• Diaphoresis
				• Apprehension
				• Hypotension
				• Tachycardia
				• Palpitations
				• Coronary artery steal causing myocardial ischemia and chest pain
				• Intrapulmonary shunt causing hypoxemia (referred to as nitroprusside-induced intrapulmonary shunt)
				• Methemoglobinemia with resultant reduction in SaO_2, SpO_2, and tissue oxygen delivery
				• Thiocyanate toxicity
					• Monitor HR, BP, urine output, neurologic status
					• Note contraindications: known hypersensitivity
					• Use cautiously in liver disease, renal disease, anemia, hypovolemia, hypothyroidism, older adult, CAD, neurologic injury
					• Discard solution after 24 hours
					• Wrap foil around bottle to protect from light
					• Discard solution if dark brown, blue, green, or red
					• Monitor for thiocyanate toxicity
					  • Thiocyanate levels should be determined daily if drugs are used longer than 72 hours
					  • Signs of thiocyanate toxicity: metabolic acidosis, confusion, hyperreflexia, seizures
					  • Treatment includes amyl nitrate, sodium nitrate, and/or sodium thiosulfate
					  • Simultaneous infusion of thiosulfate with nitroprusside may prevent thiocyanate toxicity

Continued

Table 3-25 Selected Drugs Used for Hypertensive Emergency—cont'd

Drug	Classification/ Actions	Indications	Administration	Adverse Effects	Nursing Implications
Adrenergic Blocking Agents					
Esmolol (Brevibloc): see Table 3-4					
Labetalol hydrochloride (Normodyne, Trandate)	**Alpha and Beta Adrenergic Blocker** • Blocks response to alpha and beta stimulation • Causes decrease in blood pressure without reflex tachycardia • Causes decrease in HR	• Hypertension • Hypertensive crisis	• PO: 100-400 mg every 12 hours. • IV injection: 20 mg over 2 minutes, may repeat 40 mg every 10 minutes • IV infusion: mix 300 mg in 250 mL for a total volume of 300 mg in 300 mL (1 mg/mL); usual dose is 1-2 mg/min until satisfactory response is achieved • Maximum: 300 mg	• Bradycardia • Orthostatic hypotension • Ventricular dysrhythmias • AV blocks • HF • Nausea, vomiting, diarrhea • Dizziness • Lethargy • Hypoglycemia without symptoms in type 1 DM • Hyperglycemia in type 2 DM • Agranulocytosis, thrombocytopenia • Bronchospasm in patients with COPD, asthma	• Monitor HR, BP, ECG, breath sounds, daily weight • Note contraindications: known hypersensitivity, shock, second- or third-degree AV block, sinus bradycardia, sick sinus syndrome, NYHA class IV HF, asthma • Note contraindications: known hypersensitivity, shock, second- or third-degree AV block, sinus bradycardia, HF, asthma • Use cautiously in diabetes mellitus, renal disease, hepatic disease, thyroid disease, COPD, CAD, bronchospasm, peripheral vascular disease • Keep patient supine for 3 hours after IV administration (labetalol) • Do not discontinue suddenly • Indicated for hypertension postoperatively or aortic dissection
Phentolamine (Regitine)	**Alpha Adrenergic Blocker** • Blocks response to alpha stimulation • Causes decrease in blood pressure without reflex tachycardia	• Hypertension especially autonomic dysreflexia, pheochromocytoma, monoamine oxidase inhibitor-tyramine interaction • Infiltration of vasopressor agents	• IV injection: 5-15 mg; may be repeated every 5-15 minutes • Maximum: 15 mg	• Tachycardia • Flushing • Headache	• Monitor HR, BP • Use cautiously in CAD • Beta-blocker may be given concurrently to control tachycardia

4. Assist in preparation of patient for surgical procedures to treat cause of hypertension if appropriate
   a. Angioplasty may be done for renovascular disease.
   b. Adrenalectomy is done for pheochromocytoma after tachycardia and hypertension have been adequately controlled.
5. Monitor for complications.
   a. Cerebral infarction
   b. Myocardial infarction
   c. Heart failure/pulmonary edema
   d. Dissection of aorta
   e. Renal failure
6. Provide instruction and counseling regarding lifestyle modification and need for pharmacologic therapy.
   a. Nonpharmacologic management
      1) Weight normalization
      2) Dietary modifications
         a) Low-fat, no-added-salt (2-3 g/day) diet
         b) Fresh fruits and vegetables
         c) Fish, especially fatty fish such as salmon, trout
         d) Nuts
         e) Low-fat dairy
         f) Monounsaturated fatty acids (from extra-virgin olive oil)
         g) Increase potassium, magnesium, and calcium
      3) Aerobic exercise
      4) Alcohol moderation (e.g., one glass of wine or equivalent/day)
      5) Complementary therapies: relaxation, biofeedback, acupuncture, pets
   b. Pharmacologic management
      1) Indications for pharmacologic management
         a) Mild hypertension with end-organ damage or DM
         b) Moderate hypertension that has not responded to conservative treatment
         c) Severe hypertension
      2) Choice of drug and/or combinations (Dumont & Hardware, 2009)
         a) Diuretics and beta-blockers are usually first line.
         b) If HF: thiazide diuretics and ACE inhibitor or ARB and/or beta-blocker (e.g., carvedilol [Coreg]) and/or (e.g., spironolactone [Aldactone], eplerenone [Inspra])
         c) If post-MI: beta-blocker and ACE inhibitor or ARB and/or aldosterone antagonist (e.g., spironolactone [Aldactone], eplerenone [Inspra])
         d) If DM: ACE inhibitor or ARB and/or diuretic and/or beta-blocker and/or calcium channel blocker
         e) If elderly with isolated systolic hypertension: diuretic or calcium channel blocker
         f) If hypertensive and hypercholesteremic: statin (e.g., pravastatin)
         g) If renal insufficiency: ACE inhibitor or ARB

Vascular Disease

Peripheral Arterial Disease

1. Definition: partial or total occlusion of an artery by atherosclerosis/arteriosclerosis obliterans
2. Etiology
   a. Arteriosclerosis/atherosclerosis (same risk factors as referred in discussion of coronary artery disease)
      1) Atherosclerosis: most common cause
      2) Arteriosclerosis: significant cause in older patients
   b. Hypertension
   c. Arteritis
3. Pathophysiology (Figure 3-30)
4. Clinical presentation
   a. Occlusive disease of terminal aorta and iliac
      1) Subjective
         a) Intermittent claudication in thigh and hip: pain increases with exercise and decreases with rest
         b) Impotence
      2) Objective
         a) Cool lower extremities
         b) Hair loss over lower extremities
         c) Decreased or absent iliac or femoral pulses
         d) Bruit or thrill over iliac area
   b. Occlusive disease of femoral and popliteal arteries
      1) Subjective
         a) Intermittent claudication in lower leg progressing to pain at rest
         b) Decreased sensation or paresthesia of lower extremities
      2) Objective
         a) Coolness of lower extremities
         b) Hair loss over lower extremities
         c) Pallor and mottling of lower extremities
         d) Nonhealing ulcers on toes or points of trauma
         e) Decreased motor strength in lower extremities
         f) Decreased or absent femoral and popliteal pulses
         g) Bruit or thrill over femoral or popliteal area
      3) Diagnostic
         a) Arteriography: shows partial or complete arterial occlusion
         b) Doppler and duplex ultrasonography show partial to complete vascular occlusion.
5. Collaborative management
   a. Decrease peripheral oxygen requirements
      1) Activity cessation when pain occurs

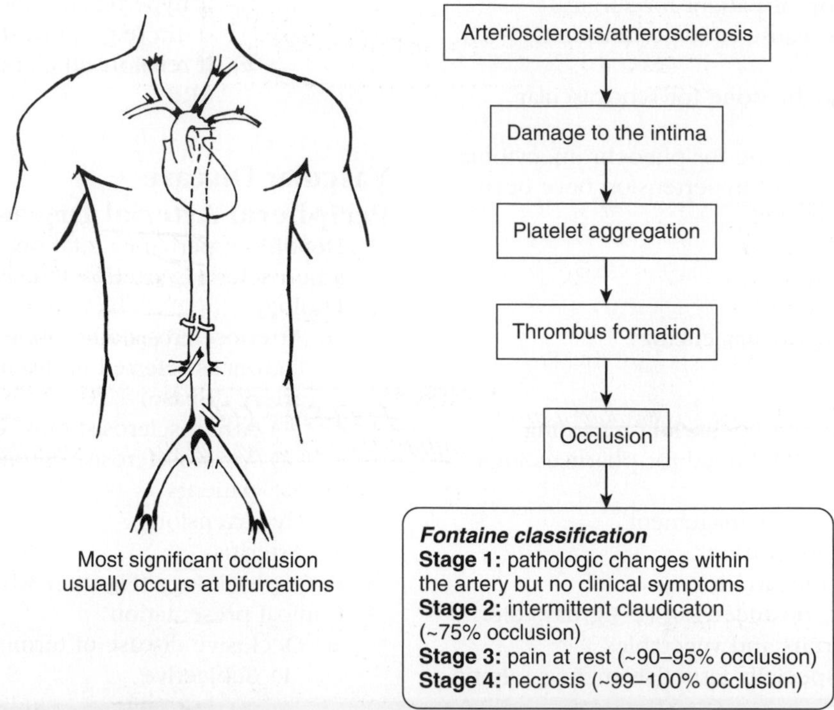

Figure 3-30 Pathophysiology of peripheral arterial disease.

2) Bed rest during acute occlusion
3) Maintenance of normothermia
4) Prevention of trauma

b. Administer appropriate pharmacologic agents to reestablish blood flow: fibrinolytics (e.g., urokinase; streptokinase; rt-PA)
   1) These agents may be administered locally by an intraarterial infusion or systemically intravenously.
   2) Followed by an anticoagulant such as heparin

c. Assist in preparation of the patient for percutaneous procedures aimed at decreasing occlusion (e.g., percutaneous balloon angioplasty, laser angioplasty, atherectomy); may be accompanied by insertion of flexible coil stent
   1) Postprocedure care as for PCI
   2) Catheter insertion site should be monitored closely for bleeding and/or hematoma formation
   3) Peripheral perfusion should be monitored closely; any indications of arterial occlusion (i.e., 6 Ps) should be reported immediately.
   4) Anticoagulants and/or platelet aggregation inhibitors as prescribed

d. Assist in preparation of the patient for surgery aimed at improving flow (Figure 3-31) and provide postoperative management.
   1) Surgical procedures
      a) Arterial embolectomy: removal of an occlusive clot from an artery; frequently accomplished with a balloon-tipped catheter
      b) Thromboendarterectomy: excision of thickened layer of artery; aortofemoral, aortoiliac, or femoral-popliteal thromboendarterectomy
      c) Bypass: Graft is anastomosed proximal and distal to the occlusion.
         i) Graft may be autologous vein (usually saphenous), human umbilical vein, or an artificial graft (Dacron or polytetrafluoroethylene [PTFE]).
         ii) Commonly performed bypasses include: aortobifemoral, femoral to femoral, femoral-popliteal, and femoral-tibial.
      d) Extraanatomical bypass (EAB): Prosthetic material is tunneled subcutaneously.
         i) May be used femoral to femoral or axillary to femoral
         ii) Used for patients who are high-risk for an open abdominal procedure or who have numerous previous surgical procedures or peritonitis (sometimes referred to as a *hostile abdomen*)
      e) Sympathectomy: interruption of sympathetic tract to decrease local vascular resistance to improve local blood flow
      f) Amputation: removal of limb performed only when attempts to revascularize the limb have failed
   2) Postoperative management

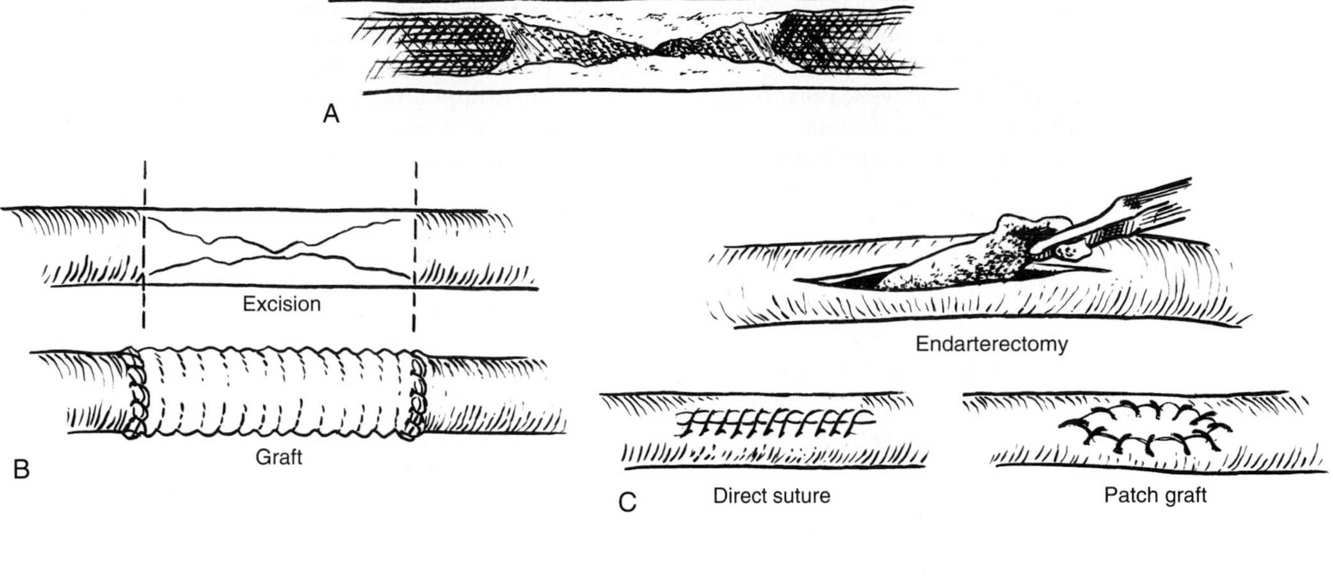

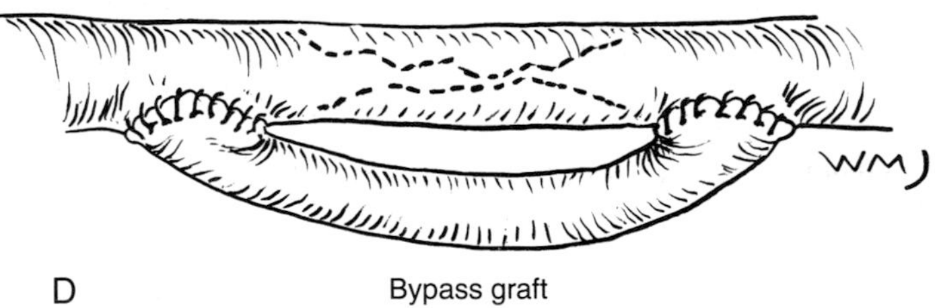

Figure 3-31 Surgical procedures for peripheral vascular disease. **A,** Occluded vessel. **B,** Excision and circumferential graft. **C,** Endarterectomy with direct suture or patch graft. **D,** Bypass graft. (Drawing by Wendy M. Johnson.)

a) Maintain airway, oxygenation, and ventilation
   i) Assess ventilatory status frequently: rate; rhythm; excursion; effort; use of accessory muscles; presence of stridor or other adventitious sounds; pulse oximetry.
   ii) Encourage deep breathing and incentive spirometry.
   iii) Assess frequently for edema, hematoma, tracheal deviation, and dysphagia.
   iv) Elevate HOB 30 degrees.
   v) Have equipment for artificial airway and suctioning.
   vi) Prevent aspiration: high-Fowler's position while eating; NPO until gag reflex returns; suction as necessary.
   vii) Administer oxygen at 2-5 L/min as prescribed.
b) Maintain adequate flow and pressure at graft site.
   i) Maintain and control systolic BP less than 120 mm Hg.
      (a) Nitroprusside (NTP)
      (b) Nicardipine (Cardene)
      (c) Analgesics as indicated
   ii) Prevent emboli by using antiembolic techniques.
      (a) Dextran 40 often used as platelet aggregation inhibitor.
      (b) Heparin may also be used.
   iii) Avoid pressure on incision sites.
      (a) Elevate HOB no greater than 30 degrees for first 72 hours.
      (b) Elevate legs 20-30 degrees.
      (c) Encourage foot and leg exercises.
      (d) Mobilize from lying to standing; avoid sitting position, flexing or crossing of legs after femoral artery revascularization.
   iv) EAB specifically
      (a) Position on nonoperative side.
      (b) Prevent external pressure on graft and avoid flexion of graft.
      (c) Feel for thrill over graft.
      (d) Assess for vascular steal: clinical indications of hypoperfusion of limb from which blood was diverted.
      (e) Monitor for brachial plexus injury if axillofemoral bypass
c) Assess for clinical indications of hypoperfusion.

i) Perform neurovascular assessment of extremities hourly; monitor for pain, pallor, pulselessness, paresthesia, paralysis, polar (cold).
ii) Measure Doppler pressures and calculate ankle-brachial index (ABI).
(a) Report any decrease in ABI of 0.15 or more.
(b) Do not measure Doppler pressure if the bypass is performed to the most distal arteries of the leg (painful for the patient and may cause graft compression).
iii) Maintain normal body temperature: heated blankets or automatic warming blanket, warming lights.

d) Treat pain.
i) Administer analgesics as indicated.
ii) Position for comfort.

e) Prevent skin breakdown related to ischemia and immobility.
i) Inspect skin, bony prominences, and affected extremities frequently.
ii) Reposition often.
iii) Utilize alternating air mattress or special bed, depending on other risk factors
iv) Keep heels elevated off bed.

f) Maintain adequate hydration.
i) Administer intravenous fluids as indicated.
ii) Monitor urine output closely, and report urine output of less than 0.5 mL/kg/hr.

g) Monitor for postoperative complications.
i) Hemorrhage
ii) Infection
(a) Assess incision and wounds for indications of infection.
(b) Monitor WBC and body temperature.
(c) Provide aseptic wound care.
(d) Administer antibiotics as prescribed.
iii) Arterial thrombosis
iv) Cerebral embolus (blood or plaque)
v) Peripheral ischemia, infarction, loss of limb
vi) Graft infection
(a) Monitor for fever, malaise, back pain, anorexia, paralytic ileus, and leukocytosis.
(b) Administer antibiotics as prescribed.
(c) Prepare patient for removal and replacement of graft as requested.

e. Provide instruction and counseling regarding lifestyle modification and need for pharmacologic therapy.
1) Nonpharmacologic therapies
a) Weight normalization
b) Dietary modifications
i) Low saturated fat
ii) ADA diet for control of blood glucose for patient with DM
c) Cessation of tobacco use
d) Regular aerobic exercise in moderation; should not exercise to the point of pain
e) Foot care: special attention to any lesions since healing may be impaired by decreased circulation
f) Avoidance of constrictive clothing
g) Complementary therapies: relaxation; imagery, biofeedback
2) Pharmacologic agents
a) Platelet aggregation inhibitors (e.g., ASA, clopidogrel [Plavix])
b) Agents that increase the flexibility of the red blood cells: pentoxifylline (Trental)
c) Peripheral vasodilators
i) Papaverine: rarely used today
ii) Cilostazol (Pletal): phosphodiesterase III inhibitor; inhibits platelet aggregation and causes vasodilation
d) Anticoagulants: warfarin (Coumadin)
e) Antihypertensives if indicated

Acute Arterial Occlusion

1. Definition: acute complete occlusion of an artery by thrombosis in an already narrowed artery, embolism, or trauma
2. Etiology
a. Arterial embolization
1) Atrial fibrillation
2) Ventricular aneurysm
3) Bacterial endocarditis
b. Injury to arterial intima causing arterial thrombosis
1) Postcardiac catheterization or angioplasty
2) IABP
3) Postarterial bypass or aneurysm
c. Compression of artery with swelling
1) Fracture (compartment syndrome)
2) Circumferential burn
3. Pathophysiology (Figure 3-32)
4. Clinical presentation
a. 6 Ps
1) Pain: severe and sudden
2) Pallor, cyanosis
3) Pulselessness
4) Paresis or paralysis
5) Paresthesia or anesthesia
6) Polar
b. Doppler stethoscope indicates diminished or absent blood flow.

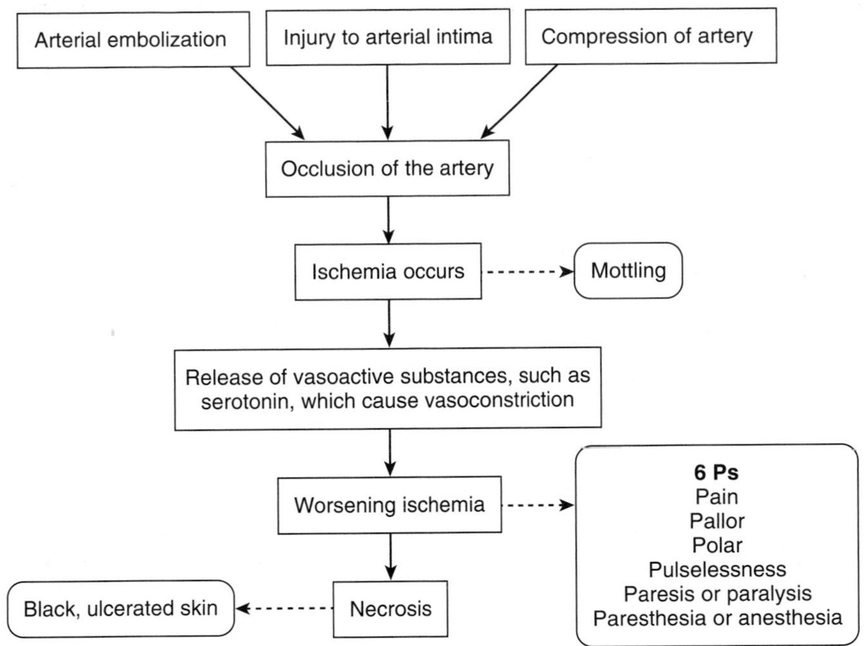

Figure 3-32 Pathophysiology of acute arterial occlusion. Dotted lines connect pathology to the clinical presentation.

c. Diagnostic study: Angiography indicates arterial occlusion.

5. Collaborative management
   a. Initiate emergency measures immediately.
      1) Oxygen at 2-5 L/min to maintain SaO_2 at 95% unless contraindicated
      2) Proper positioning of limb: keep extremity straight, warm, and dependent
      3) Notification of physician immediately of perfusion defect
      4) IV infusion of NS at KVO rate in unaffected limb
      5) Narcotics (e.g., morphine) for pain
   b. Assist in preparation of diagnostic studies: angiogram
   c. Reestablish patency of artery.
      1) Intraarterial fibrinolytic (e.g., urokinase, rt-PA) followed by anticoagulant (see Table 3-14)
      2) Preparation for surgical procedures if indicated
         a) Procedures
            i) Surgical embolectomy especially for large arteries
            ii) Balloon embolectomy
            iii) Thromboendarterectomy
            iv) Bypass grafting
      3) Postoperative care as described in Peripheral Arterial Disease section
   d. Explain procedures thoroughly to minimize stress.
   e. Monitor closely for complications.
      1) Reocclusion
      2) Loss of limb
      3) Infection
   f. Provide patient teaching as for peripheral arterial disease.

Aortic Aneurysm

1. Definition: a permanent localized dilation of the aorta with an increase of at least 1.5 times its normal diameter
2. Etiology
   a. Degenerative changes caused by aging and familial predisposition
   b. Congenital weakness of the aorta
   c. Hypertension
   d. Pregnancy: especially third trimester
   e. Coarctation of the aorta
   f. Syphilis
   g. Severe systemic infection (e.g., bacterial aneurysm, mycotic aneurysm)
   h. Marfan's syndrome
   i. Trauma: especially blunt trauma with acceleration-deceleration injury
   j. Arterial cannulation (e.g., PCI, IABP)
3. Pathophysiology (Figure 3-33)
   a. Types
      1) False: does not involve all layers of the artery; pulsating hematoma that results from arterial trauma such as arterial cannulation

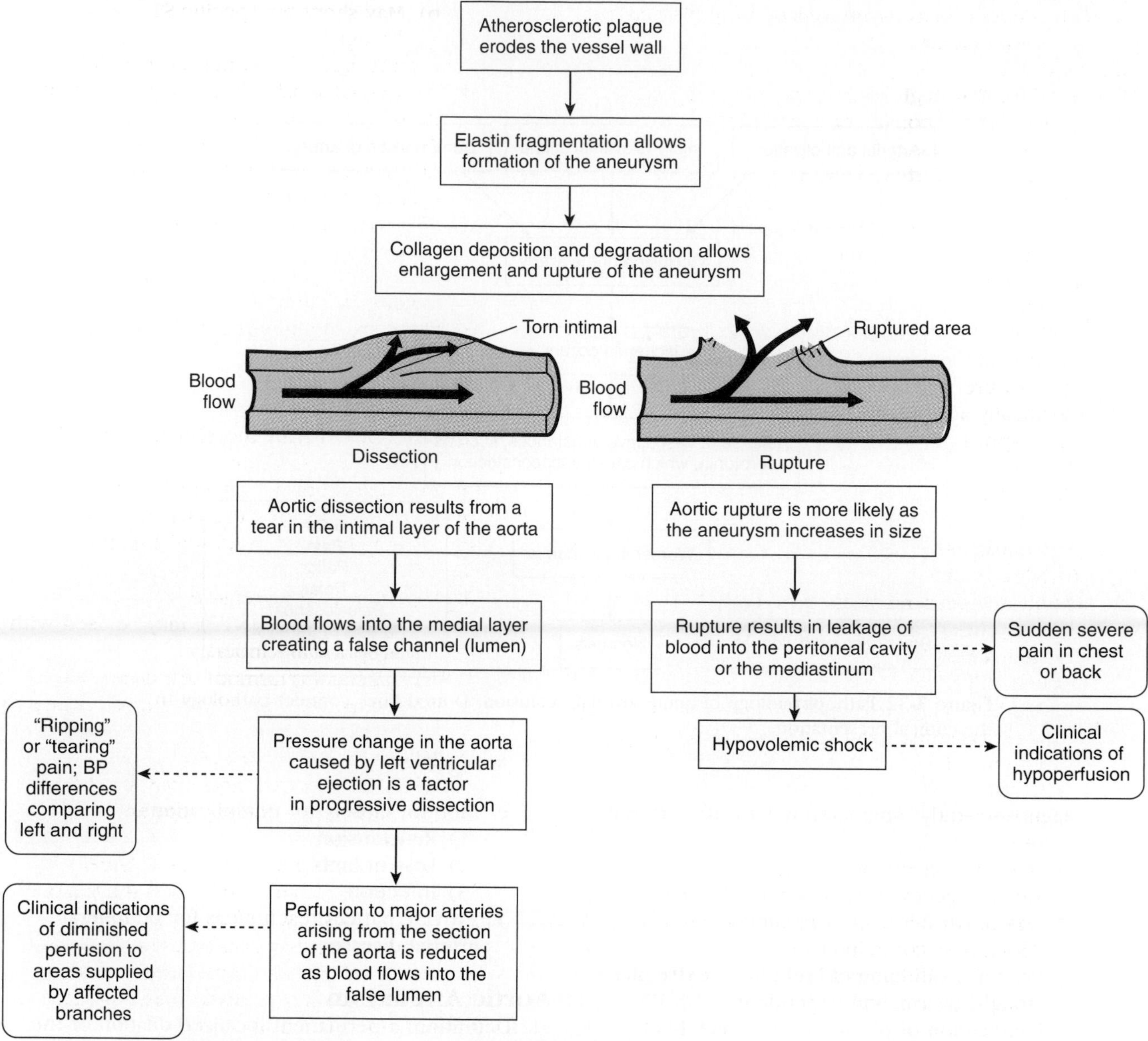

Figure 3-33 Pathophysiology of aneurysm dissection. Dotted lines connect pathology to the clinical presentation. (Drawings from Urden, L.D., et al. [2005]. *Thelan's critical care nursing: Diagnosis and management* [5th ed.]. St. Louis: Mosby.)

2) True: involves all layers of the arterial wall; usually saccular arising from a distinct portion of the wall
3) Saccular: outpouching from an artery that results from localized thinning and stretching of the media
4) Fusiform: involves the total circumference of the artery with diffuse dilatation
5) Dissecting: a cavity is formed by dissection by blood between the layers of the arterial wall
   a) Classifications
      i) DeBakey system
         (a) I: Original intimal tear begins in the ascending aorta with the dissection extending to the descending aorta.
         (b) II: Original intimal tear begins in the ascending aorta but does not extend to the descending aorta.
         (c) III: Original intimal tear begins in the descending aorta with the dissection confined in the descending aorta.
      ii) Stanford systems
         (a) A: Involves the ascending aorta
         (b) B: Involves the descending aorta
6) Rupture: Artery wall ruptures and leaks arterial blood into the mediastinum if thoracic or into abdominal cavity if abdominal.

4. Clinical presentation

a. Subjective: usually asymptomatic until dissection or rupture occur
b. Objective
   1) Normal to high BP; hypotension suggests cardiac tamponade or aortic rupture
   2) Pulsatile mass
   3) Increased aortic diameter on palpation
   4) Bruit over aorta
c. Specifically ascending thoracic aorta
   1) May be asymptomatic
   2) Dyspnea
   3) Chest pain
   4) Clinical indications of aortic regurgitation: diastolic murmur, LVF, widened pulse pressure
d. Specifically aortic arch
   1) Dyspnea
   2) Stridor
   3) Cough
   4) JVD
   5) Hoarseness
   6) Weak voice
e. Specifically descending thoracic arch
   1) Dull chest pain and upper back pain
   2) Hoarseness
f. Dissecting TAA
   1) Sudden, sharp, tearing or ripping pain in chest radiating to shoulders, neck, or back
   2) Hypotension
   3) Dyspnea
   4) Syncope
   5) Leg weakness, transient paralysis
   6) May have BP and pulse difference between arms or between arms and legs
   7) May have clinical indications of thrombotic stroke
   8) May have clinical indications of cardiac tamponade (see Cardiac Tamponade section)
g. Specifically abdominal aorta
   1) Dull abdominal and back pain
   2) Nausea and vomiting
   3) Abdominal bloating
   4) Pulsation in abdomen
h. Specifically ruptured AAA
   1) Severe, sudden, dull, continuous abdominal pain radiating to low back, hips, scrotum; unaffected by movement
   2) Feeling of abdominal fullness
   3) Nausea and vomiting
   4) Syncope and shock
   5) Pulsation in abdomen: periumbilical area
i. Diagnostic
   1) Serum: hemoglobin and hematocrit may be decreased
   2) Chest x-ray
      a) Mediastinal widening in thoracic aneurysm
      b) Aortic calcification
   3) Electrocardiography
      a) May show left ventricular hypertrophy
      b) May show nonspecific ST-T wave changes
      c) Absence of ECG indicators of MI
   4) Transesophageal echocardiography: may show aortic root dilation, intimal flap dividing true and false lumen in dissection
   5) Aortography: lumen of aneurysm; size and location of aneurysm
   6) CT scan and MRI: presence and location of aneurysm
   7) Ultrasound: presence, size, shape, and location of aneurysm
   8) Flat plate of abdomen (KUB): outline of aneurysm

5. Collaborative management
   a. Control pain
      1) Narcotics, usually morphine, are required in rupture or dissection.
      2) Extreme caution if patient is hypotensive
   b. Maintain and control mean arterial pressure at approximately 60-75 mm Hg if dissection occurs.
      1) If patient is hypertensive
         a) Nitroprusside (NTP); may be used with propranolol (Inderal)
         b) Labetalol (Normodyne); decreases contractility and the pulsatile pressure on the aorta
      2) If patient is hypotensive
         a) IV access: two large-bore, short IV catheters; blood for type and crossmatch
         b) Normal saline or lactated Ringer's by rapid infusion until blood is available; colloids (e.g., albumin, hetastarch, dextran) may also be used
         c) Blood and blood products
   c. Decrease tissue oxygenation requirements.
      1) Activity restriction
      2) Oxygen by nasal cannula at 2-6 L/min to maintain SaO_2 of 95% unless contraindicated
      3) Intubation and mechanical ventilation may be necessary.
      4) Physical comfort: temperature control, lighting, noise control
      5) Anxiolytics as prescribed: usually diazepam (Valium); lorazepam (Ativan); or alprazolam (Xanax)
   d. Assist in preparation of patient for surgical repair.
      1) Indication for surgical repair: aneurysmal dilation of 5-6 cm in diameter; indications for immediate surgical repair include:
         a) Involvement of ascending aorta; aortic insufficiency
         b) Failure of drug therapy to control progression of dissection as evidenced by continued pain and progressive symptoms
         c) Cardiac tamponade
         d) Compromise of a major branch of aorta

e) Indications of cerebral or cardiac ischemia

2) Procedures

a) Surgical procedure: resection of aneurysm and circumferential (fusiform aneurysm) or patch graft (saccular aneurysm)

i) Repair of thoracic aortic aneurysm involving the ascending aorta and/or aortic arch requires cardiopulmonary bypass; concurrent aortic valve repair or replacement may be needed for ascending thoracic aneurysms.

ii) Descending thoracic aortic aneurysms are usually repaired by thoracotomy and do not require cardiopulmonary bypass.

iii) Abdominal aortic aneurysm repairs are done through abdominal incisions; a bowel preparation is performed unless surgery is emergent.

b) Endovascular grafts (EVG) for aneurysm repair

i) Modular device that expands to fit and seal the aorta, lines the inside of the aneurysm like a sleeve providing a new path for blood flow and reducing the pressure on the aneurysm; uses either a stent or hooks to secure the sleeve

ii) Implanted through a delivery catheter inserted through the femoral artery and positioned with the use of fluoroscopy

iii) Advantages over traditional surgical aneurysm repair

(a) May be used in patients at high risk for traditional aneurysm repair; originally only used for AAA but now also used for descending thoracic aneurysms as well as Type B dissections

(b) Intubation not required; may not require critical care unit stay

(c) Fewer complications

(i) Less blood loss than open repair

(ii) Less hypothermia than with laparotomy

(d) Shorter hospital stay

(e) Lower early mortality; long-term mortality is comparable between the two options

iv) Disadvantages compared with traditional surgical repair

(a) Not all patients are candidates because the location of the aneurysm and the size of the patient's arteries above and below the aneurysm may preclude the implant

(b) May be more costly in the short-term and in the long-term because lifelong surveillance is required

3) Postoperative management

a) Maintain airway, oxygenation, and ventilation

i) Assess ventilatory status frequently: rate; rhythm; excursion; effort; use of accessory muscles; presence of stridor or other adventitious sounds; pulse oximetry

ii) Encourage deep breathing and incentive spirometry.

iii) Assess frequently for edema, hematoma, tracheal deviation, and dysphagia.

iv) Elevate HOB 30 degrees.

v) Have equipment for artificial airway and suctioning.

vi) Prevent aspiration: high-Fowler's position while eating; NPO until gag reflex returns; suction as necessary.

vii) Administer oxygen at 2-5 L/min as prescribed.

b) Maintain adequate flow and pressure at graft site.

i) Maintain and control systolic BP less than 120 mm Hg.

(a) Nitroprusside (NTP)

(b) Nicardipine (Cardene)

(c) Analgesics as indicated

ii) Prevent emboli by using antiembolic techniques.

(a) Dextran 40 often used as platelet aggregation inhibitor

(b) Heparin may also be used.

iii) Avoid pressure on incision sites.

(a) Elevate HOB no greater than 30 degrees for first 72 hours.

(b) Elevate legs 20-30 degrees.

(c) Encourage foot and leg exercises.

(d) Mobilize from lying to standing; avoid sitting position, flexing or crossing of legs after femoral artery revascularization.

c) Assess for clinical indications of hypoperfusion.

i) Perform neurovascular assessment of extremities hourly; monitor for pain, pallor, pulselessness, paresthesia, paralysis, polar (cold).

ii) Maintain normal body temperature: heated blankets or automatic warming blanket, warming lights

d) Treat pain.
   i) Administer analgesics as indicated.
   ii) Position for comfort.

e) Prevent skin breakdown related to ischemia and immobility.
   i) Inspect skin, bony prominences, and affected extremities frequently.
   ii) Reposition often.
   iii) Utilize egg crate, alternating air mattress, or special bed, depending on other risk factors.
   iv) Keep heels elevated off bed.

f) Maintain adequate hydration.
   i) Administer intravenous fluids as indicated.
   ii) Monitor urine output closely and report urine output of less than 0.5 mL/kg/hour.

g) Monitor for postoperative complications.
   i) Acute respiratory failure; monitor for all of the following:
      (a) Dyspnea
      (b) Hypoxemia
      (c) Tachypnea
      (d) Tachycardia
      (e) Fever
   ii) Hemorrhage, hypovolemia, and hematoma; monitor for all of the following:
      (a) Hypotension
      (b) Tachycardia
      (c) Clinical manifestations of hypoperfusion
      (d) Decreased RAP, PAP, PAOP
   iii) Myocardial ischemia and infarction; monitor for all of the following:
      (a) Chest pain
      (b) Dyspnea
      (c) Decreased cardiac output
      (d) Dysrhythmias
      (e) ECG: ST segment changes
   iv) Cerebral ischemia and infarction; monitor for all of the following:
      (a) Change in LOC
      (b) Pupillary change
      (c) Aphasia
      (d) Motor or sensory changes
   v) Pulmonary ischemia and infarction; monitor for all of the following:
      (a) Dyspnea
      (b) Chest pain
      (c) Pleural friction rub
      (d) Hypoxemia
   vi) Renal ischemia and infarction; monitor for all of the following:
      (a) Flank pain
      (b) Decreased urine output
      (c) Changes in BUN or creatinine
      (d) Hematuria
   vii) Mesenteric ischemia and infarction; monitor for all of the following:
      (a) Watery, bloody diarrhea
      (b) Abdominal pain
      (c) Change in bowel sounds
   viii) Splenic ischemia and infarction; monitor for all of the following:
      (a) LUQ pain radiating to left shoulder
      (b) Abdominal rigidity
   ix) Spinal cord ischemia and infarction
      (a) Monitor for all of the following:
         (i) Paralysis of lower extremities
         (ii) Bowel/bladder paralysis
      (b) Drainage of cerebral spinal fluid (CSF) naloxone, osmotic diuretics, steroids, and/or calcium channel blockers may be prescribed to prevent/treat spinal cord hyperemia/edema.
   x) Arterial thrombosis
      (a) Sudden, painful ischemia of feet (sometimes referred to as *trash foot*) and/or lower leg
      (b) Diminished or absent peripheral pulses; decreased ABI
   xi) Complications specific to endovascular aneurysm repair
      (a) Endoleak: persistence of blood flow outside the lumen of the endoluminal graft but within the aneurysmal sac
         (i) May be managed by observation, further endovascular procedures, or open repair
         (ii) Risk for continued aneurysm expansion and risk of rupture
      (b) Postimplant syndrome
         (i) Back pain and fever without a leukocytosis or other signs of infection
         (ii) May last up to 7 days
         (iii) Cause unknown
      (c) Graft limb thrombosis
         (i) Thrombectomy or embolectomy may be required.

e. Provide instruction and counseling regarding lifestyle modification and need for pharmacologic therapy as for peripheral arterial disease.

Carotid Arterial Stenosis

May be referred to as *Extracranial Cerebrovascular Disease*.

1. Etiology
   a. Atherosclerosis/arteriosclerosis: risk factors as for coronary artery disease and peripheral vascular disease
   b. Trauma
   c. Fibromuscular dysplasia
   d. Cervical irradiation
   e. Arteritis
2. Pathophysiology
   a. Atherosclerotic plaque accumulates at the bifurcation of the internal and external carotid arteries.
   b. Fragments of this plaque or associated thrombi may break away from the plaque causing cerebral emboli.
   c. Eventually, ischemia or infarction of the brain may occur.
      1) Ischemia
         a) Transient ischemic attack (TIA): focal neurologic deficit lasting less than 24 hours
      2) Infarction: a completed ischemic stroke
         a) Permanent neurologic deficit though some improvement may occur over time
         b) Carotid artery stenosis is the cause of 15-25% of strokes.
3. Clinical presentation
   a. Subjective: usually asymptomatic unless TIA, RIND, or completed stroke is experienced; symptoms may include:
      1) Visual changes: diplopia; ipsilateral monocular blindness (referred to as *amaurosis fugax*)
      2) Memory loss
      3) Vertigo
      4) Syncope
   b. Objective
      1) Bruit or thrill over one or both carotid arteries
      2) Signs of transient ischemic attacks (TIAs) or stroke may include:
         a) Slurred speech/aphasia
         b) Ataxia
         c) Paresis or paralysis
         d) Temporary loss of consciousness
   c. Diagnostic
      1) Duplex ultrasonography of the carotid arteries: initial diagnostic test for patients with known or suspected carotid stenosis
      2) Magnetic resonance angiography or computed tomography angiography: if sonography cannot be obtained or yields nondiagnostic results
      3) Cerebral arteriography
4. Collaborative management
   a. Administer pharmacologic agents as prescribed.
      1) Platelet aggregation inhibitors (e.g., ASA, clopidogrel [Plavix] OR ASA plus dipyridamole [Aggrenox]); ASA and clopidogrel together is not recommended
      2) Agents that increase the flexibility of the red blood cells: pentoxifylline (Trental)
      3) Anticoagulants: warfarin (Coumadin) for patients with atrial fibrillation or mechanical prosthetic cardiac valve to INR of 2.5
      4) Antihypertensives if indicated
   b. Prepare patient for percutaneous or surgical procedure as requested.
      1) Indications
         a) Occlusion of 70% or greater of the internal carotid artery or mild stroke within the previous 6 months
         b) No contraindications for surgery
      2) Procedures
         a) Carotid endarterectomy: removal of an atheroma at the carotid artery bifurcation
         b) Carotid artery stenting especially for patients who are high surgical risk
            i) Balloon dilation of the stenotic area and placement of a crush-resistant stent
            ii) Especially useful in patients with recurrent carotid stenosis, lesions distal in the internal carotid artery or high in the neck, or patients with history of cervical irradiation
      3) Postoperative management
         a) Maintain airway, oxygenation, and ventilation
            i) Assess ventilatory status frequently: rate, rhythm, excursion, effort, use of accessory muscles, presence of stridor or other adventitious sounds, pulse oximetry.
            ii) Encourage deep breathing and incentive spirometry.
            iii) Assess frequently for edema, hematoma, tracheal deviation, and dysphagia.
            iv) Elevate HOB 30 degrees.
            v) Have equipment for cricothyroidotomy, tracheostomy, and suction.
            vi) Prevent aspiration: high-Fowler's position while eating; NPO until gag reflex returns; suction as necessary.
            vii) Administer oxygen at 2-5 L/min as prescribed.
         b) Monitor for/prevent alteration in cerebral perfusion related to cerebral embolism, ischemia, and infarction especially after procedures.

i) Assess BP and HR frequently: BP is usually maintained within 20 mm Hg ± preoperative values.
ii) Report immediately clinical indications of cerebral hypoperfusion: change in level of consciousness, pupil changes, paresis or plegia, visual changes, dysphasia or aphasia, seizures, or headache.
iii) Check neurologic and cranial nerve function. (NOTE: There is no risk of injury to the cranial nerves with carotid artery stenting.)
   (a) LOC
   (b) Pupils
   (c) Motor function
   (d) Sensory function
   (e) Cranial nerves
      (i) CN VII: Ask patient to smile.
      (ii) CN IX, X: Check swallowing, speech, and gag.
      (iii) CN XI: Ask patient to shrug against your hands.
      (iv) CN XII: Ask patient to stick tongue out; check for midline position.
      (v) Recurrent laryngeal nerve: Check speech.
      (vi) Great auricular nerve: Note perception of sensation on face and ear.
iv) Administer antiplatelet aggregation drugs (e.g., ASA, clopidogrel [Plavix], dextran 40) as prescribed; ASA AND clopidogrel are recommended before and for at least 30 days after carotid artery stenting.

c) Monitor for hemorrhage or hematoma.
   i) Assess BP and HR frequently.
   ii) Assess neck dressing for hematoma or hemorrhage; check back of neck and assess drainage from drain if present.
   iii) Check for tracheal deviation.
   iv) Monitor hemoglobin and hematocrit.
   v) Administer antihypertensives (e.g., nitroprusside [Nipride], labetalol [Normodyne]) as prescribed to maintain BP: systolic 100-160 mm Hg, diastolic less than 100 mm Hg.

d) Monitor for complications.
   i) Myocardial infarction
   ii) Cerebral hemorrhage/embolism/infarction
   iii) Carotid hemorrhage
   iv) Hematoma
   v) Cranial nerve injury
   vi) Seizures

c. Provide instruction and counseling regarding lifestyle modification and need for pharmacologic therapy as for peripheral arterial disease.

Cardiovascular Trauma

Blunt Cardiac Injury (i.e., Myocardial Contusion)

1. Definition: transient or permanent myocardial dysfunction caused by blunt trauma to the heart and may include myocardial necrosis without coronary artery disease
2. Etiology
   a. Usually acceleration/deceleration injury sustained in motor vehicle collision; sternum may hit steering wheel or dashboard; injury may also be caused by shoulder strap of seat belt
   b. Other vehicular accidents: motorcycle collisions, auto-pedestrian collisions
   c. Kicking of chest by large animal
   d. Assault with blunt instrument
   e. Industrial crush injury
   f. Explosion
   g. Vigorous CPR
   h. Projectile objects (e.g., baseball, hockey puck)
3. Pathophysiology (Figure 3-34)
4. Clinical presentation
   a. Subjective
      1) History of events and mechanism of injury
      2) Precordial angina-like chest pain
         a) Frequently increases with inspiration, cough, and movement
         b) Unresponsive to nitroglycerin but frequently responsive to oxygen, antiinflammatory agents, or narcotics
      3) Dyspnea
      4) Palpitations
   b. Objective
      1) Tachycardia; persistent despite adequate fluid replacement
      2) Tachypnea
      3) Hypotension may occur.
      4) Ecchymosis may be present on anterior chest.
      5) Chest wall tenderness with palpation.
      6) Clinical indications of RVF: JVD, peripheral edema, hepatomegaly
      7) Clinical indications of left ventricular noncompliance: S_4
      8) Clinical indications of hypoperfusion (see Table 2-2 on page 26)
      9) Cardiac arrest as a result of fatal ventricular dysrhythmias may occur.

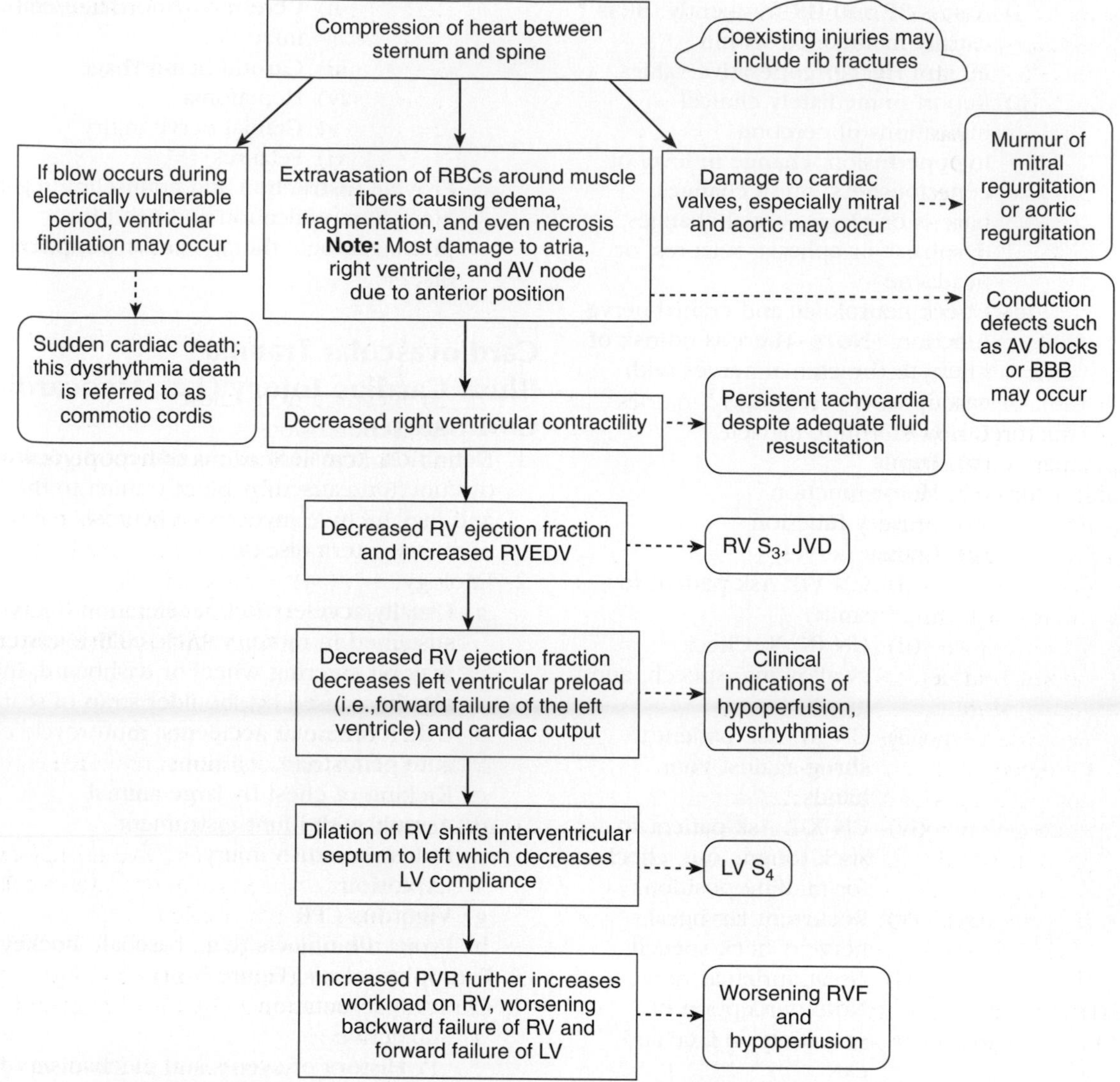

Figure 3-34 Pathophysiology of blunt cardiac injury. Dotted lines connect pathology to the clinical presentation. *BBB,* bundle branch block; *JVD,* jugular venous distention; *LV,* left ventricular; *PVR,* pulmonary vascular resistance; *RV,* right ventricular; *RVEDV,* right ventricular end-diastolic volume; *RVF,* right ventricular failure.

c. Diagnostic
   1) Serum: CK-MB and cardiac troponin may be positive depending on the severity of the injury.
   2) Electrocardiography with right ventricular leads
      a) ST segment changes, T wave inversion in V_1-V_4; Q waves may be seen if injury is severe or if a coronary artery is lacerated or thrombosed
      b) QT interval may be prolonged.
      c) Dysrhythmias
         i) Atrial dysrhythmias: PACs, atrial fibrillation, atrial flutter
         ii) Ventricular dysrhythmias: PVCs, ventricular tachycardia, ventricular fibrillation
         iii) Blocks: AV blocks, RBBB
   3) Echocardiography
      a) Decreased regional wall motion (especially right ventricular)
      b) Increased end-diastolic wall thickness
      c) Decreased RV ejection fraction
      d) May show complications (e.g., apical thrombi, pericardial effusion, cardiac tamponade)
   4) Radionuclide studies may be done: decreased RV ejection fraction.

5. Collaborative management
   a. Treat pain.
      1) Morphine sulfate usually used.
      2) Antiinflammatory agents may also be helpful.
   b. Ensure adequate right ventricular contractility, left ventricular filling, and cardiac output.
      1) Isotonic fluids as prescribed to ensure adequate left ventricular filling; avoid venous vasodilators and diuretics

2) Inotropes (e.g., dobutamine) as prescribed to improve right ventricular contractility
c. Decrease myocardial oxygen demand.
1) Bed rest
2) Oxygen by nasal cannula at 2-6 L/min to maintain SaO_2 of 95% unless contraindicated
3) Anxiolytics as prescribed and indicated
d. Treat dysrhythmias
1) Atrial: digitalis, cardioversion
2) Ventricular: usually amiodarone
3) Blocks: temporary pacemaker; permanent pacemaker may be necessary
e. Assist in assessment for other thoracic injuries (e.g., fractured ribs, sternum, clavicle, pulmonary contusion).
f. Monitor for complications.
1) Ventricular rupture
2) Cardiac tamponade
3) Coronary artery thrombosis
4) Intracardiac thrombus
5) Valve rupture
6) Conduction defects
7) Heart failure
8) Ventricular aneurysm
9) Cardiogenic shock: Monitor for clinical manifestations of hypoperfusion.
10) Systemic emboli
a) Sequential compression devices may be used on the legs.
b) Anticoagulation avoided unless there are intramural thrombi

Penetrating Cardiac Injury

1. Definition: puncture of the heart with a sharp object or rib
2. Etiology
a. Violence (e.g., knife wound, gunshot wound, ice pick)
b. Industrial accident (e.g., scaffolding)
c. Motorcycle collision (e.g., handlebar impalement)
d. Sports injury
e. Explosion
f. Crush injury
3. Pathophysiology (Figure 3-35)
4. Clinical presentation
a. Subjective
1) History of events and mechanism of injury
2) Chest pain
b. Objective
1) Visible wound; object causing penetration may be seen
2) Bleeding from chest
3) Hypotension
4) Clinical indications of hypoperfusion (see Table 2-2 on page 26)
5) Clinical indications of cardiac tamponade (see Cardiac Tamponade section)
c. Hemodynamic parameters
1) Decrease in RAP, PAP, PAOP if hemorrhage; increase in RAP, PAP, PAOP if cardiac tamponade
2) Decrease in CO, CI
3) Decrease in SvO_2
d. Diagnostic: hemoglobin and hematocrit decreased
5. Collaborative management
a. Manage cardiopulmonary arrest if indicated: manage airway, oxygenation, and circulation using BLS, ACLS if needed.
b. Control hemorrhage.
1) Do not remove an impaled object; objects may be stabilized with IV bags and dressings.
2) Apply pressure to site if the object has been removed and there is a bleeding wound.
3) Apply pressure around site if the object has not already been removed and there is bleeding around the wound.

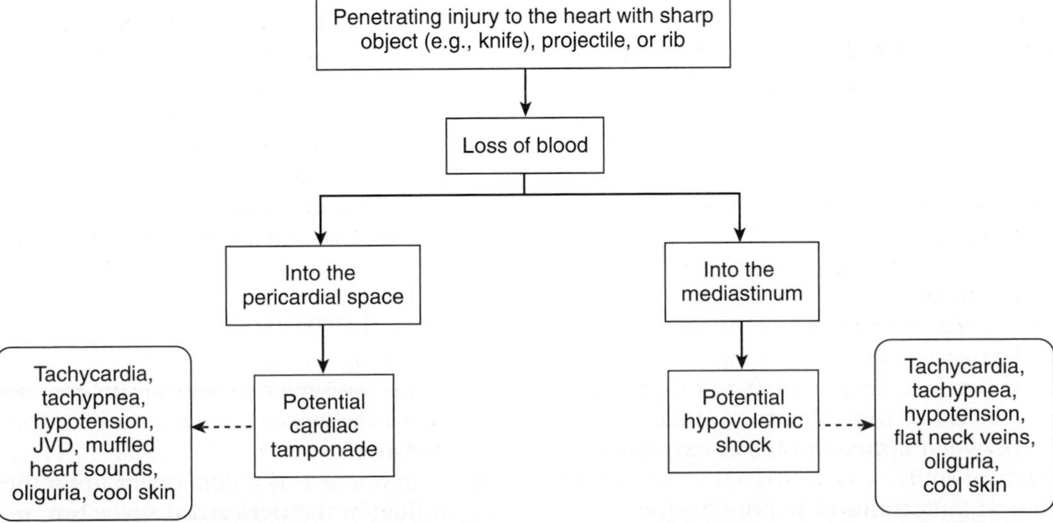

Figure 3-35 Pathophysiology of penetrating cardiac injury. Dotted lines connect pathology to the clinical presentation. *JVD,* jugular venous distention.

4) Assist in insertion of chest tube for hemothorax or pneumothorax.
5) Assist with pericardiocentesis for cardiac tamponade.

c. Improve oxygen delivery.
1) Oxygen by nasal cannula at 2-6 L/min to maintain SaO_2 of 95% unless contraindicated
2) Intubation and mechanical ventilation may be necessary.
3) IV access: 2 large-bore, short IV catheters; blood for type and crossmatch
4) Normal saline or lactated Ringer's by rapid infusion until blood is available; colloids (e.g., albumin, hetastarch, or dextran may also be used)
5) Blood and blood products

d. Assist in preparation of the patient for exploratory thoracotomy.

e. Control pain and discomfort.
1) Nonsteroidal antiinflammatory agents
2) Narcotic analgesics in doses adequate to allow patient to deep breathe and cough as indicated
3) Anxiolytics

f. Monitor for complications.
1) Hemorrhagic shock
2) Cardiac tamponade
3) Hemothorax
4) Pneumothorax

Great Vessel Injury

1. Definition: injury or tear to great vessel or vessels, usually the aorta but possibly the pulmonary artery
2. Etiology
   a. Acceleration-deceleration injury (e.g., motor vehicle collision)
   b. Compression injury
   c. Penetrating trauma
3. Pathophysiology: Disruption of major vessel integrity causes loss of effective circulating blood volume leading to shock.
4. Clinical presentation
   a. Subjective
      1) History of events and mechanism of injury
      2) Chest pain frequently radiating to back or back pain
      3) Dyspnea
      4) Dysphagia or hoarseness
      5) Sensory or motor changes in lower extremities
   b. Objective
      1) Tachycardia
      2) Blood pressure changes
         a) Hypertension or hypotension
         b) Difference between left and right arms
         c) Difference (greater than normal) between upper and lower extremities
      3) Tracheal shift
      4) Clinical indications of hypoperfusion
      5) Harsh systolic murmur may be audible along the precordium
   c. Hemodynamic parameters
      1) Decrease in RAP, PAP, PAOP
      2) Decrease in CO, CI
      3) Decrease in SvO_2
   d. Diagnostic
      1) Serum: hemoglobin and hematocrit decreased
      2) ECG: may show dysrhythmias or ST-T wave changes indicative of ischemia
      3) Chest x-ray
         a) Mediastinal widening
         b) Loss of aortic knob shadow
      4) Transesophageal echocardiography or spiral CT
      5) Aortogram: will show extravasation of dye
5. Collaborative management
   a. Manage cardiopulmonary arrest if needed: manage airway, oxygenation, and circulation using BLS, ACLS if needed.
   b. Improve oxygen delivery.
      1) Oxygen by nasal cannula at 2-6 L/min to maintain SaO_2 of 95% unless contraindicated
      2) Intubation and mechanical ventilation may be necessary.
      3) IV access: 2 large-bore, short IV catheters; blood for type and crossmatch
      4) Normal saline or lactated Ringer's by rapid infusion until blood is available; colloids (e.g., albumin, hetastarch, or dextran may also be used)
      5) Blood and blood products
   c. Control bleeding: Antihypertensive may be needed to keep MAP less than 90 mm Hg.
   d. Assist in preparation of the patient for exploratory thoracotomy as soon as possible; it is not possible to truly stabilize this patient except in the operating room with vascular repair.
   e. Control pain and discomfort.
      1) Nonsteroidal antiinflammatory agents
      2) Narcotic analgesics in doses adequate to allow patient to deep breathe and cough as indicated
      3) Anxiolytics
   f. Monitor for complications.
      1) Hemorrhagic shock
      2) Cardiac tamponade
      3) Hemothorax
      4) False aneurysm

Cardiac Tamponade

Definition

1. When fluid (blood, effusion fluid, pus) in the pericardial space compromises cardiac filling and cardiac output
2. Tamponade is not dependent upon the amount of fluid in the pericardial space but on the presence of hemodynamic consequences of pericardial fluid.

Etiology

1. Blunt or penetrating injury to heart
2. Postcardiotomy
   a. If mediastinal tube is occluded or after removal of mediastinal tube
   b. After removal of epicardial pacing wires
3. Postmyocardial infarction
   a. Pericarditis especially in the anticoagulated patient
   b. Cardiac rupture
4. Iatrogenic causes: perforation of the myocardium by transvenous pacemaker wires, invasive catheters, intracardiac injection, cardiac needle biopsy
5. Transmyocardial revascularization
6. Post-CPR, electrical cardioversion
7. Fibrinolytic or anticoagulant therapy
8. Rupture of great vessels
9. Dissecting aortic aneurysms
10. Malignancy and/or radiation therapy
11. Connective tissue disease: rheumatoid arthritis; systemic lupus erythematosus; scleroderma
12. Metabolic disease: renal failure; hepatic failure; myxedema
13. Inflammation: pericarditis
14. Infection: viral; bacterial; fungal
    a. Tuberculosis
15. Drugs: procainamide (Pronestyl); hydralazine (Apresoline); minoxidil (Loniten); phenytoin (Dilantin); daunorubicin (Cerubidine); methyldopa (Aldomet); sulfasalazine (Azulfidine); isoniazid (INH); methysergide (Sansert); sargramostim (Leukine); tetracycline derivatives

Pathophysiology

See Figure 3-36.

Clinical Presentation

1. Subjective
   a. Precordial fullness or pain
   b. Dyspnea with improvement when sitting upright
   c. Anxiety or feeling of impending doom
2. Objective
   a. Early sign is usually tachycardia but as the impairment in ventricular filling progresses, the patient may be pulseless (i.e., PEA).
   b. Hypotension, narrowed pulse pressure
      1) Pulsus paradoxus: systolic pressure decrease of 10 mm Hg or more with inspiration
   c. Increased JVD: may not be seen if patient is hypotensive
   d. Absent PMI
   e. Dullness to percussion below the left scapula (i.e., Ewart's sign)
   f. Heart sound changes
      1) Pericardial friction rub may be heard especially if tamponade associated with pericarditis
      2) Distant, muffled, or absent heart sounds
   g. Beck's triad: hypotension; distended neck veins; muffled heart sounds

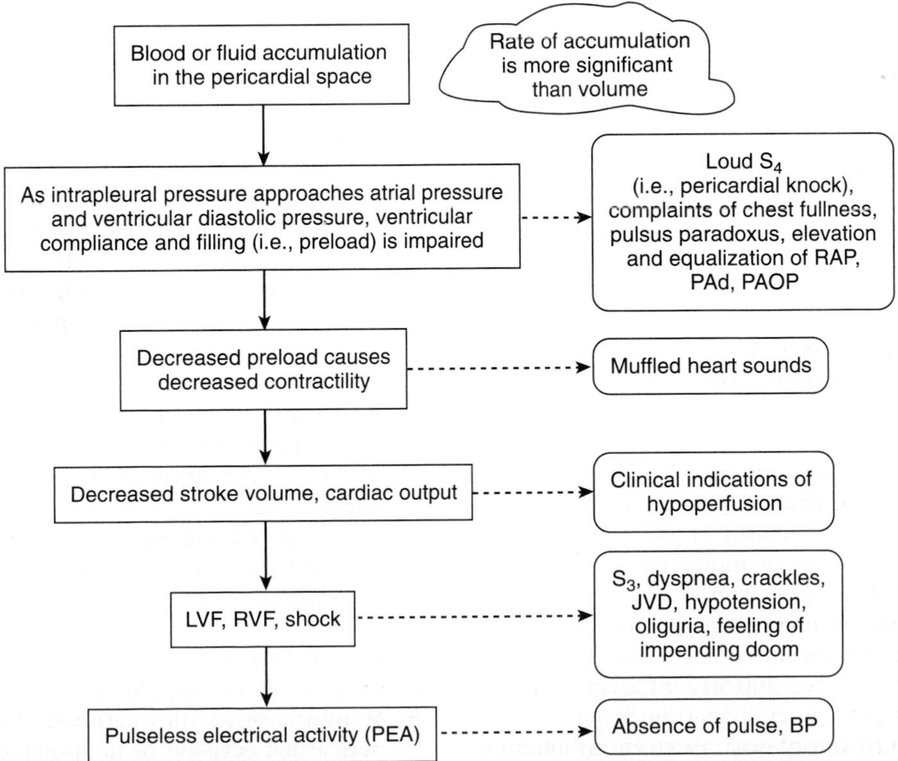

Figure 3-36 Pathophysiology of cardiac tamponade. Dotted lines connect pathology to the clinical presentation. *BP,* blood pressure; *JVD,* jugular venous distention; *LVF,* left ventricular failure; *PAd,* pulmonary artery diastolic pressure; *PAOP,* pulmonary artery occlusive pressure; *PEA,* pulseless electrical activity; *RAP,* right atrial pressure; *RVF,* right ventricular failure.

   h. Excessive mediastinal tube drainage that suddenly stops in a cardiac surgery or trauma patient
3. Hemodynamic parameters
   a. Increased CVP and RAP
   b. Pulsus paradoxus on arterial waveform
   c. Equalization of left- and right-heart filling pressures with hemodynamic monitoring: RAP, PAd, and PAOP within 5 mm Hg of each other
   d. Change in PAOP waveform: large *a* wave, large *v* wave (M sign)
   e. Decrease in CO/CI
   f. Decrease in SvO_2
4. Diagnostic
   a. CBC with differential: assess for anemia
   b. Type and crossmatch in preparation for blood administration if necessary
   c. Chest x-ray
      1) Widened mediastinum
      2) Dilated superior vena cava
      3) Enlarged heart (i.e., water-bottle silhouette)
   d. Electrocardiography
      1) Diffuse ST segment elevation across the precordial leads
      2) Decrease in the amplitude of the QRS or electrical alternans (i.e., alternating tall and small QRSs) across the precordial leads
      3) Bradycardia may indicate impending PEA
      4) Ventricular dysrhythmias
   e. Echocardiogram: 2D or transesophageal
      1) Echo-free space will be evident between the pericardium and epicardium
      2) Right atrial and ventricular collapse
      3) Respiratory variation in cardiac chamber dimension and transvalvular flow velocities
      4) Transesophageal echocardiogram or CT imaging may be required
   f. FAST – focused assessment with sonography
   g. CT of chest
   h. Fluoroscopy of chest: may be used during pericardiocentesis

Collaborative Management

1. Maintain airway, ventilation, oxygenation, and perfusion
   a. Airway, oxygenation, and circulation support using BLS, ACLS if needed
   b. 100% oxygen by face mask; intubate and mechanically ventilate as indicated
   c. Circulating volume replacement
      1) Initiate two large-bore IVs: replace vascular volume as necessary
         a) Normal saline: 200-500 mL over 10-15 minutes
         b) Fresh frozen plasma, dextran, or albumin may also be used.
         c) Blood replacement may also be necessary.
   d. Inotropes (e.g., dobutamine) as prescribed
   e. Atropine or transcutaneous pacing may be necessary for bradydysrhythmias.
2. Prepare to assist with pericardiocentesis for emergency cardiac tamponade.
   a. Place patient in semi-Fowler's position; subxiphoid or left parasternal approach are most commonly used.
   b. Apply ECG machine and electrodes.
      1) Apply limb leads.
      2) Attach chest lead wire to the exploring needle with an alligator clamp if requested; this technique is used to assess needle position because when the needle touches epicardium, ST segment elevation is seen and PVCs may occur.
   c. Have echocardiography technician available to assist with 2D echo guidance if requested; fluoroscopy may also be used.
   d. Have emergency equipment available including transcutaneous pacemaker.
   e. Assist with administration of local anesthetic.
   f. Administer sedation if the patient is anxious.
   g. Assist with slow aspiration of the fluid and send it to the laboratory department for analysis.
   h. Assist with placement of pericardial catheter if indicated; may be used for injection of sclerosing agents, corticosteroids, fibrinolytics, or chemotherapeutic agents.
   i. Monitor for complications.
      1) Laceration of coronary artery or conduction system
      2) Myocardial perforation
      3) Pneumothorax
      4) Dysrhythmias
      5) Hypotension (usually reflexogenic)
3. Administer drugs or therapies related to cause.
   a. Discontinuance of drug that contributed to the tamponade
   b. Protamine or vitamin K if patient is on anticoagulants
   c. Dialysis for patients with renal failure
   d. Antibiotics if purulent effusion
   e. Thyroid hormone replacement for myxedema
   f. Corticosteroids may be prescribed in drug-related pericardial effusions, uremia, and pericarditis
4. Assist in preparation of patient for surgical intervention.
   a. Pericardiocentesis may not resolve the tamponade if effusion is posterior; surgical drainage is indicated if purulent or hemorrhagic effusion.
   b. Subxiphoid pericardiotomy or thorascopic procedures may be necessary.
5. Monitor/assist with treatment of recurrent pericardial effusion or tamponade.
   a. Monitor for recurrence of clinical indications of tamponade.
   b. Prepare the patient for the selected procedure.
      1) Percutaneous balloon pericardiotomy

2) Intrapericardial instillation of sclerosing agent
3) Pleuropericardial or peritoneal-pericardial window

Hypovolemic Shock

Included under Cardiovascular on the CCRN Test Plan but will be covered in Chapter 11: Multisystem

Cardiogenic Shock

Included under Cardiovascular on the CCRN Test Plan but will be covered in Chapter 11: Multisystem

LEARNING ACTIVITIES

CHAPTER 3

Note: Remember that you won't see questions like these on the CCRN examination, but these activities allow you to approach the content from a different perspective to remember it better. Multiple-choice questions (like on the CCRN examination) are available on the Elsevier website.

1. Match the dysrhythmia with the most appropriate treatment summary. You may choose an answer more than once.

___ 1. Ventricular fibrillation
___ 2. Stable monomorphic ventricular tachycardia
___ 3. Asystole
___ 4. Symptomatic bradycardia
___ 5. Pulseless electrical activity
___ 6. Stable SVT
___ 7. Acute onset atrial fibrillation
___ 8. Pulseless ventricular tachycardia
___ 9. Junctional tachycardia
___ 10. Complete heart block with ventricular escape rhythm
___ 11. Sinus tachycardia
___ 12. Torsades de pointes

a. BLS, epinephrine
b. Treatment of cause, beta-blockers or sedatives
c. Cardioversion or amiodarone or ibutilide
d. Vagal maneuvers and adenosine, calcium channel blocker, beta-blocker
e. Magnesium, overdrive pacing, isoproterenol
f. BLS, defibrillation, epinephrine, amiodarone
g. Procainamide, amiodarone, or lidocaine
h. Transcutaneous pacing or atropine
i. BLS, assess for possible causes, epinephrine
j. Vagal maneuvers, withhold digoxin, administration of adenosine, calcium channel blocker, or beta-blocker

2. Complete the following table by identifying the Vaughn-Williams antidysrhythmic classification of the following drugs. Some drugs are of more than one class.

Drugs	Classification
Adenosine (Adenocard)	
Amiodarone (Cordarone)	
Atropine	
Digoxin	
Diltiazem (Cardizem)	
Dofetilide (Tikosyn)	
Esmolol (Brevibloc)	
Flecainide (Tambocor)	
Ibutilide (Corvert)	
Lidocaine (Xylocaine)	
Metoprolol (Lopressor)	
Procainamide (Pronestyl)	
Propranolol (Inderal)	
Quinidine	
Sotalol (Betapace)	
Verapamil (Calan)	

3. Complete the following calculations.

a. Drug: dobutamine
Dose: 5 mcg/kg/min
Concentration: 500 mg/500 mL
Patient's weight: 80 kg
Rate: _____

b. Drug: sodium nitroprusside
Dose: _____
Concentration: 50 mg/250 mL
Patient's weight: 70 kg
Rate: 45 mL/hr

c. Drug: dopamine
Dose: _____
Concentration: 400 mg/250 mL

Patient's weight: 70 kg
Rate: 14 mL/hr

d. Drug: dopamine
Dose: 2 mcg/kg/min
Concentration: 400 mg/500 mL
Patient's weight: 70 kg
Rate: _____

e. Drug: nitroglycerin
Dose: 50 mcg/min
Concentration: 50 mg/500 mL
Rate: _____

f. Drug: lidocaine
Dose: 3 mg/min
Concentration: 2 g/500 mL
Rate: _____

4. Complete the following table to identify the NAPSE code for the pacemaker that would have the capabilities of the others together.

AOO		VVI	a.
VVI		VAT	b.
AAI	VAT	VVI	c.

5. Complete the following puzzle on pacemaker terminology.

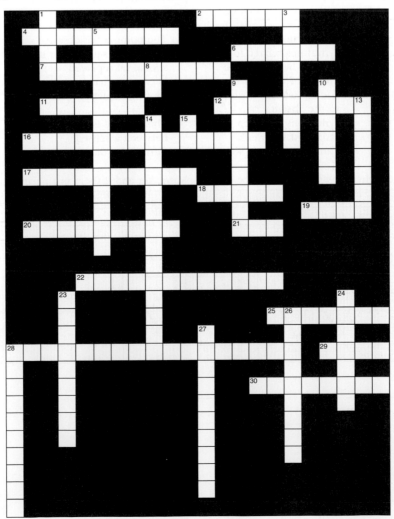

ACROSS

2. The electrical stimulus delivered by a pacemaker's pulse generator
4. The ability of the pacemaker to send information, (i.e., programmed status, measurements, signals) to the programmer
6. This type of pacemaker only discharges when the patient's heart rate drops below the preset rate for the pacemaker
7. This type of pacemaker is capable of stimulating the atria and ventricles (two words)
11. This type of beat results when an intrinsic depolarization and a paced depolarization occur simultaneously so both contribute to the depolarization
12. Inherent; belonging to or originating from the heart itself
16. The ability of a pacemaker to increase the pacing rate in response to physical activity and physiologic demand (two words)
17. A pacing parameter which allows a longer escape interval after a sensed event, allowing perpetuation of the patient's intrinsic rhythm
18. Another term for pacemaker artifact
19. This rate is the rate at which the pulse generator discharges when no intrinsic activity is detected
20. To deliver an electrical stimulus upon detecting a spontaneous depolarization
21. Radiated or conducted energy, either electrical or magnetic, which can interfere with or disrupt the function of a pulse generator (abbrev.)
22. A pulse generator with a pacing mode and/or parameters that can be changed noninvasively at any time by means of an external programmer
25. The ability of the pacemaker to detect the patient's intrinsic activity and respond appropriately by either triggering or inhibiting output
28. A collection of signs and symptoms related to the adverse hemodynamic effects of ventricular pacing, usually attributed to the absence of synchrony between the atrial and ventricular contractions (two words)
29. The manner in which a pacemaker provides artificial rate and rhythm support in the presence of dysrhythmia; identified by a three- or five-letter code
30. The spike recorded on the ECG depicting the electrical energy discharge from the pulse generator

DOWN

1. The wire or wires which carry electrical signals to and from the heart, a connector pin, and stimulating, sensing electrode(s)
3. When ventricular pacing is synchronized to sensed atrial activity
5. The unit of measurement used for electrical stimulus (i.e., output) generated by a pacemaker
8. This interval in dual-chamber pacing is analogous to the PR interval in intrinsic activity (abbrev.)
9. The point at which a pacemaker signals that it should be replaced because its battery is nearing depletion (three words)
10. This interval is the time between a sensed intrinsic cardiac event and the next pacemaker output
13. Successful depolarization of the atria and/or ventricles by an artificial pacemaker
14. This portion of the pacemaker system houses the power source and the circuitry for regulating the pacemaker (two words)
15. This interval in dual-chamber pacing is the interval between a sensed or ventricular paced event and the next atrial paced event (abbrev.)
23. The minimum amount of voltage, expressed in mA, required to obtain consistent capture
24. The lead has both positive and negative electrodes
26. The uninsulated conductive portion of a pacing lead which makes electrical contact with tissue
27. This mode of response to sensing indicates that the pacemaker output is suppressed when an intrinsic event is sensed
28. The duration of the pacing pulse expressed in millisecond; also called pulse duration (two words)

6. Analyze the following ECG rhythm strips. Identify the type of pacemaker and if there is a pacemaker malfunction.

a.

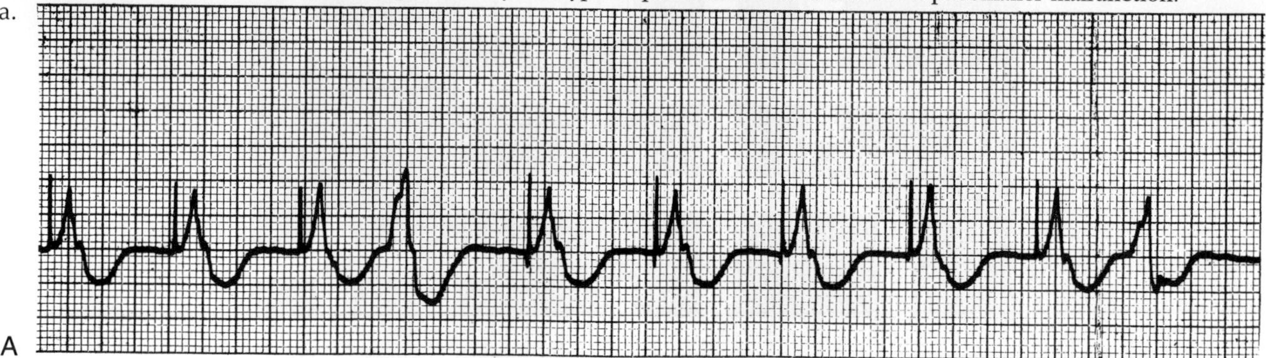

Interpretation ______________________________

b.

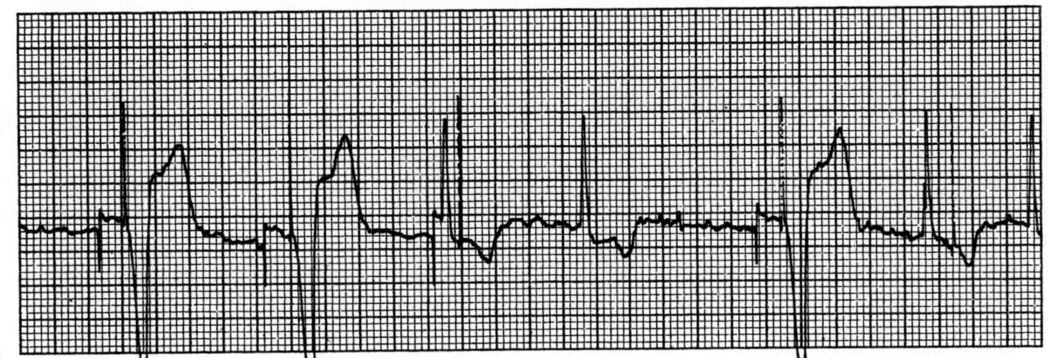

Interpretation ______________________________

c.

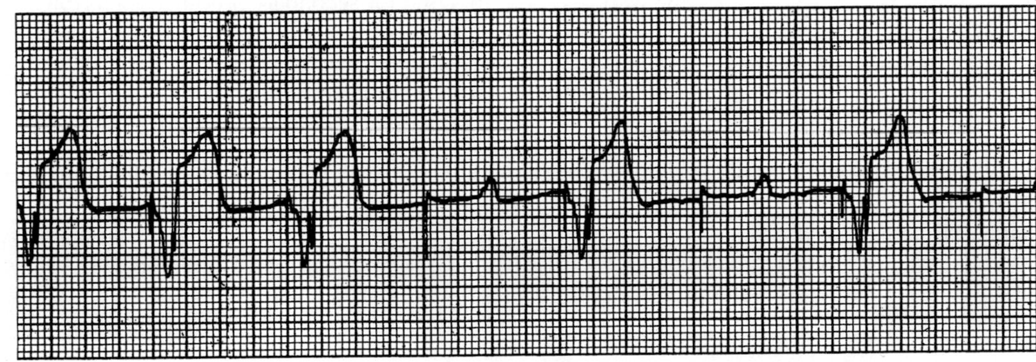

Interpretation ______________________________

7. Complete the following table differentiating cardiac risk factors as nonmodifiable or modifiable.

Nonmodifiable	Modifiable

8. **Match the following treatments for acute MI with rationales for use. More than one may apply.**

___ 1. Fibrinolytics
___ 2. Percutaneous interventional procedures (PCI)
___ 3. ACE inhibitors
___ 4. Nitroglycerin
___ 5. Calcium channel blockers
___ 6. Beta-blockers
___ 7. ASA
___ 8. Heparin
___ 9. Glycoprotein IIb/IIIa inhibitors
___ 10. Intraaortic balloon pump (IABP)

a. Increases myocardial oxygen supply by reestablishing patency of the infarct-related artery
b. Decreases myocardial oxygen demand by blocking the effects of catecholamines
c. Increases myocardial oxygen supply by reducing spasm
d. Decreases myocardial oxygen demand by reducing preload
e. Prevents extension of a clot by decreasing platelet aggregation
f. Prevents extension of a clot by preventing the conversion of prothrombin to thrombin
g. Prevents ventricular dilation and adverse remodeling of the myocardium
h. Used for secondary prevention after MI.
i. Decreases myocardial oxygen consumption by decreasing afterload
j. Increases myocardial oxygen supply by increasing coronary artery perfusion pressure

9. **Complete the following crossword puzzle dealing with coronary artery disease and acute myocardial infarction.**

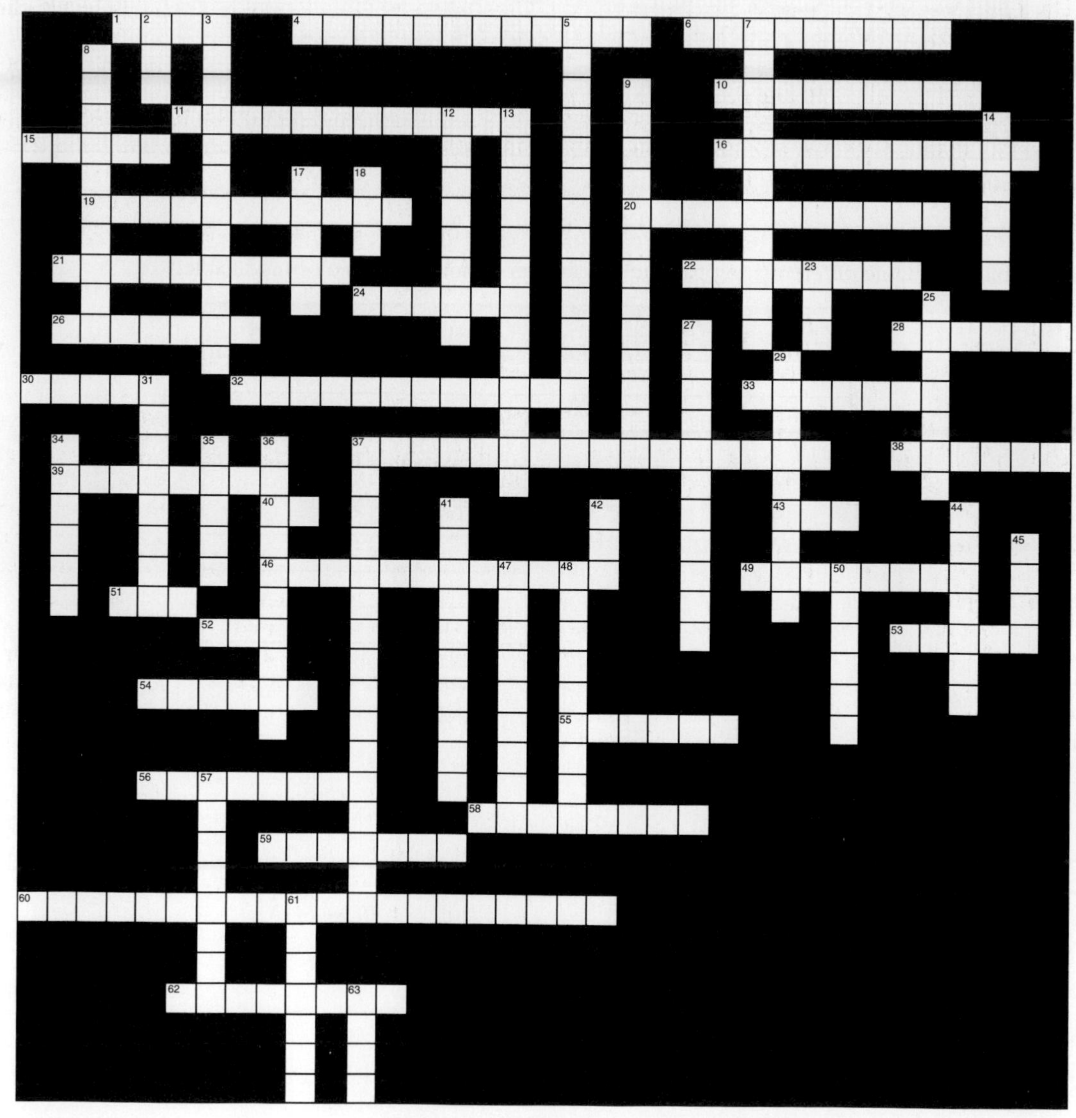

ACROSS

1. This device used to decrease afterload and increase myocardial perfusion in cardiogenic shock (abbrev.)
4. This tPA has a longer half-life than others and is administered as a single bolus
6. A GP IIb/IIIa inhibitor frequently used after PCI (generic)
10. Indicative leads for this cardiac wall are V_8 and V_9
11. The dysrhythmia most likely to cause death in MI patient is ventricular _____
15. Initial therapy for hemodynamic consequences of right ventricular MI
16. This drug is a direct thrombin inhibitor used as an alternative to heparin
19. This PCI procedure opens an occluded artery using a shaving device
20. This percutaneous coronary intervention (PCI) procedure opens an occluded artery using balloon dilation
21. This calcium channel blocker used for coronary artery spasm
22. The analgesic of choice for acute MI
24. The artery sometimes used for CABG that has a high spasm potential
26. An indirect thrombin inhibitor used to prevent extension of a clot or reocclusion
28. A new holosystolic murmur at lower sternum, increase SvO_2, and shock indicates rupture of the ___
30. Format for chest pain description
32. These drugs are used to prevent ventricular dysrhythmias post-MI and also for secondary prevention
33. Indicative leads for this cardiac wall or I and aVL and/or V_5 and V_6
37. A group of diseases characterized by thickening and loss of elasticity (calcification) of arterial walls
38. Evidenced on ECG by ST segment elevation
39. An activity that is likely to decrease body weight, BP, lipids, and stress
40. Death of myocardial tissue (abbrev.)
43. S_3, dyspnea, and crackles indicate what complication of acute MI (abbrev.)
46. The most common complication of MI
49. _____'s syndrome is a late pericarditis that is thought to be an autoimmune response
51. The preferred method of reperfusion for acute MI (abbrev)
52. Bad cholesterol (abbrev.)
53. These drugs are used to treat pericarditis (abbrev.)
54. Patients with diabetes mellitus are more likely to have this type of MI
55. Clenched fist held over the sternum with description of chest pain is referred to as _____'s sign
56. Indicative leads for this cardiac wall are V_3 and V_4
58. Indicative leads for this cardiac wall are II, III, and aVF
59. Acute chest pain and/or ST segment elevation after PCI may indicate acute ___
60. This risk factor for CAD treated with folic acid
62. New onset, crescendo, and variant are all categorized as this type of angina

DOWN

2. This platelet aggregation inhibitor is an important aspect of initial treatment of acute MI (abbrev.)
3. Elevated temperature, chest pain, and pericardial friction rub after MI indicates this complication
5. The most likely cause of acute MI
7. This oral platelet aggregation inhibitor frequently used for after PCI
8. The inotropic agent most likely to be used for cardiogenic shock with MI
9. This type of hemorrhage is a complication of fibrinolytics with dire consequences
12. Evidenced on ECG by T wave inversion
13. Nitrate used for acute chest pain
14. CABG done through small thoracotomy incision used for LIMA-LAD anastomosis (abbrev.)
17. Device used during PCI to prevent closure
18. A value of greater than 30 if considered obese (abbrev.)
23. Good cholesterol (abbrev.)
25. This syndrome is characterized by chest pain with deep T wave inversion in V_2, V_3 and associated with critical proximal LAD stenosis
27. This is evidenced by cessation of pain, ST segment return to baseline, dysrhythmias
29. Rupture of the ___ muscle causes acute mitral regurgitation; serious complication of acute MI
31. The internal mammary is now referred to as the internal ___
34. A major cause for delay in seeking assistance for chest pain
35. This coronary artery supplies RA, RV, and the inferior wall of LV
36. ACE inhibitors are used after MI to prevent this
37. A group of diseases characterized by thickening and loss of elasticity (calcification) of arterial walls
41. This cardioselective beta-blocker is often used for acute MI
42. The general term used for undifferentiated acute ischemic chest pain (abbrev.)
44. This type of angina is caused by spasm
45. Isolated right ventricular MI may be seen in patients with _____ (abbrev.)
47. A muscle protein measurement that is sensitive but not specific for MI
48. A tPA with short half-life so must be given as bolus followed by infusion
50. Indicative leads for this cardiac wall are V_1 and V_2
57. Measurement of this cardiac muscle protein is the most specific test for acute MI
61. Use of this drug may cause MI by stimulating SNS (increasing oxygen demand) and causing spasm (decreasing oxygen supply)
63. New onset occurrence of this type of block may indicate acute MI (abbrev)

10. Identify the physical findings from the following list that are seen in these pathologic conditions. More than one physical finding may be listed for each pathologic condition.

___ 1. Right ventricular failure
___ 2. Left ventricular failure
___ 3. Left ventricular MI
___ 4. Right ventricular MI
___ 5. Cardiac tamponade
___ 6. Valvular dysfunction
___ 7. Chronic arterial insufficiency

a. Jugular venous distention
b. Displaced PMI
c. S_3 at apex
d. S_3 at sternum
e. S_4 at apex
f. S_4 at sternum
g. Murmur
h. Muffled heart sounds
i. Intermittent claudication
j. Peripheral edema
k. Peripheral pallor
l. Crackles in lung bases
m. Hepatomegaly
n. Pulsus paradoxus

11. Identify whether the following causes or clinical findings are associated with left or right ventricular failure. Some may be associated with biventricular failure.

Causes	Left	Right
Aortic stenosis		
Cardiac tamponade		
Cardiomyopathy		
Mitral stenosis		
Myocardial infarction (left)		
Myocardial infarction (right)		
Pulmonary embolism		
Pulmonary hypertension		
Systemic hypertension		
Sign/Symptom	**Left**	**Right**
Abnormal liver function studies		
Ascites		
Atrial dysrhythmias		
Crackles audible over lungs		
Dyspnea		
Elevated PAOP		
Elevated RAP		
Hepatomegaly		
Jugular venous distention		
Mental confusion		
Murmur of mitral regurgitation		
Murmur of tricuspid regurgitation		
Orthopnea		
Peripheral edema		
S_3, S_4 at apex		
S_3, S_4 at sternum		
Weight gain		

12. a. List two primary effects of IABP.

1) ______________________________

____

2) ______________________________

____

b. List two major contraindications of IABP.
   1) ____
   ____
   2) ____
   ____

c. In IABP the balloon is inflated during which phase of the cardiac cycle?
   ____

d. In IABP the balloon is deflated immediately prior to which phase of the cardiac cycle?
   ____

e. List two complications caused by displacement of the balloon in the aorta.
   1) ____
   ____
   2) ____
   ____

13. Identify the labeled portions of the IABP waveform.

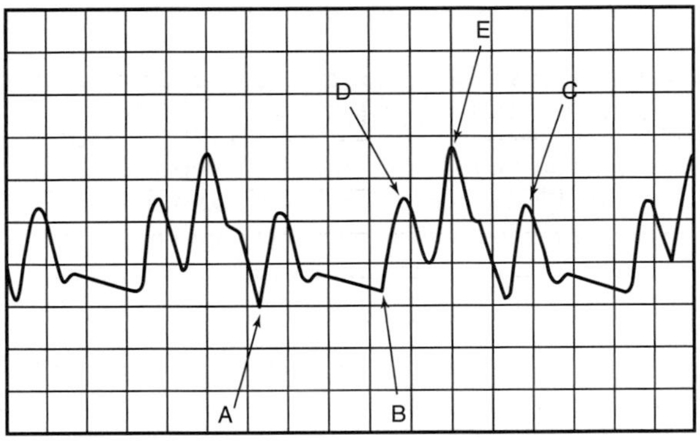

A. ______________________
B. ______________________
C. ______________________
D. ______________________
E. ______________________

14. Complete the questions following this case study.
Patient A is a 75-year-old woman admitted with complaints of increasing dyspnea and fatigue. She has a past medical history of diabetes mellitus, stable angina, and CABG approximately 10 years ago. Her blood pressure is 136/82 mm Hg and her heart rate is 92 beats/min. Her monitor shows atrial fibrillation. She has an S_3 at the apex, peripheral edema to midcalf, and JVD to 10 cm above the angle of Louis. Her current medications include captopril, carvedilol, torsemide, metformin, and warfarin. Her last measured ejection fraction was 25%.

a. Does she meet criteria for heart failure?
   ____
   ____

b. Is this systolic or diastolic dysfunction?
   ____
   ____

c. What other medications might be beneficial and why?
   ____
   ____

d. What other treatments might be helpful?
   ____
   ____

e. What ACC stage?
   ____
   ____

15. Identify whether the following vasoactive agents are arterial or venous dilators.

Drug	Arterial Dilator	Venous Dilator
Clevidipine (Cleviprex)		
Dobutamine (Dobutrex)		
Fenoldopam (Corlopam)		
Hydralazine (Apresoline)		
Milrinone (Primacor)		
Minoxidil (Loniten)		
Morphine sulfate		
Nifedipine (Procardia)		
Nitroglycerin (less than 1 mcg/kg/min)		
Nitroglycerin (greater than 1 mcg/kg/min)		
Nitroprusside (Nipride)		
Phentolamine (Regitine)		
Prazosin (Minipress)		

16. Complete the questions following this case study.
Patient B is a 65-year-old man with a 10-year history of essential hypertension who came to the emergency department with complaints of headache. He rubs the back of his head and says that it has been hurting for the last several days though he has been taking acetaminophen. He says that he had a "heart attack" 5 years ago when he was put on metoprolol (Lopressor) and enalaprilat (Vasotec). He says he has "gout" and has been on allopurinol (Zyloprim) for a number of years. He recently started taking indomethacin (Indocin) for an acute exacerbation of gout. The only other change in his health status that he reports is a weight gain of about 20 pounds over the past two months; he said he now weighs 80 kg.

He denies chest pain but he is significantly dyspneic. His BP is 220/140 mm Hg supine and 200/136 mm Hg when sitting upright. His heart rate is 62 beats/min; respiratory rate is 32/min and labored. The PMI is palpable at the anterior axillary line and the sixth left intercostal space. Cardiac auscultation reveals S_1, S_2, and an S_3. Bibasilar crackles are audible. Pulse oximeter reads 88%.

Oxygen therapy is initiated with 5 L by nasal cannula. An IV catheter is inserted and blood is collected for CBC, electrolytes, BUN, and creatinine. He voids only 50 mL of concentrated urine which is sent to the laboratory for urinalysis. Chest x-ray reveals cardiomegaly and pulmonary edema. Multiple lead ECG shows left ventricular strain pattern in V_5, V_6 and R waves in V_6 that measure 30 mm. Abnormal laboratory results included a creatinine of 3.0 mg/dL and BUN of 35 mg/dL.

a. Identify the findings that indicate hypertensive emergency.

____

b. What is the most likely cause of this abrupt increase in BP?

____

c. What organs are most likely to be affected by hypertension and hypertensive crisis?

____

d. Should he be admitted? PACU or critical care unit?

____

e. What is the therapeutic goal for BP reduction within the next 2 hours?

____

f. List a parenteral drug in each of the following categories.
Vasodilator ______________________________
ACE inhibitor ______________________________
Alpha-blocker ______________________________
Beta-blocker ______________________________
Alpha- and beta-blocker ______________________________

g. The physician prescribes nitroprusside (Nipride) to be started at 1 mcg/kg/min. Patient B weighs 80 kg. You reconstitute 50 mg of nitroprusside with 3 mL of sterile water and put it in 250 mL of normal saline. At what rate should infusion be started for the 1 mcg/kg/min prescription?

____

h. List adverse effects of nitroprusside and how to monitor for them.

____

i. Could sublingual nifedipine be used instead of the nitroprusside in this patient?

____

j. Which drug would have been most appropriate if the CT had shown cerebral hemorrhage?

____

k. What signs and/or symptoms could indicate that Patient B is experiencing thoracic aortic dissection?

____

17. Complete the following crossword puzzle dealing with cardiovascular pharmacology. Use only generic names.

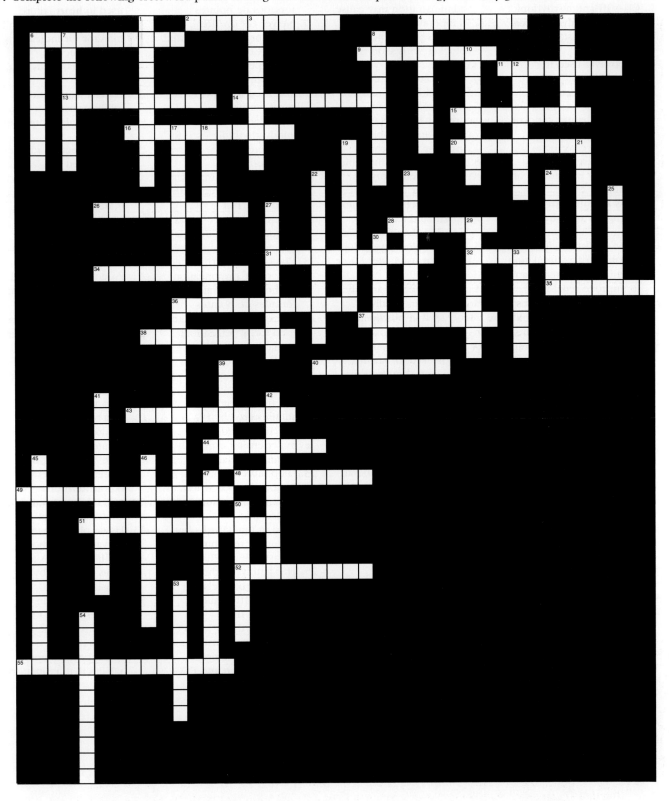

ACROSS

2. Class III antidysrhythmic; first line antidysrhythmic agent for pulseless VT or VF
4. Electrolyte used in hyperkalemia, hypermagnesemia, hypocalcemia, and calcium channel blocker toxicity
6. Cardioselective beta-blocker; used for secondary prevention of acute MI
9. Class IV antidysrhythmic; frequently used in SVT
11. Vitamin K antagonist
13. Arterial dilator with dopaminergic stimulation used in hypertension and to improve renal flow
14. Alpha- and beta-blocker used in heart failure
15. Phosphodiesterase inhibitor; more potent and with fewer side effects than inamrinone
16. Adrenergic agent used in pulseless VT, VF, asystolic, and PEA
20. Class IV antidysrhythmic agent which decreases contractility less than verapamil
26. Beta-type natriuretic hormone used in heart failure
28. Low molecular weight form used as a platelet aggregation inhibitor especially after vascular surgery
31. Intravenous ACE inhibitor that may be used for hypertension or heart failure
32. Adrenergic agent with dose dependent effects; may be inotropic or vasopressor
34. Loop diuretic; rapid administration may cause temporary deafness
35. Cardioselective beta-blocker with short half-life
36. Alpha-blocker; frequently used with vasopressor drug infiltration to prevent tissue necrosis
37. Alpha- and beta-blocker; used for hypertension
38. Class IC antidysrhythmic; used for refractory ventricular dysrhythmias
40. Loop diuretic that is more potent and longer duration than furosemide
43. Oral platelet aggregation inhibitor used after MI or stroke
44. Benzodiazepine anxiolytic
48. Electrolyte; usually included in postoperative fluid replacement
49. RBC colony-stimulating factor used for anemia
51. Pure beta stimulant; may be used in torsades de pointes to shorten repolarization
52. Nucleoside used to break reentrant mechanism in PSVT
55. Drug used in peripheral arterial disease to increase the flexibility of the RBCs

DOWN

1. Arterial selective IV calcium channel blocker used as an antihypertensive especially postoperatively
3. Adrenergic-type inotropic agent most frequently used in cardiogenic shock
4. Oral ACE inhibitor; may cause rash or cough
5. Indirect thrombin inhibitor
6. Electrolyte; indicated for torsades de pointes
7. Newer GP IIb/IIIa inhibitor; frequently used after PCI
8. Antihypertensive with dopaminergic qualities; also used to improve renal perfusion
10. Intravenous class III antidysrhythmic used for acute onset atrial fibrillation
12. The first IV GP IIb/IIIa inhibitor; still frequently used after PCI
17. Calcium channel blocker frequently used in variant angina
18. Class IA antidysrhythmic; may cause prolongation of the QT interval and torsades de pointes
19. Calcium channel blocker used for hypertension; available for IV use
21. Analgesic of choice in acute MI; venous vasodilator
22. Arterial dilator administered by IV injection; used in hypertension especially if pregnancy-related
23. Loop diuretic that is frequently used when patient is refractory to furosemide
24. Used in bradycardia but no longer recommended for asystole or PEA
25. This antidysrhythmic agent has both class II and class III qualities
27. Oral class III antidysrhythmic agent used for new onset atrial fibrillation; requires hospitalization and ECG monitoring during initiation of therapy
29. Aldosterone antagonist used in heart failure
30. Class IB antidysrhythmic; monitor for indications of toxicity such as paresthesia, confusion, seizures
33. Platelet aggregation inhibitor used for primary and secondary prevention of MI
36. Alpha selective adrenergic agent; used as a vasopressor especially when tachycardia is very undesirable
39. Cardiac glycoside; decreases ventricular response rate in atrial fibrillation and flutter
41. Predominantly arterial nitrate-type vasodilator
42. Tissue plasminogen activator with a longer half-life; given as a single bolus
45. Alpha dominant adrenergic agent; used as a vasopressor
46. Noncardioselective beta-blocker
47. Predominantly venous nitrate-type vasodilator; dose >1 mcg/kg/min causes arterial as well venous dilation
50. ACE inhibitor available in intravenous form
53. Tissue plasminogen activator with short half-life; given as a bolus followed by an infusion
54. Hormone used in pulseless VT or VF as an alternative to the first or second dose of epinephrine; longer half-life than epinephrine

The Pulmonary System: Physiology, Assessment, and Ventilatory Support

CHAPTER 4

Selected Concepts in Anatomy and Physiology

General Information

1. The pulmonary system consists of lungs, conducting air passages, muscles of ventilation, central nervous system control, thoracic cage, and alveoli.
2. Functions of the pulmonary system include the following:
   a. Allows interchange of gases between the atmosphere and the bloodstream
   b. Assists in maintenance of acid-base balance
   c. Contributes to phonation
   d. Acts as a reservoir for blood for the left atrium and ventricle
   e. Assists in metabolism

Functional Anatomy

1. Conducting airways: nose to terminal bronchioles
   a. Conduct airflow toward gas exchange units; no gas exchange occurs in these airways
      1) Consists of branching tubes with diminishing diameter
      2) Accounts for approximately 2 mL/kg of inspired tidal volume (this volume is referred to as *anatomical dead space*)
   b. Upper airway (Figure 4-1): nose or mouth to external opening of vocal cords; serves as a passageway for food and inspired gas
      1) Mouth: not as effective as the nose in conditioning the inspired air
         a) Smaller surface area
         b) No ciliated epithelium to trap dust or bacteria from inspired air
      2) Nose
         a) Structure
            i) Mucous membrane lining contains cilia and mucus-producing cells.
            ii) Rich supply of blood vessels lies under the mucous membranes to provide warmth.
            iii) Skeletal rigidity maintains patency during inspiration.
            iv) Turbinates increase surface area.
            v) Four sinuses surround and drain into the nasal cavity: frontal, maxillary, ethmoid, and sphenoid.
            vi) Septum divides the nose into two fossae.
            vii) Small inlet with larger outlet allows air to have maximal contact with the nasal mucosa.
         b) Functions
            i) Warms inspired gas to body temperature
            ii) Humidifies inspired gas to relative humidity of approximately 80-100% at body temperature; accounts for insensible water loss of 400 mL/24 hr
            iii) Protects the lower airway from foreign material; filters inspired air of particles 5 μm or larger
            iv) Prevents inspiration of potentially dangerous environmental gases
            v) Assists in production of sound in phonation
            vi) Provides sense of olfaction: olfactory area located in the superior turbinate (sniffing directs air toward this area)
         c) More resistance (2-3 times) than the mouth; this is rationale for why dyspneic patients are more likely to breathe through their mouth
      3) Pharynx: posterior nasal cavity to esophagus
         a) Structure
            i) Nasopharynx: between posterior nasal cavity to soft palate; contains the pharyngeal tonsils and eustachian tubes
               (a) Pharyngeal tonsils (also called adenoids): dense concentration of lymphatic tissue; guard entryway into respiratory and GI tracts

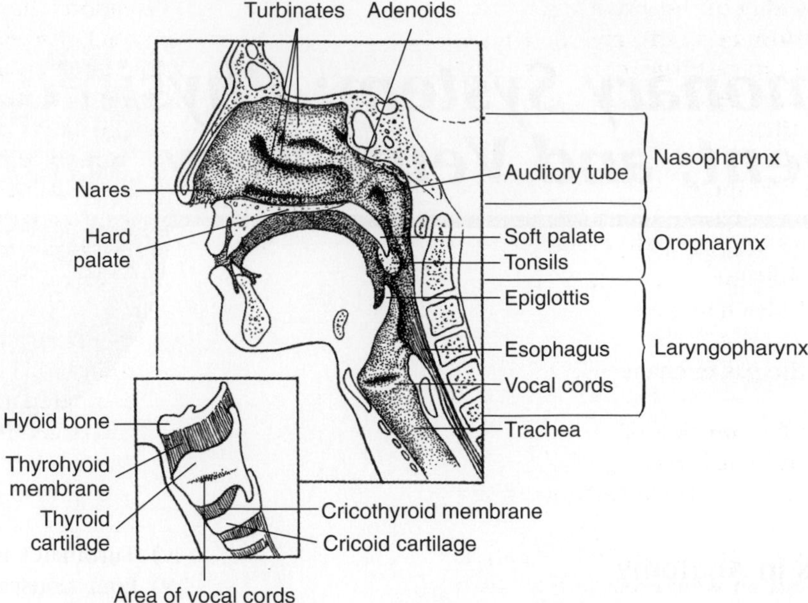

Figure 4-1 The upper airway (lateral view). (From Luce, J. M., & Pierson, D. J. [1998]. *Critical care medicine*. Philadelphia: Saunders.)

(b) Eustachian tubes: connection between nasopharynx to each middle ear; opens during swallowing to equalize pressure in the middle ear
   (i) Middle ear pain or infection may develop during upper respiratory infection if eustachian tube closes
   (ii) Nasal intubation may block eustachian tubes and cause otitis media

ii) Oropharynx: between the soft palate and base of tongue
   (a) Location of the palatine and lingual tonsils
   (b) Center of the gag reflex which defends the lower airway against aspiration; gag reflex controlled by cranial nerves IX (glossopharyngeal) and X (vagus)

iii) Laryngopharynx (also called *hypopharynx*): from base of tongue to the epiglottis

b) Functions
   i) Swallowing: Uvula and soft palate move posteriorly and superiorly to keep food and liquid from entering the nasopharynx.
   ii) Protection: Area is rich in lymphatic tissue.

4) Larynx: upper portion of the trachea; connects the laryngopharynx with the trachea

a) Structure: consists of thyroid cartilage, vocal cords, and cricoid cartilage
   i) Epiglottis: flexible cartilage attached to the thyroid cartilage which overhangs the larynx like a lid; prevents food from entering the larynx and trachea during swallowing
   ii) Thyroid cartilage: largest laryngeal cartilage
      (a) Contains the vocal cords
      (b) Also referred to as the *Adam's apple*
   iii) Vocal folds: two pairs of membranes that protrude into the lumen of the larynx; controlled by recurrent laryngeal nerve, a branch of the vagus nerve
      (a) False vocal cords: upper pair; play no part in vocalization
      (b) True vocal cords: lower pair
         (i) Form a triangular opening between them that leads to the trachea
         (ii) Change shape and vibrate in response to contraction of muscles in the larynx to result in phonation
      (c) Glottis: passage through the vocal cords
   iv) Cricothyroid membrane: avascular structure that connects the thyroid and cricoid cartilage; cricothyrotomy, an emergency

opening of the airway, is performed at this membrane
v) Cricoid cartilage: complete ring located below the thyroid cartilage
b) Functions
i) Allows speech
ii) Prevents aspiration through the valve action of epiglottis
iii) Allows for cough reflex and Valsalva maneuver

c. Lower airway (Figure 4-2): below larynx; conducts air to the gas exchange surface
1) Structure
a) Trachea: first portion of tracheobronchial tree
i) Consists of 16-20 C-shaped rings; 10-12 cm long
ii) The esophagus and trachea share a common wall; erosion through this wall (tracheoesophageal fistula) may be caused by an overinflated endotracheal tube (ET) or tracheostomy tube cuff.
b) Carina: bifurcation of trachea into left and right mainstem bronchi
i) The carina is rich in parasympathetic nervous system fibers and cough receptors.
ii) Suctioning may cause bradycardia and hypotension due to stimulation of carina with the suction catheter.
c) Bronchi
i) Right mainstem bronchus is almost straight (25 degrees) off trachea compared to the left (40-60 degrees) and larger in diameter than the left; aspiration of liquid or food, foreign bodies, suction catheter, and ET tube go to right preferentially.
ii) Conducting airways branch from mainstem bronchi branch → lobar bronchi; from lobar bronchi branch → segmental bronchi; from

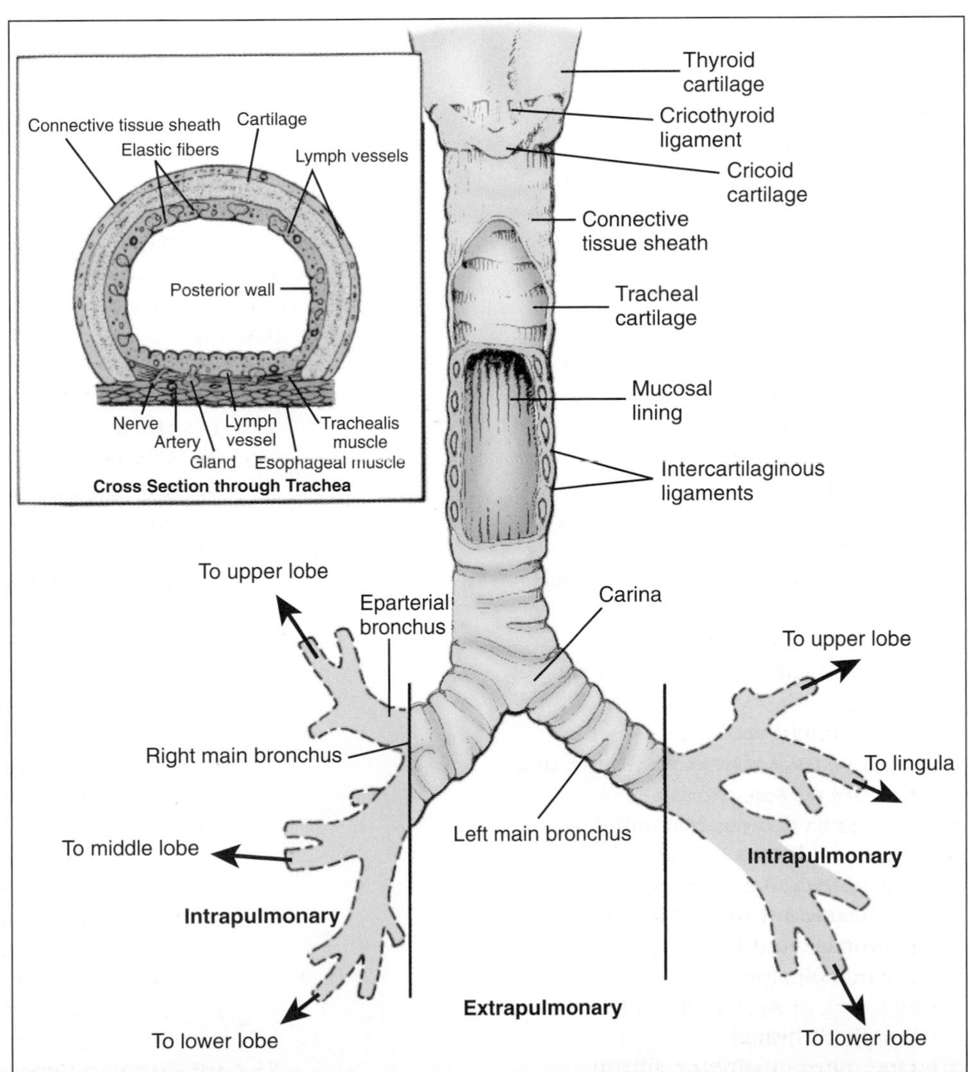

Figure 4-2 The lower airway. (From Martin, D. E. [1988]. *Respiratory anatomy and physiology*. St. Louis: Mosby.)

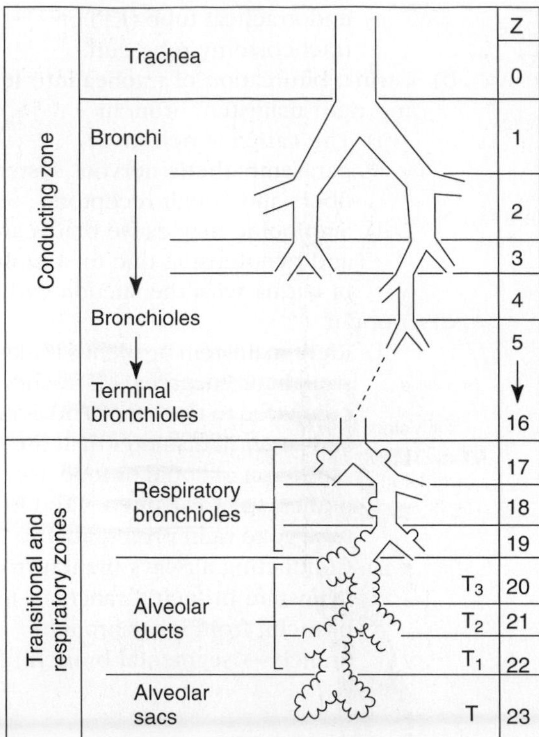

Figure 4-3 Airway generations.

segmental bronchi branch → subsegmental bronchi and so on
- (a) These branches are called generations or levels (Figure 4-3): mainstem (first level), lobar (second), segmental (third), subsegmental (fourth through ninth), bronchioles (tenth through fifteenth branches).

iii) Bronchi are supported by cartilage and smooth muscle.
iv) Mast cells lie just beneath the bronchial epithelium near the smooth muscle and blood vessels.

d) Function
- i) The lower airway conducts, warms, cleanses, and humidifies air.
- ii) The bronchi are responsible for most of total airway resistance in a healthy person.
- iii) Mast cells secrete histamine and other mediators of the inflammatory process when stimulated by antigen-antibody response.

2) Terminal bronchioles
- a) Structure
  - i) Sixteenth branch
  - ii) One mm in diameter; fibrous, elastic smooth muscle with no cartilage; no mucus glands or cilia
- b) Function
  - i) Terminal bronchioles are particularly sensitive to CO_2 and dilate in response to increased CO_2 levels
  - ii) Bronchospasm may significantly narrow the lumen and increase airway resistance

2. Lung
- a. Lobes separated by fissures
  - 1) Right: three lobes
  - 2) Left: two lobes
    - a) The upper left lobe is divided by a fissure.
    - b) The lower portion of the left upper lobe is referred to as the *lingula*; it is approximately the same size as the right middle lobe.
- b. Segments
  - 1) Right: 10 segments
  - 2) Left: eight segments
- c. Subsegments
- d. Lobules
  - 1) Primary functional units of lung
  - 2) Consists of terminal bronchiole, alveolar ducts, alveolar sacs, alveoli, and pulmonary circulation
- e. Gas exchange units: respiratory bronchioles to alveoli
  - 1) Acinus: a term used to refer to the terminal respiratory unit distal to the terminal bronchioles; has an alveolar-capillary membrane for gas exchange
  - 2) Respiratory bronchioles
    - a) Structure
      - i) Composed of the seventeenth through twentieth branches
      - ii) Less than 1 mm in diameter; bronchioles less than 1 mm are subject to collapse when compressed
    - b) Function
      - i) Increasing number of alveoli are attached.
      - ii) Gas exchange takes place here.
  - 3) Alveolar ducts, alveolar sacs, and alveoli
    - a) Structure
      - i) Alveolar ducts: twentieth through twenty-second levels;
      - ii) Alveolar sacs: level 23
      - iii) Alveoli: 300 million alveoli
        - (a) 1-2 millimicrons in size
        - (b) One-half of alveoli in ducts and one-half in alveolar sacs in grapelike clusters of 15-20 alveoli
        - (c) Surface area approximately 80 m^2
        - (d) Contain pores of Kohn: openings between alveoli in intraalveolar septa

(i) Thought to allow collateral ventilation
(ii) May also contribute to movement of microorganisms between alveoli and rapid transmission of infection

iv) Lined with alveolar epithelium: site of diffusion of oxygen and carbon dioxide between inspired air and blood

v) Type I pneumocytes
(a) Cover 90% of total alveolar surface
(b) Flat, large, squamous cells; very susceptible to injury
(c) Responsible for integumentary air-blood barrier; cytoplasmic junctions very tight and impermeable to water under normal circumstances

vi) Type II pneumocytes
(a) These small, cuboidal, granular cells cover only 5% of total alveolar surface.
(b) They produce, store, and secrete surfactant, a lipoprotein that lines the inner aspect of the alveolus.
(i) Surfactant decreases surface tension of the fluid lining the alveoli and prevents alveolar collapse at the end of expiration, especially at low volumes.
(ii) It is especially important in inferior portions of the lung where alveoli are small and distending pressures are low.
(iii) A deficiency of surfactant causes alveolar collapse, poorly compliant lungs, and alveolar edema.
(iv) The half-life of surfactant is only 14 hours; injury to these cells quickly results in massive atelectasis.
(c) If type I pneumocytes are injured, type II pneumocytes increase mitosis to replicate and form a cuboidal cell line and may differentiate to type I.

f. Alveolar-capillary membrane
1) Structure
a) Lines respiratory bronchioles to alveoli
b) Surface area of 1 m^2/kg of body weight and 0.5 μm in thickness

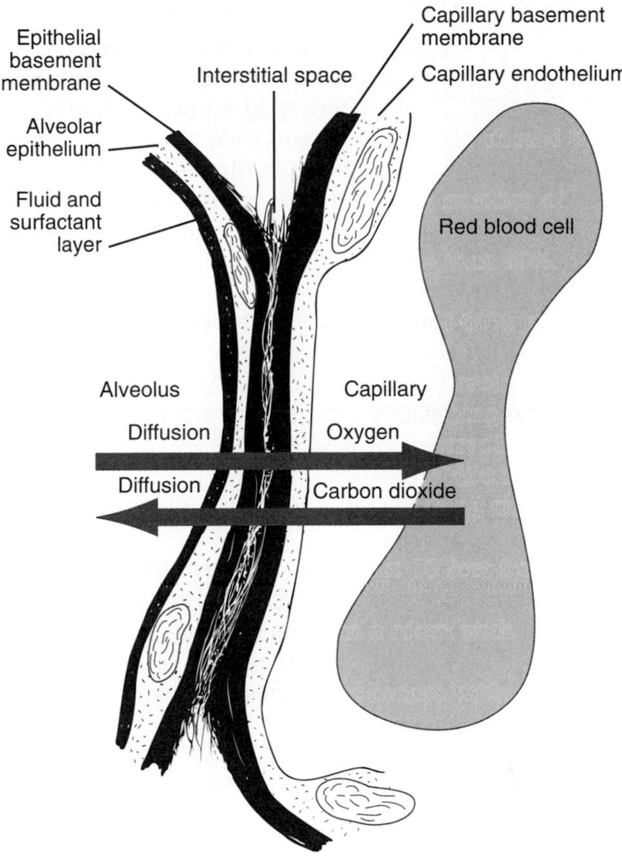

Figure 4-4 The diffusion pathway. (From Carlson, K. K. [Ed.]. [2009]. *Advanced critical care nursing.* St. Louis: Saunders.)

c) Diffusion pathway (Figure 4-4): Gases travel through the pathway from alveolus to blood (oxygen) or blood to alveolus (carbon dioxide).
i) Alveolar epithelium
ii) Epithelial basement membrane
iii) Interstitial space
iv) Capillary basement membrane
v) Capillary endothelium

2) Function
a) Immense surface area and thinness of membrane allow for rapid gas exchange by diffusion.
b) Pulmonary capillary endothelial cells produce and degrade prostaglandins, metabolize vasoactive amines, convert angiotensin I to angiotensin II, and at least partly produce coagulation factor VIII.

g. Defense mechanisms
1) Upper airway
a) Nasal cilia
b) Sneeze: reaction to irritation in the nose
c) Cough: reaction to irritation in the upper airway distal to the nose
i) Vocal cords close and intrathoracic pressure increases.
ii) Sudden opening of glottis allows propulsion of mucus.

d) Mucociliary escalator
   i) Combination of mucus and cilia
   ii) Particles not filtered by nasal cilia (smaller than 5 μm) are trapped in mucus and then propelled upward by the pulsatile motion of the cilia; this mucus is then coughed and expectorated or swallowed.
e) Lymphatics

2) Lower airway
   a) Cough: especially at level of carina
   b) Mucociliary escalator
   c) Lymphatics
3) Alveoli
   a) Immune system
   b) Lymphatics
   c) Alveolar macrophages: mononuclear phagocytes
      i) Engulf and remove bacteria and other foreign substances
      ii) Move from alveolus to alveolus through the pores of Kohn
4) Loss of normal defense mechanisms
   a) Disease
   b) Injury
   c) Anesthesia
   d) Corticosteroids
   e) Smoking
   f) Malnutrition
   g) Ethanol
   h) Uremia
   i) Hypoxia or hyperoxia
   j) Artificial airways

3. Lymphatics
   a. Structure: surround lobule
   b. Functions
      1) Remove interstitial fluid to keep lung free of excess fluid
         a) Normal lymph drainage is approximately 20 mL/hr; may be 200 mL/hr in pulmonary edema
         b) When interstitial lymphatic vessels become enlarged through increased fluid filtration such as pulmonary edema, horizontal linear opacities referred to as *Kerley-B lines* are seen on chest x-ray.
      2) Remove inhaled particles from distal areas of lung
4. Circulation (Figure 4-5)
   a. Pulmonary circulation: low-pressure, low-resistance system
      1) Lungs receive the full cardiac output (approximately 5 L/min).
      2) RV → main pulmonary artery → left and right pulmonary arteries → arterioles → capillaries which spread over the surface of the alveoli → red blood cells (RBCs) move through in single file to allow the diffusion of gases and the attachment of oxygen to hemoglobin
         a) A corresponding arteriole and venule exists for every bronchiole.

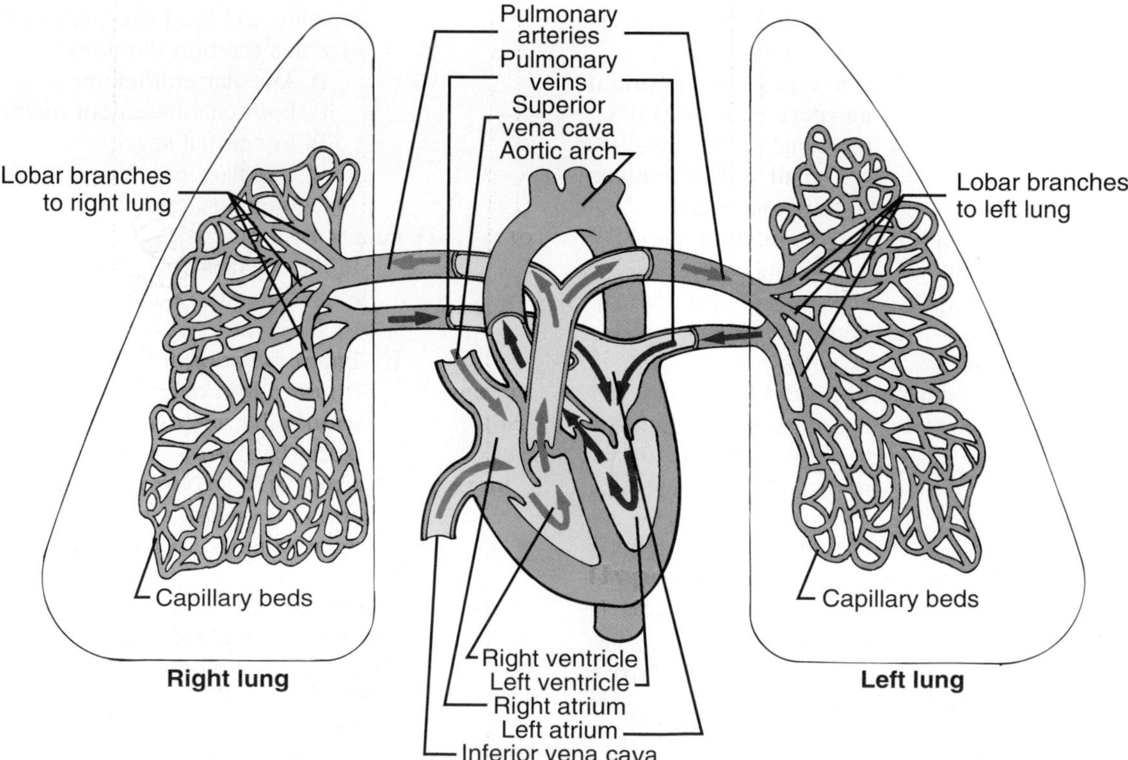

Figure 4-5 The pulmonary circulation. (From McCance, K. L., & Huether, S. E. [2010]. *Pathophysiology: The biologic basis for disease in adults and children* [6th ed.]. St. Louis: Mosby.)

b) The network of capillaries is very dense and frequently described as a sheet of blood.
c) The pulmonary capillaries are very small and will barely accommodate erythrocyte passage.

3) Veins move out of lung toward pleura.
   a) Numerous veins gradually form four pulmonary veins that empty into the left atrium.
   b) The venous system serves as an immense reservoir of blood for the left atrium and left ventricle.
4) Mean pressure in pulmonary artery: 10-20 mm Hg
   a) Pulmonary hypertension (PA_m greater than 20 mm Hg)
      i) Primary pulmonary hypertension: idiopathic
      ii) Secondary pulmonary hypertension
         (a) Passive pulmonary hypertension: result of back pressure
            (i) Mitral stenosis
            (ii) Left ventricular failure
         (b) Active pulmonary hypertension
            (i) Constriction of the pulmonary circulation is caused by decreased alveolar oxygen concentration (called *hypoxemic pulmonary hypertension*), acidosis, or endogenous agents such as epinephrine; norepinephrine; angiotensin II
            (ii) Obstruction in pulmonary circuit: pulmonary embolus
   b) Dilation of the pulmonary circulation caused by:
      i) Oxygen
      ii) Pulmonary vasodilators (e.g., isoproterenol, aminophylline, epoprostenol [Flolan], bosentan [Tracleer], nitric oxide), prostaglandins, phosphodiesterase inhibitors (e.g., sildenafil [Viagra])

b. Bronchial circulation
   1) This system consists of the nutrient and oxygen circulation for the tracheobronchial tree down to terminal bronchioles, visceral pleura, interstitial and connective tissue, some arteries and veins, lymph nodes, and nerves within the thoracic cavity.
      a) Two bronchial arteries to the left lung: directly off the aorta
      b) One bronchial artery to the right lung: from the intercostal artery that originates from the right subclavian or internal mammary artery
   2) Gas exchange units are supplied with nutrients and oxygen by the pulmonary circulation.
   3) Bronchial venous blood enters the pulmonary veins and causes some desaturation of the oxygenated blood in the pulmonary vein; this venous blood and the blood from the thebesian veins accounts for the normal physiologic shunt of 3-5%.

5. Thoracic cage (Figure 4-6)
   a. Muscular walls reinforced by bones
      1) Sternum anterior: three connected flat bones
         a) Manubrium
         b) Body
         c) Xiphoid
      2) Spine posterior: 12 pairs of ribs are attached to the vertebrae
      3) Ribs anterior, lateral, and posterior
         a) Seven pairs of ribs, called *true ribs*, are attached to sternum
         b) Five pairs of ribs are attached to the rib above it
      4) Clavicles superior
      5) Diaphragm: inferior border of the thoracic cage
   b. Properties
      1) Rigid to protect the lungs
      2) Resilient to allow expansion and reduction of lung volume that occurs during ventilation
   c. Contents
      1) Heart
      2) Lungs
      3) Esophagus

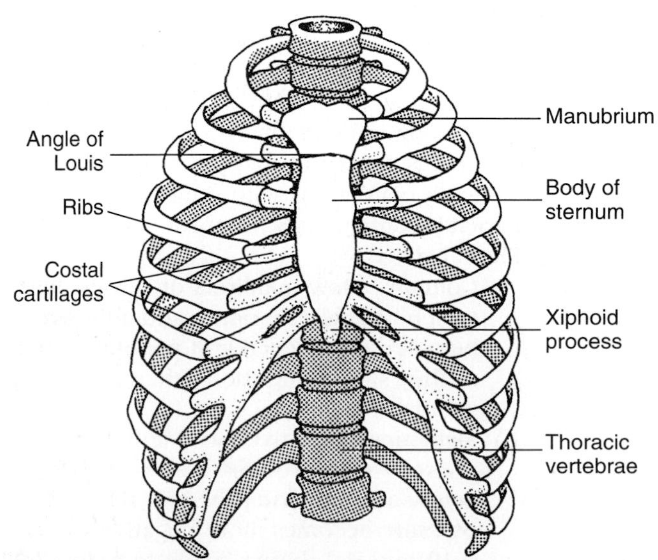

Figure 4-6 The thoracic cage. (From Scanlan, C. L., Spearman, C. B., & Sheldon, R. L. [Eds.]. [1990]. *Egan's fundamentals of respiratory care* [6th ed.]. St. Louis: Mosby.)

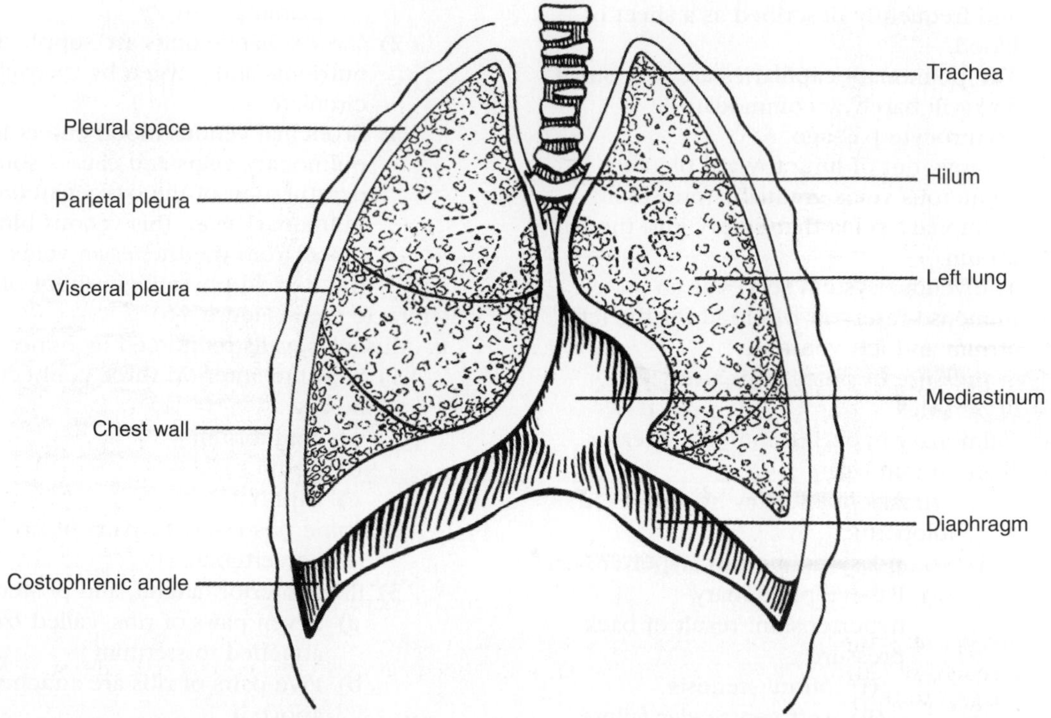

Figure 4-7 Internal structures of the thorax, including pleural cavities. (From Dettenmeier, P. A. [1992]. *Pulmonary nursing care*. St. Louis: Mosby.)

4) Great vessels
5) Liver
6) Spleen

6. Pleural cavities (Figure 4-7)
    a. Each lung hangs in its own pleural cavity attached only at the hilum; the hilum is where the two mainstem bronchi branch and where the pulmonary vessels enter and leave the thoracic space.
    b. Pleural cavities are independent of one another.
    c. The borders of pleural cavities are as follows:
        1) Chest wall lateral
        2) Mediastinum medial
        3) Diaphragm inferior
    d. Pleural linings consist of two layers.
        1) Visceral: contiguous with lung
        2) Parietal: contiguous with chest wall
        3) Pleural space
            a) Contains a few milliliters of serous fluid which acts as a lubricant and adhesive between the visceral and parietal pleura as they slide along each other with each ventilatory cycle
            b) Maintains a negative intrapleural pressure of approximately −5 mm Hg below atmospheric pressure; this pressure becomes more negative (−10 mm Hg) during inspiration; loss of this negative intrapleural pressure causes the lung to collapse (e.g., pneumothorax)
7. Mediastinum: center of thoracic cavity; contains the following:
    a. Heart and great vessels
    b. Trachea and mainstem bronchi
    c. Esophagus
    d. Phrenic, vagus, and other nerves
    e. Lymph nodes and ducts
    f. Thymus gland
8. Muscles of ventilation (Figure 4-8)
    a. Inspiratory
        1) Diaphragm
            a) Innervation occurs via phrenic nerves (C3-C5)
            b) The diaphragm consists of two hemidiaphragms connected by a central membranous tendon; this tendon is contiguous with the fibrous pericardium
            c) Contraction flattens the diaphragm
                i) Increases size of thorax superior-inferior
                ii) Normally accounts for 70% of tidal volume during quiet breathing
            d) Relaxation makes the diaphragm dome shaped and decreases the volume of the thoracic cavity
        2) External intercostals
            a) Innervation occurs from T1-T12
            b) Contraction raises the ribs, increasing the size of thorax anteroposteriorly
        3) Accessory muscles of inspiration
            a) Scalene

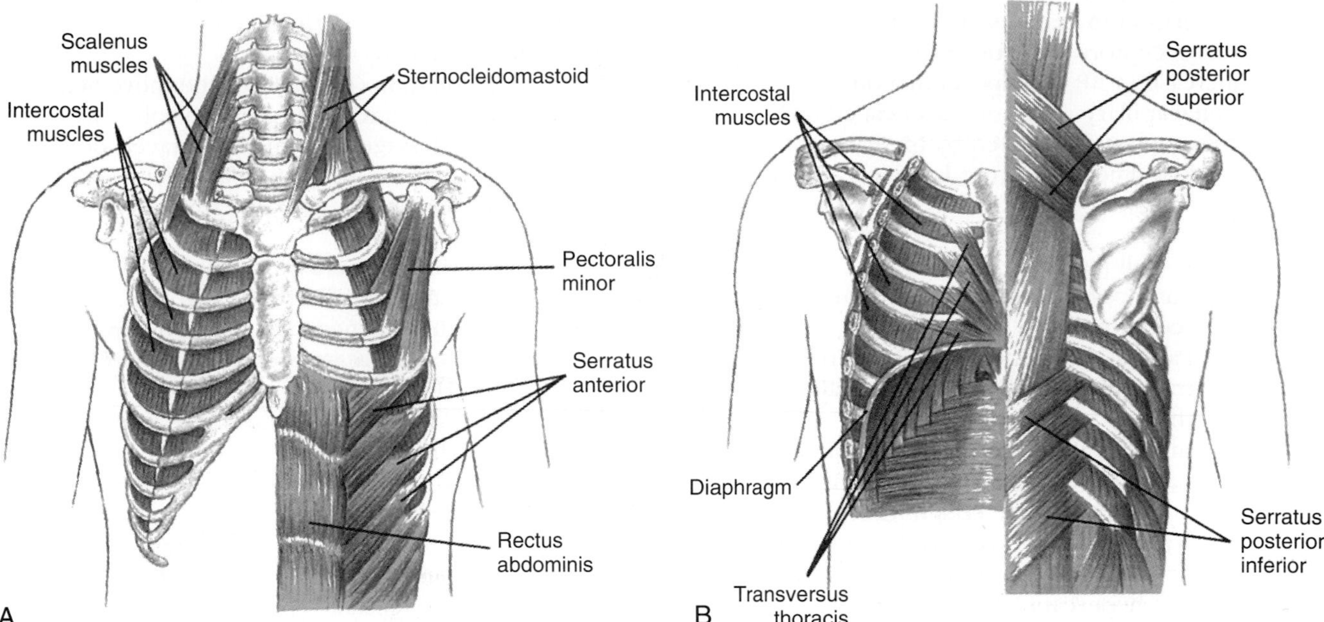

Figure 4-8 Muscles of ventilation. **A,** Anterior. **B,** Posterior. (From Urden, L., Stacy, K., & Lough, M. [2010]. *Thelan's critical care nursing: Diagnosis and management* [6th ed.]. St. Louis: Mosby.)

i) Located in the neck; stretch from the first cervical vertebrae to the first and second ribs
ii) Enlarge the upper rib cage

b) Sternocleidomastoid
i) Located in the neck; stretch from the manubrium and clavicle to the mastoid process and occipital bone
ii) Elevate the sternum to increase the anteroposterior and transverse diameter of the chest

c) Not used in normal resting ventilation but used during exercise and in respiratory distress; also used in the inspiratory phase of sneeze or cough

b. Expiratory
1) Expiration is normally passive
a) It occurs when diaphragm and external intercostals relax and return to resting position.
b) The natural tendency of the lungs is to collapse as they are made of elastic tissue; elastance is the quality of the lungs to recoil after inspiration.
2) Accessory muscles of expiration: internal oblique; external oblique; rectus abdominis, internal intercostal, and transverse abdominis
a) Depress the lower ribs and pull down the anterior portion of the lower chest
b) Increase pressure in abdominal cavity and compress the abdominal viscera up against the diaphragm
c) Used when increased levels of ventilation are needed
d) Important in forceful expiration, coughing, and sneezing

9. Neuroanatomy
a. Medulla: central chemoreceptors sensitive to cerebrospinal fluid (CSF) pH (↑ $PaCO_2$ → acidosis)
1) Primary control of ventilation is by these central chemoreceptors and $PaCO_2$ and pH levels.
2) They respond to minimal changes in $PaCO_2$ very quickly.
3) Adjustment of alveolar ventilation occurs.
a) Increase in $PaCO_2$ causes an increase in the rate and depth of ventilation.
b) Decrease in $PaCO_2$ causes a decrease in the rate and depth of ventilation.

b. Arterial chemoreceptors in aortic arch and carotid bodies: sensitive to pH, PaO_2
1) These peripheral chemoreceptors and PaO_2 levels provide secondary control of ventilation.
2) They will not respond to $PaCO_2$ levels until a 10 mm Hg change is seen.
3) They respond when PaO_2 falls below approximately 60 mm Hg; particularly important in patients with chronically elevated levels of $PaCO_2$.

c. Pontine: control rhythmic ventilation
1) Apneustic center stimulates inspiratory center.
2) Pneumotaxic center inhibits inspiratory activity.

d. Stretch receptors in alveoli (Hering-Breuer reflex): inhibit further inspiration to prevent overdistention of alveoli; may cause bronchodilation, tachycardia, vasodilation

e. Proprioceptors in muscles and tendons: increase ventilation in response to body movements
f. Baroreceptors in aortic arch and carotid bodies: increase in BP inhibits ventilation
g. Juxtacapillary receptors (also called *pulmonary J receptors*): stimulated by increase in interstitial fluid volume; may cause laryngeal constriction, hypotension, bradycardia, mucous production, dyspnea
h. Chest wall pain receptors
   1) Lung parenchyma does not have pain receptors.
   2) Parietal pleura does have pain receptors; transmit impulses via intercostal nerves and thoracic ganglia
i. Irritant receptors: stimulated by pulmonary edema, chemical or mechanical irritation; may cause bronchospasm, cough, mucus production
j. Modifying influences: drugs; brain trauma, edema, or increased intracranial pressure; chronic hypercapnia

Physiology (Figure 4-9)

1. Ventilation: movement of air between atmosphere and alveoli and distribution of air within the lungs to maintain appropriate concentrations of oxygen and carbon dioxide in the alveoli
   a. Process (Figure 4-10)
      1) Inspiration (inhalation): the movement of atmospheric air into the alveoli
         a) Message from medulla travels down phrenic nerve to diaphragm.
         b) Diaphragm and external intercostals contract.
         c) Size of thorax increases.
         d) Lungs are stretched and intrapulmonary pressure is decreased to less than atmospheric pressure (−1 cm H_2O).
         e) Air movement into lungs to equalize the difference between atmospheric and alveolar pressure
      2) Expiration (exhalation): movement of air from alveoli to the atmosphere
         a) Relaxation of diaphragm and external intercostals
         b) Recoil of lungs to their resting size and a concomitant increase in alveolar pressure above atmospheric pressure (+1 cm H_2O)

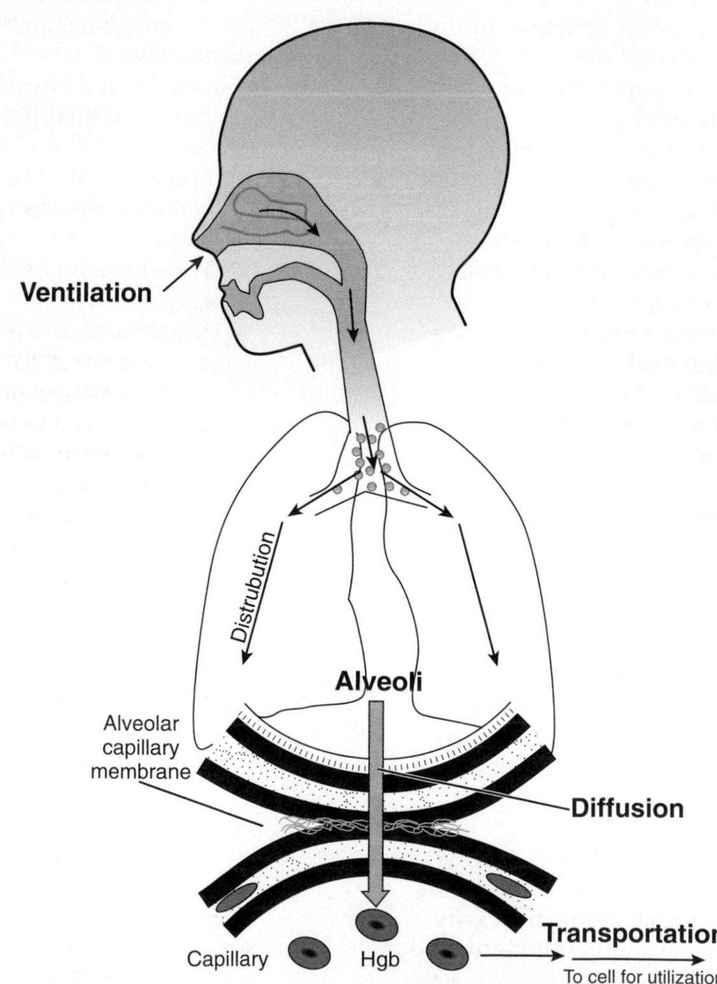

Figure 4-9 Respiratory process: ventilation, distribution, diffusion, transportation, cellular utilization. *Hgb,* Hemoglobin.

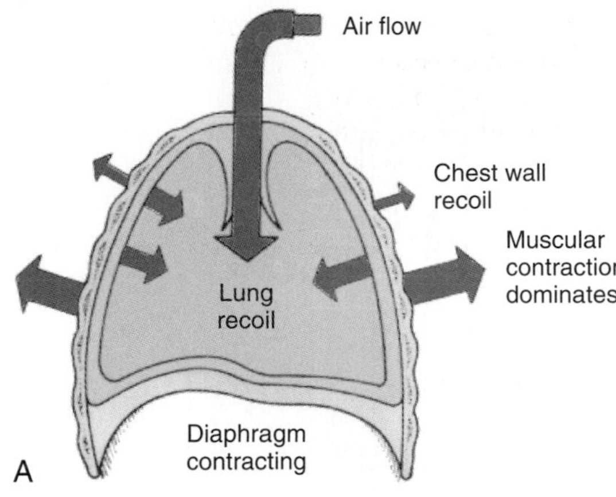

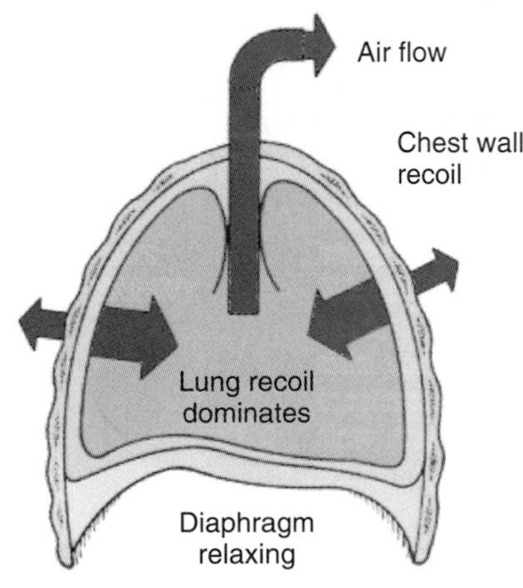

Figure 4-10 The process of ventilation. (Modified from McCance, K. L., & Huether, S. E. [2010]. *Pathophysiology: The biologic basis for disease in adults and children* [6th ed.]. St. Louis: Mosby.)

c) Air movement out of lungs to equalize the pressure difference

b. Efficiency of ventilation: evaluated by $PaCO_2$
   1) $PaCO_2$ greater than 45 mm Hg indicates hypoventilation.
   2) $PaCO_2$ less than 35 mm Hg indicates hyperventilation

c. Lung volumes (Figure 4-11 and Table 4-1)
   1) Alveolar ventilation is the volume of air per minute participating in gas exchange; it is the most important portion of minute ventilation; minute ventilation minus dead space ventilation.
   2) Dead space ventilation (Figure 4-12) is the volume of air per minute that does not participate in gas exchange.
      a) Anatomical dead space is the volume of air in conducting airways and does not participate in gas exchange; approximately 2 mL/kg of tidal volume
      b) Alveolar (pathologic) dead space is the volume of air in contact with nonperfused alveoli.
      c) Physiologic dead space is anatomical plus alveolar dead space.
         i) Calculated by:

$$\frac{V_D}{V_T} = \frac{PaCO_2 - P_ECO_2}{PaCO_2}$$

Normal: 0.2-0.4

d. Work of breathing = work of deforming the elastic system + work of producing airflow through the airways (Figure 4-13)
   1) Usually the work of breathing is negligible: 2-3% of total energy expenditure by the body
   2) Compliance
      a) Measure of expandability of lungs and/or thorax:
      b) $C = \frac{\text{Change in volume}}{\text{Change in pressure}}$
         i) Static compliance: affected by changes in compliance of chest wall or lung
         ii) Dynamic compliance: affected by changes in compliance of chest wall or lung or airway resistance
         iii) Calculation of static and dynamic compliance (Figure 4-14, Table 4-2)
      c) Factors affecting static compliance
         i) Chest wall changes
            (a) Kyphoscoliosis
            (b) Flail chest
            (c) Thoracic pain with splinting
            (d) Obesity
         ii) Lung changes
            (a) Atelectasis
            (b) Pneumonia
            (c) Pulmonary edema
            (d) Pulmonary fibrosis
            (e) Pleural effusion
            (f) Pneumothorax
      d) Additional factors affecting dynamic compliance
         i) As previously mentioned and airway resistance changes; the difference between static and dynamic compliance represents airway resistance
   3) Airway resistance
      a) Pressure differential required to produce a unit flow change; affected by airway caliber and length
      b) Factors affecting airway resistance (and dynamic compliance)
         i) Bronchospasm
         ii) Mucus
         iii) Artificial airways
         iv) Water condensation in ventilator tubing
         v) Mucosal edema
         vi) Bronchial tumor

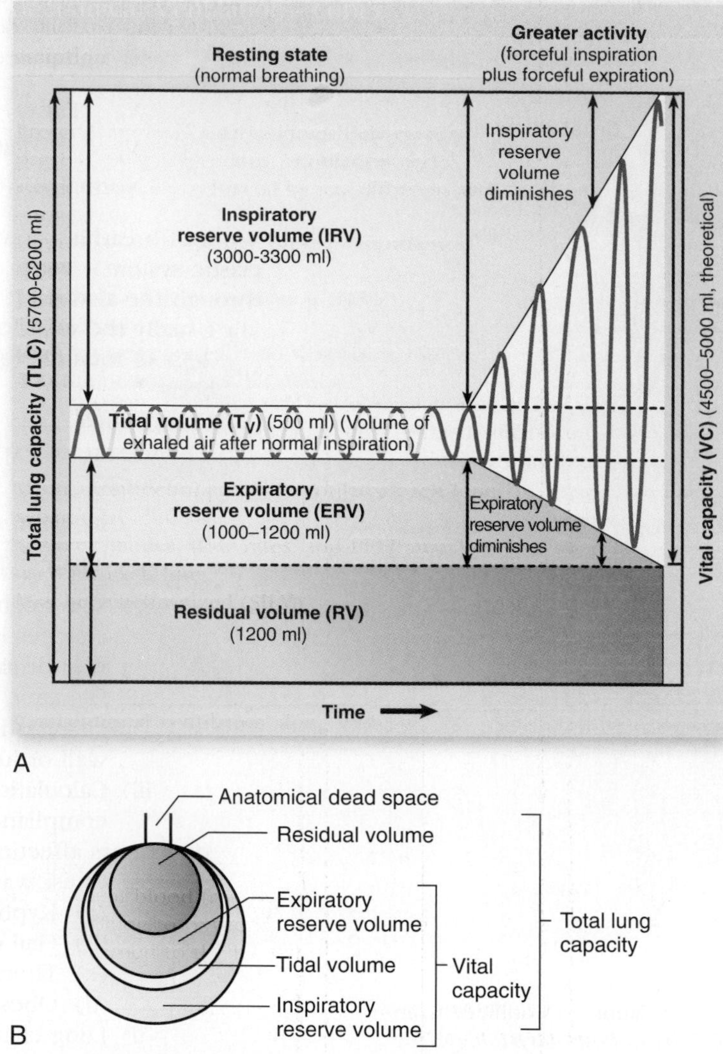

Figure 4-11 Lung volumes and capacities. Note that upward deflection reflects inspiration and downward deflection reflects expiration. **A,** Spirometry. **B,** Lung volumes. (From Patton, K. T., & Thibodeau, G. A. [2010]. *Anatomy & physiology* [7th ed.]. St. Louis: Mosby.)

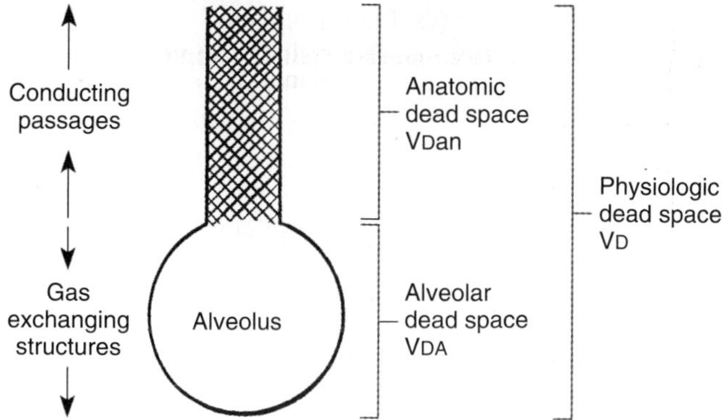

Figure 4-12 Physiologic dead space: anatomic dead space and alveolar dead space. (Drawing by Wendy W. Johnson.)

2. Perfusion: movement of blood through the pulmonary capillaries
   a. Pulmonary vasculature: resistance varies to accommodate the blood flow that it receives
   b. Distribution of perfusion
      1) Related to gravity and intraalveolar pressures
         a) Gravity causes the pressure in the capillaries in the bases to be higher than the pressure in the capillaries in the apices; preferential blood flow to the gravity-dependent areas of the lungs
         b) The intraalveolar pressures are generally equal throughout the lungs
         c) This creates the potential for intraalveolar pressure to exceed capillary hydrostatic pressure in some areas of the lung causing absence of blood flow to these areas.
      2) Zones (Figure 4-15)
         a) Zone 1: nondependent portion of the lung; potential for no perfusion;
         b) Zone 2: middle portion of the lung; varying blood flow
         c) Zone 3: gravity-dependent area of the lung; receives constant blood flow; pulmonary artery catheters ideally are

Table 4-1 Lung Volumes, Capacities, and Mechanics

Volume	Definition	Normal
Tidal Volume (V_T)	The volume of air moved in and out of the lungs with each normal breath	7 mL/kg or
Inspiratory Reserve Volume (IRV)	The volume of air that can be maximally inspired above the normal inspiratory level	3000 mL
Expiratory Reserve Volume (ERV)	The volume of air that can be maximally exhaled beyond the normal expiratory level	1000 mL
Residual Volume (RV)	The volume of air remaining in the lungs at the end of a maximal expiration	1000 mL
Inspiratory Capacity (IC)	V_T + IRC; the volume of air that can be maximally inspired from a normal expiratory level	3500 mL
Functional Residual Capacity (FRC)	RV + ERV; the volume of air remaining in the lungs at the end of normal expiration	2000 mL
Vital Capacity (VC)	V_T + IRC + ERV; the volume of air that can be maximally expired after a maximal inspiration	4500 mL
Total Lung Capacity (TLC)	V_T + IRC + ERV + RV; the volume of air that the lungs can hold with maximal inspiration	5500-6000 mL
Respiratory rate or frequency (f)	The number of breaths per minute	12-20
Minute Ventilation (M_E)	$V_T \times f$; the volume of air expired per minute	5-10 L
Dead Space (V_D)	$V_D/V_T = PaCO_2 - PeCO_2/PaCO_2$ $PaCO_2$ (arterial); $PeCO_2$ (exhaled) The volume or percentage of the V_T that does not participate in gas exchange; includes the volume of air in the conducting pathways (anatomical dead space) plus the volume of alveolar air that is not involved in gas exchange due to pathology (alveolar dead space)	V_D/V_T ratio is normally less than 0.4; V_D/V_T greater than 0.6 is usually an indication for mechanical ventilation
Alveolar Ventilation (V_A)	$V_T - V_D$; the volume of tidal air that is involved in alveolar gas exchange	350 mL
Forced Vital Capacity (FVC)	The volume of air in a forceful maximal expiration	Normally same as VC: 4500 mL
Forced Expiratory Volume (FEV)	The volume of air exhaled in a given time period; FEV_1: the volume of air exhaled in 1 second; FEV_3: the volume of air exhaled in 3 seconds	FEV_1: greater than 75% of VC FEV_3: greater than 95% of VC

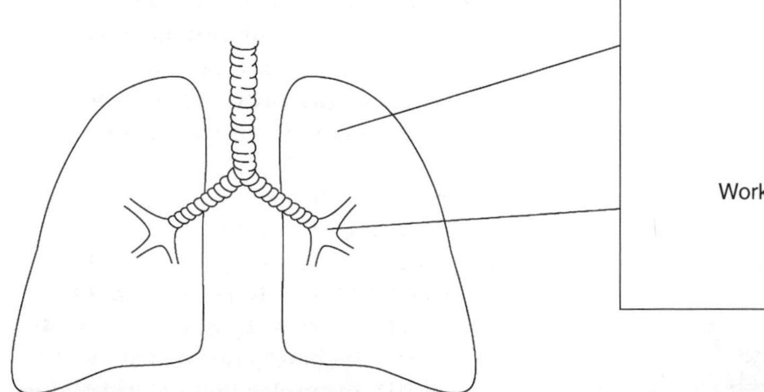

WORK OF BREATHING =

Work of deforming elastic system
(Compliance)
(Disorders known as *restrictive*)
+
Work of producing airflow through the airways
(Airway resistance)
(Disorders known as *obstructive*)

Figure 4-13 The work of breathing.

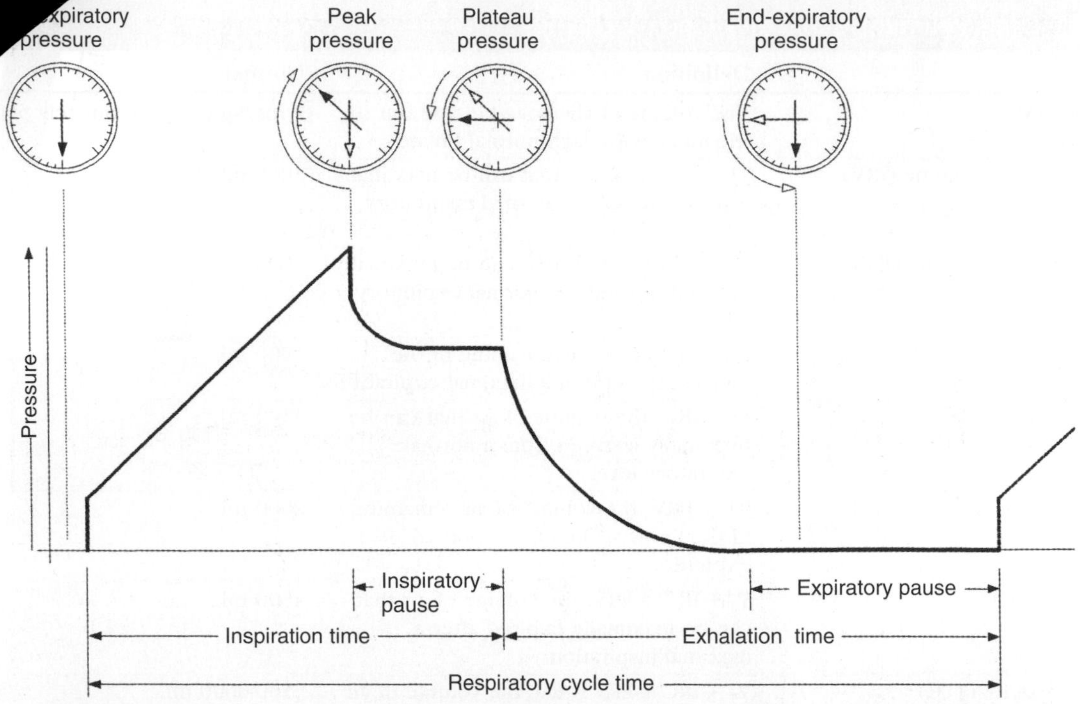

Figure 4-14 Airway pressure in a patient on positive pressure ventilation. Plateau pressure is used to calculate static compliance. Peak pressure is used to calculate dynamic compliance. The difference between static and dynamic compliance represents airway resistance. Remember that PEEP levels are subtracted from the plateau or peak pressures before calculation of compliance. (From Dupuis, Y. G [1992]. *Ventilators: Theory and clinical application* [2nd ed.]. St. Louis: Mosby-Year Book.)

Table 4-2 Types of Compliance

Type	Formula	Normal	Significance
Static compliance	$\frac{\text{Tidal volume}}{\text{Plateau pressure} - \text{PEEP}}$	50-100 mL/cm H_2O	Affected by changes in compliance of chest wall or lung
Dynamic compliance	$\frac{\text{Tidal volume}}{\text{Peak pressure} - \text{PEEP}}$	35-55 mL/cm H_2O	Affected by changes in compliance of chest wall or lung or airway resistance

placed in zone 3 for accurate reflection of left atrial pressure by the PAOP

3) Hypoxemic pulmonary vasoconstriction
   a) Localized
      i) Protective mechanism which decreases blood flow to an area of poor ventilation so that blood can be shunted to areas of better ventilation
      ii) Stimulated by decreased alveolar oxygen levels
   b) Generalized
      i) If all alveoli have low oxygen levels as occurs with alveolar hypoventilation, hypoxemic pulmonary vasoconstriction may be distributed over the lungs.
      ii) Increases pulmonary vascular resistance (PVR) and PAP
      iii) Right ventricular hypertrophy and failure (cor pulmonale) may result
         (a) Chronic cor pulmonale: chronic conditions such as COPD
         (b) Acute cor pulmonale: acute conditions such as pulmonary embolism

c. Ventilation (V)/perfusion (Q) ratio
   1) Normal (Figure 4-16): alveolar minute ventilation = ~4 L; normal cardiac output (100% goes to lungs) = ~5 L; normal V/Q ratio = 0.8
   2) Pathologic mismatch (Figure 4-17)
      a) Dead space: V greater than Q
         i) V/Q ratio greater than 0.8 (i.e., high V/Q ratio)
         ii) Examples include pulmonary embolism, shock, and decrease in

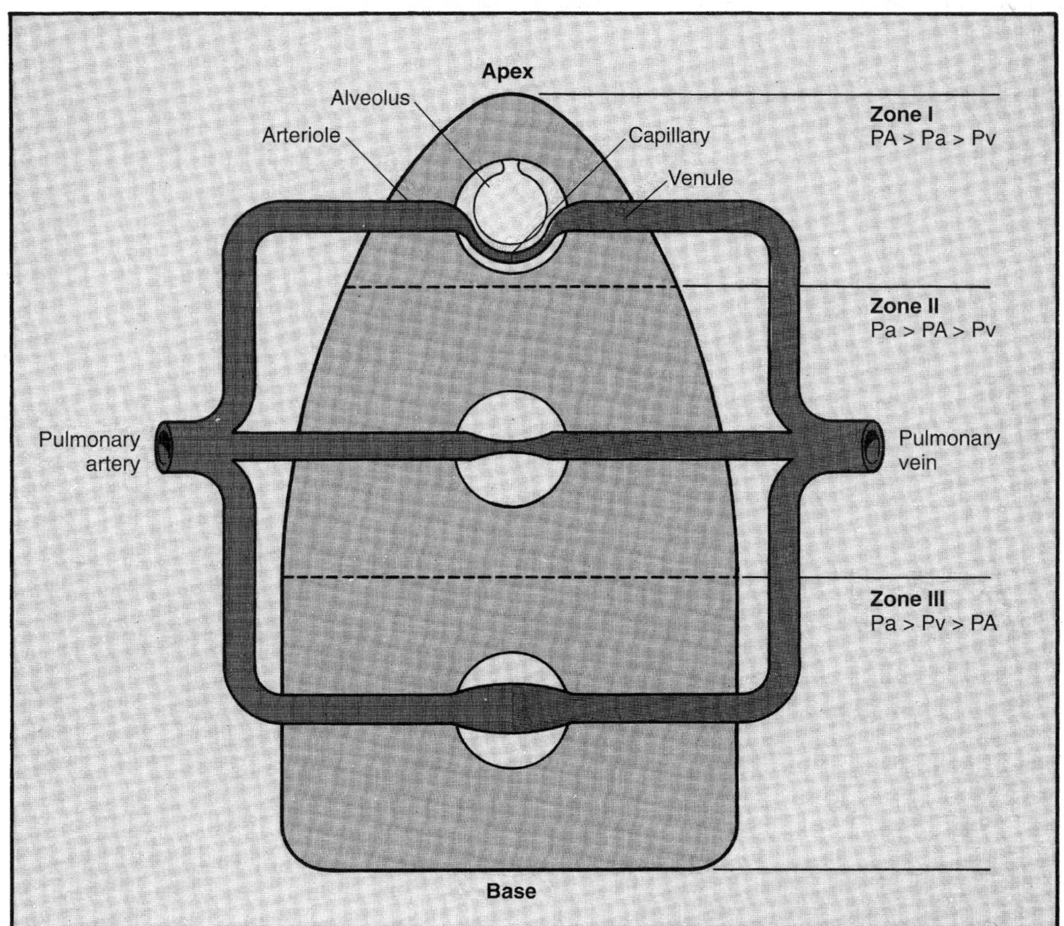

Figure 4-15 Zones of distribution of perfusion: relationship of alveolar pressure (PA) and gravitational forces to pulmonary vascular pressures and blood flow. The upright lung can be divided into three zones. In zone I, the upper third of the lung, alveolar pressure exceeds pulmonary venous (Pv) and pulmonary arterial (Pa) pressures. In zone II, the middle third of the lung, the pulmonary artery pressure is greater than alveolar pressure, which is greater than pulmonary venous pressure. In zone III, the lower third of the lung, pulmonary artery pressure is greater than pulmonary venous pressure, which is greater than alveolar pressure. NOTE: Pulmonary artery catheters are positioned in zone III for accurate measurement of PAOP as a reflection of left atrial pressure. (From McCance, K. L., & Huether, S. E. [2010]. *Pathophysiology: The biologic basis for disease in adults and children* [6th ed.]. St. Louis: Mosby.)

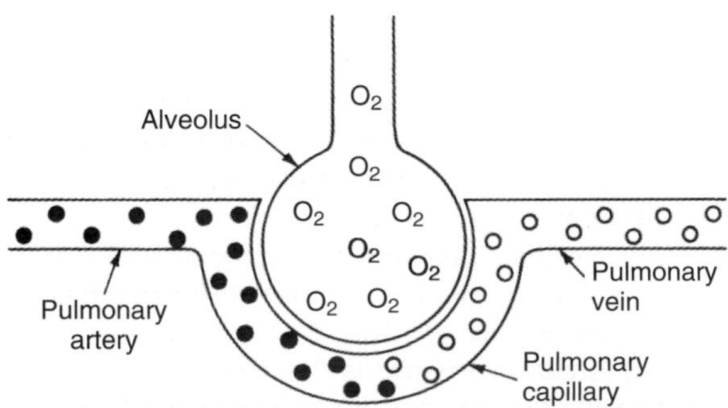

Figure 4-16 Normal V/Q ratio: normal alveolar ventilation per minute is approximately 4 L, and normal perfusion (cardiac output) is approximately 5 L/min; normal V/Q ratio is 0.8. (From Kinney, M. R., et al. [1998]. *AACN's clinical reference for critical-care nursing* [4th ed.]. St. Louis: Mosby.)

perfusion to the lung caused by excessive tidal volume or PEEP.

b) Shunt: Q greater than V
   i) V/Q ratio less than 0.8 (i.e., low V/Q ratio)
   ii) Examples include atelectasis, acute respiratory distress syndrome, and pneumonia.
   iii) PaO_2 less than 60 mm Hg with an FiO_2 of 0.5 or greater suggests clinically significant shunt.
   iv) There are several methods of estimating shunt (Table 4-3).

c) Silent: no V or Q

3) Positional mismatch (Figure 4-18)
   a) Greatest ventilation in superior areas
   b) Greatest perfusion in inferior areas

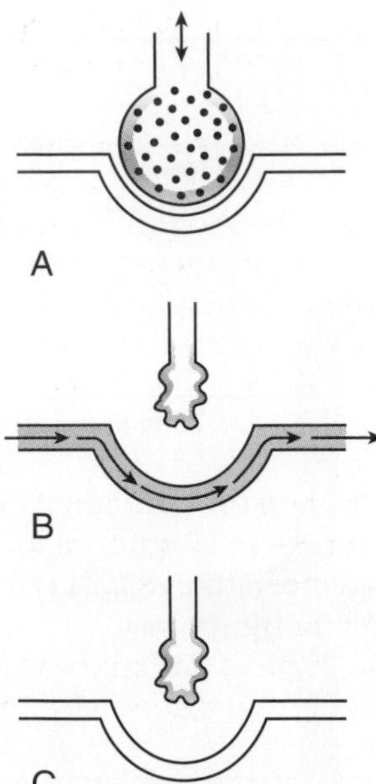

Figure 4-17 Abnormal V/Q ratio. **A,** High V/Q ratio with ventilation exceeding perfusion; also called a *dead space unit.* **B,** Low V/Q ratio with perfusion exceeding ventilation; also called a *shunt unit.* **C,** Absent ventilation and perfusion, referred to as a *silent unit.* (From Kinney, M. R., et al. [1998]. *AACN's clinical reference for critical-care nursing* [4th ed.]. St. Louis: Mosby.)

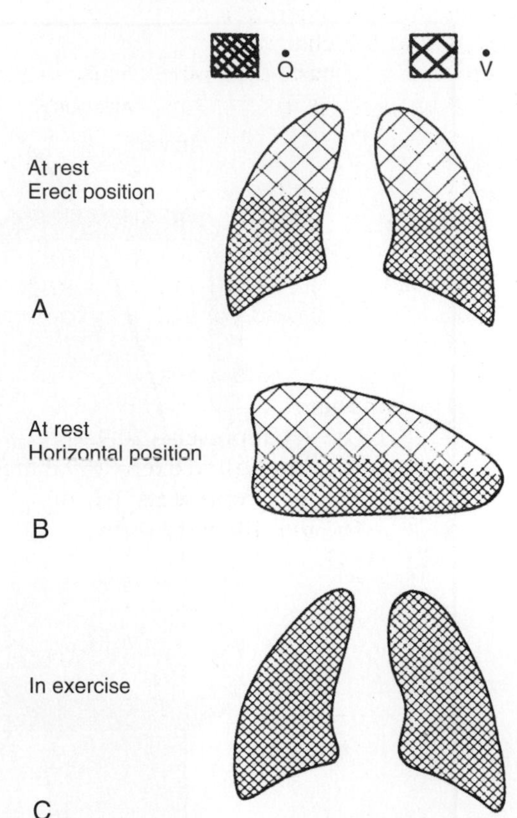

Figure 4-18 Positional changes in ventilation and perfusion. **A,** While one is sitting or standing, the upper lobes are ventilated best and the lower lobes are perfused best. **B,** While one is lying on one side, the superior lung is ventilated best and the inferior lung is perfused best. **C,** In exercise, ventilation and perfusion are increased and optimally matched throughout. (From Wade, J. F. [1982]. *Comprehensive respiratory care.* St. Louis: Mosby.)

Table 4-3 Methods of Estimating Intrapulmonary Shunt

Parameter	Formula	Normal
a/A ratio	(PaO_2/PAO_2)	• Normal: greater than 0.8 • Moderate: 0.5-0.8 • Significant: 0.25-0.5 • Critical: less than 0.25
A:a gradient	$PAO_2 - PaO_2$	• Less than 10 mm Hg • A:a gradient × 0.05 = approximate % shunt
PaO_2/FiO_2 (or P/F) ratio	$\frac{PaO_2}{FiO_2}$	• Greater than 300 • 300 = ~15% shunt • 200 = ~20% shunt
Respiratory index	$\frac{PAO_2 - PaO_2}{PaO_2}$	• Less than 1

FiO_2, Fraction of inspired oxygen (written as a decimal); *$PaCO_2$,* arterial carbon dioxide tension; *PAO_2,* alveolar oxygen tension; *PaO_2,* arterial oxygen tension; *Pb,* barometric pressure (760 mm Hg at sea level, adjust for higher altitudes).

NOTE: PaO_2 is obtained by arterial blood gas measurement. PAO_2 is calculated as: FiO_2 (Pb - 47) - ($PaCO_2$/ 0.8). The pressure of water vapor at sea level is 47 and is subtracted from barometric pressure; 0.8 is the usual respiratory quotient.

c) This is rationale for "good lung down" in unilateral lung conditions.
   i) Improves ventilation to the "bad lung" (e.g., atelectasis, pneumonia, pneumothorax) and optimizes perfusion to the "good lung"
   ii) Exception is pneumonectomy: Patient is positioned on the operative side or back so "no lung down."

3. Distribution: movement of inspired air into lobes, segments, lobules
   a. Transpulmonary pressure or distending pressure is equal to alveolar pressure minus pleural pressure.
      1) Alveolar pressure is the pressure that reaches the alveoli after resistance has been overcome.
      2) Pleural pressure is determined by gravity.
   b. Closing volume is lung volume present when a significant number of small alveoli close.
4. Diffusion: movement of gases between the alveoli, plasma, and RBCs
   a. Gases diffuse from areas of higher concentration to areas of lower concentration regardless of

medium until concentration is the same throughout the chamber.

b. Dalton's law of partial pressure (Figure 4-19): In a mixture of gases the pressure exerted by each gas is independent of the other gases and directly corresponds to the percentage of the total mixture that it represents.
   1) Atmospheric (or barometric) pressure, the pressure exerted by the weight of the atmosphere, is 760 mm Hg at sea level; adjustments should be made when at high altitudes.
      a) Components and pressures in the atmosphere
         i) Oxygen represents 20.9% of 760 mm Hg and exerts 159 mm Hg.
         ii) Nitrogen represents 79% of 760 mm Hg and exerts 597 mm Hg.
         iii) Carbon dioxide represents 0.03% of 760 mm Hg and exerts 0.2 mm Hg.
         iv) Water vapor represents 0.5% of 760 mm Hg and exerts 3.8 mm Hg.
   2) During inspiration, the upper airway warms and humidifies atmospheric air which increases the pressure of the vapor to 47 mm Hg; the partial pressures of the other gases must decrease as the total cannot exceed barometric pressure of 760 mm Hg; example:
      760 (barometric pressure at sea level)
      – 47 (pressure of water vapor at body temperature) × 0.21 (FiO_2 of room air)
      = 150 mm Hg
   3) As the inspired gas mixes with gas that was not expired, the concentrations of CO_2 and O_2 change again.

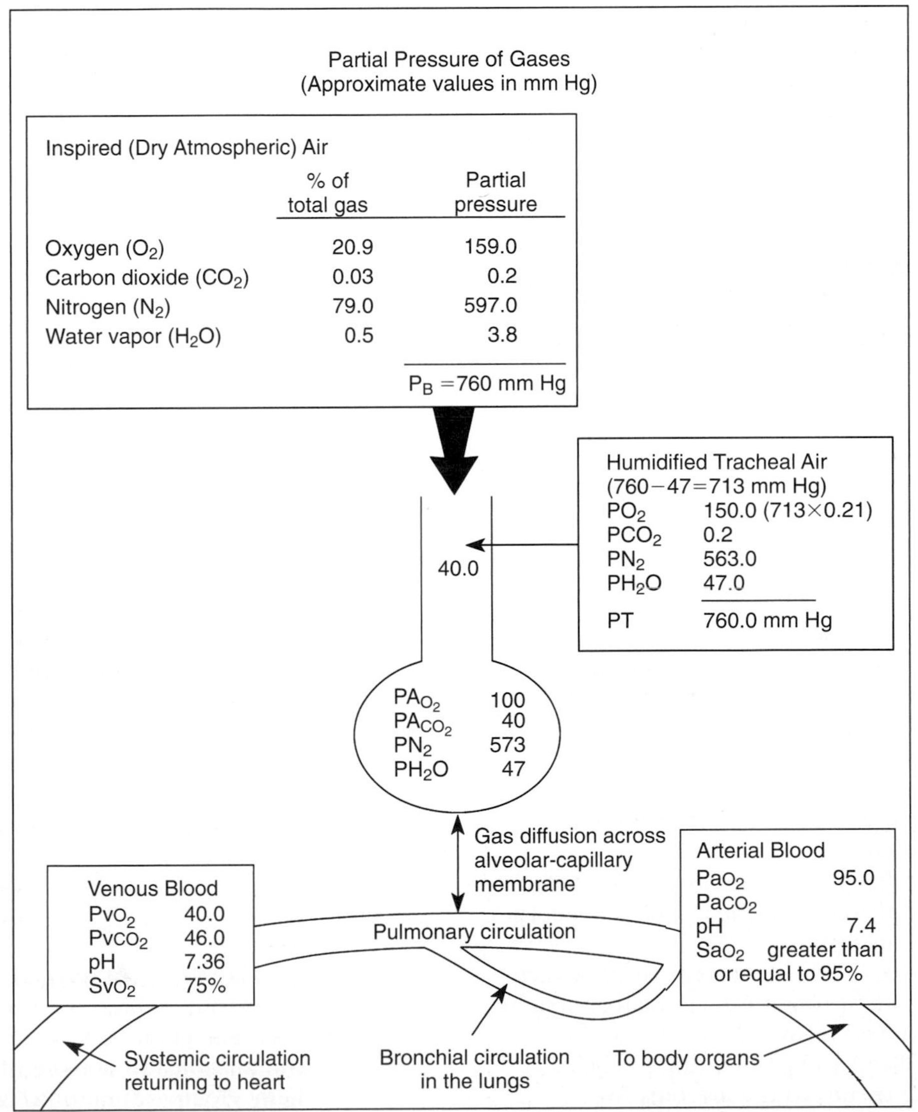

Figure 4-19 Dalton's law of partial pressure. P_T, Pressure of tracheal air; PaO_2, alveolar pressure of oxygen; $PaCO_2$, alveolar pressure of carbon dioxide; PvO_2, partial oxygen pressure in mixed venous blood; $PvCO_2$, partial carbon dioxide pressure in mixed venous blood; PH_2O, partial pressure of water vapor; PN_2, partial pressure of nitrogen; SvO_2, venous oxygen saturation; SaO_2, arterial oxygen saturation.

4) Alveolar air is high in oxygen pressure and low in carbon dioxide pressure, and the pulmonary capillary blood is high in carbon dioxide pressure and low in oxygen pressure.
5) This differential in partial pressure of oxygen and carbon dioxide causes the gases to move across the alveolar-capillary membrane toward the lower side of the respective pressure gradients (e.g., oxygen moves from the alveolus to the capillary, and carbon dioxide moves from the capillary to the alveolus).

c. Determinants of diffusion
1) Surface area available for gas transfer
   a) Fick's law of diffusion: the rate of transfer of a gas through a sheet of tissue is proportional to the tissue area; alveolar surface area is normally immense
   b) Negatively affected by pulmonary resection (e.g., lobectomy or pneumonectomy) or emphysema
2) Thickness of the alveolar-capillary membrane: negatively affected by pulmonary edema or fibrosis
3) Diffusion coefficient of gas
   a) CO_2 is 20 times more diffusible than O_2
      i) Diffusion problems cause hypoxemia but they do not cause hypercapnia.
      ii) Hypercapnia indicates hypoventilation (e.g., respiratory muscle fatigue).
4) Driving pressure
   a) Fraction of the gas × barometric pressure
   b) Negatively affected by low inspired fraction of oxygen (e.g., smoke inhalation) or low barometric pressure (e.g., high altitudes)
   c) Positively affected by higher than normal fraction of inspired oxygen (FiO_2) (e.g., supplemental oxygen) or higher than normal barometric pressure (e.g., hyperbaric oxygen chamber)
      i) CPAP and PEEP increase the driving pressure of oxygen by keeping the pressure above zero throughout the entire ventilatory cycle

5. Transport of gases in blood: movement of oxygen and carbon dioxide through the circulatory system; oxygen being moved from the alveolus to the tissues to be utilized and carbon dioxide being moved from the tissues to the alveolus for exhalation

a. Oxygen
1) Mode of transport
   a) Hgb: 97% of oxygen is combined with hemoglobin; represented by the SaO_2
      i) One molecule of hemoglobin can carry four molecules of oxygen
      ii) The amount of oxygen that the hemoglobin actually carries depends on the affinity of the hemoglobin for oxygen; there is normally more affinity at the lung level and less affinity at the tissue level due to the Bohr effect, which controls the reaction between hemoglobin and oxygen and carbon dioxide.
         (a) Oxygenated hemoglobin is a stronger acid than deoxygenated hemoglobin.
            (i) This change in pH facilitates the release of oxygen from the hemoglobin at the tissue level.
            (ii) As the hemoglobin gives up the oxygen, it becomes a weaker acid and picks up carbon dioxide for transport back to the lung.
         (b) Deoxygenated hemoglobin is a weaker acid than oxygenated hemoglobin.
            (i) This change in pH facilitates the attraction of oxygen to the hemoglobin at the lung level.
            (ii) As the hemoglobin picks up oxygen, it becomes a stronger acid and releases carbon dioxide at the lung level.
            (iii) Ability of hemoglobin to deliver oxygen to the tissues is negatively affected by:
               (1) Anemia
               (2) Abnormal hemoglobin (e.g., methemoglobinemia, carboxyhemoglobin, or hemoglobin S [sickle cell])
   b) Plasma: 3% of oxygen is dissolved in the plasma; represented by the PaO_2
2) Oxyhemoglobin dissociation curve: shows the relationship between PaO_2 and hemoglobin saturation (Figure 4-20)
   a) Critical point: PaO_2 60 mm Hg
      i) PaO_2 above 60: horizontal limb of curve; increase in PaO_2 above 60 results in minimal increases in oxygen saturation

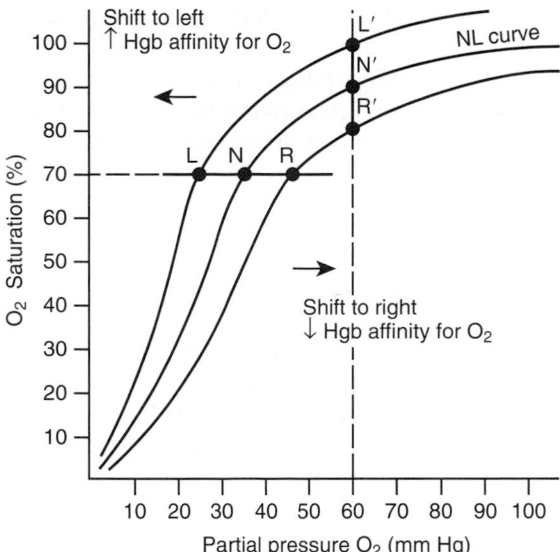

Figure 4-20 Oxyhemoglobin dissociation curve. Normal curve *(N)* optimizes pickup of O_2 at the lung and drop-off of O_2 at the tissue level; left shift *(L)* increases the affinity between O_2 and Hgb, which optimizes pickup of O_2 at the lung level but impairs drop-off of O_2 at the tissue level; right shift *(R)* decreases affinity between O_2 and Hgb, which impairs pickup of O_2 at the lung level but optimizes drop-off of O_2 at the tissue level. (From Dettenmeier, P. A. [1992]. *Pulmonary nursing care*. St. Louis: Mosby.)

ii) PaO_2 below 60: vertical limb of curve; decrease in PaO_2 below 60 mm Hg results in dramatic decreases in oxygen saturation

b) Correlation between PaO_2 and SaO_2 with a normal oxyhemoglobin dissociation curve (Table 4-4)

i) P_{50}: the partial pressure of oxygen at which hemoglobin is 50% saturated with a pH of 7.4; usually PaO_2 of 27 mm Hg

c) Shifting of the oxyhemoglobin dissociation curve

i) Decreased P_{50} and shifting of the oxyhemoglobin dissociation curve to the left

(a) Affinity of Hgb for oxygen is increased; therefore, hemoglobin is more saturated for a given PaO_2 and less oxygen is unloaded for a given PaO_2.

(b) This means that it is easier to pick up oxygen at the lung level but more difficult to drop off oxygen at the tissue level.

(c) Factors that shift the oxyhemoglobin dissociation curve to the left: alkalemia, hypothermia, hypocapnia, decreased 2,3-DPG

Table 4-4 Correlation Between PaO_2 and SaO_2 with Normal Oxyhemoglobin Dissociation Curve

PaO_2 (in mm Hg)	SaO_2 (in %)
100	98
90	97
80	95
70	93
60	90
50	85
40	75
30	57
27	50

(d) Remember: There is more LEFT over with a shift to the left.

ii) Increased P_{50} and shifting of the oxyhemoglobin dissociation curve to the right

(a) Affinity of Hgb for oxygen is decreased; therefore, hemoglobin is less saturated for a given PaO_2 and more oxygen is unloaded for a given PaO_2.

(b) This means that it is more difficult to pick up oxygen at the lung level but easier to drop off oxygen at the tissue level.

(c) Factors that shift the oxyhemoglobin dissociation curve to the right: acidemia, hyperthermia, hypercapnia, increased 2,3-DPG

(d) Remember: It is RIGHT to give it away.

iii) Discussion of 2,3-DPG (Box 4-1)

3) Oxygen capacity

a) Maximal amount of oxygen the blood can carry

b) Formula: Hgb × 1.34

i) Hemoglobin in grams/dL

ii) 1.34 represents the amount of oxygen 1 gram of hemoglobin can carry; it is a constant

4) Oxygen content in arterial blood (CaO_2)

a) Actual amount of oxygen that arterial blood is carrying

b) O_2 capacity × O_2 saturation; amount of oxygen dissolved in the plasma (.0031 × PaO_2) may be added but is such a minute factor in most situations that it is inconsequential unless the patient is hyperoxemic (e.g., hyperbaric oxygen therapy)

Box 4-1 Important Information about 2,3-Diphosphoglycerate (2,3-DPG)

What Is It?

- A substance in the erythrocyte that affects the affinity of hemoglobin for oxygen
- A chief end product of glucose metabolism and a link in the biochemical feedback control system that regulates the release of oxygen to the tissues

What Does It Do to the Oxyhemoglobin Dissociation Curve?

- Increased amounts of 2,3-DPG shift the curve to the right decreasing the affinity between hemoglobin and oxygen
- Decreased amounts of 2,3-DPG shift the curve to the left increasing the affinity between hemoglobin and oxygen

What Causes Amounts of 2,3-DPG to Increase or Decrease?

- Increased
  - Chronic hypoxemia (e.g., high altitude, congenital heart disease)
  - Anemia
  - Hyperthyroidism
  - Pyruvate kinase deficiency
- Decreased
  - Multiple blood transfusions of banked blood (i.e., total body exchange [~10 units] over minutes to hours)
  - Hypophosphatemia (e.g., malnutrition, refeeding syndrome, treatment of DKA)
  - Hypothyroidism
  - Hexokinase deficiency

c) Formula: Hgb × 1.34 × SaO_2
  i) Hemoglobin in grams/dL
  ii) 1.34 represents the amount of oxygen 1 gram of hemoglobin can carry; it is a constant
  iii) Saturation as a decimal (e.g., 95% is 0.95)
d) Normal: 18-20 mL/dL (~20 mL/dL)

5) Oxygen content in venous blood (CvO_2)
  a) Actual amount of oxygen in venous blood
  b) Formula: 1.34 × Hgb × SvO_2
    i) Hemoglobin in grams/dL
    ii) 1.34 represents the amount of oxygen 1 gram of hemoglobin can carry; it is a constant
    iii) Saturation as a decimal (e.g., 95% is 0.95)
  c) Normal: 12-16 mL/dL (~15 mL/dL)

b. CO_2: most transported as bicarbonate
  1) Carbonic acid and water in the presence of carbonic anhydrase form bicarbonate in the erythrocyte.
  2) Five percent is dissolved in plasma ($PaCO_2$).
  3) Five percent is combined with hemoglobin as carbaminohemoglobin; CO_2 attaches to hemoglobin at a different bonding site than oxygen.

c. Diffusion between systemic capillary bed and body tissues: pressure gradients allow diffusion
  1) Haldane effect: In the tissue, as O_2 leaves hemoglobin, increased CO_2 is able to be picked up by hemoglobin; in the lungs, the binding of oxygen with hemoglobin tends to displace CO_2.
  2) Oxygen diffusion to peripheral tissues is affected by the following:
    a) Quantity and rate of blood flow
    b) Difference in capillary and tissue oxygen pressures
    c) Capillary surface area
    d) Capillary permeability
    e) Intracapillary distance

6. Oxygen delivery to the tissues (see Chapter 2)
7. Cellular respiration: utilization of oxygen by the cell
  a. Estimated by the amount of carbon dioxide produced and the oxygen consumed
    1) Respiratory quotient (RQ): ratio of these two values
      a) Normally 0.8 but changes occur according to the nutritional substrate being utilized; primary carbohydrate metabolism changes the ratio to 1.0 as carbohydrate metabolism produces more carbon dioxide than does the metabolism of protein or fat
      b) Simplified Krebs cycle: food is converted by the body to H_2O and CO_2 and cellular energy (ATP)
    2) Variables affecting oxygen consumption
      a) Increased oxygen consumption
        i) Increased work of breathing
        ii) Hyperthermia
        iii) Trauma
        iv) Sepsis
        v) Anxiety
        vi) Hyperthyroidism
        vii) Muscle tremors or seizures
      b) Decreased oxygen consumption
        i) Hypothermia
        ii) Sedation
        iii) Neuromuscular blockade
        iv) Anesthesia
        v) Hypothyroidism
        vi) Inactivity
  b. Oxygen is utilized by the mitochondria in the production of cellular energy; oxygen deficit may result in lethal cell injury if prolonged.
8. Metabolic functions of the lung
  a. Synthesis of interferon and tumor inhibiting factor
  b. Production, conversion, or removal of many vasoactive substances in the pulmonary circulation; bradykinin, serotonin, heparin, histamine, prostaglandins E, F, and certain polypeptides such as angiotensin I

Pulmonary Assessment

Interview

1. Chief complaint: why the patient is seeking help and duration of the problem; possible symptoms related to pulmonary disorders which may be identified as chief complaint may include any of the following
   a. Dyspnea or shortness of breath
      1) Onset
      2) Duration
      3) Frequency
      4) Timing: time of day; weather or season; activity; eating; talking; deep breathing
      5) Position (e.g., orthopnea)
      6) Severity
         a) Subjective scale
            i) Grade 1: shortness of breath with mild exertion, such as running a short distance or climbing a flight of stairs
            ii) Grade 2: shortness of breath while walking a short distance at a normal pace on level grade
            iii) Grade 3: shortness of breath with mild daily activity such as shaving or bathing
            iv) Grade 4: shortness of breath while sitting at rest
            v) Grade 5: shortness of breath while lying down
         b) Effect on ability to do activities of daily living (ADL)
         c) Frequently accentuated by anxiety
      7) Palliation: what is effective in relieving dyspnea
      8) Accompanying symptoms
         a) Cough
         b) Chest pain
         c) Wheezing
   b. Cough
      1) Onset
      2) Duration
      3) Frequency
      4) Timing: time of day, weather or season, activity, eating, talking, deep breathing
      5) Position
      6) Pattern: regular or occasional
      7) Dry or productive
      8) Accompanying symptoms
         a) Sputum production
         b) Hemoptysis
         c) Chest pain
         d) Wheezing
         e) Dyspnea
      9) Medication history: may be side effect of ACE inhibitors (e.g., captopril [Capoten], enalapril [Vasotec])
   c. Sputum production
      1) Duration
      2) Frequency
      3) Amount: use household measurements (e.g., teaspoons, tablespoons, shot glass, Dixie cup, iced tea glass)
      4) Color
      5) Consistency
      6) Odor
      7) Hemoptysis
      8) Usual treatment (e.g., expectorants, cough drops, a cigarette)
   d. Hemoptysis
      1) May be related to tuberculosis, lung cancer, bronchiectasis, pneumonia, pulmonary embolism
      2) Character
         a) Grossly bloody
         b) Blood-tinged
         c) Blood-streaked
         d) Hematest positive
      3) Differentiation from hematemesis
         a) Hemoptysis: frothy, alkaline, accompanied by sputum
         b) Hematemesis: nonfrothy, acidic, dark red or brown, accompanied by food particles
   e. Chest pain: (information regarding Differentiation of Chest Pain is located in Table 2-5)
      1) P
         a) Provocation: Pulmonary pain is frequently provoked by trauma, coughing, deep breathing, or movement.
         b) Palliation: Pulmonary pain may be relieved by sitting upright or by narcotics.
      2) Q
         a) Quality: Pulmonary pain is most frequently sharp and increased by coughing, inspiration, movement.
      3) R
         a) Region: Pulmonary pain is usually located at lateral chest.
         b) Radiation: Pulmonary pain may radiate to shoulder or neck.
      4) S
         a) Severity: Pulmonary pain is usually moderate but may be severe.
      5) T
         a) Timing
            i) Onset: Pulmonary pain onset is usually gradual.
            ii) Duration: Pulmonary pain duration is usually days to weeks.
   f. Wheezing
      1) Onset
      2) Duration
      3) Timing: time of day, weather or season, activity, eating, talking, deep breathing, position, inspiratory or expiratory or both
      4) Identified triggers (e.g., dust, pollen, propellants)

5) Usual treatment

g. Nasal or sinus problems
   1) Epistaxis
   2) Nasal stuffiness
   3) Postnasal drip
   4) Sinus pain

h. Hoarseness: Chronic hoarseness may be related to cancer of larynx.

i. Ascites: may be related to cor pulmonale

j. Abdominal pain: may be related to cor pulmonale

k. Edema or weight gain: may be related to cor pulmonale

l. Fatigue or weakness: may be related to cor pulmonale

m. Fever: may be related to pulmonary infections

n. Night sweats: may be related to tuberculosis

o. Anorexia: may be related to cor pulmonale, dyspnea, or drug side effects (e.g., xanthine bronchodilators)

p. Weight loss: may be related to dyspnea, fatigue (preventing food preparation), or hypermetabolism

q. Sleep disturbances: may be related to dyspnea or coughing

2. History of present illness
   a. PQRST
   b. Associated symptoms

3. Past medical history
   a. Childhood diseases
      1) Frequent respiratory infections
      2) Allergies
      3) Asthma
      4) Scarlet fever
   b. Past illnesses
      1) Recurrent respiratory infections
      2) Pneumonia
      3) Cystic fibrosis
      4) Asthma
      5) Chronic obstructive pulmonary disease (COPD)
         a) Possible components
            i) Chronic bronchitis: Dominant reported symptom is coughing with sputum production.
            ii) Emphysema: Dominant reported symptom is dyspnea.
            iii) Patients with COPD often also have asthma: Dominant reported symptom is wheezing.
         b) Most patients have two, if not all three, of these components.
      6) Tuberculosis
      7) Lung cancer
      8) Pulmonary fibrosis: frequently related to occupational lung disease
         a) Pneumoconiosis (coal worker's lung disease)
         b) Asbestosis
         c) Silicosis
      9) Fungal disease (e.g., histoplasmosis)
      10) Pulmonary embolism
      11) Pneumothorax
      12) Granulomatous diseases (e.g., sarcoidosis)
      13) Connective tissue disorders (e.g., lupus, scleroderma)
      14) Immunosuppression
      15) Cor pulmonale: right ventricular hypertrophy and/or failure as a result of pulmonary disease
   c. Past injury: chest trauma
   d. Past surgical procedures: thoracotomy
   e. Allergies and type of reaction
   f. Past diagnostic studies
      1) Allergy testing
      2) Tuberculin and/or fungal skin tests
      3) Chest x-ray
      4) Pulmonary function studies
      5) Bronchoscopy
      6) Laryngoscopy

4. Family history of genetically predisposed disease
   a. Asthma
   b. Emphysema: particularly alpha$_1$-antitrypsin deficiency-related emphysema
   c. Tuberculosis
   d. Cystic fibrosis
   e. Cancer

5. Social history
   a. Work environment
      1) Occupation
      2) Environmental hazards: chemicals, vapors, dust, pulmonary irritants, allergens
      3) Use of protective devices
   b. Home environment
      1) Allergens: pets, plants, trees, molds, dust mites
      2) Type of heating
      3) Use of air conditioner and/or humidifier
   c. Recreational habits: exposure to inhalants and allergens
   d. Exercise habits
   e. Tobacco use: present and past
      1) Type of tobacco
      2) Duration and amount
         a) Cigarettes: Record as pack-years (number of packs per day times the number of years the patient has been smoking)
         b) Chewing or rubbing tobacco: type and amount per day
         c) Marijuana: joints per day
      3) Efforts to quit: previous and current desire to quit
      4) Second-hand smoke exposure
   f. Fluid consumption
      1) Volume of water/day
      2) Caffeine-containing beverages
      3) Alcohol-containing beverages: alcoholic beverages per day or per week
   g. Eating habits
      1) Quality and quantity of meals
      2) Number of meals/day

3) Pulmonary symptoms during meals: dyspnea, cough, wheezing
6. Medication history
   a. Prescribed drug, dose, frequency, time of last dose
   b. Nonprescribed drugs
      1) Over-the-counter drugs, including herbs
         a) St. John's Wort can worsen asthma symptoms if taken with theophylline or amitriptyline (Elavil).
         b) Guarana can increase the likelihood of side effects if taken with respiratory medications because it contains theophylline.
         c) Ginseng reduces the effectiveness of beta-blockers.
         d) Licorice elimination is reduced if taken with corticosteroids.
         e) Blue cohosh and lobelia may increase the side effects of nicotine patches.
         f) Ma hang can increase toxicity of methylxanthines in asthmatics.
      2) Substance abuse
   c. Patient's understanding of drug actions, side effects; knowledge of how to use and clean an inhaler if prescribed

Landmarks (see Figure 2-29)

1. Anatomical
   a. Clavicle
   b. Sternum
   c. Ribs
   d. Intercostal spaces
   e. Angle of Louis: sternal angle between manubrium and body of sternum
   f. Xiphoid process
   g. Costal margin
   h. Costal angle
2. Imaginary
   a. Midsternal line
   b. Midclavicular line (MCL)
   c. Anterior axillary line (AAL)
   d. Midaxillary line (MAL)
   e. Posterior axillary line (PAL)
   f. Scapular line
   g. Midspinal line
3. Location of lungs (Figure 4-21)
   a. The apex of the lungs extends 2-4 cm above the inner third of the clavicle.
   b. The inferior border anteriorly is at the sixth rib at the MCL and at the eighth rib at the MAL, posteriorly at T10 on expiration and at T12 with deep inspiration.
   c. Fissure dividing upper and lower lobes is at T3 posteriorly.
   d. Upper lobes primarily anterior; lower lobes primarily posterior
   e. Trachea bifurcates at the angle of Louis anteriorly or T4 posteriorly.

Inspection and Palpation

1. Vital signs
   a. Blood pressure
   b. Heart rate
   c. Respiratory (ventilatory) rate
   d. Temperature
   e. Height
   f. Weight
2. General survey
   a. Apparent health status: Compare apparent age relative to chronological age.
   b. Level of consciousness: Note restlessness and/or confusion (frequently the first sign of hypoxia).
   c. Increased work of breathing: Note use of accessory muscles.

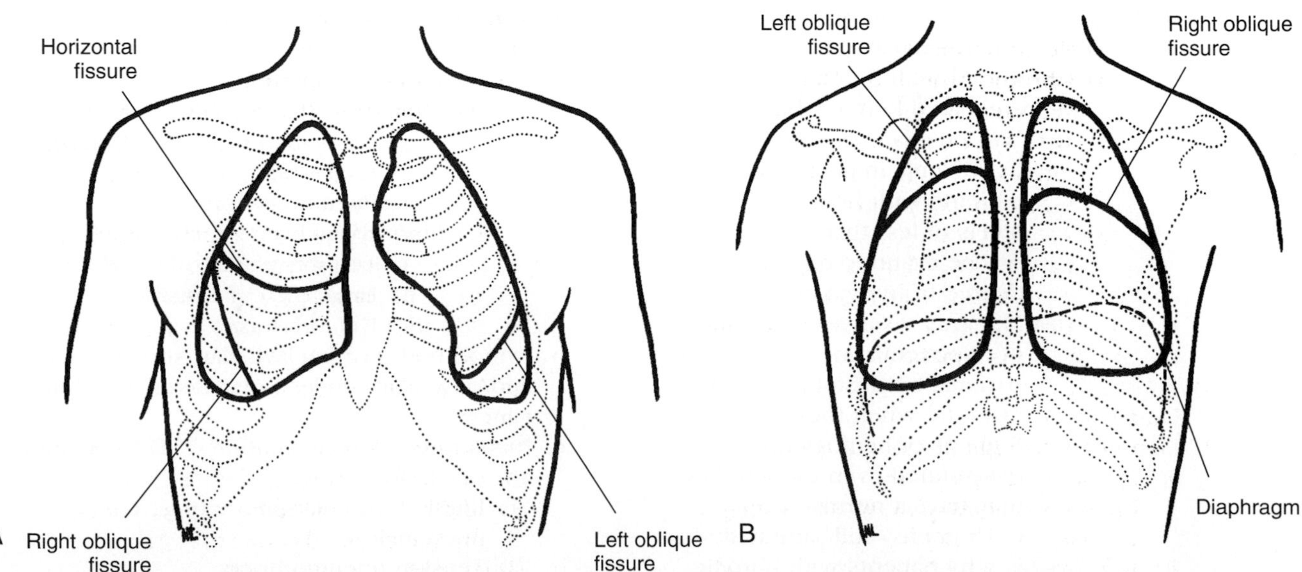

Figure 4-21 Location of the lungs. **A,** Anterior. **B,** Posterior. (From Wilkins, R. L., Sheldon, R. L., & Krider, S. J. [1994]. *Clinical assessment in respiratory care*. St Louis: Mosby.)

d. Speech pattern: Note pausing midsentence to take a breath.
e. Presence of injury, abrasion, or deformity
f. Nutritional status
g. Stature/posture

3. Mouth or nose
   a. Pursed-lip breathing: may be instinctive or the patient may have been taught to use this technique during times of dyspnea
   b. Artificial airway
      1) Type
      2) Size
      3) Placement (e.g., cm mark at teeth for oral endotracheal tube)
      4) Cuff pressure (measured with a cuff pressure gauge or sphygmomanometer with three-way stopcock)
   c. Oxygen therapy
      1) Administration device and flow rate
      2) FiO_2
   d. Nasogastric, nasointestinal tube, orogastric, or orointestinal tube
      1) Size
      2) Placement confirmation
         a) Aspiration of gastric (acidic) or intestinal (alkaline) contents
         b) Radiologic confirmation
   e. Condition of nasal or oral mucosa
   f. Presence of halitosis: suggests poor oral hygiene, poor dental health, or sinus infection
4. Skin, mucous membranes, and appendages
   a. Color
      1) Pallor: may indicate anemia
      2) Rubor: may indicate hypercapnia or polycythemia
      3) Cyanosis
         a) Peripheral (or cold) cyanosis
            i) Seen on fingertips and toes
            ii) Associated with peripheral hypoperfusion or vasoconstriction
         b) Central (or warm) cyanosis
            i) Seen on lips and mucous membranes
            ii) Associated with 5 grams of deoxygenated hemoglobin
               (a) Will be a late sign of hypoxemia in anemic patients; patients with hemoglobin levels of less than 5 g/dL will not be cyanotic regardless of degree of hypoxemia
               (b) May be a relatively early sign of hypoxemia in polycythemic patients because they will be cyanotic when they have 5 grams of hemoglobin desaturated even though they may have a normal level (~15 grams) still saturated; this is why patients with chronic bronchitis are nicknamed "blue bloaters"
                  (i) Blue due to chronic cyanosis
                  (ii) Bloaters due to chronic RVF
         c) In dark-skinned patients, cyanosis appears as an ashen color.
      4) Cherry-red: may indicate carbon monoxide intoxication
      5) Tobacco stains on fingertips
   b. Scars: especially thoracic
   c. Petechiae: may indicate any of the following:
      1) Blood dyscrasias affecting platelets
         a) Disseminated intravascular coagulation (DIC)
         b) Platelet aggregation inhibitors (e.g., ASA, nonsteroidal antiinflammatory agents, clopidogrel [Plavix])
      2) Liver disease
      3) Fat embolism
   d. Edema: may be associated with cor pulmonale
   e. Nailbeds
      1) Color: note cyanosis
      2) Clubbing
         a) Indicates chronic decrease in oxygen supply to body tissues
            i) Especially indicative of restrictive lung diseases (e.g., pulmonary fibrosis, lung cancer)
            ii) Also indicative of right-to-left cardiac shunting (e.g., cyanotic heart disease)
            iii) May be seen in late obstructive lung disease
         b) Normal angle between nailbed and nail less than 180 degrees
         c) Early clubbing angle equal to 180 degrees
         d) Late clubbing greater than 180 degrees
5. Neck
   a. Tracheal deviation
      1) Local causes: hematoma, goiter
      2) Mediastinal causes
         a) Shifts toward affected side
            i) Spontaneous pneumothorax
            ii) Atelectasis
            iii) Pneumonectomy
         b) Shifts away from affected side
            i) Tension pneumothorax
            ii) Large pleural effusion
            iii) Hemothorax
   b. Lymph nodes (infraclavicular, supraclavicular, and/or axillary nodes): may be enlarged in lung cancer
   c. Jugular neck vein distention (JVD): may indicate any of the following:
      1) Right ventricular failure (e.g., cor pulmonale)
      2) Tension pneumothorax
      3) Cardiac tamponade
      4) Superior vena cava syndrome

a) Edema of neck, eyelids, hands also seen
b) May occur in lung cancer

d. Accessory muscle use: indicates respiratory distress

6. Thorax
   a. Posture: tripod position
      1) Sitting up and leaning forward (e.g., over bedside table)
      2) Position for optimal ventilation
      3) Indicates respiratory distress
   b. Contour
      1) Normal
         a) Slope of ribs: Ribs are normally at 45-degree angle to vertebrae.
         b) Costal angle: normally less than 90 degrees
         c) Anterior-posterior (A-P) diameter: normally one-half of lateral diameter so that normal ratio of anterior-posterior to lateral diameter is 1:2
         d) Symmetrical
      2) Abnormalities
         a) Pectus excavatum (funnel chest)
            i) Sternum pushed inward
            ii) May cause hypoventilation or restrictive lung disease
         b) Pectus carinatum (pigeon chest)
            i) Sternum pushed outward
            ii) May cause hypoventilation or restrictive lung disease
         c) Scoliosis
            i) "S" curvature to spine
            ii) May cause hypoventilation or restrictive lung disease
         d) Kyphosis (hunchback)
            i) Frequently occurs with aging due to osteoporosis
            ii) May cause hypoventilation or restrictive lung disease
         e) Increased A-P diameter (also referred to as *barrel chest*): indicates obstructive lung disease
   c. Intercostal spaces
      1) Retraction of interspaces during inspiration
         a) Tracheal obstruction
         b) Asthma
      2) Bulging of interspaces during expiration
         a) Asthma
         b) Tension pneumothorax
         c) Pleural effusion
   d. Chest movement
      1) Impaired movement
         a) Thoracic pain with splinting
         b) Restrictive lung disease
      2) Unequal expansion
         a) Massive unilateral atelectasis
         b) Massive pleural effusion
         c) Pneumonia
         d) Pneumothorax
         e) Pulmonary resection: lobectomy, pneumonectomy
         f) Right mainstem intubation (no movement on left)
         g) Flail chest
      3) Respiratory excursion: normally 3-6 cm during normal breathing
   e. Respiratory rate, rhythm, quality
      1) Rate and rhythm (Table 4-5)
      2) Type
         a) Abdominal: males or supine females
         b) Thoracic or costal: upright females
      3) Inspiration to expiration (I:E) ratio
         a) Normally 1:2 with expiration lasting twice as long as inspiration
         b) Obstructive lung diseases cause prolonged expiratory time with ratios 1:3 or greater
   f. Chest wall
      1) Point of maximal impulse
         a) Normally palpated at fifth LICS at MCL
         b) Frequently shifted medially in patients with chronic lung disease and pulmonary hypertension due to right ventricular hypertrophy
         c) May be shifted in either direction with mediastinal shift depending on side and type of condition creating mediastinal shift
      2) Heave: right ventricular heave may be felt at the sternum or in epigastric area due to right ventricular hypertrophy and/or failure
      3) Tenderness: may be caused by any of the following:
         a) Fracture
         b) Tumor
         c) Costochondritis
      4) Fremitus
         a) Vocal fremitus
            i) Evaluated by asking the patient to say "99" while the patient's thorax is palpated with the ball of the examiner's hand
            ii) Decreased vocal fremitus
               (a) Thick chest wall
               (b) Bronchial obstruction
               (c) Pleural effusion
               (d) Pleural thickening
               (e) Pneumothorax
               (f) Emphysema
            iii) Increased vocal fremitus
               (a) Over large airways
               (b) Pneumonia
               (c) Tumor
               (d) Pulmonary fibrosis
               (e) Pulmonary infarction
         b) Pleural friction fremitus: grating sensation that occurs with pleural inflammation
         c) Rhonchal fremitus: vibration felt with movement of secretions through the tracheobronchial tree

Table 4-5 Respiratory Rhythms

Rhythm	Description	Possible Causes
Eupnea	Rate 12-20/min and normal depth of ventilation; regular with occasional sigh	• Normal
Bradypnea	Slow (less than 10/min), regular ventilation	• Depression of respiratory center with opium, alcohol, or tumor • Sleep • Increased intracranial pressure • CO_2 narcosis • Metabolic alkalosis
Tachypnea	Rapid (greater than 30/min) ventilation; depth may be normal or decreased	• Restrictive lung disease • Pneumonia • Pleurisy • Chest pain • Fear • Anxiety • Respiratory insufficiency
Hypopnea	Shallow ventilation, normal rate	• Deep sleep • Heart failure • Shock • Meningitis • Central nervous system depression • Coma
Hyperpnea	Deep ventilation; rate may be normal or increased	• Exercise • Hypoxia • Fever • Hepatic coma • Midbrain or pons lesions • Acid-base imbalance • Salicylate overdosage
Cheyne-Stokes	Increasing and decreasing rate and depth of ventilation followed by apnea lasting 20-60 seconds	• Increased intracranial pressure • Heart failure • Renal failure • Meningitis • Cerebral hemisphere damage • Drug overdosage
Kussmaul	Deep, gasping, rapid (usually greater than 35/min) ventilation	• Metabolic acidosis (e.g., diabetic ketoacidosis; renal failure) • Peritonitis
Apneustic	Prolonged gasping inspiration followed by short inefficient expiration	• Lesion of pons
Biot's	Periods of apnea alternating with a series of breaths of equal depth; breathing may be slow and deep or rapid and shallow	• Meningitis • Encephalitis • Head trauma • Increased intracranial pressure
Ataxic	Lack of any pattern to ventilation	• Brainstem lesion
Obstructive	I : E ratio of 1 : 4 or greater	• Asthma • Emphysema • Chronic bronchitis
Apnea	Cessation of ventilation for longer than 15 seconds	• Central nervous system damage • Sleep apnea

5) Subcutaneous emphysema (air in subcutaneous tissue)
   a) Assess for subcutaneous emphysema around tracheostomy, chest tube, or stab wound
   b) Assess for subcutaneous emphysema after bronchoscopy; indicates perforation of tracheobronchial tree
6) Chest tubes
7) Central venous catheters

a) Location
b) Patency
c) Rate and type of solutions
8) Wounds
7. Abdomen
   a. Liver
      1) May be palpable in patients with normal liver but hyperinflated lungs because liver is pushed downward
      2) May be enlarged and tender due to cor pulmonale
   b. Abdominal muscles (accessory muscles of expiration): frequently used by patients with obstructive lung disease to help push the air out of the lungs
8. Ventilatory support
   a. Mode
   b. Tidal volume
   c. Rate
   d. FiO_2
   e. PEEP
   f. Peak inspiratory pressure and calculated dynamic compliance
   g. Plateau pressure and calculated static compliance
9. Clinical indications of respiratory distress (Box 4-2)
10. Clinical indications of hypoxemia/hypoxia
   a. Hypoxemia (decreased oxygen in the blood): noted by PaO_2 less than 80 mm Hg and SaO_2 less than 95% on ABGs or SaO_2 less than 95% by pulse oximetry
   b. Hypoxia (decreased oxygen in the tissues): noted by clinical indications of hypoxia (Box 4-3) and increased serum lactate level
11. Clinical indications of hypercapnia (increased CO_2 in the blood): noted by increased $PaCO_2$ on ABGs and clinical indications of hypercapnia (Box 4-4)

Percussion

1. Description of percussion tones (Table 4-6)
2. Thorax
   a. Percussion tones normally heard
      1) Lung: resonance
      2) Diaphragm: flat
      3) Heart: dull
   b. Abnormal percussion tones over thorax
      1) Hyperresonant: asthma, emphysema, pneumothorax
      2) Dull: atelectasis, pneumonia, tumor
      3) Flat: pleural effusion
   c. Diaphragmatic excursion
      1) Evaluated by percussing the position of the diaphragm at expiration and then during full inspiration
      2) Normal diaphragmatic excursion is 3-5 cm
      3) May be decreased by the following:
         a) Increased intrathoracic volume: emphysema
         b) Increased intraabdominal volume and pressure:
            i) Ascites
            ii) Hepatomegaly
            iii) Pregnancy
            iv) Gaseous abdominal distention

Box 4-2 Clinical Indications of Respiratory Distress

Pursed lip breathing
Tripod positioning
Speaking only one or two words between breaths
Cough
Use of accessory muscles
Intercostal retractions

Box 4-3 Clinical Indications of Hypoxia

Restlessness → confusion → lethargy → coma
Tachycardia → dysrhythmias
Tachypnea
Dyspnea
Use of accessory muscles
Mild hypertension (early) → hypotension (late)
Cyanosis may be present (depending on hemoglobin level)

Box 4-4 Clinical Indications of Hypercapnia

Headache
Irritability
Confusion
Inability to concentrate → somnolence → coma
Bradypnea
Tachycardia → dysrhythmias
Hypotension
Facial rubor (plethora)

Table 4-6 Percussion Tones

Tone	Intensity	Pitch	Duration	Quality	Normal Location
Tympanic	Loud	High	Medium	Drumlike	Stomach, bowel
Hyperresonant	Loud	Low	Long	Booming	Hyperinflated lungs
Resonant	Medium	Low	Long	Hollow	Normal lung
Dull	Soft	High	Medium	Thudlike	Liver, spleen, heart
Flat	Soft	High	Short	Extreme dullness	Muscle, bone

c) Decreased chest excursion and tidal volume: thoracic or abdominal pain
d) Phrenic nerve injury

3. Abdomen
   a. Liver
      1) Normal liver span in the right MCL is 6-12 cm
      2) Hepatomegaly (i.e., liver span greater than 12 cm in left MCL) may be seen in cor pulmonale
         a) Assessment by percussion is necessary before specifying hepatomegaly because patients with hyperinflated lungs may have a palpable normal liver because it is pushed downward.

Auscultation

1. Method of lung auscultation
   a. Use diaphragm of stethoscope.
   b. Ask patient to take deep breaths through his or her mouth.
   c. Listen to at least one full breath at each location.
   d. Compare symmetrical areas.
2. Breath sounds
   a. Intensity
      1) Increased
         a) Hyperventilation
         b) Anything that decreases the distance between the lung and your stethoscope (e.g., thin chest wall)
      2) Decreased
         a) Hypoventilation
            i) Emphysema
            ii) Thoracic pain
            iii) Restrictive lungs (e.g., atelectasis, pulmonary fibrosis)
         b) Anything that increases the distance between the lung and your stethoscope
            i) Muscular or obese chest
            ii) Pneumothorax (may be diminished or absent)
            iii) Hemothorax (may be diminished or absent)
            iv) Pleural effusion
      3) Absent
         a) Severe bronchospasm
         b) Massive atelectasis
         c) Pneumonectomy
         d) Pneumothorax
         e) Hemothorax
         f) Malpositioned endotracheal tube (absent breath sounds over left lung)
   b. Quality
      1) Descriptions and normal locations (Figure 4-22 and Table 4-7)
      2) Implications
         a) Bronchial in areas other than normal location: consolidation (e.g., atelectasis, pneumonia, tumor)
         b) Bronchovesicular in areas other than normal location: partial consolidation, partial aeration
   c. Adventitious sounds (Table 4-8): pathologic extra sounds which may be heard at points in the ventilatory cycle or throughout the ventilatory cycle
   d. Voice sounds: abnormal and indicative of consolidation

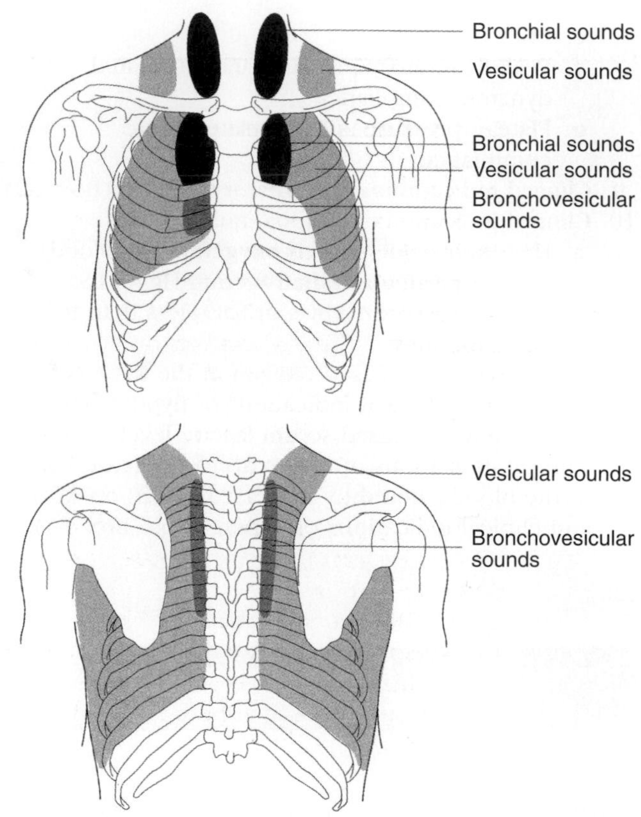

Figure 4-22 Breath sounds: normal locations. (From Barkauskas, V. H., et al. [1994]. *Health and physical assessment*. St. Louis: Mosby.)

Table 4-7 Breath Sounds: Quality

Quality	I:E Ratio	Intensity	Pitch	Description	Normal Location
Bronchial	I less than E	Loud	High	Hollow	Trachea
Bronchovesicular	I = E	Medium	Medium	Breezy	Mainstem bronchi
Vesicular	I greater than E	Soft	Low	Swishy	Peripheral lung

Table 4-8 Breath Sounds: Adventitious Sounds

Sound	Alternative Terms	Phase	Description	Cause
Stridor	Croupy	Inspiratory	High-pitched whistle audible without a stethoscope	• Upper airway obstruction • Epiglottis • Foreign body • Laryngospasm • Laryngeal edema

Wheezes	Whistles; sibilant rhonchi	Inspiratory or expiratory	High-pitched whistling sound	• Decrease in airway lumen
				  • Bronchospasm
				  • Mucus plug
				  • Tumor

Crackles	Rales	Inspiratory	Discontinuous crackling sound; similar to rubbing hair between fingers	• Pulmonary edema • Atelectasis • Pulmonary fibrosis
Rhonchi	Gurgles, sonorous rhonchi, coarse crackles	Expiratory	Continuous gurgling sound	• Fluid or mucus in airways
Pleural friction rub		Inspiratory and expiratory	Grating or scratching sound	• Pulmonary infarction • Pleurisy • Tuberculosis • Lung cancer

1) Bronchophony: increase in clarity of voice sounds
   a) Ask patient to say "99."
   b) Voice sounds are normally muffled.
   c) If voice sounds are clear over a particular area, bronchophony is present.
2) Egophony: "e" to "a" conversion of voice sounds
   a) Ask patient to say "e."
   b) Muffled "e" should be heard over normal lung.
   c) If "a" is heard over a particular area, egophony is present.
3) Whispered pectoriloquy: increase in clarity of whispered sounds
   a) Ask the patient to whisper "99."
   b) Whispered sounds are normally muffled.
   c) If whispered sounds are clear over a particular area, whispered pectoriloquy is present.

Bedside Assessment of Pulmonary Function

1. Bedside parameters (also referred to as *ventilatory mechanics*)
   a. Spirometry: measured with Wright respirometer
      1) Tidal volume (V_T)
         a) Amount of air moved in and out each breath
         b) Normal: 7 mL/kg
            i) Tidal volume less than 5 mL/kg indicates need for artificial airway and/or mechanical ventilation.
            ii) Tidal volume greater than 5 mL/kg indicates that the patient can be weaned and/or extubated.
      2) Vital capacity (VC)
         a) Maximal amount of air that can be exhaled after a maximal inspiration
         b) Normal: 15 mL/kg
            i) Vital capacity less than 10 mL/kg indicates need for artificial airway and/or mechanical ventilation.
            ii) Vital capacity greater than 10 mL/kg indicates that the patient can be weaned and/or extubated.
      3) Minute ventilation
         a) $f \times V_T$
         b) Normal: 5-10 L/min
      4) Maximal voluntary ventilation (MVV)
         a) Volume of air moved into and out of the lungs with maximal effort over a short period of time (usually 10-15 seconds)
         b) Normal is 170 L/min (NOTE: One-quarter of this total is actually measured in the 15-second period; patients are not asked to ventilate at this intensity for an entire minute.)
         c) Reflects the status of the ventilatory muscles, compliance of the lung and thorax, and airway resistance; may provide a quick assessment of the patient's ventilatory reserve prior to surgery
   b. Maximal inspiratory pressure (MIP): measured with negative inspiratory pressure meter
      1) Also referred to as *negative inspiratory force* (NIF)
      2) Normal is greater than (more negative than) −60 to −80 cm H_2O.
         a) MIP of less than −25 cm H_2O indicates need for artificial airway and/or mechanical ventilation.

b) MIP of greater than −25 cm H_2O indicates that the patient can be weaned and/or extubated.

c. Rapid shallow breathing index (RSBI)

1) Calculated as: f/V_T (in liters) using frequency in 1 minute and average tidal volume over 1 minute

2) Provides an indication of the brain's perception of how well the respiratory muscles tolerate the work of breathing; if the brain senses that the workload is too high for the respiratory muscles to tolerate, the reflex ventilatory pattern is rapid shallow breathing

3) RSBI of less than or equal to 105 breaths/min/L indicates readiness for weaning.

2. Capnography (may also be referred to as *end-tidal CO_2 monitoring*)

a. Continuous noninvasive method for evaluating the adequacy of CO_2 exchange in the lungs; assesses $PaCO_2$ indirectly by detecting the level of CO_2 in the exhaled air

1) Measurement of expired carbon dioxide tension

2) Display of the carbon dioxide waveform from breath to breath (Figure 4-23)

b. Indications

1) Verification of tracheal intubation

a) Esophageal intubation is reflected by decreased $P_{et}CO_2$ or an abnormal waveform

b) Inexpensive, disposable, colorimetric CO_2 indicators are frequently used for this purpose; they do not display waveform.

2) Verification of adequacy of chest compression during CPR

a) In the absence of pulmonary blood flow, $P_{et}CO_2$ decreases rapidly because no CO_2 is being returned to the lungs.

b) $P_{et}CO_2$ is decreased when chest compressions are inadequate, and $P_{et}CO_2$ increases when effectiveness of compression is increased.

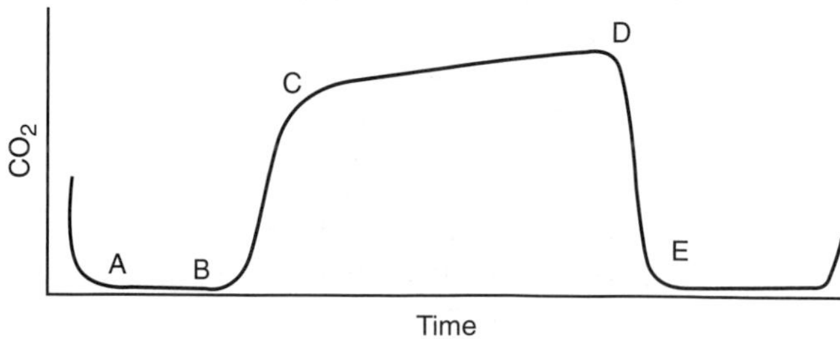

Figure 4-23 Typical normal CO_2 waveform. *A to B,* Exhalation of CO_2-free gas from dead space. *B to C,* Combination of dead space and alveolar gases. *C to D,* Exhalation of mostly alveolar gas. *D,* Exhalation of CO_2 at maximal point (end-tidal point). *D to E,* Inspiration begins and CO_2 concentration rapidly falls to baseline or zero. (From St. John, R. E. [2004]. Airway management. *Crit Care Nurse,* 24[2], 93-96.)

3) Evaluation of ventilation and $PaCO_2$

a) This use is limited in critically ill patients because the relationship between $PaCO_2$ and $P_{et}CO_2$ is affected by changes in pulmonary dead space and perfusion.

b) $PaCO_2$ - $P_{et}CO_2$ gradient may be used as an indication of changes in pulmonary dead space or a drop in cardiac output.

c) May be used during procedural sedation to monitor for changes in ventilation

4) Monitoring during weaning: progressive rise indicates increased work of breathing

c. Description

1) The CO_2 in the expired air is measured; the end tidal ($P_{et}CO_2$) is assumed to represent alveolar gas and may be used to estimate the $PaCO_2$; because this relationship is dependent on the ventilation-perfusion ratios throughout the lung, this assumption may be particularly erroneous in critically ill patients.

d. Normal value: The $P_{et}CO_2$ is usually 1-6 mm Hg below the $PaCO_2$ or approximately 38 mm Hg.

1) Increased $P_{et}CO_2$ assumes hypoventilation.

2) Decreased $P_{et}CO_2$ assumes hyperventilation.

e. Implication: Changes in $P_{et}CO_2$ indicates that the patient requires prompt assessment and arterial blood gases for analysis.

3. Pulse oximetry (SpO_2)

a. Continuous noninvasive method of monitoring arterial oxygen saturation

b. Indications

1) Assessment of adequacy of oxygenation (do not adequately evaluate ventilation because $PaCO_2$ increases with hypoventilation, but PaO_2 and O_2 saturation do not decrease until much later)

2) Recovery from anesthesia

c. Description

1) Sensor with light source is placed on the fingertip, toe, bridge of nose, forehead, or earlobe; care must be taken to use the appropriate sensor for the location (i.e., a finger sensor should not be attached to the earlobe).

2) The amount of arterial hemoglobin that is saturated with oxygen is determined by beams of light passed through the tissue.

d. Normal value: greater than 95%; moderate to severe hypoxemia should be suspected if less than 90%; causes of decreased SpO_2:

1) Decrease in SaO_2 and PaO_2

2) Decrease in cardiac output

e. Limitations

1) Inadequate pulsations may result from the following:

a) Significant hypotension

b) Vasopressor use

c) Severe hypothermia

d) Arterial compression

2) Tends to overestimate SaO_2 by 2-5%; accuracy of SpO_2 below 70% is questionable; the lower the SaO_2, the larger the difference between it and the SpO_2
3) Does not accurately reflect oxygen tissue delivery in patients with anemia or abnormal hemoglobins
   a) Carboxyhemoglobin
      i) Results in overestimation of oxygen saturation reading because hemoglobin is saturated but with carbon monoxide
      ii) Smokers may have elevated carboxyhemoglobin levels
   b) Methemoglobin
      i) Results in overestimation of SaO_2
      ii) Methemoglobin is a form of hemoglobin that cannot carry oxygen.
      iii) May be related to the administration of nitroglycerin, nitroprusside, sulfonamides, local anesthetics
   c) Hemoglobin S: sickle cell anemia
4) Other variables may impair accuracy.
   a) Intravenous dyes (e.g., methylene blue, indocyanine green): result in inaccurate readings
   b) Increased bilirubin (greater than 20 mg/dL): results in inaccurately low readings
   c) Ambient light: may affect accuracy
   d) Motion artifact: may affect accuracy
   e) Edema: may result in inaccurately low readings
   f) Nail polish: blue, green, gold, black, or brown nail polish needs to be removed
   g) Pierced earlobe: results in inaccurate reading

f. Implication: Changes in SpO_2 indicate that the patient requires prompt assessment and arterial blood gases for analysis.

4. Transcutaneous PaO_2 ($P_{tc}O_2$) monitoring
   a. Continuous noninvasive method of monitoring PaO_2
   b. Indications: as for pulse oximetry
   c. Description
      1) Sensor is placed on the skin; electrode has a heating element to warm skin and cause capillaries to dilate and increase blood flow.
   d. Normal value: greater than 80 mm Hg; moderate to severe hypoxemia should be suspected if less than 60 mm Hg
   e. Limitations
      1) Affected by skin blood flow, thickness, temperature, skin oxygen consumption, subcutaneous emphysema, edema
      2) Tends to underestimate PaO_2
      3) Less reliable in adults than in infants
   f. Implications
      1) PaO_2 will always be equal to or greater than $P_{tc}O_2$.
      2) Changes in $P_{tc}O_2$ indicate that the patient requires prompt assessment and arterial blood gases for analysis.
5. Mixed venous oxygen saturation (SvO_2)
   a. Oxygen saturation of the blood as it returns to the lung for reoxygenation; reflects how well the body's demand for oxygen is met by the amount of oxygen supplied
   b. Normal SvO_2: 60-80%
   c. Complete discussion of SvO_2 monitoring in Hemodynamic Monitoring section of Chapter 2
6. Continuous airway pressure monitoring (CAPM)
   a. Noninvasive technique for displaying the patient's airway pressure waveforms on a bedside monitoring system; provides a visual representation of the patient's own spontaneous effort and the function of the ventilator
   b. Description
      1) Air-filled (i.e., not primed with fluid) pressure tubing is connected to the ventilator tubing at the Y connector.
      2) Tubing is connected to a transducer and the transducer is attached to a channel of the bedside monitor.
      3) Zeroing is at any level.
      4) Positive waveform deflections indicate positive pressure ventilation, and negative deflections indicate spontaneous inspiratory effort.
   c. Implications
      1) Assessment of asynchrony between patient and ventilator
      2) Identification of ventilator mode
      3) Detection of PEEP, including auto-PEEP
      4) Improvement of accuracy of hemodynamic waveforms
      5) Identification of respiratory efforts when muscle paralysis and/or sedation is inadequate

Basic Chest X-ray Interpretation

1. Basic principles
   a. Density: Denser tissues absorb more of the x-rays, and less dense tissues absorb less of the x-rays.
      1) Air is radiolucent and appears black.
      2) Water (e.g., heart, muscle, blood, diaphragm, liver, spleen) appears gray.
      3) Fat (e.g., breasts) appears whitish-gray.
      4) Bone is radiopaque and appears white.
         a) Bullets, teeth, and wires are also radiopaque.
2. Initial steps
   a. Check the patient's name and date on the x-ray.
   b. Check for the "R" or "L" marker and orient the film appropriately on the view box.
   c. Ensure the quality of the inspiratory effort: The middle of the right hemidiaphragm should be at the tenth rib posteriorly.

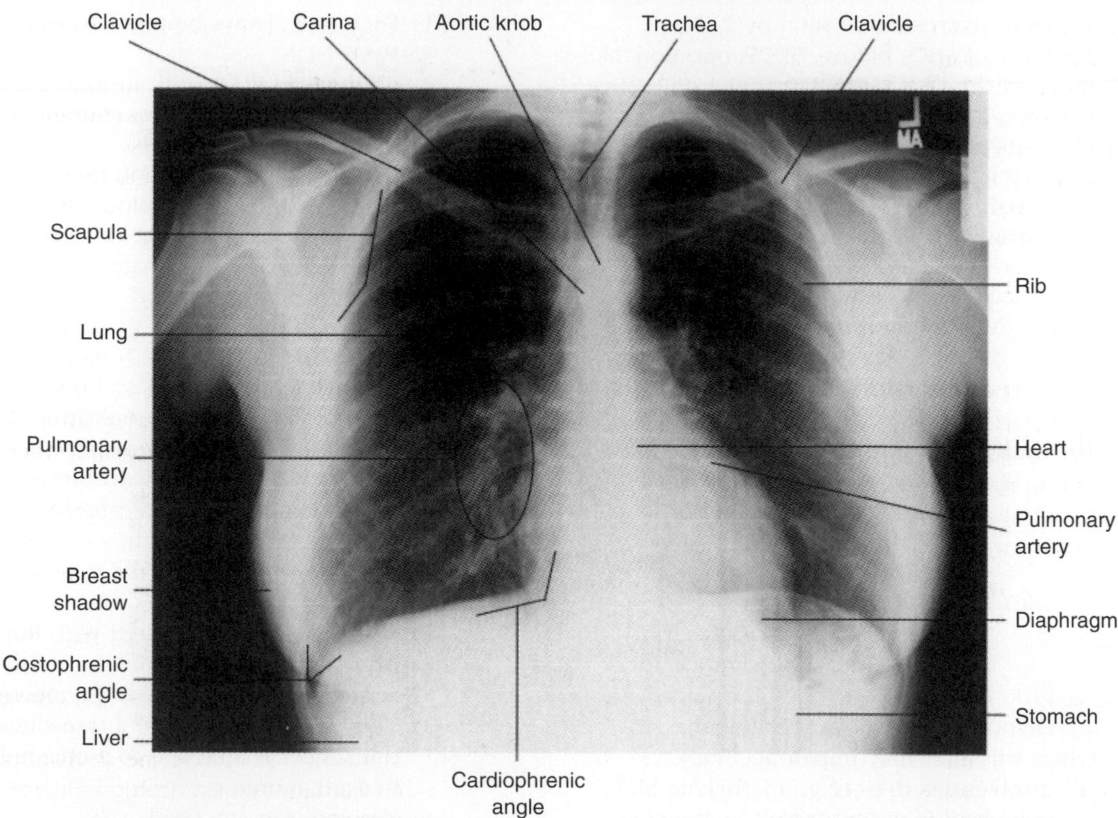

Figure 4-24 Anatomical landmarks on chest x-ray. (From Dettenmeir, P. A. *Radiographic assessment for nurses* [1995]. St Louis: Mosby.)

d. If there are previous films, view side by side with the new film.

3. Steps for interpretation (Urden et al., 2010)
   a. Evaluate the different densities to determine air, fluid, tissue, and bone.
   b. Evaluate the shape of each density to determine what normal anatomic structure the shape represents.
   c. Compare the left and right sides to determine if there are physiologic and/or pathophysiologic differences (Figure 4-24)
      1) A: airway including large airways, lung, pleura
      2) B: bones including clavicles, ribs, spine
      3) C: circulation including heart, mediastinum, and vascular markings
      4) D: diaphragm
   d. Evaluate all structures for abnormalities
      1) Cardiomegaly: heart size more than half the lateral diameter of the chest
      2) Atelectasis
         a) Area of atelectasis appears whitish-gray.
         b) Areas around the atelectasis appear darker than normal due to compensatory hyperinflation.
         c) Elevation of the hemidiaphragm on affected side
         d) Deviation of mediastinal structures toward the affected side
      3) Pneumonia
         a) Cloudlike infiltrates which may be localized or diffuse and may involve one or both lungs
         b) May be difficult to differentiate from pulmonary edema so clinical and diagnostic (e.g., BNP) profiles are crucial
      4) Hydrothorax (e.g., hemothorax or pleural effusion)
         a) Upright film shows a pleural air-fluid level with air (i.e., black) on top and fluid (i.e., gray) below the level
      5) Pneumothorax
         a) Area that is blacker than normal lung without vascular markings
         b) Pleura may appear as a fine, white line that separates the pleural space from the aerated lung
      6) Emphysema
         a) Hyperinflated (i.e., very black) lungs with flattened diaphragms
      7) ARDS: depends on stage
         a) I: Normal
         b) II: Fine, diffuse infiltrates commonly referred to as "*ground glass infiltrates*"
         c) III: Diffuse patchy, scattered infiltrates as atelectasis progresses to "white outs."
         d) IV: White-out areas may appear blacker as hyaline membranes have developed.
   e. If there are wires, tubes and/or lines, determine if they are in the proper place (Siela, 2008).

1) ET tube: 3-5 cm above the carina
2) Central venous catheter: in superior vena cava
3) Pulmonary artery catheter: in left or right pulmonary artery with tip about 2 cm from the hilum
4) IABP: Tip should be distal to the origin of the left subclavian artery.
5) NG tube: Tip should extend to about 10 cm into the stomach.
6) Dobbhoff feeding tube: Tip should be in duodenum.

Diagnostic Studies

1. Serum chemistries
   a. Sodium: normal 136-145 mEq/L
   b. Potassium: normal 3.5-5.5 mEq/L
   c. Chloride: normal 96-106 mEq/L
   d. Calcium: normal 8.5-10.5 mg/dL
   e. Phosphorus: normal 3-4.5 mg/dL
   f. Magnesium: normal 1.5-2.2 mEq/L or 1.8-2.4 mg/dL
   g. Glucose: normal 70-115 mEq/L
   h. BUN: normal 5-20 mg/dL
   i. Creatinine: normal 0.7-1.5 mg/dL
   j. Lactate: 1-2 mmol/L
2. Arterial blood gases
   a. pH: normal 7.35-7.45
   b. $PaCO_2$: normal 35-45 mm Hg
   c. HCO_3^-: normal 22-26 mEq/L
   d. PaO_2: normal 80-100 mm Hg
   e. SaO_2: greater than 95%
3. Hematology
   a. Hematocrit: normal 40-52% for males; 35-47% for females
   b. Hemoglobin: normal 13-18 g/dL for males; 12-16 g/dL for females
   c. White blood cells (WBC): normal 3500-11,000 mm^3
   d. D-dimer: normal negative
4. Sputum analysis: may be obtained by AM specimen by cough, induced tracheobronchial aspiration, transtracheal aspiration, or bronchoscopy
   a. Characteristics: color, odor, viscosity, presence of blood
   b. Culture and sensitivity tests: identifies infecting organism and effective antibiotic agent
   c. Gram's stain: differentiates between gram-negative or gram-positive bacteria
   d. Acid-fast stain: determines presence of acid-fast bacilli (tuberculosis)
   e. Cytology studies: determine presence of malignant cells
5. Pleural fluid analysis
   a. Total protein: differentiates between exudative pleural effusion and transudative pleural effusion
   b. Gram's stain: differentiates between gram-negative or gram-positive bacteria
   c. Acid-fast stain: determines presence of acid-fast bacilli (tuberculosis)
   d. Cytology studies: determine presence of malignant cells
6. Skin tests
   a. Type I hypersensitivity tests ("allergy tests")
   b. Type II hypersensitivity tests: purified protein derivative (PPD) for tuberculosis
   c. Fungal diseases (e.g., *Candida*)
7. Other diagnostic studies (Table 4-9)

Acid-Base Balance and Arterial Blood Gas Interpretation

Physiology Review

1. Acid: a substance that can give up an H^+ ion; acids are produced by the body as a result of cellular metabolism
   a. Volatile (e.g., carbonic acid)
      1) Exhalable
      2) Results from aerobic metabolism of glucose
      3) Eliminated by the lungs
   b. Nonvolatile (also called fixed) (e.g., sulfuric, phosphoric, uric)
      1) Nonexhalable and cannot be converted into a gas
      2) Results from aerobic metabolism of protein and fat and the anaerobic metabolism of glucose
      3) Eliminated by the kidney
   c. Elimination or neutralization necessary
2. Acidemia: the condition of the blood with a pH of below 7.35
3. Acidosis: the process that causes the acidemia
4. Base: a substance that can accept an H^+ (the primary base in the body is bicarbonate)
5. Alkalemia: the condition of the blood with a pH of above 7.45
6. Alkalosis: the process that causes the alkalemia
7. pH
   a. Indirect measurement of hydrogen ion concentration
   b. Reflection of the balance between carbonic acid (acid regulated by the lungs) and bicarbonate (base regulated by the kidneys)
   c. Inversely proportional to hydrogen ion concentration
      1) Increase in H^+ concentration: lower pH, more acid
      2) Decrease in H^+ concentration: higher pH, more base
   d. Must be maintained within a narrow range to allow functioning of enzymatic systems in the body
      1) pH below 6.8 or above 7.8 is incompatible with life
      2) Note that this is a 0.6 change toward acidosis but only a 0.4 change toward alkalosis (from midline normal of 7.4); this is because the shift of the oxyhemoglobin dissociation curve caused by alkalosis affects tissue oxygenation more adversely than does the shift caused by acidosis

Table 4-9 Pulmonary Diagnostic Studies

Study	Evaluation	Comments
Bronchography	• Detects obstruction or malformation of the tracheobronchial tree	• Patient inspires radiopaque substance and then x-rays are taken • Inquire about possibility of pregnancy
Chest x-ray	• Detects lung pathology (e.g., pneumonia, pulmonary edema, atelectasis, tuberculosis, etc.) • Determines size and location of lung lesions and tumors • Verifies placement of endotracheal tube, central venous catheters, chest tubes	• Noninvasive test with minimal radiation exposure • Inquire about possibility of pregnancy • Posteroanterior (PA) and lateral films are done most commonly, but in critical care areas anteroposterior (AP) portable films are frequently necessary due to inability to transport patient • Lateral decubitus films aid in identification of pleural effusion
Exercise testing	• Identifies early disability • Differentiates between cardiac and pulmonary disease	• Monitor for changes in SpO_2 during exercise • Monitor closely for exercise-induced hypotension or ventricular dysrhythmias
Laryngoscopy, bronchoscopy, mediastinoscopy	• Obtain cytology specimen or biopsy • Identify tumors, obstructions, secretions, foreign bodies in tracheobronchial tree • Locate a bleeding site • May be used therapeutically to remove secretions, foreign bodies, other contaminants	• Patient is sedated prior to the procedure, usually with a benzodiazepine (e.g., diazepam, midazolam) • Monitor the patient for subcutaneous emphysema after study; indicates tracheal or bronchial tear • Monitor for hemoptysis; some blood in sputum is normal after biopsy but frank hemoptysis requires immediate attention
Lung biopsy Transthoracic needle lung biopsy Open lung biopsy	• Obtain specimen for Cytology evaluation	• Transthoracic needle biopsy performed under fluoroscopy; inquire about possibility of pregnancy • Open lung biopsy requires thoracotomy
Magnetic resonance imaging (MRI)	• Distinguishes tumors from other structures (e.g., tumor, pleural thickening, fibrosis)	• Noninvasive test • Contraindicated for patients with pacemakers or implanted metallic devices
Pulmonary angiography	• Detects changes in lung tissue (e.g., masses) • Diagnoses abnormalities in pulmonary vasculature including thrombi and emboli • Identifies congenital abnormalities of the circulation	• Invasive test • Inquire about possibility of pregnancy • Contrast media injected into pulmonary artery; ensure adequate hydration after study • Monitor arterial puncture point for hematoma or hemorrhage
Pulmonary function studies (See Table 4-1 for lung volumes and parameters with normal values) Spirometry: volumes and capacities RV, FRC, TLC requires nitrogen washout technique Ventilatory mechanics Flow-volume loop studies Diffusing capacity	• Measure lung volumes, capacities, and flow rates • Identify features of restrictive or obstructive lung disease • Evaluate responsiveness to bronchodilator therapy • Aid in evaluation of surgical risk • Document a disability or cause of dyspnea	• Noninvasive study • Frequently repeated after bronchodilator therapy
Sleep studies	• Diagnose and differentiate between obstructive sleep apnea, central sleep apnea, and cardiac sleep apnea	• Restrict caffeine prior to testing • Usually done during normal sleep hours
Thoracentesis (may include pleural biopsy)	• Obtain pleural fluid and/or tissue specimen • May be used therapeutically to remove pleural fluid	• Monitor patient for indications of pneumothorax • Monitor for leakage from puncture point

Table 4-9 Pulmonary Diagnostic Studies—cont'd

Study	Evaluation	Comments
Thoracic computerized tomography (CT)	• Defines lesions, masses, cavities, or shadows seen on a normal chest x-ray • Evaluates tracheal or bronchial narrowing • Aids in planning radiation therapy	• X-rays taken at different angles
Ultrasonography	• Evaluates pleural disease • Visualizes diaphragm and detects disease around diaphragm (e.g., subphrenic hematoma or abscess)	• Noninvasive test
Ventilation scan Lung perfusion scan Ventilation/perfusion (V/Q) scan	• Diagnose ventilation and/or perfusion abnormalities including emphysema, pulmonary emboli	• Invasive test: radioisotope inspired and injected intravascularly • Inquire about possibility of pregnancy • Nuclear scan study: assure patient that amount of radioactive material is minimal

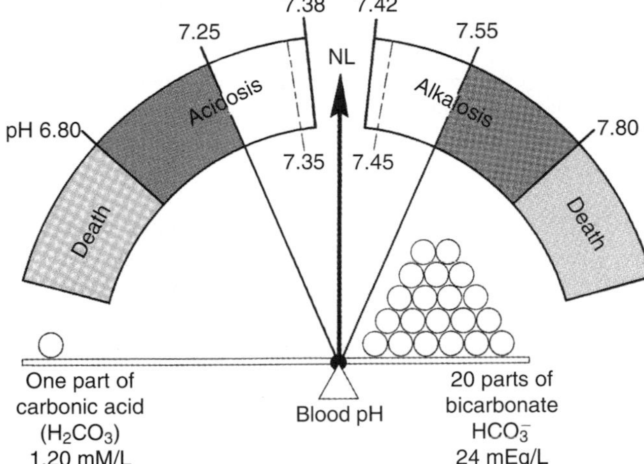

Figure 4-25 Acid-base balance. Twenty parts of HCO_3^- are required to buffer one part carbonic acid; pH normally is maintained within the narrow range (*NL*) of 7.35-7.45; pH below 6.8 or above 7.8 is incompatible with life. (From Price, S. A., & Wilson, L. M. [2003]. *Pathophysiology: Clinical concepts of disease processes* [6th ed.]. St. Louis: Mosby.)

8. Henderson-Hasselbalch equation
   a. pH is determined by the logarithm of the ratio of bicarbonate concentration to arterial $PaCO_2$
      1) $pH = \dfrac{pK\ (\text{constant of } 6.1) + \log HCO_3^-}{PaCO_2}$
   b. Ratio of 20 bicarbonate:1 carbonic acid maintains normal pH (Figure 4-25)

Acid-Base Regulation

1. Physiologic buffers
   a. Weak acid and its salt
   b. Immediate response when a change in acid-base status occurs by combining with excess acid or base
   c. Buffer systems
      1) Bicarbonate-carbonic acid buffer system
         a) The most important buffer system
         b) Bicarbonate is generated by the kidney and aids in the elimination of H^+
         c) $CO_2 + H_2O \Leftrightarrow H_2CO_3 \Leftrightarrow H^+ + HCO_3^-$
            LUNGS KIDNEYS
      2) Phosphate system: aids in excretion of H^+ by the kidney
      3) Ammonium: H^+ is added to ammonia (NH_3) in the renal tubule to form ammonium (NH_4); allows greater excretion of H^+ by the kidney
      4) Hemoglobin and other proteins: aid in buffering extracellular fluid
2. Respiratory system
   a. Regulates the excretion or retention of carbonic acid
      1) If pH decreases, the rate and depth of ventilation increase.
      2) If pH increases, the rate and depth of ventilation decrease.
   b. Responds within minutes: fast but weak
3. Renal system
   a. Regulates the excretion or retention of bicarbonate and the excretion of hydrogen and nonvolatile acids
      1) If pH decreases, the kidney retains bicarbonate.
      2) If pH increases, the kidney excretes bicarbonate
   b. Responds within 48 hours: slow but powerful

Acid-Base Imbalances (Figure 4-26)

1. Acidemia: pH below 7.35
   a. Acidosis: the process causing acidemia
      1) Caused by acid gain
         a) If acid is volatile (reflected by increase in $PaCO_2$): respiratory acidosis
         b) If acid is nonvolatile (reflected by decrease in HCO_3^-): metabolic acidosis
      2) Caused by base loss or metabolic acid gain (reflected by decrease in HCO_3^-): metabolic acidosis

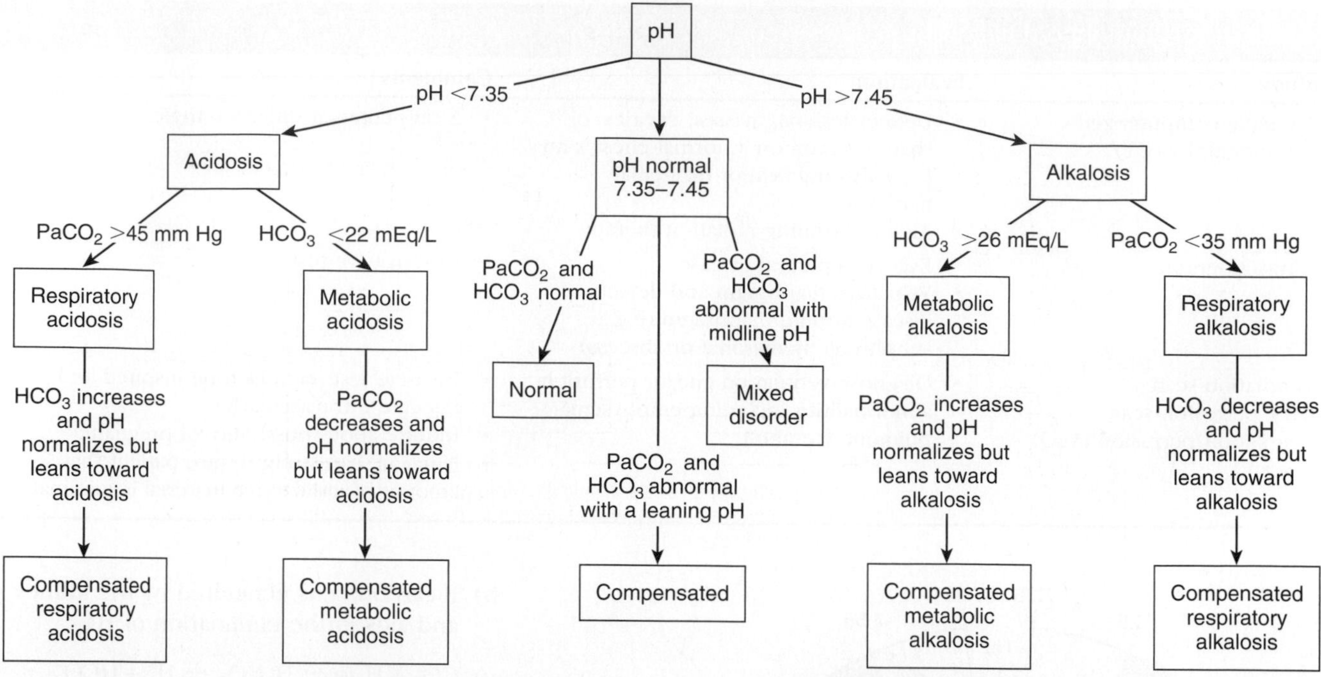

Figure 4-26 Determination of acid-base balance or imbalance.

3) Anion gap is used to differentiate between metabolic acid gain or base loss as cause of metabolic acidosis
   a) Calculated: $(Na^+ + K^+) - (Cl^- + CO_2^-)$
   b) Normal: 5-15
   c) If anion gap is normal (between 5-15), metabolic acidosis is due to a base loss.
   d) If anion gap is increased (greater than 15), metabolic acidosis is due to acid gain.
      i) Memory aid for causes of increased anion gap
         (a) M: methanol or ethanol ingestion
         (b) U: uremia
         (c) D: diabetic ketoacidosis or alcoholic ketoacidosis or starvation
         (d) P: paraldehyde ingestion
         (e) I: iron or isoniazid (INH)
         (f) L: lactic acidosis
         (g) E: ethylene glycol ingestion
         (h) S: salicylate toxicity

2. Alkalemia: pH above 7.45
   a. Alkalosis: the process causing alkalosis
      1) Caused by acid loss
         a) If acid is volatile (reflected by decrease in $PaCO_2$): respiratory alkalosis
         b) If acid is nonvolatile (reflected by increase in HCO_3^-): metabolic alkalosis
      2) Caused by base gain or metabolic acid loss (reflected by increase in HCO_3^-): metabolic alkalosis
3. Compensation
   a. Respiratory acidosis
      1) The kidneys reabsorb more bicarbonate or excrete more H^+.
      2) The bicarbonate and base excess levels increase.
      3) This change will be slow and may take as long as 2-3 days.
   b. Respiratory alkalosis
      1) The kidneys excrete more bicarbonate.
      2) The bicarbonate and base excess levels decrease.
      3) This change will be slow and may take as long as 2-3 days.
         a) Because respiratory alkalosis is almost always a short-term process (e.g., hyperventilation anxiety syndrome), compensation for respiratory alkalosis is rarely seen because it takes too long and the problem would be resolved.
   c. Metabolic acidosis
      1) The lungs increase the rate and depth of ventilation.
      2) The $PaCO_2$ level decreases.
      3) This change will be rapid, usually within minutes to hours.
   d. Metabolic alkalosis
      1) The lungs decrease the rate and depth of ventilation.
      2) The $PaCO_2$ level increases.
      3) This change will be rapid, usually within minutes to hours.
   e. Correction versus compensation
      1) Correction may be a physiologic process or the result of appropriate therapeutic measures; correction is achieved when the

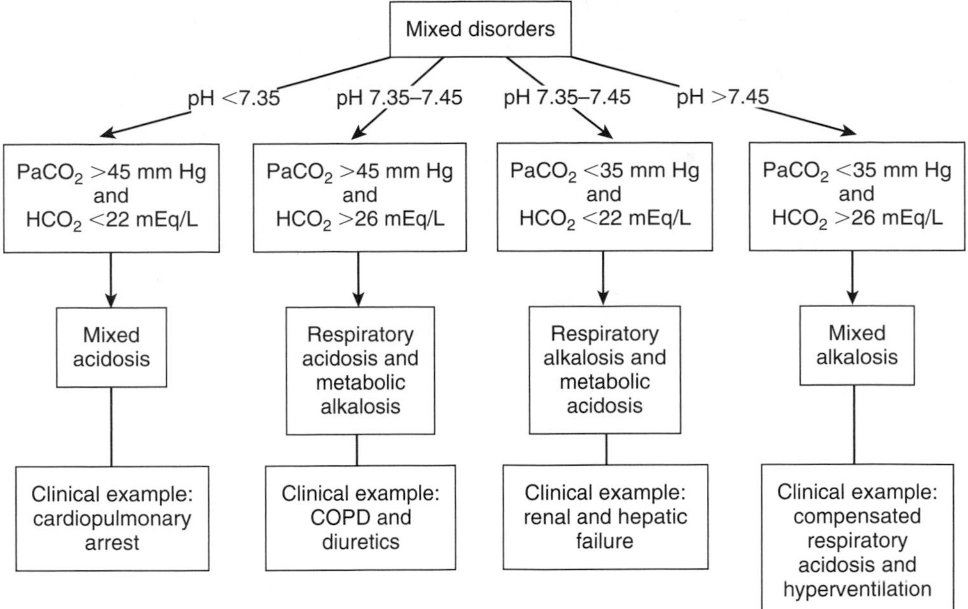

Figure 4-27 Mixed disorders and clinical examples.

*pH and HCO_3 move in the same direction

pH is normal and both indicators ($PaCO_2$, HCO_3^-) are normal.

2) Compensation is a physiologic process; the pH is normal and both indicators are abnormal.
   a) Partial compensation: pH is still abnormal but the secondary parameter is outside normal range in the direction to move the pH toward normal
   b) Full compensation: pH is normal and the secondary parameter is outside normal range in the direction to move the pH toward normal

4. Mixed disorders (Figure 4-27)
   a. More than one disorder may coexist.
   b. The degree of respiratory component versus metabolic component can be calculated utilizing these formulas.
      1) As the $PaCO_2$ changes by 10 mm Hg (from normal of 40), it is associated with a change in pH of .08 in the opposite direction.
      2) As the pH changes by 0.15 (from normal of 7.4), it is associated with a change in base of 10 mEq.
   c. Compensation cannot exist in mixed disorders because each system is independently abnormal and cannot help the other.

Analysis of Arterial Blood Gases

1. Purposes of arterial blood gases
   a. Evaluate ventilation: $PaCO_2$
   b. Evaluate acid-base status: pH; to determine the cause of the acid-base imbalance, determine which parameter is abnormal
      1) Respiratory: $PaCO_2$
      2) Metabolic: HCO_3^-
   c. Evaluate oxygenation: PaO_2

Box 4-5 Arterial Blood Gas Normal Values

pH	7.35-7.45
$PaCO_2$	35-45 mm Hg
HCO_3^-	22-26 mEq/L
PaO_2	80-100 mm Hg

2. Parameters and normals (Box 4-5)
   a. pH: negative logarithm of hydrogen ion concentration in arterial blood
      1) Normal pH is 7.35-7.45
      2) Levels below 7.35 indicate an acidosis
      3) Levels above 7.45 indicate an alkalosis
   b. $PaCO_2$: partial pressure of carbon dioxide in arterial blood
      1) Normal $PaCO_2$ is 35-45 mm Hg
      2) Levels below 35 indicate a respiratory alkalosis or respiratory compensation for a metabolic acidosis
      3) Levels above 45 indicate a respiratory acidosis or respiratory compensation for a metabolic alkalosis
   c. HCO_3^-: bicarbonate ion level in arterial blood
      1) Normal HCO_3^- is 22-26 mEq/L
      2) Levels below 22 indicate a metabolic acidosis or metabolic compensation for respiratory alkalosis
      3) Levels above 26 indicate a metabolic alkalosis or metabolic compensation for respiratory acidosis
   d. Base excess (BE): difference between acid and base levels in arterial blood
      1) Normal BE is +2 to −2
      2) Levels below −2 (actually a base deficit) indicate a metabolic acidosis or metabolic compensation for respiratory alkalosis

3) Levels above +2 indicate a metabolic alkalosis or metabolic compensation for respiratory acidosis
e. PaO_2: partial pressure of oxygen in arterial blood
1) Normal PaO_2 is 80-100 mm Hg
2) Levels above 100 indicate hyperoxemia
3) Levels below 80 indicate mild hypoxemia
4) Levels below 60 indicate moderate hypoxemia
5) Levels below 40 indicate severe hypoxemia
f. SaO_2: saturation of hemoglobin by oxygen
1) Normal SaO_2 is 95% or greater
2) Levels below 95% indicate mild desaturation of hemoglobin
3) Levels below 90% indicate moderate desaturation of hemoglobin
4) Levels below 75% indicate severe desaturation of hemoglobin
3. Steps in analysis
a. Is pH acidotic, alkalotic, or normal?
b. Which parameter is abnormal?
1) $PaCO_2$: respiratory
2) HCO_3^-: metabolic
c. If the pH is normal, is it leaning? If so, consider compensation.
1) Compensation causes a leaning pH; the pH leans toward the initial disorder.
a) The body never overcompensates; a normal nonleaning pH with two abnormal indicators ($PaCO_2$ and HCO_3^-) suggests a mixed disorder (e.g., one alkalotic process + one acidotic process).
2) For compensation to be occurring, one parameter change must help the other.
a) Full compensation: normal pH with both indicators abnormal
b) Partial compensation
i) pH is still abnormal
ii) Both indicators ($PaCO_2$ and HCO_3^-) are abnormal with the secondary indicator moving in the direction to help normalize the pH
d. Assess oxygenation
1) PaO_2 less than 80 mm Hg is hypoxemia.
2) PaO_2 less than 60 mm Hg on room air is usually an indication for oxygen administration.
3) Acceptable PaO_2 should be adjusted for age; one method is to subtract 1 mm Hg for each year greater than 60 years from 80 mm Hg; this gives acceptable PaO_2 on room air for a patient of that age.
4. Technical problems that may affect accuracy of arterial blood gas values
a. Too much heparin: decrease in $PaCO_2$, decrease in HCO_3^-, increase in base excess except with point of care analyzers (e.g., ISTAT)
b. Air bubble: increase in pH, decrease in $PaCO_2$, increase in PaO_2
c. Not chilled immediately: decrease in pH, decrease in PaO_2, increase in $PaCO_2$ except with point of care analyzers (e.g., ISTAT)
d. Inadequate discard volume when drawing from catheter with flush solution: decreased $PaCO_2$

Discussion of Acid-Base Imbalances

See Table 4-10.

Airway Management

Etiology of Airway Obstruction

1. Upper airway
a. Relaxation of tongue against hypopharynx: primary cause of obstruction in unconscious patient
b. Foreign body aspiration
1) Aspiration of food: primary cause of obstruction in conscious patient
2) Vomitus
3) Dentures
c. Tumor
d. Hematoma
e. Laryngeal spasm, edema
f. Vocal cord paralysis
g. Infection (e.g., epiglottis)
h. Trauma (e.g., fractured trachea)
i. Inflammation (e.g., angioedema, ingestion of caustic agents)
2. Lower airway
a. Foreign bodies
b. Secretions
c. Hemorrhage
d. Pneumonia
e. Space-occupying lesions, tumors
f. Bronchospasm

Clinical Presentation of Airway Obstruction

1. Partial obstruction
a. Presence of air movement
b. Restlessness, agitation, anxiety
c. Respiratory distress: tracheal tug; intercostal retractions; use of accessory muscles
d. Cyanosis
e. Coughing
f. Altered speech
g. Inspiratory sounds: snoring; stridor
h. Breath sound changes: wheezes; rhonchi
2. Complete obstruction
a. Lack of air movement
b. Extreme anxiety in conscious patient
c. Respiratory distress: tracheal tug; intercostal retractions; use of accessory muscles
d. Cyanosis
e. Inability to speak, cough, or produce any sound
f. Universal sign of choking: patient clutches throat with hand
g. Unconsciousness within seconds

Table 4-10 Discussion of Acid-Base Imbalances

Imbalance	Etiology	Clinical Presentation	Collaborative Management

Respiratory acidosis: pH low; $PaCO_2$ high	Hypoventilation
	• Airway obstruction
	• CNS depression from drugs, injury, or disease
	• Chest wall injury (e.g., flail chest)
	• Obstructive lung disease (e.g., chronic bronchitis, emphysema, late asthma)
	• Restrictive lung disease (e.g., kyphoscoliosis, obesity hypoventilation syndrome)
	• Oxygen-induced hypoventilation in patients with chronic hypercapnia
	• Neuromuscular abnormality (e.g., Guillain-Barré syndrome, myasthenia gravis, multiple sclerosis)
	• Atelectasis, pneumonia
	• Pulmonary edema
	• Respiratory arrest
		Initially
		• Sympathetic nervous system stimulation symptoms (e.g., tachycardia, tachypnea, diaphoresis)
		Later
		• Bradypnea
		• Hypotension
		• Dysrhythmias
		• Confusion
		• Headache
		• Blurred vision
		• Flushed face (plethora)
		• Somnolence leading to coma
		(These late symptoms are also referred to as *CO_2 narcosis*)
			Increase ventilation and treat cause
			• Maintain patent airway
			• Position for optimal ventilation
			• Implement bronchial hygiene measures
			• Administer drug therapy (e.g., bronchodilators, mucolytics, antibiotics)
			• Mechanical ventilation may be necessary
			• If patient is on mechanical ventilation
			  • Increase rate
			  • Increase tidal volume

Respiratory alkalosis: pH high; $PaCO_2$ low	Hyperventilation
	• Anxiety or hysteria
	• Thoracic pain
	• Early asthma
	• Pneumothorax
	• Pulmonary embolus
	• Early salicylate intoxication
	• Hyperthyroidism
	• Hepatic failure
	• Fever
	• Gram-negative septicemia
	• CNS infection or injury
	• Excessive mechanical ventilation
		• Tachycardia
		• Palpitations
		• Dry mouth
		• Anxiety
		• Profuse perspiration
		• Paresthesia around mouth and extremities
		• Dizziness, vertigo, syncope
		• Increased muscle irritability, twitching
		• Tetany
		• Inability to concentrate
		• Seizures
		• Coma
			Decrease ventilation and treat cause
			• Provide reassurance and maintain a calm attitude
			• Administer sedatives (frequently given intravenously)
			• Ask patient to breathe into and out of a paper bag or use a rebreathing mask
			• If patient is on mechanical ventilation
			  • Decrease rate
			  • Decrease tidal volume
			  • Change from assist-control to IMV
			  • Consider sedation
			  • Consider addition of dead space tubing

Metabolic acidosis: pH low; HCO_3^- low	Acid gain (increased anion gap)
	• Tissue hypoxia (e.g., shock [lactic acidosis])
	• Ketoacidosis (diabetic ketoacidosis or starvation)
	• Renal failure
	• Drugs and toxins (e.g., salicylates; methanol, ethylene glycol)
	Bicarbonate loss (normal anion gap)
	• Bile drainage
	• Pancreatic fistula
	• Diarrhea
	• Acetazolamide (Diamox) therapy
		• Nausea, vomiting, abdominal discomfort
		• Weakness
		• Tremors
		• Malaise
		• Headache
		• Tachypnea progressing to Kussmaul's
		• Hypotension
		• Dysrhythmias
		• Confusion
		• Lethargy → coma
			• Treat cause as appropriate
			  • Improve oxygenation and/or perfusion (lactic acidosis)
			  • Give insulin for DKA
			  • Initiate dialysis for renal failure
			  • Administer antidiarrheals for diarrhea
			Administer buffer
			  • Bicarbonate IV or orally for pH 7 or less

Continued

Table 4-10 Discussion of Acid-Base Imbalances—cont'd

Imbalance	Etiology	Clinical Presentation	Collaborative Management

Metabolic alkalosis: pH high; HCO_3^- high	Acid loss
	• Nasogastric suction or severe vomiting
	• Potassium-wasting diuretic therapy
	• Steroid therapy
	• Cushing's disease
	• Hyperaldosteronism
	• Hepatic disease
	• Hypokalemia, hypochloremia
	Bicarbonate gain
	• Bicarbonate administration
	• Excess infusion of lactated Ringer's solution
	• Lactate administration in dialysis solution
		• Bradypnea
		• Nausea, vomiting, diarrhea
		• Paresthesia around mouth and extremities
		• Confusion
		• Dizziness
		• Increased muscle irritability
		• Tetany
		• Seizures
		• Coma
			• Treat cause
			  • Antiemetic
			  • Electrolyte replacement: potassium and/or chloride
			  • Discontinuance of sodium bicarbonate or lactated Ringer's solution
			• Administer carbonic anhydrase inhibitor
			  • Acetazolamide (Diamox)
			• Administer buffer
			  • Arginine monohydrochloride
			  • Ammonium chloride
			  • Weak HCl acid solution

Collaborative Management of Airway Obstruction and/or Respiratory Distress

1. Evaluate the patency of the airway: look, listen, feel for airflow
2. Maintain optimal airway and thoracic position
   a. Use head tilt–chin lift (also called *sniffing*) position for optimal airway position.
      1) True hyperextension should be avoided.
      2) Contraindicated if cervical spine fracture possible (instead use jaw thrust)
   b. Position head of bed for optimal chest excursion: semi-Fowler's to high Fowler's position
3. Remove any obstruction.
   a. Inspect the mouth for blood, teeth, loose dentures, food, or anything else that may cause obstruction.
   b. Remove any visible obstruction.
      1) Use fingers to remove visible foreign bodies; blind sweeps are not recommended due to concern that the obstruction may be pushed deeper into the airway.
      2) Magill forceps may be used, but care must be taken to prevent pushing the obstruction deeper into the airway.
   c. Use abdominal thrusts (also referred to as *Heimlich maneuver*): subxiphoid thrusts to relieve upper airway obstruction
      1) Alternate five abdominal thrusts with attempts to ventilate in unconscious patient.
      2) Avoid abdominal thrusts (use chest thrusts) in any of the following situations:
         a) Patient is too obese for you to get your arms around him or her.
         b) Patient has had recent abdominal surgery.
         c) Patient is pregnant.
   d. Place in recovery position: side-lying on left side
4. Encourage deep breathing: sustained inspiratory effort
   a. Purposes of deep breathing include the following:
      1) Increases air in the alveoli, preventing atelectasis
      2) Makes coughing more effective
   b. Incentive spirometry may also be used to provide graded incentives for sustained inspiration.
5. Remove secretions as required.
   a. Cough: forceful expiration to dislodge and remove secretions from the tracheobronchial tree
      1) Indications
         a) Breath sound changes: especially rhonchi; wheezes caused by mucus plugs may also clear with coughing
         b) With postural drainage: between position changes but never in a head-down position
         c) NOTE: While coughing should be encouraged in the previously identified situations, routine coughing may increase the incidence of atelectasis; preventive measures (e.g., for postoperative patients) should focus on deep breathing with sustained inspiration rather than forced expiration (e.g., coughing)
      2) Technique for effective coughing
         a) Assist patient to a comfortable position.
         b) Instruct patient to do the following:
            i) Inhale deeply.
            ii) Cough two to three times with mouth open.
            iii) Expectorate any sputum.
            iv) Inhale slowly and deeply.
      3) Special techniques
         a) Huff coughing

i) Forced expiration with glottis open
ii) May be helpful for patients with COPD to keep airways open

b) Augmented coughing
i) Requires an assistant to deliver a subxiphoid thrust during expiration
ii) May be necessary for patients with abdominal muscle weakness or paralysis

c) Use of a flutter valve (Warren & Livesay, 2006)
i) Small plastic handheld device that consists of a small plastic cone containing a steel ball
ii) Instruction to patient should include the following:
(a) Inhaling deeply, hold the breath for 2-3 seconds, and then exhale into the flutter valve.
(b) Use it 3-4 times daily with 10-15 repetitions each session.
(c) Use any prescribed bronchodilator before use of the flutter valve.
iii) Promotes airway clearance in the following ways:
(a) Vibration of airways to loosen secretions
(b) Maintenance of open airways during exhalation
(c) Creation of mini-coughs

b. Suctioning of oropharynx: removal of secretions from the oropharynx through the use of a suction catheter and negative pressure
1) Performed before deflation of endotracheal tube cuff to prevent oropharyngeal secretions from draining into tracheobronchial tree
2) Performed routinely after suctioning of tracheobronchial tree to prevent accumulation of oropharyngeal secretions that can be silently aspirated around endotracheal tube cuff
3) Yankauer suction device usually used; if suction catheter that was used to suction the tracheobronchial tree is used, suction oropharynx only **after** suctioning the tracheobronchial tree and rinsing the catheter
4) Specialized endotracheal tube to allow for continuous aspiration of subglottic secretions (CASS) has been shown to reduce the incidence or delay the onset of ventilator-associated pneumonia (see Pneumonia in Chapter 5)
a) Upper airway secretions pool above the ET tube cuff and cause microaspiration and ventilator-associated pneumonia.
b) Multiple studies have established effectiveness of CASS, and a recent study (Speroni et al., 2011) also demonstrated cost effectiveness.

c. Suctioning of tracheobronchial tree: removal of secretions from the tracheobronchial tree through the use of a suction catheter and negative pressure
1) Clinical indications for the need to suction; suctioning of the airway should not be "routine" but should be performed when indicated
a) Sympathetic nervous system stimulation (tachycardia, tachypnea)
b) Change in BP: increased or decreased
c) Dyspnea
d) Noisy or shallow ventilation
e) Rhonchi
f) Obvious visible secretions
g) Frequent or sustained coughing especially during inspiratory cycle of ventilator
h) High-pressure alarm on ventilator
i) Clinical indications of hypoxia (Box 4-3), hypercapnia (Box 4-4)
2) Technique for suctioning the tracheobronchial tree utilizing principles to prevent complications
a) Suction only if indicated and limit number of passes to minimum required.
b) The outer diameter of the catheter should be no more than half the inner diameter of the ET tube or tracheostomy.
c) Utilize closed suction system if possible.
i) Advantages of closed suction system include the following:
(a) Continued oxygenation and reduction in loss of PEEP so decreased incidence of hypoxemia
(b) Decreased cost and nursing time
(c) Decreased chance of aerosolization of secretions, which protects patient's and nurse's eyes
(d) Decreased risk of introducing bacteria into airway
ii) If closed suction system is not available, utilize special adaptor for patients on therapeutic PEEP because these patients frequently have significant oxygen desaturation during suctioning.
iii) Special curved-tip catheter (Coude′ catheter) is required to enter the left mainstem bronchus; it is usually adequate to use a regular suction catheter to suction the right mainstem bronchus and the

trachea because the coughing stimulated effectively clears the left mainstem bronchus into the trachea.

d) Sterile technique is used if suctioning through endotracheal tube or tracheostomy; aseptic technique is used if suctioning nasotracheally
   i) Two gloves should be used.
   ii) Goggles should be worn to protect the nurse's eyes.
e) Explain procedure to the patient; protect the patient's eyes if not using a closed suction system.
f) Hyperoxygenation (100% oxygen) before, during, and after suctioning; ensure that SpO_2 reflects this increase in oxygen prior to initiating suctioning
g) If doing nasotracheal suctioning, place patient in "sniffing" position while sitting up, or place towel roll between shoulders if patient is supine and use water-soluble lubricant to lubricate the catheter
h) Advance catheter to no farther than 1 cm past the end of the ET tube to avoid contact with the trachea and carina.
   i) The previous technique of advancing the catheter to the point of obstruction, then pulling back slightly before applying suction, should be avoided.
   ii) Shallow suctioning decreases mucosal damage, decreases mucus production, and results in less mucosal inflammation
i) Limit suctioning to 10 seconds; there is no difference in patient outcomes with intermittent versus continuous suction as long as the duration is limited to 10 seconds.
j) Avoid excessive negative pressure; keep pressure 100 mm Hg or less unless closed suction system; 120 mm Hg is recommended if closed suction system
k) Liquefy secretions through humidification and hydration.
   i) Instillation of saline (also referred to as *saline lavage*) has been proven ineffective and potentially harmful; contributes to hypoxemia and ventilator-associated pneumonia
   ii) If increased oral or parenteral fluids cannot be given (e.g., renal failure), either of the following may be prescribed.
      (a) Saline by inhalation (small particle size allows deeper penetration into tracheobronchial tube and liquefies mucus)
      (b) Acetylcysteine (Mucomyst) given by inhalation (breaks down disulfide bonds to liquefy mucus); concurrent bronchodilator is frequently required
l) Rinse catheter and appropriately discard disposable catheter; if closed suction system, rinse the catheter after pulling it back to black line and then injecting saline into irrigation port while applying suction (note that this is irrigation, not lavage), and then close irrigation port and suction valve.
m) Monitor complications during and after suctioning.
   i) SpO_2 during suctioning for oxygen desaturation
   ii) ECG during and after suctioning for vagal stimulation (bradycardia) as well as dysrhythmias related to hypoxemia (PVCs)
n) Stop suctioning if: change in heart rate, ECG rhythm, or skin color; significant change in SpO_2 or SvO_2
o) Assess breath sounds after suctioning to evaluate effectiveness.

3) If doing nasotracheal suctioning in a patient who does not have an endotracheal or tracheostomy tube
   a) Provide oxygen with a non-rebreathing mask prior to suctioning.
   b) Place patient in "sniffing" position while sitting up, or place towel roll between shoulders if patient is supine.
   c) Lubricate catheter with water-soluble lubricant prior to insertion.
   d) Prevent injury to the nasal mucosa.
      i) Placement of a nasopharyngeal airway may be done to prevent injury to the nasal mucosa if frequent suctioning is required.
      ii) Endotracheal intubation or tracheostomy may also be required if frequent suctioning is required.
   e) Ask the patient to cough and advance the catheter during that time because the glottis is open; if the patient cannot follow commands, advance the catheter during inspiration.
   f) Note indications that the catheter is in the trachea.
      i) Patient becomes anxious
      ii) Patient cannot speak
   g) Complete suctioning as for a patient with an endotracheal or tracheostomy tube.
4) Advantages of closed suction system

a) Continued oxygenation and reduction in loss of PEEP so decreased incidence of hypoxemia
b) Decreased cost and nursing time
c) Decreased chance of aerosolization of secretions, which protects patient's and nurse's eyes
d) Decreased risk of introducing bacteria into airway

5) Specialized endotracheal tube to allow for continuous aspiration of subglottic secretions (CASS) has been shown to reduce the incidence or delay the onset of ventilator-associated pneumonia (see Pneumonia in Chapter 5).
a) Upper airway secretions pool above the ET tube cuff and cause microaspiration and ventilator-associated pneumonia.
b) Multiple studies have established effectiveness of CASS, and a recent study (Speroni et al., 2011) also demonstrated cost effectiveness

6. Provide chest physiotherapy (chest PT) as indicated.
a. Purposes
1) To promote bronchial hygiene
2) Improve breathing efficiency
3) Promote physical reconditioning
b. Postural drainage (PD): sequential positioning of the patient
1) Purpose: Utilize gravity to drain secretions from peripheral areas into the major bronchi or trachea so that they can be coughed and expectorated or suctioned.
2) Indication: prevention and treatment of respiratory complications
a) Lobar atelectasis
b) Disorders with significant mucus production (e.g., cystic fibrosis, bronchiectasis, COPD)
3) Technique
a) Administer bronchodilator prior to PD if prescribed.
b) Turn off enteral feedings for 30 minutes prior to postural drainage; ensure that cuff of endotracheal or tracheostomy tube is inflated.
c) Place patient in position to drain selected segment of lung or alternate through the following positions.
i) Left side with hips higher than head
ii) Right side with hips higher than head
iii) Supine with hips higher than head
iv) Prone with hips higher than head
d) Maintain each position for 10-30 minutes.
e) Cough between position changes but never in a head-down position.
f) Avoid PD for at least 1.5 hours after meals
4) Contraindications
a) Obesity
b) Spinal fracture, rib fracture, flail chest
c) Pulmonary hemorrhage, embolism, malignancy
d) Pneumothorax, empyema, large pleural effusion
e) Tuberculosis
f) Asthma, acute bronchospasm
g) Bleeding disorder
h) Seizures, intracranial hypertension
i) Acute myocardial infarction, heart failure, hemodynamic instability
j) Recent pacemaker insertion
k) Increased risk of aspiration
c. Percussion: clapping the chest with cupped hands
1) Purpose: Mechanically dislodge secretions from the bronchial walls into the major bronchi or trachea so that they can be coughed and expectorated or suctioned.
2) Technique
a) If using hands:
i) Cup hands as if holding water.
ii) Tap chest with cupped hands listening for a cupping, not slapping, sound.
b) If using vibropercussion bed function:
i) Set timing.
ii) May be used in conjunction with continuous lateral rotation therapy (CLRT)
c) Avoid: spine, liver, kidneys, spleen, and female patient's breasts
3) Contraindications
a) Known bleeding disorder
b) Lung cancer
c) Pneumothorax
d) Extreme caution in elderly patients with osteoporosis after thoracotomy
d. Vibration: during expiration of areas of the chest with either an open hand or a vibrating device
1) Purpose: Loosen secretions from the bronchial walls into the major bronchi or trachea so that they can be coughed and expectorated or suctioned.
2) Technique
a) Hold hand flat against chest and vibrate hand during expiration.
b) Hand vibrator may also be used.
3) Contraindications: as for percussion

7. Turn patient at least every 2 hours; utilize special bed as appropriate.
a. Consider "good lung down" principle for patients with unilateral lung conditions (exception: pneumonectomy when the rule is "no lung down")

b. Consider kinetic therapy through the use of continuous lateral rotational therapy bed if appropriate.
   1) Effect: promotes redistribution of ventilation, promotes redistribution of perfusion, and optimizes ventilation/perfusion matching
   2) Indications
      a) Acute lung injury (ALI)/acute respiratory distress syndrome (ARDS) or high risk for ALI/ARDS
      b) Pneumonia
      c) Prevention of ventilator-associated pneumonia (VAP) and lobar atelectasis
   3) Guidelines
      a) Start as early as possible.
      b) Explain the process to the patient prior to turning.
      c) Monitor blood pressure and SpO_2 frequently especially initially until acclimation.
   4) Contraindications
      a) Table rotational beds
         i) Severe claustrophobia, though most of these patients will be sedated
         ii) Uncontrolled diarrhea
         iii) Weight of greater than 500 pounds
      b) Cushion-based beds and mattress replacement beds
         i) Severe claustrophobia, though most of these patients will be sedated
         ii) Uncontrolled diarrhea
         iii) Weight of greater than 300 pounds
         iv) Unstable spinal cord injury
         v) Skeletal traction
c. Consider placing the patient in prone position periodically if appropriate; frequently used in acute lung injury (ALI) and acute respiratory distress syndrome (ARDS)
   1) Effects
      a) Improved compliance of the dorsal chest wall which increases reexpansion of dependent lung regions which optimizes V/Q matching
      b) Reduction in the amount of lung volume compressed by the heart
      c) Lessening of the compression on the lower lobes by the pressure of the abdominal contents against the diaphragm, which improves ventilation of the lower lobes
      d) Reduction of the gradients of pleural and transpulmonary pressures causing more even distribution of ventilation
      e) PEEP is more likely to result in more homogeneous perfusion in the lung in prone position; PEEP tends to redistribute blood flow away from well-ventilated ventral areas of the lung in supine position.
   2) Contraindications
      a) Intracranial hypertension
      b) Unstable fractures, especially cervical, thoracic, or lumbar fractures
      c) Cervical or skeletal traction
      d) Left ventricular failure
      e) Hemodynamic instability
      f) Active intraabdominal process
      g) Pregnancy
      h) Weight greater than 300 pounds may be a contraindication depending on method of turning and/or special bed
   3) Complications
      a) Skin breakdown, particularly the face, ears, nose, eyes, mouth, shoulders, elbows, hips, knees, genitalia, and breasts
         i) Extra care must be taken with breast and penile implants
      b) Dependent edema
      c) Corneal abrasions
      d) Inadvertent extubation or removal of catheters
      e) Obstructed chest tube
      f) Nerve injury
      g) Transient supraventricular tachycardia
      h) Aspiration
   4) Methods
      a) Requires three to four personnel depending on patient size; one person should be at the head to stabilize endotracheal tube, central venous catheters, etc.
      b) Explain the procedure to the patient and administer sedation and/or analgesia
      c) Withhold enteral feedings for the hour prior to turning to prone but continue feedings once in prone position
      d) Equipment
         i) Use of pillows to position patient in swimming position and elevate abdomen off the bed to prevent impairment in diaphragmatic excursion
         ii) KCI's RotoProne bed
         iii) Use of special bed with pronating capability (e.g., KCI's TriaDyne II with proning accessory)
         iv) Use of Hillrom's Vollman Prone Positioner
      e) Monitor blood pressure and SpO_2
      f) Frequent repositioning is still required to prevent pressure ulcers.
   5) Though dramatic improvement in oxygenation frequently occurs, improved survival has not been demonstrated.

8. Utilize artificial airways safely and appropriately.
   a. General principles

1) Provide humidification because natural humidification mechanisms are bypassed.
2) Use aseptic technique with upper airway artificial airways; use sterile technique with lower airway artificial airways.
3) Suction as indicated; because endotracheal tubes splint the epiglottis open, effective coughing is impaired.
4) Provide method of communication; this is the most significant stressor experienced by intubated patients.
   a) Picture communication board, alphabet board, magic slate, felt-tip pen or marker and paper may be used; avoid pencils and ballpoint pens, which require more pressure.
   b) Fenestrated or Passy-Muir tracheostomy tubes may be used in some patients; these allow air to leak over the vocal cords.
   c) Lip reading is usually *not* an acceptable method especially if oral tube is in place.

b. Selection of appropriate artificial airway (Table 4-11)
c. Summary of artificial airways (Table 4-12)
   1) Upper airway artificial airways
      a) Oropharyngeal airway
      b) Nasopharyngeal airway
      c) Cricothyrotomy
   2) Lower airway artificial airways
      a) Esophageal-tracheal Combitube
      b) Laryngeal mask airway (LMA)
      c) Endotracheal tube
         i) Nasotracheal tube
         ii) Orotracheal tube
         iii) Continuous subglottic secretion (CASS) ET tube (Figure 4-28)
      d) Tracheostomy

d. Endotracheal intubation
   1) Indications
      a) Tidal volume less than 5 mL/kg
      b) Vital capacity less than 10 mL/kg
      c) Maximal inspiratory pressure less than -20 cm H_2O
      d) Inability to adequately cough and clear airway
      e) Loss of protective reflexes
      f) Need for sealed airway (e.g., mechanical ventilation, risk for aspiration)
   2) Insertion of endotracheal tube
      a) Prepare the oxygen delivery system to be used after intubation: usually T-piece with nebulizer or mechanical ventilator; manual resuscitation bag with reservoir bag with 100% oxygen may be used during cardiac arrest or until mechanical ventilator is ready.
      b) Collect supplies and select tube size.
         i) Tube: females usually 7.5-8; males usually 8-8.5
         ii) Equipment to insert and secure tube: laryngoscope with straight (Miller) and curved (MacIntosh) blades with working lights, stylet, Magill forceps, lubricant, syringe, tape or device for stabilization of tube
         iii) Suction equipment including suction catheter and Yankauer suction device
      c) Monitor ECG and SaO_2 during intubation
      d) Hyperoxygenate with 100% oxygen for at least 2 minutes
      e) Place patient in head tilt–chin lift position
      f) Intubation should be performed by the most qualified person available who has been trained in endotracheal intubation and frequently performs the procedure (usually physician or nurse anesthetist).
      g) Intubation should be completed within 30 seconds; if not, attempts should be ceased and the patient should again be hyperoxygenated.
      h) Confirm placement of endotracheal tube.
         i) Feel air movement through tube.
         ii) Assess bilateral chest excursion.
         iii) Auscultate bilateral breath sounds; if breath sounds are audible on the right but not on the left, right mainstem intubation has occurred; pull the tube back slightly and then recheck breath sounds.

Table 4-11 Selection of Appropriate Artificial Airway

Problem	Preferred Artificial Airway
Tongue against hypopharynx	Oropharyngeal or nasopharyngeal
Need for frequent nasotracheal suctioning	Nasopharyngeal
Inability to open mouth (e.g., seizure)	Nasopharyngeal
Facial or jaw fracture	Nasopharyngeal or nasotracheal tube
Complete upper airway obstruction when endotracheal intubation is impossible (e.g., laryngeal edema or spasm, tracheal fracture)	Cricothyrotomy or tracheostomy
Need for sealed airway (e.g., mechanical ventilation or potential for aspiration)	Endotracheal tube or tracheostomy
Need for long-term lower airway access and sealed airway	Tracheostomy

Table 4-12 Summary of Artificial Airways

Type of Airway	Advantages	Disadvantages	Miscellaneous

Oropharyngeal airway	• Easy to insert
	• Inexpensive
	• Effectively holds tongue away from pharynx
		• Improper insertion technique can push tongue back and occlude airway
		• Easily dislodged
		• Poorly tolerated by conscious patients as it may stimulate gag reflex
		• Causes increased oral secretions
		• Contraindicated in patients with trauma to lower face, recent oral surgery, loose or avulsed teeth
			• Determine appropriate size: with flange at teeth, end of airway should not extend beyond the angle of the jaw
			  • Large adult: usually 100 mm (size 5)
			  • Medium adult: usually 90 mm (size 4)
			  • Small adult: usually 80 mm (size 3)
			• Insert by holding tongue down with tongue blade and sliding into place; alternative method: insert upside down and turn over when into pharynx; take care not to traumatize palate
			• Do not use as a bite block; likely to cause vomiting and potential aspiration in conscious patients
			• Remove, wash, and give mouth care every 4 hours; check mucous membranes for ulcerations

Nasopharyngeal airway (also called a *trumpet airway*)	• Easy to insert
	• Inexpensive
	• Effectively holds tongue away from pharynx
	• May be used in conscious or unconscious patients
	• Prevents trauma to nasal mucosa during nasotracheal suctioning
	• May be inserted when mouth cannot be opened (e.g., during seizures, jaw fractures)
		• May cause nosebleeds, pressure necrosis, or sinus infection
		• Kinks and clogs easily
		• Contraindicated in patients predisposed to nosebleeds, nasal obstruction, bleeding disorder, sepsis and in patients with basal skull fracture
			• Determine appropriate size: 1 inch longer than nose to earlobe; lumen smaller than naris
			  • Large adult: usually 8-9 internal diameter
			  • Medium adult: usually 7-8 internal diameter
			  • Small adult: usually 6-7 internal diameter
			• Insert with bevel against septum
			• Use viscous Xylocaine as a lubricant for insertion to decrease discomfort
			• Do not use in patients receiving anticoagulants
			• Provide humidification of inspired air
			• Confirm placement by visualizing the tip of the airway next to the uvula
			• Rotate naris to naris every 8 hours
			• Limit the duration of use to reduce risk of sinus infection

Esophageal-tracheal Combitube	• Allows ventilation whether the tube is inserted into the trachea or the esophagus • Reduces risk of aspiration over mask ventilation • Permits easier placement over endotracheal tube because visualization of the vocal cords is not necessary • Provides comparable ventilation and oxygenation to that achieved with an endotracheal tube	• Incorrect identification of the position of the distal lumen may result in absence of ventilation • May cause esophageal trauma • Cannot mechanically ventilate the patient with a Combitube	• Use of an end-tidal CO_2 or esophageal detector device is recommended to confirm placement as either being in the trachea or esophagus

Table 4-12 Summary of Artificial Airways—cont'd

Type of Airway	Advantages	Disadvantages	Miscellaneous
Laryngeal mask airway (LMA)	• Permits easier placement than endotracheal tube because visualization of the vocal cords is not necessary • Provides comparable ventilation and oxygenation to that achieved with an endotracheal tube • Allows placement when there is a possibility of unstable neck injury or when appropriate positioning of the patient for tracheal intubation is impossible • Reduces risk of aspiration over mask ventilation • Permits coughing and speech	• Small proportion of patients cannot be ventilated with an LMA so an alternative strategy is needed • Cannot prevent aspiration because it does not separate the GI tract from the respiratory tract • May cause laryngospasm or bronchospasm • May be difficult to ventilate patients who require high airway pressures to attain adequate tidal volumes	• If lubrication is required, only the posterior aspect of the airway should be lubricated • If used for mechanical ventilation, an audible air leak may occur

Endotracheal tube (general)	• Provides relatively sealed airway for mechanical ventilation and prevention of aspiration
	• Permits easy suctioning
	• Prevents gastric distention with air during CPR
		• Requires skilled personnel for insertion
		• Splints epiglottis open and prevents effective cough
		• Causes loss of physiologic PEEP because epiglottis is splinted open; patient should receive 3-5 cm PEEP to reestablish physiologic PEEP
		• May kink and clog
		• Causes aphonia
		• May cause laryngeal or tracheal damage
		• Contraindicated in patients with laryngeal obstruction caused by tumor, infection, or vocal cord paralysis
			• Determine appropriate size
			  • Females: usually 7.5-8 internal diameter
			  • Males: usually 8-8.5 internal diameter
			  • Tube may need to be 0.5-1 smaller if to be inserted nasally
			• Provide humidification of inspired air
			• Mark tube at corner of mouth or at naris to assess any movement
			• Use minimal occlusive volume or minimal leak volume for cuff inflation; insure that cuff pressure does not exceed 25 mm Hg (if pressure greater than 25 mm Hg required to achieve seal, tube is too small and needs to be replaced with larger tube)
			• Confirm placement by chest x-ray: tip of tube should be 3-5 cm above carina
			• Provide mouth care every 4 hours; observe oral or nasal mucosa for signs of ulcerations or necrosis
			• Position to prevent kinking; utilize mechanical ventilator's support arms to support ventilator tubing

Continued

Table 4-12 Summary of Artificial Airways—cont'd

Type of Airway	Advantages	Disadvantages	Miscellaneous
Oral (specific) endotracheal tube	• Easier insertion than nasal intubation • Permits larger tube than nasal intubation	• Less stable and comfortable than nasal tube • May stimulate gag reflex • May be bitten or chewed • May cause necrosis at corner of mouth • Increases oral secretions; makes mouth care more difficult • Contraindicated in patients with acute unstable cervical spine injury due to need for neck extension (blind nasotracheal intubation may be attempted in these patients)	• Reposition tube from one side of the mouth to the other and reapply tape when indicated; avoid unnecessary manipulation of tube
Nasal (specific) endotracheal tube	• More comfortable for patient than oral endotracheal tube • Permits good oral hygiene • Cannot be bitten or chewed	• More difficult insertion than oral intubation • May cause pressure necrosis or sinus infection • Requires smaller size • Contraindicated in patients with nasal obstruction, fractured nose, sinusitis, bleeding disorder, basal skull fracture	• Monitor for clinical indications of sinus infection: fever; increased pharyngeal drainage; halitosis; leukocytosis; sinus pain or headache
Cricothyrotomy	• Provides immediate airway access, especially helpful if complete upper airway obstruction	• May cause bleeding • Only temporary; very small opening if established with large needle; larger if airway opened with scalpel and small tracheostomy tube used	• Provide humidification of inspired air • Use large bore over-the-needle catheter; adaptor required to attach to manual resuscitation bag • Physician may use scalpel and insert small tracheostomy tube • Monitor for bleeding, subcutaneous emphysema
Tracheostomy	• Provides long-term airway access • Minimizes risk of vocal cord damage from an endotracheal tube during long-term airway maintenance • Decreases dead space and decreases work of breathing • Provides a relative seal to prevent aspiration • Allows the patient to eat and swallow • Allows easier suctioning • Permits Valsalva maneuver and effective cough • Is more comfortable for patient • Is less likely to be dislodged than endotracheal tube • Bypasses upper airway obstruction	• May require surgery but may be performed percutaneously • Causes aphonia • May cause false passage anterior to trachea in patients with thick necks • May cause erosion of innominate artery with tip of tube or low stoma • Causes scar • May cause tracheocutaneous or tracheoesophageal fistula	• Usually considered if artificial airway is required longer than 2-3 weeks • Determine appropriate size: usually 5-6 • Requires humidification of inspired air • Preferred if airway obstruction (e.g., tumor or laryngeal edema or spasm) • Provide tracheostomy care that includes cleaning stoma and tube every 8 hours with saline; keep stoma dry (if 4 × 4-inch gauze used, change often if secretions present) • Keep obturator, extra tracheostomy tube, and tracheal spreader at bedside

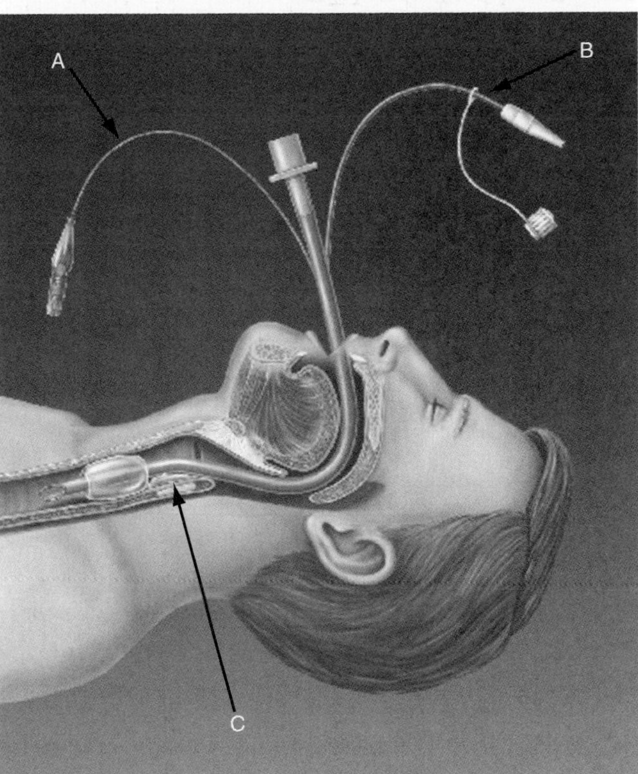

Figure 4-28 Specialized endotracheal tube used for continuous aspiration of subglottic secretions (CASS). *A,* Lumen for inflation of cuff. *B,* Lumen for aspiration of subglottic secretions. *C,* Opening of aspiration port. (Courtesy Nellcor Puritan Bennett Inc., Pleasanton, CA.)

iv) Use a capnometer to confirm consistent exhalation of CO_2.
v) Auscultate over epigastrium: Air movement should not be audible.
vi) Confirm tube positioning by chest x-ray; distal tip of tube should be 3-5 cm above the carina.

i) Inflate the cuff using either minimal occlusive volume or minimal leak volume.
   i) Cuffs in current use are high-volume, low-pressure cuffs; these cuffs distribute the low pressure over a larger area of the trachea and decrease the incidence of tracheal ischemia and stenosis; laryngectomy patients may have uncuffed (and longer) laryngectomy tube.
   ii) Cuffed tubes provide **relative** seal for patients receiving mechanical ventilation and aid in prevention of aspiration; note that cuffs do not establish an absolute seal, and silent aspiration of oropharyngeal or gastric secretions is common in critically ill patients.
   iii) Inflate cuff using minimal occlusive volume or minimal leak volume.
      (a) Minimal occlusive volume
         (i) Listen over trachea with stethoscope.
         (ii) Inflate cuff until no air leak is audible during the inspiratory cycle of the ventilator.
      (b) Minimal leak volume
         (i) Listen over trachea with stethoscope.
         (ii) Inflate cuff until no air leak is audible during the inspiratory cycle of the ventilator.
         (iii) Remove 0.1 cm of air or until a minimal leak is audible during the inspiratory cycle of the ventilator.

j) Intracuff pressure should not exceed capillary filling pressure but should be adequate to prevent the drainage of excessive subglottic secretions.
   i) Measure and record cuff pressure every 8 hours with a cuff pressure gauge or a mercury manometer and three-way stopcock.
      (a) Continuous monitoring of cuff pressure is currently being advocated because cuff pressures change over time and with some clinical activities such as endotracheal suctioning, coughing, and patient-ventilator dyssynchrony (Sole et al., 2009).
   ii) Recommended pressure is between 20-25 mm Hg (24-30 cm H_2O)

k) Routine deflation is not necessary with high-volume, low-pressure cuffs and may contribute to nosocomial pneumonia by allowing oropharyngeal secretions to drain into the tracheobronchial tree.

l) Tape tube in place.
   i) Secure tape to minimize pressure areas on the face; tape with tension to both sides to avoid excessive pressure on corner of mouth if oral tube.
   ii) If a commercial stabilization device is used, monitor oral mucosa carefully for evidence of excessive pressure.

m) Note the depth marking on the side of the tube.
   i) Usually at 19-23 cm for an average adult or 3 times the tube size so that a size 7 should be at ~21 cm, a size 7.5 should be at ~22.5, etc.
   ii) Cut tube so that only 2-3 inches of tube extends beyond mouth or

nose to decrease airway resistance and potential for kinking.

n) Attach oxygen delivery system or mechanical ventilator.

e. Extubation of intubated patients
   1) Criteria
      a) Patient awake and oriented or able to keep airway open
         i) Protective reflexes must be intact (e.g., gag).
         ii) Patient should not be paralyzed or excessively narcotized or sedated.
      b) Vital signs stable; acceptable hemoglobin and hemodynamics
      c) ABGs within acceptable limits after a trial of 30 minutes on nebulizer (T-piece) at 40% oxygen: PaO_2 60 mm Hg or greater, SaO_2 90% or greater, $PaCO_2$ 35-45 mm Hg or consistent with patient's normal values
      d) Acceptable bedside ventilatory parameters:
         i) Tidal volume 5 mL/kg or greater
         ii) Vital capacity 10 mL/kg or greater
         iii) Maximal inspiratory pressure (MIP) of −20 cm H_2O or greater
   2) Technique
      a) Have postextubation oxygen delivery system ready; intubation kit should also be available.
      b) Suction trachea, then pharynx.
      c) Deflate cuff.
      d) Remove tube during expiration.
      e) Apply oxygen delivery system.
      f) Encourage patient to cough; suction if needed.
      g) Repeat blood gases 20-30 minutes after extubation and as indicated thereafter.
      h) Observe for laryngospasm: stridor, dyspnea, tachypnea; treatment may include high humidity, steroids, racemic epinephrine, or reintubation.
      i) Monitor patient's tolerance to extubation by clinical observation, ventilatory measurements, and blood gas studies.

f. Weaning patients from tracheostomy tube
   1) Indications same as for endotracheal extubation
   2) Techniques
      a) Progression to a smaller size uncuffed (or cuff not inflated) trach tube
         i) Allows the patient to use his or her upper airway and the opening of the trach tube
         ii) Increases airway resistance and work of breathing
      b) Change to fenestrated tube: opening at the top of tube allows air to leak upward so that the patient can use the upper airway (and can speak)
      c) Deflate cuff
         i) Allows the patient to use his or her upper airway and the opening of the trach tube
         ii) Increases airway resistance and work of breathing
      d) Trach button
         i) Closes the opening in the trachea so that the patient uses his or her upper airway
         ii) Increases airway resistance and work of breathing

g. Complications of airway intubation
   1) Physiologic alterations created by airway diversion
      a) Inadequate humidification of inspired air
      b) Increased risk of nosocomial pneumonia caused by accumulation of secretions
         i) Increased mucus caused by tube because it is a foreign body
         ii) Impaired ciliary movement
      c) Aphonia: most significant stressor identified by patients
      d) Ineffective cough: Endotracheal tubes splint the epiglottis open preventing effective intrathoracic pressure to achieve an effective cough; patients can cough with a tracheostomy because the epiglottis is not splinted open.
      e) Loss of physiologic PEEP
         i) Endotracheal tubes splint the epiglottis open and remove physiologic PEEP.
         ii) Physiologic PEEP is reestablished with 3-5 cm H_2O of PEEP for intubated patients. (NOTE: may be contraindicated with thoracotomy patients)
   2) During placement
      a) Endotracheal intubation
         i) Trauma: damage to teeth, mucous membranes, perforation or laceration of pharynx, larynx, trachea
         ii) Aspiration
         iii) Laryngospasm, bronchospasm
         iv) Tube malposition: esophageal or endobronchial intubation
         v) Hypoxia or anoxia if attempts are prolonged
      b) Tracheostomy
         i) Barotrauma: pneumothorax or pneumomediastinum
         ii) Hemorrhage
         iii) Tracheoesophageal fistula
         iv) Laryngeal nerve injury
         v) Cardiopulmonary arrest
   3) While tube is in place
      a) Tube obstruction or displacement
      b) Cuff rupture

c) Disconnection between tracheal tube and ventilator including self-extubation
d) Pressure necrosis
    i) At corners of mouth if oral endotracheal tube
    ii) At superior nasal concha if nasal endotracheal tube
e) Local infection; otitis media; sinus infection with nasotracheal tubes
f) Bronchospasm
g) Leaks due to broken cuff balloon
h) Trauma: laryngeal injury; tracheal ischemia, necrosis, dilation
i) Transition from ET to tracheostomy usually occurs approximately 2 weeks after intubation, but several studies have shown benefit (e.g., decreases length of mechanical ventilation, shorter critical care and hospital stay) in earlier tracheostomy (within 3 days when it is anticipated that the patient will require prolonged mechanical ventilation).

4) Postextubation
  a) Endotracheal tube
    i) Acute laryngeal edema
    ii) Hoarseness (common)
    iii) Aspiration if swallowing is impaired
    iv) Stenosis of larynx or trachea (late complication)
  b) Tracheostomy
    i) Difficulties with decannulation of a tracheostomy
    ii) Tracheoesophageal fistula
    iii) Tracheoinnominate artery fistula
    iv) Tracheocutaneous fistula
    v) Tracheal stenosis

9. Provide oral care for patient comfort and to aid in prevention of nosocomial pneumonia.
  a. Recognize factors contributing to poor oral hygiene.
    1) Artificial airways
    2) Poor nutrition
    3) Nothing by mouth status
    4) Mouth breathing or tachypnea
    5) Oxygen administration
    6) Anxiety
    7) Drugs such as antihistamines, antiemetics, antibiotics
  b. Assess the lips, oral mucosa, tongue, gums, teeth, and soft and hard palate at least twice daily.
  c. Provide oral care periodically.
    1) Every 2-4 hours
      a) Use suction foam swabs over teeth, tongue, and oral mucosa followed by moisturizing swabs and water-soluble lip balm.
        i) Foam swabs stimulate the oral mucosa.
        ii) Avoid lemon glycerin swabs, which are drying to the oral mucosa.
      b) Suction oropharynx
        i) Rinse catheter (e.g., Yankauer) with sterile water or saline after each use.
        ii) Store oropharyngeal suction catheter in an unsealed bag when not in use.
        iii) Replace oropharyngeal suction device, tubing, and suction canister every 24 hours.
    2) Twice daily
      a) Brush teeth to prevent dental plaque colonization.
        i) Brushing the teeth with a toothbrush removes dental plaque and reduces the number of oral microorganisms.
        ii) A soft-bristle pediatric toothbrush should be used along with toothpaste, preferably with an alkaline pH.
        iii) Removable partial dentures should be removed and thoroughly cleaned.
      b) Administer chlorhexidine gluconate (Peridex) by spray or rinse as prescribed.
        i) Chlorhexidine: broad-spectrum antibacterial agent, which is not absorbed through the skin or mucous membranes
          (a) Concentration recommendations vary from 0.12-0.2%
        ii) Effectiveness in prevention of ventilator-associated pneumonia inconclusive
        iii) Initiated preoperatively if surgical patient

Oxygen Therapy

Definitions

1. Hypoxemia
  a. Decrease in arterial blood oxygen tension
  b. Diagnosis by arterial blood gases
  c. Decrease in PaO_2 and SaO_2
    1) Mild hypoxemia: PaO_2 less than 80 mm Hg (~SaO_2 95%)
    2) Moderate (significant) hypoxemia: PaO_2 less than 60 mm Hg (~SaO_2 90%)
    3) Severe hypoxemia: PaO_2 less than 40 mm Hg (~SaO_2 75%)
2. Hypoxia
  a. Decrease in tissue oxygenation
  b. Diagnosis by clinical indications (Box 4-3)
  c. Affected by PaO_2 and SaO_2, hemoglobin, cardiac output, patent vessels, cellular demand

Etiologies of Oxygen Deficiencies

1. Hypoxemia
   a. Low inspired oxygen concentration (e.g., high altitudes, smoke)
   b. Pulmonary causes (Figure 4-29)
      1) Hypoventilation (e.g., asthma)
      2) V/Q mismatch
         a) Low V/Q mismatch (i.e., shunt) (e.g., acute respiratory distress syndrome)
         b) High V/Q mismatch (i.e., dead space) (e.g., pulmonary embolism)
      3) Diffusion abnormalities (e.g., pulmonary edema, pulmonary fibrosis)
2. Hypoxia
   a. Hypoxemic hypoxia: secondary to a gas exchange problem (e.g., ventilation-perfusion mismatch, shunt, diffusion abnormalities)
   b. Anemic hypoxia: secondary to reduced oxygen-carrying capacity of the blood (e.g., anemia, carbon monoxide poisoning, methemoglobinemia)
   c. Circulatory hypoxia: secondary to a reduced blood flow in the body or a reduction in cardiac output (e.g., shock)
   d. Histotoxic hypoxia: secondary to the inability of the cells to utilize oxygen (e.g., cyanide poisoning)

Pathophysiology

1. Decrease in PaO_2 initially stimulates the sympathetic nervous system (SNS).
2. Oxygen extraction at tissue level increases.
3. As PaO_2 becomes critically low, tissue oxygenation becomes inadequate and hypoxia occurs.
4. Nutrient metabolism changes from aerobic to anaerobic which results in 20 times less ATP than aerobic metabolism and lactic acid as a waste product.
5. Acidosis and decreased cellular energy results.

Assessment

1. Evidence of altered perfusion
   a. Tachycardia
   b. Hypotension
   c. Changes in skin color and temperature
2. Evidence of anaerobic metabolism: lactic acidosis (serum arterial lactate level greater than 2 mmol/L)
3. Evidence of organ dysfunction
   a. Cerebral: altered sensorium

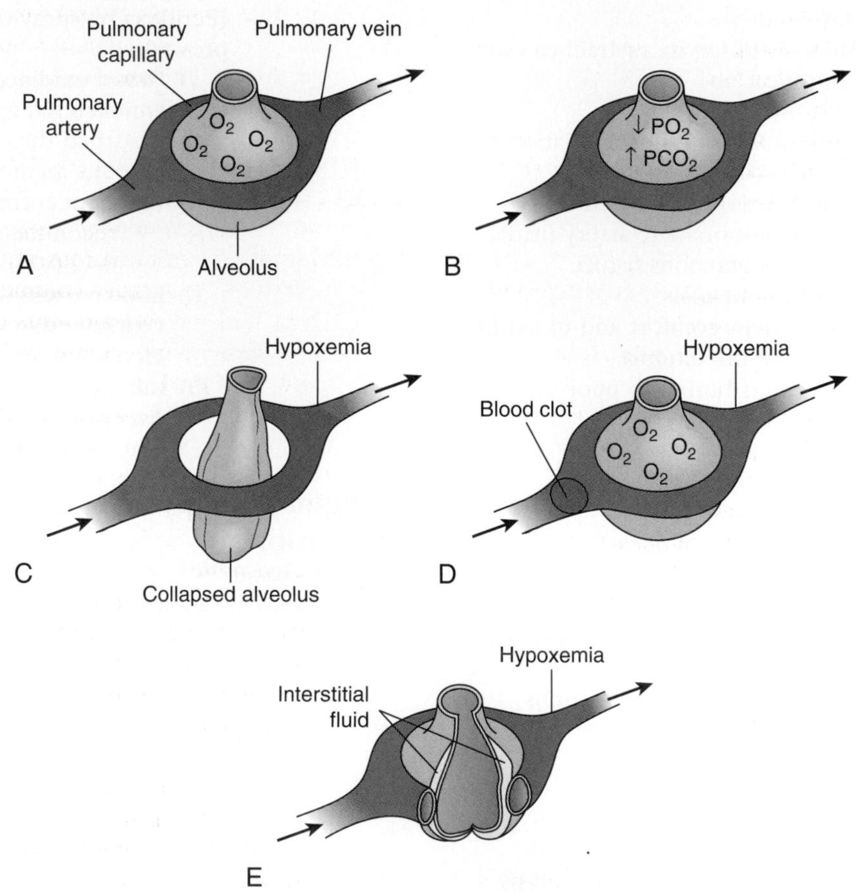

Figure 4-29 Pulmonary causes of hypoxemia. **A,** Normal alveolar-capillary unit. **B,** Hypoventilation. **C,** Low V/Q (i.e., shunt). **D,** High V/Q (i.e., dead space). **E,** Diffusion abnormality. (From Sole, M. L., Klein, D. G., & Moseley, M. J. [2009]. *Introduction to critical care nursing* [5th ed.]. Philadelphia: Saunders.)

b. Myocardial: decreased cardiac output or dysrhythmias
c. Renal: decreased urine output
4. Parameters of oxygen delivery
 a. PaO_2, SaO_2, SpO_2
 b. Hemoglobin or hematocrit
 c. Cardiac output or cardiac index
5. Hemodynamic monitoring parameters
 a. Cardiac output
 b. Venous oxygen saturation (SvO_2)
  1) Measured by SvO_2 port of a fiberoptic oximetric pulmonary artery catheter (PAC) or by mixed venous blood gas analysis
  2) Normal: 60-80%
 c. $ScvO_2$
  1) Measured by fiberoptic oximetric central venous catheter
  2) Normal: 60-80%

Indications for Oxygen Therapy

1. Significant hypoxemia: PaO_2 less than 60 mm Hg; SaO_2 or SpO_2 less than 90% on room air (i.e., 21%)
2. Suspected hypoxemia (e.g., asthma, pulmonary embolism, aspiration, drug overdose, seizure or postictal state, pneumothorax, trauma)
3. Any acute care situation in which hypoxemia is likely
 a. Increased myocardial workload (e.g., heart failure, hypertensive crisis, MI)
 b. Decreased cardiac output (e.g., shock, hypotension, cardiopulmonary arrest)
 c. Increased oxygen demand (e.g., sepsis, increased ventilatory work, trauma)
 d. Prior to procedures that may cause hypoxemia (e.g., suctioning, during and after anesthesia, transportation of unstable patient, bronchoscopy)
4. Decreased oxygen carrying capacity (e.g., carbon monoxide or cyanide poisoning, methemoglobinemia, sickle cell disease, anemia)

Principles of Oxygen Therapy

1. Airway is always the first priority; oxygen is useless without an adequate airway.
2. Oxygen is a potent drug which is administered as prescribed; may be prescribed as flow rate, oxygen concentration (expressed as a %), or fraction of inspired oxygen (FiO_2) (expressed as a decimal)
3. The objective is to improve tissue oxygenation.
 a. Maintain PaO_2 at least 60 mm Hg and SaO_2 at 90%; serial serum lactate levels are also helpful in monitoring progression or improvement of hypoxia and degree of anaerobic metabolism.
 b. Determine the effectiveness of oxygen therapy: determined by pathology
  1) Oxygen therapy is ineffective for shunt; alveoli must be opened (also referred to as *alveolar recruitment*) to get the oxygen to the alveolar-capillary membrane; PEEP is required in these cases.
4. If high concentrations are necessary, limit duration to prevent oxygen toxicity.
 a. Frequent ABGs are mandatory if FiO_2 is above 0.4.
 b. Exact concentration of inspired O_2 should be measured with O_2 analyzer.
5. FiO_2 can be estimated by counting number of reservoirs.
 a. Nose and pharynx only (1) less than 40%: example, nasal cannula
 b. Nose and pharynx + mask (2) 40-60%: example, simple face mask
 c. Nose and pharynx + mask + reservoir bag (3) 60-80%: example, partial rebreathing mask
 d. Nose and pharynx + mask + reservoir bag + one-way valves (3 + decrease in dilution) 80-100%: example, non-rebreathing mask
6. Safety guidelines
 a. Keep oxygen source at least 10 feet from open flame.
 b. Do not allow smoking in a room with supplemental oxygen.
 c. Do not use electrical appliances within 5 feet of oxygen source.
 d. Do not use petroleum-based products around oxygen source; use only water-soluble lubricants and creams.
 e. Turn the oxygen off when not in use.
 f. Secure the oxygen tanks to prevent accidental dropping; keep oxygen source away from heat or direct sunlight.

High-Flow Versus Low-Flow Oxygen Delivery Systems

1. Low-flow oxygen delivery systems
 a. Do not provide total inspired gas; remainder of patient's inspiratory volume is met by patient breathing varying amounts of room air.
 b. FiO_2 dependent on rate and depth of ventilation and fit of device
  1) If minute ventilation increases, oxygen concentration decreases because the amount of room air (diluent) increases in relation to the amount of oxygen via the oxygen delivery system.
  2) If minute ventilation decreases, oxygen concentration increases.
 c. Does not necessarily mean low FiO_2
 d. Criteria indicating that low-flow O_2 delivery system is acceptable
  1) Normal or near-normal tidal volume (~7 mL/kg of IBW)
  2) Respiratory rate normal or near normal (~15-25/min)
  3) Regular respiratory rhythm
  4) Specific oxygen concentration not critical to patient's care
 e. Devices
  1) Nasal cannula
  2) Reservoir systems

a) Simple face mask
b) Partial rebreathing mask
c) Non-rebreathing mask
2. High-flow oxygen delivery systems
   a. Provide the entire inspired gas by high flow of gas or entrainment of room air.
   b. Provide a predictable FiO_2.
   c. Does not necessarily mean high FiO_2
   d. Criteria indicating that high-flow O_2 delivery system is needed
      1) Tidal volume is significantly less than or more than normal (~7 mL/kg of IBW)
      2) Respiratory rate less than 15/min or more than 25/min
      3) Irregular respiratory rhythm
      4) Specific oxygen concentration is critical to patient's care.
      5) Evidence of alveolar hypoventilation with hypercapnia
   e. Devices
      1) Venturi mask
      2) T-piece: may be high or low flow depending on flow rate
      3) Trach collar: may be high or low flow depending on flow rate
      4) Mechanical ventilator

Oxygen Delivery Systems

See Table 4-13.

Hazards of Oxygen Therapy

1. Oxygen-induced hypoventilation
   a. Greatest risk if $PaCO_2$ greater than 50 mm Hg because low PaO_2 becomes primary stimulus to breath
      1) Airway obstruction
      2) COPD
      3) Respiratory center depression
   b. Use O_2 with caution but remember low PaO_2, not FiO_2, is stimulus to breathe; use only enough oxygen to bring PaO_2 up to approximately 60 mm Hg or SaO_2 or SpO_2 up to approximately 90%.
2. Absorptive atelectasis
   a. Causes
      1) High concentrations of oxygen (an absorbable gas) washes out the nitrogen (a nonabsorbable gas) that normally holds the alveoli open at the end of expiration.
      2) Effects of oxygen on pulmonary surfactant
      3) Depression of ciliary function
   b. Prevention: Do not administer oxygen that is not indicated.
3. Oxygen toxicity
   a. Cause: too high a concentration over too long a period of time (hours to days)
   b. Pathophysiology
      1) Overproduction of oxygen free radicals
      2) Large numbers of oxygen free radicles overwhelm the supply of neutralizing enzymes.
      3) Injury to capillary endothelium and increase in interstitial edema
      4) Injury to Type I pneumocytes and intraalveolar edema
      5) Proliferation of Type II pneumocytes
      6) Thickening of alveolar-capillary membrane
      7) Scarring and pulmonary fibrosis
   c. Clinical indications
      1) Early
         a) Substernal chest pain that increases with deep breathing
         b) Dry cough and tracheal irritation
         c) Dyspnea
         d) Upper airway changes (e.g., nasal stuffiness, sore throat, eye and ear discomfort)
         e) Anorexia, nausea, vomiting
         f) Fatigue, lethargy, malaise
         g) Restlessness
      2) Late
         a) Chest x-ray changes: atelectasis or patches of pneumonia
         b) Progressive ventilatory difficulty: decreased vital capacity; decreased compliance; hypercapnia
         c) Increased intrapulmonary shunt: increasing A:a gradient and decreased PaO_2/FiO_2 ratio; hypoxemia
   d. Prevention:
      1) Use the lowest FiO_2 possible to maintain a PaO_2 of at least 60 mm Hg (SaO_2 90%).
         a) Limit duration of 1 FiO_2 (i.e., 100%) to 24 hours if at all possible.
         b) Limit the use of FiO_2 above 0.6 to 2-3 days if at all possible.
         c) Assess arterial blood gases frequently if FiO_2 is above 0.4 to ensure that high concentration is still required.
         d) FiO_2 of less than or equal to 0.4 is considered relatively safe.
      2) Utilize PEEP to increase the driving pressure of oxygen; use of PEEP achieves the following:
         a) The same PaO_2 at a lower FiO_2
         b) A better PaO_2 at the same FiO_2
      3) Remember hypoxia is far more common than O_2 toxicity and must be corrected; **actual** hypoxemia should never be allowed to persist because of concern regarding **potential** oxygen toxicity.

Hyperbaric Oxygenation

1. Definition: administration of high concentration (usually 100%) oxygen under greatly increased pressure (usually 2-3 atmospheres)
2. Indications: carbon monoxide or cyanide poisoning, air embolism, radiation therapy, gas gangrene, burns, nonhealing wounds, necrotizing fasciitis, decompression illness, osteomyelitis, intracranial abscess, anaerobic infection

Table 4-13 Summary of Oxygen Delivery Systems

System	Advantages	Disadvantages	Miscellaneous
Nasal cannula 1 lpm = ~24% 2 lpm = ~28% 3 lpm = ~32% 4 lpm = ~36% 5 lpm = ~40% 6 lpm = ~44%	• Safe and simple • Comfortable • Effective for low oxygen concentration • Allows eating and talking • Inexpensive	• Contraindicated in nasal obstruction • May cause drying and irritation of nasal mucosa • May cause necrosis at ears • Cannot be used when patient has nasal obstruction • Variable concentrations of oxygen depending on tidal volume, ventilatory rate, flow rate, and nasal patency	• Ensure that flow rates do not exceed 6 L/min • Provide humidification if flow rates exceed 4 L/min • Use gauze pads under cannula at tops of ears to prevent pressure ulceration • Give oral and nasal care every 8 hours; moisten lips and nose with water-soluble lubricant
Reservoir nasal cannula; mustache-style or pendant-style Delivers greater than or equal to 50% oxygen	• As for nasal cannula • Captures water vapor with patient exhalation and returns the moisture during inhalation so no need for humidification	• As for nasal cannula • Pendant-style may weigh down the ear loops	• As for nasal cannula • Must be replaced regularly • Used most often in home care • Conserves oxygen use
Simple face mask 5 lpm = ~40% 6 lpm = ~45-50% 7 lpm = ~50-55% 8 lpm = ~55-60%	• Delivers high oxygen concentration • Doesn't dry mucous membranes of nose and mouth • Can be used in patients with nasal obstruction	• Hot, confining, uncomfortable • Tight seal necessary • Frequently poorly tolerated in dyspneic patient • Interferes with eating and talking • May cause CO_2 retention if flow rate is less than 6 L/min • Variable concentrations of oxygen depending on tidal volume, ventilatory rate, and flow rate • Can't deliver less than 40% • Potential for oxygen toxicity • Impractical for long-term therapy	• Place pads between mask and bony facial parts • Wash and dry face every 4 hours • Clean mask every 8 hours • Ensure flow rate of at least 5 L/min • Check ABGs frequently • Watch for signs of oxygen toxicity
Partial rebreathing mask 6 lpm = ~35-40% 8 lpm = ~45-50% 10 lpm = ~60%	• Delivers high oxygen concentrations • Doesn't dry mucous membranes	• As for face mask • May cause CO_2 retention if reservoir bag is allowed to collapse	• Ensure that bag does not totally deflate during inhalation (increase flow rate) • Keep mask snug • Check ABGs frequently • Watch for signs of oxygen toxicity
Non-rebreathing mask 6 lpm = ~60% 7 lpm = ~70% 8 lpm = ~70% 9 lpm = ~90% 10 lpm = close to 100%	• As for other masks • One-way valves prevent rebreathing of CO_2 and increases oxygen concentrations	• As for other masks except does not cause CO_2 retention	• As for partial rebreathing mask • Check ABGs frequently • Watch for signs of oxygen toxicity
Venturi mask 4 lpm = ~24-28% 8 lpm = ~35-40% 12 lpm = ~50%	• Delivers accurate oxygen concentration depending on flow rate and diluter jet inserted despite changes in patient's respiratory pattern • Oxygen concentration can be changed • Doesn't dry mucous membranes	• FiO_2 can be lowered if mask doesn't fit snugly, if tubing is kinked, if oxygen intake ports are blocked, or if less than recommended liter flow is used • Hot, confining, and uncomfortable • Tight seal necessary • Frequently poorly tolerated in dyspneic patient • Interferes with eating and talking	• Check ABGs frequently • Watch for signs of oxygen toxicity • As for other masks

Continued

Table 4-13 Summary of Oxygen Delivery Systems—cont'd

System	Advantages	Disadvantages	Miscellaneous
Trach collar • Delivers 21-70% at 10 L or to provide visible mist	• Does not pull on tracheostomy • Elastic ties allow movement of mask away from tracheostomy without removing it	• Oxygen diluted by room air • Increased likelihood of infection and skin irritation around stoma because of high humidity • Condensation can collect in the tubing and drain into patient's airway especially during turning	• Ensure that oxygen be warmed and humidified • Empty condensation from tubing frequently; empty into water trap or container for appropriate discard; do not empty water back into humidifier
T-piece or tube • Delivers 21-100% with flow rate set at 2.5 times patient's minute ventilation	• Delivers variable concentrations • Less moisture around tracheostomy than with tracheostomy collar	• May cause CO_2 retention at low flow rates • Weight of T-piece can pull on tracheostomy tube • Condensation can collect in the tubing and drain into patient's airway especially during turning	• Requires heated nebulizer • Use extension on open side to act as a reservoir and increase oxygen concentration as prescribed • Empty condensation from tubing frequently • Check ABGs frequently • Watch for signs of oxygen toxicity
Mechanical ventilation • Delivers 21-100%	• Delivers predictable, constant concentrations of oxygen • Supports ventilation as well as oxygenation • Addition of positive end-expiratory pressure (PEEP) augments the driving pressure of oxygen; this aids in the achievement of acceptable PaO_2 levels at lower oxygen concentrations	• Requires skilled personnel • Requires electricity and backup power generator (plug into red outlet) • Condensation can collect in the tubing and drain into patient's airway especially during turning	• Requires heated humidifier • Empty condensation from tubing frequently • Check ABGs frequently • Watch for signs of oxygen toxicity

3. Actions: can cause a 22-fold increase in PaO_2, which increases the amount of oxygen dissolved in the blood to enhance tissue oxygenation
4. Complications: oxygen toxicity; absorptive atelectasis; acute respiratory distress syndrome, bleeding and edema of eustachian tubes, rupture of tympanic membrane

Mechanical Ventilation

Indications for Mechanical Ventilation

1. Acute ventilatory failure with respiratory acidosis not relieved by ordinary methods
2. Hypoxemia despite maximum oxygen therapy
3. Relief of hypoxemia causes increased CO_2 retention
4. Apnea: consideration needs to be given to the reversibility of the situation (i.e., mechanical ventilation is not indicated to prolong a terminal condition).
5. Physiologic indications
   a. Vital capacity less than 10 mL/kg or twice predicted tidal volume
   b. Unable to achieve maximal inspiratory force of −25 cm H_2O
   c. PaO_2 less than 60 mm Hg with FiO_2 greater than 0.6
   d. Arterial $PaCO_2$ below 30 or above 50 mm Hg
      1) Hypercapnia alone is not an indication for mechanical ventilation and must be accompanied by acidosis to be an indication for mechanical ventilation: for example, a patient with COPD has chronic hypercapnia (not an indication for mechanical ventilation) but develops an even greater $PaCO_2$ level and decompensated respiratory acidosis with acute respiratory infection (a potential indication for mechanical ventilation).
   e. Dead space/tidal volume ratio (V_D/V_T) greater than 0.6
   f. Respiratory rate greater than 30-35/min
6. May also be used for the following purposes:
   a. Reduce oxygen consumption by reducing the work of breathing (e.g., shock).
   b. Stabilize the chest wall (e.g., flail chest).
   c. Allow sedation and neuromuscular paralysis.

Types of Ventilators

1. Negative pressure ventilators
   a. Types: iron lung, chest cuirass, poncho style, body wrap
   b. Ventilatory process
      1) Negative pressure generated outside of body excluding the upper airway
      2) Negativity transmitted to intrapleural and intraalveolar spaces
      3) Pressure gradient occurs and air moves into lungs.
      4) Expiration passively occurs by removing negative pressure around the chest wall.
   c. Uses
      1) Restricted to nonpulmonary (e.g., neuromuscular) problems
      2) Long-term ventilator support without an artificial airway
      3) Primarily in home or rehabilitation settings
   d. Advantages
      1) Artificial airway not required
      2) Normal breathing mechanics maintained so avoids harmful changes in intrathoracic pressure caused by positive pressure ventilators
   e. Disadvantages
      1) Not helpful for patients with lung disease
      2) Not possible to precisely regulate tidal volume and alveolar ventilation
      3) Large size required (e.g., iron lung)
      4) Restriction of patient movement
      5) Patient care difficult because body is enclosed in ventilator
      6) Difficulty obtaining a seal around chest
      7) May cause venous pooling in the abdomen leading to decreased cardiac output particularly in hypovolemic patients
2. Positive pressure ventilators
   a. Ventilatory process
      1) Inspiration is created by positive pressure being pushed into the airway.
      2) Expiration occurs passively when the positive pressure stops.
   b. Cycling classifications
      1) Time-cycled: deliver inspiratory flow until preset time interval has ended; used in neonates and children
      2) Pressure-cycled: deliver inspiratory flow until preset pressure is met; pressure is set and tidal volume varies
         a) Advantages
            i) Relatively inexpensive
            ii) Mobile
            iii) Run on compressed air or oxygen
         b) Disadvantages
            i) Tidal volume varies dependent upon compliance of the lung and the integrity of the ventilatory circuit
            ii) Sealed airway (e.g., cuffed endotracheal tube or tracheostomy tube) required
            iii) Positive intrathoracic pressure decreases venous return to the right heart and may decrease cardiac output especially in hypovolemic patients.
            iv) Risk of ventilator-induced lung injury (VILI)
      3) Volume-cycled: deliver inspiratory flow until preset volume is met; tidal volume is set and pressure varies
         a) Advantages: deliver the set tidal volume regardless of changes in lung compliance
         b) Disadvantages
            i) Sealed airway required
            ii) Positive intrathoracic pressure decreases venous return to the right heart and may decrease cardiac output especially in hypovolemic patients.
            iii) Risk of ventilator-induced lung injury (VILI)

Inspiratory Modes (Table 4-14)

1. Volume cycled modes end inspiration when a preset volume is achieved.
2. Pressure cycled modes end inspiration when a preset pressure is achieved.

Expiratory Maneuvers

1. Positive end-expiratory pressure (PEEP)
   a. Definition: maintenance of pressure above atmospheric at airway opening at end-expiration
      1) Physiologic: 3-5 cm H_2O
      2) Therapeutic: greater than 5 cm H_2O
         a) Adjustment of PEEP
            i) Begin with 3-5 cm H_2O of PEEP
            ii) Increase in increments of 3-5 cm H_2O until SaO_2 (or SpO_2) of 90% is achieved
         b) Though there is no true upper limit, the higher the level, the greater the chance of barotrauma
         c) Levels greater than 20 cm H_2O may be referred to as super-PEEP
      3) Best (or optimal) PEEP: PEEP that provides SaO_2 of at least 90% without compromising cardiac output (remember that tissue oxygen delivery is affected by SaO_2, Hgb, and CO; if SaO_2 is increased but CO is decreased, no true gains in tissue oxygen delivery are achieved and tissue oxygen delivery may even be decreased)
      4) Auto-PEEP (also called *occult PEEP* or *intrinsic PEEP*): adds to therapeutic PEEP (Figure 4-30)

Table 4-14 Modes of Mechanical Ventilation

Mode	Description	Comments
Volume Modes		
Control	• Preset tidal volume and rate; the ventilator delivers the tidal volume at the rate, and the circuit is closed in between these mandatory breaths	• Patients must be apneic or paralyzed or they "fight" the ventilator • Guarantees ventilation with a specific minute ventilation • Allows ventilatory muscle rest
Assist/control (also called *assisted mandatory ventilation*)	• Preset tidal volume, minimum rate (control rate), and inspiratory effort required to "trigger" the ventilator to cycle to assist breaths (sensitivity); the ventilator delivers the control breaths of the specified tidal volume and responds by cycling additionally if the patient's inspiratory effort (negative pressure) is adequate	• More comfortable than control mode • Less work of breathing for patient than spontaneous breathing or IMV • Allows ventilatory muscle rest • Risk for hyperventilation because each assisted breath is delivered at same tidal volume as mandatory breaths; sedation may be necessary to decrease number of spontaneously triggered breaths
Synchronized intermittent mandatory ventilation (SIMV)	• Preset tidal volume and minimum rate; the ventilatory circuit is open between the mandatory breaths so that the patient may take additional breaths; since the ventilator does not cycle to assist these breaths, the tidal volume of these breaths varies • Mandatory breaths are synchronized so that they do not occur during the patient's ventilatory efforts	• Allows muscle reconditioning better than control or assist/control • Less potential for hyperventilation since patient-initiated breaths are at the tidal volume determined by the patient • More work of breathing for patient than assist-control because patient-initiated breaths are not assisted • Less need for sedation than assist/control or control modes • Does not decrease cardiac output as much as assist/control or control modes • Frequently used for weaning
Pressure Modes		
Pressure support ventilation (PSV)	• Preset inspiratory support pressure level; when the patient initiates a breath, this positive pressure flows to assist the patient's spontaneous breaths; tidal volume and rate is patient controlled	• Low level (5-10 cm H_2O) helps to eliminate the increased work of breathing associated with an endotracheal tube; higher levels help to augment the patient's own intrinsic tidal volume • Lessens work of breathing but also allows use of respiratory muscles to lessen muscular atrophy • Lower mean airway pressures than volume ventilation • May be used with IMV or alone; if used alone, patient must be spontaneously breathing • There is no preset ventilatory rate, and apnea occurs if the patient does not initiate a breath; newer models provide a volume ventilation backup (called *volume-assured pressure support ventilation [VAPSV]*)
Pressure-controlled ventilation (PCV)	• Preset inspiratory pressure limit, rate, and I : E ratio; the ventilator delivers air until the pressure limit is reached and maintains this pressure throughout inspiration • Tidal volumes vary due to changes in the patient's lung compliance, inspiratory time, and airway resistance	• Lower mean airway pressures than volume ventilation • Allows more even distribution of air and improves arterial oxygenation at lower FiO_2 levels • Does not provide a guaranteed tidal volume • Requires sedation

Table 4-14 Modes of Mechanical Ventilation—cont'd

Mode	Description	Comments
Pressure-controlled/ inverse ratio ventilation (PC/IRV)	• Preset I:E ratio with inspiratory time to be greater than expiratory time; I:E ratio of 2:1 or greater; may be volume controlled or pressure controlled • Combination of pressure support ventilation and inverse ratio ventilation	• Improves oxygenation and allows reduction of FiO_2 • Improves distribution of ventilation • Prevents collapse of alveoli • Increases PaO_2 and SaO_2 • Increases mean airway pressure without further increases in peak inspiratory pressures • May decrease cardiac output • Makes the patient uncomfortable; patients require sedation to decrease discomfort and anxiety; muscle paralysis may be required along with sedation • May be used in ARDS with refractory hypoxemia • May cause auto-PEEP which, when added to therapeutic PEEP, increases risk of barotrauma • Do not use in patients with COPD
Volume-Guaranteed Pressure Modes		
Volume-assured pressure support ventilation (VAPSV)	• Preset inspiratory pressure limit, target tidal volume, and terminal flow rate • When the preset tidal volume has been achieved, inspiratory flow ends; if the preset tidal volume has not been achieved, inspiratory time is extended at the terminal flow rate until the set tidal volume is achieved • Starts as a pressure breath but ends as a volume breath if the preset tidal volume is not achieved	• Provides guarantee of adequate tidal volume lacking from PSV
Pressure-regulated volume-controlled (PRVC) (may also be referred to as *adaptive pressure ventilation* or *autoflow*)	• Preset target tidal volume and pressure limit; the ventilator automatically sets the initial flow rate and flow waveform to deliver the desired volume at the desired pressure • Inspiratory pressure changes breath to breath to augment the tidal volume delivery of subsequent breaths accounting for changes in compliance, resistance, and patient effort • Measurement of compliance at predetermined intervals and adjusts the flow rate and pressure support to deliver the set tidal volume at or below the maximal pressure	• Preferred mode for patients with high airway pressures • Produces a guaranteed tidal volume but minimizes the risk of barotrauma and volutrauma • Requires special ventilator
Airway pressure release ventilation (APRV)	• PSV with short (1-1.5 seconds) releases from higher CPAP pressure to lower CPAP pressure to allow further expiration and CO_2 elimination	• Prevents lung overdistention while maintaining inflation of newly recruited alveoli • Maintains lower mean and peak airway pressures • Less hemodynamic compromise than traditional modes • Contraindicated in patients with obstructive lung disease
Bi-level	CPAP with two different levels; CPAP-high and CPAP-low	

Continued

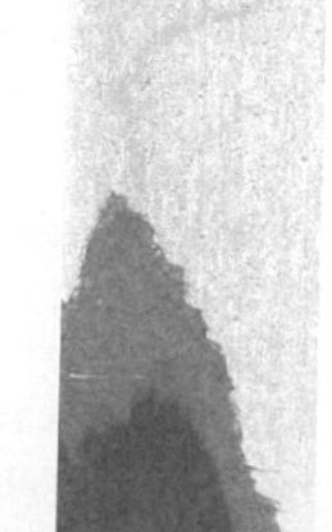

Table 4-14 Modes of Mechanical Ventilation—cont'd

Mode	Description	Comments
High-Frequency Ventilation		
High-frequency ventilation (HFV)	• Preset (very low) tidal volumes delivered at present (very high) rates; ventilation and oxygenation are achieved by gas diffusion and convection • High-frequency positive pressure ventilation (HFPPV): 60-120 bpm • High-frequency jet ventilation (HFJV): 120-600 bpm • High-frequency oscillation ventilation (HFO): 500-1200 oscillations per minute	• May be used in some cases of chest trauma, bronchopleural fistula, or ARDS • Causes lower airway and intrathoracic pressures than traditional mechanical ventilation; may reduce the incidence of barotrauma and decreased cardiac output • Muscle paralysis along with sedation required • May cause increased oral secretions • Auscultation of heart and lung sounds is difficult • Requires special ventilator
Miscellaneous		
Independent lung ventilation (ILV) (also called ***differential lung ventilation*** or ***split-lung ventilation)***	• Ventilation technique that ventilates each lung separately • Separate modes, flow rates, and PEEP may be used for each lung • May be synchronized (SILV)	• Used for unilateral pathology or thoracic trauma • Requires double lumen tube and separate ventilators to each lumen (and a synchronizer if SILV) • Asynchronous lung ventilation is better tolerated hemodynamically in most patients • Patient requires sedation and/or paralysis
Liquid ventilation	• Conventional ventilation along with the substitution of nitrogen with inert perfluorochemical fluids	• Perfluorochemical fluids serve as a liquid PEEP recruiting alveoli and as a local antiinflammatory • Fluids are replaced as evaporation occurs • Chest x-ray interpretation is complicated by the fluid
Extracorporeal membrane oxygenation	• Transfer of blood from the patient through an artificial lung to oxygenate the blood which is then returned to the body	• Provides blood oxygenation while allowing the lung to rest and heal • Not available in all medical centers and no survival benefit shown thus far

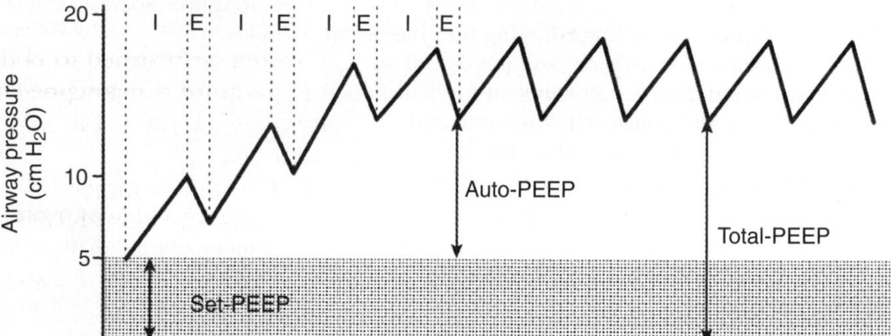

Figure 4-30 Auto-PEEP (positive end-expiratory pressure) as frequently is seen in inverse ratio ventilation. Insufficient expiratory time permits the trapping of gases in the lung. This trapped gas creates pressure, which is known as auto-PEEP. This PEEP is added to therapeutic PEEP for total PEEP. *I,* Inspiration; *E,* expiration. (From Pierce, L. [1995]. *Guide to mechanical ventilation and intensive respiratory care.* Philadelphia: Saunders.)

a) Cause: inadequate emptying of the lungs
   i) May be caused by airway obstruction or decreased compliance
   ii) May be inherent in modes with very rapid rates and/or short expiratory time

b) Adverse effects
   i) Increased risk of barotrauma and volutrauma
   ii) Accentuation of hemodynamic compromise
   iii) Increased work of breathing
   iv) Patient anxiety

c) Measurement: difference between the mean alveolar pressure and external airway pressure at end-expiration
    i) Newer ventilators may provide automated assessment
    ii) May be manually determined
        (a) Place patient on assist-control
        (b) Occlude airway at end-expiration
        (c) Observe increase in airway pressure
d) Goal: reduce auto-PEEP to the lowest practical level
    i) Reduce bronchospasm
    ii) Adjust flow rates and I:E ratio

b. Actions of PEEP
    1) Increases driving pressure of oxygen
        a) Improves the PaO_2 without increasing the FiO_2
        b) Allows the use of lower FiO_2 to achieve the same PaO_2, thereby decreasing risk of oxygen toxicity
    2) Decreases surface tension to prevent alveolar collapse at end-expiration
    3) Decreases intrapulmonary shunt by opening alveoli that are collapsed (referred to as *alveolar recruitment*); increases functional residual capacity
    4) Minimizes the risk of VILI by stabilizing the lung units and reducing the repeated opening and collapsing of alveoli
c. Uses of PEEP
    1) Acute respiratory distress syndrome (ARDS) (also referred to as *noncardiac pulmonary edema*)
    2) Cardiac pulmonary edema
    3) Acute respiratory failure with persistent hypoxemia
    4) Occasionally used to increase intrapulmonic pressure in patients with intrathoracic bleeding
    5) Physiologic PEEP is used to mimic the positive end-expiratory pressure exerted by the closed glottis in intubated patients
d. Maintaining prescribed levels of PEEP
    1) Patients with an inspiratory effort pull a negative pressure and negate the level of PEEP; these patients require sedation and/or muscle paralysis to maintain the therapeutic effects of PEEP
e. Adverse effects of PEEP
    1) Hemodynamic consequences of positive pressure ventilation are accentuated.
        a) Decreased venous return
        b) Increased right ventricular afterload
        c) Decreased left ventricular distensibility
        d) Decreased cardiac output
    2) Barotrauma
    3) Increased intracranial pressure (ICP)
f. Contraindications of PEEP
    1) Untreated hypovolemia
    2) Extreme caution in hypotensive states
    3) Increased risk of barotrauma in patients with COPD

Mechanical Ventilator Parameters

1. Mode
2. Tidal volume: 5-10 mL/kg of ideal body weight; 4-8 mL/kg of ideal body weight in patients with ALI/ARDS
3. Respiratory rate: varies according to ventilator flow rate, I:E ratio, and whether ventilator is on control or assist mode; usually 4-20/min with slower rates used for weaning
4. FiO_2
    a. Initially 1 (i.e., 100%) for 20 minutes especially if cardiac arrest
    b. Adjusted so that PaO_2 is 60 mm Hg
    c. Use lowest FiO_2 that achieves desired PaO_2 (usually at least 60 mm Hg) and SaO_2 (usually 90-95%).
    d. PEEP may be added to maintain acceptable PaO_2 with lower FiO_2 to reduce the risk of oxygen toxicity.
5. PEEP or CPAP
6. Sensitivity: if assist mode is used
    a. Amount of inspired effort required to initiate an assisted breath
    b. Usually set at −1 to −2 cm H_2O
7. Sigh
    a. Volume: 1.5-2 times the inspired tidal volume
    b. Frequency: 10-15 times/hr
    c. Though sighing was done infrequently when large tidal volumes were used, they may be helpful in preventing atelectasis now that more physiologic tidal volumes are being used.
8. Humidification
    a. Continuous humidification is required with inspired air warmed to body temperature; temperature is maintained at 32-37° C and humidity at 100%; purposes include the following:
        1) Prevent hypothermia.
        2) Thin secretions to prevent airway obstruction
    b. Methods of adding moisture; may be active or passive
        1) Humidifiers
            a) Active
                i) Bubble humidifiers pass the inhaled gas through a water reservoir.
                ii) Passover humidifiers pass the inhaled gas over a large surface area water-soaked membrane; capillary action draws water from the reservoir.
                iii) While active humidifiers do provide more humidification than passive systems, they allow more condensation (may be referred to as *rainout*).

(a) Increases risk of ventilator circuit contamination and ventilation airflow obstruction
(b) Must be emptied frequently into a water trap or container for discard

b) Passive
i) These devices trap the heat and humidity from the patient's exhaled air and then return some of the heat and humidity in the inhaled air.
(a) Heat and moisture exchanger (HME)
(b) Hygroscopic condenser humidifier (HCH)
ii) Disadvantages of these devices
(a) Increased mechanical dead space which increases work of breathing
(b) Increased the risk of obstruction since they do provide less humidity than active devices; usually used for short-term ventilation
(c) Aerosol treatment cannot be given through an HME so the ventilator circuit must be interrupted and risks contamination
iii) Primary advantage is lower risk of ventilator circuit contamination.

2) Nebulizers: High-frequency sound waves (ultrasonic) or a gas-powered airstream (pneumatic) focused on a water source produces an aerosol.

c. Methods of adding warmth
1) Heated wire circuit
a) An electrically heated wire runs through the ventilator circuit to warm the inspired gas to the desired temperature.
b) Eliminates water condensation in ventilator tubing because the wire heats the tubing so that it is the same temperature as gas leaving the ventilator
2) Servomechanism: A thermal sensor at the patient "Y" sends information to the ventilator humidity system so that the humidifier is adjusted to match the desired temperature.

9. Flow rate
a. Usually 40-80 L/min but adjusted so that inspiratory volume can be completed in time allowed, based on desired ventilatory rate and I:E ratio
1) Slower the flow rate, better distribution in normal lung
2) Faster the flow rate, better for patients with COPD so that more time is allowed for expiration
b. Patient comfort is also a consideration: Does the patient feel like he or she is getting enough air?

10. I:E ratio
a. Usually 1:1.5 or 1:2
b. Inverse ratio ventilation: more time for inspiration than expiration; thought to improve distribution of inspired air, especially in ARDS

11. Alarm settings: all alarms should be ON
a. High pressure alarm: Set alarm 10-20 cm H_2O above the patient's peak inspiratory pressure.
1) Causes for high-pressure alarm
a) Increased airway resistance: secretions; bronchospasm; kink in tubing; displacement of artificial airway; patient coughing during inspiration; patient biting on ET tube; water condensation in tubing
b) Decreased compliance: pneumothorax (sudden increase); development of pulmonary edema, atelectasis, pneumonia, ARDS (gradual increase)
b. Low exhaled volume alarm: Set alarm at 50-100 mL below inspired tidal volume; causes for low exhaled volume alarm:
1) Disconnection
2) Cuff leak
3) Leak in circuitry
4) Overbreathing: occurs when the patient deeply inspires as the ventilator is delivering inspiration; the ventilator senses low pressure; this patient may require sedation to prevent recurrent ventilator alarms
c. Apnea: ON
1) Patient fatigue
2) Overmedication
3) Decrease in level of consciousness
d. Low FiO_2: ON
1) Oxygen disconnect
2) Break in inspiratory circuit

12. Power: The mechanical ventilator must be plugged into a grounded electrical outlet that is backed up by the emergency generator; this outlet is usually red.

Assessment of the Mechanically Ventilated Patient

1. Pulmonary
a. Airway: type, size, position, and cuff pressure
b. Chest excursion and use of accessory muscles
c. Breath sounds
d. Secretions: amount, color, consistency, and odor
e. Spontaneous ventilatory mechanics: at least every 24 hours without sedation (i.e., sedation vacation) though sedation withdrawal is contraindicated for some patients (e.g., neurologically injured patients)
1) Respiratory rate
2) Patient's own tidal volume
3) Vital capacity
4) Minute ventilation
5) Maximal inspiratory pressure
6) Rapid shallow breathing index: best single index for assessing readiness for weaning
a) Calculated: f/V_T

b) RSBI less than or equal to 105 indicates readiness to wean
f. Ventilator parameters
1) Mode: as set
2) Tidal volume as set and exhaled
3) Respiratory rate: ventilator and patient initiated
4) FiO_2: confirmed with oxygen analyzer
5) PEEP: airway pressure at the end of expiration (on pressure gauge not just what it is set to be)
6) Peak inspiratory pressure: airway pressure at the peak of inspiration; calculate dynamic compliance
7) Plateau pressure: airway pressure with an inflation hold; calculate static compliance
8) Alarms: Check that all are ON.
g. Ventilator circuitry: leaks, condensation, and temperature of inspired air
h. Pulse oximetry: SpO_2
i. Chest x-ray: usually done daily unless chronic situation
j. Arterial blood gases: usually done daily and 20-30 minutes after any ventilator changes and as indicated by change in patient status

2. Cardiovascular
   a. Heart rate
   b. ECG rhythm
   c. Heart sounds
   d. Blood pressure: direct (arterial catheter) or indirect (auscultated)
   e. Hemodynamic parameters: RAP; PAP; PAOP; CO/CI; SVR/SVRI; PVR/PVRI; SvO_2
3. Neurologic
   a. Level of consciousness
   b. Airway reflexes: gag, swallowing, and corneal
   c. Sedation level
4. Renal/Metabolic
   a. Urine output
   b. Urine specific gravity
   c. Serum electrolytes
5. Gastrointestinal
   a. Abdominal distention
   b. Bowel sounds
   c. Guaiac testing: NG aspirate; vomitus; stools
6. Nutritional status
   a. Daily weight
   b. Total protein, albumin, and serum transferrin levels
   c. Calorie counts and nutrient balance
7. Immunologic
   a. Temperature
   b. Sputum cultures
   c. White blood cell count
8. Psychological
   a. Complaints of pain or anxiety
   b. Clinical indicators of pain or anxiety

Collaborative Management

1. Ensure patient safety
   a. Frequent assessment for change in status
      1) SpO_2
      2) Arterial blood gases
      3) End-tidal CO_2
      4) Breath sounds
      5) Heart sounds
      6) Neurologic status
      7) Peak inspiratory pressure and plateau pressure
      8) Cuff pressure
      9) Airway and need for suctioning
   b. Close monitoring of ventilator settings, ventilator connections, peak and plateau pressures, ventilator alarms on
   c. Empty condensation for water traps as indicated.
   d. Discontinue gastric feedings during chest physiotherapy and as indicated.
2. Assist with ventilator changes according to ABGs and patient's clinical status (Table 4-15)
   1) Note that only one change should be made at a time.
3. Reduce patient discomfort and anxiety.
   a. Communication with patient to orient to place and time, inform the patient regarding what is happening, and his or her needs using communication aids
   b. Distraction (e.g., music, television, radio)
   c. Nonpharmacologic comfort measures (e.g., massage, aromatherapy)

Table 4-15 Mechanical Ventilator Parameter Changes to Make According to Arterial Blood Gases

If $PaCO_2$ is greater than 45 mm Hg (or above the patient's normal if patient has COPD)	• Increase ventilation • Increase rate • Increase tidal volume (if it does not currently exceed 10 mL/kg)
If $PaCO_2$ is less than 35 mm Hg	• Decrease ventilation • Decrease rate • Decrease tidal volume • If patient is on assist/control mode: change mode from AC to IMV • Consider sedation and/or analgesia • Mechanical dead space may be considered (tubing which acts as a rebreathing device)
If PaO_2 is less than 60 mm Hg	• Increase FiO_2 • Add or increase PEEP (especially if FiO_2 is already greater than 0.6 [60%])
If PaO_2 is greater than 100 mm Hg	• Decrease FiO_2 • Decrease PEEP (especially if FiO_2 is less than 0.4 [40%])

d. Analgesics: Morphine intermittently or infusion may be needed especially in patients who have chest trauma or surgery.
e. Sedatives as indicated
   1) Types of sedatives (Table 4-16 and Table 4-17)
      a) Benzodiazepines (e.g., diazepam [Valium], lorazepam [Ativan], midazolam [Versed])
         i) Midazolam is benzodiazepine of choice for short-term (less than 24 hours) sedation of critically ill patients
         ii) Lorazepam is benzodiazepine of choice for long-term (greater than 24 hours) sedation of critically ill patients
      b) Sedative-hypnotics (e.g., propofol [Diprivan])
         i) Provides advantage of reversibility to allow for short-term breathing trial daily for patients on mechanical ventilation (i.e.,. "sedation vacation")
      c) Alpha$_2$-adrenoceptor agonist (e.g., dexmedetomidine [Precedex]): increasingly popular due to lack of respiratory depression
   2) Nursing management principles of sedation (Park et al., 2001)
      a) Always treat pain first.
      b) Ensure patient safety.
      c) Talk to the patient, assess orientation, and reorient as required.
      d) Identify and treat cause of agitation (e.g., pain, anxiety, sleep deprivation, alcohol or drug withdrawal).
      e) Complement medication use with provision of comfort, control of environment, music.
      f) Determine the need for sedation.
      g) Select and treat to a target level of sedation; use the smallest effective dose of drug.
         i) Ramsay sedation scale (Table 4-18)
         ii) Sedation-agitation scale (Table 4-19)
         iii) Motor activity assessment scale (Table 4-20)
         iv) Bispectral index (BIS) monitoring
            (a) An EEG parameter developed to specifically measure patient's response to sedation and anesthesia
            (b) Method
               (i) A sensor pad is placed on the patient's forehead to detect electrical activity in the brain.
               (ii) The EEG signals are transmitted to the BIS module, and it is processed to provide a measure of level of consciousness.
               (iii) Changes reflect changes in the effects of sedative and anesthetic agents.
            (c) Evaluation: Usual goal is a BIS of 60-70.
               (i) Value of close to 100 corresponds to a fully awake state.
               (ii) Value of greater than 80 corresponds to anxiolysis with response to normal voice.
               (iii) Value of 60-80 corresponds to a light hypnotic state with response to loud commands or gentle shaking.
               (iv) Value of 40-60 corresponds to a deep level of sedation; unresponsive to verbal stimuli.
               (v) Value of 40 or less corresponds to a deep hypnotic state or barbiturate
      h) Continually reassess the need for analgesics and sedatives.

4. Provide adequate nutritional support.
   a. Enteral route is preferred.
   b. High protein/low carbohydrate (e.g., Pulmocare) is preferred especially during weaning since

Table 4-16 Comparison of Selected Sedative Agents

	Propofol (Diprivan)	Midazolam (Versed)	Lorazepam (Ativan)	Diazepam (Valium)	Dexmedetomidine (Precedex)
Elimination half-life	1-8 hours	1-12 hours	10-20 hours	20-80 hours	2 hours
Onset	1 minute	2-5 minutes	5-20 minutes	2-5 minutes	2-6 minutes
Active metabolites	No	Yes	No	Yes	No
Continuous infusion	Yes	Yes	Yes	No	Yes

Table 4-17 Selected Sedative Agents

Drug	Administration	Adverse Effects	Nursing Implications
Diazepam (Valium) and other benzodiazepines	Diazepam (Valium) • PO: 2-10 mg every 6-8 hours • IV injection: 1-15 mg at rate no faster than 2 mg/min; may repeat every 2-4 hours • Maximum: 60 mg • Do not mix with any other drugs or dextrose solution Other benzodiazepines Lorazepam (Ativan) • PO: 2-6 mg/day in divided doses • IV injection: 1-4 mg slowly every 2-4 hours • IV infusion: 1-10 mg/hr adjusted to desirable sedation level Alprazolam (Xanax) • PO: 0.25-0.5 mg three times daily	• Tachycardia • Hypotension (IV) • Nausea, vomiting • Urinary retention • Drowsiness • Dizziness, ataxia • Blurred vision • Slurred speech • Confusion • Respiratory depression (IV) • Drug dependence may occur	• Monitor HR, BP, ECG, respiratory rate and depth • Note contraindications: known hypersensitivity, glaucoma, psychosis • Use cautiously in liver disease, renal disease, older adult • Use large veins for IV injection • Administer flumazenil (Romazicon), a benzodiazepine antagonist, if necessary and prescribed
Midazolam hydrochloride (Versed)	• IM injection: 0.07-0.35 mg/kg • IV injection: 0.15-0.35 mg/kg • IV infusion: mix 150 mg in 250 mL (0.6 mg/mL); usual dose is 0.05-0.25 mg/kg/hr	• Bradycardia • Dysrhythmias • Hypotension • Nausea, vomiting, hiccoughs • Headache • Agitation • Bronchospasm • Respiratory depression, apnea • Pain and tenderness at injection site	• Monitor HR, BP, respiratory rate and depth • Note contraindications: known hypersensitivity, shock, coma, acute alcohol intoxication, glaucoma • Use cautiously in COPD, HF, renal failure, older adult, debilitated person • Use large muscle mass if given IM; use large vein if given IV, avoid infiltration • Administer flumazenil (Romazicon), a benzodiazepine antagonist, if necessary and prescribed
Propofol (Diprivan)	• IV injection: 5 mcg/kg initially then increase dose by 5-10 mcg/kg/min every 5-10 minutes until level of sedation is reached; followed by IV infusion • IV infusion: premixed in 10 mg/mL concentration, infuse 5-50 mcg/kg/min • Maximum: 150 mcg/kg/min • Use strict aseptic technique; discard tubing and unused solution at least every 12 hours	• Bradycardia • Hypotension • Decreased cardiac output • Nausea, vomiting • Headache • Twitching • Rash • Green urine • Respiratory depression • Reactions such as agitation, hyperactivity, combativeness may occur • Burning/pain at injection site • Hypertriglyceridemia with prolonged infusion • Metabolic acidosis with prolonged infusion • Pancreatitis • Sepsis	• Monitor HR, BP, ECG, respiratory rate • Note that this drug allows for faster weaning process and faster time to extubation than neuromuscular paralytics • Note contraindications: known hypersensitivity to propofol or lipid emulsion, hyperlipidemia and disorders of lipid metabolism, intracranial hypertension • Use cautiously in respiratory depression, dysrhythmias, pancreatitis, hypotension, hypovolemia, and in older adult • Correct hypovolemia before administration of propofol • Administer with analgesics if needed since this drug provides n[illegible] analgesia • W[illegible]an by reducing the rate by 5[illegible]0 mcg/kg/min every 10-15 m[illegible]utes; stop when patient r[illegible]hes baseline consciousness a[illegible]rientation

Continued

Table 4-17 Selected Sedative Agents—cont'd

Drug	Administration	Adverse Effects	Nursing Implications
Dexmedetomidine HCl (Precedex)	• IV injection: 1 mcg/kg over 10 minutes followed by IV infusion • IV infusion: 0.2-0.7 mcg/kg/hr titrated to patient response for up to 24 hours	• Hypotension or hypertension • Bradycardia or tachycardia • Dysrhythmia especially atrial fibrillation • Nausea, vomiting • Fever • Hypoxia • Anemia	• Monitor HR, BP, SaO_2 • Arousability and alertness with stimulation does not necessarily indicate lack of efficacy in the absence of other clinical findings • Use caution in patients with advanced heart block • Coadministration with other anesthetics, sedatives, hypnotics, and opioids is likely to lead to enhancement of the effects of those drugs • Avoid contact of dexmedetomidine with rubber because it may interact with natural rubber
Pentobarbital (Nembutal)	For intracranial hypertension • IV injection: 3 mg/kg IV slowly • IV infusion: mix 2 grams in 500 mL (4 mg/mL); usual dose is 1-3 mg/kg/hr For status epilepticus • IV injection: 2-8 mg/kg IV slowly • IV infusion: mix 2 grams in 500 mL (4 mg/mL); usual dose is 1-3 mg/kg • Therapeutic blood level: 25-40 mg/dL	• Bradycardia • Hypotension • Rash • Agranulocytosis, thrombocytopenia, anemia • Myocardial depression; may induce HF • Respiratory depression	• Monitor HR, BP, respiratory rate, neurologic status • Note that ICP monitoring is recommended because the most important indicator of neurologic status (level of consciousness) is eliminated by induced coma • Monitor for clinical indications of heart failure • Note contraindications: known hypersensitivity, respiratory depression, liver failure, renal failure • Use cautiously in anemia, liver disease, renal disease, hypertension, older adult

Table 4-18 Ramsay Sedation Scale

Score	Description
1	Anxious, agitated or restless, or both
2	Cooperative, oriented, tranquil
3	Responding to commands only
4	Asleep but with brisk response to light glabellar tap or loud auditory stimulus
5	Asleep with sluggish response to light glabellar tap or loud auditory stimulus
6	Asleep, nonresponsive

From Ramsay, M., Savege, T., Simpson, B., & Goodwin, R. (1974). Controlled sedation with alphaxalone-alphadolone. *Br Med J, 2*, 656.

high carbohydrates cause an increase in CO_2 production.

5. Prevent, assess for, and manage patient-ventilator asynchrony.
   a. Neuromuscular blockers (Table 4-21)
      1) Actions
         a) Block the transmission of nerve impulses at the skeletal neuromuscular junction.
         b) Cause paralysis of all striated muscle.
         c) Do not affect consciousness, cerebration, or relieve pain.
      2) Indications
         a) Patient-ventilator asynchrony
            i) High-frequency ventilation
            ii) Pressure-controlled inverse-ratio ventilation
         b) Poor lung/chest wall compliance
         c) Poor gas exchange
         d) Increased ICP
         e) Tetanus
         f) Need to decrease O_2 consumption
         g) Need to facilitate procedures (e.g., intubation)
         h) Need to eliminate shivering
      3) Assessment of degree of neuromuscular blockade
         a) Use of a peripheral nerve stimulation device to evaluate train-of-four (Figure 4-31)
            i) Method
               (a) Attach leads to ulnar nerve at the wrist.
               (b) Attach peripheral nerve stimulator to leads.

Table 4-19 Sedation-Agitation Scale

Score	Definition	Description
7	Dangerous agitation	Pulling at ET tube, trying to remove catheters, climbing over bed rail, striking at staff, thrashing side to side
6	Very agitated	Does not calm despite frequent verbal reminding of limits; requires physical restraints, biting ET tube
5	Agitated	Anxious or mildly agitated, attempting to sit up, calms down to verbal instructions
4	Calm and cooperative	Calm, wakes easily, follows commands
3	Sedated	Difficult to rouse, awakens to verbal stimuli or gently shaking but drifts off again, follows simple commands
2	Very sedated	Arouses to physical stimuli but does not communicate or follow commands, may move spontaneously
1	Unarousable	Minimal or no response to noxious stimuli, does not communicate or follow commands

From Riker, R., Picard, J., & Fraser, G. (1999). Prospective evaluation of the Sedation-Agitation Scale for adult critically ill patients. *Crit Care Med, 27*, 1325.

(Remember: Negative is black; positive is red).

(c) Evaluate voltage required prior to paralysis if possible.
  (i) Turn voltage dial to 2 to start. Increase as necessary.
  (ii) Turn unit on and push train-of-four.
  (iii) Look for thumb twitch, eyelid twitch, foot

Table 4-20 Motor Activity Assessment Scale

Score	Definition
0	Unresponsiveness
1	Responsive only to noxious stimuli
2	Responsive to touch
3	Calm and cooperative
4	Restless and cooperative
5	Agitated
6	Dangerously agitated

From Devlin, J. W., Boleski, G., Mlynarek, M., Nerenz, D. R., Peterson, E., Jankowski, M., et al. (1999). Motor activity assessment scale: A valid and reliable sedation scale for use with mechanically ventilated patients in an adult surgical intensive care unit. *Crit Care Med, 27*(7), 1271-1275.

Table 4-21 Selected Neuromuscular Blocking Agents

Drug	Administration	Adverse Effects	Nursing Implications
Pancuronium (Pavulon)	• IV injection: 0.1-0.2 mg/kg initially followed by 1-2 mcg/kg/min Other neuromuscular blockers • Atracurium (Tracrium): IV injection 0.2-0.5 mg/kg followed by IV infusion of 4-12 mcg/kg/min • Cisatracurium (Nimbex): IV injection 0.1-0.2 mg/kg followed by IV infusion of 1-3 mcg/kg/min • Doxacurium (Nuromax): IV injection of 0.05-0.1 mg/kg; IV infusion is not typical • Mivacurium (Mivacron): IV injection 0.1-0.25 mg/kg followed by IV infusion of 8-10 mcg/kg/min • Pipecuronium (Arduan): IV injection 0.1-0.2 mg/kg followed by IV infusion of 0.5-2 mcg/kg/min • Rocuronium (Zemuron): IV injection 0.6-1.2 mg/kg followed by IV infusion of 10-12 mcg/kg/min • Vecuronium bromide (Norcuron): IV injection 0.08-0.1 mg/kg followed by IV infusion of 1-2 mcg/kg/min	• Tachycardia or bradycardia • Hypertension or hypotension • Wheezing • Residual muscle weakness • Prolonged use may make weaning difficult due to muscle reconditioning	• Monitor heart rate, BP, serum electrolyte (especially potassium, magnesium), inspiratory effort, and nerve stimulation • Use this drug only with intubated patients • Note contraindications: known hypersensitivity • Use cautiously in CAD, renal disease, electrolyte imbalance, neuromuscular disease, pulmonary disease • Store in refrigerator • Inform patient that paralysis is temporary and always give analgesic and/or sedative concurrently • Provide eye care with artificial tears or Lacri-Lube to prevent corneal abrasion because the patient cannot blink • Evaluate dose by using peripheral nerve stimulation train-of-four; one to two twitches out of four indicates sufficient but not excessive dose; if no twitches out of four, decrease dose; if three to four twitches, increase dose

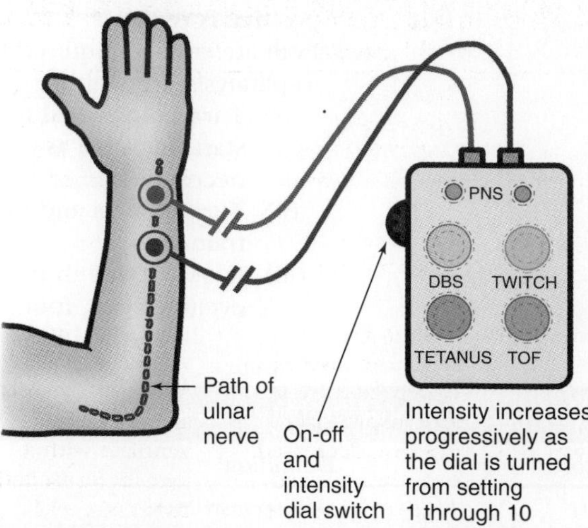

Figure 4-31 Peripheral nerve stimulator. Note placement of electrodes along ulnar nerve. If train-of-four is used, one or two twitches of the thumb is a desirable result. Absence of any thumb twitch indicates overparalysis (reduce dosage of paralytic agent). Three or four twitches of the thumb indicates underparalysis (increase dosage of paralytic agent). (From Urden, L., Stacy, K., & Lough, M. [2009]. *Critical care nursing: Diagnosis and management* [6th ed.]. St. Louis: Mosby.)

dorsiflexion, or plantar flexion of great toe.

(iv) Increase voltage if necessary.

ii) Evaluation
  (a) Desired response is one to two twitches out of four stimuli if the patient is receiving the adequate dose for neuromuscular blockade.
  (b) Underparalysis
    (i) Three or four responses of four stimuli indicates underparalysis.
    (ii) Dosage should be increased.
  (c) Overparalysis
    (i) No response even with the voltage at maximum indicates overparalysis.
    (ii) Dosage should be decreased.

4) Types of neuromuscular blockers and duration of action
  a) Depolarizing
    i) Succinylcholine (Anectine): 8-10 minutes
  b) Nondepolarizing
    i) Mivacurium (Mivacron):15-30 minutes
    ii) Rocuronium (Zemuron): 20-30 minutes
    iii) Atracurium (Tracrium): 20-35 minutes
    iv) Vecuronium (Norcuron): 25-30 minutes
    v) Cisatracurium (Nimbex): 30-50 minutes
    vi) Tubocurarine (Curare): 30-100 minutes
    vii) Pancuronium (Pavulon): 60-75 minutes
    viii) Pipecuronium (Arduan): 60-140 minutes
    ix) Doxacurium (Nuromax): 100-150 minutes

5) Nursing management principles of neuromuscular blockage
  a) Give sedative and/or analgesics concurrently with paralytics.
    i) Clinical signs of inadequate sedation in a patient receiving neuromuscular blocking agents
      (a) Hypertension
      (b) Tachycardia
      (c) Diaphoresis
      (d) Lacrimation
  b) Explain the situation to the patient prior to paralysis.
  c) Protect the patient's corneas, skin, joints; DVT prophylaxis is indicated.
  d) Evaluate dose by evaluating train-of-four and adjust accordingly.
  e) Prevent, assess for, and manage potential complications of positive pressure ventilation (Table 4-22)
    i) Bundles to prevent complications
      (a) Bundle concept: evidence-based interventions "bundled" together to improve patient outcomes; a small number of interventions (3-5) is recommended (Institute for Healthcare Improvement, 2005)
      (b) Interventions typically included in a "vent" bundle (IHI, 2005)
      (c) Elevation of the head of the bed
      (d) Daily "sedation vacations" and assessment of readiness to wean or extubate
      (e) Peptic ulcer disease prophylaxis
      (f) Deep venous thrombosis prophylaxis
      (g) Daily oral care with chlorhexidine

Weaning (also Referred to as *Liberation*)

1. Definition: the gradual withdrawal of ventilatory support for patients who have been mechanically ventilated more than 24 hours
2. Phases of weaning

Table 4-22 Complications of Mechanical Ventilation

Complication	Causes	Prevention	Clinical Presentation	Treatment
Decreased cardiac output	• Increased intrathoracic pressures which • Decrease venous return to the right heart • Increased RV afterload • Decreased LV distensibility	• Ensure adequate preload prior to mechanical ventilation • Avoid excessive tidal volumes • Adjust PEEP carefully	• Tachycardia, hypotension • Cool, clammy skin • Decrease in urine output • Change in level of consciousness	• Administer fluids to increase preload • Administer inotropes as prescribed
Ventilator-induced lung injury (VILI)	• Barotrauma: high inflation pressures may cause pneumothorax, pneumomediastinum, subcutaneous emphysema • Volutrauma: high inflation volumes and repeated end-expiratory collapse followed by repeated reopening during inspiration may cause release of inflammatory mediators, injury to the lung ultrastructure, and ALI/ARDS • Oxygen toxicity • High end-inspiratory lung volume, such as occurs with high levels of PEEP, auto-PEEP (e.g., IRV), and high functional residual capacity, such as elderly patients (i.e., senile emphysema) or patients with COPD	• Avoid excessive tidal volumes; now recommended to be within 5-10 mL/kg of IBW with even lower tidal volumes for patients with ALI/ARDS (~6 mL/kg of IBW) • Keep plateau pressure less than 30 cm H_2O • Keep FiO_2 less than 0.6 (60%) • Adjust PEEP carefully	• Pneumothorax: chest pain, dyspnea, sudden increase in peak inspiratory pressure, decreased breath sounds and chest movement on affected side, tracheal shift, hypotension, JVD if tension pneumothorax, clinical indications of hypoxia, decreased SpO_2, chest x-ray changes • ALI/ARDS: high peak and plateau pressures, refractory hypoxemia (P/F ratio less than 300 mm Hg), noncardiac (PAOP less than 18 mm Hg) pulmonary edema, patchy atelectasis on chest x-ray	• If pneumothorax is suspected: take patient off ventilator and manually ventilate with a manual resuscitation bag; assist with insertion of chest tube for pneumothorax • Decrease tidal volume or PEEP if possible to decrease mean airway pressure and prevent alveolar overdistention
Fluid retention	• Decrease in insensible loss via respiratory system • Overhydration by humidification • Decreased urine output due to ADH and aldosterone secretion	• Avoid decrease in cardiac output which stimulates renin-angiotensin-aldosterone system	• Weight gain • Intake greater than output • Crackles • Decreased compliance	• Utilize therapies above to prevent decrease in cardiac output

Continued

Table 4-22 Complications of Mechanical Ventilation—cont'd

Complication	Causes	Prevention	Clinical Presentation	Treatment
Atelectasis	• Airway obstruction • Small tidal volumes or lack of sighing • Infrequent turning of patient	• Use periodic sighing • Turn frequently • Provide adequate humidification • Perform tracheal suctioning as indicated • Provide chest physical therapy (PT) as indicated • Reposition frequently	• Diminished breath sounds • Crackles • Abnormal chest x-ray • Increased A:a gradient • Decreased compliance	• Provide periodic sighing • Provide chest PT
Hypercapnia; hypocapnia	• Inadequate or excessive ventilation • Hypermetabolism may contribute to hypercapnia	• Initiate ventilation with tidal volume at 10-15 mL/kg and rate of 8-12 • Make ventilator changes after initial ABGs	• Increased (greater than 45 mm Hg) or decreased (less than 35 mm Hg) $PaCO_2$	• Hypercapnia: increase tidal volume (or rate) • Hypocapnia: decrease rate (or tidal volume); change to IMV or PSV
Oxygen toxicity	• Too high a concentration of O_2 over too long a time	• Maintain FiO_2 as low as possible to maintain a SaO_2 (or SpO_2) of 90% and limit duration of FiO_2 of greater than 0.4 if possible; addition of PEEP allows reduction of FiO_2 while maintaining the same SaO_2 • **Remember:** hypoxemia is far more common than O_2 toxicity and must be corrected	• Substernal distress • Paresthesias in extremities • Anorexia, nausea, vomiting • Fatigue, lethargy, malaise • Restlessness • Dyspnea, progressive respiratory difficulty • Decreased compliance • Increased A:a gradient	• Decrease O_2 concentration as soon as possible • Provide supportive management
Aspiration	• Stomach contents • Tube feedings • Oral secretions • Gastric distention • Impaired gastric emptying • Esophageal reflux	• Maintain cuff inflation using minimal occlusive volume • Keep head of bed elevated 30-45 degrees • Check for gastric retention at least every 4 hours • Check NG tube placement at least every 4 hours	• Increased tracheal secretions • Fever • Rhonchi, wheezes • Signs/symptoms of hypoxemia/ hypoxia • Infiltrate on chest x-ray	• Provide supportive management • Administer antibiotics as prescribed • Administer steroids as prescribed
GI effects: stress ulcer, ileus, gastric dilation	• Hyperacidity • Endogenous or exogenous steroids • Gastric or mesenteric ischemia • Inadequate nutrition	• Utilize enteral feedings • Administer antacids; H_2 receptor antagonists (e.g., cimetidine [Tagamet]); barrier agents (e.g., sucralfate [Carafate]) as prescribed	• NG aspirate, vomitus, or stools positive for blood • Decreased bowel sounds • Gastric distention • Increased gastric retention	• Note effect of hemoglobin loss of tissue oxygenation; blood administration may be necessary • Administer antacids, sucralfate, H_2 receptor antagonists, and/or PP, as prescribed

Table 4-22 Complications of Mechanical Ventilation—cont'd

Complication	Causes	Prevention	Clinical Presentation	Treatment
Infection	• Immunosuppression • Artificial airways bypass normal upper airway defense mechanisms • Ventilatory equipment: warm, moist environment is good for bacterial growth • Suctioning procedure • Silent aspiration of GI bacteria when PPIs, H_2 antagonists, or antacids used for ulcer prophylaxis; controversial issue • Cross-contamination may be cause	• Use good hand-washing techniques • Use sterile technique for suctioning • Provide aseptic airway management, tubing changes, etc. • Avoid change in usual acidic gastric pH; use enteral feedings for ulcer prophylaxis if gastric mobility adequate • Keep head of bed elevated during tube feedings • Keep ET tube or trach cuff inflated to 20-25 mm Hg • Drain humidifier condensation into water trap or container and not back into humidifier • Routine change of ventilator circuit is no longer indicated, but the circuit should be changed if visibly soiled or malfunctioning • Additional information in Pneumonia section of Chapter 5	• Tachycardia, tachypnea • Fever • Crackles, rhonchi, or wheezes • Hypoxemia • Change in color or character of sputum • Positive cultures • Infiltrate on chest x-ray	• Administer antibiotic specific to culture
Patient-ventilator asynchrony (patient "fighting" ventilator)	• Incorrect ventilator setup for the patient's needs • Acute change in patient's status • Obstructed airway • Ventilator malfunction • Anxiety	• Ensure proper setup of ventilator equipment; monitor settings every hour • Monitor peak inspiratory pressure • Suction as indicated • Talk to patient, keep him or her informed • Administer anxiolytics as indicated	• Anxiety, agitation • Increase in peak inspiratory pressure • Ventilator alarm sounding • Change in pulse oximetry or ABGs	• Perform rapid check of patient and ventilator • Disconnect patient from ventilator and provide manual ventilation via manual resuscitation bag • Check vital signs, breath sounds, pulse oximetry • Assess ABGs • Suction airway • Check patency of endotracheal or tracheostomy tube

Continued

Table 4-22 Complications of Mechanical Ventilation—cont'd

Complication	Causes	Prevention	Clinical Presentation	Treatment
Anxiety	• Loss of autonomy over vital body function (breathing) • Inability to communicate • Sensory overload (e.g., alarms, repeated interruptions for vital signs, noise of ventilator) • Sensory deprivation (e.g., separation from family, work, meaningful activities) • Discomfort (e.g., arterial punctures, endotracheal tube, nasogastric tube, Foley catheter, etc.)	• Explain to patient why he or she can't speak; provide method of communication • Explain all procedures thoroughly; keep patient informed regarding progress and plans • Add familiar objects to patient's environment (e.g., family photos, cards) • Have calendar and clock in room; have window shades or curtains open to orient patient to light and dark • Allow uninterrupted time for rest and sleep • Put eyeglasses and hearing aid on patient if appropriate • Encourage expression of fears • Be available; answer call bell promptly • Promote as much independence as possible • Provide emotional support to the family • Avoid uncomfortable or painful procedures if possible (e.g., arterial catheter instead of arterial punctures) • Use complementary therapies such as music, aromatherapy	• High-pressure alarm because the patient is breathing out of synch with ventilator • Tachycardia • Tachypnea, excessive triggering of ventilator is on assist/control, potentially causing hypocapnia and respiratory alkalosis • Complaints of being "nervous"	• Stay with patient during times of extreme anxiety • Use therapeutic touch (e.g., hold hand) • Utilize soft restraints only as necessary to prevent self-extubation • Encourage family visitation and participation if appropriate
Inability to wean	• COPD: occurs when $PaCO_2$ is corrected instead of pH • Malnutrition: catabolism and muscle breakdown • Neuromuscular blocking agents: disuse syndrome	• Correct pH instead of $PaCO_2$ in patients with COPD • Provide adequate calories to prevent catabolism; adequate protein and high calories are given; adequate calories must be given to prevent the protein from being utilized for energy; calories given are predominantly fat because CHO metabolism produces more CO_2 • Avoid neuromuscular blocking agents if possible; limit duration of use	• Increased $PaCO_2$, increased ventilatory rate, tachycardia with weaning efforts	• COPD: allow $PaCO_2$ to increase so that the kidney will hold on to bicarbonate to compensate; keep PaO_2 close to patient's normal (e.g., 60-65 mm Hg) • Provide adequate protein and calories; avoid high carbohydrate feedings during weaning • Discontinue several days prior to weaning

a. Preweaning phase: assessment to determine if the patient is capable of attempting spontaneous ventilation
  1) Respiratory factors
    a) Resolution or improvement of disease process that necessitated mechanical ventilation
    b) Oxygenation
      i) Patient does not require more than 5 cm of PEEP or FiO_2 greater than 0.5 to maintain acceptable PaO_2 (PaO_2 60 mm Hg) and SaO_2 (SaO_2 of 90%)
      ii) P/F ratio greater than or equal to 150 mm Hg
    c) Ventilation
      i) Respiratory rate less than 30 breaths/min
      ii) $PaCO_2$ less than 45 mm Hg or equal to the patient's baseline $PaCO_2$
      iii) Tidal volume greater than 5 mL/kg
      iv) Vital capacity greater than 10 mL/kg
      v) Minute ventilation less than 10 L/min
    d) Lung mechanics
      i) Maximal inspiratory pressure greater than −25 cm H_2O
      ii) Rapid shallow breathing index less than or equal to 125 breaths/min/L
  2) Nonrespiratory factors
    a) Neurologic status: conscious
    b) Hemodynamics: stable
    c) Hemoglobin: adequate
    d) Fluid and electrolytes: corrected and normal
    e) Nutrition: adequate nutritional status
    f) Psychological factors: psychologically prepared and cooperative
    g) Medications: cessation of deep sedation and muscle paralytics

b. Weaning phase
  1) Methods of weaning
    a) Spontaneous breathing trial (SBT) with T-piece for short-term mechanical ventilation (i.e., less than 72 hours)
      i) Spontaneous breathing for 120 minutes through ventilator with PSV of 0; CPAP of up to 5 cm H_2O allowed
        (a) If successful, extubation
        (b) If unsuccessful, allow patient to rest and try again the next day; tracheostomy may also be considered.
      ii) Advantage: may be able to wean patient more quickly than IMV or PSV methods
      iii) Disadvantage: Recurrent ventilatory failures discourage and frighten the patient.
    b) IMV
      i) Gradually reduce IMV rate.
      ii) Advantages
        (a) Provides exercise for ventilatory musculature
        (b) More physiologic $PaCO_2$ may be achieved
        (c) Large ventilator-provided breaths help to prevent atelectasis.
        (d) Safer than trial-and-error method
        (e) Good acceptance by patients
      iii) Disadvantages: may take longer than T-piece method
    c) Pressure support ventilation (PSV) method
      i) Gradually decrease the amount of pressure support assisting the patient
        (a) Usually started at 15-25 cm H_2O
        (b) Gradually decreased by 3-6 cm H_2O every 1-3 days as long as maintaining a satisfactory minute ventilation
        (c) When the patient can maintain adequate ventilation with the PSV at 5 cm H_2O, extubation is considered.
      ii) Advantages
        (a) Patient comfort frequently greater with PSV
        (b) Less work of breathing than with IMV or T-piece method
    d) CPAP
      i) May be used for patients whose PaO_2 is PEEP-dependent; the patient is weaned from the ventilator by one of the previously noted methods but left on CPAP to provide the improved driving pressure needed to maintain an adequate PaO_2.
  2) Criteria used to stop a weaning trial
    a) Neurologic
      i) Change in level of consciousness
      ii) Extreme anxiety
    b) Pulmonary
      i) Respiratory rate greater than 35/min or less than 10/min
      ii) Use of accessory muscle of ventilation
      iii) Paradoxical chest wall motion
      iv) Complaints of dyspnea, fatigue, or pain
      v) SaO_2 less than 90%
      vi) Increase in $PaCO_2$ of 5-8 mm Hg and/or pH of less than 7.3
    c) Cardiovascular
      i) Systolic BP greater than 180 mm Hg or less than 90 mm Hg

ii) Heart rate greater than 140/min or sustained increase 20% above baseline
iii) PVCs greater than 6/min, couplets, or runs of ventricular tachycardia
iv) ST segment changes

3) Therapies to facilitate weaning
a) Coordination and communication among disciplines: flow sheets and communication boards
b) Multidisciplinary weaning protocol
c) Multidisciplinary rounds
d) Recognition of likely reasons for failure to wean
i) Underlying illness has not resolved sufficiently
ii) Malnutrition
iii) Excessive secretions
iv) Presence of auto-PEEP
v) Impaired muscle function secondary to electrolyte imbalance (e.g., hypokalemia, hypophosphatemia, hypomagnesemia)
vi) Respiratory muscle fatigue

c. Weaning outcomes phase
1) Complete weaning: The patient is able to maintain a normal respiratory rate and tidal volume while breathing spontaneously.
2) Partial weaning: The patient is able to maintain spontaneous ventilation for short periods.
3) Terminal weaning followed by death

3. General guidelines
a. Position for optimal ventilation: usually semi-Fowler's to high Fowler's
b. Avoid depressing the patient's ventilatory drive and muscle strength by avoiding sedatives and muscle paralytics; treat pain but do not overnarcotize.
c. Reduce carbohydrates if indicated; equivalent calories can be provided in the form of fats.
1) Utilize Pulmocare if being fed enterally: high fat and protein but low carbohydrates
2) Decrease glucose and increase fat (Intralipids) if being fed parenterally.
d. Begin weaning attempts in the early morning; do not attempt to wean the patient at night.
e. Complementary therapies such as biofeedback and music may be helpful.
f. Since the mechanical ventilator may provide security for the patient, it may be helpful to leave ventilator in room with patient for 24 hours after weaning.
g. Monitor closely for clinical indicators of fatigue and ventilatory failure and abort if necessary.

Noninvasive Positive Pressure Ventilation (NPPV)

Description

Positive pressure ventilation (usually CPAP or Bi-PAP) of a nonintubated spontaneous breathing patient, primarily with a face or nasal mask attached to a standard ventilator or a machine specifically for NIV with the purpose of augmenting alveolar ventilation

1. Modes
a. CPAP: preset positive airway pressure during spontaneous breaths
b. Bi-PAP: preset positive pressure to be delivered during inspiration and preset pressure to be maintained during expiration; combination of PSV (I-PAP) and CPAP (E-PAP)
2. Patient-ventilator interface
a. Types
1) Nasal mask
2) Facial mask
3) Nasal prongs
4) Helmet
b. Considerations
1) Patient preference
2) Facial shape
3) Patient acuity
4) Patient anxiety level

Indications

1. Acute respiratory failure especially in COPD
2. Cardiac pulmonary edema
3. Weaning of a patient from traditional mechanical ventilation and/or PEEP
4. Sleep apnea
5. Terminal care to avoid intubation, such as a patient with end-stage COPD

Advantages over Traditional Mechanical Ventilation

1. Avoidance of intubation and complications of intubation such as VAP
2. Improved patient comfort
3. Lower incidence of nosocomial pneumonia
4. Lower sedation requirements
5. Shorter critical care unit stays
6. Can be initiated, discontinued, and reinitiated if only required intermittently

Disadvantages

1. Uncomfortable because mask requires a seal
2. Seal difficult to obtain if orogastric or nasogastric tube in place
3. Cannot eat due to high risk of aspiration

Contraindications

1. Absolute
a. Hemodynamic instability
b. Problems with airway patency (e.g., copious secretions)
c. Risk for aspiration

d. Altered level of consciousness (i.e., patient without airway protective reflexes)
e. Recent upper airway or esophageal surgery

2. Relative
   a. Uncooperative patient
   b. Morbid obesity
   c. Unstable angina or acute MI
   d. Inability to fit mask
   e. Agitation

Complications

1. Facial skin breakdown
2. Nasal congestion
3. Conjunctivitis
4. Gastric distention
5. Aspiration
6. Pneumothorax

Reasons to Switch to Invasive Ventilation (Bauman, 2009)

1. Worsening of $PaCO_2$ and respiratory acidosis
2. Worsening PaO_2 and SaO_2
3. Severe tachypnea
4. Hemodynamic instability
5. Altered level of consciousness
6. Inability to clear airway secretions
7. Inability to tolerate face mask

Chest Tubes

Purposes of Chest Tubes (also Called *Thoracostomy Tube* or *Thoracic Catheter*)

1. Pleural tubes
   a. To remove free air: tube placed anterior and superior (usually at second ICS at MCL)
      1) Pneumothorax (i.e., air in the pleural space)
         a) Chest tube is indicated if pneumothorax is greater than 15% or on mechanical ventilator
         b) Small spontaneous pneumothorax will be resolved without chest tube.
   b. To drain the intrapleural space: tube placed lateral and inferior (usually at fifth or sixth ICS at midaxillary line)
      1) Hemothorax (i.e., blood in the pleural space): Chest tube is indicated if greater than 500 mL.
      2) Pleural effusion: liquid in the pleural space; may be transudate or exudate
         a) Transudate: occurs if there is a rise in pulmonary venous pressure (e.g., HF) or hypoproteinemia (e.g., malnutrition, cirrhosis); tends to accumulate at the base of the lungs
         b) Exudate: occurs as a result of increased capillary permeability or impaired lymphatic absorption (e.g., involvement of the pleura by inflammation or malignancy); the fluid has a higher specific gravity and protein content than a transudate
      3) Empyema (also called pyothorax): pus in the pleural space
      4) Chylothorax: chyle (lymph fluid and triglyceride fat) in the pleural space
      5) Hydrothorax: water (e.g., IV fluid) in the pleural space
   c. To reestablish negative pressure in pleural space
2. Mediastinal tubes: to drain air and blood from the mediastinum after cardiac or other mediastinal surgery

Insertion

1. Chest tubes may be inserted in surgery when the thoracic cavity must be invaded during the surgical procedure, in the interventional radiology department, or at the bedside.
2. Informed consent is required.
3. Explanation to patient and family should be given by physician and reinforced by nurse.
4. Chest drainage system is set up prior to insertion of tube.
5. Local anesthetic is used but pressure is felt.
6. The tube is sutured in place and then the insertion site is dressed and the tube is taped securely to avoid tugging.
7. Chest x-ray is obtained to confirm placement.

Chest Drainage System

1. Components
   a. Drainage collection bottle or chamber collects liquid drainage.
   b. Water-seal bottle or chamber provides a one-way valve to allow air to escape but does not allow atmospheric air to go into the pleural space.
   c. Suction control bottle or chamber controls the amount of suction.
2. Systems (Figure 4-32)
   a. Three-bottle system
      1) The drainage collection bottle is the bottle closest to the patient; this bottle is connected to the water-seal bottle.
      2) The water-seal bottle is filled so that the tube from the chest tube is submerged 2 cm under the water.
      3) The water-seal bottle must have a vent open at the top of the bottle to allow air to escape.
      4) The third bottle is the suction control bottle.
         a) It has one tube to connect it to the water-seal bottle.
         b) Another tube connects it to the suction device (usually wall suction but it may be a free-standing Emerson-type suction device).
         c) The third tube is submerged under water to the prescribed suction amount in water (usually 20 cm H_2O); the other end of this tube is open to air.

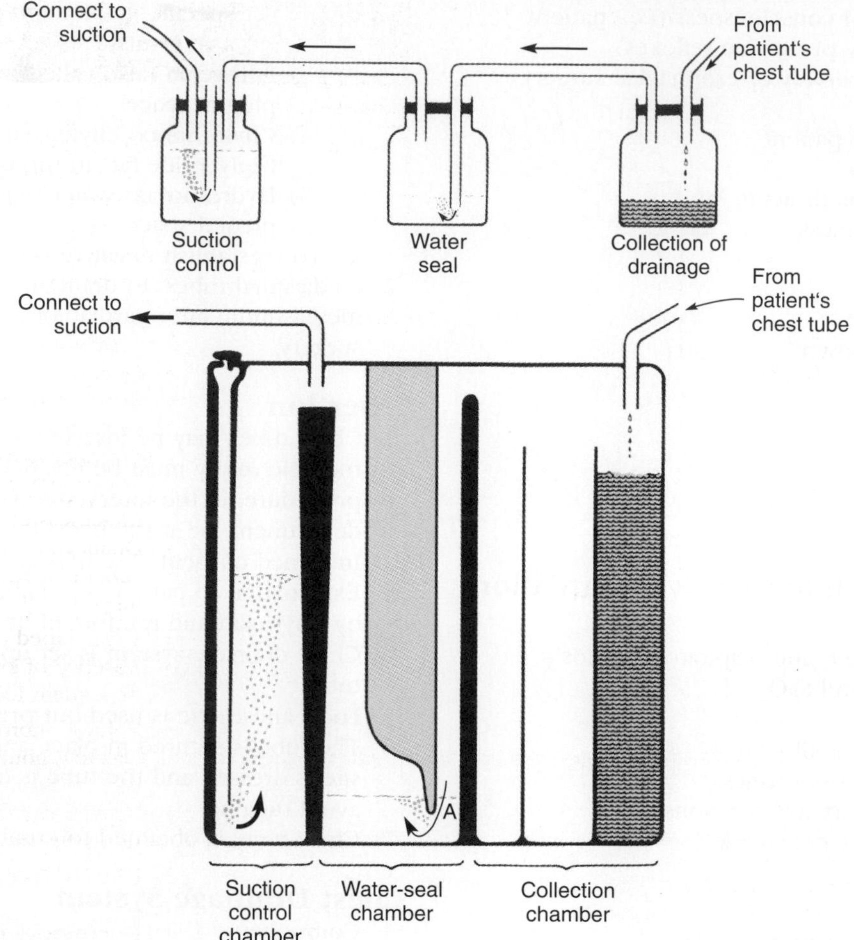

Figure 4-32 Comparison of a commercially available chest tube drainage system with a three-bottle system. (From Urden, L. D., Stacy, K. M., & Lough, M. E. [2006]. *Thelan's critical care nursing: Diagnosis and management* [5th ed.]. St. Louis: Mosby.)

d) Suction is adjusted so that a gentle bubbling occurs in this bottle.
   i) Remember vigorous bubbling just makes it evaporate more quickly so that you must keep refilling it.
   ii) The actual amount of suction is determined by the depth that the tube is submersed minus the water seal.
   iii) Suction is not necessary to remove air and free-flowing fluid; if the pleural air or liquid does not respond to gravity water-seal drainage, suction may be applied.

b. All-in-one system
   1) More convenient
   2) Only the water-seal and drainage collection chambers may be used or all three will be used if suction is desired
   3) In a wet system (e.g., Atrium, Pleur-evac, Thora Seal, Aqua Seal, Medi-Vac): Adjust the amount of suction by filling the water level in the suction control chamber; adjust wall suction so that gentle bubbling occurs in the suction control chamber.
      a) Again, remember the actual amount of suction is the height of the suction control chamber minus the height of the water-seal chamber
   4) In a dry system (e.g., Sentinel Seal, Thora-Klex, Argyle Altitude, Pleur-evac Sahara, Atrium Oasis): Adjust the amount of suction until the indicator appears.

c. Portable chest drainage system (e.g., Atrium Express)
   1) Only one chamber to collect chest drainage
   2) Has a dry seal
   3) Usually used as a gravity drain only but may be used with suction; automatically regulated to −20 cm H_2O when connected to wall suction

d. Heimlich valve (Figure 4-33)
   1) One-way flutter valve made of rubber tubing encased in a clear, plastic chamber
   2) Used for uncomplicated pneumothorax with little or no liquid drainage
      a) May be connected to a small drainage bag to the valve but usually not used if more than 50 mL of fluid

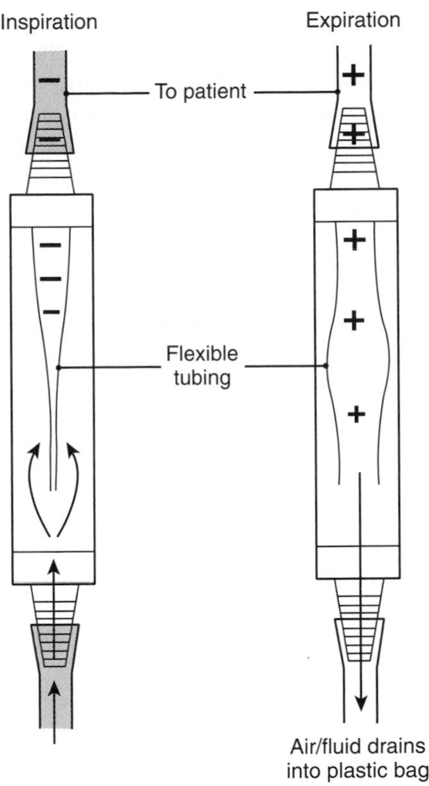

Figure 4-33 Heimlich one-way valve. **A,** During inspiration, negative pressure collapses the flexible tubing and prevents outside air from entering the pleural space. **B,** During expiration, positive pressure opens the flexible tubing and allows air and fluid to drain into an attached plastic bag. (From Kersten, L. D. [1989]. *Comprehensive respiratory nursing: A decision-making approach.* Philadelphia: Saunders.)

b) May be connected to wall suction (but is not usually)
c) Note fluttering of the valve as air escapes from the pleural space.

3) Advantages: small, lightweight, and allows the patient to move around more easily; patient may be discharged with a chest tube attached to a Heimlich valve

Table 4-23 Assessment Parameters for the Patient with a Chest Tube

Parameter	Note
Patient	• Ventilatory effort • Chest discomfort or pain • Anxiety • Level of understanding • Cough • Sputum production
Breathing	• Rate • Regularity • Depth • Breath sounds (disconnection of suction from suction control chamber is required for accurate assessment of breath sounds)
Entry site	• Intactness of dressing • Drainage on dressing • Subcutaneous emphysema around insertion site
Tubing	• Tight, taped connections • Absence of kinks, compressions, or dependent loops
Drainage collection chamber	• Volume (normal 50-100 mL/hr for first few hours after thoracotomy, then 10-20 mL/hr) • Type: color; consistency; odor • Bottle below chest level
Water-seal chamber	• Filled to 2 cm or prescribed amount • Fluctuations with respirations (also referred to as *tidaling*) • Any bubbling • If not on suction: air vent open
Suction control chamber	• Filled to prescribed amount (usually −20 cm H_2O) • Gentle, continuous bubbling
Suction source	• If no control bottle: suction set at ordered level • If control bottle: suction set so gentle, continuous bubbling occurs

Assessment (Table 4-23)

1. Patient parameters
2. Tube and drainage system

Collaborative Management

1. Control pain.
   a. Administer analgesics and/or local anesthetics as prescribed to relieve pain and encourage deep breathing.
   b. Instruct the patient how to splint chest when coughing; instruct the family how to assist.
2. Maintain airway patency and adequate oxygenation and ventilation.
   a. Position the patient for optimal ventilation/perfusion matching.
      1) HOB elevated to 30-45 degrees.
      2) "Good lung down" optimizes ventilation to encourage reexpansion of the surgical lung and optimizes perfusion to the unaffected "good" lung.
         a) Exception: Pneumonectomy patients are positioned on their operative lung or back (i.e., no lung down).
   b. Assess the position of the trachea; report immediately any shift from the normal midline.
   c. Encourage deep breathing and use of the incentive spirometer.
      1) Note that air is removed from the pleural space by the positive pressure of expiration and the negative pressure of suction on the chest tube; deep breathing is *very* important in reexpansion of the lung.
   d. Maintain airway clearance.
      1) Focus on sustained inspiration maneuver; this frequently stimulates the patient to cough if coughing is needed.

2) Suction only if the patient is unable to clear secretions.

e. Administer oxygen as indicated by arterial blood gases and SpO_2.

f. Assist with weaning from mechanical ventilation and extubation as soon as possible as positive pressure ventilation increases risk of air leak.

3. Maintain water-seal drainage system and patency of chest tubes.

a. Assess chest drainage system hourly.

1) Ensure that connections are spiral taped.

2) Position tubing to prevent kinks and dependent loops.

3) Maintain suction level at prescribed level; water may need to be added to the suction control chamber as water evaporates in wet chest drainage systems

4) Assess the water-seal chamber for fluctuation with ventilation (also referred to as *tidaling*); if no tidaling, it may be caused of any of the following:

a) The lung is reexpanded; confirm by assessment of chest x-ray.

b) The tube is kinked; follow the tube from chest to chest drainage system and position tube to prevent kinking.

c) The tube is occluded.

i) The risk of an occluded tube, especially in a patient on mechanical ventilation, is tension pneumothorax, mediastinal shift, and potential tearing of great vessels.

ii) Though routine milking or stripping is not recommended, efforts should be made to reestablish patency of an occluded tube (and prevent tension pneumothorax).

(a) Milk the tube first: if unsuccessful in reestablishing fluctuation in the water-seal chamber, strip short sections.

(i) Milking is hand-over-hand squeezing of the chest tube; stripping is to clamp with the thumb and forefinger of the nondominant hand while pulling the tube between the thumb and forefinger of the dominant hand followed by release of the thumb and forefinger of the nondominant hand.

(ii) Milking and stripping chest tubes create negative pressure within the pleural space; while it may help to move a clot along, it may create trauma to the pleura.

(b) If milking or stripping short sections is unsuccessful in reestablishing fluctuation in the water-seal chamber, notify the physician; a new tube may be required.

5) Assess for air leak and differentiate between expected removal of air from pleural space (occasional bubble) and a break in the chest tube system.

a) An occasional bubble indicates that the tube is still needed because air is still escaping from the pleural space.

b) Excessive bubbling indicates the need to search for a leak in the system.

i) Brief clamping with hemostats moving from the chest drainage system to the insertion site can be helpful in identifying the location of the leak.

ii) Ensure that all connections are connected and spiral taped.

iii) Assess the insertion site for displacement of the tube so that the proximal eyelet is outside the skin; notify the physician so that the tube can be repositioned.

iv) Suspect bronchopleural fistula if no external air leak can be identified.

b. Keep the chest drainage system lower than the patient's chest.

c. Avoid intentionally occluding (e.g., clamping) the tube.

1) Clamp the tube only if one of the following occurs:

a) The chest drainage system must be lifted above the level of the chest (e.g., putting patient in helicopter for transport) so that chest drainage does not drain back into the pleural space; clamp as briefly as possible.

i) NOTE: Heimlich valves or portable chest drainage systems (gravity drainage) are frequently used for transports.

b) If the drainage collection is full (e.g., large pleural effusions), have the new chest drainage system ready, clamp as briefly as possible while connecting the chest tube to the new chest drainage system.

c) If specifically instructed to by the physician prior to chest tube removal

i) This is done to see if the patient is likely to tolerate not having the chest tube.

ii) Monitor closely for clinical indications of tension pneumothorax.

2) If there has been a significant air leak and the chest drainage system breaks, submerse the tube about 2 cm into a bottle of sterile water or sterile saline; if a bottle of sterile water or saline is not available, put tap water into a clean Styrofoam cup and submerse the tube about 2 cm into the cup.
    a) NOTE: The patient is better off with an open pneumothorax than a tension pneumothorax.
3) If there has been a significant air leak and the tube accidentally comes out of the chest: Apply a dressing to the chest with your hand or tape it on three sides (i.e., as you would for a sucking chest wound) and notify the physician immediately.

4. Assist with removal of chest tube: usually removed when there has been no air leak from anterior tube or less than 100 mL/24 hr for posterior tube.
    a. Clamp tube for up to 24 hours before removal as requested.
    b. Administer analgesics prior to chest tube removal; music may also be helpful.
        1) Recommended analgesics include the following:
            a) Ketorolac (Toradol) 30 mg IV 60 minutes before
            b) Morphine 4 mg IV 20 minutes before
    c. Instruct the patient to hold his or her breath when requested.
        1) There is no difference in the rate of post chest tube removal pneumothoraces using either end-inspiration or end-expiration (Bell, Ovadia, Abdullah, Spector, & Rabinovici, 2001).
    d. Apply occlusive dressing after the physician removes the tube at the end of expiration.
    e. Monitor the patient for clinical indications of recurrent pneumothorax: dyspnea, chest pain, asymmetrical chest excursion, diminished breath sounds.
    f. Obtain chest x-ray for confirmation of reexpansion.

LEARNING ACTIVITIES

CHAPTER 4

1. Complete the following crossword puzzle to review pulmonary anatomy, physiology, and assessment.

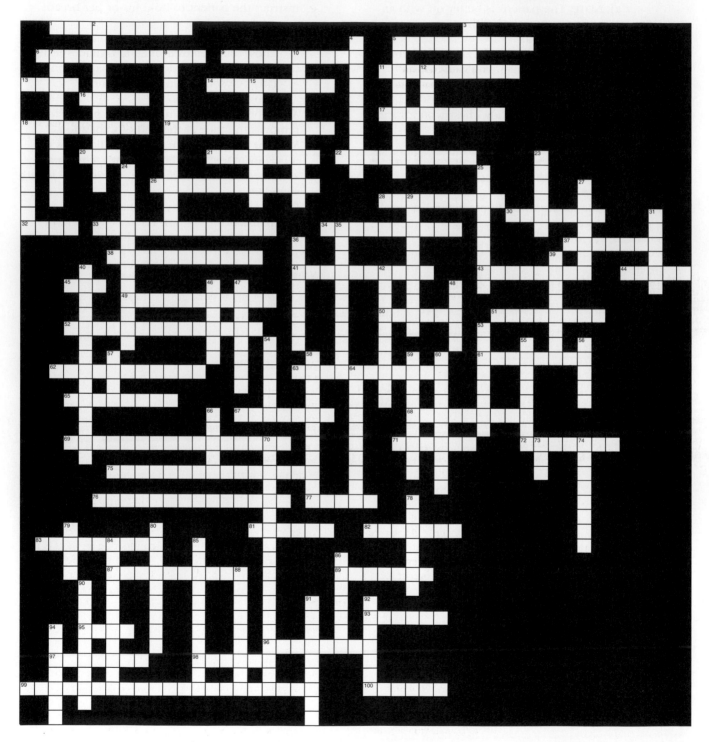

ACROSS

1. These structures increase the surface area in the nose
5. The flexible cartilage attached to the thyroid cartilage; closes to protect the larynx
6. The avascular membrane that can be punctured or opened with a scalpel to provide an emergency airway
9. The change in pressure for a given change in volume
11. Measurement of lung volumes
13. The type of cell that secretes histamine
14. This acid-base imbalance would cause the oxyhemoglobin dissociation curve to shift to the left
16. When deoxygenated blood comes in contact with nonventilated alveoli; V less than Q
17. Rapid breathing
18. A pulmonary embolism would decrease _____ relative to ventilation
19. These cellular organelles use oxygen and nutrients to make ATP
20. A decrease in surfactant would cause a decrease in compliance and an increase in _____ (abbrev.)
21. Alkalosis increases the _____ between hemoglobin and oxygen which impairs oxygen drop-off at the tissue
22. A phagocyte in the alveoli
26. In this type of acid-base imbalance, one system (i.e., respiratory or renal) changes as a result of an abnormality in the other system
28. These normal breath sounds are heard over peripheral lung
30. The passage through the vocal cords
32. A shift of the oxyhemoglobin dissociation curve to the ____ would improve pick-up at the lung but impair drop-off to the tissues
33. This gas is 20 × more diffusible than oxygen (2 words)
34. The area between the soft palate and the base of the tongue; the center for the gag reflex is located here
37. The area of the left lung that corresponds to the right middle lobe
38. The movement of air into and out of the lungs
41. Airway _____ affects the work of breathing
43. This nailbed change is associated with chronic hypoxia
44. Decreased compliance of the chest wall occurs in _____
45. This adventitious breath sound is associated with pleurisy
49. The eustachian tubes open into the ____
50. A dense concentration of lymphatic tissue which guards entryways into the GI or respiratory tracts
51. Noninvasive method of measuring arterial oxygen saturation
52. The lowest portion of the pharynx
61. The type of dead space which describes the air in the alveoli that are not perfused; V greater than Q
62. Measurement of expired carbon dioxide tension
63. This type of disorder is when expansion of the alveolus, lung, or chest wall is impaired and compliance is decreased
65. An enzyme that breaks down elastic tissue
67. These chemoreceptors are primarily sensitive to blood carbon dioxide levels
68. A decrease in blood oxygen; manifested by a decrease in PaO_2 and SaO_2
69. These normal breath sounds are heard over the mainstem bronchi
71. The first portion of the trachea
72. Shift of this structure is seen with mediastinal shift
75. The cause of hypoxemia in myasthenia gravis would be alveolar _____
76. These receptors cause an increase in ventilation rate in response to body movement
77. In this type of acid-base imbalance, there are two disorders occurring concurrently
81. The area at the bifurcation of the trachea; rich in parasympathetic fibers
82. These sounds are heard when listening with a stethoscope to a patient with pneumonia or chronic bronchitis
83. The nutrient circulation of the lung is supplied by this artery
87. Surfactant is produced by the type II _____
89. A decrease in tissue oxygen; manifested by SNS innervation, cyanosis, restlessness or confusion
93. A cause for hypoxia even though the patient has a normal PaO_2
95. Percussion tone heard over pleural effusion
96. This acid-base imbalance causes vasodilation resulting in headache, flushed face, and hypotension
97. Shortness of breath
98. The terminal respiratory unit which has an alveolar-capillary membrane for the exchange of oxygen and carbon dioxide
99. This is caused most commonly by hypoxemia (2 words)
100. Respiratory pattern with normal rate and depth

DOWN

2. A procedure to view the bronchioles with a fiber optic scope
3. This structure is primarily responsible for warming, humidifying, and filtering inspired air
4. These chemoreceptors are primarily sensitive to blood oxygen levels
5. The passive phase of ventilation
7. The first bronchial branch which is part of the gas exchange unit is the _____ bronchiole
8. The _____ dissociation curve shows the relationship between PaO_2 and SaO_2
10. The active phase of ventilation
12. A shift of the oxyhemoglobin dissociation curve to the ___ would decrease the affinity between hemoglobin and oxygen
15. The main accessory muscles of expiration are the internal intercostal and _____ muscles
18. The pleural layer that is contiguous with the chest wall
23. _____'s law is why the PaO_2 goes down if the $PaCO_2$ goes up (assuming room air)
24. Percussion tone heard over hyperinflated lung
25. Area of ventilation without perfusion (2 words)
27. This pressure is calculated by multiplying the FiO_2 (as a decimal) by the barometric pressure (760 mm Hg at sea level)
29. A lipoprotein that decreases surface tension and keeps the alveoli open at low distending pressure
31. The type of compliance which reflects the compliance of the lung and the chest wall
35. Air and gas are _____ and appear black on chest x-ray
36. The last branch of the conducting airways is the _____ bronchiole
39. The pleural layer that is contiguous with the lung
40. These receptors are stimulated by an increase in interstitial fluid volume
42. The type of dead space which describes the air in conducting pathways
46. Obstructive lung disease, such as emphysema, causes the chest to be shaped like a _____
47. Bluish skin color associated with at least 5 gm of desaturated hemoglobin
48. Hairlike projections which move mucus with

entrapped particles upward to be coughed out
53. These sounds are heard when listening with a stethoscope to a patient with atelectasis, pulmonary edema, and ARDS
54. The primary responsibility of the pulmonary system is to ensure the delivery of _____ to the tissues
55. Percussion tone heard over normal lung
56. This cycle converts food to ATP
57. The area of the brain which controls rhythmic ventilation; contains both the apneustic and pneumotaxic centers
58. The center of the thoracic cavity
59. The primary muscle of inspiration
60. Bloody sputum; may be seen in lung cancer or tuberculosis
64. Metal and bone are _____ and appear white on chest x-ray
66. pH, $PaCO_2$, temperature, and 2, 3-DPG cause the oxyhemoglobin dissociation curve to _____ to the left or right
70. This diagnostic study is used to evaluate the adequacy of ventilation (3 words)
73. This may be caused by pulmonary hypertension (abbrev.)
74. The primary function of the nose is to filter, warm, and _____ inspired air
78. The type of compliance which reflects both compliance of the lung and airway resistance
79. These openings between the alveoli are called pores of _____
80. This type of chest pain is sharp pain which occurs with deep inspiration
84. Increased $PaCO_2$
85. Most carbon dioxide is transported in the blood as _____
86. These sounds are heard when listening with a stethoscope to a patient with asthma (plural)
88. The ability of the lung to return to its original size after inspiration
90. The process by which oxygen and carbon dioxide move across the alveolar-capillary membrane
91. Respiratory pattern with rate less than 10 breaths/min
92. Transfusion of greater than 10 units which causes decreased 2,3-DPG and impaired oxygen release from hemoglobin
94. Central chemoreceptors are located in this area of the brain

2. Fill in the primary and accessory muscles of inspiration and expiration.

	Primary	Accessory
Inspiration		
Expiration		

3. Identify whether the following factors cause a shift of the oxyhemoglobin curve to the left or right.

	Left	Right
Increased 2,3-DPG		
Hypothermia		
Hypercapnia		
Hyperthermia		
Acidosis		
Decreased 2,3-DPG		
Hypocapnia		
Alkalosis		
Hypophosphatemia		
Massive blood transfusion		

4. Your patient with ARDS has pronounced hypoxemia despite 100% oxygen. His PaO_2 is 60 mm Hg and his $PaCO_2$ is 40 mm Hg at sea level. Calculate the driving pressure of oxygen, PAO_2, the A:a gradient, estimated shunt, and the P/F ratio.

____

____

5. Identify the following conditions as restrictive or obstructive. Remember: If compliance of the lung or chest wall is affected, the condition is restrictive; if airway resistance is affected, the condition is obstructive.

	Restrictive	Obstructive
Obesity hypoventilation syndrome		
Asthma		
Pneumothorax		
Atelectasis		
Pneumonia		
Kyphoscoliosis		
Pulmonary edema		
Mucus plugs		
Lung cancer (bronchial)		
Lung cancer (parenchymal)		
Chronic bronchitis		
Artificial airway		
Bronchospasm		

6. Identify the primary breath sound change that occurs in the following conditions.

Condition	Breath Sound Change or Changes
Emphysema	
Atelectasis	
Pneumonia	
Chronic bronchitis	
Pneumothorax	
Pulmonary fibrosis	
Asthma	
Pulmonary edema	
Pleurisy	
Hemothorax	
Pleural effusion	
Pulmonary embolism	

7. Match the abnormal clinical finding with the associated pathology. You may use choices more than once.

____ 1. Nailbed clubbing
____ 2. Stridor
____ 3. Crackles on auscultation
____ 4. Hyperresonance to percussion
____ 5. Dullness to percussion
____ 6. Absent breath sounds
____ 7. Increased tactile fremitus on palpation
____ 8. Rhonchi on auscultation
____ 9. Pleural friction rub on auscultation
____ 10. Bronchovesicular breath sounds auscultated over peripheral lung
____ 11. Wheezes on auscultation

a. Air trapping such as emphysema
b. Chronic hypoxia
c. Partial obstruction of larynx or trachea
d. Inflammation of the pleura
e. Consolidation
f. Bronchial narrowing
g. Fluid or mucus in the airways
h. Sudden opening of peripheral airways
i. Pneumothorax

8. Match the following volumes, capacity, and indices to their description.

___ 1. V_T
___ 2. TLC
___ 3. FVC
___ 4. RV
___ 5. FEV_1
___ 6. VC
___ 7. FRC
___ 8. RSBI

a. Volume of air exhaled in the first second of forced vital capacity
b. Volume of air inhaled and exhaled with each breath
c. Maximum volume that can be exhaled after a maximal inspiration
d. Maximum volume of air that the lungs can contain
e. Amount of air that can be quickly and forcefully exhaled after a maximum inspiration
f. Volume of air remaining in the lungs after forced expiration
g. Respiratory rate divided by tidal volume
h. Volume of air remaining in the lungs at the end of a normal exhalation

9. Identify normal values for the following patient parameters.

Tidal volume	
Vital capacity	
Maximal inspiratory pressure	
PaO_2	
SaO_2	
SvO_2	

10. Identify the acid-base imbalance likely to occur in each of these situations.

a. A patient is admitted to your unit with epidural analgesia being delivered. Her ventilatory rate is 8/min.	
b. A patient has had large volumes of NG drainage for the last several shifts.	
c. A postoperative patient has a history of COPD. He is now having problems with retained secretions.	
d. A postoperative patient has a history of HF. She has been on diuretics before and after surgery.	
e. A postoperative thoracotomy patient is complaining of chest pain and has a RR of 32/min. She is complaining of tingling around her mouth and fingertips.	
f. A postoperative patient has large volumes of ileal drainage from the new ileostomy.	

11. Analyze the following arterial blood gases. Identify any acid-base imbalance, any partial or total compensation, and the presence of hypoxemia. Assume all patients to be under 60 years of age.

	pH	$PaCO_2$	HCO_3^-	PaO_2	Answer
1.	7.30	54	26	64	
2.	7.48	30	24	96	
3.	7.30	40	18	85	
4.	7.50	40	33	92	
5.	7.35	54	30	55	
6.	7.21	60	20	48	
7.	7.54	25	30	95	
8.	7.40	58	33	72	
9.	7.40	30	18	89	
10.	7.40	40	24	98	
11.	7.33	40	21	62	
12.	7.34	60	34	70	
13.	7.29	32	15	98	
14.	7.52	28	22	95	
15.	7.49	48	38	72	

12. Answer the following questions.

a. What is the difference between hypoxemia and hypoxia?

____

____

b. What are the indications of hypoxemia?

____

____

c. What are the indications of hypoxia?

____

____

d. Can hypoxemia occur without hypoxia? If so, how?

____

____

e. Can hypoxia occur without hypoxemia? If so, how?

____

____

13. Identify the type of artificial airway in each of the following situations. More than one may be listed.

Problem	Preferred Artificial Airway
Tongue against hypopharynx	
Need for frequent nasotracheal suctioning	
Inability to open mouth (e.g., seizure)	
Facial or jaw fracture	
Complete upper airway obstruction when endotracheal intubation is impossible (e.g., laryngeal edema or spasm, tracheal fracture)	
Need for sealed airway (e.g., mechanical ventilation or potential for aspiration)	
Need for long-term lower airway access and sealed airway	

14. Match the type of oxygen delivery with the description.

___ 1. Non-rebreathing mask
___ 2. Venturi mask
___ 3. Nasal cannula
___ 4. Tracheostomy collar
___ 5. Partial rebreathing mask

a. Most comfortable method of oxygen administration
b. May cause aspiration of condensed fluid
c. Delivers approximately 40-60% oxygen concentration
d. Provides the highest oxygen concentration
e. Ensures a reliable oxygen concentration regardless of change in respiratory rate and/or depth

15. Match ventilator mode, setting, or parameter with the correct description.

___ 1. Control
___ 2. Assist-control
___ 3. Synchronized intermittent mandatory ventilation
___ 4. Pressure support ventilation
___ 5. Pressure-controlled ventilation
___ 6. Independent lung ventilation
___ 7. High-frequency ventilation
___ 8. Pressure-regulated volume-controlled
___ 9. Bi-PAP
___ 10. Airway pressure release ventilation
___ 11. Tidal volume
___ 12. Positive end-expiratory pressure
___ 13. Sigh
___ 14. Peak inspiratory pressure
___ 15. FiO_2
___ 16. Plateau pressure
___ 17. Continuous positive airway pressure

a. Augments a patient-initiated breath by using positive pressure to reduce the work of breathing
b. Pressure measured at inflation hold which is used to calculate static compliance
c. Combines pressure support ventilation (PSV) and continuous positive airway pressure (CPAP)
d. Useful for patients with unilateral lung disease, such as a pulmonary contusion
e. Ventilator delivers a mandatory number of breaths per minute but allows the client to breathe spontaneously between set rate
f. Varies the flow rate and flow waveform to deliver the desired volume at the desired pressure
g. Provides short periods of lower pressure during CPAP to allow further expiration
h. Uses small tidal volumes and rapid rates to keep airway pressures lower
i. Maintains a closed circuit between control breaths so the patient cannot take additional breaths
j. Ends inspiration when a preset pressure is reached; tidal volume is variable
k. Occasional breaths with volume 1.5-2 times the tidal volume
l. Positive pressure throughout the entire ventilatory process in a spontaneously breathing patient
m. Volume of air given with each breath
n. Percentage of oxygen expressed as a decimal
o. Positive pressure maintained through the expiratory phase in a mechanically ventilated patient
p. Pressure measured at the peak of inspiration which is used to calculate a dynamic compliance
q. Allows the patient to trigger additional assisted breaths between control breaths

16. Identify four physiologic effects of PEEP and CPAP.

a. ______________________________
b. ______________________________
c. ______________________________
d. ______________________________

17. Identify if the following factors will cause a high pressure or low exhaled volume alarm.

	High Pressure	Low Exhaled Volume
Cuff leak		
Bronchospasm		
Need for suctioning		
Disconnect		
Water condensation in tubing		
Pneumothorax		
ARDS		

18. Identify the values for the following parameters that indicate that the patient may be successfully weaned from mechanical ventilation.

a. Spontaneous tidal volume_____
b. Spontaneous vital capacity_____
c. Maximal inspiratory pressure_____
d. PaO_2 of at least _____ on an FiO_2 of no greater than ____ with no more than _____cm H_2O PEEP.
e. Rapid shallow breathing index _____

19. Complete the following table and determine if either of these patients is ready for weaning from mechanical ventilation.

	Patient A	Patient B
Age	38	64
Gender	F	M
Diagnosis	Asthma	ARDS
IBW	60 kg	75 kg
ABGs	FiO_2 of 0.28	FiO_2 of 0.6 with 10 cm H_2O PEEP
	pH 7.42	pH 7.32
	$PaCO_2$ 39 mm Hg	$PaCO_2$ 50 mm Hg
	HCO_3 25 mEq/L	HCO_3 23 mEq/L
	PaO_2 88 mm Hg	PaO_2 55 mm Hg
	SaO_2 98%	SaO_2 88%
Spontaneous V_T	350 mL	300 mL
Spontaneous Vital Capacity	650 mL	600 mL
Spontaneous Minute Ventilation		
NIF	−40 cm H_2O	−20 cm H_2O
Spontaneous Respiratory Rate	20/min	36/min
Rapid Shallow Breathing Index (RSBI)		
Ready for weaning?		

The Pulmonary System: Pathologic Conditions

Chest Surgery and Chest Tubes

Surgical Procedures

1. Bronchoplastic reconstruction (sleeve resection): removal of a mass that involves or protrudes into the airway; a section of the airway and lung is removed and then reanastomosis of the airway proximal and distal to the resected area is performed
2. Bullectomy: removal of cysts or bullae in lung; may be performed with laser to avoid thoracotomy
3. Chest trauma surgery: repair of penetrating or nonpenetrating trauma; drainage of pleural cavity and control of hemorrhage
4. Closed thoracostomy: insertion of chest tube through intercostal space into pleural space; tube is connected to chest drainage system
5. Decortication of lung: removal of fibrinous membrane covering visceral and parietal pleura; used for recurrent spontaneous pneumothorax
6. Diaphragmatic hernia repair: repositioning of the abdominal contents back into the abdominal cavity and closure of diaphragm with suture or patch
7. Esophagogastrectomy: resection of a part of the esophagus and upper portion of the stomach with end-to-end anastomosis; colon interposition using a portion of the large intestine may be performed as an alternative to end-to-end anastomosis; for cancer of esophagus or corrosive esophagitis
8. Exploratory thoracotomy: opening of the thorax in order to perform a biopsy or locate bleeding
9. Lobectomy: removal of one or more lobes of the lung
10. Open thoracostomy: insertion of chest tube during rib resection; usually used in empyema when pleural space is fixed
11. Pleurodesis: process of fusing the two layers of the pleura through the use of agents (e.g., doxycycline, monocycline, sterile talc) which cause a fibrotic reaction to prevent pleural fluid formation; used for recurrent malignant pleural effusion
12. Pneumonectomy: removal of an entire lung with or without mediastinal lymph node resection; indicated when tumor is centrally located at hilus or bronchus
13. Reduction pneumoplasty (lung volume reduction surgery): resection of hyperinflated areas of lung to allow more normal function of diaphragm and expansion of more normal areas of the lung
14. Removal of mediastinal masses: removal of cysts, tumors, abscesses from mediastinum
15. Segmental resection: removal of segment(s) of a lobe
16. Thoracoplasty: surgical collapse of a portion of chest wall by multiple rib resections to decrease volume in the hemithorax; may be used after pulmonary resection if lung can not reexpand to fill thoracic space or after pneumonectomy: reduces the size of the thoracic cavity on the operative side and decreases the chance of mediastinal shift toward that side
17. Thoracotomy: opening into the thorax or pleural cavity
18. Thymectomy: removal of the thymus; frequently performed for myasthenia gravis
19. Tracheal resection: resection of a portion of the trachea with end-to-end anastomosis; removal of stenotic area of trachea or tumor
20. Video-assisted thoracotomy: use of two or more small incisions in the chest for visualization and instrumentation; may be used for exploration, biopsy, or resection
21. Wedge resection: removal of a small peripheral section of the lung without regard to segments

Collaborative Management

1. Maintain airway patency and adequate oxygenation and ventilation.
   a. Position the patient for optimal ventilation/perfusion matching.
      1) HOB elevated to 30-45 degrees
      2) "Good lung down" optimizes ventilation to encourage reexpansion of the surgical lung and optimizes perfusion to the unaffected "good" lung.

a) Exception: Pneumonectomy patients are positioned on their operative lung or back; remember "no lung down."
3) Frequent turning
4) Early ambulation

b. Encourage deep breathing and use of the incentive spirometer.
1) Note that air is removed from the pleural space by the positive pressure of expiration and the negative pressure of suction on the chest tube; deep breathing is *very* important in reexpansion of the lung.

c. Maintain airway clearance.
1) Encourage sustained inspiration through deep breathing and incentive spirometry.
a) Coughing will occur if needed but routine coughing is not indicated because of the following:
i) Coughing is forceful expiration which may actually increase the risk of atelectasis.
ii) Coughing causes pain and may cause splinting and decrease in chest excursion and increase the risk of atelectasis.
2) Suction only if the patient is unable to clear secretions.
a) Utilize caution when suctioning the patient because leakage from the bronchial stump may occur (especially with pneumonectomy patients).

d. Assess the position of the trachea; report immediately any shift from the normal midline.
e. Administer bronchodilators as prescribed.
f. Prevent gastric distention; gastric suction may be required.
g. Administer oxygen as indicated by arterial blood gases and SpO_2.
h. Assist with weaning from mechanical ventilation and extubation as soon as possible because positive pressure ventilation increases risk of air leak.

2. Control pain.
a. Administer analgesics and/or local anesthetics as prescribed to relieve pain and encourage deep breathing.
1) Intravenous analgesia: by regularly scheduled IV injection or by patient-controlled analgesia (PCA)
2) Interpleural analgesia: local anesthetic (e.g., bupivacaine [Marcaine]) injected into pleural space during surgery; may use chest tube with injection port for periodic lidocaine
3) Epidural analgesia: opiate and/or local anesthetic injected into epidural space; basal rate and PCA
4) Nonsteroidal antiinflammatory agent (e.g., ketorolac [Toradol]) to augment the pain relief of narcotics

b. Instruct the patient how to splint chest when coughing; instruct the family how to assist.

3. Maintain water-seal drainage system and patency of chest tubes (see Chest Tubes section of Chapter 4).
a. Monitor drainage.
1) Should progress from bloody to serosanguineous to serous over 2-3 days
2) Expected drainage is 100-300 mL for the first 2 hours and then less than 50 mL/hr for the next several hours with negligible drainage within 2 days.
b. Assess for air leak and differentiate expected removal of air from pleural space (occasional bubble) from a break in the chest tube system.

4. Monitor for common complications.
a. Hemorrhage/shock
1) Replace blood and fluid volume as prescribed; thoracic surgery patients generally receive less fluid than nonthoracic surgery patients in early postoperative period to prevent ARDS and pulmonary edema.
2) Monitor for clinical indications of hypoperfusion (see Table 2-2).
b. Infection
1) Utilize sterile technique while dressing the insertion site, setting up the chest drainage system, and replacing the system.
2) Monitor for fever, purulent drainage, leukocytosis, and other clinical indications of infection.
3) Assess the incision and the chest tube insertion site for redness, induration, and drainage; culture drainage if purulent.
4) Monitor sputum and chest drainage for signs of infection; culture as necessary.
5) Administer antibiotics as prescribed.
c. Tension pneumothorax
1) Maintain patency of the chest tube and functioning of chest drainage system.
2) Avoid clamping chest tube except for reasons identified earlier.
3) Monitor for clinical indications of tension pneumothorax: dyspnea; chest pain; tracheal shift away from affected side; hyperresonance to percussion; decreased breath sounds on affected side
d. Dysrhythmias: especially atrial dysrhythmias
1) Most likely in patients having pneumonectomy
2) Prophylactic antidysrhythmics may be initiated preoperatively
e. Pulmonary edema: related to capillary leak and pulmonary hypertension
1) Use caution with fluid administration.
2) Hemodynamic monitoring may be necessary.
f. ARDS
1) Devastating after pneumonectomy
2) Monitor for changes in ventilatory effort, SpO_2.
g. Pulmonary embolism

1) Have patient sit on edge of bed the evening of surgery, out of bed into chair within 24-36 hours.
2) Ambulate as soon as possible until contraindicated by hemodynamic instability.

h. Bronchopleural fistula: usually related to empyema
   1) Very small tidal volumes used with mechanical ventilation (e.g., high frequency jet ventilation)

i. Empyema: Treat infection with drainage and antimicrobials.

j. Frozen shoulder: impairment in shoulder mobility
   1) Encourage range of motion to shoulder on operative side.
   2) Administer analgesics to allow movement.
   3) Encourage use of arm for self-care activities.

Acute Respiratory Failure

Definitions

1. Acute respiratory failure: failure of the respiratory system to provide for the exchange of oxygen and carbon dioxide between the environment and tissues in quantities sufficient to sustain life
   a. Hypoxemic normocapnic respiratory failure (Type I): low PaO_2 with normal $PaCO_2$
   b. Hypoxemic hypercapnic respiratory failure (Type II): low PaO_2 with high $PaCO_2$
2. Chronic obstructive pulmonary disease (COPD) with acute exacerbation: acute process in a patient with a chronic condition; usually caused by respiratory infection
   a. Chronic obstructive pulmonary disease (COPD), also known as *chronic obstructive lung disease (COLD)*: a disease state characterized by the presence of airflow obstruction due to chronic bronchitis or emphysema; the airflow obstruction is progressive, may be accompanied by airway hyperactivity, and may be partially reversible (American Thoracic Society)
      1) Chronic bronchitis: defined clinically by excessive mucus secretion in the bronchi
      2) Emphysema: defined pathophysiologically by enlargement of the air spaces distal to the terminal bronchioles with destruction of alveolar walls
      3) Many of these patients have some degree of asthma.
   b. Acute exacerbation of COPD: worsening dyspnea, increase in sputum volume, and increase in sputum purulence

Etiology

1. Type I respiratory failure
   a. Pneumonia
   b. Pulmonary edema
   c. Pulmonary fibrosis
   d. Pleural effusion
   e. Pneumothorax
   f. Asthma
   g. Atelectasis
   h. Aspiration pneumonitis
   i. ARDS (early)
   j. Smoke inhalation
   k. Pulmonary embolism
   l. Kyphoscoliosis
   m. Fat embolism
2. Type II respiratory failure (may also be called *acute ventilatory failure*)
   a. COPD with acute exacerbation
   b. Status asthmaticus
   c. CNS depressant drugs
   d. Anesthesia
   e. Neuromuscular blocking drugs
      1) Muscle paralytics
      2) Aminoglycosides
      3) Organophosphate poisoning
   f. Head trauma
   g. Poliomyelitis
   h. Amyotrophic lateral sclerosis
   i. Spinal cord injury
   j. Guillain-Barré syndrome
   k. Myasthenia gravis
   l. Multiple sclerosis
   m. Muscular dystrophy
   n. Morbid obesity
   o. Chest trauma
   p. Surgery: especially thoracic, abdominal, flank incision
   q. Sleep apnea
   r. Tracheal obstruction
   s. Epiglottitis
   t. Cystic fibrosis
   u. Near-drowning

Pathophysiology (Table 5-1)

1. Hypoventilation
2. Ventilation-perfusion mismatching
3. Shunting
4. Diffusion defects

Clinical Presentation

1. Subjective
   a. History of precipitating factor
   b. Clinical indications of respiratory distress (see Box 4-2)
   c. Clinical indications of hypoxia (see Box 4-3)
   d. Clinical indications of hypercapnia (see Box 4-4)
2. Objective
   a. Clinical indications of respiratory distress (see Box 4-2)
   b. Hypoxemia: decrease in SpO_2, SaO_2, PaO_2
   c. Clinical indications of hypoxia (see Box 4-3)
   d. Clinical indications of hypercapnia (see Box 4-4)
3. Diagnostic
   a. Arterial blood gas changes
      1) PaO_2 less than 50-60 mm Hg
      2) $PaCO_2$ greater than 50 mm Hg with a pH of less than 7.3
   b. Chest x-ray: may identify cause

Table 5-1 Mechanisms of Acute Respiratory Failure

Mechanism	Pathophysiology	Etiology	Diagnosis	Treatment

Hypoventilation	Hypoventilation causes CO_2 retention and hypoxemia	Damage to/depression of the neurologic control of ventilation:
		• Head injury
		• Cerebral thrombosis or hemorrhage
		• CNS depressant drugs
		• Oxygen-induced hypoventilation
		Neuromuscular defects in the ventilatory mechanism:
		• Myasthenia gravis
		• Multiple sclerosis
		• Muscular dystrophy
		• Guillain-Barré syndrome
		• Poliomyelitis
		• Spinal cord injuries
		• Botulism
		• Tetanus
		• Neuromuscular blocking drugs
		Obstructive lung conditions
		• Asthma
		• Chronic bronchitis
		• Emphysema
		• Airway obstruction
		• Cystic fibrosis
		Restrictive lung conditions
		• Kyphoscoliosis
		• Obesity hypoventilation syndrome
		• Recent thoracic, abdominal, or flank incision
		• Lung cancer
		• Flail chest
		• Pleural effusion
		• Pneumothorax
			• Physical examination
			  • Neurologic status may be altered
			  • Abnormal chest wall motion
			  • Abnormal breath sounds
			  • Clinical indications of hypoxemia, hypercapnia
			• ABGs: hypoxemia with increased $PaCO_2$ and normal A:a gradient
			• May have abnormal chest x-ray, PFTs
				• Improve oxygenation by increasing alveolar ventilation (e.g., positioning, bronchial hygiene, drug therapy)
				• Specific therapy is dependent upon the specific etiology

V/Q mismatching	Low V/Q units, with perfusion in excess of ventilation, result in hypoxemia because the blood traversing these alveolar units is not fully oxygenated
	High V/Q units, with ventilation in excess of perfusion, result in oxygenated alveolar units which are not perfused
		Regional ventilation abnormalities
		• Asthma
		• Chronic bronchitis
		• Emphysema
		• Atelectasis
		• Pneumonia
		• Bronchospasm
		• Mucus plugs
		• Foreign bodies
		• Tumor
		Regional perfusion abnormalities
		• Pulmonary embolus
		• Decreased cardiac output/index
		• Excessive PEEP
			• Physical examination
			  • Abnormal chest wall motion
			  • Abnormal breath sounds
			  • Clinical indications of hypoxemia
			• ABGs: hypoxemia with a widened A:a gradient; $PaCO_2$ dependent on ventilation status
			• Abnormal chest x-ray, PFTs, and/or V/Q scan
				• Oxygen
				• Specific therapy dependent upon the specific etiology

Continued

Table 5-1 Mechanisms of Acute Respiratory Failure—cont'd

Mechanism	Pathophysiology	Etiology	Diagnosis	Treatment

Shunt	Blood transverses from the right heart to the left heart without being oxygenated: anatomical shunt is when the blood bypasses the alveolar-capillary unit, and physiologic shunt is when the blood goes through the alveolar-capillary unit but it is nonfunctional	Anatomic shunts
		• Normal anatomic shunts: bronchial, pleural, thebesian veins
		• Intrapulmonary shunts: pulmonary A-V fistula
		• Intracardiac shunts: tetralogy of Fallot
		• Other pathologic shunts (e.g., shunts associated with neoplasms)
		Physiologic shunts
		• Alveolar collapse
		  • Atelectasis
		  • Pneumothorax
		  • Hemothorax
		  • Pleural effusion
		• Alveoli filled with a fluid or foreign material
		  • Cardiac pulmonary edema
		  • Noncardiac pulmonary edema (e.g., near-drowning, ARDS)
		  • Pneumonias
			• Physical examination
			  • Abnormal breath sounds
			  • Clinical indications of hypoxemia
			• ABGs: hypoxemia with a normal or decreased $PaCO_2$
			  • Widened A:a gradient
			  • Shunt greater than 6%
			• May have abnormal chest x-ray, PFTs
				• Oxygen administration has little or no effect
				• Specific therapy dependent upon the specific etiology
				• Positive end-expiratory pressure is frequently used for physiologic shunt

Diffusion abnormalities	Increased diffusion pathway: diffusion between alveolar oxygen and pulmonary capillary blood is impaired; blood exiting the gas exchange unit is hypoxemic
	Decreased diffusion area: decrease in alveolar-capillary membrane surface area available for diffusion and/or loss of pulmonary capillary bed
		Increased diffusion pathway
		• Accumulation of fluid
		• Pulmonary edema: cardiac or noncardiac
		• Accumulation of collagen in the pulmonary interstitium
		• Pulmonary fibrosis
		• Sarcoidosis
		• Collagen-vascular disease
		Decreased diffusion area
		• Pulmonary resection (e.g., lobectomy, pneumonectomy)
		• Destructive lung diseases
		  • Emphysema
		  • Tumor
		  • Obliterative pulmonary vascular diseases
			• History and physical exam findings are compatible with the diagnosis
			• ABGs: hypoxemia with normal or low $PaCO_2$
			  • Widened A:a gradient
			  • Further decrease in PaO_2 with exercise
			• PFTs: decreased diffusing capacity for CO
			• Chest x-ray may show cause
				• Oxygen
				• Home oxygen therapy is frequently indicated

Collaborative Management

1. Treat the cause.
2. Maintain patient airway and optimal ventilation.
   a. Position the patient for optimal ventilation.
      1) Head of bed to 30-45 degrees
      2) Overbed table for patient to lean on
      3) "Good lung down" if unilateral lung condition exists
      4) Continuous lateral rotation therapy especially if P/F ratio is less than 250 mm Hg
      5) Prone position especially in ARDS
   b. Maintain adequate hydration: usually 2-3 L/24 hr unless contraindicated by cardiac or renal disease.
      1) Oral fluids: noncaffeinated
      2) Intravenous fluids: usually D_5NS
   c. Provide bronchial hygiene and chest physiotherapy as indicated.
      1) Inspiratory maneuvers
         a) Examples include deep breathing, incentive spirometry, flutter valve.
         b) These methods encourage reexpansion of alveoli and generate cough if needed.
      2) Analgesics in doses adequate to allow patient to deep breathe and cough as indicated
      3) Suctioning if the patient is unable to clear airways
      4) Ambulation
      5) Postural drainage, percussion, and vibration may be necessary.
      6) Bronchoscopy may be necessary if airway clearance techniques are inadequate.
      7) Noninvasive ventilation may be used to avert intubation.
         a) May be either CPAP or bi-PAP mode
         b) If the patient requires nocturnal CPAP or bi-PAP, the family should be asked to bring in the equipment.
      8) Intubation and mechanical ventilation may be necessary if $PaCO_2$ continues to rise and acidosis develops.
         a) The goal of mechanical ventilation is to normalize the pH, not necessarily the $PaCO_2$.
         b) It is not appropriate to normalize the $PaCO_2$ in patients with COPD and chronic hypercapnia (this causes metabolic alkalosis, eventual excretion of sodium bicarbonate, and weaning difficulties).
   d. Administer appropriate drug therapy.
      1) Bronchodilators may be indicated.
         a) Action: smooth muscle relaxation and bronchodilation
         b) Indications
            i) Asthma (i.e., reactive airway disease)
            ii) Acute bronchospasm related to anaphylaxis
            iii) Pulmonary hypertension (specifically xanthines)
         c) Types of bronchodilators and specific actions (Table 5-2)
            i) Sympathomimetics (beta adrenergic agents) (e.g., epinephrine, isoproterenol [Isuprel], albuterol [Proventil], isoetharine [Bronkosol], metaproterenol [Alupent], terbutaline sulfate [Brethine], salmeterol [Serevent])
               (a) Beta2-adrenergic agonists: these agents are preferred over nonrespiratory-selective beta stimulants like epinephrine and isoproterenol because they cause fewer cardiovascular side effects
               (b) These respiratory selective agents include albuterol (Proventil), isoetharine (Bronkosol), metaproterenol (Alupent), turbutaline sulfate (Brethine), salmeterol (Serevent), and levalbuterol (Xopenex)
            ii) Anticholinergics (e.g., ipratropium [Atrovent])
               (a) Combivent is a combination of albuterol and ipratropium given by inhalation.
            iii) Methylxanthines (e.g., aminophylline [Aminophyllin], oxtriphylline [Choledyl], theophylline [Theo-Dur])
            iv) Electrolytes (e.g., magnesium)
      2) Corticosteroids (e.g., betamethasone [Vanceril])
      3) Expectorants (e.g., guaifenesin [Robitussin], potassium iodide [SSKI]) may be used but hydration is most important
      4) Mucolytics (e.g., acetylcysteine [Mucomyst]) may be used to decrease the tenacity of the mucus; frequently causes bronchospasm so given with a bronchodilator
      5) Sedatives: generally avoided unless patient is very agitated
      6) Antitussives: Avoid use of antitussives unless nonproductive cough is causing patient fatigue.
3. Optimize oxygen delivery and decrease oxygen consumption.
   a. Administer oxygen as indicated for hypoxemia.
      1) Nasal cannula or mask
         a) Masks are contraindicated in hypercapnic patients because the high concentration of oxygen provided by these delivery systems would likely eliminate the hypoxic drive.

Table 5-2 Bronchodilators

Drug	Administration	Adverse Effects	Nursing Implications
Short-Acting Beta$_2$ Adrenergic Agents*			
Albuterol (Proventil, Ventolin)	• PO: 2-4 mg every 6-8 hours • Hand-held inhaler: 1-2 inhalations every 4-6 hours • Nebulizer: 0.5 mL (2.5 mg) in 3-5 mL of normal saline over 10-15 minutes every 6 hours	• Tachycardia • Palpitations • Nausea, vomiting • Anxiety • Tremor • Headache	• Monitor HR, BP, breath sounds • Note contraindications: known hypersensitivity, glaucoma, tachydysrhythmias; do not give with MAO inhibitors • Use cautiously in older adults and patients with diabetes mellitus, hypertension, hyperthyroidism, cardiac disease, seizure disorder, prostatic hypertrophy • Do not administer with beta-blockers (they block effect)
Metaproterenol (Alupent, Metaprel)	• PO: 20 mg every 6-8 hours • Hand-held inhaler: 2-3 inhalations every 3-4 hours • Nebulizer: 0.2-0.3 mL of undiluted 5% solution or 2.5 mL of a 6% solution every 6-8 hours	• Tachycardia • Palpitations • Nausea, vomiting • Anxiety • Tremor • Headache	• Monitor HR, BP, breath sounds • Note contraindications: known hypersensitivity, glaucoma, tachydysrhythmias; do not give with MAO inhibitors • Use cautiously in older adults and patients with diabetes mellitus, hypertension, hyperthyroidism, cardiac disease, seizure disorder, prostatic hypertrophy • Do not administer with beta-blockers (they block effect)
Anticholinergic Agents			
Ipratropium (Atrovent)	• PO: 20 mg every 6-8 hours • Handheld inhaler: 2-3 inhalations every 3-4 hours • Nebulizer: 0.2-0.3 mL of undiluted 5% solution or 2.5 mL of a 6% solution every 6-8 hours	• Tachycardia • Palpitations • Anxiety • Restlessness • Dizziness • Headache • Cough • Blurred vision • Gastrointestinal distress • Dry mouth	• Monitor HR, BP, ECG, respiratory rate and rhythm, breath sounds, urine output, and fluid status • Note contraindications: known sensitivity, cardiac dysrhythmias • Use cautiously in older adults and patients with acute MI, HF, hypertension
Methylxanthines			

Aminophylline (Theophylline, Elixophyllin, Tedral, Quibron, Choledyl)	• PO: 250-500 mg every 6-8 hours
	• IV: loading dose of 5-6 mg/kg (250-500 mg) over 20 minutes followed by infusion
	• IV infusion: mix 500 mg in 250 mL (2 mg/mL) and infuse at 0.1-0.9 mg/kg/hr
	  • HF, liver disease: ~0.1-0.2 mg/kg/hr
	  • COPD: ~0.3 mg/kg/hr
	  • Smokers: ~0.8 mg/kg/hr
	• Therapeutic blood level 10-20 mcg/mL
		• Tachycardia
		• Hypotension
		• Palpitations
		• Anxiety
		• Restlessness
		• Insomnia
		• Dizziness
		• Tremors
		• Headache
		Signs of toxicity
		• Anorexia, nausea, vomiting
		• Ventricular dysrhythmias
		• Agitation, seizures
			• Monitor HR, BP, ECG, respiratory rate and rhythm, breath sounds, urine output, and fluid status
			• Note contraindications: known sensitivity, cardiac dysrhythmias
			• Use cautiously in older adults and patients with acute MI, HF, hypertension, hepatic disease, acute peptic ulcer, hyperthyroidism, diabetes mellitus
			• Administer PO drug with meals to decrease GI adverse effects

Table 5-2 Bronchodilators—cont'd

Drug	Administration	Adverse Effects	Nursing Implications
Electrolytes			
Magnesium sulfate	• IV infusion: mix 1-2 grams in 100 mL and infuse over 1-4 hours • May also be given by inhalation	• Bradycardia • Hypotension • Diaphoresis • Flushing • Hypermagnesemia resulting in respiratory muscle weakness and arrest	• Monitor HR, BP, respiratory rate, ECG, urine output, deep tendon reflexes, mental status • Note contraindications: renal disease • Use cautiously in renal insufficiency, patients on digitalis • Monitor closely for clinical indications of hypermagnesemia: hypotension, AV block, CNS depression, depressed or absent DTR, muscle weakness or paralysis, respiratory arrest • Administer calcium IV as prescribed for hypermagnesemic effects • Have intubation equipment and mechanical ventilator available

*Additional short-acting $beta_2$ adrenergic agents include terbutaline (Brethine, Brethaire), levalbuterol (Xopenex), pirbuterol (Maxair), bitolterol (Tornalate). Long-acting $beta_2$ stimulants include: salmeterol (Serevent), formoterol (Foradil)

2) Flow rate or oxygen concentration to keep SpO_2 approximately 95% unless contraindicated
   a) In patients with chronic hypercapnia, adjust flow rate or oxygen concentration to keep SpO_2 approximately 90%.

b. Utilize positive end-expiratory pressure (PEEP) as necessary to maintain adequate SaO_2, PaO_2.
c. Ensure rest periods especially after meals or activities.
d. Provide a quiet, restful environment.
e. Treat fever (controversial because pyrogens are helpful in mobilizing the immune system)
   1) Antipyretics (e.g., acetaminophen [Tylenol])
   2) Cooling blankets may be used, but shivering should be avoided due to effect on oxygen consumption.
f. Improve delivery of oxygen to the tissues.
   1) Improve SaO_2: oxygen, PEEP as required
   2) Improve CI: fluid administration, inotropes, intraaortic balloon pump, vasoactive agents, etc., as required
   3) Increase hemoglobin: packed red blood cells as required
   4) Utilize extracorporeal membrane oxygenator as indicated and available: viewed primarily as a rescue therapy when other therapies have failed

4. Treat infection if present.
   a. Administer antimicrobials as indicated: empirically or specific to cultured microorganism
   b. Utilize bronchial hygiene techniques.
5. Monitor for/prevent complications
   a. Dysrhythmias
   b. Pulmonary infections: pneumonia
   c. Pulmonary edema
   d. Pulmonary embolism
   e. Barotrauma (e.g., pneumothorax)
   f. Pulmonary fibrosis
   g. Oxygen toxicity
   h. Renal failure
   i. Acid-base imbalance
      1) Respiratory acidosis
      2) Respiratory alkalosis occurs in patients with chronic hypercapnia when $PaCO_2$ is normalized rather than the pH due to long-term renal retention of bicarbonate.
   j. Electrolyte imbalance
   k. GI complications: abdominal distention, ileus, ulcer, hemorrhage
   l. Thromboembolism
   m. Disseminated intravascular coagulation (DIC)
   n. Sepsis or septic shock
   o. Psychologic responses: psychosis or depression
6. Provide patient and family instruction.
   a. Smoking cessation
   b. Clinical indications of infection

Acute Respiratory Distress Syndrome

Definitions

1. Acute lung injury
   a. A syndrome of lung inflammation and increased alveolar-capillary permeability characterized by hypoxemia resistant to oxygen therapy
   b. The less severe end of the spectrum of the pulmonary component of systemic inflammatory response syndrome (SIRS)
   c. PaO_2/FiO_2 ratio less than 300 mm Hg
2. Acute respiratory distress syndrome
   a. A syndrome of acute respiratory failure characterized by noncardiac pulmonary edema and manifested by refractory hypoxemia caused by intrapulmonary shunt
   b. May be considered the severe end of the spectrum of the pulmonary component of

systemic inflammatory response syndrome (SIRS)
   c. PaO_2/FiO_2 ratio less than or equal to 200 mm Hg
   d. Synonyms: shock lung, pump lung (postperfusion lung), Da Nang lung, wet lung, posttraumatic lung, respirator lung, congestive atelectasis, pulmonary fat embolism syndrome, alveolar-capillary leak syndrome, noncardiac pulmonary edema

Etiology: Risk Increases if More than One Occurs Simultaneously

1. Direct injury
   a. Chest trauma: pulmonary contusion
   b. Near-drowning
   c. Hypervolemia or pulmonary edema
   d. Inhalation of toxic gases and vapors
      1) Smoke
      2) Chemicals
      3) Oxygen toxicity
   e. Pneumonia: viral, bacterial, or fungal
   f. Aspiration pneumonitis
   g. Radiation pneumonitis
   h. Pulmonary embolism: particularly fat or amniotic fluid
   i. Radiation
   j. Drugs: bleomycin
2. Indirect injury
   a. Sepsis: most likely cause
   b. Shock or prolonged hypotension
      1) Septic shock
      2) Hypovolemic shock
      3) Cardiogenic shock
      4) Anaphylactic shock
      5) Neurogenic shock
   c. Multisystem trauma especially multiple fractures
   d. Blood transfusion (i.e., transfusion-related acute lung injury)
   e. Burns
   f. Cardiopulmonary bypass
   g. Disseminated intravascular coagulation (DIC)
   h. Toxemia of pregnancy
   i. Acute pancreatitis
   j. Diabetic coma
   k. Central nervous system (CNS) injury
   l. Drug overdosage: heroin, methadone, barbiturates, aspirin, thiazide diuretics
   m. Abdominal trauma

Pathophysiology

See Figure 5-1.

Clinical Presentation

1. Phases of ARDS (Table 5-3)
2. Criteria used in ARDS diagnosis
   a. Presence of a predisposing condition
   b. Severe oxygenation defect: Hypoxemia is the hallmark of ARDS.
      1) PaO_2 less than 60 mm Hg on FiO_2 greater than 0.5
      2) PaO_2/FiO_2 ratio less than or equal to 200
   c. Chest x-ray: diffuse bilateral parenchymal infiltrates
   d. Static compliance: significantly less than the normal of 50-100 mL/cm H_2O (usually 15-25 mL/cm H_2O)
   e. PAOP: less than 18 mm Hg
   f. No other explanation for the previous findings
3. Recommended criteria for acute lung injury and ARDS (adapted from NIH [2008]) (Table 5-4)
4. Hemodynamic parameters: invasive monitoring may be used for the following:
   a. Differentiation of cardiac from noncardiac pulmonary edema
      1) ARDS (noncardiac pulmonary edema) causes elevated PAP with normal PAOP.
      2) Cardiac pulmonary edema causes elevated PAP and PAOP.
   b. Determination of degree of pulmonary hypertension
      1) PAd greater than 5 mm higher than PAOP
      2) PAm greater than 25 mm Hg
      3) PVR greater than 250 dynes/sec/cm^{-5}
   c. Guide fluid management to avoid overhydration during resuscitation and fluid conservation after resuscitation.
5. Diagnostic
   a. May give clues to cause
   b. Arterial blood gases (see Table 5-3): refractory hypoxemia (hypoxemia despite high concentration of oxygen); PaO_2 of less than 55 mm Hg despite FiO_2 0.5 or greater for 24 hours
   c. Sputum analysis: tracheal protein/plasma protein ratio greater than 0.7 (cardiac pulmonary edema less than 0.5)
   d. Pulmonary function studies
      1) Lung volumes decreased: tidal volume; vital capacity
      2) Functional residual capacity decreased
      3) Static and dynamic compliance decreased
   e. Chest x-ray
      1) May be normal initially
      2) Bilateral diffuse interstitial and alveolar infiltrates
      3) Ground glass appearance
      4) "White-out" due to massive atelectasis
      5) Heart size is normal (one factor that differentiates ARDS from cardiac pulmonary edema).
   f. CT of thorax
      1) Gravity-dependent infiltrates
      2) Lack of homogeneity of infiltrates
   g. Bronchoalveolar lavage: prevalent polymorphonuclear leukocytes

Collaborative Management

1. Prevent ALI/ARDS or detect ALI/ARDS as early as possible.
   a. Utilize standard infection control measures (sepsis is the most common etiology).

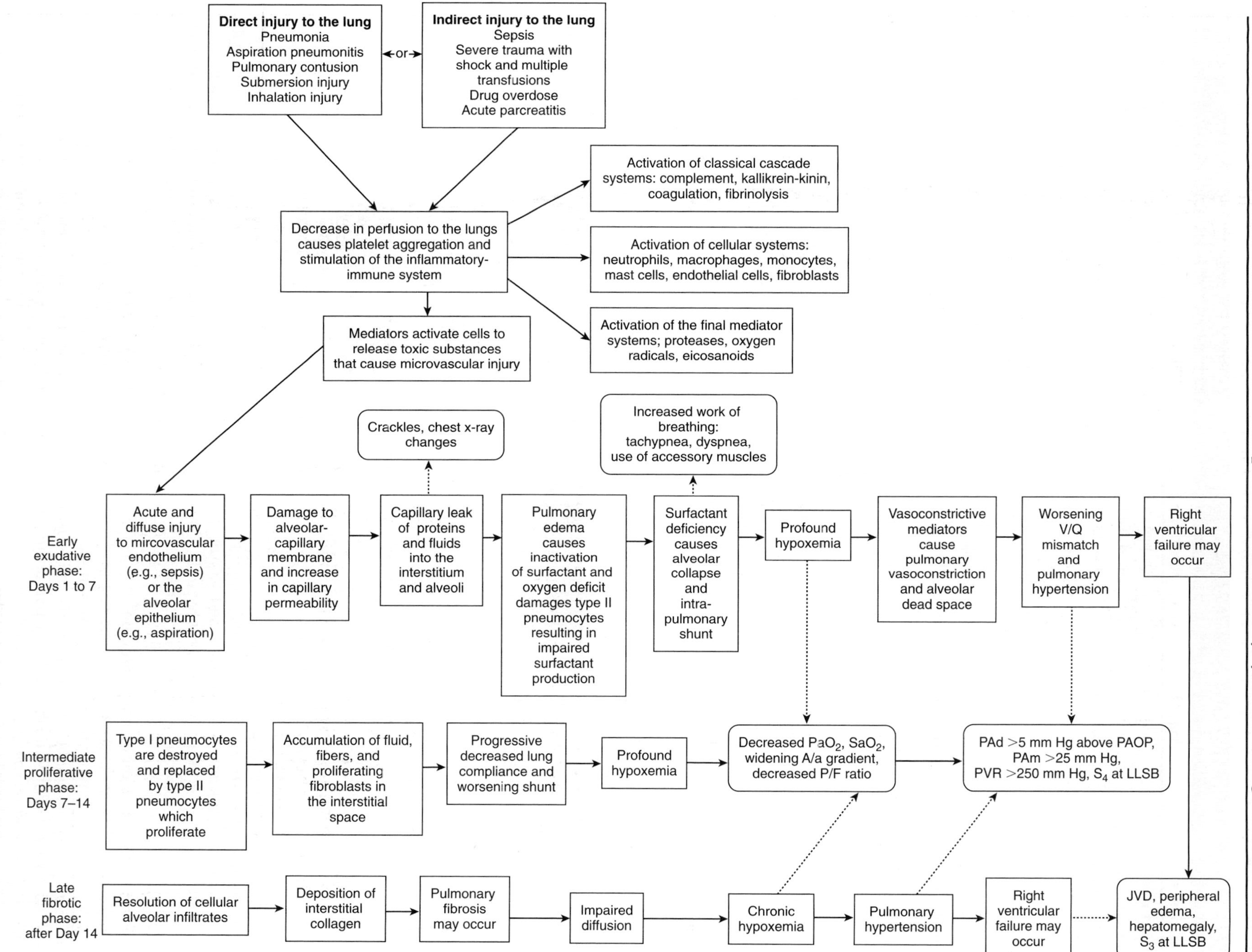

Figure 5-1 Pathophysiology of ARDS. Dotted lines connect pathology to clinical presentation.

Table 5-3 Phases of ARDS

Parameter	Phase I	Phase II	Phase III	Phase IV
Heart rate	Tachycardia	Tachycardia	Tachycardia	Bradycardia
Cardiac index	Normal	Increased	Increased	Decreased
Tidal volume/min ventilation	Increased	Increased	Normal or decreased	Decreased
$PaCO_2$	Decreased	Decreased	Normal or increased	Increased
Acid-base	Respiratory alkalosis	Respiratory alkalosis	Metabolic (and possibly respiratory) acidosis	Respiratory and metabolic acidosis
PaO_2 on room air	Normal	Normal or slightly decreased (~60 mm Hg)	Significantly decreased (~40 mm Hg)	Severely decreased (~25 mm Hg)
Shunt	Less than 6%	10%	20%	Greater than 30%
Compliance	Normal	Slightly decreased	Moderately decreased	Severely decreased
Pulmonary clinical manifestations	Dyspnea	Dyspnea; fatigue; retractions	Dyspnea; fatigue; retractions; cyanosis	Dyspnea; fatigue (may have had respiratory arrest); cyanosis; rusty sputum
Breath sounds	Clear	Fine crackles	Coarse crackles and/or wheezes	Crackles, rhonchi, and/or wheezes
Chest x-ray	Normal	Patchy infiltrates usually in dependent areas	Diffuse infiltrates	Consolidation
Other signs/symptoms	Tachycardia	Tachycardia	Tachycardia; dysrhythmias; decreasing sensorium	Bradycardia; dysrhythmias; hypotension; decreasing sensorium

Table 5-4 Criteria for Acute Lung Injury (ALI) and Acute Respiratory Distress Syndrome (ARDS)

	Onset	Oxygenation: PaO_2/FiO_2 Ratio	Frontal Chest X-ray	PAOP
Acute lung injury	Acute	Less than 300 mm Hg (regardless of PEEP)	Bilateral (patchy, diffuse, or homogenous) infiltrates	Less than 18 mm Hg or no clinical evidence of left atrial enlargement
Acute respiratory distress syndrome (ARDS)	Acute	Less than or equal to 200 mm Hg (regardless of PEEP)	Bilateral (patchy, diffuse, or homogenous) infiltrates	Less than 18 mm Hg or no clinical evidence of left atrial enlargement

b. Treat precipitating factors (e.g., antimicrobials if infection is present).
c. Provide nutritional support.
   1) Enteral feeding preferred
      a) Effects of enteral nutritional support significant to ARDS, SIRS, and MODS
         i) Prevents villous atrophy and increases blood flow to the GI tract
         ii) Retards transmigration (translocation) of bacteria or lipopolysaccharides, which play a significant role in sepsis and MODS
      b) Orogastric feeding tube or percutaneous endoscopic gastroscopy tube is preferred in order to avoid the complications of nasogastric tube, such as sinusitis and epistaxis.
   2) Parenteral nutrition if enteral feeding is contraindicated
      a) Dedicated intravenous catheter (or lumen of multilumen catheter) for parenteral nutrition
      b) Selective decontamination of digestive tract (SDD) may be used in patients who cannot be fed enterally to prevent bacterial translocation from the GI tract.
d. Monitor patients at high risk for ALI/ARDS closely.
   1) Assess patient for indications of respiratory distress (e.g., tachypnea, use of accessory muscles)
   2) Monitor pulse oximetry for drop in SpO_2.
   3) Monitor static and dynamic compliance in patients on a mechanical ventilator.

2. Maintain airway, oxygenation, and ventilation; the goal is to maintain acceptable oxygenation (SaO_2 of at least 90%) with nontoxic FiO_2 levels (less than 60%) and acceptable plateau pressures (less than or equal to 30 mL H_2O).

a. Position the patient for optimal ventilation.
   1) Elevate HOB 30-45 degrees.
   2) Turn the patient every 2 hours; kinetic therapy with 60-degree lateral rotation may be used.
   3) Position the patient in prone or semiprone position periodically.
      a) Recommended frequency has not been established, but the patient is likely to be kept prone for 4-8 hours with frequent repositioning to reduce pressure injury.

b. Provide bronchial hygiene and chest physiotherapy as indicated.
   1) Encourage the patient to deep breathe to facilitate cough and/or suction as indicated.
   2) Chest physiotherapy may be indicated.

c. Administer oxygen as indicated.
   1) May require high concentrations (up to 100%) with non-rebreathing mask prior to intubation and mechanical ventilation
   2) FiO_2 should be maintained as low as possible to prevent oxygen toxicity; positive pressure (CPAP or PEEP) will increase driving pressure allowing the use of a lower FiO_2 to maintain an acceptable oxygenation.
      a) Noninvasive ventilation via mask may be utilized prior to intubation.
      b) Mechanical ventilation with PEEP; sedation and/or muscle paralysis may be necessary to maintain PEEP
      c) NOTE: These patients are usually very PEEP-dependent and will quickly desaturate when PEEP is temporarily discontinued; utilize closed suction system or PEEP valve on a manual resuscitation bag prior to and after suctioning.

d. Ensure adequate ventilation.
   1) Noninvasive positive pressure ventilation (e.g., CPAP, bi-PAP) with face mask prior to need for intubation as prescribed
   2) Endotracheal intubation: indicated to deliver mechanical ventilation and PEEP when FiO_2 greater than 0.50 is required to maintain acceptable oxygenation or as patient fatigues
   3) Mechanical ventilation to maintain adequate ventilation and oxygenation while preventing lung-induced ventilation injury (VILI)
      a) Modes: PC-IRV, PRVC, APRV, or high frequency ventilation may be used.
      b) Tidal volume: Limitation of peak inspiratory pressure and reduction of regional lung overdistention by the use of low tidal volumes with permissive hypercapnia may reduce ventilator-induced lung injury and improve outcome in severe ARDS (Brower et al., 2004).
         i) Tidal volume at 4-8 mL/kg (~6 mL/kg) of ideal body weight (IBW).
            (a) Large tidal volumes are avoided because the ARDS lung is like a "baby lung" and large tidal volumes have been shown to cause increased alveolar edema and worsening of lung injury.
               (i) Volutrauma results from large tidal volumes though it is unclear as to whether the volume or the distending pressures are responsible for the lung injury (Burns, 2005).
            (b) Lung injury occurs as the result of the following:
               (i) Overdistention and shearing of open alveoli
               (ii) Repeated reopening of collapsed alveoli (atelectrauma)
            (c) Initially 8 mL/kg predicted body weight is recommended and then the VT is reduced at 1 mL/kg approximately every 2 hours until 6 mL/kg (NIH, 2008).
               (i) Predicted body weight (see Appendix C)
      c) Rate: usually less than 30 per minute to reduce the risk of dynamic hyperinflation and auto-PEEP
      d) Flow rates and tidal volume are adjusted to keep plateau pressure at less than or equal to 30 cm H_2O:
         i) Peak inspiratory flow rate usually 70-80 L/min
         ii) Flow taper may be used to lower peak inspiratory flow rates.
      e) Permissive hypercapnia
         i) Limitation of the tidal volume and minute ventilation may permit the accumulation of carbon dioxide.
         ii) Permissive hypercapnia stems from the hypothesis that the adverse effects of alveoli overdistention is more detrimental to patient outcome than the adverse effects of respiratory acidosis
            (a) Overdistention of the alveoli causes the following:
               (i) Ventilator-induced lung injury (i.e., volutrauma and barotrauma)
               (ii) Release of inflammatory cytokines
               (iii) Decrease in surfactant production

iii) Contraindication: intracranial hypertension

iv) Treatment of resultant respiratory acidosis

(a) Bicarbonate may be used if pH is less than 7.2

(b) $ECCO_2R$: similar to ECMO; used to remove carbon dioxide

(c) Tracheal gas insufflation: gas flow near the carina to wash carbon dioxide out of the large airways during expiration

4) CPAP or PEEP

a) Effects of CPAP or PEEP in the ARDS patient

i) Decreases surface tension so alveoli are open at low distending pressures at the end of expiration (i.e., alveolar recruitment and the prevention of alveolar derecruitment)

ii) Aids in reopening collapsed alveoli to reduce intrapulmonary shunt

iii) Increases the driving pressure of oxygen to allow achievement of same PaO_2 on a lower FiO_2 or a higher PaO_2 on the same FiO_2; this effect therefore decreases risk of oxygen toxicity

iv) Prevents shearing forces from reopening and collapsing alveoli (i.e., atelectrauma)

b) Levels

i) Minimum level is 5 cm H_2O

ii) Usual level is 5-15 cm H_2O, but higher levels may be needed to maintain SaO_2 and PaO_2; titrated upward in increments of 2 cm H_2O until oxygenation ceases to improve and/or cardiac index is decreased despite adequate circulating blood volume

iii) Oxygenation goal is PaO_2 of 55-80 mm Hg or SpO_2 of 88-95%.

c) Adverse effects in the ARDS patient, particularly with high levels of CPAP or PEEP

i) Ventilator-induced lung injury

ii) Decreased cardiac output related to decrease in venous return

(a) Ensure adequate preload.

(b) Remember that a decrease in cardiac output is more detrimental to tissue oxygenation than is borderline hypoxemia.

e. Administer aerosolized surfactant (e.g., colfosceril [Exosurf] or beractant [Survanta]) as prescribed.

1) Effects

a) Recognition that surfactant is deficient and dysfunctional in ARDS; so surfactant replacement is intended to decrease surface tension, allow more equitable distribution of tidal volume among the alveoli to decrease VILI, and aid in the prevention of alveolar collapse along with reinflation of already collapsed alveoli

2) Administration by aerosolization; direct instillation into the endotracheal tube being studied

3) Though an oxygenation benefit has been demonstrated, no survival benefit has been proven in adults.

a) New delivery methods, such as instilling surfactant directly into the lungs, have shown some promise but they are laborious and time-consuming (Kesecioglu, 2010).

f. Utilize partial liquid ventilation with perfluorocarbon (PFC) (e.g., perflubron) as prescribed.

1) Effects: PFC is a noncompressible liquid with a low surface tension and high solubility for oxygen and carbon dioxide.

a) Allows for effective gas transfer

b) Reduces surface tension of surfactant-deficient lung tissue which increases pulmonary end-expiratory volume and improves lung compliance; acts as a liquid PEEP

c) Accumulates in dependent regions of the lung (because heavier than water) which concentrates their action in areas of the lung most susceptible to ventilator-induced lung injury

d) Redistributes pulmonary blood flow to nondependent lung issues which allows more effective gas exchange through fully aerated alveoli

e) Reduces lung inflammation by reduction of proinflammatory cytokines

f) Mobilizes mucus and purulent secretions from the alveoli; they float to the top of the PFC layer and can be easily removed

2) Method

a) PFC is instilled via endotracheal tube to replace all or some of the functional residual capacity, and conventional mechanical ventilation is maintained.

b) Sedation and neuromuscular blockade are required.

3) Complication: mucus plugging of the airways and endotracheal tube

4) Though an oxygenation benefit has been demonstrated, no survival benefit has been proven and at least one randomized controlled trial showed an increase in mortality (Kacmarek et al., 2006).

g. Decrease intraalveolar fluid
   1) Administer volume as indicated by CVP readings: maintain CVP ~4 mm Hg after fluid resuscitation achieved (i.e., MAP of at least 60 mm Hg without vasopressors) (Wiedemann et al., 2006).
      a) Conservative fluid administration has been shown to improve lung function, shorten duration of mechanical ventilation, and reduce critical care unit stay (Wiedemann et al., 2006).
      b) Pulmonary artery catheter is not routinely required for ALI/ARDS (Wheeler et al., 2006) but may be required by precipitating event (e.g., trauma, shock).
      c) Overhydration, such as may occur in fluid resuscitation of trauma patients, must be avoided but conservative.
      d) Crystalloids versus colloids debate
         i) Colloids will leak across the alveolar-capillary membrane as readily as crystalloids in this patient due to damage to the alveolar-capillary membrane
         ii) There is no advantage of one over the other in these patients; balanced amounts may be used or crystalloids may be used because they have a cost benefit (Alderson et al., 2004; Hartog et al., 2011).
   2) Administer diuretics as prescribed.
      a) May be given to prevent further fluid sequestration into the alveoli
      b) Guided by PAOP: Maintain PAOP at ~12 mm Hg.
      c) May be given along with albumin in patients with hypoproteinemia with fluid retention
   3) Utilize CPAP or PEEP to increase intraalveolar pressure and aid in prevention of further fluid sequestration into the alveoli.
   4) Administer beta$_2$ agonists as prescribed.
      a) Intravenous albuterol has been shown to decrease alveolar-capillary permeability in patients with ARDS; though the mechanism is unclear, it may stimulate alveolar epithelial repair
h. Maintain cardiac output and tissue oxygenation.
   1) Administer volume as required to ensure adequate circulating volume but avoid overhydration, which would contribute to intraalveolar fluid and worsening diffusion defect.
   2) Ensure adequate hemoglobin levels.
      a) Blood if hemoglobin is less than 7 g/dL but may be necessary at hemoglobin 8-10 g/dL if there is impaired oxygen delivery as evidenced by SvO_2 or $ScvO_2$ (Napolitano et al., 2009)
         i) There is a known relationship between transfusion and ALI/ARDS, so blood transfusion should be avoided in patients at risk of ALI/ARDS after completion of resuscitation (Napolitano et al., 2009).
      b) Erythropoietin (Epogen) may be used.
   3) Administer inotropes as indicated by LVSWI and CI; dobutamine is usually first choice.
   4) Utilize hemodynamic monitoring, including SvO_2, to guide therapy if indicated.
      a) Volume or diuretics
      b) Inotropic therapy
      c) Best PEEP: level of PEEP to achieve SaO_2 of at ~90% but without decreasing the CI
   5) Utilize extracorporeal membrane oxygenation (ECMO) when available and indicated.
      a) Form of cardiopulmonary bypass in which the blood is removed from the patient, passed through large membrane lungs, and then placed back into circulation; mechanical ventilation can be maintained without the high levels of FiO_2 and PEEP that may cause VILI
      b) Effects
         i) Provides oxygenation of blood along with removal of carbon dioxide
         ii) Allows time for the lungs to heal
         iii) Prevents possible VILI and oxygen toxicity
      c) May be used as a salvage therapy in patients with life-threatening respiratory failure without multiple organ dysfunction in tertiary centers with capability and experience
      d) Studies have not demonstrated a survival benefit.
   6) Utilize extracorporeal carbon dioxide removal ($ECCO_2OR$) when available and indicated.
      a) Similar to ECMO and may be used to correct pH especially in patients with significant hypercapnia
      b) No survival benefit has been demonstrated.
i. Decrease oxygen consumption.
   1) Eliminate unnecessary activity.
   2) Provide rest periods after meals and other activities that increase oxygen consumption.
   3) Decrease anxiety: anxiolytics or sedatives
      a) Neuromuscular blockers reduce oxygen requirements and may be necessary to maintain adequate ventilation especially in a restless patient.
   4) Treat fever using antipyretics (acetaminophen [Tylenol]) and cooling blanket.

a) Debate continues regarding the benefits of fever reduction because the pyrogens are thought to be essential in mobilizing the immune system.
b) Reduction of fever does reduce oxygen requirements and may be necessary be reduce the tissue oxygen deficit.
c) Care must be taken while using cooling blanket to prevent shivering.

3. Treat pulmonary hypertension.
   a. Utilize oxygen and CPAP or PEEP to reduce hypoxemia which causes hypoxemic pulmonary vasoconstriction.
   b. Administer pulmonary vasodilators as prescribed. (Table 5-5)
      1) Nitric oxide: endogenously synthesized by vascular endothelium and acts as a natural local vasodilator; exogenously administered by inhalation
         a) Nitroglycerin and nitroprusside work by a nitric oxide-activated pathway; however, these drugs given intravenously would dilate all vessels (including vessels to nonventilated alveoli), interfere with hypoxemic vasoconstriction, and lead to increased intrapulmonary shunting; systemic hypotension would also likely occur
         b) Effects of nitric oxide by inhalation
            i) Dilates vessels only to ventilated alveoli
            ii) Reduces pulmonary hypertension
            iii) Acts as a potent bronchodilator
         c) Nitric oxide is likely to have best results when used at an earlier, less severe stage of acute lung injury; effect also augmented by prone position.
         d) Note that a recent Cochrane review concluded that inhaled nitric oxide cannot be recommended for patients with ALI/ARDS and that though it results in a transient improvement in oxygenation, it does not reduce mortality and may be harmful (Afshari, 2010B).
      2) Prostacyclin (epoprostenol [Flolan]): Note that a recent Cochrane review could not support nor refute the use of aerosolized prostacyclin for ALI/ARDS (Afshari, 2010A).
4. Modify mediator release and effect (under continuing investigation).
   a. Administer corticosteroids as prescribed.
      1) While not effective in preventing the onset of ARDS, may be helpful during the fibroproliferative phase; reduces duration of mechanical ventilation and critical care unit stay (Bream-Rouwenhorst et al., 2008)
      2) Reduces some proinflammatory cytokines
      3) Methylprednisolone usually used
   b. Administer antioxidants as prescribed.
      1) Toxic oxygen radicals produced by activated neutrophils, macrophages, and endothelial cells play a key role in lung injury.
      2) Action: may shorten the duration of lung injury
      3) Examples: N-acetylcysteine (NAC) or procysteine (OTZ)
   c. Administer antiinflammatory agents: anticytokines; antiprostaglandins (e.g., ketorolac [Toradol], ibuprofen [Motrin], indomethacin [Indocin]) as prescribed
   d. Administer ketoconazole (Nizoral) as prescribed.
      1) Actions
         a) Inhibits the production of leukotrienes and thromboxane by the alveolar macrophages
         b) May prevent ARDS in patients with sepsis
      2) Administered through enteral tube
5. Provide nutritional support to prevent respiratory muscle atrophy.
   a. Utilize enteral route if possible.
   b. Administer high-protein and high-calorie diet rich in omega 3 and omega 6.
      1) 1 to 2 g/kg of ideal body weight (IBW) of protein
         a) Conditionally essential amino acids glutamine and alanine may be particularly helpful in reducing endotoxemia and should be included.
      2) 20 to 25 kcal/kg of IBW of nonprotein calories to prevent exogenous protein and muscle tissue from catabolism to meet nutritional requirements
      3) Nonprotein carbohydrate calories increase carbon dioxide production; reduced carbohydrate formulas, such as Pulmocare, may be preferable, especially in patients with hypercapnia
   c. Replace multivitamins and minerals: vitamins A, C, E, zinc, selenium.
6. Monitor for complications.
   a. Secondary infections: nosocomial pneumonia
   b. Sepsis
   c. Shock
   d. Multiple organ dysfunction syndrome (MODS)
   e. Airway trauma
   f. Dysrhythmias
   g. Pulmonary embolism
   h. Pulmonary fibrosis
   i. Pneumothorax
   j. GI hemorrhage
   k. Disseminated intravascular coagulation (DIC)
   l. Heart failure
   m. Renal failure

Pulmonary Arterial Hypertension/ Pulmonary Hypertension

Definition

Abnormal elevation of the pressure in the blood vessels of the lungs

Table 5-5 Pulmonary Vasodilators

Drug	Administration	Adverse Effects	Nursing Implications
Calcium Channel Blocker			
Nifedipine (Procardia)	• PO immediate release: 10-30 mg tid or qid; maximum 180 mg/24 hr • PO sustained release: 30-120 mg/daily	• Tachycardia • Dysrhythmias • Hypotension • Nausea, vomiting, heartburn • Diarrhea or constipation • Headache • Flushing • Fatigue • Dizziness • Rash • Pedal edema • Hypokalemia	• Monitor HR, BP, potassium • Note contraindications: known hypersensitivity, severe aortic stenosis • Use caution in HF, sick sinus syndrome, second- or third-degree AV block, systolic BP less than 90 mm Hg, liver disease, renal insufficiency or failure, and in the elderly
Methylxanthines			
Aminophylline (Theophylline, Elixophyllin, Tedral, Quibron, Choledyl): see Table 5-2			
Direct Vasodilators			
Nitric oxide (NO)	• Inhalation along with inspired air delivered by mechanical ventilator: 2-80 ppm; usual dose range is 5-40 ppm; low dosages seem to have best effects	• Methemoglobinemia • Lung injury as a result of nitrogen dioxide (NO_2): nitric oxide and oxygen can combine to form nitrogen dioxide, which is injurious to the lung; risk is greatest with high levels of NO and high FiO_2 • Renal dysfunction	• Monitor heart rate, BP, ECG, SpO_2 • Monitor closely for tachycardia, pulmonary hypertension, and hypoxemia with dosage reduction; weaning usually occurs over a 24-hour period
Prostanoids			
Epoprostenol (Flolan)	• IV infusion by central venous catheter: 2-15 ng/kg/min titrated, based on symptoms and adverse effects • Inhalation	• Flushing • Hypotension • Headache • Nausea/vomiting • Diarrhea • Anxiety • Skeletal pain • Jaw pain • Flulike symptoms • Thrombocytopenia • Central venous catheter infections	• Monitor heart rate, BP, and for clinical indications of central venous catheter infection and/or sepsis • Requires refrigeration • Administered by central venous catheter if given IV • Do not stop abruptly; can lead to worsening of PH • Monitor for indications of platelet dysfunction (i.e., petechiae, bleeding)
Iloprost (Ventavis)	• PO: 50-300 mcg bid • IV infusion by central venous catheter: 2-4 ng/kg/min • Inhalation: 2.5-5 mcg 6-9 times/day but not more than every 2 hours	• Flushing • Hypotension • Supraventricular tachycardia • Headache • Insomnia • Nausea/vomiting • Flulike symptoms • Cough (from inhalation) • Infusion site pain	• Monitor heart rate, BP, and for clinical indications of central venous catheter infection and/or sepsis • Administered by central venous catheter if given IV
Treprostinil (Remodulin [IV], Tyvaso [inhalation])	• IV or subcutaneous infusion: 1.25 ng/kg/min (or 0.625 ng/kg/min if it is not tolerated or the patient has mild to moderate hepatic insufficiency); dose should be increased, based on clinical response in increments of 1.25 ng/kg/min per week for the first 4 weeks of treatment and 2.5 ng/kg/min per week after that. • Inhalation: 3 breaths (18 mcg of treprostinil) per treatment session, qid	• Rash • Flushing • Headache • Nausea • Diarrhea • Jaw pain • Thrombocytopenia • Pain at infusion site • Cough, throat irritation with inhalation	• Monitor heart rate, BP, ECG • Administered IV by central venous catheter; continuous subcutaneous administration is preferred • Monitor for indications of platelet dysfunction (i.e., petechiae, bleeding) • Use cautiously in patients with hepatic insufficiency

Continued

Table 5-5 Pulmonary Vasodilators—cont'd

Drug	Administration	Adverse Effects	Nursing Implications
Endothelin Receptor Antagonist			
Bosentan (Tracleer)	• PO: start at 62.5 mg bid for 4 weeks and then increase to 125 mg bid	• Elevation of liver enzymes, hepatotoxicity • Anemia • Headache • Flushing • Hypotension • Chest pain • Syncope • Respiratory tract infections • Peripheral edema	• Monitor heart rate, BP, ECG, liver function studies • Requires liver function studies monthly and hematocrit every 3 months
Ambrisentan (Letairis)	• PO: 5-10 mg daily	• Elevation of liver enzymes • Anemia • Peripheral edema • Headache • Flushing • Hypotension • Syncope	• Monitor heart rate, BP, ECG, liver function studies • Requires liver function studies monthly and hematocrit every 3 months
Phosphodiesterase Type 5 Inhibitors			
Sildenafil (Viagra, Revatio)	• PO: 20 mg tid	• Headache • Dyspepsia • Flushing • Dyspnea • Epistaxis • Hearing loss	• Monitor heart rate, BP, ECG • Should not be administered with nitrates
Tadalafil (Adcirca)	• PO: 2.5-40 mg daily	• Headache • Flushing • Hypotension • Myalgias • Nasopharyngitis • Respiratory tract infections • Hearing or vision loss	• Monitor heart rate, BP, ECG • Should not be administered with nitrates

Classification and Etiology (Simonneau et al., 2009)

1. Pulmonary arterial hypertension: primary disease of small- to medium-size arteries in the vascular bed of the lung which causes high pulmonary vascular pressures
   a. Idiopathic; risk factors include the following:
      1) Usually seen in women 20-40 years old
      2) Oral contraceptives, elevated catecholamines, and hepatic dysfunction are contributing factors.
   b. Heredity
   c. Drug or toxin-induced (e.g., fen-phen)
   d. Pulmonary veno-occlusive disease or pulmonary capillary hemangiomatosis
   e. Other associated conditions such as connective tissue disease, HIV, portal hypertension, congenital heart disease, chronic hemolytic anemia, schistosomiasis (parasite)
2. Secondary: high pulmonary vascular pressures secondary to another pathologic state
   a. Left heart disease
   b. Lung disease and/or hypoxia
   c. Chronic thromboembolic disease
   d. Unclear multifactorial mechanisms (e.g., thyroid disorders, chronic renal failure, sarcoidosis, vasculitis)

Pathophysiology

See Figure 5-2.

Clinical Presentation

1. Subjective
   a. Dyspnea; initially exertional progressing to dyspnea with mild exertion to dyspnea at rest
   b. Fatigue, lethargy
   c. Chest discomfort
   d. Palpitations
   e. Syncope
   f. Cyanosis may be present.
2. Objective
   a. Tachypnea
   b. Use of accessory muscles
   c. Cough; may exhibit hemoptysis

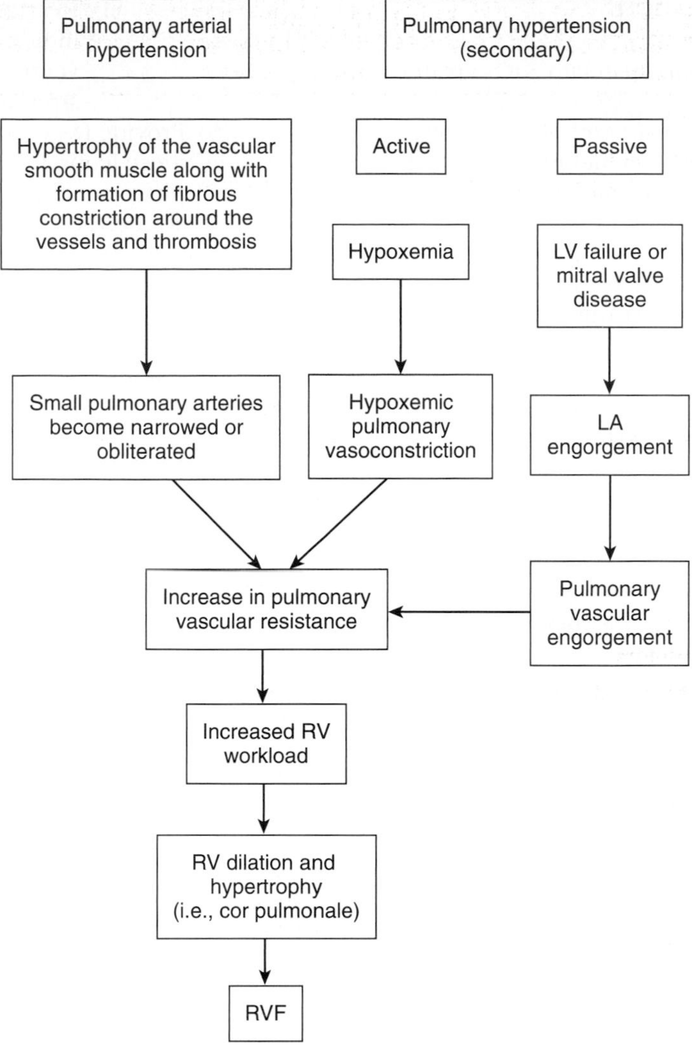

Figure 5-2 Pathophysiology of pulmonary arterial hypertension and pulmonary hypertension.

d. Accentuated P_2: the second component of S_2
e. May have clinical indications of right ventricular hypertrophy (RVH): right ventricular heave; right-sided S_4
f. May have clinical indications of RVF: JVD, peripheral edema, hepatomegaly, murmur of tricuspid regurgitation

3. Diagnostic
   a. Hemodynamic monitoring
      1) PA diastolic more than 5 mm Hg greater than PAOP
      2) PAP greater than 30/15 mm Hg
      3) PA mean greater than 25 mm Hg at rest or greater than 30 mm Hg with activity with a normal PAOP
      4) Pulmonary vascular resistance more than 250 dynes/sec/cm^{-5}
   b. Serum
      1) Hemoglobin and hematocrit may be elevated; polycythemia is caused by erythropoietin release triggered by hypoxemia.
      2) Liver function studies may be elevated.
      3) Arterial blood gases: may be normal at rest but hypoxemia occurs with exertion; eventually hypoxemia at rest
   c. Chest x-ray: may show cardiomegaly, dilated central pulmonary vessels
   d. Electrocardiography: right atrial enlargement, right ventricular strain and hypertrophy
   e. Echocardiograms: used to evaluate heart size, function, and blood flow
   f. Ventilation-perfusion scan: used to evaluate for presence of pulmonary embolism
   g. Cardiac catheterization: elevated right heart and pulmonary pressures
   h. Vasodilator testing for pulmonary arterial hypertension
      1) Performed in the cardiac catheterization lab with IV adenosine or epoprostenol or inhaled nitric oxide
      2) An acute response is defined as a decrease in PAm of greater than or equal to 10 mm Hg to a PAm of less than 40 mm Hg

Collaborative Management

1. Treat cause if possible.
   a. Oxygen for hypoxemia; maintain SaO_2 greater than 90%
   b. Fibrinolytics or pulmonary embolectomy and anticoagulants if caused by pulmonary emboli
   c. Phlebotomy may be performed for patients with significant polycythemia.
   d. Discontinue any causative drug.
2. Decrease pulmonary vascular pressures.
   a. Anticoagulants: warfarin (Coumadin) to maintain INR between 2 and 3
   b. Pulmonary vasodilators
      1) Action: relax the smooth muscle of the pulmonary vascular system
      2) Indications
         a) Pulmonary arterial hypertension
         b) Secondary pulmonary hypertension
            i) Remember that the most common cause of secondary pulmonary hypertension is hypoxemia; oxygen is the first treatment.
            ii) Secondary pulmonary hypertension caused by left ventricular failure requires treatment of the heart failure.
      3) Types of pulmonary vasodilators (Table 5-5)
         a) Calcium channel blockers (e.g., nifedipine)
         b) Methylxanthines (e.g., aminophylline)
         c) Nitric oxide: administered by inhalation so that only vessels to ventilated alveoli are dilated
         d) Prostanoids (e.g., epoprostenol, iloprost, treprostinil)
         e) Endothelin receptor antagonists (e.g., bosentan, ambrisentan)
         f) Phosphodiesterase type 5 inhibitors (e.g., sildenafil, tadalafil)
      4) Provide treatment for heart failure if present.
         a) Diuretics may be required for congestive symptoms.
         b) Digoxin if concurrent LVF is present
         c) Sodium restriction to 2-3 g/day
      5) Prepare patient for surgery as requested.
         a) Surgery for treatment of cause (e.g., valve repair or replacement)
         b) Balloon dilation atrial septostomy
            i) Palliative treatment for patients with primary PH refractory to vasodilator therapy
            ii) Atrial septal defect is created; right-to-left shunting that occurs improves left ventricular filling and cardiac output, offsetting the desaturation of the blood that bypassed the lung.
         c) Lung transplant or heart-lung transplant
            i) Single or double lung transplant is indicated for patients with primary PH who fail to respond to therapy.
            ii) Heart-lung transplantation is indicated for patients with left ventricular disease or congenital structural abnormalities.
      6) Provide instruction and counseling regarding lifestyle modification and need for pharmacologic therapy
         a) Oxygen therapy
            i) Usually recommended for continuous use
            ii) Avoidance of high altitude which would decrease the driving pressure of oxygen and worsen hypoxemia; oxygen should be used when flying
         b) Low (2-3 grams) sodium diet
         c) Cessation of nicotine use
         d) Moderate exercise avoiding overexertion
         e) Energy conservation methods
         f) Avoidance of drugs that may accentuate PH, cause thrombogenesis, or interfere with anticoagulant therapy: oral anticoagulants (pregnancy should be avoided so another method of birth control is recommended); decongestants; aspirin and NSAIDs, herbal medications

Pneumonia

Definitions

1. Pneumonia: inflammatory process of the lung parenchyma, including alveolar spaces and interstitial tissue, produced by an infectious agent
2. Community-acquired pneumonia: infection of the lungs in individuals who have not been recently hospitalized
3. Health care-associated pneumonia (HCAP): acute infection of the lungs that develops after 48 hours of hospitalization; also referred to as *nosocomial pneumonia* or *hospital-acquired pneumonia*
   a. Assumption of a more virulent organism; these organisms are often resistant to multiple antibiotics
   b. Ventilator-associated pneumonia (VAP): subtype of HCAP associated with intubation and mechanical ventilation
      1) Early-onset: develops within 4 days of intubation and mechanical ventilation
      2) Late-onset: develops 5 or more days after intubation and mechanical ventilation

Etiology

1. Causative agents
   a. Bacteria
      1) Community-acquired pneumonia (CAP)
         a) *Streptococcus pneumoniae*: most common
         b) *Haemophilus influenzae*
         c) *Staphylococcus aureus*
         d) *Enterobacter* species
         e) *Streptococcus pyogenes*

f) *Chlamydia pneumoniae*
g) *Legionella pneumophila*
h) *Mycoplasma pneumoniae*
i) *Moraxella catarrhalis*
j) *Bacteroides fragilis*
k) *Mycobacterium tuberculosis*
2) Health care-acquired pneumonia (HCAP)
a) *Pseudomonas* species
b) *Staphylococcus aureus*
c) *Enterobacter* species
d) *Klebsiella pneumoniae*
e) *Escherichia coli*
f) *Haemophilus influenzae*
g) *Serratia marcescens*
h) *Streptococcus* species
i) *Proteus mirabilis*
j) *Acinetobacter* species
k) *Legionella pneumophila*
3) Ventilator-associated pneumonia (VAP)
a) Early onset
i) *Staphylococcus aureus*
ii) *Streptococcus pneumoniae*
iii) *Haemophilus influenzae*
iv) *Moraxella catarrhalis*
v) *Proteus* species
vi) *Serratia marcescens*
vii) *Klebsiella pneumoniae*
viii) *Escherichia coli*
b) Late onset: more likely to be antibiotic resistant
i) Methicillin-resistant *Staphylococcus aureus*
ii) *Pseudomonas aeruginosa*
iii) *Klebsiella pneumoniae*
iv) *Acinetobacter* species
v) *Enterobacter* species
b. Viruses
1) Adenovirus
2) Hantavirus
3) Influenza types A and B
4) Respiratory syncytium virus (RSV)
c. Fungi
1) *Histoplasma capsulatum*
2) *Coccidioides immitis*
3) *Candida* species
4) *Aspergillus* species
d. Parasites (e.g., *Pneumocystis carinii*)
e. Mycoplasma: *Mycoplasma pneumoniae*
2. Predisposing factors
a. Patient-related
1) Advanced age
2) History of smoking
3) Periodontal disease
4) Altered level of consciousness
5) Chronic illness
a) COPD
b) Diabetes mellitus
c) Cardiovascular disease
d) Malignancy
6) Severe acute illness
a) Shock
b) Head injury
c) Chest trauma
7) Malnutrition: alcoholism, malignancy, eating disorder, poverty
8) Immunocompromise
a) Patients with neutropenia resulting from acute leukemia or cytotoxic agents usually have gram-negative bacilli as a source.
b) Severely immunocompromised patient may also develop pneumonia caused by
i) Gram-negative aerobic bacteria
(a) *Haemophilus influenzae*
(b) *Klebsiella pneumoniae*
(c) *Legionella pneumophila*
(d) *Escherichia coli*
(e) *Pseudomonas aeruginosa*
(f) *Proteus mirabilis*
(g) *Klebsiella pneumoniae*
(h) *Enterobacter* species
ii) Viruses
(a) Cytomegalovirus
(b) Varicella-zoster
(c) Herpes simplex
iii) Fungi
(a) *Candida albicans*
(b) *Aspergillus fumigatus*
(c) *Cryptococcus neoformans*
iv) Protozoa: *Pneumocystis carinii*
9) Chronic immobility
b. Treatment-related
1) Surgery, especially if the following:
a) Thoracic, abdominal, or flank incisions
b) Craniotomy
c) Long anesthesia time
d) Prolonged hospitalization
2) Artificial airway, especially self-extubation or reintubation
3) Saline lavage during suctioning of endotracheal tube or tracheostomy
a) Ineffective in liquefying secretions
b) Dislodges 5 times the number of bacterial colonies than suction catheter alone (Hagler & Traver, 1994)
c) Not completely removed with suctioning allowing colonized saline to lie in lungs
4) Bronchoscopy
5) Mechanical ventilation
6) Nasogastric tube
7) Aspiration of colonized material related to therapies
a) Oropharyngeal colonization
i) Previous or concurrent antibiotic therapy: predisposes the patient to colonization of the oropharynx
ii) Leakage of pharyngeal flora around the ET tube cuff
b) Gastric colonization
i) Gastric colonization likely with a gastric pH of greater than 4;

bacteria in the stomach then migrate upward to be silently aspirated into the lungs
(a) Effects of drugs on gastric pH
(i) H_2 receptor antagonist, proton pump inhibitors (PPIs), and antacids alter the pH of the stomach (normally 1-3)
(ii) Sucralfate (Carafate) does not significantly alter the pH and is associated with a lower incidence of pneumonia than PPIs, H_2 receptor antagonists, or antacids.
(b) Continuous enteral feedings may also alter gastric pH
ii) Pneumonia rates of patients receiving mechanical ventilation correlate directly with increased gastric pH levels (Daschner et al., 1988).
8) Supine position
9) Broad-spectrum antibiotic therapy, especially cephalosporins
c. Infection control-related
1) Poor hand washing
2) Failure to change gloves between contacts with patients
3) Failure to wear appropriate protective equipment especially when antibiotic-resistant bacterial strains have been identified
4) Inadequate disinfection/sterilization of devices
5) Contaminated water for humidification
6) Contaminated respiratory therapy or anesthesia equipment
7) Changing of ventilator tubing more often than every 48 hours

Pathophysiology (Figure 5-3)

1. Nosocomial pneumonia specifically
a. Cross-colonization
b. Altered defenses of intubated and mechanically ventilated patient
1) Normal anatomic barriers are bypassed.
2) Impairment of cough reflex
3) Increase in mucus production
4) Stagnation of mucus
5) Impairment of mucociliary apparatus
c. Contaminated aerosol generation
1) Inadequate disinfection/sterilization of devices
2) Contaminated water for humidification

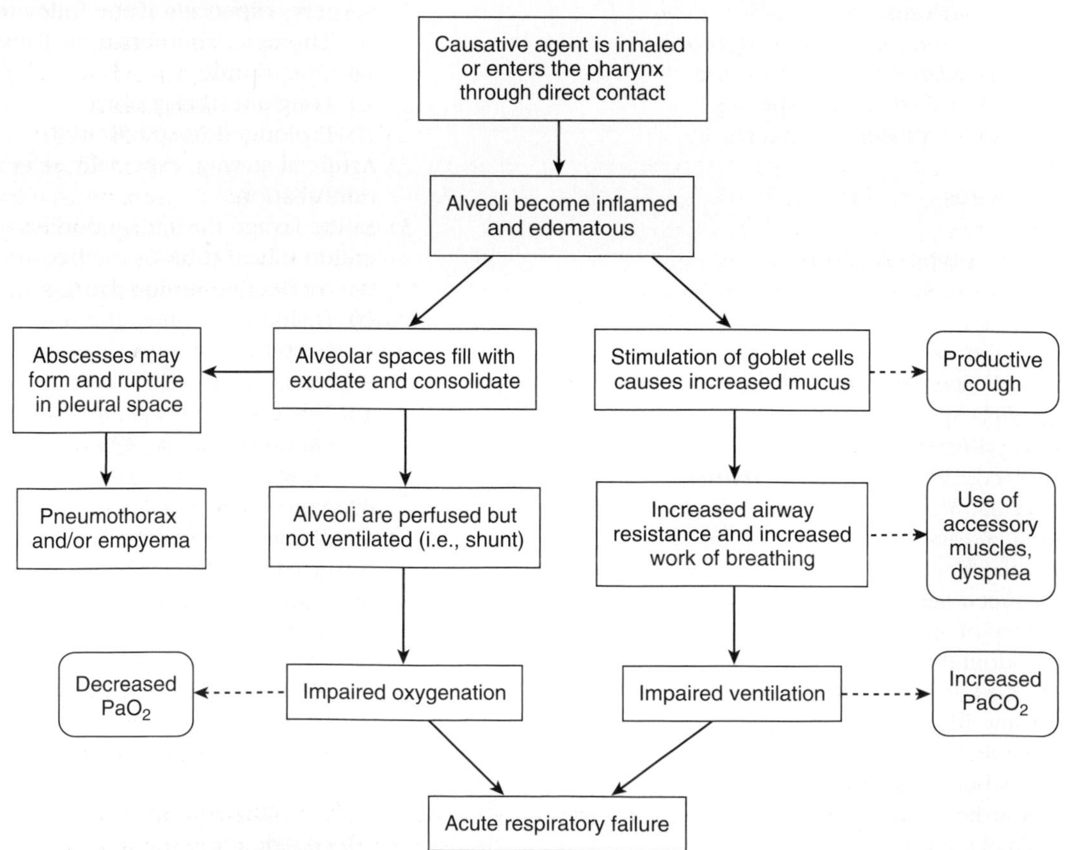

Figure 5-3 Pathophysiology of pneumonia. Dotted lines connect pathology to the clinical presentation.

3) Contaminated respiratory therapy or anesthesia equipment
4) Saline lavage during suctioning of endotracheal tube or tracheostomy

d. Aspiration of colonized material
   1) Oropharyngeal colonization
      a) Concurrent antibiotic therapy: predisposes the patient to colonization of the oropharynx
      b) Leakage of pharyngeal flora around the ET tube cuff
   2) Gastric colonization
      a) Gastric colonization is likely with a gastric pH of greater than 4
      b) H_2 receptor antagonist, proton pump inhibitors (PPIs), and antacids contribute to alter the normal acidic pH of the stomach, allowing proliferation of bacteria in the stomach which then migrate upward to be silently aspirated into the lungs; sucralfate (Carafate) is associated with a lower incidence of pneumonia than PPIs, H_2 receptor antagonists, or antacids.
      c) Pneumonia rates of patients receiving mechanical ventilation correlate directly with increased gastric pH levels (Daschner et al., 1988).
      d) Agents that alter gastric pH have been shown to increase the incidence of CAP, HCAP, and VAP (Herzig et al., 2009).

e. Hematogenous spread from another site

Clinical Presentation

1. Subjective
   a. Frequently begins with cold or flulike symptoms; infectious symptoms: chills, fever, malaise, tachycardia, headache, myalgia
   b. Chest pain (frequently pleuritic-type pain)
   c. Confusion: especially in elderly patients
2. Objective
   a. Tachycardia
   b. Tachypnea
   c. Fever though elderly patients may be hypothermic
   d. Productive cough; sputum mucoid, rusty, bloody, or purulent; may have foul odor
   e. Diaphoresis
   f. Cyanosis may be seen (dependent on hemoglobin and SaO_2 levels).
   g. Splinting of chest; decreased chest excursion
   h. Use of accessory muscles
   i. Increased tactile fremitus
   j. Clinical indications of dehydration
   k. Dullness to percussion over areas of consolidation
   l. Breath sound changes: diminished; bronchial breath sounds; crackles and/or rhonchi; rub may be audible
   m. Voice sounds: egophony, bronchophony, whispered pectoriloquy
3. Diagnostic
   a. Serum
      1) WBC
         a) Elevated with shift to left if bacterial but may be normal in elderly patient, immunocompromised patient, or in overwhelming infection
         b) Normal or decreased if viral
      2) Arterial blood gases: decreased PaO_2 with clinical indications of hypoxemia; $PaCO_2$ may be increased, decreased, or normal depending on ventilation
   b. Blood culture: positive for specific organism in bacteremia
   c. Sputum: may be induced or obtained through bronchoscopy with either protected specimen brush (PSB) or bronchoalveolar lavage (BAL)
      1) Gram stain
      2) Acid-fast stain
      3) Culture and sensitivity to identify specific organism if bacterial
      4) Acid-fast: to rule out tuberculosis
      5) *Legionella*
   d. PPD skin test for tuberculosis
   e. Chest x-ray
      1) Localization and pattern
         a) Bronchopneumonia: inflammation of the bronchioles and alveoli
         b) Interstitial pneumonia: inflammation of the tissue around alveoli
         c) Alveolar pneumonia: inflammation of the alveoli; usually caused by a virus
         d) Necrotizing pneumonia: necrosis of a portion of lung tissue
      2) Viral pneumonias cause diffuse changes.
      3) Pleural effusion may indicate empyema.
   f. Percutaneous needle aspiration of infiltrate: especially in immunocompromised patient not responding to antibiotics
   g. CURB-65 scoring method for CAP (Lim et al., 2003)
      1) Criteria
         a) **C**onfusion
         b) **U**remia (BUN greater than 20 mg/dL)
         c) **R**espiratory rate (greater than or equal to 30 breaths/min)
         d) Low **B**lood pressure (systolic BP less than 90 mm Hg or diastolic BP less than or equal to 60 mm Hg
         e) Age greater than or equal to **65** years
      2) Recommendation for site of care
         a) One criterion: outpatient treatment
         b) Two criteria: inpatient unit
         c) Three or more criteria: often requires critical care admission

Collaborative Management

1. Prevent nosocomial pneumonia or spread of infection
   a. Prevent cross-contamination

1) Maintain standard precautions; other specific precautions may be indicated depending on the type of pneumonia.
2) Wash hands with soap and water or waterless antiseptic agent.
   a) Before and after any contact with the patient
   b) After contact with mucous membranes, respiratory secretions, or objects contaminated with respiratory secretions
3) Wear gloves for handling respiratory secretions or any object contaminated by respiratory secretions.
4) Avoid jewelry, artificial nails or tips, and nail polish.

b. Prevent colonization.
1) Avoid unnecessary antibiotics (e.g., prophylactic antibiotics in situations where not warranted).
2) Avoid unnecessary stress ulcer prophylaxis, and use sucralfate (Carafate) rather than agents which reduce the acidity of gastric secretions (Kollef, 2004); agents that alter the pH of gastric secretions, such as H_2 receptor antagonists, and proton pump inhibitors, have been shown to increase the risk of HAP and CAP (Herzig et al., 2009).
3) Provide oral care.
   a) Every 2-4 hours
      i) Use suction foam swabs to clean teeth and tongue followed by moisturizing swabs and water-soluble lip balm.
      ii) Suction the oropharynx.
         (a) Rinse catheter (e.g., Yankauer) with sterile water or saline after each use.
         (b) Store oropharyngeal suction catheter in an unsealed bag when not in use.
         (c) Replace oropharyngeal suction device, tubing, and suction canister every 24 hours.
   b) Twice daily
      i) Brush teeth to prevent dental plaque colonization.
         (a) A soft-bristle pediatric toothbrush should be used along with toothpaste, preferably with an alkaline pH.
         (b) Removable partial dentures should be removed and thoroughly cleaned.
      ii) Chlorhexidine gluconate (Peridex) 0.12% by spray or rinse as prescribed
         (a) Has been shown to be effective in the prevention of nosocomial pneumonia
         (b) Chlorhexidine is a broad-spectrum antibacterial agent that is not absorbed through the skin or mucous membranes.
         (c) Initiate this oral care preoperatively for surgical patients.
4) Use special silver-coated endotracheal tube to prevent biofilm formation (Kollef et al., 2008).
5) Use continuous lateral rotation therapy to prevent VAP in mechanically ventilated patients (Staudinger et al., 2010).
6) Use aseptic preparation and maintenance of enteral feedings to prevent contamination and gastric colonization.
7) Utilize selective decontamination of the digestive tract as prescribed.
   a) Topical antibiotics such as polymyxin, tobramycin, and amphotericin B (Fungizone) or nystatin
   b) May allow emergence of bacterial resistance

c. Prevent aspiration of contaminated secretions.
1) Avoid intubation by using NIPPV if possible.
2) Prevent accidental extubation by adequately securing endotracheal tube.
3) Avoid nasal tubes if possible: nasotracheal or nasogastric, nasopharyngeal airways
   a) May cause sinusitis and/or potentiate gastric reflux
   b) Orotracheal tube is preferred over nasotracheal tube.
   c) Orogastric tube is preferred over nasogastric but risk of gastric reflux is still present because it also causes incompetence of the gastroesophageal sphincter; percutaneous endoscopic gastrostomy tube is preferred if it is anticipated that the need for enteral feeding will be prolonged.
      i) Remove nasogastric or orogastric tube as soon as possible.
4) Limit the duration of intubation and mechanical ventilation if possible.
   a) Evaluate appropriateness for weaning at least daily by evaluating spontaneous ventilatory parameters after a "sedation vacation."
   b) Use weaning protocols.
5) Maintain endotracheal or tracheostomy cuff pressure at 20-25 mm Hg (25-35 cm H_2O).
6) Maintain continuous aspiration of subglottic secretions (CASS) using a specialized endotracheal tube (see Figure 4-28 on page 291); a dorsal lumen allows continuous suctioning of pooled secretions above the cuff of the endotracheal tube.
7) Suction only as necessary and avoid saline lavage during suctioning of endotracheal tube or tracheostomy.
   a) Ineffective in liquefying secretion

b) Accentuates oxygen desaturation during suctioning
c) Dislodges 5 times the number of bacterial colonies than suction catheter alone
d) Not completely removed with suctioning allowing colonized saline to lie in lungs
8) Rinse the suction catheter after suctioning (catheter pulled back to black line, saline injected into irrigation port while suction is maintained).
9) Elevate the head of bed to 30-45 degrees; turn and reposition every 2 hours.
10) Prevent gastric distention and regurgitation.
a) Ensure correct placement of tube.
b) Evaluate gastric retention for patients receiving enteral feedings; duodenal or jejunal feedings may be beneficial in prevention of aspiration.
c) Utilize gastric suction if necessary.
11) Avoid ventilator circuit changes/ manipulation; change ventilator circuit and closed-suction systems when contamination of the circuit with blood, emesis, or purulent secretions is noted.
a) Ventilator tubing change more often than every 48 hours has been shown to increase the risk of nosocomial pneumonia.
12) Empty water condensation in ventilator or nebulizer tubing into water trap, never back into humidifier reservoir.
13) Change humidification system every week or when contaminated.
14) Prevent aspiration of enteral feedings (see Aspiration Lung Disorder).

d. Encourage the patient to breathe deeply and use incentive spirometry, especially in postoperative patients; adequate analgesia must be achieved so that the patient will breathe deeply.

2. Detect HCAP and VAP (Wood & Swanson, 2009).
a. Obtain a culture for any patient with a new or changing infiltrate on chest x-ray who also exhibits at least two of the following:
1) Fever
2) Leukocytosis
3) Purulent sputum
b. Participate in the acquisition of high quality cultures such as bronchoalveolar lavage (BAL) or protected specimen brush (PSB) cultures if indicated because these provide the highest quality cultures; nonbronchoscopic collection of endotracheal aspirates from the lower airways or nonbronchoscopic bronchoalveolar lavage may be used but produce a lower quality culture.

3. Maintain airway and improve ventilation.
a. Position the patient for optimal ventilation.
1) Elevate head of bed to 30-45 degrees.
2) Turn from "good lung down" to back; use of a 60-degree lateral rotation bed is also advocated.
b. Administer antimicrobials as prescribed.
1) Antibiotics for bacterial infection
a) CAP: should be started within 4 hours of arrival to hospital; broad-spectrum antibiotic prescribed initially empirically (i.e., most likely organism(s) as determined by experience); antibiotic prescription changed if necessary depending on patient response and/or culture
b) Critically-ill patients usually put on a beta-lactam (e.g., amoxicillin, penicillin, piperacillin [Pipracil]) and either a macrolide (azithromycin [Zithromax], clarithromycin [Biaxin], dirithromycin [Dynabac]) or a fluoroquinolone (levofloxacin [Levaquin]), moxifloxacin [Avelox], sparfloxacin [Zagam])
2) Antivirals (e.g., amantadine [Symmetrel], zanamivir [Relenza], oseltamivir [Tamiflu]) for viral infection
3) Other antimicrobials as prescribed
c. Provide adequate hydration: 2-3 L/24 hr unless contraindicated by cardiac or renal disease
1) Oral fluids: noncaffeinated
2) Intravenous fluids: usually D_5NS
d. Maintain bronchial hygiene and provide chest physiotherapy as indicated.
1) Inspiratory maneuvers: deep breathing; incentive spirometry
2) Humidified air and/or oxygen
3) Encouragement to cough or suctioning if the patient is unable to clear airways
4) Postural drainage, percussion, vibration if necessary
5) Bronchodilators as prescribed
6) Expectorants (e.g., guaifenesin [Robitussin], potassium iodide [SSKI]) may be used but hydration is most important; water is the best expectorant.
7) Mucolytics (e.g., acetylcysteine [Mucomyst]) may be used to decrease the tenacity of the mucus
8) Sedatives: generally avoided unless patient is very agitated or on mechanical ventilation
9) Antitussives: Avoid use of antitussives unless the cough is nonproductive and causing fatigue.
e. Prepare the patient for bronchoscopy as requested: may be necessary if airway clearance techniques are inadequate
f. Ensure intubation and mechanical ventilation as indicated.
1) If $PaCO_2$ continues to rise and acidosis develops
2) The goal of mechanical ventilation is to normalize the pH, not necessarily the $PaCO_2$.

4. Optimize oxygen delivery and decrease oxygen consumption.
a. Administer oxygen.

1) Nasal cannula or mask; masks are contraindicated in chronically hypercapnic patients because the high concentration of oxygen provided by these delivery systems would likely eliminate the hypoxic drive.
2) Flow rate or oxygen concentration to keep SpO_2 approximately 95% unless contraindicated; in patients with chronic hypercapnia, adjust flow rate or oxygen concentration to keep SpO_2 approximately 90%

b. Provide rest periods especially after meals or activities.
c. Treat fever.
   1) Antipyretics (acetaminophen [Tylenol])
   2) Use cooling blankets with attention to the prevention of shivering

5. Treat chest pain: analgesics in doses adequate to allow patient to deep breathe and cough as indicated.
6. Provide appropriate nutritional support.
7. Monitor for complications.
   a. Acute respiratory failure
   b. Acute respiratory distress syndrome
   c. Pleural effusion
   d. Empyema
   e. Lung abscess
   f. Sepsis, septic shock
8. Provide instruction and counseling regarding lifestyle modification and need for pharmacologic therapy.
   a. Importance of immunizations (e.g., influenza, *Pneumococcus*, *Haemophilus*)
   b. Hydration
   c. Nutrition
   d. Smoking cessation
   e. Hand-washing techniques, disposal of tissues, prevention of cross-contamination
   f. Recognition of symptoms to report to the physician
   g. Prescribed antimicrobials and the importance of taking the entire prescription

Aspiration Lung Disorder

Definitions

1. Aspiration lung disorder: lung injury related to the inhalation of gastric contents, oropharyngeal secretions, food, or other foreign material into the tracheobronchial tree
2. Aspiration pneumonitis (also referred to as Mendelson's syndrome): chemical injury of the lung caused by aspiration of gastric contents, oropharyngeal secretions, or exogenous liquids
3. Aspiration pneumonia: lung infection caused by aspiration of colonized oropharyngeal or gastric contents

Etiology

1. Altered consciousness and/or gag reflex
   a. Older age
   b. Sedation
   c. Anesthesia especially emergency surgery when the patient has eaten recently
   d. CNS disorders
      1) Cerebral infarction or hemorrhage
      2) Seizures
      3) Neuromuscular diseases
   e. Drug or alcohol intoxication
2. Altered anatomy
   a. Endotracheal tube keeps the epiglottis splinted open.
   b. Tracheostomy tube impairs swallowing mechanism.
   c. Nasogastric or orogastric tube causes incompetence of the gastroesophageal sphincter.
   d. GI tamponade (e.g., Sengstaken-Blakemore tube)
   e. Facial, neck, or oral trauma
   f. Poor oral hygiene
3. GI conditions
   a. Esophageal abnormalities (e.g., tracheoesophageal fistula or stricture)
   b. Gastroesophageal reflux
      1) Obesity
      2) Hiatal hernia
      3) Pregnancy
   c. Decreased GI motility (e.g., diabetic gastroparesis)
   d. GI hemorrhage
   e. Vomiting
   f. Intestinal obstruction
      1) Functional (e.g., ileus)
      2) Structural (e.g., tumor, volvulus)
4. Enteral nutritional support
   a. Impaired gastric motility: a frequent problem in critically ill patients due to perfusion deficits, sepsis, drugs (e.g., propofol, opioids)
   b. Improper positioning of patients especially if on enteral feedings
5. Drugs that decrease gastroesophageal sphincter tone: anticholinergics (e.g., atropine), adrenergics (e.g., dopamine), nitrates, caffeine, calcium channel blockers (e.g., nifedipine), estrogen

Pathophysiology

See Figure 5-4.

Clinical Presentation

1. Subjective
   a. Dyspnea
   b. Cough
   c. Chest pain: pleuritic in nature
   d. Anxiety
   e. May have history of witnessed vomiting or aspiration
2. Objective
   a. Tachycardia
   b. Tachypnea
   c. Fever
   d. Increased work of breathing: use of accessory muscles; intercostal retractions
   e. Productive cough or suctioned material

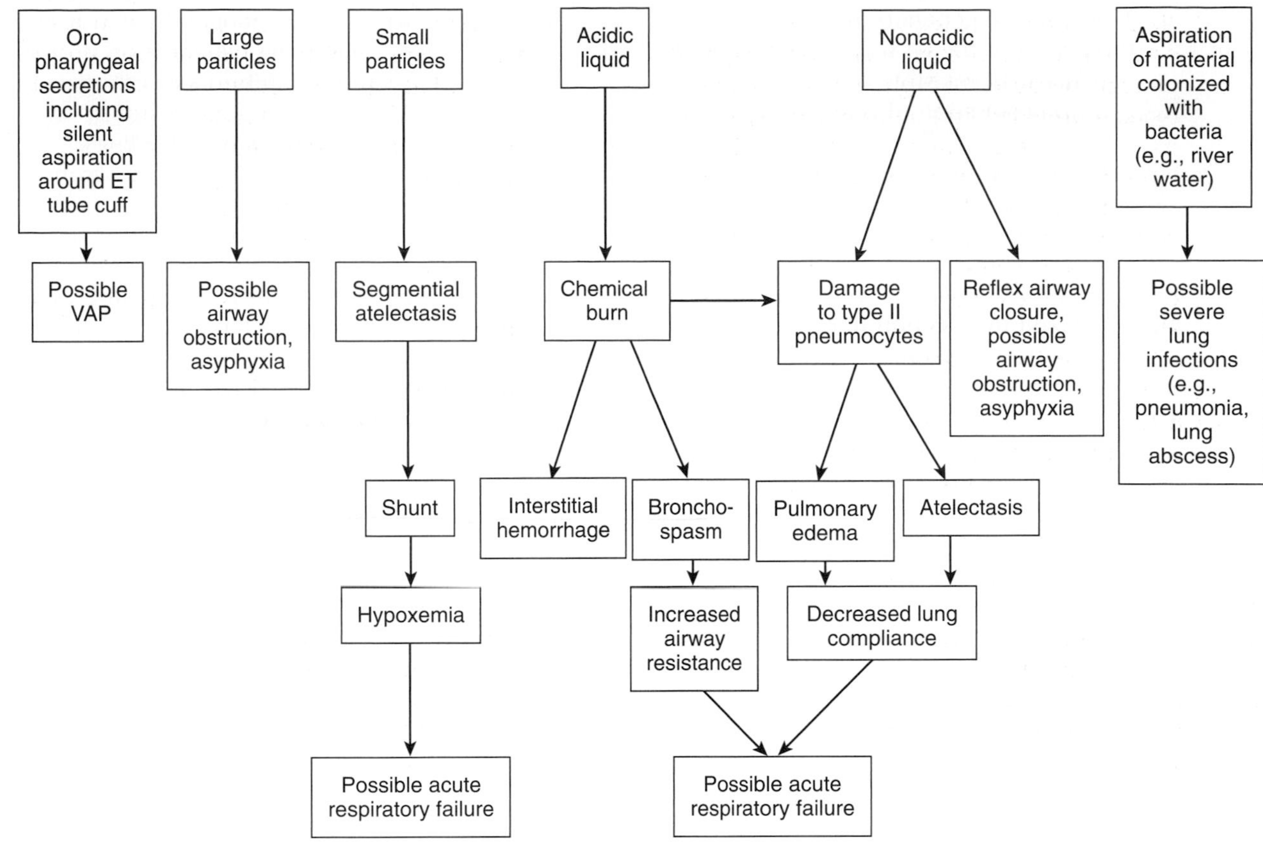

Figure 5-4 Pathophysiology of aspiration lung disorder.

1) Foul-smelling sputum
2) Food or stomach contents may be seen in secretions suctioned from lungs.
   a) If aspirated, enteral feedings will test positive for glucose.
3) Pink, frothy sputum may occur with acidic aspiration.

f. Breath sounds
1) Stridor if obstruction of the upper airway occurs
2) Diminished breath sounds
3) Adventitious sounds: crackles, rhonchi, wheezing

g. Hypoxemia (decreased SpO_2, SaO_2, PaO_2) and clinical indications of hypoxia (see Box 4-3)

h. Compliance: decreased static and dynamic compliance; increased peak inspiratory pressures

3. Diagnostic
a. Serum
1) WBC increased
2) Arterial blood gases
   a) PaO_2 and SaO_2 decreased
   b) $PaCO_2$ may be normal, decreased, or increased depending on ventilation pattern (e.g., may be low due to hyperventilation or high due to hypoventilation)

b. Tracheal aspirate: visualization or analysis to determine if aspiration has occurred
1) Pepsin: a proxy for gastric contents
   a) Likely the most sensitive indicator of aspiration
2) pH: continuous monitoring of tracheal pH
   a) A sensitive instrument to detect acid aspirate in the trachea
3) Glucose: use of glucose oxidase reagent strips to detect presence of glucose
   a) More sensitive than dye method
   b) Some potential problems (Bowman et al., 2005)
      i) Blood in tracheal secretions may cause a positive test result (false-positive).
      ii) Low glucose formulas may not cause a positive result.
      iii) Concerns regarding specificity because some patients not being enterally-fed had positive results
      iv) Concerns about validity of using strips intended for blood or urine for tracheal aspirate
4) Dye: visual assessment of tracheal aspirate for discoloration caused by blue dye (usually blue food coloring) that was added to enteral feeding; it is no longer recommended to add blue food coloring to enteral feedings for the following reasons:

a) May result in generalized absorption of the dye from the GI tract; more likely in patients with multiple organ failure
   i) Discoloration of body fluids and tissues
   ii) May cause fatal liver toxicity
   iii) Causes questionable specificity because discoloration of tracheal secretions may have occurred by systemic route
b) May result in infection due to contamination of the food coloring
c) Interferes with occult blood testing
d) Causes allergic reactions in some people due to presence of FD&C yellow No. 5
e) Has relatively low sensitivity

c. Sputum: presence of polymorphonuclear leukocytes
   1) Culture and sensitivity: infecting organism if pneumonia present

d. Chest x-ray
   1) Bilateral patchy infiltrates or atelectasis
   2) Pulmonary edema may be present.

Collaborative Management

1. Prevent aspiration of gastric contents.
   a. Utilize appropriate positioning to reduce risk of aspiration and reduce volume of aspiration should vomiting occur.
      1) Place unconscious patient in side-lying position; endotracheal intubation may be necessary.
      2) Avoid flat position especially in patients receiving enteral feedings; keep head of bed elevated to 45 degrees continuously for patients on continuous feedings and for at least 30 minutes after intermittent feedings.
         a) Stop continuous enteral feedings at least 30 minutes prior to any procedure that requires that the head of bed must be lowered.
         b) If the head of bed cannot be elevated, position the patient on his or her right side as much as possible to facilitate movement of gastric contents through the pylorus and allow drainage of emesis out of the mouth rather than be aspirated.
      3) Do not restrain in such a way as the patient cannot protect his or her airway if vomiting occurs.
   b. Maintain proper functioning of nasogastric, orogastric, or intestinal tube utilized for gastric suctioning or enteral feeding.
      1) Confirm proper placement: More than one method to verify tube placement should be utilized (Metheny, 2009).
         a) During the procedure
            i) Note any indications of respiratory distress.
            ii) Utilize capnography if available unless the patient is on proton pump inhibitors or other acid-suppressing medications, or continuous tube feedings.
            iii) Measure pH of aspirate from tube; gastric secretions have a pH of 4 or less unless the patient is receiving acid-suppressing medications or continuous feedings; intestinal secretions have a pH of greater than 7.
            iv) Observe visual characteristics of the aspirate.
         b) Radiographic confirmation is the recommended practice for blindly inserted gastrointestinal tubes; the x-ray should be read by a radiologist.
         c) Auscultatory (air bolus) and water bubbling methods can be unreliable.
      2) Reassess placement every 4 hours.
         a) Be alert to change in length of tubing outside of patient during the markings on the tube.
         b) Note change in the volume of aspirate from the tube.
         c) Obtain x-ray to confirm position if location of tube is in question.
   c. Prevent aspiration in patients with artificial airways.
      1) Keep the cuff of endotracheal or tracheostomy tube inflated to 20-30 cm H_2O.
         a) If the patient is not on a mechanical ventilator, inflate the cuff during meals and suction mouth and oropharynx before deflating the cuff.
      2) Suction oropharynx to reduce oropharyngeal secretions that accumulate above the cuff of an endotracheal tube.
         a) Subglottic suctioning is advocated to prevent pneumonia associated with this silent aspiration; involves specialized endotracheal tubing with a port above the cuff that allows continuous suction to remove accumulated secretions
   d. Select appropriate tube and site for enteral feeding.
      1) Use intragastric feedings when GI motility is normal because they are easier and less expensive to place than small intestinal tubes.
         a) Small lumen feeding tubes cause less gastroesophageal incompetence than do larger lumen nasogastric tubes.
         b) Tubes that do not go through the gastroesophageal sphincter (e.g., percutaneous endoscopic gastrostomy [PEG] or needle jejunostomy tubes) are best for long-term enteral feeding.
      2) Use small intestinal tubes and feedings when GI motility is impaired.

a) Because these feedings do increase gastric secretions and duodenal feedings may reflux back into the stomach, aspiration is still possible.
b) A nasogastric or orogastric tube may be inserted to monitor gastric volume or for gastric decompression.

e. Monitor for gastric retention in patients on gastric enteral feedings.
   1) Check for retention before each feeding if intermittent enteral feedings are being administered and every 4-6 hours if continuous enteral feedings are being administered.
      a) If more than 250 mL are aspirated, consider the following:
         i) Changing to continuous feedings if bolus or intermittent feedings being used
         ii) Changing the enteral feeding site to the duodenum or jejunum (though this does not completely eliminate the risk)
         iii) Administering metoclopramide (Reglan) or erythromycin as prescribed to increase gastric motility
         iv) Do not hold feedings but reassess in 1 hour.
      b) If more than 500 mL, withhold feeding for 1 hour and then recheck for retention.
         i) Holding or discontinuing feedings can result in malnutrition so consider changes stated earlier.
   2) Aspiration of small-lumen feeding tubes is difficult because they tend to collapse with suction; increase in abdominal girth, absent bowel sounds, and nausea are indications of retention, and causes of delayed gastric emptying need to be evaluated.

f. Monitor the secretions suctioned or expectorated: Glucose testing may be performed to confirm presence of enteral feeding in sputum.

g. Keep appropriate equipment at bedside.
   1) Airway suctioning equipment
   2) Wire cutters for patients with wired jaws
   3) Scissors for patients with Sengstaken-Blakemore tube

h. Prepare patient for surgery for intractable aspiration as requested: tracheoesophageal diversion or laryngotracheal separation

2. Maintain airway, ventilation, and oxygenation if aspiration does occur.
   a. Position the bed in a slight Trendelenburg position with the patient in a right lateral decubitus position.
   b. Suction the airway immediately; provide adequate oxygenation during suctioning.
      1) Endotracheal intubation may be necessary.
      2) Bronchoscopy for removal of large particles if indicated
   c. Stop enteral feeding if being administered.
   d. Monitor arterial blood gases and pulse oximetry: A decrease in SpO_2, SaO_2, and PaO_2 may indicate the development of acute respiratory distress syndrome.
   e. Administer oxygen therapy if hypoxemia is present.
      1) CPAP or PEEP may be necessary to maintain adequate oxygenation.
   f. Initiate mechanical ventilation as prescribed if hypercapnia develops.
   g. Administer bronchodilators as prescribed.
   h. Administer antibiotics as prescribed (prophylactic antibiotics are not recommended but antibiotics specific to positive sputum or blood cultures are indicated).
   i. Prepare the patient for pulmonary resection if abscess develops.

3. Monitor for complications.
   a. Acute respiratory failure
   b. Acute respiratory distress syndrome
   c. Pneumonia
   d. Lung abscess
   e. Empyema

Status Asthmaticus

Definitions

1. Asthma: a recurrent, reversible airway disease characterized by increased airway responsiveness to a variety of stimuli that produces airway narrowing
2. Status asthmaticus: exacerbation of acute asthma characterized by severe airflow obstruction that is not relieved after 24 hours of maximal doses of traditional therapy

Etiology

1. Extrinsic: when a specific allergy can be related to the attack
   a. Dust and dust mites
   b. Animal dander or feathers
   c. Pollen
   d. Mold
   e. Smoke
   f. Propellants
   g. Air pollution
   h. Preservatives (e.g., bisulfites)
   i. Food such as nuts, legumes (e.g., peanuts), chocolate, eggs, shellfish, and food additives
   j. Alcohol
   k. Changes in inspired air such as cold or hot air, very high or very low humidity
   l. Medications
      1) Aspirin
      2) Nonsteroidal noninflammatory drugs (NSAIDs)
      3) Beta-blockers
2. Intrinsic: when the attack is seemingly unrelated to a specific allergen

a. Infection, such as bacterial or viral pneumonia, bronchitis, or sinusitis
b. Stress
c. Exercise
d. Gastroesophageal reflux disease (GERD)
e. Aspiration
f. Fear, anger, crying, or laughing
g. Menstrual cycle

Pathophysiology

See Figure 5-5.

Clinical Presentation

1. Subjective
   a. History of a slow, progressive worsening of airflow obstruction over the course of several days or weeks
   b. Anxiety
   c. Dyspnea
   d. Chest tightness
   e. Fatigue
   f. Insomnia
   g. Anorexia
2. Objective
   a. Tachycardia
   b. Tachypnea; inability to speak in full sentences due to dyspnea
   c. Cough with thick tenacious sputum production
   d. Use of accessory muscles
   e. Intercostal retractions
   f. Prolonged expiration (more than 1 to 3 I:E ratio)
   g. Diaphoresis
   h. Peak expiratory flow rate (PEFR) below 80% of patient's personal or predicted best; frequently below 50% of patient's personal best
   i. Clinical indications of dehydration: poor skin turgor; dry mucous membranes; increased specific gravity of urine
   j. Clinical indications of hypoxemia (see Box 4-3)
   k. Clinical indications of hypercapnia (see Box 4-4)

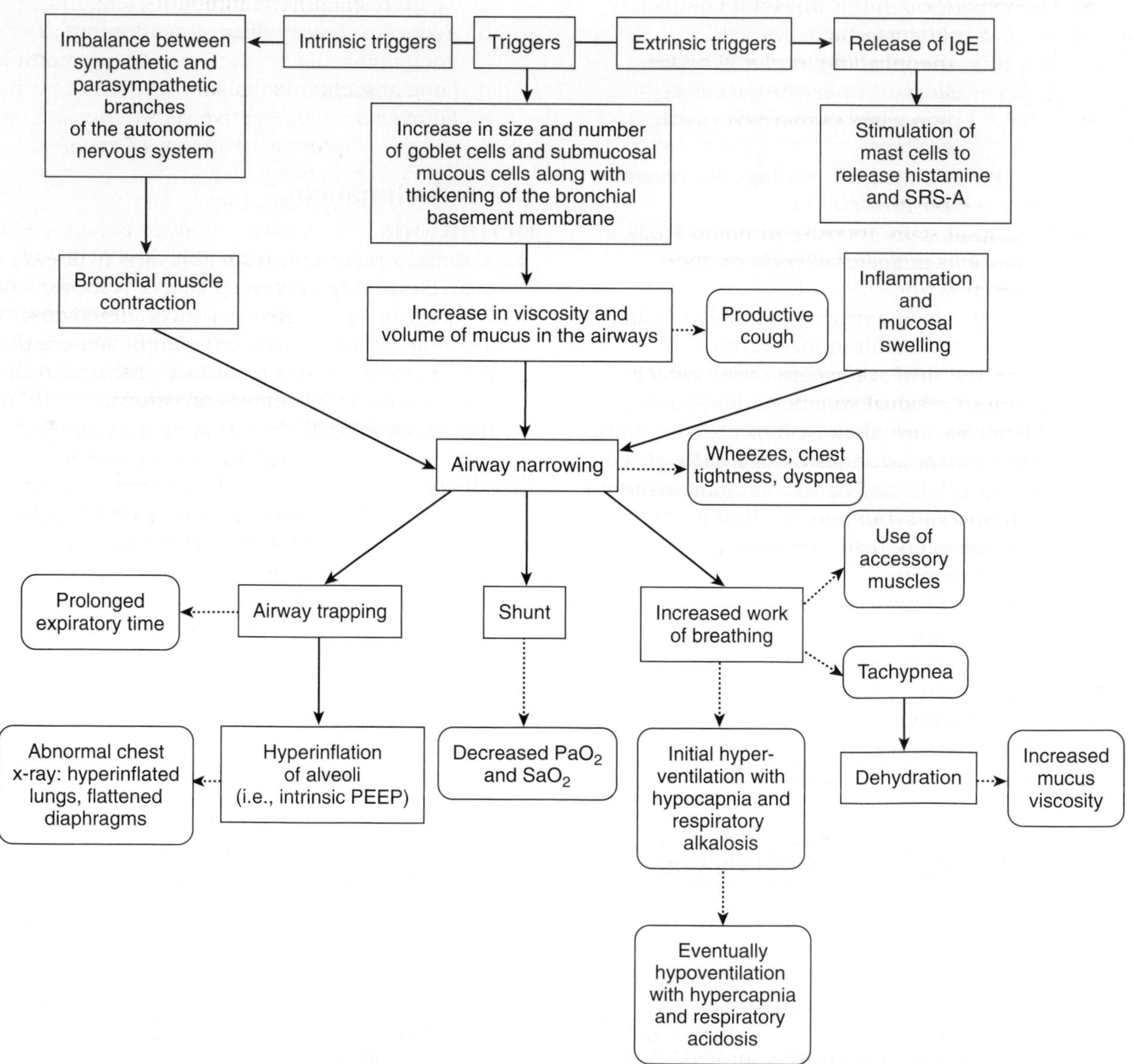

Figure 5-5 Pathophysiology of asthma. Dotted lines connect pathology to the clinical presentation.

l. Breath sound changes: rhonchi and wheezing
m. Indications of potential imminent respiratory arrest
   1) Change in consciousness: drowsiness or confusion
   2) Paradoxical thoracoabdominal movement
   3) Absence of rhonchi and wheezes may occur in critical stages; indication of absence of airflow
   4) Bradycardia
   5) Pulsus paradoxus greater than 20 mm Hg

3. Diagnostic
   a. Serum
      1) WBC count may be increased if infection is the cause.
      2) Eosinophil count may be increased if patient is not receiving steroids.
      3) Hematocrit may be increased due to dehydration.
      4) Electrolytes: Potassium and/or magnesium may be low during an acute attack.
      5) Theophylline level: if therapeutic 10-20 mcg/dL; if patient has not been taking the drug, theophylline level will be less than therapeutic
      6) Arterial blood gases (Table 5-6)
   b. Sputum
      1) Increased viscosity
      2) May have positive culture
      3) Eosinophil stain: Increase in number of eosinophils indicates allergic reaction.
   c. Pulmonary function studies (may be impossible to do during attack because the patient is so dyspneic)
      1) Decreased tidal volume and vital capacity
      2) Increased residual volume
      3) PEF or FEV_1 are diminished with improvement after bronchodilators.
         a) A combination of best FEV_1 and patient report of symptoms is a better predictor of mortality than best peak expiratory flow in patients with asthma.
   d. ECG: sinus tachycardia
   e. Chest x-ray
      1) Normal or hyperinflated lungs with flattened diaphragms
      2) Helpful to rule out foreign body, aspiration, pulmonary edema, pulmonary embolism, pneumonia, or pneumothorax

Collaborative Management

1. Assess predisposing factors; eliminate and/or treat cause.
   a. Antibiotics to promptly treat infection
   b. Avoidance of exposure to pulmonary irritants and pollutants
   c. Avoidance of drugs or foods that may trigger an attack
   d. Cromolyn sodium (Intal) or nedocromil (Tilade) are inhaled mast cell stabilizers which prevent the release of histamine from the mast cells; these agents have no direct bronchodilation or antiinflammatory effect and are not helpful during an acute attack.
2. Maintain airway and improve ventilation.
   a. Elevate head of bed to 30 to 45 degrees; overbed table may be helpful for patient to lean on.
   b. Administer pharmacologic agents as prescribed.
      1) Bronchodilators to relax bronchial smooth muscle
         a) Leukotriene inhibitors/leukotriene receptor antagonists (e.g., zafirlukast [Accolate], zileuton [Zyflo], montelukast sodium [Singulair]) may have been used as a preventative agent; they are not helpful for treatment of acute bronchospasm.
         b) $Beta_2$ stimulants
            i) Action: stimulate $beta_2$ receptors to cause smooth muscle relaxation
            ii) Long-acting (e.g., salmeterol [Serevent]) by metered-dose inhaler will likely have been used long-term by the patient with a diagnosis of asthma.
            iii) Short-acting $beta_2$ agonists (e.g., metaproterenol [Alupent, Metaprel], albuterol [Proventil, Ventolin], pirbuterol [Maxair], bitolterol [Tornalate], terbutaline [Brethaire], epinephrine)
               (a) Metered-dose inhaler is usually used and may be as effective as nebulizers when used with a spacing device.
               (b) Nebulizer is frequently used if the PEFR is less than 50% of the patient's personal best; the

Table 5-6 Asthma: ABG Analysis

Stage	PaO_2	$PaCO_2$	pH	Acid-Base Imbalance
I	Normal	Decreased	Increased	Respiratory alkalosis
II	Decreased	Decreased	Increased	Respiratory alkalosis Mild to moderate hypoxemia
III	Very low	Normal	Normal	Significant hypoxemia
IV	Extremely low	Elevated	Decreased	Respiratory acidosis Critical hypoxemia

beta-agonist is administered by nebulizer every 20 minutes or continuously for 1 hour.
  (i) Continuous nebulizers have been shown as effective with no more side effects than intermittent nebulizers and require less clinician time
(c) Intravenous beta-agonists are not recommended if inhalation therapy is possible because they do not result in better results but increase adverse effects significantly.
iv) Monitor closely for adverse effects such as significant tachycardia, dysrhythmias, hypertension, headache, tremor, anxiety, or hypokalemia.

c) Anticholinergic (e.g., ipratropium bromide [Atrovent]) may be used in severe attacks to augment the effects of beta$_2$ agonists.
  i) Action: block parasympathetic stimulation (making sympathetic stimulation dominant) to cause smooth muscle relaxation
  ii) May be especially helpful for asthma stimulated by an intrinsic trigger
  iii) Administered as a metered-dose inhaler or nebulizer
  iv) May be administered as a combination agent with beta agonist (e.g., ipratropium bromide and albuterol sulfate [Combivent])

d) Xanthines (e.g., theophylline, aminophylline) may be given intravenously for refractory attack.
  i) Actions
    (a) Smooth muscle relaxation causing bronchodilation though less effective than nebulized beta agonists; also more adverse effects than beta agonists
    (b) Immune-modulating effects including inhibition of T lymphocytes and other inflammatory cells and inhibition of cytokine release
  ii) No longer first-line agent primarily because of the narrow therapeutic window and interactions with other commonly prescribed drugs but should be continued in patients on xanthine therapy at home
    (a) Obtain a theophylline level for patients who have been receiving xanthines at home.
    (b) Monitor closely for indications of theophylline toxicity.
      (i) GI: anorexia, nausea, vomiting
      (ii) Cardiac: dysrhythmias
      (iii) Neurologic: restlessness or seizures
  iii) Administration orally for long-term therapy but usually by intravenous infusion in acute asthma

e) Magnesium: used in acutely ill asthmatic patients with severe exacerbation
  i) Actions: smooth muscle relaxation, bronchodilation, improved airflow
    (a) Considered for patients who have not responded to other bronchodilators after 1 hour
  ii) Administered as intravenous infusion: Usual dose is 1-2 grams over 20 minutes.
  iii) Contraindicated in hypotension or renal failure
  iv) Monitor blood pressure during infusion; note and report significant hypotension or loss of deep tendon reflexes.

2) Corticosteroids to reduce inflammation
  a) Actions
    i) Decrease mucosal swelling and release of histamine by the mast cells
    ii) Potentiates bronchodilators
  b) Administration
    i) Patient has usually administered steroids (e.g., beclomethasone [Vanceril, Beclovent], flunisolide [Aerobid], triamcinolone [Azmacort], fluticasone [Flovent]) via metered-dose inhaler prior to hospitalization.
      (a) Steroids by inhalation diminish (but do not completely avoid) the systemic effects of steroid administration.
    ii) Steroids may be initially administered intravenously (e.g., methylprednisolone [Solu-Medrol]) or orally (prednisone and prednisolone) in status asthmaticus.
      (a) Initial large doses are titrated downward over days to weeks.
      (b) Alternate-day oral dosing decreases the potential for adrenal suppression.
    iii) Steroid-resistant asthma: Intravenous immunoglobulin may be administered.

3) Expectorants (e.g., guaifenesin [Robitussin], potassium iodide [SSKI]) may be used but hydration is most important; water is the best expectorant.
4) Mucolytics (e.g., acetylcysteine [Mucomyst]) are generally contraindicated because of the adverse effect of bronchospasm.
5) Antitussives: Avoid use of antitussives.
6) Antibiotics: indicated only if infection

c. Maintain bronchial hygiene.
   1) Abdominal (i.e., deep) breathing
   2) Effective coughing
   3) Suctioning only if coughing is ineffective
   4) Chest physical therapy is not generally recommended and may be unnecessarily stressful for a patient with status asthmaticus.

d. Utilize noninvasive ventilatory methods (CPAP, Bi-PAP) as prescribed.
   1) May be used with a mask if the patient is not intubated
   2) May prevent further deterioration and intubation and mechanical ventilation by unloading the respiratory muscles and reducing the work of breathing
   3) May improve survival rates (Young, 2010)

e. Ensure intubation and mechanical ventilation as necessary.
   1) Indicated if $PaCO_2$ continues to rise and acidosis develops
   2) The goal of mechanical ventilation is to normalize the pH, not necessarily the $PaCO_2$.
      a) Mode: AC or PRVC
      b) Tidal volume: 4-8 mL/kg
      c) Respiratory rate: 10-12 breaths/min and adjust to normalize pH though $PaCO_2$ may still be elevated
         i) Permissive hypercapnia, expected and accepted hypercapnia, results from the deliberate attempt to decrease alveolar ventilation by reducing tidal volumes and alveolar pressures
         ii) Contraindicated in intracranial hypertension or cerebral anoxia
         iii) Sedation may be required.
            (a) Morphine is avoided because it causes histamine release.
            (b) Propofol and fentanyl OR ketamine (causes bronchodilation) and midazolam
         iv) Bicarbonate infusions may be utilized to keep the pH above 7.2.
      d) Flow rate: 60-100 L/min; higher inspiratory flow rate shortens inspiration to allow more time for expiration to reduce air trapping and auto-PEEP
         i) I:E ratio: 1:3 or 1:4 to allow longer expiratory times
      e) Peak inspiratory pressure should be kept under 40 cm H_2O, and plateau pressure should be kept below 35 cm H_2O if possible.
      f) FiO2: adjusted to maintain SpO_2 of approximately 90%
      g) PEEP should be avoided or less than or equal to 5 cm H_2O if possible since the patient is at high risk for barotrauma.
         i) Monitor levels of auto-PEEP caused by air trapping

3. Optimize oxygen delivery and decrease oxygen consumption.
   a. Administer oxygen as indicated.
      1) Uncontrolled high-flow oxygen should be avoided in acute asthma; oxygen concentration should be adjusted to keep SpO_2 ~90%.
   b. Teach and encourage relaxation techniques.
   c. Teach and encourage abdominal breathing though difficult for the patient when dyspneic and tachypneic.
   d. Provide rest periods especially after meals or activities.
   e. Administer antipyretics if indicated.
   f. Utilize heliox as prescribed.
      1) Helium is a light gas that decreases work of breathing when it replaces nitrogen in the inspired air.
         a) Oxygen percentage is prescribed and helium replaces nitrogen to make up the remainder (e.g., 80% helium/20% oxygen, 70% helium/30% oxygen, 60% helium/40% oxygen).
      2) Actions
         a) Decreases airway resistance and work of breathing
         b) Decreases hypercapnia and need for intubation and mechanical ventilation
      3) Administration
         a) By face mask
         b) By mechanical ventilator: requires recalibration for this lighter gas

4. Provide adequate rehydration.
   a. Oral fluids: noncaffeinated
   b. Intravenous fluids: usually D_5NS or $D_5{}^1/_2NS$

5. Provide instruction and counseling regarding lifestyle modification and need for pharmacologic therapy.
   a. Recognition and avoidance of triggers; allergy testing and desensitization may be needed
   b. Symptom monitoring
      1) To measure PEFR twice daily
      2) When to call the physician
         a) PEFR drops by 20% or more below its usual level
         b) Increase in symptoms such as dyspnea
         c) Indications of respiratory infection
   c. Drug therapy
      1) Inhaled bronchodilators and corticosteroids

a) How to use and clean a metered-dose inhaler or nebulizer
b) To use corticosteroids after the bronchodilator
c) To rinse mouth after inhaled corticosteroids to avoid oral fungal infection (e.g., candidiasis)
2) Cromolyn may be prescribed.
3) Antimicrobials
d. Breathing exercises: slow abdominal breathing and pursed-lip breathing
e. Importance of immunizations (e.g., influenza, *Pneumococcus*, *Haemophilus*)
f. Control of GERD
1) H_2 receptor antagonists or proton-pump inhibitors (e.g., omeprazole [Prilosec], lansoprazole [Protonix], rabeprazole)
2) Avoidance of large meals and supine position after eating
3) Normalization of body weight
6. Monitor for complications.
a. Asphyxia
b. Acute respiratory failure
c. Barotrauma/volutrauma (e.g., pneumothorax)
d. Pneumonia
e. Dysrhythmias
f. Hypovolemia
g. Hypotension related to hypovolemia, lung hyperinflation decreasing venous return to the heart, tension pneumothorax, oversedation

Pulmonary Embolism/Infarction

Definition

Obstruction of blood flow to one or more arteries of the lung by a thrombus lodged in a pulmonary vessel; other types of emboli include fat, air, amniotic fluid, tumor, and foreign body (e.g., catheter fragment)

1. Massive: more than 50% occlusion of pulmonary blood flow; caused by occlusion of a lobar artery or larger artery
2. Submassive: less than 50% occlusion of pulmonary blood flow; in patients with preexisting heart or lung disease, hemodynamic deterioration occurs with less than 50% pulmonary vascular obstruction

Etiology

1. Risk factors for thrombus formation (Virchow's triad)
a. Hypercoagulability
1) Malignancy: especially breast, lung, pancreas, or GI or GU tracts
2) Estrogen, especially in smokers
a) Oral contraceptives
b) Postmenopausal hormone replacement therapy
3) Dehydration and hemoconcentration
4) Fever
5) Sickle-cell anemia
6) Pregnancy and postpartum period
7) Polycythemia vera
8) Abrupt discontinuance of anticoagulants
9) Sepsis
10) Protein C, protein S, or antithrombin III deficiency
b. Alterations in the vessel wall
1) Trauma
2) IV drug use
3) Aging
4) Vasculitis
5) Varicose veins
6) Diabetes mellitus
7) Atherosclerosis
8) Inflammatory process
c. Venous stasis
1) Prolonged bed rest or immobilization
2) Obesity
3) Advanced age
4) Burns
5) Pregnancy
6) Postpartum period
7) Heart failure
8) Myocardial infarction
9) Bacterial endocarditis
10) Recent surgery especially legs, pelvis, or abdomen
11) Thrombus formation in heart (AF)
12) Cardioversion
2. Risk factors for fat embolism
a. Long bone (e.g., femur) fracture, pelvic fracture, multiple fractures
b. Orthopedic surgery with intramedullary manipulation
c. Trauma to adipose tissue or liver
d. Osteomyelitis
e. Sickle cell crisis
f. Burns
g. Acute pancreatitis
h. Liposuction
3. Risk factors for air embolism
a. Recent surgical procedure
b. Insertion of deep vein catheter
c. Cardiopulmonary bypass
d. Hemodialysis
e. Endoscopy

Pathophysiology (Figure 5-6)

1. Fat emboli specifically
a. Most likely to develop 1-3 days after injury but may occur up to a week after injury
b. Fat globules enter the bloodstream and form emboli.
c. Presence of fat emboli in the bloodstream causes interactions with platelets and free fatty acids along with release of vasoactive substances.
d. Cerebral ischemia
2. Air emboli specifically
a. Activation of the clotting cascade
b. Interruption of circulation

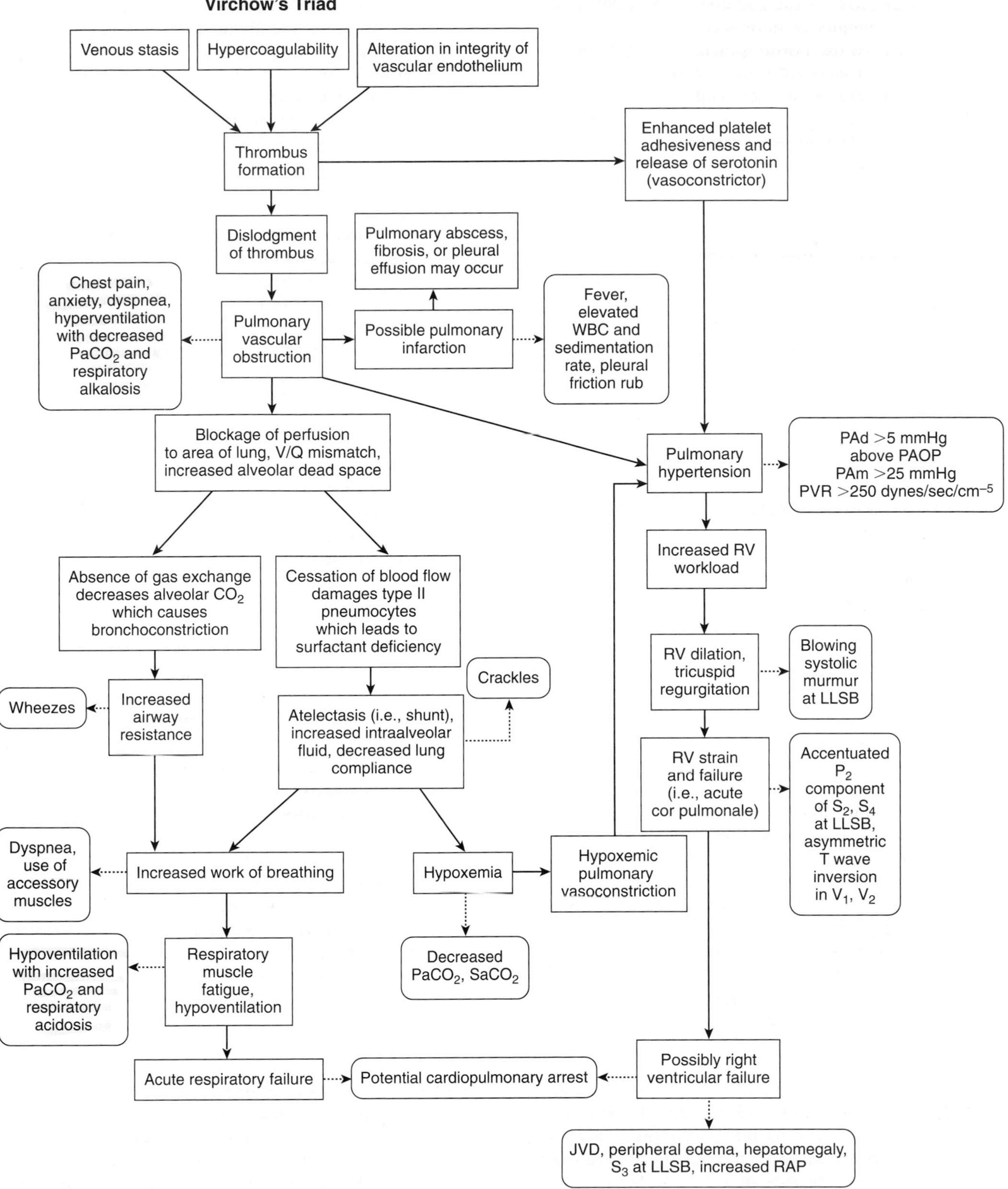

Figure 5-6 Pathophysiology of pulmonary embolism. Dotted lines connect pathology to clinical presentation.

Clinical Presentation

1. Small embolus: Patient is asymptomatic.
2. Small to medium embolus
   a. Anxiety
   b. Dyspnea
   c. Tachypnea
   d. Tachycardia
   e. Chest pain
   f. Cough
   g. Accentuated P_2 (pulmonic component of S_2; the second component of S_2)

h. Right-sided S_3 or S_4 (audible at sternum)
i. Breath sound changes: crackles

3. Large to massive: Massive PE is when 50% of pulmonary artery bed is occluded.
   a. Feeling of impending doom
   b. Dyspnea
   c. Tachypnea
   d. Tachycardia
   e. Chest pain
   f. Mental clouding and/or syncope
   g. Cyanosis
   h. Clinical indications of RVF: JVD, hepatomegaly, murmur of tricuspid regurgitation, right ventricular heave
   i. Hypotension or sudden shock
   j. May present as pulseless electrical activity (PEA)
4. If pulmonary infarction develops (hours to days after embolism), the patient will also have
   a. Fever
   b. Pleuritic chest pain
   c. Hemoptysis
   d. Pleural friction rub
5. Hemodynamic monitoring
   a. Elevated CVP and RAP
   b. Elevated PA pressures with normal PAOP (increased PAd-PAOP gradient)
   c. Elevated PVR
   d. Decreased CO/CI in massive PE
6. Diagnostic
   a. Laboratory
      1) D-dimer
         a) Elevated in almost all patients with PE because of endogenous fibrinolysis (i.e., high negative predictive value)
         b) High sensitivity but low specificity; 99% negative predictive value
         c) Indeterminate V/Q and a positive D-dimer is an indication for pulmonary angiogram
      2) Troponin I: may be elevated; indicates right ventricular microinfarction
      3) BNP: may be elevated with right ventricular overload
      4) ABGs
         a) If thrombotic
            i) Decreased PaO_2, SaO_2, and SvO_2; PaO_2 less than 50 mm Hg in a patient with previously normal ABGs indicates greater than 50% obstruction of the pulmonary tree and that pulmonary hypertension is present
            ii) Decreased $PaCO_2$
            iii) Respiratory alkalosis initially; may have metabolic acidosis if severe hypoxemia; respiratory acidosis may develop with significant atelectasis or fatigue
         b) If fat or air embolism
            i) Decreased PaO_2 and SaO_2
            ii) Increased $PaCO_2$
            iii) Respiratory acidosis; may have metabolic acidosis if severe hypoxemia
   b. ECG
      1) Dysrhythmias
         a) Sinus tachycardia
         b) Atrial dysrhythmias, especially atrial fibrillation, are common.
         c) Ventricular dysrhythmias may occur in hypoxemia.
      2) Blocks: New RBBB may be seen.
      3) Tall, peaked P waves in lead II (P-pulmonale)
      4) Right axis deviation may be seen (QRS complex negative in I, positive in aVF).
      5) Right ventricular strain: ST segment elevation in V_1 and V_2
      6) Helpful to rule out MI as cause of signs/symptoms
   c. Chest x-ray
      1) Almost always normal initially but may be helpful to rule out other sources of patient symptoms
      2) If thrombotic
         a) Initially normal
         b) After 24 hours: small infiltrates may be seen secondary to atelectasis; elevated hemidiaphragm on affected side; decreased pulmonary vascularity
         c) If pulmonary infarction: Infiltrates and pleural effusion may be seen.
      3) If fat embolism
         a) Diffuse extensive interstitial and alveolar infiltrates
   d. Echocardiography
      1) Usually normal but may show right ventricular dilation, hypokinesis, and tricuspid regurgitation
      2) May show bulging of interventricular septum into LV which reduces LV size with D-shaped LV
      3) Also helpful to rule out cardiac tamponade, dissection of the aorta, and acute myocardial infarction
   e. V/Q scan
      1) Shows perfusion defect with normal ventilation
      2) Positive predictive value of high probability V/Q scan is 96% when supported by high clinical suspicion of PE; negative predictive value of negative V/Q scan is also excellent with a normal V/Q scan accurately ruling out PE 98% of the time; unfortunately, 75% of patients fall within the indeterminate category
      3) Intermediate or low probability V/Q scan with positive D-dimer is indication for pulmonary angiography.
   f. Spiral (helical) CT
      1) Widely available

2) Easier study to obtain than a V/Q scan or pulmonary angiogram
3) Capable of demonstrating a variety of thoracic pathologies that can mimic PE
4) Sensitivity greatly affected by generation of scanner used; significantly better sensitivity with new scanners; excellent specificity

g. Magnetic resonance angiography
1) Gadolinium-enhanced MRA allows high-resolution angiography during a single breath.
2) Fast but accurate test that does not involve nephrotoxic contrast agents

h. Pulmonary angiography
1) Shows cutoff of a vessel or a filling defect within 24-72 hours
2) Continues to be the "gold standard" but not without risks
3) Indicated in patients with a high probability of having a PE and nondiagnostic noninvasive studies
4) Excellent sensitivity and specificity
5) Disadvantages: risk of significant bleeding, provides a relative contraindication for fibrinolytic therapy because of the risk of bleeding from the puncture site

i. The Wells score (Wells & Ginsberg, 1995)
1) Scores for factors that increase likelihood that PE exists
a) Clinically suspected DVT: 3 points
b) The alternative diagnosis is less likely than PE: 3 points
c) Tachycardia: 1.5 points
d) Immobilization or surgery within previous 4 weeks: 1.5 points
e) History of DVT or PE: 1.5 points
f) Presence of hemoptysis: 1 point
g) Treatment for malignancy within 6 months or palliative management: 1 point
2) Interpretation of summative score
a) Score greater than 6: high probability of PE
b) Score 2-6: moderate probability of PE
c) Score less than 2: Low probability of PE
3) Testing recommendations
a) Score greater than 4: PE likely so consider diagnostic imaging
b) Score 4 or less: PE unlikely so consider D-dimer to rule out PE

7. If fat embolism: may have no symptoms for 12-48 hours
a. Subjective
1) Restlessness, agitation, irritability, and confusion
2) Dyspnea
3) Delirium
b. Objective
1) Tachypnea
2) Tachycardia
3) Fever
4) Petechiae on conjunctivae, anterior chest, neck, or axilla
5) Retinal hemorrhages with emboli present on the retina
6) Breath sound changes: stridor, wheezes, or crackles
7) Lethargy, coma
8) Seizures
9) Hypoxemia: decreased SpO_2, SaO_2, and PaO_2
10) Clinical indications of hypoxia (see Box 4-3)
c. Diagnostic
1) Serum
a) Elevated lipase
b) Elevated triglycerides
c) Increased free fatty acids
d) Elevated sedimentation rate
e) Decreased hemoglobin or hematocrit
f) Thrombocytopenia
g) Elevated fibrin split products
2) Arterial blood gases: hypoxemia
3) Urinalysis: fat globules in the urine
4) Sputum: fat globules in the sputum

8. If air embolism
a. Subjective
1) Feeling of impending doom
2) Lightheadedness
3) Weakness
4) Nausea
5) Chest pain
6) Dyspnea
7) Palpitations
8) Confusion
b. Objective
1) Pallor
2) Tachypnea
3) Tachycardia
4) Hypotension
5) Churning noise ("mill wheel murmur") may be audible.
6) Hypoxemia: decreased SpO_2, SaO_2, and PaO_2
7) Clinical indications of hypoxia (see Box 4-3)
8) Clinical indications of pulmonary edema: S_3 or crackles
9) Seizures
c. Diagnostic
1) Serum: arterial blood gases: hypoxemia; hypercapnia
2) Chest x-ray: may show evidence of right ventricular failure and/or pulmonary edema
3) Ventilation/perfusion scan: similar to PE but may resolve within 24 hours
4) Echocardiography: shows air in right ventricle, right ventricular dilation, and/or pulmonary hypertension

Collaborative Management

1. Prevent emboli formation.
a. All patients
1) Deep breathing exercises hourly for postoperative patients
2) Ambulation as soon as possible

3) Leg exercises, especially for patients who cannot be ambulated; passive range of motion of all extremities for patients who cannot do leg exercises
4) Frequent repositioning; avoid extreme knee or hip flexion; instruct patient not to cross legs
5) Adequate fluid intake to prevent dehydration and hypercoagulability
6) Careful venipuncture and IV care
   a) Avoidance of venipunctures in legs
   b) Atraumatic venipuncture; avoid multiple sticks

b. Patients with moderate risk for deep vein thrombosis (DVT) also require elastic stockings or intermittent pneumatic compression devices.
   1) Elastic stockings: Care must be taken to prevent constriction and tourniquet effect of stockings.
   2) Intermittent pneumatic compression devices: also referred to as *sequential compression devices*
      a) Stimulates endogenous fibrinolytic activity in addition to direct physical stimulation of increased venous blood return

c. Patients with high risk for DVT are likely to have subcutaneous low-dose unfractionated heparin (UFH) or low-molecular-weight heparin (LMWH) be prescribed if not contraindicated.
   1) Enoxaparin (Lovenox): 30 or 40 mg every 12 hours
   2) Unfractionated heparin: 5000 units every 8 to 12 hours
   3) Dalteparin sodium (Fragmin): 2500 IU daily

d. Patients with documented deep vein thrombosis (DVT) require low-dose unfractionated heparin (UFH) or low-molecular-weight heparin (LMWH).

2. Prevent dislodgment of clot.
   a. Monitor closely for clinical indications of DVT.
      1) Low-grade fever
      2) Calf pain or tenderness
      3) Unilateral edema, erythema, warmth, or dilated collateral veins
      4) Positive venography, venous duplex, and/or compression ultrasonography
   b. Instruct the patient regarding avoidance of Valsalva maneuver.
   c. Maintain steady IV flow rates.
   d. Avoid leg massage.
   e. Avoid bed rest for DVT unless there is substantial pain and swelling (Tapson, 2008).

3. Maintain adequate airway, ventilation, and oxygenation.
   a. Administer oxygen to maintain SpO_2 greater than 90%.
      1) Nasal cannula at 5 L/min unless contraindicated
      2) High concentrations of O_2 via non-rebreathing mask may be required to maintain an SpO_2 greater than ~90%.
   b. Administer analgesics as prescribed to prevent splinting and encourage deep breathing.
   c. Provide quiet, restful environment.
   d. Ensure intubation and mechanical ventilation if required.
      1) The primary initial problem in PE is diffusion due to the perfusion defect; the patient is generally ventilating adequately initially (frequently even excessively as evidenced by a low $PaCO_2$) but may require intubation and mechanical ventilation as respiratory muscle fatigue occurs.

4. Arrest thrombosis and reestablish perfusion.
   a. Obtain baseline clotting profile.
   b. Administer fibrinolytic therapy as prescribed.
      1) Indications
         a) Hypodynamic instability
         b) Acute right ventricular failure
         c) Significant hypoxemia despite optimal oxygen therapy
      2) Actions
         a) Dissolves recent clots promptly to speed pulmonary tissue reperfusion
         b) Reverses right ventricular failure
         c) Improves pulmonary capillary blood volume
      3) Possible agents and typical dose (van Es et al., 2010)
         a) Tissue plasminogen activator (tPA): alteplase (Activase) 100 mg over 2 hours
         b) Streptokinase: 250,000 units IV during the initial 30 minutes, then 100,000 units/hr for 24 hours
         c) Urokinase: 4400 units/kg IV during the initial 10 minutes, then 4400 units/kg/hr for 12 hours
      4) Contraindications and nursing management as in MI section of Chapter 3
      5) Anticoagulation follows fibrinolytic therapy.
   c. Administer anticoagulants as prescribed for stable patients.
      1) Action: prevents extension of the clot and reocclusion
      2) Parenteral agents: usually maintained for 7-10 days
         a) Fondaparinux (Arixtra): a factor Xa inhibitor
            i) Dose administered subcutaneously
               (a) Body weight less than 50 kg: 5 mg
               (b) Body weight 50-100 kg: 7.5 mg
               (c) Body weight greater than 100 kg: 10 mg
            ii) Advantages
               (a) Lower risk of heparin-induced thrombocytopenia (HIT) than with heparin
               (b) Lower risk of major bleeding than with heparin
         b) Low-molecular-weight heparin (LMWH): indirect thrombin inhibitor

i) Agents
(a) Enoxaparin (Lovenox): 1 mg/kg subcutaneously every 12 hours
ii) Advantages
(a) Longer plasma half-life than unfractionated heparin (UFH)
(b) More predictable anticoagulant response to weight-adjusted doses than UFH
(c) No need to monitor clotting studies though monitoring is indicated in patients who are morbidly obese, have renal insufficiency, or who weigh less than 50 kg
(d) Lower incidence of heparin-induced thrombocytopenia (HIT)
iii) Potential disadvantage: longer half-life and lesser reversibility with protamine than UFH
c) Unfractionated heparin (UFH): indirect thrombin inhibitor
i) Dose: bolus 70-80 units/kg initially, followed by 15-20 units/kg/hr to maintain aPTT 60-80 seconds; higher doses may be necessary initially due to low antithrombin III levels after PE
d) For patients with heparin-induced thrombocytopenia (HIT) (also referred to as *heparin-associated thrombocytopenia* or *white clot syndrome*)
i) Lepirudin (Refludan)
ii) Argatroban
3) Oral agent: warfarin
a) Started 3-4 days before parenteral anticoagulants are discontinued and continued for up to 6 months
b) Usual starting dose is 5 mg daily and adjusted to maintain INR 2-3
d. Prepare patient for pulmonary embolectomy as requested: indicated for patient with massive PE with hemodynamic instability (e.g., cardiogenic shock) and cannot receive fibrinolytic therapy
1) Surgical embolectomy
a) Complication rates for pulmonary embolectomy are relatively very high
b) Requires cardiopulmonary bypass
2) Catheter embolectomy
a) Clot fragmentation using pigtail catheter
b) Rheolytic thrombectomy using high-velocity saline jet (e.g., AngioJet)
c) Clot aspiration (e.g., transluminal extraction catheter)
e. Prepare patient for insertion of inferior vena cava filter as requested.
1) Indications
a) Recurrent PE despite effective anticoagulation
b) Anticoagulants are contraindicated.
c) Note that these are effective in protecting the lung from successive emboli but they do not do anything about the current PE.
2) Types
a) Vena caval umbrella
b) Greenfield filter
c) Bird's nest filter (does not require precise axial orientation)
f. Provide treatment of pulmonary hypertension and acute right ventricular failure as prescribed.
1) First priority is elimination of the pulmonary vascular obstruction and reduction of PVR: fibrinolytics, embolectomy
2) Inotropes (e.g., dobutamine [Dobutrex]) and fluids may also be prescribed to ensure adequate left ventricular contractility and filling volume.
g. Administer antibiotics as prescribed for septic emboli (rather than fibrinolytics and anticoagulants).
5. Monitor for complications.
a. Pulmonary infarction
b. Cerebral infarction
c. Myocardial infarction
d. Right ventricular failure
e. Dysrhythmias or blocks
1) Atrial dysrhythmias are common if RVF occurs.
2) Ventricular dysrhythmias may occur in hypoxemia.
3) RBBB may occur but is usually transient.
f. Hepatic congestion and necrosis
g. Pneumonia
h. Pulmonary abscess
i. Acute respiratory distress syndrome
j. Disseminated intravascular coagulation
k. Shock
l. Complications of therapy
1) Bleeding related to fibrinolytic or anticoagulant therapy
2) Oxygen toxicity related to high concentrations of oxygen
6. Specific to fat embolism
a. Prevention: early immobilization of long-bone fractures
b. Treatment
1) Oxygen via nasal cannula at 5 L/min unless contraindicated; 100% non-rebreathing mask may be necessary to maintain SpO_2 of at least 95%
2) Intubation and mechanical ventilation may be necessary.
3) Steroids (e.g., hydrocortisone) to decrease inflammatory response (controversial)
4) Fluids to flush the fatty acids and prevent renal damage

5) Osmotic diuretics: if pulmonary edema is present
6) Red blood cells and/or platelets may be necessary
7. Specific to air embolism
a. Prevention
1) Priming of intravenous tubing and central catheters with fluid to remove air prior to connection or insertion
2) Use of intravenous pumps with air detectors
3) Use of twist-lock connections on central venous catheters to prevent accidental disconnections
4) Positioning of patient in Trendelenburg position for the insertion of central venous catheters or treatment of chest trauma unless contraindicated (e.g., head trauma)
5) Instruction of the patient to hold his or her breath and bear down (i.e., Valsalva maneuver) during tubing changes and catheter removal
6) Use of pressure dressing to central venous site at time of catheter removal
b. Treatment
1) Left lateral decubitus position with head down (referred to as *Durant's maneuver*) if air embolism suspected
2) Attempt to aspirate the air embolus
3) External cardiac compressions push air out of the right ventricle into the pulmonary circulation, fragmenting the air bolus into smaller air bubbles.
4) Oxygen via 100% non-rebreathing mask; hyperbaric oxygen is indicated for arterial embolization and clinical deterioration
5) Anticoagulants may be administered.

Chest Trauma

General Information

1. Types of trauma
a. Blunt trauma leaves the body surface intact.
b. Penetrating trauma disrupts the body surface.
c. Perforating trauma leaves both entrance and exit wounds as an object passes through the body.
2. Etiology
a. Motor vehicle collision
b. Motorcycle collision
c. Vehicle/pedestrian collision
d. Fall
e. Assault
f. Explosion (blast injury)
g. Projectiles: bullet, knives, impalement
3. Mechanisms of injury
a. Blunt chest trauma
1) Rapid acceleration/deceleration: Shearing force causes stretching of tissue, organs, blood vessels with resultant tearing, leaking, or rupture.
2) Direct impact: Object striking chest or chest striking object causes rib, sternal, or scapular fractures, injury to the heart or lung parenchyma.
3) Compression: Force of rapid deceleration as tissues hit a fixed object, such as the sternum or rib cage, causes concussion, contusion, bleeding, or rupture of an organ.
b. Penetrating chest trauma
1) Penetration of lung, heart, great vessel, or diaphragm causes bleeding and may cause loss of intactness of an organ or vessel.

Pulmonary Contusion

1. Definition: damage to the lung parenchyma that results in localized edema and hemorrhage
2. Etiology
a. High-velocity blunt trauma dispersed across the chest; occurs in approximately 75% of blunt trauma patients
b. Crush injuries
c. Chest compressions during cardiopulmonary resuscitation
d. Frequently associated with other chest injuries (e.g., flail chest)
3. Pathophysiology
a. Blunt trauma causes deceleration injury to chest wall and compression of thoracic cavity.
b. Diminished thoracic size compresses lung tissue, and decompression causes capillary rupture and subsequent hemorrhage.
c. Initial hemorrhage due to bruising, pulmonary tears, lacerations
1) Interstitial and alveolar edema at site of contusion
2) Massive interstitial edema with general inflammation
3) Damaged or closed alveolar-capillary units cause ventilation/perfusion mismatch and shunt.
4) Increased pulmonary vascular resistance (PVR), decreased lung compliance, and decreased pulmonary blood flow occur.
5) Atelectasis may occur due to retained secretions and infection.
d. Severe pulmonary lacerations may cause concurrent hemothorax.
e. Pulmonary contusion may accompany flail chest and may be masked by the obvious ventilation difficulties seen in flail chest.
4. Clinical presentation (may be delayed 24-48 hours)
a. Subjective
1) Anxiety, restlessness
2) Dyspnea
3) Chest tenderness
b. Objective
1) Tachycardia
2) Tachypnea
3) Increased work of breathing: use of accessory muscles; tripod position
4) Ecchymosis at site of impact
5) Ineffective cough, guarding
6) Hemoptysis

7) Crepitus or deformity noted on palpation if rib fractures
8) Subcutaneous emphysema: suggests concurrent pneumothorax or upper airway injury
9) Dullness to percussion on affected side
10) Breath sound changes: crackles, wheezes

c. Diagnostic
1) Arterial blood gases
a) Decreased PaO_2
b) $PaCO_2$ may be normal or decreased depending on ventilation pattern (e.g., may be low due to hyperventilation or high if pain or fatigue causes hypoventilation).
2) Chest x-ray
a) Changes may take 2-24 hours to develop on chest x-ray: patchy, poorly defined areas of increased parenchymal density reflecting intraalveolar hemorrhage; linear and irregular infiltrates in the bronchioles
b) If severe, extensive areas of increased parenchymal density within one or both lungs
c) Diaphragm may be lower on affected side as injured lung is bigger.
d) To differentiate ARDS from pulmonary contusion
i) Pulmonary contusion is usually localized and occurs near the site of external trauma.
ii) ARDS causes diffuse bilateral changes.
3) CT scan: assesses damage to pulmonary parenchyma and pleural cavity

5. Collaborative management
a. Establish and maintain airway, ventilation, and oxygenation.
1) Oxygen per nasal cannula at 2-6 L/min to achieve a SpO_2 greater than 95% unless contraindicated; if patient has history of COPD, administer oxygen to achieve an oxygen saturation of ~90% by pulse oximetry
2) Analgesics in doses adequate to allow patient to turn and deep breathe
3) Airway clearance
a) Suctioning if patient cannot cough adequately to clear airways
b) Bronchoscopy may be necessary if airway clearance techniques are inadequate.
4) Endotracheal intubation and mechanical ventilation with PEEP may be necessary.
a) Synchronous independent lung ventilation may be necessary to prevent the detrimental effects of PEEP on the normal alveoli (e.g., increased alveolar pressure and decreased blood flow).
i) Requires double-lumen endotracheal tube and two mechanical ventilators
5) Positioning with good lung down
6) Careful fluid administration to prevent pulmonary edema
a) Goal is usually to maintain RAP ~4 mm Hg and PAOP ~10 mm Hg.
b) Diuretics may also be given.
7) Steroids were given frequently in the past but are no longer recommended due to the risk of resultant immunosuppression and infection.

b. Control pain.
1) Narcotics given on a regular schedule
2) Intercostal nerve block
3) Epidural analgesic with a basal rate and PCA

c. Monitor for complications.
1) Pneumonia: very common complication
a) Prophylactic antibiotics are not recommended; antibiotics are indicated only if infection is present.
b) Culture sputum as indicated
2) Lung abscess
3) Empyema
4) Pulmonary edema
5) Pulmonary embolism
6) Acute respiratory distress syndrome

Closed (Noncommunicating) Pneumothorax (Figure 5-7)

1. Definition: Air enters the intrapleural space through the lung, causing partial or total collapse of the lung.
a. Small: less than 15%
b. Medium: 15-60%
c. Large: greater than 60%

2. Etiology
a. Primary: related to congenital bleb (common in endomorphic males, age 20-40 years)
b. Secondary
1) Emphysematous bullous
2) Tuberculosis
3) Lung cancer
c. Traumatic
1) Blunt trauma caused by motor vehicle collision, falls, blows to chest, blast injuries
2) Cardiopulmonary resuscitation
3) Positive pressure mechanical ventilator
d. Iatrogenic causes: central venous catheterization via subclavian or low jugular vein puncture; intracardiac injection; thoracentesis; positive pressure ventilation

3. Pathophysiology
a. Disruption of normal negative intrapleural pressure
1) Lung laceration by rib fracture or needle
2) Compression of the lung at the height of inspiration when alveolar pressure is high

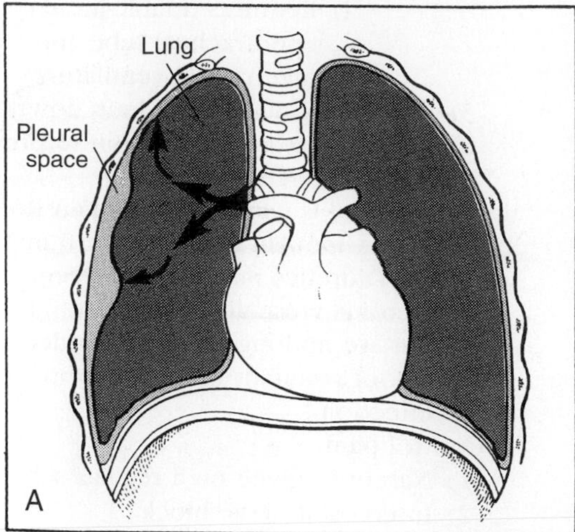

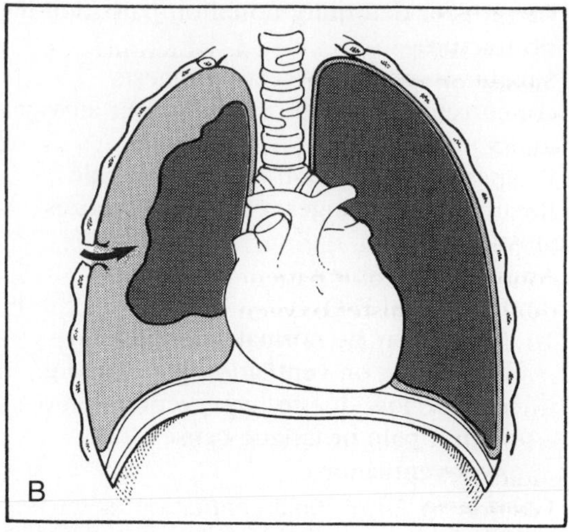

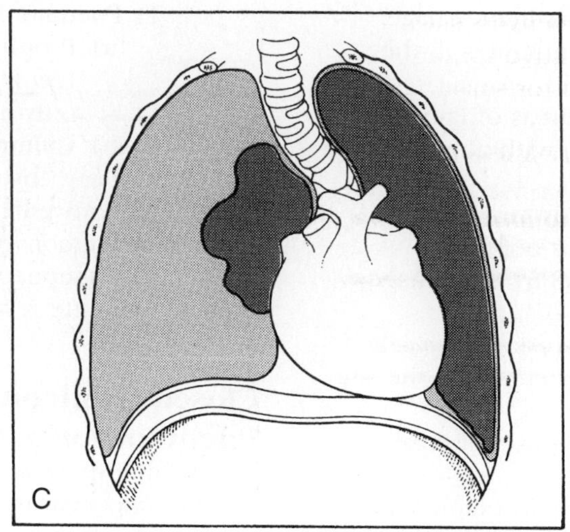

Figure 5-7 Pneumothorax. **A,** Closed. **B,** Open. **C,** Tension. (From Wilson, T. [1990]. *Respiratory disorders [Mosby's clinical nursing series].* St. Louis: Mosby.)

3) Rupture of weak alveolus, bleb, or bullous

b. Lung collapse
c. Decreased surface area for exchange of gases
d. Acute respiratory failure

4. Clinical presentation
   a. Subjective
      1) Dyspnea
      2) Chest pain: sudden, sharp, may be referred to corresponding shoulder, across chest, or abdomen
   b. Objective
      1) Tachycardia
      2) Tachypnea
      3) Cough: dry, nonproductive
      4) Asymmetrical chest excursion with limited motion of affected hemithorax
      5) Subcutaneous emphysema possible
      6) Decreased fremitus on affected side
      7) Hyperresonance to percussion on affected side
      8) Diminished to absent breath sounds on affected side
      9) Clinical indications of hypoxemia may be present
      10) If patient on mechanical ventilator
         a) Dramatic increase in peak inspiratory pressures
         b) High pressure alarm
   c. Diagnostic
      1) Arterial blood gases
         a) Decreased PaO_2
         b) Increased $PaCO_2$
      2) Chest x-ray
         a) Air in pleural space and lung collapse on affected side
         b) May show mediastinal shift toward unaffected side

3) CT of thorax: better at detecting very small or anterior pneumothorax, which may be missed on chest x-ray

5. Collaborative management
   a. Establish and maintain airway, ventilation, and oxygenation.
      1) Oxygen per nasal cannula at 1-6 L/min to achieve a SpO_2 greater than 95% unless contraindicated; if patient has history of COPD, administer oxygen to achieve an oxygen saturation of ~90% by pulse oximetry
      2) Analgesics in doses adequate to allow patient to deep breathe and cough as indicated
      3) Positioning for optimal ventilation: semi-Fowler's or Fowler's position
         a) If supine: position with good lung down
      4) Sustained inspiratory maneuvers such as deep breathing and incentive spirometry; only necessary treatment for small (less than 15%) pneumothorax
      5) Chest tube (not necessary if less than 15% and asymptomatic)
         a) Inserted into fourth to fifth intercostal space at midaxillary line
         b) Connected to a Heimlich flutter valve or chest drainage system
   b. Control pain: narcotics given on a regular schedule
   c. Monitor for complications
      1) Recurrent pneumothorax
         a) Avoidance of IPPB in patients with COPD
         b) If positive pressure mechanical ventilation: careful adjustment of tidal volume and PEEP; close monitoring of peak inspiratory pressures
         c) Careful placement of subclavian or jugular venous catheters
         d) Decortication may be performed for patients with recurrent spontaneous pneumothorax; involves the stripping of the parietal pleura from the apex of the lung to allow the visceral pleura to adhere to the chest wall
      2) Atelectasis
      3) Pneumonia, abscess

Tension Pneumothorax (Figure 5-8)

1. Definition: accumulation of air in pleural space without means of escape causing complete collapse of lung and potential mediastinal shift
2. Etiology
   a. Blunt or penetrating trauma
   b. Positive pressure mechanical ventilation, especially if patient:
      1) Has emphysematous bullae or congenital blebs
      2) Receiving large tidal volumes and/or PEEP
   c. Nonfunctional (e.g., clotted or clamped) chest drainage system
   d. Occlusive dressing on an open pneumothorax
3. Pathophysiology
   a. Air rushes into, but not out of, the pleural space.
   b. Disruption of negative intrapleural pressure; creation of a positive pressure in the pleural space
   c. Ipsilateral lung collapses
   d. If tear does not seal, a one-way valve effect may be produced, allowing air to enter during inspiration but not to escape during exhalation.
   e. Increasing positive intrapleural pressure may cause mediastinal shift leading to compression of the contralateral lung, thoracic aorta, vena cava, and heart.
   f. Decreased right ventricular filling, decreased cardiac output
   g. Acute respiratory failure and shock may occur.
4. Clinical presentation
   a. Subjective
      1) Dyspnea
      2) Chest pain

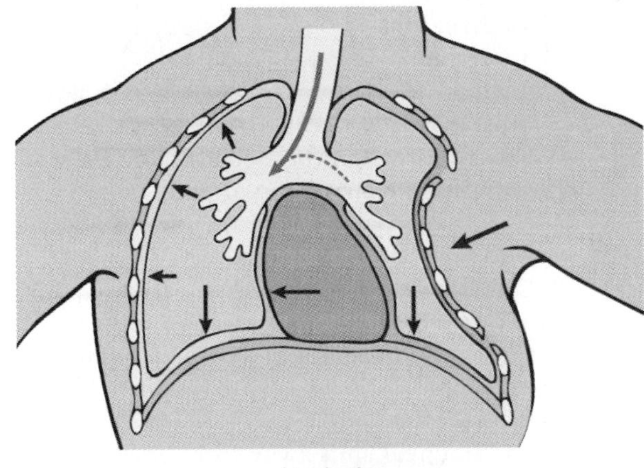

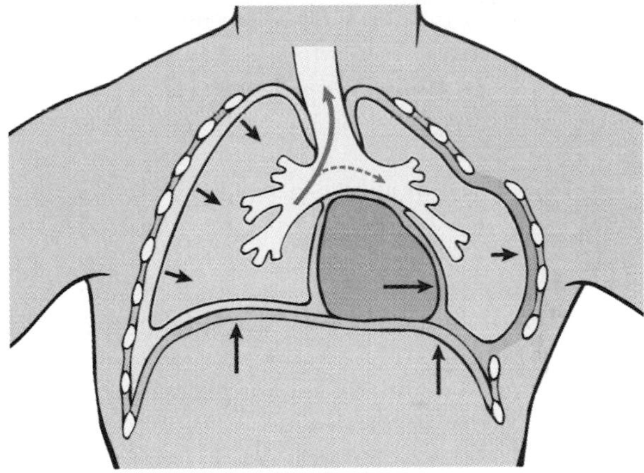

Figure 5-8 Flail chest produces paradoxical chest excursion. On inspiration, the flail section sinks in. On expiration, the flail section bulges outward.

b. Objective
   1) Tachycardia
   2) Tachypnea
   3) Asymmetrical chest excursion with limited motion of affected hemithorax
   4) Subcutaneous emphysema possible
   5) Decreased fremitus on affected side
   6) Hyperresonance to percussion on affected side; may even be tympanic
   7) Diminished to absent breath sounds on affected side
   8) Clinical indications of hypoxemia may be present.
   9) If mediastinal shift:
      a) Tracheal shift away from affected side
      b) Point of maximal impulse (PMI) shift away from affected side
      c) Jugular venous distention
      d) Hypotension
c. Diagnostic
   1) Arterial blood gases
      a) Decreased PaO_2
      b) Increased $PaCO_2$
   2) Chest x-ray
      a) Absence of lung marking on the affected side
      b) Widening of the intercostal spaces on the affected side
      c) Mediastinal shift (away from the affected side) may be present.

5. Collaborative management
   a. Establish and maintain airway, ventilation, and oxygenation.
      1) Oxygen per nasal cannula at 2-5 L/min to achieve a SpO_2 greater than 95% unless contraindicated; if patient has history of COPD, administer oxygen to achieve an oxygen saturation of ~90% by pulse oximetry
      2) Emergency decompression with perpendicular insertion of a large-bore needle (or IV catheter [e.g., Angiocath]) into second anterior interspace at the midclavicular line on the affected side until a chest tube can be inserted; a flutter valve (e.g., Heimlich valve, finger cot with a slit cut at the end) may be placed on the needle to allow air to escape but prevent atmospheric air from entering the pleural space
      3) Chest tube and chest drainage system
      4) Analgesics in doses adequate to allow patient to deep breathe and cough as indicated
      5) Position for optimal ventilation: semi-Fowler's or Fowler's position
      6) If supine: position with good lung down
   b. Control pain: narcotics given on a regular schedule or by patient-controlled analgesia
   c. Monitor for complications.
      1) Shock
      2) Cardiopulmonary arrest
      3) Atelectasis
      4) Pneumonia, abscess

Open (Communicating) Pneumothorax (Also Called *Sucking Chest Wound*) (Figure 5-8)

1. Definition: Air enters the interpleural space through the chest wall.
2. Etiology: penetrating trauma
3. Pathophysiology
   a. Communication between the intrathoracic space and the atmosphere results in equilibrium between intrathoracic and atmospheric pressures.
   b. Air movement in and out of opening in chest wall
   c. If opening in chest wall is smaller than diameter of trachea, patient may tolerate condition well.
   d. If opening is larger, more air enters pleural space than enters lungs through trachea.
   e. During inspiration, the affected lung collapses, resulting in ineffective gas exchange.
   f. May cause tension pneumothorax
4. Clinical presentation
   a. Subjective
      1) Dyspnea
      2) Chest pain
   b. Objective
      1) Tachycardia
      2) Tachypnea
      3) Obvious wound with noise of air moving in and out of pleural space
      4) Subcutaneous emphysema is usually present.
   c. Other subjective, objective, and diagnostic findings as for closed pneumothorax
5. Collaborative management
   a. Establish and maintain airway, ventilation, and oxygenation.
      1) Oxygen per nasal cannula at 2-5 L/min to achieve a SpO_2 greater than 95% unless contraindicated; if patient has history of COPD, administer oxygen to achieve an oxygen saturation of ~90% by pulse oximetry
      2) Positioning for optimal ventilation: semi-Fowler's or Fowler's position; good lung down or back
      3) Closure of open sucking chest wound with gauze dressing taped on three sides so that air can escape during expiration
      4) Chest tube and water-seal drainage
      5) Analgesics in doses adequate to allow patient to deep breathe and cough as indicated
      6) Surgical intervention may be needed to explore and débride the wound.
   b. Control pain: narcotics given on a regular schedule

c. Monitor for complications.
   1) Tension pneumothorax
   2) Atelectasis
   3) Pneumonia, abscess

Hemothorax

1. Definition: accumulation of blood in pleural space, causing compression and collapse of the lung
2. Etiology
   a. Blunt or penetrating trauma to chest wall, lung tissue, or mediastinum
   b. Pleural or pulmonary neoplasm
   c. Anticoagulant therapy
   d. Iatrogenic causes: subclavian vein puncture (e.g., insertion of deep vein catheter), lung biopsy
3. Pathophysiology
   a. Hemorrhage into pleural space compresses and collapses lung.
   b. Ventilation and oxygenation are impaired.
   c. Hemorrhage may lead to shock.
4. Clinical presentation
   a. Subjective
      1) Chest pain may be present.
      2) Dyspnea
   b. Objective
      1) Tachycardia
      2) Hypotension
      3) Asymmetrical chest excursion with limited motion of affected hemithorax
      4) Dullness to percussion on affected side
      5) Diminished or absent breath sounds on affected side
      6) May have clinical indications of shock if greater than 400 mL
   c. Diagnostic
      1) Serum
         a) Hemoglobin and hematocrit: may be decreased but remember that changes may occur for up to 6 hours after blood loss
         b) Arterial blood gases
            i) Decreased PaO_2
            ii) Increased $PaCO_2$
      2) Chest x-ray
         a) Fluid in pleural space and lung compression
         b) Blunting of costophrenic angle if greater than 250 mL
         c) Hazy appearance over the lower chest
5. Collaborative management
   a. Establish and maintain airway, ventilation, and oxygenation.
      1) Oxygen per nasal cannula at 2-5 L/min to achieve a SpO_2 greater than 95% unless contraindicated; if patient has history of COPD, administer oxygen to achieve an oxygen saturation of ~90% by pulse oximetry
      2) Chest tube with chest drainage system may be adequate treatment if bleeding is self-limiting.
      3) Indications for surgery for isolation and repair of source of hemorrhage
         a) Initial drainage of more than 1500 mL of blood after placement of chest tube
         b) Drainage of blood at rate greater than 250 mL/hr for more than 2 hours after placement of chest tube
         c) Hemodynamic instability despite fluid resuscitation
      4) Positioning for optimal ventilation
         a) Semi-Fowler's or Fowler's position unless patient has significant hypotension with head of bed elevated
         b) After thoracotomy, nonoperative ("good") lung down or supine with regular turning
   b. Maintain perfusion and adequate circulating volume.
      1) Fluids and/or blood transfusion may be necessary.
      2) Autotransfusion may be indicated if blood loss is greater than 400 mL.
   c. Control pain: narcotics given on a regular schedule
   d. Monitor for complications
      1) Atelectasis
      2) Shock

Rib Fracture/Sternal Fracture/Flail Chest

1. Definition
   a. Rib fracture: break in the bony continuity of the ribs
   b. Sternal fracture: break in the bony continuity of the sternum
   c. Flail chest: instability of chest wall as a result of multiple rib or sternal fractures causing paradoxical movement of the chest wall during ventilation
      1) Two or more ribs broken in two or more places
      2) Fractured sternum
      3) Sternotomy that hasn't healed
2. Etiology
   a. Blunt trauma from motor vehicle collision, assault
   b. Relatively minor trauma in patients with the following:
      1) Osteoporosis
      2) Total sternectomy
      3) Multiple myeloma
3. Pathophysiology
   a. Rib fracture
      1) Fracture of the first and second rib is rare and requires extreme force so suspect underlying injury to great vessel, lungs, and spine
      2) If left lower rib fractures, suspect spleen injuries
      3) If right lower rib fractures, suspect hepatic injury

4) Elderly patients are more likely to have complications because they are likely to have senile emphysema and concurrent cardiopulmonary disease.

b. Sternal fracture
  1) Tremendous force (i.e., impact with steering wheel) required to cause sternal fracture
    a) This force may also cause myocardial contusion or cardiac tamponade.
  2) Most common location is the junction of the manubrium and body of the sternum.

c. Flail chest (Figure 5-8)
  1) Fractured segment is free of the bony thorax and moves independently in response to intrathoracic pressure.
    a) During inspiration, atmospheric pressure exceeds intrathoracic pressure on affected side, causing chest wall to move inward.
    b) On expiration, intrathoracic pressure exceeds atmospheric pressure, causing chest wall to move outward until the thorax contracts.
  2) The bellows effect of the thorax is lost; intrapleural pressure is less negative than normal.
  3) Ventilation is diminished; tidal volume is decreased, causing hypercapnia and resultant hypoxemia; atelectasis may occur.
  4) Increased work of breathing causes fatigue.
  5) Note related injuries: pulmonary contusion frequently accompanies flail chest; pneumothorax, pleural effusion may also be present

4. Clinical presentation
  a. Subjective
    1) Dyspnea
    2) Chest pain: related to inspiration, movement, coughing
    3) Chest tenderness to palpation
  b. Objective
    1) Tachycardia
    2) Tachypnea
    3) Diminished air movement at mouth and nose
    4) Ineffective cough
    5) Ecchymosis over thorax
    6) Paradoxical movement of flail segment
    7) Palpable detached segment, bony crepitation at fracture sites
    8) Subcutaneous emphysema with pneumothorax or laryngeal injury
    9) Breath sound changes: diminished breath sounds on affected side
    10) Clinical indications of hypoxia (see Box 4-3)
  c. Diagnostic
    1) Arterial blood gases
      a) Decreased PaO_2
      b) Decreased SaO_2
      c) Increased $PaCO_2$
    2) Spirometry: decreased tidal volume and vital capacity
    3) ECG: to assess for indications of myocardial contusion if sternal fracture
    4) Echocardiography: to assess for cardiac tamponade if sternal fracture
    5) Chest x-ray: rib and/or sternal fractures
    6) CT scan of chest: shows fractures

5. Collaborative management
  a. Establish and maintain airway, ventilation, and oxygenation.
    1) Oxygen per nasal cannula at 2-5 L/min to achieve a SpO_2 greater than 95% unless contraindicated; if patient has history of COPD, administer oxygen to achieve an oxygen saturation of ~90% by pulse oximetry
    2) Reestablishment of the thoracic bellows effect
      a) Stabilization of flail segment with hand or tape (temporary); avoid binding or constricting chest excursion
      b) Position on affected side if cervical spine fracture has been ruled out.
      c) Intubation and internal stabilization with mechanical ventilation may be necessary if patient cannot maintain adequate ventilation despite adequate analgesia.
        i) Indications: respiratory rate greater than 35, PaO_2 less than 60 mm Hg with supplemental oxygen; $PaCO_2$ greater than 50 mm Hg
        ii) Mechanical ventilation may need to be maintained for 3 weeks or longer
      d) Surgical internal fixation of rib and sternal fragments with plates and screws may be done for multiple rib fractures or flail chest, especially if thoracotomy is needed for another reason.
      e) Surgical reduction of displaced sternal fracture
    3) Chest physiotherapy
      a) Deep breathing and incentive spirometry
      b) Positioning for optimal ventilation: semi-Fowler's or Fowler's position
      c) Postural drainage, percussion, vibration
        i) Do not percuss over fractured areas.
      d) Coughing; suctioning if coughing is ineffective and rhonchi are present
      e) Bronchoscopy may be necessary if airway clearance is inadequate.
  b. Provide adequate analgesia to encourage deep breathing (and coughing if indicated).
    1) Epidural analgesia
    2) Intravenous narcotics
    3) Intercostal nerve blocks
    4) Intrapleural analgesia
  c. Assist in insertion of chest tube and establish water-seal drainage if pneumothorax is also present.

d. Monitor for complications.
   1) Pain
   2) Nonunion
   3) Permanent chest wall deformity
   4) Atelectasis
   5) Pneumonia, abscess

Diaphragmatic Rupture

1. Definition: rupture of the diaphragm allowing the movement of abdominal contents into the thorax
2. Etiology: injury below nipple line, in flanks, or lateral chest wall
   a. Blunt trauma from motor vehicle collision, assault, fall against an immobile object
   b. Penetrating injury such as from a gunshot or knife wound
   c. There may be a latent period after the injury.
3. Pathophysiology
   a. Opening in the diaphragm
      1) Blunt trauma
         a) More common on the left side because the left hemidiaphragm is weaker than the right and the right hemidiaphragm is somewhat protected by the liver
         b) A sudden, dramatic increase in abdominal or thoracic pressure causes a tear in the diaphragm.
      2) Penetrating trauma causes a perforation in the diaphragm.
   b. The intrathoracic pressure is negative while the intraabdominal pressure is positive.
   c. The size of the rupture determines the extent to which the organs migrate upward: the stomach and/or loops of intestine may enter the chest and compromise lung expansion.
   d. Ventilation problems are most evident if the left hemidiaphragm is affected because when the right hemidiaphragm is affected the liver is fixed and cannot move upward into the thorax.
      1) Abdominal contents compress the lung on the affected side and may even cause mediastinal shift.
      2) The decrease in the effectiveness of the diaphragm causes ineffective ventilatory excursion.
4. Clinical presentation
   a. Subjective
      1) Dyspnea
      2) Dysphagia
      3) May have nausea, eructation
      4) Pain in shoulder, chest or abdomen
         a) Kehr's sign: pain radiates to left shoulder (as a result of injury to the phrenic nerve)
         b) Exacerbated by supine position
   b. Objective
      1) Obvious injury to chest, abdomen
      2) Ecchymosis
      3) Tachypnea
      4) Tachycardia, hypotension
      5) Crepitus or deformity on palpation
      6) JVD if a mediastinal shift occurs
      7) Heart sounds may be shifted to opposite side of the injury.
      8) Diminished or absent breath sounds on the affected side
      9) Abdominal distention
      10) Bowel sounds audible over the affected side of the chest
      11) If chest tubes are placed for another condition, may see fecal matter or undigested food in the chest drainage system
   c. Diagnostic
      1) Chest x-ray
         a) Normal if no abdominal contents displaced in chest
         b) May have unilateral elevation of hemidiaphragm
         c) May have hollow or solid mass above the diaphragm (the stomach) may be visible
         d) May have mediastinal shift away from affected side
         e) May place nasogastric tube prior to x-ray, and tube will be seen in the chest
      2) CT of the chest and abdomen
         a) Confirms rupture of the diaphragm and any movement of abdominal contents into the thorax
         b) Focused assessment sonography trauma (FAST): indicates if intraabdominal fluid is present
5. Collaborative management
   a. Establish and maintain airway, ventilation, and oxygenation.
      1) Oxygen by nasal cannula at 2-6 L/min to maintain SpO_2 of 95% unless contraindicated; in patients with COPD, use pulse oximetry to guide oxygen administration to SpO_2 of 90%
      2) Elevation of head of bed to 30-45 degrees; overbed table may be helpful for patient to lean on.
      3) Surgical intervention to pull the abdominal organs back into the abdomen and repair the diaphragm; prophylactic antibiotics will be prescribed
      4) Chest tube and drainage system as required for pneumothorax
      5) Deep breathing and incentive spirometry to prevent atelectasis
      6) Nasogastric tube placement to decompress the stomach
   b. Maintain adequate circulation.
      1) IV access for fluid and medication administration
      2) Hydration
         a) Intravenous fluids: usually 0.9% saline
         b) Avoidance of overhydration because the patient may have associated pulmonary contusion and be at risk for ARDS

c. Control pain, discomfort, and anxiety.
 1) Nonsteroidal antiinflammatory agents and/or narcotic analgesics in doses which will allow patient to deep breathe and cough may be indicated.
 2) Anxiolytics may be indicated.
d. Monitor for complications.
 1) Atelectasis
 2) Pneumonia, abscess
 3) Bowel strangulation
 4) Tension viscerothorax: chest tube is indicated
 5) Sepsis
 6) Shock

Tracheobronchial Injury

1. Definition: disruption in the integrity of the tracheobronchial tree; usually occurs at the proximal trachea or near the carina
2. Predisposing factors
 a. Blunt trauma (e.g., MVC, clothesline injury): most common cause resulting in a partial or complete tear of the tracheal or bronchial wall
 b. Deceleration injuries: can cause shearing forces between the fixed carina or proximal bronchus
 c. Rapid anteroposterior compression of the chest: can cause lateral traction on the lungs resulting in a tearing of the bronchus from the fixed carina
  1) Rupture can occur from an abrupt increase in pressure against a closed glottis.
 d. Compression of the trachea between the sternum and spinal column
 e. Penetrating trauma
3. Pathophysiology
 a. Injury causes a tear of the bronchial tree
 b. Ineffective ventilation as inspired air escapes into the thoracic cavity and does not reach the lungs
 c. Swelling can cause airway obstruction.
 d. Severity of symptoms related to the level of the injury, degree of injury, and airflow changes that occur
4. Clinical presentation
 a. Subjective
  1) History of trauma; injury may go unrecognized for 3-4 days
  2) Pain that increases with breathing and swallowing
  3) Dyspnea
 b. Objective
  1) Tachycardia
  2) Tachypnea
  3) Clinical indications of respiratory distress (see Box 4-2)
   a) Sitting up and leaning forward
   b) Use of inspiratory accessory muscles in neck and shoulders
  4) Hoarse voice
  5) May have stridor
  6) Hemoptysis
  7) Chest contusion, ecchymosis, or wound
  8) Altered level of consciousness
  9) Subcutaneous emphysema palpated in the chest, face, neck, and/or suprasternal area
  10) Breath sound changes: decreased or absent on the affected side
  11) Hamman's sign: mediastinal crunch associated with pneumomediastinum
  12) Persistent air leak from chest tube
 c. Diagnostic
  1) ABGs: may show hypoxemia
  2) Radiography
   a) Soft tissue lateral neck films
   b) Chest: pneumomediastinum below the carina
  3) Bronchoscopy: direct visualization of injury
5. Collaborative management
 a. Establish and maintain airway, ventilation, and oxygenation.
  1) Once tracheobronchial injury confirmed, prepare for RSI and intubation even if no evidence of respiratory compromise
   a) Placement of endotracheal tube below the level of injury
   b) Cricothyrotomy or emergent tracheostomy may be required.
  2) Oxygen by nasal cannula at 2-6 L/min to maintain SpO_2 of 95% unless contraindicated; in patients with COPD, use pulse oximetry to guide oxygen administration to SpO_2 of 90%
  3) Elevation of head of bed to 30 to 45 degrees
  4) Open chest wounds should be covered; remove if clinical indications of tension pneumothorax occur.
  5) Thoracotomy for surgical repair
  6) Deep breathing and incentive spirometry to prevent atelectasis
  7) Nasogastric tube placement to decompress the stomach
 b. Maintain adequate circulation.
  1) IV access for fluid and medication administration
  2) Hydration
   a) Intravenous fluids: usually 0.9% saline
   b) Warming of fluids, especially if patient is hypothermic
 c. Control pain, discomfort, and anxiety.
  1) Nonsteroidal antiinflammatory agents and/or narcotic analgesics in doses which will allow patient to deep breathe and cough may be indicated.
  2) Anxiolytics may be indicated.
 d. Monitor for complications.
  1) Airway obstruction
  2) Acute respiratory failure
  3) Shock

LEARNING ACTIVITIES

1. Complete the following crossword puzzle regarding thoracic surgery and trauma.

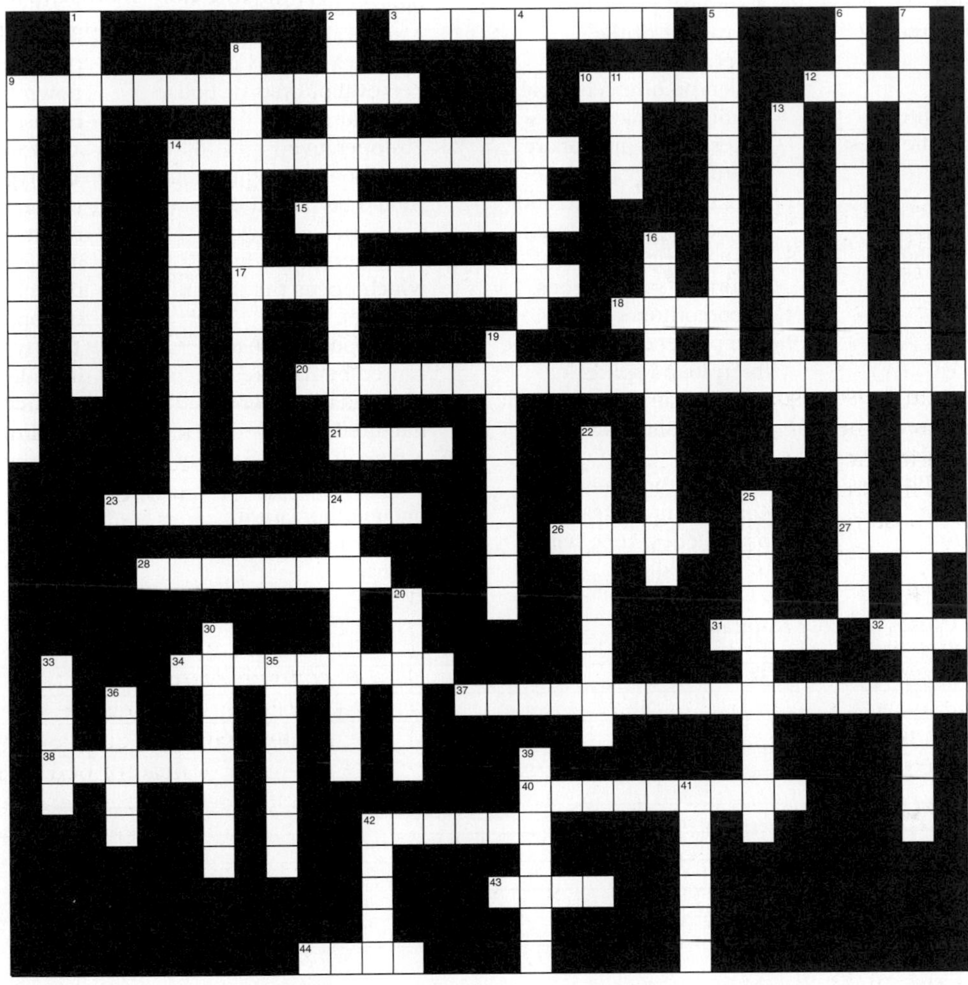

ACROSS

3. Rupture of this structure may cause bowel sounds to be heard over the thorax
9. A surgical procedure to remove an entire lung
10. This type of trauma can cause injury due to acceleration/deceleration, direct impact, or compression
12. Patients with unilateral lung conditions (except pneumonectomy) should be placed on their _____ lung or their back
14. A surgical procedure to decrease the volume in a hemithorax after lung resection to prevent mediastinal shift
15. Edema and hemorrhage of the lung parenchyma caused by trauma is referred to as a pulmonary _____
17. The presence of lymph fluid in the interpleural space
18. _____'s sign may be evident in diaphragmatic rupture
20. A connection between the bronchus and the pleura which causes a persistent air leak (2 words)
21. Another term for reduction pneumoplasty; used for emphysema (abbrev.)
23. A surgical procedure used in patients with myasthenia gravis
26. When two or more ribs are fractured or the sternum is fractured, a _____ chest results
27. The type of pneumothorax that creates a sucking sound as the patient breathes
28. Patients with diaphragmatic rupture may have referred pain to the left _____
31. A type of sonography frequently used for trauma patients to quickly identify possible injuries (abbrev.)
32. A chest tube that is placed anterior and superior is intended to remove _____
34. A surgical procedure to remove a segment of the lung is referred to as a *segmental* _____
37. The presence of air and blood in the interpleural space; frequently surgically induced

38. This type of dysrhythmia is common after pneumonectomy
40. Crepitus around the chest tube insertion site indicates subcutaneous _____
42. Arm and shoulder exercises after thoracotomy are recommended to reduce the chance of _____ shoulder
43. To successively squeeze and then release the chest tube tubing to try to improve patency
44. Patients with pulmonary contusion are at high risk for _____ (abbrev.)

DOWN

1. A surgical procedure to remove hyperinflated areas of the lung done for patients with COPD; may also be called *lung volume reduction surgery*
2. Internal air leak indicates _____ fistula
4. The presence of blood in the interpleural space
5. This type of analgesia involves injection of a local anesthetic through a thoracostomy tube or catheter
6. A surgical procedure for cancer of the esophagus
7. This type of mechanical ventilation may be necessary in pulmonary contusion because one lung may be injured and the other not (3 words)
8. Pleural stripping for recurrent spontaneous pneumothorax
9. The presence of air in the interpleural space
11. Bubbling in the water-seal chamber indicates an air _____
13. _____ in the water-seal chamber indicates a patent chest tube with transmission of interpleural pressures to the chamber
14. The process of inserting a chest tube; may be open or closed
16. The process of fusing the two layers of the pleura by injecting an agent such as sterile talc into the interpleural space
19. A surgical procedure to remove a lobe of a lung
22. Removal of cysts or bullae in the lung
24. Postoperative pneumonectomy patients should be placed on their _____ side or back
25. A surgical procedure which opens the thorax
29. The type of pneumothorax that is caused by rupture of a congenital bleb or a fractured rib
30. A type of valve that may be used for pneumothorax with little or no liquid drainage
33. Epidural analgesia after thoracotomy should include a _____ rate as well as patient-controlled analgesia
35. The presence of pus in the interpleural space
36. To hold the chest tube with thumb and forefinger of one hand and then slide the other thumb and forefinger down the tube and then release the first thumb and forefinger
39. The type of pneumothorax that results when pressure in the chest increases and the mediastinum shifts to the opposite side
41. This type of resection includes anastomosis of the airway proximal and distal to where the mass was removed
42. A chest tube that is placed lateral and inferior is intended to remove _____

2. List 10 possible causes of acute respiratory failure.

a. ______________________________

b. ______________________________

c. ______________________________

d. ______________________________

e. ______________________________

f. ______________________________

g. ______________________________

h. ______________________________

i. ______________________________

j. ______________________________

3. Match the cause of acute respiratory failure to the primary treatment.

___ 1. Upper airway obstruction	a. Antimicrobials
___ 2. Airway secretions	b. Deep breathing and incentive spirometry
___ 3. Overdosage of narcotics	c. Chest tube
___ 4. Bronchospasm	d. Positioning and airway placement
___ 5. Pneumothorax	e. Cholinergic drugs and mechanical ventilator
___ 6. Pneumonia	f. Encouragement of coughing; suctioning if cannot effectively cough
___ 7. Postoperative pain	g. PEEP
___ 8. ARDS	h. Bronchodilators
___ 9. Myasthenic crisis	i. Naloxone (Narcan)
___ 10. Atelectasis	j. Analgesics

4. Answer the following questions and explain your logic with a clinical example.
   a. If the PaO_2 is decreased, must the $PaCO_2$ be increased?

   ____

   ____

   b. If the $PaCO_2$ is increased, must the PaO_2 be decreased?

   ____

   ____

5. List five pulmonary and five nonpulmonary causes for acute respiratory distress syndrome (ARDS).

Pulmonary	Nonpulmonary
a.	f.
b.	g.
c.	h.
d.	i.
e.	j.

6. Match the treatment to the pathophysiology of ARDS. Choices may be used more than once.

____ 1. Pulmonary hypertension	a. PEEP
____ 2. Intrapulmonary shunt	b. Nitric oxide
____ 3. Ventilation/perfusion mismatch	c. Fluid restriction and diuretics
____ 4. Diffusion defect	d. High concentrations of oxygen
____ 5. Pulmonary edema	e. Prone positioning

7. Identify whether the following microorganisms are associated with community-acquired pneumonia (CAP) or health care-acquired pneumonia (HCAP). Choices may be used more than once.

Staphylococcus aureus	
Serratia marcescens	
Escherichia coli	
Legionella pneumophila	
Proteus mirabilis	
Bacteroides fragilis	
Hantavirus	

8. List four nursing interventions to prevent aspiration in a patient on enteral feedings.

   1. ____

   ____

   2. ____

   ____

   3. ____

   ____

9. Complete the following table describing arterial blood gas changes in asthma using ↑ for increased, ↓ for decreased, or ↔ for no change.

Stage	PaO_2	$PaCO_2$	pH	Acid-Base Imbalance
I				
II				
III				
IV				

10. List four classifications of bronchodilators and an example of each.

Classification	Example
1.	
2.	
3.	
4.	

11. List three causes of pulmonary embolism in each of the following categories.

Hypercoagulability	Alteration In Blood Vessel	Venous Stasis

12. Match the treatment to the pathology in pulmonary embolism. Choices may be used more than once.

____ 1. Forward failure of left ventricle
____ 2. Pulmonary hypertension
____ 3. Occlusion of pulmonary blood supply
____ 4. Backward failure of right ventricle
____ 5. Low levels of antithrombin III
____ 6. V/Q mismatch

a. Pulmonary embolectomy
b. Dobutamine
c. Heparin
d. Tissue plasminogen activator (tPA)
e. Fluids
f. Oxygen

13. Identify whether the parameters in this case study are decreased, normal, or increased. Discuss implications and treatment goals.

The patient is a 65-year-old female admitted with a fractured hip. She had surgery 2 weeks ago. Earlier today she complained about chest pain, shortness of breath, and a feeling of doom. ABGs revealed respiratory alkalosis and hypoxemia. After she was transferred to the critical care unit, the physician inserted a pulmonary artery catheter to aid in diagnosis and evaluation of therapy. The patient's BSA is 1.6 m^2.

Parameter	↑, ↓, or Normal	Parameter	↑, ↓, or Normal
BP: 112/84 mm Hg		SV: 40 mL/beat	
MAP: 93 mm Hg		SI: 25 mL/m^2/beat	
HR 110 beats/min		SVR: 1364 dynes/sec/cm^{-5}	
RAP: 18 mm Hg		SVRI: 2182 dynes/sec/cm^{-5}	
PAP: 55/32 mm Hg		PVR: 618 dynes/sec/cm^{-5}	
PAm: 40 mm Hg		PVRI: 989 dynes/sec/cm^{-5}	
PAOP: 6 mm Hg		LVSWI: 30 g • m/m^2	
CO: 4.4 L/min		RVSWI: 7 g • m/m^2	
CI: 2.75 L/min/m^2		SvO_2: 58%	
SaO_2: 85% on 5 L/min by nasal cannula		DO_2I: 470 mL/min/m^2	

Implications and treatment goals: ____________________

____

____

____

____

____

____

14. Match the clinical presentation to the type of chest trauma.

___ 1. Pulmonary contusion
___ 2. Flail chest
___ 3. Simple pneumothorax
___ 4. Hemothorax
___ 5. Tension pneumothorax
___ 6. Diaphragmatic rupture

a. Chest pain, dyspnea, diminished breath sounds on affected side, hyperresonance to percussion, tracheal shift away from affected side
b. Chest pain, dyspnea, diminished breath sounds on affected side, hyperresonance to percussion, tracheal shift toward affected side
c. Ecchymosis at site of impact, chest tenderness, dyspnea, hemoptysis
d. Epigastric pain, dyspnea, dysphagia, bowel sounds audible over affected side of chest
e. Chest pain, dyspnea, diminished breath sounds on affected side, dullness to percussion
f. Chest tenderness, dyspnea, paradoxical chest movement

15. Complete the following crossword puzzle to review pulmonary drugs and therapies.

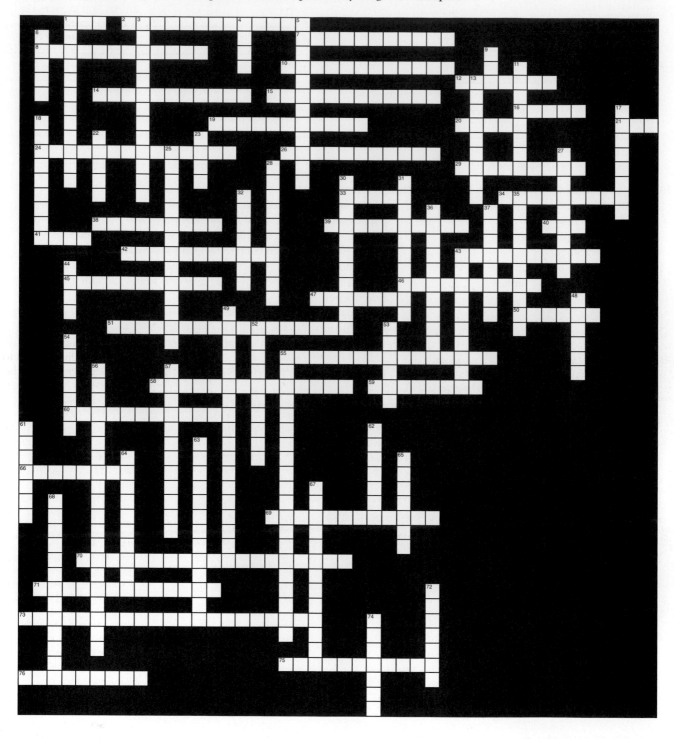

ACROSS

1. $PaCO_2$ of greater than 50 mm Hg and/or PaO_2 of less than 50-60 mm Hg (abbrev)
2. A drug that may be given in metabolic alkalosis; may cause metabolic acidosis
7. Inflammatory mediators including leukotrienes are released by _____ in ARDS
8. Pulmonary _____ is when the pulmonary vascular pressures are elevated
10. Results from release of erythropoietin in response to chronically low oxygen levels
12. A drug used to prevent extension or recurrence of a clot in patients with pulmonary embolism (generic)
14. Collapse of alveoli; frequently seen in postoperative patients
15. Pulmonary edema in ARDS is caused by increased capillary _____
16. The first treatment for asthma is the elimination of _____
19. This type of disorder is when expansion of the alveolus, lung, or chest wall is impaired and compliance is decreased
20. The most likely cause of ARDS
21. This may be caused by pulmonary hypertension (abbrev.)
24. A steroid that is frequently given by inhalation in patients with asthma (generic)
26. A $beta_2$ stimulant that may be given orally, subcutaneously, or by inhalation (generic)
29. Antibiotic _____ gram-positive bacterial strains have increased the mortality of health care-acquired pneumonia
33. Patient position recommended to optimize ventilation/perfusion matching in patients with ARDS
34. A pulmonary embolism would decrease _____ relative to ventilation
38. A drug used in patients with pulmonary embolism with acute right ventricular failure or refractory hypoxemia to break down the clot (generic)
39. Surfactant is produced by the type II _____
40. A decrease in surfactant would cause a decrease in compliance and an increase in _____ (abbrev)
41. Type of heparin that may be administered subcutaneously to prevent deep vein thrombosis and pulmonary embolism (abbrev)
42. Complication caused by hyperventilation in status asthmaticus
43. More likely to occur in the right lung
45. Treatment of pneumonia includes oxygen, bronchial hygiene, and _____
46. Drug used for stress ulcer prophylaxis that does not support gastric colonization (generic)
47. These sounds are heard when listening with a stethoscope to a patient with pneumonia or chronic bronchitis
50. Indicated when SaO_2 is less than 90%
51. This condition is characterized by an increase in the number and size of mucous and goblet cells
55. The cause of hypoxemia in myasthenia gravis would be alveolar _____
58. These receptors cause an increase in ventilation rate in response to body movement
59. A feeling of impending doom is a symptom of massive pulmonary _____
60. A prostanoid-type pulmonary vasodilator (generic)
66. Most community-acquired pneumonia caused by gram _____ bacteria
69. A procedure to view the bronchioles with a fiberoptic scope
70. This is caused by histamine
71. A diagnostic study to obtain fluid from the pleural space for analysis
73. This is caused by the decrease in PaO_2 in COPD, ARDS, and PE (2 words)
75. This type of disorder is when airway resistance is increased
76. This type of chest pain is sharp pain which occurs with deep inspiration

DOWN

1. IV antifungal (generic)
3. Fibrous exudate causes the _____ in pneumonia which is manifested by crackles, bronchial breath sounds, egophony, and whispered pectoriloquy
4. A form of noncardiac pulmonary edema caused by inflammatory mediators and surfactant deficiency (abbrev)
5. This type airway provides a relative seal to allow mechanical ventilation without the surgical risks of tracheostomy
6. When deoxygenated blood comes in contact with nonventilated alveoli; V less than Q
9. The most common pneumonia in AIDS patients (abbrev.)
11. These sounds are heard when listening with a stethoscope to a patient with atelectasis, pulmonary edema, and ARDS
13. This disorder is a chronic obstructive lung disease associated with the breakdown of elastic tissue, air trapping, and dyspnea
17. Chronic air _____ cause the shape of the thorax to change to be barrel-shaped
18. A $beta_2$ stimulant which is administered orally or by inhalation
22. Two common symptoms of pulmonary conditions are dyspnea and _____
23. The goal of oxygen therapy in this condition is to keep the SaO_2 at around 90% (abbrev.)
25. A drug that breaks down the disulfide bonds in mucus (generic)
27. Inflammation of the alveoli and bronchioles
28. A muscle paralytic that may be administered by IV infusion in patients on mechanical ventilation (generic)
30. This type of pneumothorax is most often associated with rupture of a congenital bleb
31. Bloody sputum; may be seen in lung cancer or tuberculosis
32. This habit is the No. 1 cause of COPD
35. Patients with obstructive disease have prolonged _____
36. Increased $PaCO_2$
37. A sedative frequently used in mechanically ventilated patients (generic)
43. Group of drugs that should be administered to allow a patient to breathe deeply after thoracotomy
44. The type of cell that secretes histamine
48. A gas which may be used in place of nitrogen in inspired air for patients with increased airway resistance
49. This diagnostic study is used to evaluate the adequacy of ventilation and oxygenation (3 words)
52. Another name for health care-acquired pneumonia
53. Also referred to as restrictive airway disease; mucosal swelling and smooth muscle spasm cause wheezing and increased airway resistance
54. These sounds are heard when listening with a stethoscope to a patient with asthma (plural)
55. Another term for type I acute respiratory failure (2 words)
56. Another term for type II acute respiratory failure (2 words)
57. An antibiotic which may be used to increase gastric motility (generic)
61. Shortness of breath
62. Placing a patient with an air embolism in a left lateral decubitus position

with his or her head down is referred to as _____ maneuver (possessive)

63. This level increases in asthma, causing bronchospasm and increased mucus secretion
64. Airway _____ affects the work of breathing
65. Testing sputum for _____ is a common method to check for aspiration of enteral feeding
67. Impaired _____ is the risk factor most commonly associated with aspiration
68. A xanthine bronchodilator; also dilates pulmonary vasculature (generic)
72. Shift of this structure is seen with mediastinal shift
74. _____'s triad are three things that predispose to clot formation: hypercoagulability, venous stasis, and vascular injury

The Neurologic System

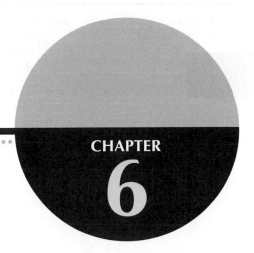

Selected Concepts in Anatomy and Physiology

General Information

1. Functions of the neurologic system
   a. Receiving stimuli from the internal and external environment over sensory pathways
   b. Communicating information between the body periphery and the central nervous system
   c. Processing information received at reflex or conscious levels to determine appropriate responses
   d. Transmitting information over motor pathways to organs responsible for responding to the stimuli
2. Components of the neurologic system
   a. Central nervous system (CNS)
      1) Brain
      2) Spinal cord
   b. Peripheral nervous system
      1) Cranial nerves
      2) Spinal nerves
      3) Peripheral nerves
   c. Autonomic nervous system (ANS)
      1) Sympathetic nervous system (SNS)
      2) Parasympathetic nervous system (PNS)

Microscopic Anatomy and Physiology

1. Nerve cells
   a. Neuroglia (also called *glial cells*)
      1) Neuroglia are more numerous than neurons (85% of the cells in the CNS are neuroglial).
      2) These cells provide support, nourishment, and protection to the neurons.
      3) Most tumors of the CNS are neuroglial since they are mitotic and can replicate themselves.
      4) Types
         a) Microglia
            i) Part of the reticuloendothelial system
            ii) Relatively rare in normal CNS tissue
            iii) Become mobile and travel to the area of damage when the neurons become damaged; microglia then enlarge and phagocytize tissue debris
         b) Oligodendroglia: responsible for myelin formation in the CNS
         c) Astrocytes
            i) May provide nutrients and regulate chemical environment for neurons
            ii) Form the blood-brain barrier with the endothelium of the blood vessels
            iii) Provide structure and support for nerve cells
            iv) May have indirect role in synaptic transmission
         d) Ependyma
            i) Line the ventricles of brain and central canal of spinal cord
            ii) Aid in secretion of CSF
   b. Neurons (Figure 6-1)
      1) Transmit nerve impulses
      2) Ten billion in CNS; most are in the cerebral cortex
      3) Cannot regenerate in the CNS; can regenerate in peripheral nervous system by growing within the myelin if the cell body is intact
      4) Components
         a) Cell body (soma)
            i) Nucleus: controls metabolic processes of cell
            ii) Cytoplasm: contains organelles to carry out metabolic functions
         b) Axons
            i) Conduct impulses away from cell body to other neurons or to end organs
            ii) One axon per neuron
            iii) May be myelinated or unmyelinated
         c) Dendrites

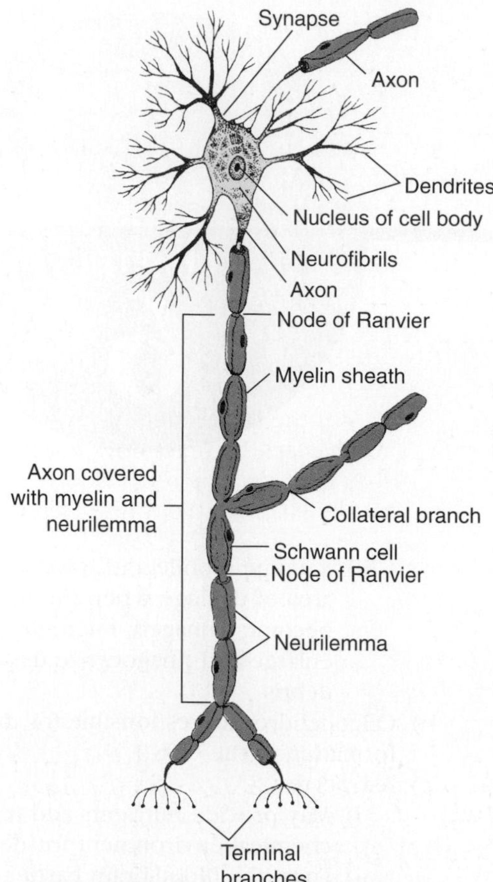

Figure 6-1 The neuron. (From Black, J. M., & Hawks, J. A. [2009]. *Medical-surgical nursing: Clinical management for positive outcomes* [8th ed.]. Philadelphia: Saunders.)

i) Conduct impulses toward cell body, which receives nerve impulses from the axons of other neurons
ii) May be more than one dendrite

d) Neurofibrils: thin, threadlike fibers forming a network in the cytoplasm

e) Nissl bodies
i) Specialize in protein synthesis with RNA
ii) Maintain and regenerate neuronal processes

f) Myelin sheath
i) In some neurons, the axons covered with myelin, a white lipid substance, between the nodes of Ranvier
ii) Acts as insulation to speed conduction of impulses down the axon sheath
iii) Accounts for white color found in parts of brain and spinal cord
iv) Made by oligodendroglia in CNS and by Schwann cell in PNS

g) Nodes of Ranvier
i) Constrictions occurring periodically along the axon where it is not covered by myelin
ii) Allows rapid conduction of impulses by saltatory conduction (node to node)

h) Neurilemma
i) Outer coating of the neurons in the peripheral nervous system
ii) Provides for peripheral nerve regeneration

i) Synaptic knobs: contain vesicles which store neurotransmitter substances

5) Categorization
a) Direction of impulse formation
i) Afferent sensory neurons transmit impulses to the spinal cord or brain.
ii) Efferent motor neurons transmit impulses away from the brain or spinal cord.
iii) Remember SA ME (sensory afferent, motor efferent).
iv) Interneurons transmit impulses from sensory neurons to motor neurons.

b) Number of processes
i) Unipolar neurons have one process coming from the cell body; it bifurcates into an axon and a dendrite.
ii) Bipolar neurons have two processes (one axon and one dendrite) coming from the cell body.
iii) Multipolar neurons have one axon and more than one dendrite.

c) Location
i) Upper motor neurons originate above the brainstem.
ii) Lower motor neurons originate below the brainstem.

2. Neurophysiology
a. Impulse transmission
1) Initiated by a stimulus: chemical, electrical, mechanical, thermal
2) Change in permeability of the cell membrane to sodium
3) Depolarization of the cell caused by sodium influx; initiation of an action potential
4) Repolarization and return to normal resting polarized (ready) state occurs
5) Synaptic transmission
a) Unidirectional conduction of an impulse from one neuron to the next
b) As the impulse nears the end of the axon, a release of neurotransmitter from the synaptic vesicles
c) Diffusion of neurotransmitter across the synaptic gap changing the permeability

of the cell membrane of the adjoining cell
   d) Continuation of the impulse to its end-organ or cell
   e) Types of synapses
      i) Axosomatic: the axon of one neuron synapses with the cell body of another neuron
      ii) Axodendritic: the axon of one neuron synapses with the dendrite of another neuron
      iii) Axoaxonic: the axon of one neuron synapses with the axon of another neuron
  b. Refractory periods
   1) Absolute: period of time when the nerve cannot be stimulated again
   2) Relative: period of time when the nerve can only be stimulated by a strong impulse
3. Cerebral neurotransmitters (Table 6-1)
  a. Function
   1) Neurotransmitters are released from the presynaptic vesicles and act as a chemical bridge for the transmission of impulses from one neuron to another.
   2) After synaptic transmission, the neurotransmitter is inactivated by an enzyme (e.g., cholinesterase deactivates acetylcholine).
  b. Types
   1) Excitatory neurotransmitters promote conduction of the impulse from one cell to the next.
   2) Inhibitory neurotransmitters increase resistance to depolarization.
4. Cerebral metabolism
  a. Oxygen requirements
   1) The brain weighs 2% of body weight but receives 20% of the cardiac output and uses 20% of oxygen delivered.
   2) The brain, especially the cerebral cortex, is very susceptible to change in oxygen delivery; the brainstem is the most resistant to hypoxic damage.
   3) Anoxia causes brain edema and neuron death.
  b. Nutrient requirements
   1) The brain has high metabolic energy needs.
   2) Glucose is the main source of cellular energy (ATP).
      a) Triggered by the SNS, gluconeogenesis is a very important process because it causes the conversion of protein and fat to glucose; the brain does not require insulin to use glucose.
      b) Hypoglycemia is associated with neurologic symptoms.
         i) Confusion usually occurs if blood glucose is less than 50 to 70 mg/dL.
         ii) Coma occurs if blood glucose is less than 20 mg/dL.
      c) Although hyperglycemia does not cause direct neurologic effects, the osmotic effect may cause hyperosmolality and brain dehydration (e.g., HHS).
   3) Vitamins
      a) Thiamine (B_1) is important in the Krebs cycle; deficiency of B_1 causes Wernicke's encephalopathy.
      b) Vitamin B_{12} is important in the spinal cord and peripheral nervous system; deficiency of B_{12} causes pernicious anemia and gradual deterioration of the CNS and peripheral nerves.
      c) Pyridoxine (B_6) is a coenzyme that participates in many enzymatic reactions in the CNS; deficiency of B_6 causes neuropathy and seizures.

Table 6-1 Neurologic System Neurotransmitters

Name	Type	Region	Predominant Effect
Acetylcholine	Cholinergic	• Basal ganglia • Pyramidal cells • Parasympathetic branch of ANS	Excitatory
Norepinephrine	Amine	• Hypothalamus • Brainstem • Sympathetic branch of ANS	Inhibitory/excitatory
Dopamine	Amine	• Basal ganglia • Brainstem	Inhibitory
Serotonin	Amine	• Hypothalamus • Brainstem	Inhibitory
Gamma-aminobutyric acid (GABA)	Amino acid	• Basal ganglia • Cerebellum • Spinal cord	Inhibitory
Glycine	Amino acid	• Spinal cord	Inhibitory
Beta-endorphins	Peptide	• Spinal cord	Inhibitory
Substance P	Peptide	• Pain fibers in spinal cord	Excitatory

d) Niacin (nicotinic acid) is needed for the synthesis of coenzymes; deficiency of niacin causes pellagra.

5. Blood-brain barrier
   a. Not a true structure but a special permeability characteristic of the brain capillaries and choroid plexus
   b. Functions
      1) Acts to limit transfer of certain substances into extracellular fluid (ECF) or cerebral spinal fluid (CSF) of brain
      2) Prevents toxic substances from readily entering the extracellular space of the nervous system; may hinder the effective use of certain drug therapies in the treatment of neurologic system problems
      3) May be altered by trauma, induction of some toxic elements, intracranial tumor, or brain irradiation

Macroscopic Anatomy and Physiology

1. Scalp: skin covering the cranium
   a. Made of five layers
      1) **Skin**: thicker than anywhere else in the body
      2) **Cutaneous tissue**
      3) **Adipose tissue**
      4) **Ligament layer referred to as** *galea aponeurotica*; moves freely over the skull
      5) **Pericranium**
   b. Blood vessels located in the subcutaneous tissue
      1) The scalp is very vascular.
      2) Blood vessels here do not contract well when injured.
      3) Scalp laceration can result in significant blood loss.
2. Skull (Figure 6-2): bony structure of the head, consisting of the cranium and the skeleton of the face
   a. The skull is composed of an inner table and outer table separated by cancellous (spongy) bone; this structure allows for maximum strength and minimal weight.
   b. The cranium is a body vault that holds and protects the brain from external forces; volume capacity is approximately 1500 mL.
   c. The cranium consists of 8 bones
      1) Frontal: 1
      2) Parietal: 2
      3) Temporal: 2
      4) Occipital: 1
      5) Ethmoid: 1
      6) Sphenoid: 1

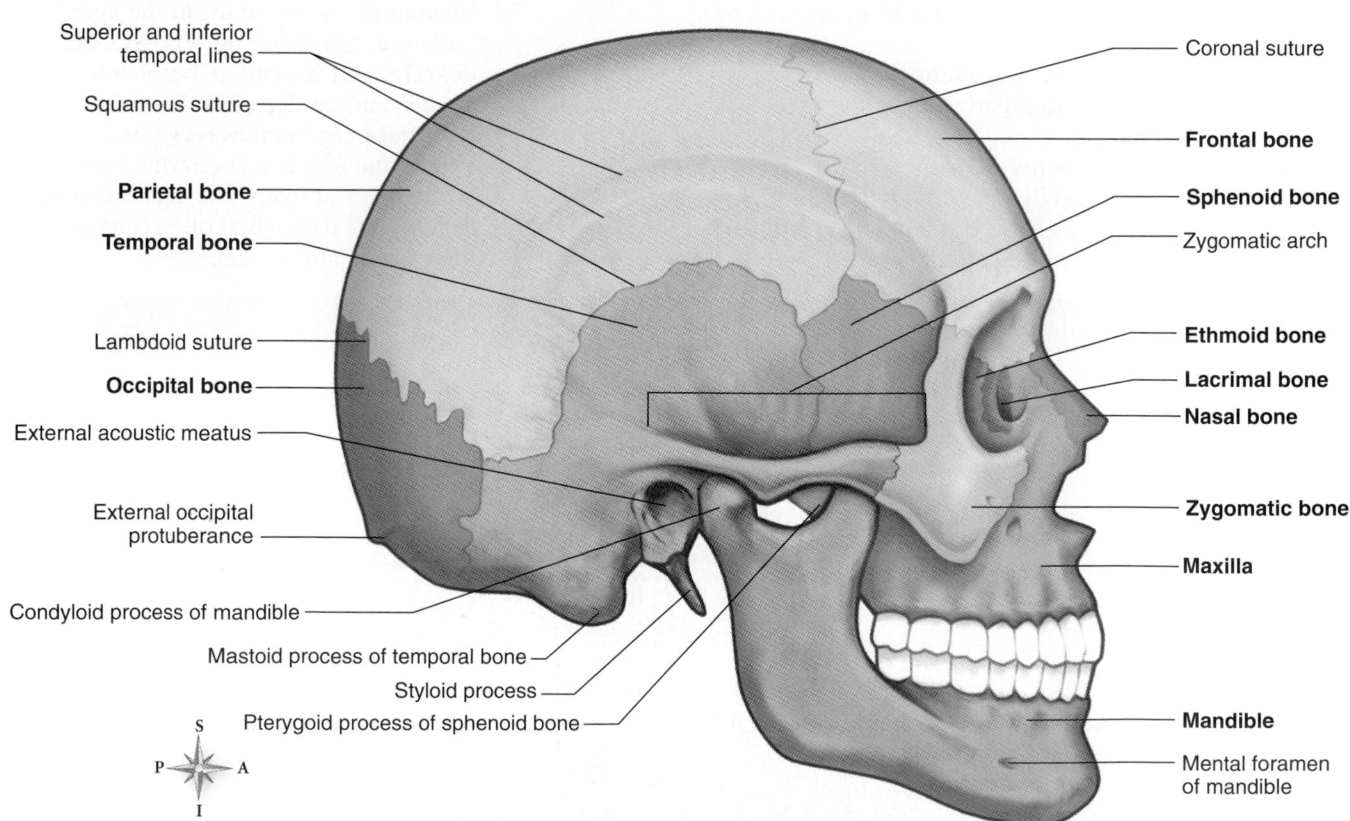

Figure 6-2 Lateral view of skull. (From Patton, K. T., & Thibodeau, G. F. [2013]. *Anatomy & physiology* [8th ed.]. St. Louis: Mosby.)

d. The sphenoid bone divides interior of skull into 3 fossae. (Figure 6-3)
   1) Anterior fossa: contains the frontal lobes
   2) Middle fossa: contains the temporal, parietal, and occipital lobes
   3) Posterior fossa: contains the cerebellum
e. The foramen magnum is a large oval-shaped opening at the base of the skull; this is the location of the connection of the brain and spinal cord.

3. Meninges (Figure 6-4): protective coverings of the brain and the spinal cord

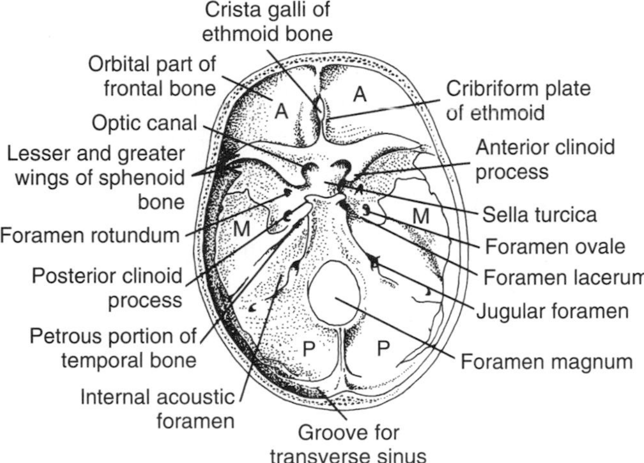

Figure 6-3 Bones that form the floor of the cranial cavity and the three fossae formed by these bones. (From Kinney, M.R., et al. [1998]. *AACN's clinical reference for critical care nursing* [4th ed.]. St. Louis: Mosby.)

a. Pia mater
   1) This is the delicate layer that adheres to surface of brain and spinal cord.
   2) This layer follows sulci and gyri of brain and carries branches of cerebral arteries with it.
      a) Sulci: shallow grooves or invaginations on the surface of the brain (deep sulci are referred to as *fissures*)
      b) Gyri: convolutions on the surface of the brain
   3) Blood vessels of pia form the choroid plexus.
b. Arachnoid mater
   1) This is the middle layer of the meninges.
   2) The subarachnoid space is between the arachnoid mater and the pia mater.
      a) Contains larger blood vessels of brain
      b) Contains CSF
      c) Contains arachnoid villi (i.e., projections of arachnoid mater that serve as channels for absorption of CSF into venous system)
c. Dura mater
   1) This is the outermost layer of meninges.
   2) Meningeal arteries and venous sinuses lie within clefts formed by separation of inner and outer layers of dura.
   3) The epidural space is between the skull and the dura mater.
      a) Only a potential space
      b) Site of epidural hemorrhage or hematoma
   4) The subdural space is between the dura mater and the arachnoid mater
      a) Only a potential space
      b) Site of subdural hemorrhage or hematoma

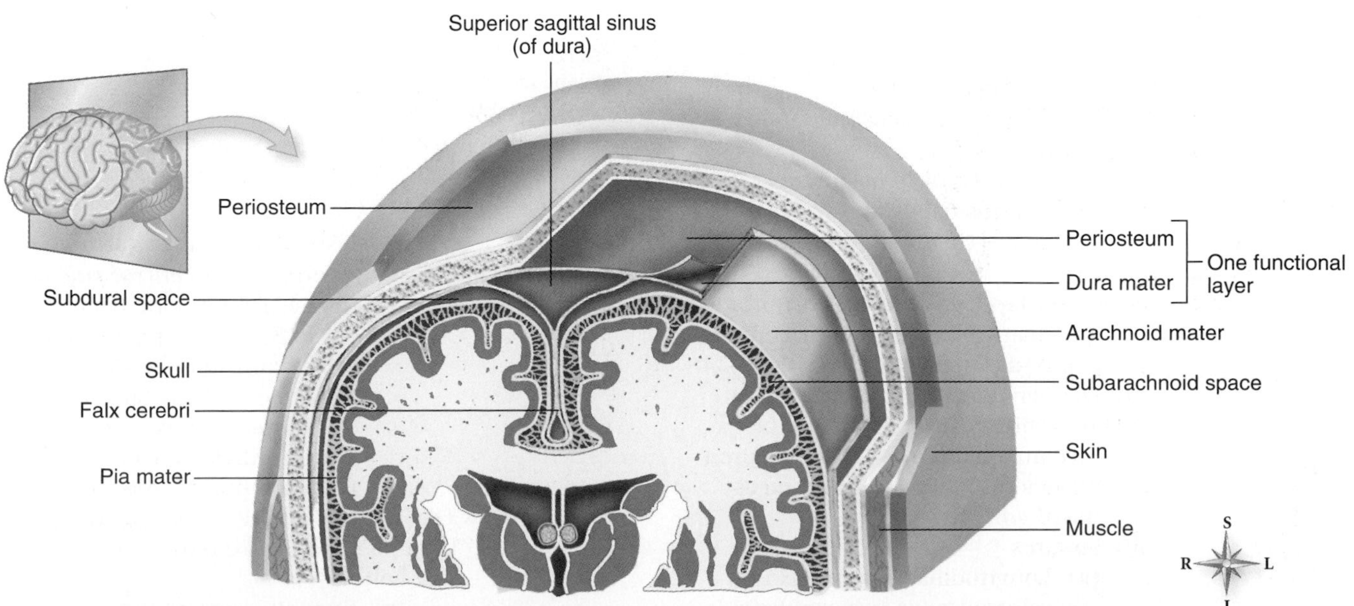

Figure 6-4 Coverings of the brain. (From Patton, K. T., & Thibodeau, G. F. [2013]. *Anatomy & physiology* [8th ed.]. St. Louis: Mosby.)

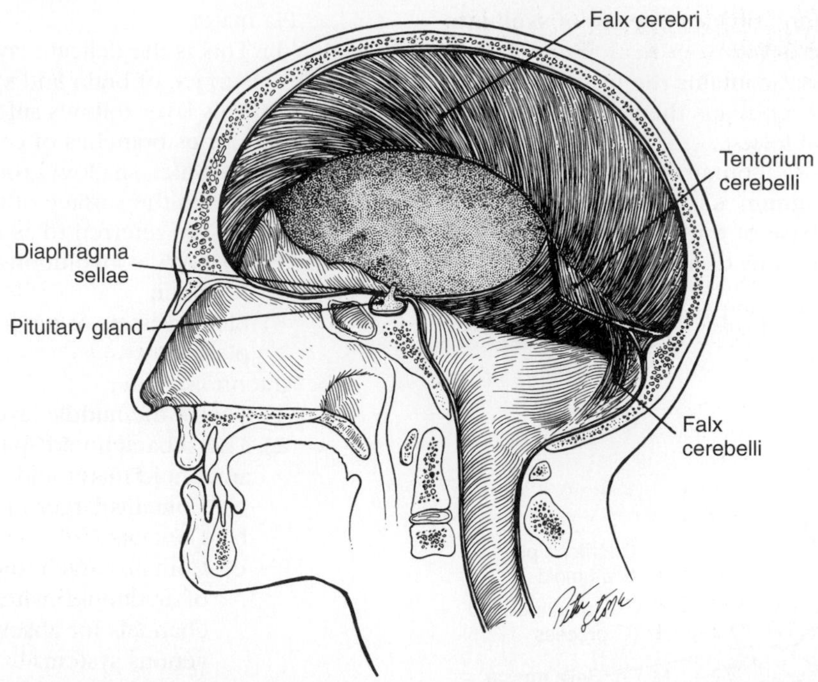

Figure 6-5 Folds of the dura. (From Kinney, M.R., et al. [1998]. *AACN's clinical reference for critical care nursing* [4th ed.]. St. Louis: Mosby.)

5) There are several folds of the dura mater. (Figure 6-5)
   a) The falx cerebri separates the two cerebral hemispheres.
   b) The falx cerebelli separates the two cerebellar hemispheres.
   c) The tentorium cerebelli separates the cerebral hemispheres from the cerebellum.
   d) The diaphragma sella canopies the sella turcica (where pituitary gland is located) and encloses the pituitary gland.

4. Brain
   a. General information
      1) Weighs approximately 1.5 kg
      2) Divided into cerebrum, brainstem, and cerebellum
   b. Telencephalon: two cerebral hemispheres connected by the corpus callosum
      1) Cerebrum (Figure 6-6)
         a) Structure
            i) Outer layer of cerebral cortex is gray matter consisting of neuron cell bodies (six cell layers thick).
            ii) Deeper layers of each hemisphere are white matter consisting of myelinated axons with four paired masses of gray matter known as *basal ganglia.*
            iii) Fissures
               (a) Longitudinal fissure (also referred to as *falx cerebri*): divides the left and right cerebral hemispheres

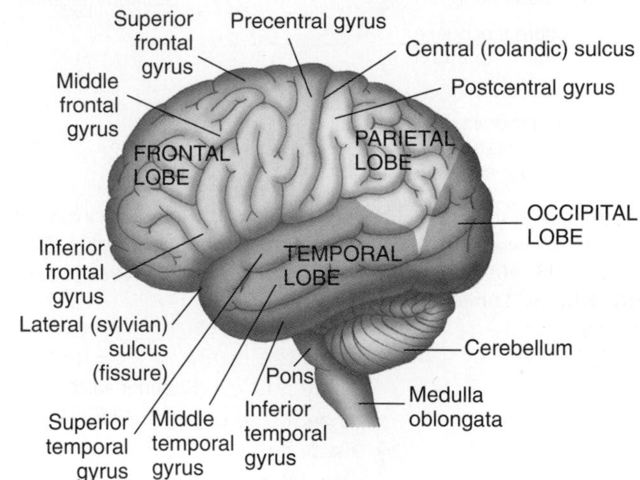

Figure 6-6 Cerebral hemispheres. (From McCance, K. L., & Huether, S. E. [2009]. *Pathophysiology: The biologic basis for disease in adults and children* [6th ed.]. St. Louis: Mosby.)

               (b) Fissure of Rolando (also referred to as *central sulcus*): divides frontal lobe from parietal lobes; separates the motor and sensory strips
               (c) Fissure of Sylvius (also referred to as *lateral sulcus or Sylvian fissure*): divides frontal lobe from temporal lobes
         b) Cerebral cortical areas and functions (Table 6-2 and Figure 6-6)
            i) Lobes
               (a) Frontal: contains the precentral gyrus (also referred to as the *motor strip*)

Table 6-2 Cerebral Cortical Areas and Functions

Cerebral Cortical Area	Functions

Frontal lobe	• Personality
	• Behavior: ethical; moral; social
	• Intellectual functions
	  • Conscious thought
	  • Abstract thinking
	  • Judgment and foresight
	• Short-term memory
	• Voluntary motor function
	• Motor speech (Broca's area in dominant hemisphere)

Parietal lobe	• Localization of sensory information to the body surface • Sensory integration and discrimination • Object recognition • Position sense • Body awareness • Body image
Temporal lobe	• Emotion • Long-term memory • Processing of olfactory, gustatory, auditory input • Sensory speech (Wernicke's area in dominant hemisphere)
Occipital lobe	• Processing of visual input

(b) Parietal: contains the postcentral gyrus (also referred to as the *sensory strip*)
(c) Temporal
(d) Occipital

ii) Cerebral hemispheres
(a) Each hemisphere of the brain receives sensory information from the opposite side of the body and controls skeletal muscles of the opposite side
(b) Each hemisphere has specialization
(i) The left cerebral hemisphere is specialized for analysis, problem solving, language, mathematics, abstract reasoning, and interpretation of symbols.
(ii) The right cerebral hemisphere is specialized for visuospatial patterns, nonverbal communication, music, and artistic ability.
(c) Hemispheric dominance
(i) Ninety percent of right-handed people are left hemisphere dominant.
(ii) Sixty percent of left-handed people are right hemisphere dominant.
(iii) Language centers are located in dominant hemisphere; lesions in dominant hemisphere frequently cause aphasia.

c) Corpus callosum: path for fibers to cross from one cerebral hemisphere to the other

d) Basal ganglia
i) Major center of the extrapyramidal system
ii) Functions
(a) Regulates and controls motor integration
(b) Influences posture
(c) Allows fine voluntary movements

c. Diencephalon
1) Thalamus: relay of incoming messages to appropriate areas of the brain
2) Hypothalamus
a) Temperature regulation
b) Regulation of food and water intake
c) Sleep patterns
d) Autonomic responses
e) Control of hormonal secretion of pituitary gland
3) Limbic system
a) Self-preservation behaviors, including aggression
b) Basic drives (e.g., food, sex)
c) Affective aspect of emotional behavior
d) Some aspects of memory

d. Brainstem
1) Functions
a) Relays messages between the brain and lower levels of the nervous system
b) Is the origin of all cranial nerves except first and second
2) Divisions
a) Mesencephalon (midbrain)
i) Is the origin of third and fourth cranial nerves
ii) Contains motor and sensory pathways
iii) Location of reticular activating system (RAS); responsible for arousal from sleep, wakefulness, and focusing of attention
b) Pons
i) Is the origin of fifth, sixth, and seventh cranial nerves
ii) Connects cerebral cortex and cerebellum
iii) Contains motor and sensory pathways

iv) Contains respiratory centers

c) Medulla oblongata

i) Is the origin of eighth, ninth, tenth, eleventh, and twelfth cranial nerves

ii) Connect motor and sensory tracts of spinal cord to medulla

iii) Contains cardiac and respiratory centers

e. Cerebellum

1) Coordinates muscle movement with sensory input

2) Controls balance

3) Influences muscle tone in relation to equilibrium

4) Affects locomotion and posture

5) Controls nonstereotyped movements

6) Synchronizes muscle action

5. Cerebral circulation (Table 6-3)

a. The brain receives 20% of cardiac output

b. Arterial system (Figure 6-7)

1) External carotid system: arises from common carotid arteries

a) Occipital arteries: supply the posterior fossa

b) Temporal arteries: supply the temporal area

c) Maxillary arteries: form the middle meningeal arteries

d) Meningeal arteries: branches of external carotid arteries that supply dura mater

Table 6-3 Cerebral Artery Distribution

Artery	Areas
Anterior Circulation: Internal Carotid System	
Anterior cerebral arteries	• Superior surface of the frontal and parietal lobes • Medial surface of cerebral hemispheres • Basal ganglia • Corpus callosum • Hypothalamus
Middle cerebral arteries	• Lateral surfaces of frontal, parietal, and temporal lobes • Superior surface of temporal lobe • Subcortical structures (e.g., thalamus, hypothalamus, basal ganglia) • Precentral (motor) gyri • Postcentral (sensory) gyri
Posterior Circulation: Vertebrobasilar System	
Basilar artery	• Most of brainstem • Cerebellum
Posterior cerebral arteries	• Thalamus • Medial portion of occipital lobe • Inferior portion of temporal lobe • Vestibular organs • Cochlear apparatus

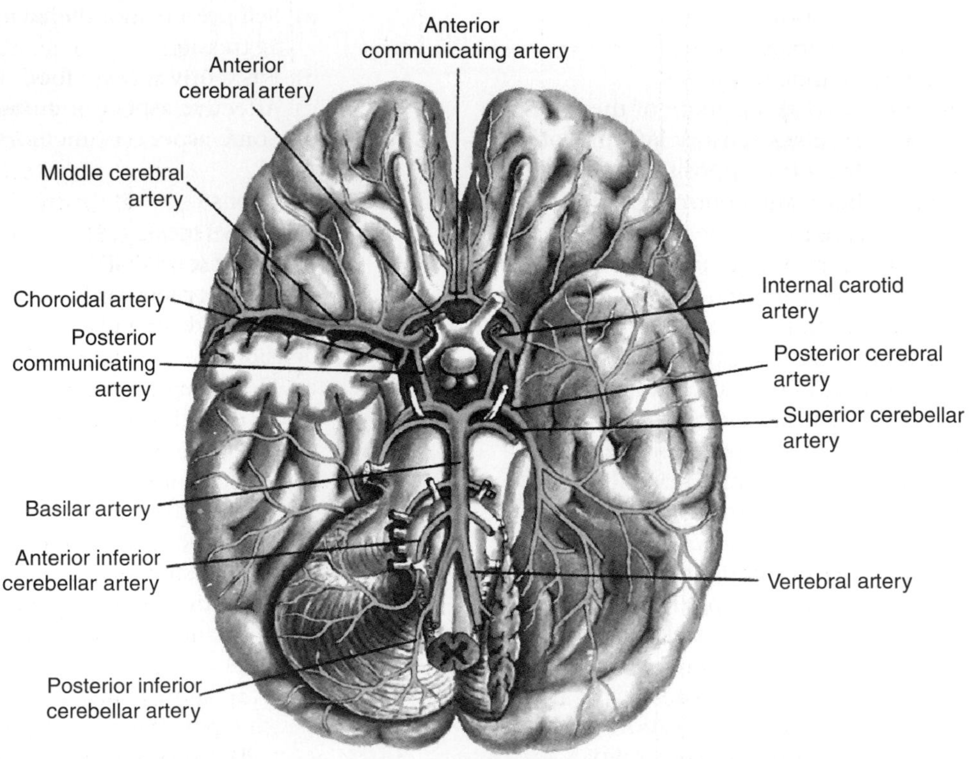

Figure 6-7 Arterial system of the brain. (From Urden, L., Stacy, K., & Lough, M. [2010]. *Critical care nursing: Diagnosis and management* [6th ed.]. St. Louis: Mosby.)

(internal carotid and vertebral arteries supply pia and arachnoid mater)
   - i) Anterior meningeal artery: supplies anterior portion of dura
   - ii) Middle meningeal artery: supplies most of dura
   - iii) Posterior meningeal artery: supplies occipital area of dura

2) Anterior circulation: internal carotid system
   - a) Arises from common carotid arteries
   - b) Accounts for 80% of cerebral perfusion
   - c) Includes the following:
     - i) Anterior cerebral arteries
     - ii) Anterior communicating artery
       - (a) Connects right and left anterior cerebral arteries
       - (b) Forms anterior section of circle of Willis
     - iii) Middle cerebral arteries
     - iv) Posterior communicating arteries
       - (a) Connect posterior cerebral arteries with the anterior circulation
       - (b) Form posterior portion of circle of Willis

3) Posterior circulation: Vertebrobasilar system
   - a) Arises from subclavian arteries and joins at lower border of pons to form basilar artery
   - b) Includes the following:
     - i) Posterior cerebral arteries
     - ii) Basilar artery
     - iii) Anterior spinal artery: supplies anterior half of three quarters of spinal cord and medial aspect of brainstem
     - iv) Posterior spinal arteries: traverse the cord along the dorsal roots

4) Circle of Willis
   - a) Formed by internal carotids and vertebral arteries
   - b) Permits collateral circulation if one of the carotid or vertebral arteries becomes occluded; unfortunately, many people have an incomplete circle of Willis which prevents this collateral flow when injury or occlusion occurs
   - c) Prone to aneurysmal formation due to multiple bifurcations

c. Cerebral blood flow

1) Brings oxygen and nutrients to the brain tissue for cellular energy production; waste products are removed from the blood

2) Cerebral blood flow (CBF) varies with changes in cerebral perfusion pressure (CPP) and diameter of the cerebrovascular bed
   - a) Normal cerebral blood flow is approximately 50 mL/100 g/min.
   - b) Normal cerebral oxygen extraction ratio is between 25 and 35%; an oxygen extraction ratio greater than 40% indicates an imbalance between oxygen supply and demand and impending cerebral ischemia.
     - i) Calculated by SaO_2 - SjO_2 / SaO_2 where SaO_2 is oxygen saturation of arterial blood by arterial blood gases or pulse oximetry and SjO_2 is the saturation of the venous blood from the jugular vein by a fiberoptic catheter placed in the jugular bulb

3) CPP = mean arterial pressure (MAP) – mean intracranial pressure (ICP)
   - a) Changes in MAP or ICP will affect CPP.
   - b) Normal MAP is 70-105 mm Hg; normal ICP is 5-15 mm Hg; so normal CPP is 60-100 mm Hg.
   - c) CPP less than 50 mm Hg is associated with impaired neuronal functioning.

4) Autoregulation is the ability of the brain to alter the diameter of the arterioles to maintain cerebral blood flow at a constant level despite changes in CPP.
   - a) When ICP approaches MAP, CPP decreases to the point where autoregulation is impaired and CBF decreases.
   - b) Limits of autoregulation are CPP between 50 and 150 mm Hg.
     - i) CPP less than 50 mm Hg causes hypoperfusion (e.g., cardiopulmonary arrest, shock) causing anoxic encephalopathy.
     - ii) CPP greater than 150 mm Hg causes hyperperfusion (e.g., hypertensive crisis) causing brain edema and hypertensive encephalopathy.

5) Factors affecting CBF
   - a) Increase in CBF
     - i) Hypercapnia
     - ii) Hypoxemia
     - iii) Decreased blood viscosity
     - iv) Hyperthermia
     - v) Drugs: vasodilators
   - b) Decrease in CBF
     - i) Hypocapnia
     - ii) Hyperoxemia
     - iii) Increased blood viscosity
     - iv) Hypothermia
     - v) Intracranial hypertension
     - vi) Drugs: vasopressors
     - vii) Cerebral vasospasm
   - c) Drugs which are often used therapeutically to optimize CO, BP, and CPP and/or minimize oxygen consumption may result in decreased CO, BP, CPP, and CBF when used inappropriately or in excess.

i) Negative inotropes (e.g., beta-blockers, barbiturates)
ii) Vasodilators (e.g., nitroprusside, nitroglycerin)
iii) Anesthetic agents

d) Therapies utilized to manage intracranial hypertension, which are aimed at lowering $PaCO_2$ (i.e., hyperventilation) result in vasoconstriction, thereby reducing cerebral blood flow and oxygenation.

d. Venous system
1) The cerebrum has external veins that lie in subarachnoid space on surfaces of hemispheres and internal veins that drain the central core of cerebrum and lie beneath corpus callosum.
2) Both external and internal venous systems empty into venous sinuses that lie between dural layers.
a) Superior sagittal sinus drains venous blood from the anterior portions of the brain.
b) Cavernous sinus drains venous blood from the inferior portions of the brain.
c) Transvenous sinus drains venous blood from the posterior portion of the brain.
3) The internal jugular veins collect blood from dural venous sinuses.

6. Cerebrospinal fluid (CSF)
a. Characteristics
1) Functions
a) Cushions brain and spinal cord
b) Allows for compensation for changes in ICP; displacement of CSF out of cranial cavity compensates for increases in intracranial volume to prevent increase in intracranial pressure
2) Volume: 120-150 mL
a) Distribution: 90 mL in lumbar subarachnoid space, 25 mL in ventricles, 35 mL in rest of subarachnoid space
b) Daily synthesis: 500 mL
3) Pressure: less than 200 mm H_2O, measured at lumbar level, with patient in side-lying position

b. CSF production and reabsorption
1) CSF is a transudate of plasma formed by choroid plexus in ventricles
a) Choroid plexus: sheets of epithelial cells that project into the lumen of the ventricular spaces
b) Majority (95%) of CSF produced in lateral ventricles
2) CSF is absorbed via arachnoid villi, which return it to systemic circulation by the internal jugular veins; hydrostatic pressure gradient between CSF and venous sinus is one factor that determines CSF absorption.

c. CSF communication system within brain (Figure 6-8)
1) Ventricles: hollow spaces that are lined with ependyma; contain specialized epithelium called choroid plexus, which produce CSF
a) The lateral ventricles are the largest of the ventricles; one lies in each cerebral hemisphere.
b) The third ventricle lies midline between the two lateral ventricles.
c) The fourth ventricle lies in posterior fossa.
2) Pathway of CSF circulation (Figure 6-9)

7. Spine and spinal cord
a. Structure
1) Vertebral column: composed of 7 cervical, 12 thoracic, 5 lumbar, 5 sacral, and 4 coccygeal vertebrae
2) Spinal cord: 42-45 cm extending from superior border of atlas to upper border of second lumbar vertebrae (L2); continuous with the brainstem
a) Meninges: pia mater, arachnoid mater, and dura mater
b) Central canal: opening in the center of the spinal cord that contains CSF; communicates with the fourth ventricle
c) Central gray horns that form an "H": contain mostly cell bodies (Figure 6-10)
i) The anterior (or ventral) horn of gray matter contains cell bodies of efferent or motor fibers.
ii) The posterior (or dorsal) horn of gray matter contains cell bodies of afferent or sensory fibers.
iii) The lateral horns of gray matter contain preganglionic fibers of autonomic system.
d) Columns of white matter that are fiber tracts surround the gray matter: contain mostly myelinated axons
i) Posterior tracts (dorsal columns) and the anterior and lateral spinothalamic tracts are ascending tracts that conduct sensory impulses from the spinal cord to the thalamus and cerebral cortex.
ii) Lateral tracts (the corticospinal and pyramidal) are descending tracts that conduct motor impulses from the brain to motor neurons in the anterior horn.
iii) Spinal tracts are named by column, origin, and termination (e.g., lateral corticospinal tract is located in the lateral column, originates in the cortex, and terminates in the spine; it is therefore a descending tract [cortex to spine]); Table 6-4 describes clinically significant tracts.

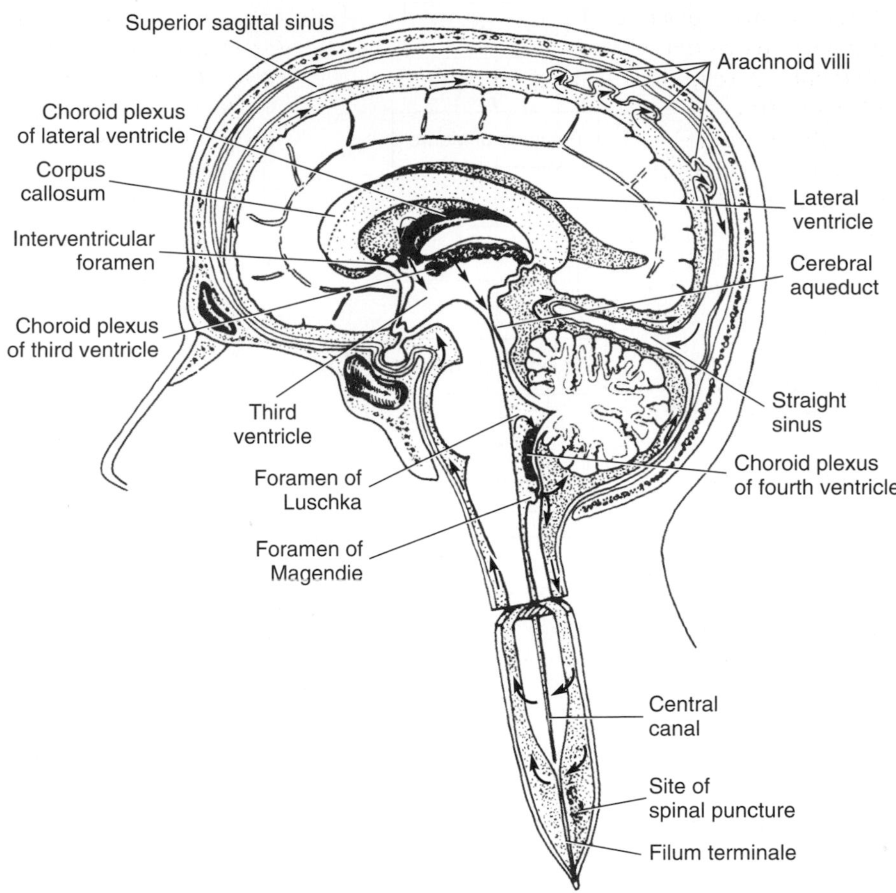

Figure 6-8 Lateral view of the ventricular system. Arrows show direction of CSF circulation. (From Kinney, M.R., et al. [1998]. *AACN's clinical reference for critical care nursing* [4th ed.]. St. Louis: Mosby.)

3) Upper and lower motor neurons
   a) Upper motor neurons (UMNs): located in the cerebral cortex and brainstem
      i) Cell bodies lie in the motor area of the cerebral cortex
      ii) Axons pass through the spinal cord to synapse with the lower motor neurons
      iii) Damage to UMN causes spastic paralysis and hyperactive reflexes
   b) Lower motor neurons (LMNs): located in the spinal cord
      i) Cell bodies lie in the anterior horn of gray matter in the spinal cord
      ii) Axons directly innervate striated muscle fibers
      iii) Damage to LMN causes flaccid paralysis and areflexia

b. Function
   1) Mediates the reflex arc (Figure 6-11)
      a) An involuntary response to a stimulus (e.g., touching hot stove causes reflex withdrawal of hand)
      b) Does not go beyond the spinal cord to the brain; does not require cerebral interpretation
      c) Components
         i) Receptor organ
         ii) Afferent neuron
         iii) Effector neuron
         iv) Effector organ
   2) Serves as the communicating pathway between the brain and the peripheral nervous system

8. Peripheral nervous system
   a. Spinal segments consist of 31 pairs of spinal nerves: 8 cervical (C1-C8), 12 thoracic (T1-T12), 5 lumbar (L1-L5), 5 sacral (S1-S5), and 1 coccygeal
      1) Fibers of spinal nerve
         a) Motor fibers
            i) Originate in anterior gray column of spinal cord
            ii) Form ventral root of spinal nerve and pass to skeletal muscles
         b) Sensory fibers
            i) Originate in spinal ganglia of dorsal roots
            ii) Peripheral branches distribute to visceral and somatic structures as mediators of sensory impulses to CNS

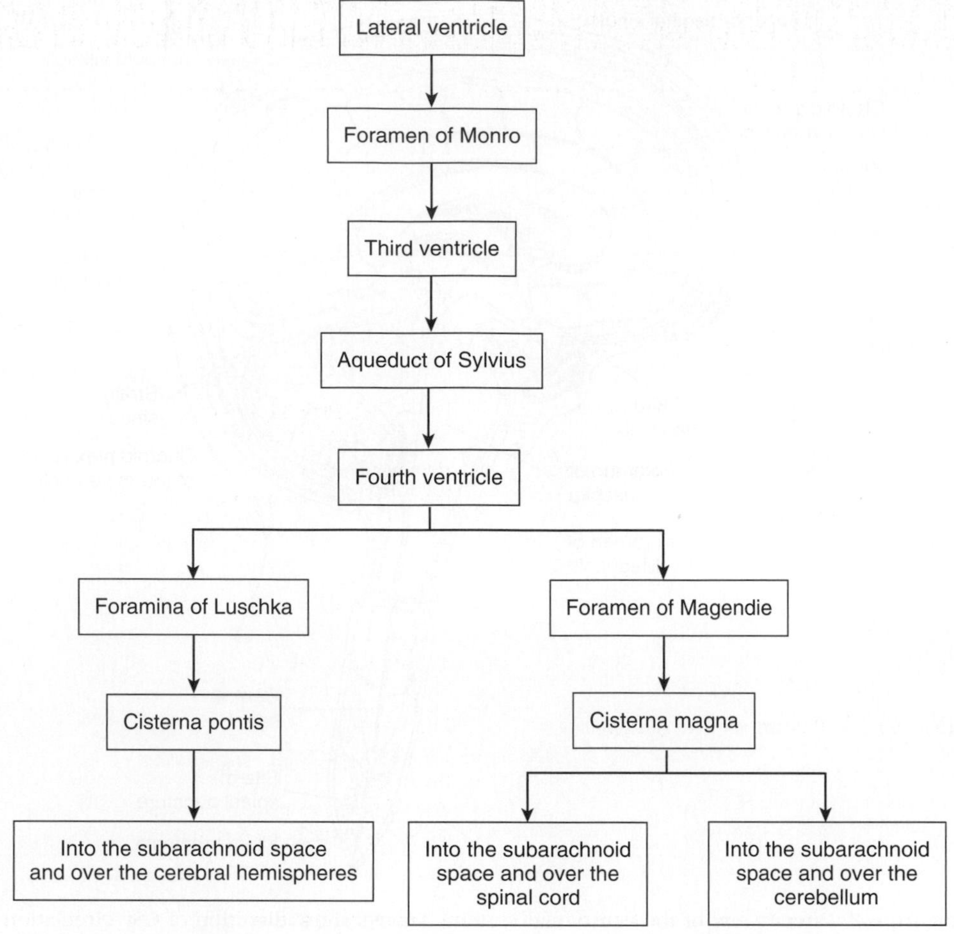

Figure 6-9 Circulation of CSF.

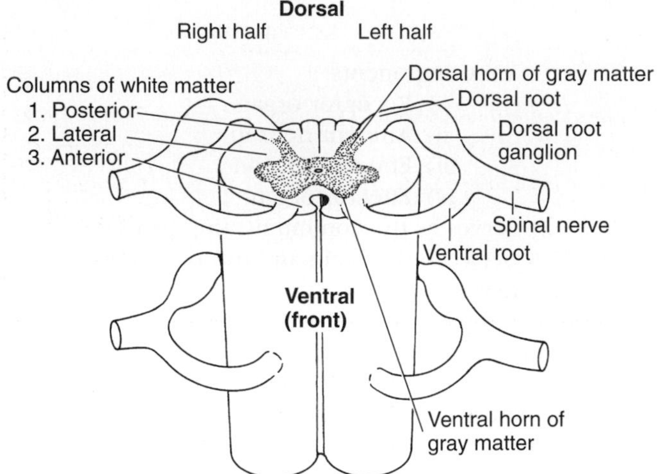

Figure 6-10 Segment of the thoracic spinal cord in cross section. (From Kinney, M.R., et al. [1998]. *AACN's clinical reference for critical care nursing* [4th ed.]. St. Louis: Mosby.)

2) Dermatomes: each spinal nerve innervates a specific portion of the skin identified as the dermatome for that spinal nerve (Figure 6-12 and Table 6-5)
3) Spinal nerves form various nerve plexuses that innervate the skin and muscles throughout the body (Figure 6-12).
   a) Cervical plexus: C1-C4
   b) Brachial plexus: C5-C8, T1
   c) Lumbar plexus: L1-L4
   d) Sacral plexus: L4-L5, S1-S4

b. Cranial nerves (Table 6-6) consist of 12 pairs of nerves that carry impulses to and from the brain

9. Autonomic nervous system (ANS)
   a. Structure
      1) ANS consists of two neuron chains that carry information from the central nervous system to peripheral effector organs.
      2) Preganglionic neuron has cell body in the CNS.
         a) Sympathetic branch: Cell bodies are located in the spinal cord from T1 to L2.
         b) Parasympathetic branch: Cell bodies are located in the nuclei of cranial nerves III, VII, IX, X or in the spinal cord from S2-S4.
      3) The preganglionic neuron axon terminates on the postganglionic neuron cell bodies that are located throughout the body in autonomic ganglia.
      4) The postganglionic neuron axon terminates and innervates the specific effector organs of the autonomic nervous system.
      5) Neurotransmitters form a chemical bridge in transmission of a nerve impulse.

Table 6-4 Spinal Cord Tracts and Functions

Tract	Column	Direction	Functions	Sidedness
Spinothalamic				
Lateral spinothalamic	Lateral	Ascending	• Pain • Temperature	Contralateral
Anterior spinothalamic	Anterior	Ascending	• Light touch • Pressure • Pain • Temperature	Contralateral
Spinotectal	Lateral	Ascending	• Tactile stimulation arousing consciousness	Contralateral
Spinocerebellar				
Dorsal spinocerebellar	Lateral	Ascending	• Reflex proprioception • Muscle tone and synergy	Ipsilateral
Ventral spinocerebellar	Lateral	Ascending	• Reflex proprioception • Muscle tone and synergy	Contralateral
Medial Lemniscal System				
Fasciculus gracilis	Posterior	Ascending	• Position sense • Vibratory sense • Pressure • Tactile localization • Two-point discrimination	Ipsilateral
Fasciculus cuneatus	Posterior	Ascending	• Position sense • Vibratory sense • Pressure • Tactile localization • Two-point discrimination	Ipsilateral
Pyramidal				
Lateral corticospinal	Lateral	Descending	• Voluntary movement	Contralateral
Ventral corticospinal	Lateral	Descending	• Voluntary movement	Ipsilateral
Corticobulbar		Descending	• Facial expression • Swallowing • Speech	Contralateral
Extrapyramidal				
Rubrospinal	Lateral	Descending	• Synergy and muscle tone	Contralateral
Lateral vestibulospinal	Anterior	Descending	• Posture and equilibrium	Ipsilateral
Medial vestibulospinal	Anterior	Descending	• Posture and equilibrium	Contralateral
Lateral reticulospinal	Lateral	Descending	• Muscle tone	Ipsilateral
Medial reticulospinal	Anterior	Descending	• Muscle tone	Ipsilateral
Tectospinal	Anterior	Descending	• Vision and hearing	Contralateral

a) Sympathetic branch: epinephrine; norepinephrine
b) Parasympathetic branch: acetylcholine

b. Function
  1) Controls activities of the viscera at an unconscious level
  2) Consists of two parallel systems that regulate visceral organs by acting in opposing manners (Table 6-7)
    a) Sympathetic branch (also called *adrenergic*)
      i) Dominates in crisis situations and is frequently referred to as *fight or flight system*
      ii) Innervated by physiologic or psychological stressors
      iii) Promotes activities that prepare the body for crisis situations
    b) Parasympathetic branch (also called *cholinergic*)
      i) Dominant in moments of calm or "steady state"
      ii) Promotes activities that restore the body's energy sources

Neurologic Assessment

Interview

1. Chief complaint: why the patient is seeking help and duration of the problem
  a. Symptoms related to neurologic problems
    1) Head or spinal cord trauma

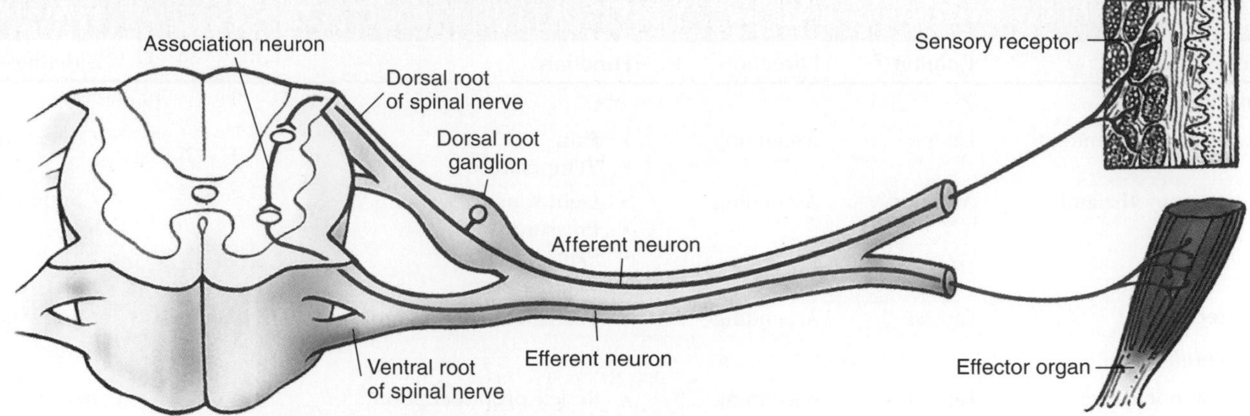

Figure 6-11 Basic diagram of a reflex arc, including the sensory receptor, afferent neuron, association neuron, efferent neuron, and effector organ. (From Lewis, S. M., Heitkemper, M. M., & Dirksen, S. R. [2000]. *Medical-surgical nursing* [5th ed.]. St Louis: Mosby.)

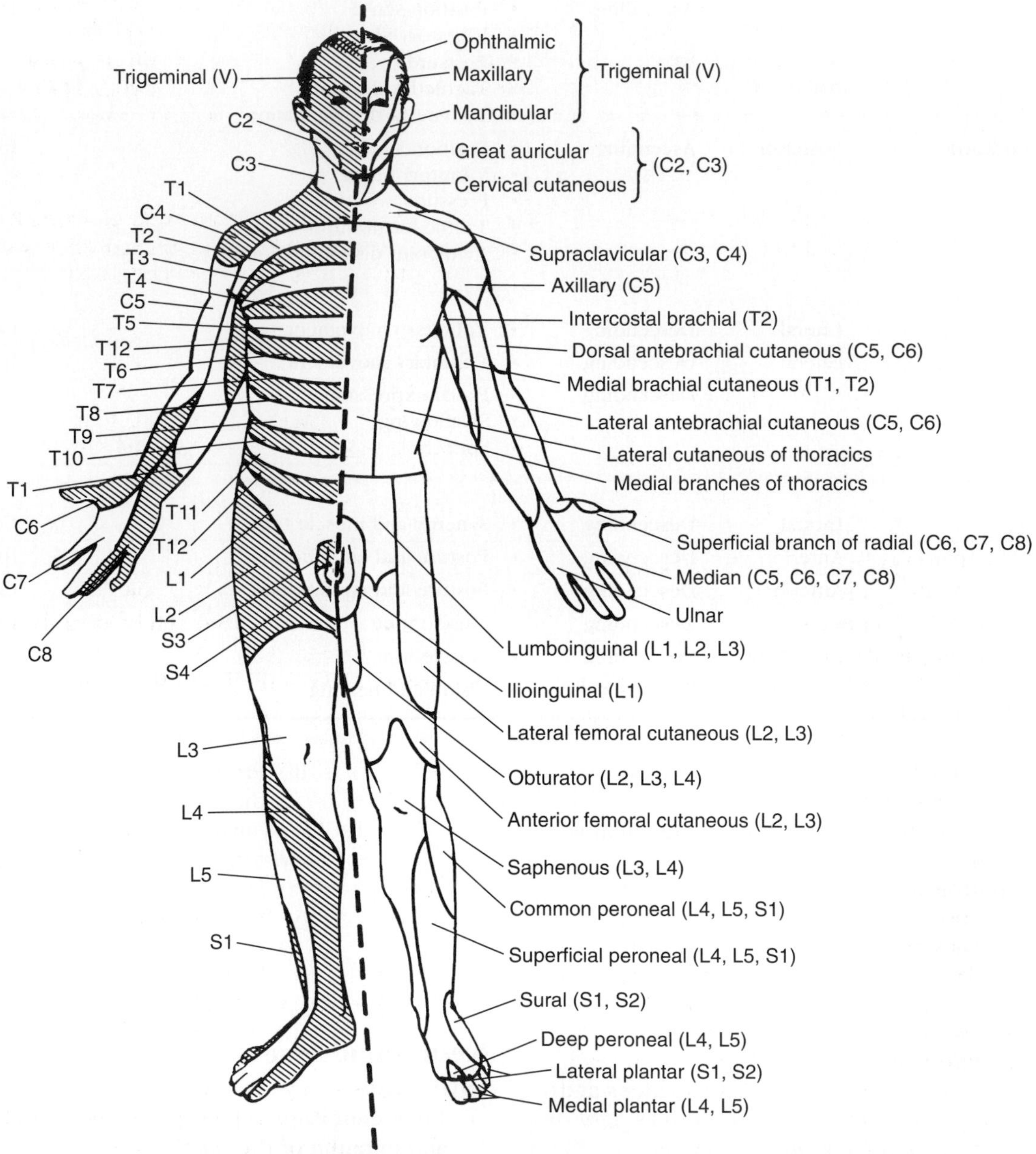

Figure 6-12 *Left:* Dermatome distribution. *Right:* Peripheral distribution of cutaneous nerves. (From Long, B. C., Phipps, W. J., & Cassmeyer, V. L. [1993]. *Medical-surgical nursing: A nursing process approach* [3rd ed.], St Louis: Mosby.)

Table 6-5 Relationship of Spinal Cord Segments to Peripheral Nerves, Muscles, and Functional Ability

Spinal Cord Segment	Peripheral Nerves	Muscles	Functional Ability
C3-5	• Phrenic nerve	• Diaphragm	• Diaphragmatic chest excursion
C5	• Spinal accessory nerve	• Trapezius	• Shoulder shrug
C5-6	• Axillary nerve • Musculocutaneous nerve • Radial nerve	• Deltoid • Biceps • Brachioradialis	• Arm elevation • Forearm flexion
C6-8	• Radial nerve	• Triceps • Extensor carpi radialis and ulnaris • Flexor carpi radialis and ulnaris	• Forearm extension • Wrist extension • Wrist flexion
C8, T1	• Median nerve • Ulnar nerve	• Adductor pollicis • Dorsal interossei	• Handgrip • Finger spreading
T1-T12	• Thoracic and lumbosacral branches	• Intercostals • Rectus abdominis and obliques	• Intercostal chest excursion • Rotation at waist
L1-L3	• Femoral nerve	• Iliopsoas • Quadriceps	• Hip flexion • Knee extension
L2-4	• Deep peroneal nerve • Sciatic nerve	• Extensor hallucis and digitorum • Biceps femoris and hamstrings	• Foot dorsiflexion • Knee flexion
L5-S2	• Inferior gluteal nerve • Tibial nerve	• Gluteus maximus • Gastrocnemius	• Hip extension • Plantar flexion

a) Sequence of events
b) Mechanism of injury
c) Elapsed time
d) Extent of injury
e) Previous treatment
f) Current status

2) Change in consciousness (e.g., difficulty staying awake)
3) Headache
   a) Focal or generalized
   b) Unilateral or bilateral
   c) With or without fever
      i) Headache with fever: infectious process (e.g., meningitis, encephalitis)
      ii) Headache without fever: intracerebral hemorrhage or tumor
   d) Time of day: early morning headache suggestive of tumor
4) Seizures
   a) New onset
   b) Increased frequency if patient has history of epilepsy
5) Visual changes
   a) Loss of a portion of the visual field
   b) Diplopia
   c) Photophobia: may be experienced with increased ICP or meningitis
   d) Nystagmus
6) Impaired speech (e.g., dysarthria, aphasia)
7) Change in mood (e.g., depression, euphoria, emotional lability)
8) Change in thought processes (e.g., hallucinations, delusions, illusions, paranoia) and cognition
9) Change in behavior (e.g., hygiene habits, inappropriate laughter, frequent crying)
10) Change in motor function
    a) Tremor
    b) Paresis
    c) Paralysis
11) Change in gait
12) Dizziness, syncope, vertigo
13) Change in sensory function
    a) Pain
    b) Paresthesia
    c) Anesthesia
14) Memory changes
15) Swallowing difficulties
16) Difficulties with activities of daily living (ADL)

2. History of present illness: determine PQRST
   a. P
      1) Provocation: What provokes or worsens the pain?
      2) Palliation
         a) What relieves the pain?
         b) What was used but did not relieve pain?
   b. Q
      1) Quality: What does the pain feel like?
   c. R
      1) Region: Where is the pain located?
      2) Radiation: If the pain radiates, where does the pain radiate?
   d. S
      1) Severity: How severe is the pain on a 0-10 scale with 0 being no pain and 10 being the most severe pain?
   e. T
      1) Timing

Table 6-6 Cranial Nerve Summary

Number	Name	Memory Jogger: Name	Memory Jogger: Motor/Sensory/Both	Functions
I	Olfactory	On	Some	Sensory • Smell
II	Optic	Old	Say	Sensory • Vision
III	Oculomotor	Olympus	Marry	Motor • Upward, lateral eye movement • Pupillary constriction • Eyelid elevation
IV	Trochlear	Towering	Money	Motor • Downward, medial eye movement
V	Trigeminal	Tops	But	Sensory • Sensation of scalp and face • Sensation of cornea of eye Motor • Temporal and masseter muscles
VI	Abducens	A	My	Motor • Lateral eye movement
VII	Facial	Fin	Brother	Sensory • Taste on anterior two thirds of tongue Motor • Muscles of facial expression • Eyelid closure • Lacrimal and salivary glands
VIII	Acoustic	And	Says	Sensory • Hearing • Equilibrium and balance
IX	Glossopharyngeal	German	Bad	Sensory • Taste on posterior one third of tongue • Pharynx Motor • Parotid gland
X	Vagus	Viewed	Business	Sensory • Pharynx, larynx, neck Motor • Palate, larynx, pharynx • Swallowing • Cardiac muscle • Secretory glands of pancreas and GI tract
XI	Spinal Accessory	Some	Marry	Motor • Shoulder and neck movement • Sternocleidomastoid and trapezius muscles
XII	Hypoglossal	Hops	Money	Motor • Tongue

a) Intermittent or continuous
b) Relationship to other events or activities
c) Time last seen normal: important in stroke assessment and determination of candidacy for fibrinolytic therapy

3. Past medical history
   a. Congenital disorders
      1) Spina bifida
      2) Cerebral palsy
      3) Down syndrome
   b. Childhood diseases: poliomyelitis
   c. Epilepsy
   d. Head trauma
   e. Infectious neurologic conditions
      1) Encephalitis
      2) Meningitis
   f. Neuromuscular disease
      1) Multiple sclerosis
      2) Myasthenia gravis
      3) Amyotrophic lateral sclerosis (ALS)
      4) Parkinson's disease
   g. Spinal cord injury

Table 6-7 Autonomic Nervous System: Sympathetic and Parasympathetic Branch Function

	Sympathetic (Adrenergic)	Parasympathetic (Cholinergic)
Eyes	• Pupils dilate	• Pupils constrict
Heart	• Heart rate increases • Contractility increases • Coronary arteries dilate	• Heart rate decreases • Contractility decreases • No effect on coronary arteries
Lungs	• Bronchodilation	• Bronchoconstriction
Liver	• Glycogenolysis and lipolysis	• Glycogenesis
GI	• Salivary flow decreases • Gastric mobility and secretion decreases • Intestinal motility decreases	• Salivary flow increases • Gastric mobility and secretion increases • Intestinal motility increases
Urinary bladder	• Bladder relaxes • Sphincter closes	• Bladder contracts • Sphincter opens
Adrenal glands	• Secrete epinephrine, norepinephrine	• No effect
Skin	• Piloerection (goose pimples) • Increased perspiration	• No effect

h. Alzheimer's disease
i. Cancer
j. Cardiovascular disease
  1) Coronary artery disease: angina; myocardial infarction
  2) Valvular heart disease
  3) Hypertension
  4) Hyperlipidemia
  5) Dysrhythmia especially atrial fibrillation
  6) Ventricular aneurysm
  7) Endocarditis
k. Cerebrovascular disease
  1) Ischemic stroke
  2) Hemorrhagic stroke
  3) Carotid artery disease: bruit; prior carotid endarterectomy
l. Diabetes mellitus
m. Renal insufficiency/failure
n. Pulmonary embolism
o. Impairment of vision: use of eyeglasses, contact lenses, prosthesis
p. Impairment of hearing: use of hearing aid

4. Family history
  a. Epilepsy
  b. Diabetes mellitus
  c. Cardiac disease
  d. Hypertension
  e. Cerebrovascular disease
    1) Ischemic stroke
    2) Hemorrhagic stroke
  f. Cancer
  g. Neurologic disorders
    1) Amyotrophic lateral sclerosis (ALS)
    2) Huntington's disease
    3) Muscular dystrophy
    4) Neurofibromatosis
    5) Tay-Sachs disease
    6) Myasthenia gravis
    7) Multiple sclerosis
    8) Alzheimer's disease
    9) Tremor
    10) Dementia
  h. Psychiatric disorders
5. Social history
  a. Relationship with spouse or significant other; family structure
  b. Occupation: exposure to toxins (e.g., solvents, pesticides, arsenic, lead)
  c. Educational level
  d. Stress level and usual coping mechanisms
  e. Recreational habits
  f. Exercise habits
  g. Dietary habits
  h. Caffeine intake
  i. Tobacco use: Record as pack-years (number of packs per day times the number of years the patient has been smoking).
  j. Alcohol use: Record as alcoholic beverages consumed per month, week, or day.
  k. Drug use or abuse
  l. Toxin exposure
  m. Travel
  n. Handedness: left or right
6. Medication history
  a. Prescribed drug, dose, frequency, time of last dose
  b. Nonprescribed drugs
    1) Over-the-counter remedies
    2) Substance abuse
    3) Herbs
  c. Patient understanding of drug actions, side effects
  d. Drugs frequently used for neurologic problems
    1) Tranquilizers
    2) Sedatives
    3) Aspirin
    4) Anticonvulsants
    5) Antihypertensives
    6) Platelet aggregation inhibitors

e. Drugs that may cause neurologic problems
 1) Tranquilizers
 2) Sedatives
 3) Aspirin
 4) Anticoagulants
 5) Alcohol

Vital Signs

1. Cushing's triad: increased systolic BP with a decreased diastolic BP (widened pulse pressure), bradycardia, and abnormal respiratory pattern; late sign of increased intracranial pressure and impending herniation
2. BP
 a. Hypotension
  1) Hemorrhage
   a) Because the cranium is an inexpansible vault, intracranial hemorrhage cannot result in hypotension since herniation would result before significant hypotension.
   b) Consider other sources of bleeding (e.g., lacerated liver, ruptured spleen, thoracic trauma).
  2) General neurologic deterioration
  3) Of great concern because CPP = MAP − ICP
 b. Hypertension
  1) Systolic hypertension may be seen as a component of Cushing's triad, a late sign of intracranial hypertension.
  2) May indicate a change in arterial resistance and associated with vessel occlusion (e.g., stroke)
 c. Pulse pressure: difference between systolic and diastolic
  1) Normal is 30-40 mm Hg.
  2) Increased pulse pressure is a component of Cushing's triad, a late sign of intracranial hypertension.
3. Pulse
 a. Sinus bradycardia: a component of Cushing's triad, a late sign of intracranial hypertension
 b. Sinus tachycardia
  1) Hypoxia
  2) Hemorrhage
  3) General neurologic deterioration
 c. Atrial dysrhythmias (e.g., premature atrial contractions, atrial fibrillation, atrial flutter) may be etiologic factor in ischemic stroke.
4. Ventilatory rate and rhythm (Figure 6-13)
 a. Bradypnea
  1) Description: regular rhythm with rate less than 12/min
  2) Caused by CNS depression by injury, disease, or drugs
 b. Cheyne-Stokes
  1) Increasing rate and depth of ventilation followed by decreasing rate and depth of ventilation and then apnea
  2) Causes
   a) Bilateral lesions of cerebral hemispheres
   b) Lesion of basal ganglia
   c) Cerebellar lesion
   d) Lesion of upper brainstem
   e) Metabolic condition
 c. CNS hyperventilation
  1) Sustained increased rate and depth of ventilation
  2) Causes
   a) Lesions of lower midbrain or upper pons
   b) May be secondary to transtentorial herniation

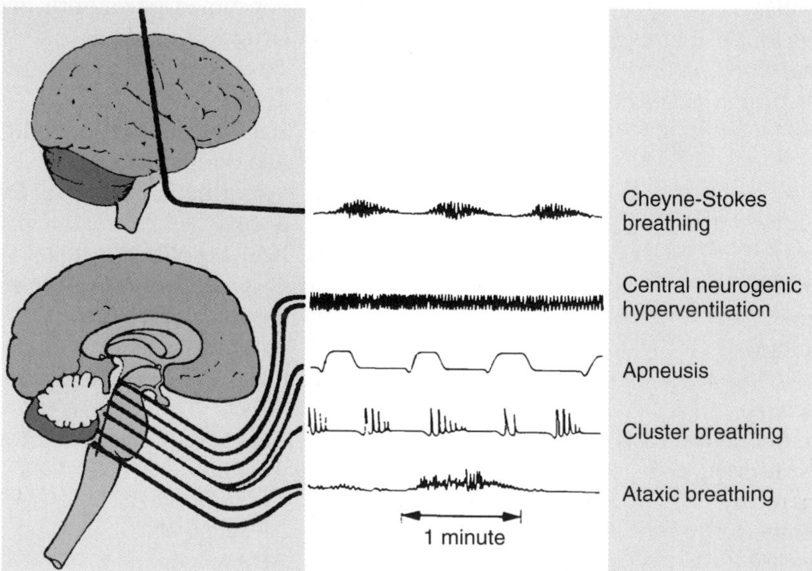

Figure 6-13 Abnormal respiratory patterns with corresponding level of central nervous system activity. (From McCance, K. L., & Huether, S. E. [2010]. *Pathophysiology: The biologic basis for disease in adults and children* [6th ed.]. St. Louis: Mosby.)

d. Apneustic
   1) Apnea with inspiration followed by exhalation
   2) Cause: lesions of mid to lower pons
e. Cluster
   1) 3-4 breaths of identical rate and depth followed by apnea, sequence repeated
   2) Cause: lesions of lower pons or upper medulla
f. Ataxic
   1) No pattern to ventilation; completely irregular with mostly apnea
   2) Cause: lesion of the medulla

5. Temperature
   a. Decreased (subnormal)
      1) Shock
      2) Drug overdose
      3) Metabolic coma (e.g., myxedema coma)
      4) Terminal stages of neurologic disease
   b. Increased
      1) Infection
         a) Systemic infection
         b) CNS infection
      2) Subarachnoid hemorrhage
      3) Seizures
      4) Restlessness
      5) Injury to hypothalamus: especially if inordinately elevated

General Appearance

1. Attire: appropriateness to age, environment
2. Grooming
   a. Hair
   b. Teeth
   c. Hygiene
   d. Nails
3. General behavior
   a. Demeanor
   b. Affect: facial expressions; body language
   c. Mood: euphoria; anger; depression; suicidal thoughts
4. Posture: gestures; fidgeting; restlessness; tremor; rigidity
5. Gait: Ataxia is uncoordinated movements of the body.
6. Obvious physical defects
   a. Hemiparesis or hemiplegia
   b. Facial asymmetry
   c. Ptosis
   d. Tremor
   e. Amputations
   f. Mass response: decorticate or decerebrate posturing

Mental Status and Cognition

1. Level of consciousness: the most sensitive clinical indicator of a change in neurologic status
   a. Consciousness is a state of awareness: self; environment; responses to environment
      1) Arousal
         a) Measure of being awake
         b) Function of the reticular activating system (RAS) in the midbrain
      2) Awareness
         a) Involves interpreting sensory input and giving an appropriate response
         b) Requires both an intact RAS and cerebral hemispheres
   b. Evaluate the degree of stimulus to get a response
      1) Verbal stimuli
         a) Call the patient by name, speaking at normal voice volume.
         b) Ask the patient to make a fist with his or her hand; when performed, ask the patient to open the fist.
         c) Use increased volume ("yelling") if the patient does not respond to normal voice volume
      2) Tactile stimuli: Touch or shake the patient.
      3) Painful stimuli: Utilize only if the other methods are unsuccessful; avoid trauma and bruising caused by pinching.
         a) Techniques to elicit a pain response
            i) Central: Brain responds.
               (a) Pressure to trapezius muscle: Squeeze large muscle mass between thumb and index finger; do not pinch skin.
               (b) Pressure to Achilles tendon: Squeeze large muscle mass between thumb and index finger; do not pinch skin.
               (c) Supraorbital pressure
                  (i) Push up against the supraorbital ridge with thumb; exert gentle upward pressure.
                  (ii) Do not push into the eye socket; injury to the eye or vagal response may occur.
                  (iii) Do not use this technique in patients with facial fracture or cranial fracture.
               (d) Sternal rub: Rub sternum gently with knuckle; if bruising results, discontinue using this technique.
            ii) Peripheral: Spine responds.
               (a) Nailbed pressure: Apply pressure to the nailbed, using the flat surface of a pen or pencil.
                  (i) Useful in determining sensory and motor function but should not be used as the only method of evaluation of pain response

c. Levels of consciousness (Haymore, 2004)
   1) Normal: arouses easily, maintains wakefulness, speaks coherently, responds appropriately to stimuli
   2) Hypersomnia: prolonged sleeping time with normal sleep pattern
   3) Lethargy, obtundation, stupor
      a) These are confusing terms indicating diminishing levels of consciousness.
      b) It is recommended to describe the patient's response to stimuli and behavior rather than use these labels.
   4) Coma: absence of awareness and responsiveness caused by structural lesion or metabolic condition
   5) Persistent vegetative state: unaware of self and surroundings
      a) Sleep-wake patterns occur along with eye opening but no response to stimuli occurs.
      b) Brainstem and hypothalamic function intact
   6) Locked-in syndrome: consciousness with near-complete paralysis
      a) Able to answer questions with eye blink
      b) Vision and hearing are preserved.
      c) Due to lesion of midbrain or pons
   7) Brain death: absence of all cortical and brainstem function
d. Glasgow coma scale (Table 6-8)
   1) Developed as a method to standardize observation of responsiveness in patients with traumatic brain injury
   2) Best or highest response is recorded; E (eye), M (motor), V (verbal) may be recorded separately along with a quantitative score.

Table 6-8 Glasgow Coma Scale

Parameter	Response	Score
Eye opening	Spontaneous	4
	To speech	3
	To pain	2
	None	1
	Untestable	U
Best motor response	Obeys commands	6
	Localizes pain	5
	Withdraws from pain	4
	Abnormal flexion (decorticate posturing)	3
	Abnormal extension (decerebrate posturing)	2
	None	1
	Untestable	U
Best verbal response	Oriented	5
	Confused	4
	Inappropriate	3
	Incomprehensible	2
	None	1
	Untestable	U

   3) Note if certain responses cannot be evaluated because of any of the following:
      a) Endotracheal intubation or tracheostomy
      b) Aphasia
      c) Eyes swollen shut
   4) Parameters
      a) Minimum: 3
      b) Maximum (normal): 15
      c) Clinically significant: change of 2 points or more
e. National Institutes of Health Stroke Scale (NIHSS) (Table 6-9)
   1) Used to assess the severity of presenting signs and symptoms
   2) Score over 22 indicates severe neurologic deficit
   3) Baseline assessment completed at admission; repeat assessments 2 hours after treatment, 24 hours post onset of symptoms, 7-10 days post onset of symptoms, and 3 months post onset of symptoms

2. Cognitive function
a. Orientation: Patient may be alert but confused.
   1) Orientation to time
      a) Ability to give today's date (e.g., What is today's date?)
      b) Ability to state the year (e.g., What year is it?)
   2) Orientation to place
      a) Ability to identify surroundings (e.g., Where are you now?)
      b) Ability to state address (e.g., Where do you live?)
   3) Orientation to person
      a) Ability to identify self by name (e.g., Who are you? What is your name?)
      b) Recognition of friends, family
   4) Orientation to situation: ability to identify why they are in the hospital (e.g., Why are you here?)
b. Memory
   1) How old are you?
   2) Remote memory: What is your birthday? Where were you born?
   3) Recent memory: What did you have for breakfast? What is your doctor's name?
c. Short-term recall: Can the patient repeat three or four objects after 3 to 5 minutes?
d. General knowledge: Ask a question about a current event.
e. Attention span: Is the patient able to stay on a subject?
f. Thought content: Note evidence of illusions, hallucinations, delusions, paranoia.
g. Calculation skills: Can you count backwards from 20 to 1?
h. Judgment: Why are you here?; What would you do if there were a fire in the wastebasket?
i. Abstraction: Ask the patient to spell the word "world" backward.

Table 6-9 National Institutes of Health Stroke Scale

Item/Domain	Response	Score
1A Level of consciousness	• Alert, keenly responsive • Obeys, answers or responds to minor stimulation • Responds only to repeated stimulation or painful stimulation (excludes reflex response) • Responds only with reflex motor or totally unresponsive	0 1 2 3
1B Orientation Ask the month and patient age; must be exactly right.	• Answers both correctly • Answers one correctly or patient unable to speak due to any reason other than aphasia or coma • Answers neither correctly, or too stuporous or aphasic	0 1 2
1C Response to commands Ask patient to open and close eyes and then grip and release nonparetic hand	• Performs both tasks correctly • Performs 1 task correctly • Performs neither task correctly	0 1 2
2 Gaze Only horizontal movements tested	• Normal • Partial gaze palsy • Forced deviation or total gaze paresis not overcome by oculocephalic maneuver	0 1 2
3 Visual field Tested by confrontation	• No visual loss • Partial hemianopia • Complete hemianopia • Bilateral hemianopia (blind from any cause including cortical blindness)	0 1 2 3
4 Facial movement Encourage patient to smile and close eyes, or note symmetry of grimace in response to noxious stimuli if poorly responsive	• Normal symmetrical movement • Minor paralysis (flattened nasolabial fold, asymmetry on smiling) • Partial paralysis (total or near-total lower face paralysis) • Complete paralysis (absence of facial movement upper/lower face)	0 1 2 3
5a Left arm motor function Extend left arm palm down at 90 degrees (sitting) or 45 degrees (supine)	• No drift—holds for full 10 seconds • Drifts down before 10 seconds but does not hit bed/support • Some effort against gravity, but cannot get up to 90 (or 45 if supine) degrees • No effort against gravity; limb falls • No movement	0 1 2 3 4
5b Right arm motor function Extend right arm palm down at 90 degrees (sitting) or 45 degrees (supine)	• No drift—holds for full 10 seconds • Drifts down before 10 seconds but does not hit bed/support • Some effort against gravity, but cannot get up to 90 (or 45 if supine) degrees • No effort against gravity; limb falls • No movement	0 1 2 3 4
6a Left leg motor function Extend left leg and flex at hip to 30 degrees	• No drift—holds for full 5 seconds • Drifts down before 5 seconds but does not hit bed/support • Some effort against gravity • No effort against gravity; limb falls • No movement	0 1 2 3 4
6b Right leg motor function Extend right leg and flex at hip to 30 degrees	• No drift—holds for full 5 seconds • Drifts down before 5 seconds but does not hit bed/support • Some effort against gravity • No effort against gravity; limb falls • No movement	0 1 2 3 4
7 Limb ataxia Finger/nose and heel/shin done on both sides; not ataxia if hemiplegic or unable to comprehend; ataxia must be out of proportion to any weakness present	• Absent • Present in one limb • Present in two limbs	0 1 2
8 Sensory	• Normal • Pinprick less sharp or dull on affected side • Severe to total sensory loss; patient unaware of being touched	0 1 2

Continued

Table 6-9 National Institutes of Health Stroke Scale—cont'd

Item/Domain	Response	Score
9 Best language Name items; read short sentences	• No aphasia • Some loss of fluency or comprehension • Severe aphasia—fragmentary communication; listener carries burden of communication • Mute, global aphasia. No usable speech or auditory comprehension	0 1 2 3
10 Dysarthria If not obviously present, have patient read	• Normal • Slurs some words • So slurred as to be unintelligible, or mute	0 1 2
11 Extinction/inattention	• No abnormality • Inattention to any sensory modality or extinction to bilateral simultaneous stimulation in one sensory modality • Profound hemi-inattention or hemi-inattention to more than one modality; does not recognize own hand	0 1 2

From National Institutes of Health. (2008). NIH stroke scale. Retrieved August 2, 2011, from http://www.ninds.nih.gov/doctors/NIH_Stroke_Scale_Booklet.pdf

3. Speech and language
   a. Note punctuation, rhythm, stream of talk, sentence structure, appropriate use of words; speech should be fluent with expression of connected thoughts.
   b. If patient cannot utilize or understand verbal communication
      1) Can the patient understand or utilize gestures?
      2) Can the patient understand written language or write messages?
   c. Identify the presence of speech disorders.
      1) Dysphonia: difficulty producing sound
      2) Dysarthria: difficulty with articulation
      3) Dysprosody: lack of inflection while talking
      4) Aphasia: impaired understanding or expression of verbal and/or written language
         a) Receptive (sensory) aphasia: lesion in Wernicke's area in temporal area
         b) Expressive (motor) aphasia: lesion in Broca's area in frontal area
         c) Global: both

Motor Function

1. Muscle size
   a. Symmetry
   b. Atrophy or hypertrophy
2. Symmetrical movement and strength of extremities
   a. Movement
      1) Spontaneous movement and symmetry of movement
      2) Assumption of a position of comfort
   b. Muscle strength (Table 6-10)
      1) Arm strength
         a) Test flexor and extensor muscle groups by evaluating strength against resistance.
         b) Pronator drift
            i) Detection: Have patient hold his or her arms out in front with palms up and eyes closed.
            ii) Normal: Patient should be able to hold arms even for at least 20 seconds.
            iii) Abnormal: The weak arm begins to drift and pronate (turn palm downward).
      2) Leg strength
         a) Test flexor and extensor muscle groups by evaluating strength against resistance.
         b) Ask the patient to raise legs one at a time to 30 degrees off the bed from supine position and hold in place for a count to 5; observe for drift.
3. Muscle tone
   a. Flaccidity: no resistance to passive movement; flaccid paralysis is generally associated with lower motor neuron lesions but may also occur early in upper motor neuron lesions
   b. Hypotonia: little resistance to passive movement
   c. Hypertonia: increased muscle resistance to passive movement
   d. Rigidity: increased muscle resistance to passive movement of a rigid limb that is uniform through both flexion and extension (paratonic rigidity may occur in coma and is a sign of diffuse cerebral dysfunction)

Table 6-10 Muscle Strength Grading Scale

Grade	Description
0/5	No movement or muscle contraction
1/5	Trace; no movement but evidence of muscle contraction
2/5	Not greater than gravity; movement with gravity eliminated
3/5	Greater than gravity; movement against gravity
4/5	Slight weakness; movement against some resistance
5/5	Normal; movement against full resistance

e. Spasticity: gradual increase in tone causing increased resistance until tone is suddenly reduced
   1) Clonus, continued rhythmic contraction of a muscle after the stimulus has been applied, may be evident
   2) Spastic paralysis is associated with upper motor neuron lesions and emerges after resolution of the early flaccidity stage.

f. Upper motor neuron versus lower motor neuron (Table 6-11)

4. Coordination
   a. Point-to-point movements
      1) Finger-nose test: Ask patient to touch his or her nose with the finger with eyes closed.
      2) Finger-finger test: Ask patient to touch your finger with his or her finger with eyes closed.
      3) Heel-knee test: Ask patient to run the heel of one foot down the opposite leg from the knee to the foot.
   b. Rapid, rhythmic alternating movements
      1) Pronation-supination test: Ask patient to rapidly pronate and supinate his or her hand.
      2) Patting test: Ask patient to rapidly pronate and supinate his or her hand against a leg.
   c. Figure-of-eight test: Ask patient to draw a figure of eight in the air with his or her great toe.
5. Gait
   a. Tandem gait: patient asked to walk heel-to-toe in a straight line
      1) Normal: ability to walk heel-to-toe without difficulty
      2) Abnormal: loss of balance indicates cerebellar dysfunction
   b. Abnormal gaits
      1) Spastic: Leg is held stiff and moved slowly; toes and lateral aspect of foot scrape the floor as the leg is moved; this indicates corticospinal tract lesion.
      2) Steppage: Foot is lifted very high for each step with a distinctive slapping sound as it hits the floor; this indicates peripheral nerve injury.
      3) Ataxic: Feet are broad-based and steps are unsteady and staggering; this indicates cerebellar or dorsal column lesions.
      4) Propulsive: Body is bent forward, steps are short, momentum is increased, and falls are common; this indicates basal ganglia dysfunction (e.g., Parkinson's disease).
      5) Waddling: Pelvis opposite the weight-bearing hip drops and the trunk inclines, causing a waddle; this indicates proximal muscle weakness (e.g., muscular dystrophy).
      6) Scissors: Thighs are held together and each foot is alternately brought forward; this indicates upper motor neuron lesion.
6. Station: tested by Romberg test
   a. Method: patient asked to stand with feet together and arms extended in front with eyes closed
   b. Normal: patient able to stand erect and steady; slight swaying may be seen
   c. Abnormal: Patient loses balance; this indicates loss of position sense and/or cerebellar dysfunction.
7. Involuntary movements
   a. Posturing may occur spontaneously or to pain in comatose patients; may also be considered a "mass response"
      1) Abnormal flexion (Figure 6-14)
         a) Also called decorticate posturing
         b) Arms are flexed toward the body, legs are extended
         c) Indicates cerebral lesion
      2) Abnormal extension (Figure 6-14)
         a) Also called decerebrate posturing
         b) Arms are extended, wrists are externally rotated, and legs are extended.
         c) Indicates midbrain or brainstem lesion

Table 6-11 Locating Site of Motor Problems

		Upper Motor Neuron	
	Lower Motor Neuron	**Pyramidal Tract**	**Extrapyramidal Tract**
Effect	Flaccid paralysis Areflexia	• Spastic paralysis with hyperactive reflexes • Positive Babinski's reflex	• No paralysis • Altered muscle tone and abnormal movements
Muscle appearance	Atrophy Small muscular contractions (fasciculation)	Mild atrophy from disuse	Tremor when at rest
Muscle tone	Decreased	Increased	Increased
Muscle strength	Decreased or absent	Decreased or absent	Normal
Coordination	Absent or poor	Absent or poor	Slowed
Examples	• Poliomyelitis • ALS • Guillain-Barré syndrome	• Stroke • Spinal cord injury • Multiple sclerosis • ALS	• Parkinson's disease

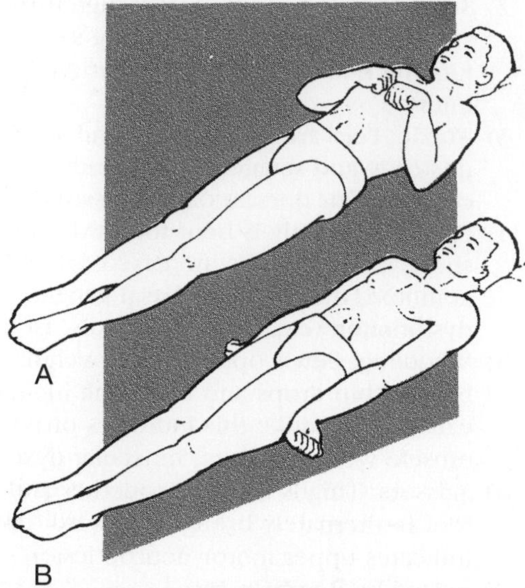

Figure 6-14 A, Abnormal flexion (decorticate) posturing. **B,** Abnormal extension (decerebrate) posturing. (From Urden, L., Stacy, K., & Lough, M. [2010]. *Critical care nursing: Diagnosis and management* [6th ed.]. St. Louis: Mosby.)

3) Opisthotonos
   a) Also referred to as arching
   b) Extension of arms, legs and arching of the back and neck
   c) May indicate brainstem injury
4) Flaccid posture: Entire body is flaccid even with painful stimulation.

b. Tremor
   1) Resting: Parkinson's disease
   2) Intentional: cerebellar disease
   3) Flapping: metabolic encephalopathy (e.g., hepatic or renal failure)
   4) Physiologic: stress induced
   5) Senile: age induced

c. Seizure: Describe.
   1) Preceding events: aura?
   2) Initial cry or sound
   3) Onset
      a) Initial body movements
      b) Deviation of head and eyes
      c) Chewing and salivation
      d) Posture of body
      e) Sensory changes
   4) Tonic and clonic phases
      a) Progression of movements of body
      b) Skin color and airway
      c) Pupillary changes
      d) Incontinence
      e) Duration of each phase
   5) Level of consciousness during seizure
   6) Postictal phase
      a) Duration
      b) General behavior
      c) Memory of events
      d) Orientation
      e) Pupillary changes
      f) Headache
      g) Aphasia
      h) Injuries
   7) Duration of entire seizure
   8) Medications given and response
   9) Findings on diagnostic studies
      a) Serum electrolytes
      b) Diagnostic imaging (e.g., CT, MRI)
      c) EEG

Sensory Function

1. Ability to perceive sensation
   a. Superficial sensation
      1) Light touch: wisp of cotton on skin
      2) Superficial pain: light pinprick on skin (use sterile needle and discard appropriately after testing)
      3) Skin temperature: hot and cold test tubes on skin; rarely performed
   b. Deep sensation
      1) Vibration: vibration of tuning fork on bony surface
      2) Position sense: position of great toe, thumb with eyes closed
      3) Deep pain: pressure on Achilles tendon, calf muscles, upper arm muscles
   c. Cortical/discriminatory sensation: requires cortical interpretation
      1) Two-point discrimination: ability to distinguish between one or two points; touch patient with two points at varying degrees of separation to see if the patient feels only one point or two points
      2) Stereognosis: ability to distinguish common objects placed in the hand with eyes closed
      3) Topognosis: ability to distinguish which finger is being touched with eyes closed
      4) Graphesthesia: ability to recognize numbers or letters traced on the skin with eyes closed
      5) Double simultaneous stimulation (tactile inattention testing): ability to differentiate between one point and two points when being touched by one or two points on opposite sides of the body in corresponding locations
   d. Ability to recognize objects through the special senses; inability referred to as *agnosia*
      1) Visual: occipital lobe
      2) Auditory: temporal lobe
      3) Tactile: parietal lobe
      4) Body parts and relationships: parietal lobe
   e. Distribution of sensory loss
      1) Entire side of body: parietal or thalamic lesion
      2) Dermatomal (Table 6-12 and Figure 6-12)
         a) Dermatome: skin area supplied by sensory fibers of a single spinal nerve
         b) Sensory loss below a dermatomal level: spinal cord lesion

Table 6-12 Dermatomal Levels for Bedside Assessment

Anatomical Location	Spinal Level
Front of neck	C3
Thumb	C6
Ring and little fingers	C8
Nipple line	T4
Umbilicus	T10
Groin crease	L1
Knee	L3
Anterior ankle and foot	L5
Lateral foot and heel	S1
Genitalia	S3, S4

c) Sensory loss along a dermatome: spinal nerve lesion
3) Peripheral nerve distribution (see Figure 6-12)
f. Degrees of sensory loss
1) Anesthesia: loss of sensation
2) Dysesthesia: impaired sensation
3) Hyperesthesia: increased sensation
4) Hypesthesia: decreased sensation
5) Paresthesia: burning, tingling sensation

Cranial Nerve Function

1. Olfactory (I)
a. Test: patient's ability to identify familiar odors (e.g., coffee, cloves, tobacco, alcohol) tested; each nostril tested separately with eyes closed; rarely performed in acute care
b. Normal: able to identify familiar odors
c. Abnormal: unable to identify familiar odors; referred to as *anosmia*
2. Optic (II)
a. Visual acuity: test by the following:
1) Snellen chart
a) Ask patient to read lines of the Snellen chart from a distance of 20 feet or use a pocket Snellen card for patients who are bed-bound.
b) Record the number on the lowest line that the patient can read with 50% accuracy.
c) Test with glasses or contact lenses.
2) If patient cannot see well enough to read the Snellen chart, ask how many fingers you are holding up.
3) If the patient cannot see well enough to tell you how many fingers you are holding up, assess whether he or she blinks to visual threat.
b. Visual fields
1) Test by confrontation: comparison of patient's visual field to examiner's visual field with eye on same side covered
2) Loss of vision or portion of visual field
a) Unilateral blindness: lesion of eye, retina, or optic nerve
b) Bitemporal hemianopsia: lesion of optic chiasm or lesion causing pressure on optic chiasm (e.g., pituitary tumor)
c) Left homonymous hemianopsia: lesion of right optic tract
d) Right homonymous hemianopsia: lesion of left optic tract
e) Left homonymous hemianopsia with macular sparing: lesion of right geniculocalcarine tract
f) Right homonymous hemianopsia with macular sparing: lesion of left geniculocalcarine tract
c. Near vision
1) Test: Ask the patient to read newsprint at a distance of 12 inches or use pocket Snellen card.
2) Normal: Patient should be able to read newsprint at 1 foot.
d. Funduscopic examination with ophthalmoscope to detect papilledema
1) Optic disk is pushed forward.
2) Disk margins are blurry.
3) Indication of intracranial hypertension
a) May be late in acute intracranial hypertension
b) May be first sign in chronic intracranial hypertension (e.g., tumor)
3. Oculomotor (III), trochlear (IV), abducens (VI)
a. Eyelids: Elevation of the eyelid is controlled by cranial nerve III; ptosis may indicate cranial nerve III injury.
b. Pupils
1) Size
a) Normal 2 to 6 mm
b) Abnormal: Clinically significant change is change of more than 1 mm.
i) Pinpoint (and nonreactive)
(a) Pontine lesion
(b) Medication effect
(i) Opiates (e.g., morphine)
(ii) Miotics (e.g., pilocarpine)
ii) Midsize (2 to 6 mm) but nonreactive: midbrain lesion
iii) Unilateral large (greater than 6 mm) and nonreactive (may be referred to as *blown or Hutchinsonian pupil*): pressure on oculomotor nerve on same side
iv) Bilateral large (greater than 6 mm) and nonreactive
(a) Brainstem lesion
(b) Medication effect
(i) Parasympatholytics (e.g., atropine)
(ii) Sympathomimetics (e.g., epinephrine)
2) Equality
a) Normal: equal

b) Abnormal: unequal (referred to as *anisocoria*)
   i) Normal variation: 15-20% of the population has slightly unequal pupils (1 mm or less difference)
   ii) Abnormal: difference of more than 1 mm or change from baseline
   iii) Injury effects
      (a) Injury to parasympathetic fibers of the oculomotor nerve: ipsilateral (same side) pupil dilation
      (b) Injury to sympathetic fibers of the oculomotor nerves (e.g., Horner's syndrome: ipsilateral pupil constriction)

3) Shape
   a) Normal: round
   b) Abnormal
      i) Oval
         (a) May precede dilated pupil as a sign of pressure on the oculomotor nerve
         (b) Associated with intracranial pressure of 18-35 mm Hg
      ii) Irregular (e.g., keyhole shaped may be seen in patients after cataract removal due to concurrent iridectomy)

4) Position
   a) Normal: midposition
   b) Abnormal
      i) Both eyes deviated toward one side
         (a) Unilateral pontine lesion
         (b) Fixed lesion such as tumor, stroke, or hemorrhage: toward the lesion and away from the hemiparesis
         (c) Seizure: away from the seizure focus and toward the hemiparesis
      ii) Downward deviation of both eyes (frequently with inward convergence): thalamic lesion
      iii) Downward deviation of 1 eye: cranial nerve III palsy
      iv) Medial deviation of 1 eye: cranial nerve IV palsy

5) Reactivity to light
   a) Test
      i) Darken the room if pupils are small.
      ii) Use a small, bright penlight in front of each eye.
      iii) Note pupil constriction as the direct reaction.
      iv) Note pupil constriction of the opposite pupil as consensual reaction.
   b) Normal: brisk bilateral direct and consensual reaction to light
   c) Abnormal
      i) Sluggish or absent reaction; indicative of any of the following:
         (a) Cranial nerve III pressure or injury
         (b) Hypothermia
         (c) Barbiturate intoxication
      ii) Hippus: pupil initially reacts briskly, then followed by an exaggerated rhythmic contraction and dilation of the pupil; may be normal but may be indicative of any of the following:
         (a) Early cranial nerve III pressure or injury
         (b) Midbrain injury
         (c) Barbiturate intoxication

6) Accommodation
   a) Test: Ask the patient to focus on a distant object and accommodate as the object moves closer.
   b) Pupils dilate when focusing on a far object.
   c) Pupils constrict when focusing on a near object.

7) Ciliospinal reflex
   a) Test: Squeeze trapezius muscle and observe reaction of pupil on same side.
   b) Normal: ipsilateral pupil dilation with trapezius squeeze
   c) Abnormal: no response; indicative of interruption of sympathetic fibers of cranial nerve III

c. Extraocular movements (EOMs)
   1) Test: patient asked to keep head straight and follow your finger with eyes; move your finger in the direction of the six cardinal positions of gaze (Figure 6-15)
   2) Normal: Both eyes move conjugately in the direction of your finger.
   3) Abnormal: one or both eyes do not move to follow finger; indicative of cranial nerve injury or isolated muscular dysfunction

d. Abnormal eye movements
   1) Nystagmus: jerky eye movement that oscillates the eye back and forth quickly; may be seen in lesions of vestibular system or brainstem
   2) Dysconjugate eye movement: may indicate damage to the brainstem
   3) Conjugate eye movement: may indicate cerebral hemispheric damage

4. Trigeminal (V)
   a. Sensory branch
      1) Test
         a) Three branches (ophthalmic, maxillary, mandibular) tested on both sides with a wisp of cotton (light touch) and pinprick (superficial pain)

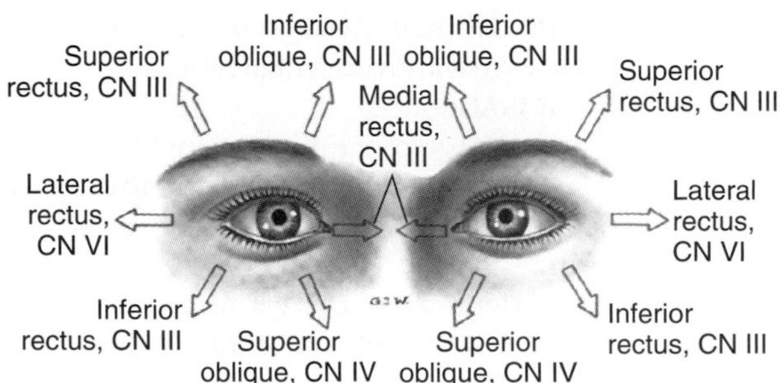

Figure 6-15 The six cardinal positions of gaze. (From Seidel, H. M., et al. [1991]. *Mosby's guide to physical examination* [2nd ed.]. St Louis: Mosby.)

i) Normal: detection of touch and pain
ii) Abnormal: no detection of touch or pain

b) Corneal blink reflex
i) Detection: corneal touched with a wisp of cotton
ii) Normal: bilateral blink; indicates intactness of cranial nerves V and VII
iii) Abnormal: decreased or absent blink; may indicate cranial nerve V injury (NOTE: Contact lens wearers have diminished corneal blink reflex.)

b. Motor branch
1) Test: face inspected for muscle atrophy, tremor; the masseter muscle palpated while the patient clenches teeth; the temporal muscles palpated as the patient squeezes eyes closed
2) Normal: symmetry of muscle strength, no atrophy or tremor
3) Abnormal: asymmetry of muscle strength; may indicate cranial nerve V injury

5. Facial (VII)
a. Motor branch
1) Test: symmetry of facial expressions noted while patient raises eyebrows, frowns, smiles, and closes eyelids tightly
2) Abnormal: asymmetry of facial expression; loss of nasolabial fold, eye remaining open; indicates cranial nerve VII injury (Bell's palsy)

b. Sensory branch
1) Test: ability to taste sour and bitter on posterior tongue tested; rarely performed in acute care
2) Normal: ability to taste
3) Abnormal: inability to taste; indicates cranial nerve VII injury

6. Acoustic (VIII)
a. Cochlear branch: hearing acuity
1) Whisper test
a) Test: face turned away and examiner whispers to see if patient can hear what is whispered
b) Test each ear separately.
c) This test differentiates between hearing and lip reading

2) Weber test
a) Test: tuning fork placed at the midline vertex of skull
b) Normal: Patient hears equally on both sides.
c) Abnormal: patient indicates difference between the two ears; will hear the sound better with the "good" ear

3) Rinne test
a) Test: tuning fork placed on the mastoid; when the patient can no longer hear the sound by bone, the tuning fork is moved to in front of the ear
b) Normal: Air conduction is usually better than bone conduction so the patient should still be able to hear the sound when the tuning fork is moved in front of the ear after the patient reports not being able to hear the sound any longer by bone.
c) Abnormal: inability to hear the sound by air after the cessation of the sound by bone; diminished air conduction is associated with middle ear infection or disease

b. Vestibular branch
1) Not tested directly; problems may be detected by symptoms such as nystagmus, vertigo, nausea, vomiting, pallor, sweating, and hypotension
2) Reflexes: vestibular branch of cranial nerve VIII and connections with cranial nerves III and VI provide information regarding integrity of the brainstem
a) Oculocephalic reflex (also called *doll's eyes reflex*) (Figure 6-16)
i) Prerequisites
(a) Cervical spine has been radiologically cleared.
(b) Patient must be unconscious.
(c) Eyes are held open so that eye movement can be observed.
ii) Test: head rotated side to side
iii) Normal: eyes move in the opposite direction of the head (presence of doll's eyes: like an expensive china doll); indicates supratentorial cause for the coma
iv) Abnormal: eyes stay midline or turn to the same direction as the head (absence of doll's eyes); indicates compression in the midbrain-pontine area

b) Oculovestibular reflex (also called *caloric testing*) (Figure 6-16)
i) Prerequisites
(a) Intact tympanic membrane
(b) Absence of basal skull fracture

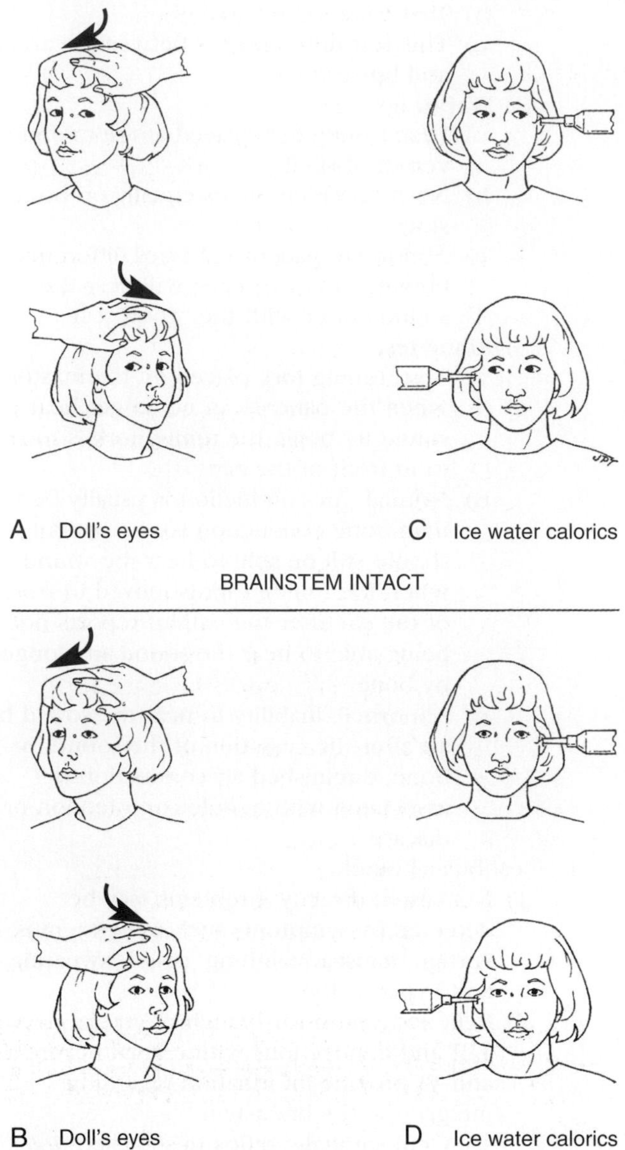

Figure 6-16 A, Oculocephalic (doll's eyes) reflex with normal response: eyes move in the direction opposite the direction that the head is turned. **B,** Oculocephalic (doll's eyes) reflex with abnormal response: eyes either move in the same direction as the head is being turned or stay midline. **C,** Oculovestibular (caloric) reflex with normal response: nystagmus is present, and there may be conjugate movement toward the irrigated ear. **D,** Oculovestibular (caloric) reflex with abnormal response: no nystagmus or dysconjugate movement of the eyes. (From Beare, P. G., & Myers, J. L. [1994]. *Principles and practice of adult health nursing* [2nd ed.]. St Louis: Mosby.)

ii) Test
(a) Elevation of the head of bed 30 degrees
(b) Injection of 20-50 mL of iced water into the ear canal and against the tympanic membrane

iii) Normal: nystagmus with deviation toward the irrigated ear
iv) Abnormal
(a) No eye movement
(b) Dysconjugate eye movement

7. Glossopharyngeal (IX), vagus (X)
   a. Phonation
      1) Test: patient asked to say "Ah"
      2) Normal: bilateral elevation of palate
      3) Abnormal: no elevation of palate on one side
   b. Speech
      1) Test: speech assessed; any hoarseness detected
      2) Normal: voice clear with ability to change volume and pitch
      3) Abnormal: hoarseness; indicates damage to the laryngeal branch of cranial nerve X
   c. Taste
      1) Test: ability to taste sour and bitter on posterior tongue tested; rarely performed in acute care
      2) Normal: ability to taste
      3) Abnormal: inability to taste sour or bitter
   d. Swallowing
      1) Test
         a) Hold tongue down with a tongue blade and touch each side of the pharynx with a cotton swab.
         b) Palpate elevation of larynx with swallow.
         c) If patient is conscious, give sip of water.
      2) Normal: involuntary swallow or gag when palate is stroked, elevation of larynx with swallow; effective swallow; indicates intactness of cranial nerves IX and X
      3) Abnormal
         a) No swallow or gag; do not give fluids; position on side; have suction equipment available
         b) Cough on water swallow: Request evaluation by speech and language pathologist.
   e. Gag
      1) Test: palate stroked with a tongue blade (NOTE: Do not perform this test within 2 hours after eating.)
      2) Normal: involuntary gag; indicates intactness of ninth and tenth cranial nerves
      3) Abnormal: no gag (NOTE: Do not give fluids; position on side; and have suction equipment available.)
   f. Cough
      1) Test: Touch hypopharynx with suction catheter.
      2) Normal: involuntary cough; indicates intactness of cranial nerves IX and X
      3) Abnormal: no cough
8. Spinal accessory (XI)
   a. Test

1) Sternocleidomastoid and trapezius muscles inspected for size and symmetry
2) Patient asked to shrug shoulders as you push down with your hands on the shoulders
3) Patient asked to turn head to each side against resistance

b. Normal: symmetry; adequate muscle strength
c. Abnormal: asymmetry; poor muscle strength

9. Hypoglossal (XII)
   a. Test
      1) Tongue inspected for atrophy, fasciculations, alignment
      2) Tongue strength tested with your index finger when the patient pushes his or her tongue against the cheek
   b. Normal: no atrophy, fasciculations, midline alignment when protrudes, normal strength
   c. Abnormal: atrophy, fasciculations, or deviation from midline; decreased strength

Reflexes

1. Deep tendon (also called *muscle-stretch reflexes*)
   a. Test: tendon tapped with a reflex hammer
   b. Normal: contraction of the muscle and a jerk of affected limb
   c. Abnormal
      1) Hyporeflexia
         a) Less than normal contraction
         b) May be seen in hypocalcemia, hyperphosphatemia, hypomagnesemia, lower motor neuron lesion
      2) Hyperreflexia
         a) More than normal contraction; may be associated with clonus
         b) May be seen in hypercalcemia, hypophosphatemia, hypermagnesemia, and upper motor neuron lesion
   d. Grading scale (Table 6-13)
   e. Locations and spinal levels
      1) Jaw: cranial nerve V (trigeminal)
      2) Biceps: elbow flexion; C5-6
      3) Brachioradialis: wrist extension; C5-6
      4) Triceps: elbow extension; C7-8
      5) Patellar: knee extension; L2-4
      6) Achilles: foot extension; S1-2
2. Superficial reflexes
   a. Abdominal reflexes
      1) Test: abdomen stroked toward umbilicus with blunt end of cotton-tipped applicator
      2) Normal: Umbilicus moves toward the quadrant that is stroked.
      3) Abnormal: no response; indicates lesion at T7-9 for upper abdomen; T11-12 for lower abdomen
   b. Cremasteric reflex
      1) Test: inner thigh stroked
      2) Normal: Testis on stimulated side elevates.
      3) Abnormal: no response: indicates lesion at L1-2
   c. Plantar reflex
      1) Test: sole of the foot stroked with a blunt instrument (Figure 6-17)
      2) Normal: Toes curl downward.
      3) Abnormal (Babinski's reflex): extension of great toe and fanning of other toes; indicates upper motor neuron lesion
3. Pathologic reflexes
   a. Babinski's: described earlier
   b. Grasp
      1) Test: something (frequently finger) placed in the patient's hand
      2) Normal: releases grasp on command
      3) Abnormal: will not release grasp on command; infantile reflex: indicates diffuse cerebral dysfunction

Table 6-13 Grading Scale for Deep Tendon Reflexes

Grade	Description
0	Absent
1+	Diminished
2+	Normal
3+	More brisk than average but may be normal
4+	Hyperactive with clonus

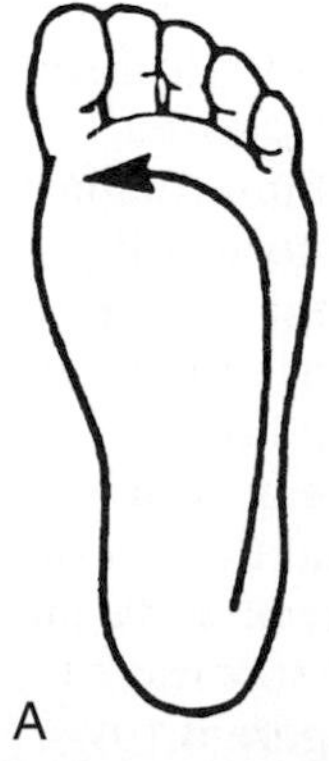

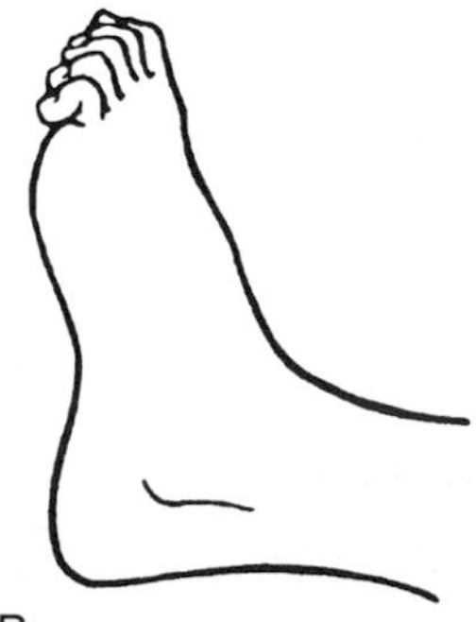

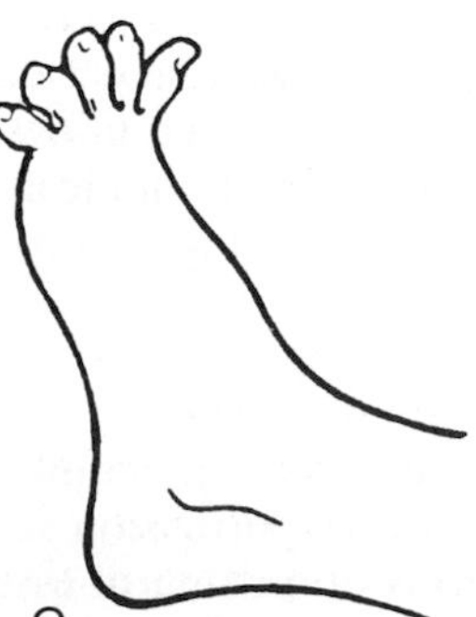

Figure 6-17 Babinski's reflex. **A,** Method of stroking sole of foot. **B,** Normal response (absence of Babinski's reflex). **C,** Abnormal response (presence of Babinski's reflex).

c. Sucking
   1) Test: corner of the patient's mouth touched
   2) Normal: no response
   3) Abnormal: patient purses lips and starts to suck; infantile reflex: indicates diffuse cerebral dysfunction
d. Glabellar
   1) Test: patient's forehead tapped
   2) Normal: no response
   3) Abnormal: patient repeatedly blinks; indicates diffuse cerebral dysfunction

Miscellaneous

1. Clinical indications of neurologic trauma
   a. Scalp: tears or swelling
   b. Head and face
      1) Face, maxilla, and mandible should be palpated for fractures.
      2) Note Battle's sign: bruising of mastoid (behind ear); indicative of basal skull fracture (Figure 6-18)
   c. Eyes
      1) Eye orbits should be palpated; note complaints of pain
      2) Visual acuity should be evaluated if corneal burn or trauma
      3) Note raccoon eyes: bruising around eyes indicative of basal skull fracture (Figure 6-18)
   d. Nose
      1) Nose should be palpated; note complaints of pain.
      2) Note CSF leak: may be seen in basal skull fracture; referred to as *rhinorrhea*
         a) Differentiation of CSF from mucus by testing for significant glucose
            i) CSF glucose is normally 60% of serum glucose
            ii) Low levels of glucose may be seen with mucus
         b) CSF also leaves a "halo" on 4 × 4-inch gauze or linens; this refers to blood settling in the middle with a lighter-colored concentric ring around the blood (Figure 6-18)
   e. Ears
      1) Note edema and trauma to external ear or ear canal
      2) Note blood in external ear canal or blood behind ear drum: seen in basal skull fracture
      3) Note cerebrospinal fluid leak from ear: seen in basal skull fracture; referred to as *otorrhea*
   f. Injury to teeth, tongue, gums, mucosa
   g. Alteration in consciousness
   h. Clinical indications of intracranial hypertension (see Intracranial Hypertension section)
2. Clinical indications of meningeal irritation
   a. Nuchal rigidity: indicative of meningeal irritation (e.g., infection or hemorrhage)
   b. Brudzinski's sign (Figure 6-19)

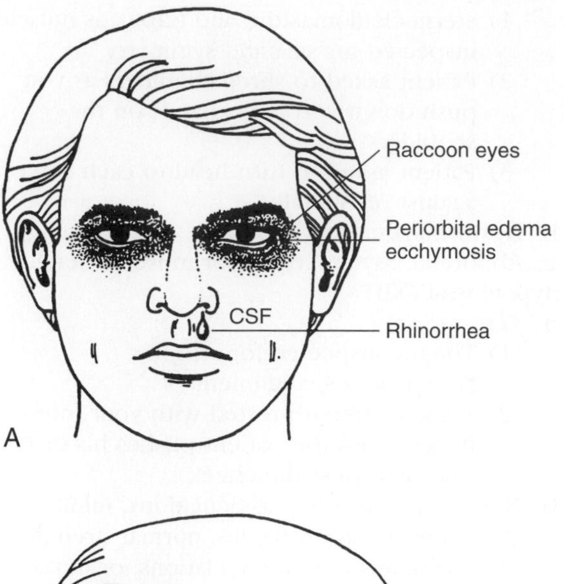

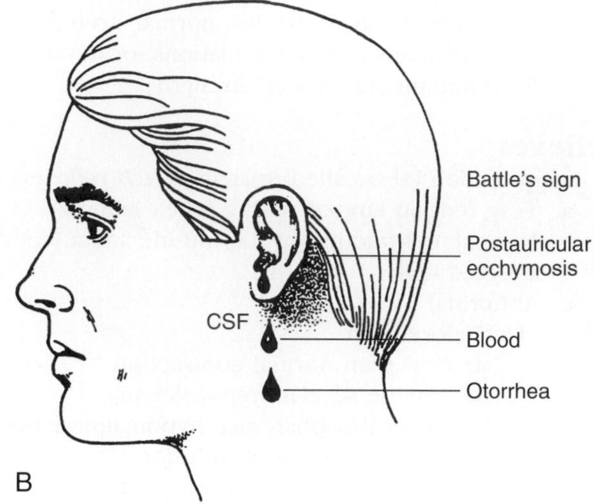

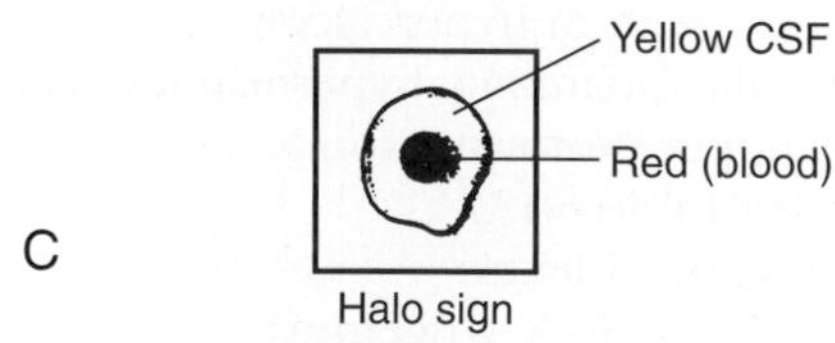

Figure 6-18 **A,** Raccoon eyes and rhinorrhea. **B,** Battle's sign with otorrhea. **C,** Halo sign. (From Barker, E. [2008]. *Neuroscience nursing: A spectrum of care* [3rd ed.]. St. Louis: Mosby.)

      1) Prerequisite: Cervical spine must be radiologically cleared.
      2) Detection: chin brought toward chest and head moved forward
      3) Normal: absence of neck pain and absence of involuntary adduction and flexion of knees toward body
      4) Abnormal: neck pain and involuntary adduction and flexion of legs with attempts to flex the neck; indicates irritation of the meninges by infection or blood
   c. Kernig's sign (Figure 6-19)
      1) Detection: patient placed on his or her back and assisted to flex thigh toward chest until

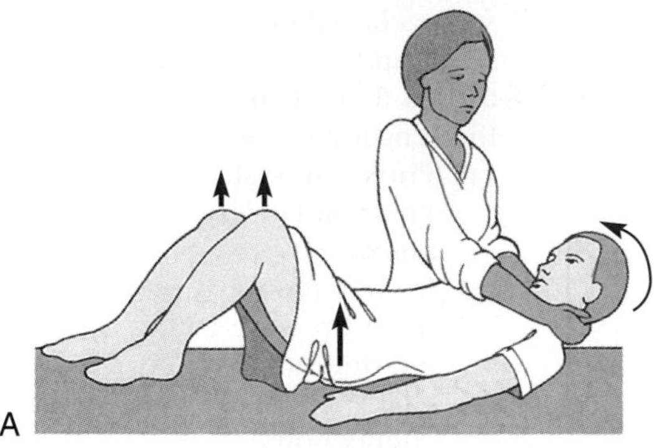

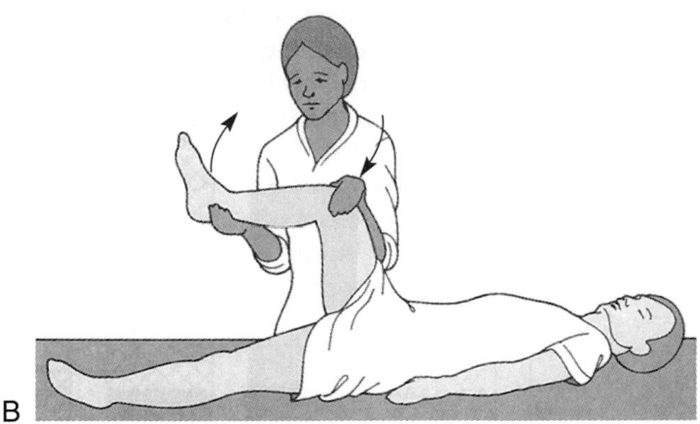

Figure 6-19 **A,** Brudzinski's sign. **B,** Kernig's sign. (From Barker, E. [2008]. *Neuroscience nursing: A spectrum of care* [3rd ed.]. St. Louis: Mosby.)

hip is at 90-degree angle; then leg extended at knee
2) Normal: ability to fully extend leg without pain
3) Abnormal: inability to fully extend leg when thigh is flexed toward abdomen; neck pain may also occur; indicates irritation of the meninges by infection or blood

3. Clinical indications of brain death
   a. Criteria: irreversible cessation of all functions of the entire brain, including the brainstem; note that specific requirements for declaration of brain death may be affected by state law and hospital policy
      1) Recognizable cause of coma (e.g., severe traumatic brain injury, intracranial hemorrhage or infarction, anoxic encephalopathy following cardiac arrest, drowning, asphyxiation)
      2) Exclusion of potentially reversible causes of coma (sedative drugs including alcohol, neuromuscular blocking agents, hypothermia, metabolic or endocrine disturbance)
         a) BP greater than 90 mm Hg
         b) Temperature greater than 32° C (90° F)
      3) Clinical examination
         a) Absence of responsiveness to noxious stimuli
         b) Absence of movement, including posturing, shivering, and seizures, either spontaneously or to central pain stimulation in the absence of sedation and neuromuscular blockade; spinal reflexes and Babinski's reflex may be present even in the presence of brain death
         c) Absence of brainstem function
            i) No pupillary light reflex
            ii) No corneal reflex
            iii) No oculocephalic reflex (i.e., doll's eyes)
            iv) No oculovestibular reflex (caloric)
            v) No gag or cough reflexes
         d) Absence of spontaneous ventilation when tested for a sufficient time; usually 3-5 minutes of $PaCO_2$ of greater than 60 mm Hg; apnea testing is performed by doing the following:
            i) Disconnect the mechanical ventilator.
            ii) Deliver 100% oxygen.
            iii) Monitor for ventilatory effort.
            iv) Measure arterial blood gases to confirm $PaCO_2$ greater than 60 mm Hg.
            v) Reconnect the ventilator.
      4) Optional confirmatory diagnostic and laboratory studies
         a) EEG: no electrical activity during a period of at least 30 minutes
         b) Cerebral angiography: no intracerebral filling in circle of Willis or at carotid bifurcation
         c) Cerebral blood flow scan: no uptake of radionuclide in brain parenchyma, indicating no cerebral blood flow
         d) Transcranial Doppler: reverberating flow signals
   b. Repeat evaluation in 6 hours is recommended.
   c. Signature of two physicians required for determination of brain death with one of the physicians not involved in the care of the patient; note that neither of the physicians should be involved in organ transplantation

Neurologic Monitoring

1. Intracranial pressure
   a. Indications
      1) The need for ICP monitoring usually correlates with a GCS of 8 or less.
      2) All of the following are potential diagnoses when ICP monitoring may be needed.
         a) Severe head trauma especially if abnormal findings on admission CT scan
         b) Intracerebral masses
         c) Subarachnoid hemorrhage
         d) Intracerebral hemorrhage (e.g., massive stroke)
         e) Infectious processes (e.g., encephalitis, meningitis)
         f) Encephalopathy

i) Anoxic encephalopathy (e.g., postcardiac arrest)
ii) Reye's syndrome
g) Hydrocephalus
h) Postcraniotomy
3) ICP monitoring should be used if deep sedation, paralysis, or barbiturate coma is being utilized because LOC as an assessment parameter is eliminated.

b. Purposes
1) Diagnose intracranial hypertension.
2) Allow drainage of CSF to maintain pressure.
3) Observe effects of medical or nursing management.
4) Predict outcomes: Patients who sustain an ICP greater than 50 mm Hg for longer than 20 minutes have a very poor prognosis.

c. General information
1) CSF is considered the most accurate indication of ICP.
a) The most accurate devices measure the pressure of CSF and are in contact with CSF.
b) This contact with CSF creates an infection risk.
c) Intraparenchymal devices: There is a linear relationship between intraventricular and intraparenchymal pressure measured with fiberoptic transducer-tipped probe.
2) There are several types of ICP measuring devices (Figure 6-20 and Table 6-14)
a) Insertion of all of these devices is either during craniotomy or through a small burr hole made with a twist drill utilizing strict aseptic technique.
3) There are three types of monitoring systems.
a) Fluid-filled system
i) Sensor: fluid-filled catheter or bolt that communicates the subarachnoid or interventricular space and the transducer
ii) Closed fluid-filled system between the sensor and the transducer
(a) Prime the system using preservative-free isotonic saline.
(b) Do not add heparin; do not use a pressure bag or intermittent flush device.
(c) Utilize Luer-Lok connections.
(d) Do not routinely irrigate; subarachnoid bolts may be irrigated if specifically ordered with approximately 0.1 mL every 2 hours; dilute antibiotic solution may be prescribed as irrigation solution.
iii) Transducer: converts the pressure signal to an electrical signal that can be recorded
(a) Position the transducer at the level of the foramen of Monro; this correlates externally to the tragus of ear.
(b) Connect the transducer cable to the pressure module of the bedside monitor.
b) Continuous drainage system (Figure 6-21)
i) Place the drip chamber at the prescribed height above foramen of Monro; height is based on the desired upper limit for controlling the ICP.
ii) Utilize commercial systems that have one-way flow valves and micropore filters on air vents.
c) Fiberoptic transducer

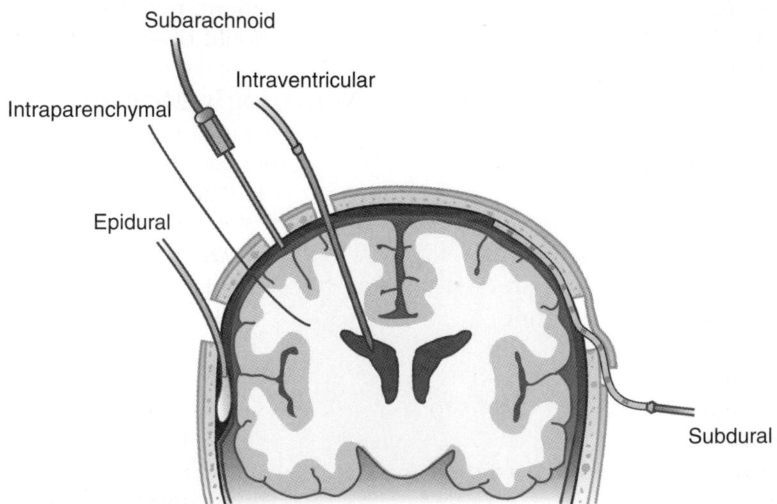

Figure 6-20 Devices for the measurement of intracranial pressure. (From Carlson, K. K. [Ed.]. [2009]. *Advanced critical care nursing.* St. Louis: Saunders.)

Table 6-14 ICP Measuring Devices

Device	Location	Accuracy	Comments
Intraventricular catheter	Lateral ventricle nondominant hemisphere is used if possible but location of skull fracture and trauma may limit placement possibilities	Excellent; can test VPR	• Preferred since most accurate and reliable, low cost, and provides opportunity to drain CSF for specimen or treatment of intracranial hypertension • May be difficult to insert especially if ventricles are small or displaced • Therapeutic or diagnostic removal of CSF possible • Provides access for determination of volume-pressure relationship • May permit CSF leakage, but rapid CSF drainage may result in collapsed ventricle or subdural hematoma • May cause intracerebral bleeding or edema at cannula track • Infection rate 2-5% • Fluid-filled system utilized if intraventricular catheter is placed
Subarachnoid bolt	Subarachnoid space	Fair; unreliable at high ICP	• Easy to insert; especially useful if ventricles are small • Inexpensive • Does not penetrate brain • Requires intact skull • Bolt can become occluded with clots or tissue; may require irrigation • Needs to be recalibrated frequently • Unable to drain CSF or to test VPR • Infection rate 1-2% • Fluid-filled system used
Epidural sensor or transducer	Between the skull and the dura	Variable	• Easy to insert • Does not penetrate brain or dura • Unable to drain CSF or to test VPR • Infection rate less than 1% • Head position has no effect on pressure reading • Cannot be re-zeroed once in place • Epidural pressure is slightly higher than intraventricular pressure
Intraparenchymal transducer	1 cm into brain tissue	Excellent	• Easy to insert • Unable to drain CSF or to test VPR • Catheter relatively fragile; avoid sharp kinks or pulls • Head position has no effect on pressure reading • Cannot be re-zeroed once in place • Risk of intracerebral bleeding and infection

i) A fluid-filled system is not necessary.
ii) The catheter is plugged directly into the monitor.
iii) This system requires a special monitor module.

d. Measurement guidelines
1) Explain procedure to patient and/or family.
2) Re-level and zero with each head position change if fluid-filled system.
3) Do not stimulate patient prior to measures.
4) Evaluate trends instead of one measurement.
5) Assist with volume-pressure response (VPR) test (or *pressure-volume index*) as requested.
a) Inject 1 mL of preservative-free isotonic saline in 1 second into an intraventricular catheter.
b) Normal: increase in ICP of 2 mm Hg or less
c) Low compliance: increase in ICP of 3 mm Hg or more
6) If the ICP does not return to normal within 4 minutes after activity, compliance is poor

e. ICP values
1) Normal: 5-15 mm Hg
2) Slightly elevated: 16-20 mm Hg
3) Moderately elevated: 21-40 mm Hg
4) Severely elevated: greater than 40 mm Hg

f. ICP waveforms (Table 6-15)
1) Normal actual time waveform (Figure 6-22)
a) P_1
i) Percussion wave
ii) Reflects ejection of blood from the heart transmitted through the choroid plexus

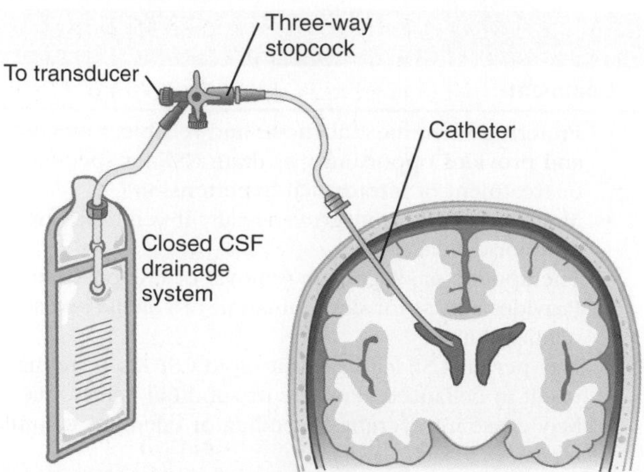

Figure 6-21 Continuous drainage system. Continuous drainage involves placing the drip chamber of the drainage system at a specified level above the foramen of Monro (usually 15 cm). The system is left open to allow continuous drainage of CSF into the chamber (which drains into a collection bag) against a pressure gradient that prevents excessive drainage and ventricular collapse. (From Carlson, K. K. [Ed.]. [2009]. *Advanced critical care nursing.* St. Louis: Saunders.)

b) P_2
   i) Tidal wave
   ii) Reflects elastic recoil during reduced systolic ejection phase of the cardiac cycle and arterial compliance within the brain
   iii) Normally P_2 is approximately 60% of the height of P_1; when the amplitude of P_2 is greater than 60% of P_1 or becomes lost in the tracing, it is indicative of a decrease in compliance.

c) P_3
   i) Dicrotic wave
   ii) Reflects closure of aortic valve

2) Trend waveforms (Figure 6-23)
   a) C waves (NOTE: remember that C waves are cool)
      i) Rapid, rhythmic oscillation of pressure without any relevance
      ii) Small spikes as high as 20 mm Hg at 6 per minute

Table 6-15 ICP Waveforms

Waveforms	Description	Significance	Comments
Normal	• Low-amplitude fluctuations in ICP with pressure less than 15 mm Hg	• Normal	
C waves	• Rapid, rhythmic oscillation of pressure • Small spikes as high as 20 mm Hg at 6 per minute	• Not significant • Associated with changes in arterial BP, ventilation	
B waves	• Sharp, sawtooth appearance waves • Pressures as high as 50 mm Hg lasting 30 seconds to 2 minutes	• Probably not clinically significant but may precede A waves	• Do not perform any activities that may further increase ICP • Assess for reversible causes of increased ICP (e.g., jugular vein compression by cervical collar or tight tracheostomy ties, compromised airway, restlessness) • May indicate decreased brain compliance
A waves or plateau waves	• Elevations on top of baseline elevation of ICP • Pressures reach 50-100 mm Hg and last 5-20 minutes	• Most significant • Pathologic waves produced by secondary changes in cerebral blood volume • Ominous sign of decreasing cerebral compliance and rapidly progressing decompensation • Usually occur only in advanced stages of intracranial hypertension	• Requires treatment • Irreversible brain damage will occur if not resolved within 15 minutes
Terminal wave	• Flat wave with pressure of 50-100 mm Hg	• MAP = ICP, and CBF ceases • Indicative of brain death	
Dampened waveform	• Low-voltage wave with pressure notches	• May be caused by tubing kinks, blood in line, or stopcock positioned incorrectly	

iii) Associated with changes in arterial BP and ventilation

b) B waves (NOTE: remember that B waves are bad)
   i) Sharp, sawtooth-appearance waves
   ii) Pressures as high as 50 mm Hg lasting 30 seconds to 2 minutes
   iii) Related to changes in cerebral blood flow
   iv) Though not significant alone, may precede A waves

c) A waves (NOTE: remember that A waves are awful)

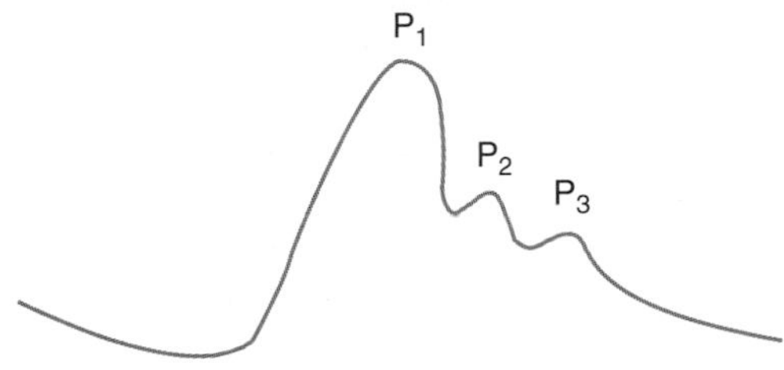

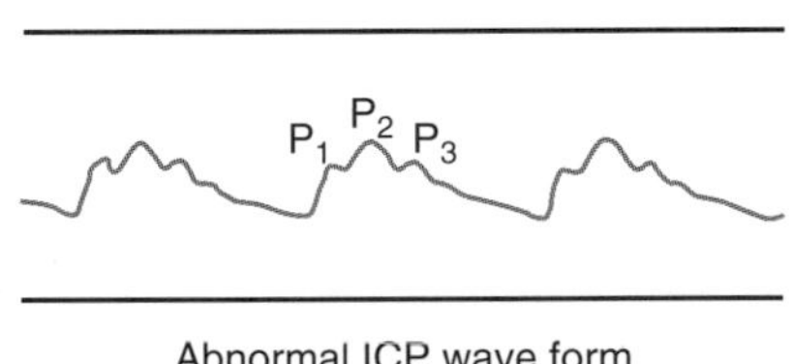

Figure 6-22 Actual time intracranial pressure (ICP) waveforms. **A,** Normal ICP waveform. **B,** Abnormal waveform. Note that P_2 is more than 60% of P_1. (**A** from Barker, E. [2008]. *Neuroscience nursing: A spectrum of care*. [3rd ed.]. St. Louis: Mosby. **B** from Sole, M. L., Klein, D. G., & Moseley, M. J. [2009]. *Introduction to critical care nursing* [5th ed.]. Philadelphia: Saunders.)

   i) Elevations on top of baseline elevation of ICP
   ii) Pressures reach 50-100 mm Hg and last 5-20 minutes
   iii) Pathologic waves produced by secondary changes in cerebral blood volume
   iv) Require immediate treatment

g. Prevent/detect/treat complications of ICP monitoring
   1) Infection (e.g., bacterial meningitis, bacterial ventriculitis)
      a) Risk factors associated with ICP monitoring-related infection
         i) Intracerebral hemorrhage with intraventricular blood
         ii) Open head trauma
         iii) Postcraniotomy
         iv) ICP greater than 20 mm Hg
         v) Elderly patient
         vi) Burr hole larger than necessary
         vii) Nonsterile technique for insertion
         viii) Device that penetrates dura
         ix) Monitoring for greater than 3-5 days
         x) Irrigation of ICP monitoring system
         xi) Opening of system for CSF specimen collection, VPR testing, irrigation
      b) Prevention
         i) Change dressing according to hospital policy utilizing sterile technique.
         ii) Maintain closed system; limit irrigation; use strict aseptic technique if system must be interrupted (e.g., VPR test)
         iii) ICP monitoring is typically maintained for 3-7 days; the risk of infection increases the longer the catheter is in place.

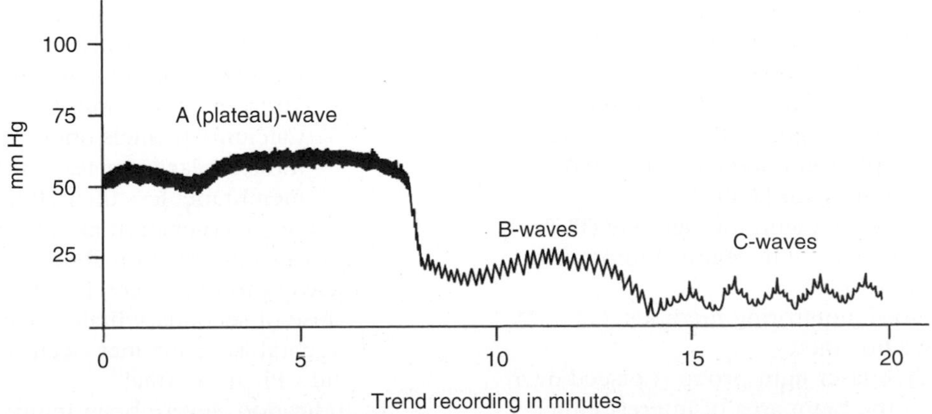

Figure 6-23 Trend intracranial pressure waveforms. Remember that C waves are "Cool," B waves are "Bad," and A waves are "Awful." (See text for more complete description). (From Barker, E. [2008]. *Neuroscience nursing: A spectrum of care* [3rd ed.]. St. Louis: Mosby.)

c) Detection
   i) Monitor for clinical indications of infection.
      (a) Fever
      (b) Leukocytosis
      (c) Cloudy CSF
   ii) Monitor for laboratory findings indicating infection through routine CSF sampling.
      (a) Elevated CSF protein
      (b) Low CSF glucose (normal CSF glucose is ~60% of serum glucose)
      (c) Positive CSF bacterial culture
d) Treatment: Administer antibiotics as prescribed.
   i) Intravenous antibiotic
   ii) Intrathecal antibiotic (usually aminoglycosides)
   iii) Irrigation of ICP catheter with very small volume (e.g., 0.1-0.2 mL) of antibiotic solution

2) Intercerebral hemorrhage, hematoma
   a) Monitor for change in color of CSF, change in neurologic status
   b) Maintain the air-fluid meniscus of the transducer at the level of the foramen of Monro; do not allow drainage bag to be lowered below the head.
3) CSF leak
   a) Use Luer-Lok connections.
   b) Maintain closed system.
4) CSF overdrainage
   a) Do not drain CSF below a pressure of 15-20 mm Hg unless specifically instructed.
   b) Ventricular collapse may cause hemorrhage.
5) Dislodgement or occlusion of catheter
6) CSF leakage around insertion site
7) Pneumoencephalopathy

2. Cerebral blood flow (CBF)
   a. Techniques
      1) Diagnostic tests which provide a snapshot in time
         a) Stable-xenon-enhanced computed tomography (XeCT),
         b) Perfusion computed tomography
         c) Perfusion magnetic resonance imaging
         d) Single photon emission computed tomography (SPECT)
         e) Positron emission tomography (PET) all provide excellent regional information about CBF
      2) Continuous monitoring methods
         a) Laser flowmetry
            i) A laser light probe is placed over the brain area of interest either during craniotomy or by burr hole.
            ii) The light deflection is transformed into a CBF measurement.
            iii) Risks: infection, bleeding, displacement
            iv) Advantage: Small size allows the probe to be placed in an ICP monitor.
         b) Thermal diffusion flowmetry
            i) A catheter with both a heat source and a thermistor is placed over the brain area of interest either during craniotomy or by burr hole.
            ii) CBF is determined by the difference between the temperature of the heat source and the thermistor; the greater the temperature difference, the lower the blood flow.
            iii) Risks: infection, bleeding, displacement
         c) Disadvantage: CBF is measured in a local area of the brain that may not reflect the global state of the brain or a specific region of interest.
      3) Intermittent measurement of CBF: transcranial Doppler ultrasound
         a) Doppler ultrasound probe placed over the skin on the cranium in temporal window, which allows assessment of blood flow velocity through the anterior and middle cerebral arteries
         b) Normal flow velocity: less than 120 cm/second
            i) Increase in flow velocity indicates that blood is flowing through a restricted area (e.g., vasospasm, stenosis) upstream from the probe.
            ii) Decrease in flow velocity indicates obstruction downstream (e.g., carotid stenosis) from the probe.
         c) Disadvantage: need for technical expertise
   b. CBF values
      1) Normal: 50-60 mL/100 g/min
      2) Altered level of consciousness and EEG: 20-25 mL/100 g/min
      3) Isoelectric EEG and neurotransmitter failure: 15-20 mL/100 g/min
      4) Ion pump failure and cytotoxic brain edema: 10-15 mL/100 g/min
      5) Calcium channels open, activation of intracellular enzymes, alterations of cell membrane: less than 10 mm Hg

3. Brain tissue oxygenation monitoring ($PbtO_2$)
   a. Provides information about cerebral oxygen delivery to detect cerebral ischemia, a potential cause of secondary brain injury; secondary cerebral ischemia may occur even through ICP and CPP are normal
   b. Indication: severe brain injury with risk of cerebral ischemia
   c. Technique: A probe is placed into the white matter of the brain for global brain assessment

or the penumbra of an injury for regional assessment.

  d. Normal value: 20-50 mm Hg in uninjured tissue; less than 15 mm Hg is correlated with a poor outcome and increased chance of death
  e. Risks: infection, hematoma

4. Jugular venous oxygen saturation (SjO_2) monitoring
   a. Provides a global measure of oxygen reserve for the brain as a whole
   b. Technique
      1) Fiberoptic catheter placed into the jugular vein bulb to continuously monitor the oxygen saturation of the blood returning from the brain and intermittently sample venous blood gases
      2) Comparison between arterial oxygen saturation and jugular venous oxygen saturation allows calculation of arteriovenous oxygen difference
   c. Normal value: 55-75%; saturation less than 55% indicates brain ischemia
   d. Limitations
      1) May not be reliable if performed unilaterally since the oxygen content of each jugular bulb may differ
      2) Normal values do not ensure adequate perfusion to all brain areas
      3) Prone to technical artifact and will not detect causes such as arteriovenous shunting
5. IN-Vivo Optical Spectroscopy (INVOS)
   a. Technique
      1) A sensor is placed on the forehead, either right or left of midline.
      2) Low-intensity near-infrared light is passed into the patient's forehead where it penetrates the skull and passes through the cerebral cortex.
      3) The returned light at 2 distances from the light source allows determination of the regional oxygen saturation index (rSO_2), which is a measure of the oxygen saturation of the mixed arterial and venous blood in the brain cortex.
   b. Interpretation: used for trending
      1) Change in rSO_2 of 12-20 points or 20-30% correlates with changes in the neurologic status
      2) rSO_2 index less than 50 is associated with poor outcome
6. Continuous EEG monitoring
   a. Detects ischemia, severe metabolic and anoxic encephalopathy, drug intoxication, and seizures, including subclinical seizures
   b. Technique: five electrodes are used to monitor two EEG leads
7. Bispectral Index (BIS): an EEG parameter developed to specifically measure patient's response to sedation and anesthesia
   a. Electrodes are placed across the patient's forehead to detect electrical activity in the brain; changes reflect changes in the effects of sedative and anesthetic agents.
   b. Values
      1) Value of close to 100 corresponds to an awake state
      2) Value of 70-90 corresponds to light to moderate sedation
      3) Value of 40-70 corresponds to a moderate to deep level of sedation
      4) Value of 40 or less corresponds to a deep hypnotic state or barbiturate coma
   c. Advantage over traditional sedation scales (e.g., Ramsay, Riker): provides objective and reproducible data

Diagnostic Studies

1. Serum
   a. Chemistries
      1) Sodium: normal 136-145 mEq/liter
      2) Potassium: normal 3.5-5.0 mEq/liter
      3) Chloride: normal 96-106 mEq/liter
      4) Calcium: normal 8.5-10.5 mg/dL
      5) Phosphorus: normal 3.0-4.5 mg/dL
      6) Magnesium: normal 1.5-2.2 mEq/liter or 1.8-2.4 mg/dL
      7) Glucose: normal 70-110 mEq/liter
      8) BUN: normal 5-20 mg/dL
      9) Serum osmolality: normal 285-295 mmol/kg
      10) Creatinine: normal 0.7-1.5 mg/dL
      11) Lactate: negative
      12) Enzymes
          a) Total CK: normal 55-170 units/L for males; 30-135 units/L for females
          b) LDH: 90-200 IU/L
   b. Arterial blood gases
      1) pH: normal 7.35-7.45
      2) $PaCO_2$: normal 35-45 mm Hg
      3) HCO_3 : normal 22-26 mEq/L
      4) PaO_2: normal 80-100 mm Hg
      5) SaO_2: greater than 95%
   c. Hematology
      1) Hematocrit: normal 40-52% for males; 35-47% for females
      2) Hemoglobin: normal 13-18 g/dL for males; 12-16 g/dL for females
      3) White blood cells (WBC): normal 3500-11,000 mm^3
      4) Erythrocyte sedimentation rate: normal up to 15 mm/hr for males; up to 20 mm/hr for females
   d. Clotting profile
      1) Prothrombin time (PT): normal 12-15 seconds; therapeutic 1.5-2.5 times normal
      2) Partial thromboplastin time (PTT): normal 60-90 seconds; therapeutic 1.5-2.5 times normal
      3) Activated partial thromboplastin time (aPTT): normal 25-38 seconds; therapeutic 1.5-2.5 times normal
      4) Activated clotting time (ACT): normal 70-120 seconds; therapeutic 150-190 seconds

5) Thrombin time: normal 10-15 seconds
6) Bleeding time: normal 1-9.5 minutes
7) International normalized ratio (INR): normal less than 2.0
   a) Therapeutic range for atrial fibrillation: 1.5-2.5
   b) Therapeutic range for deep vein thrombosis (DVT) or pulmonary embolus (PE): 2-3
   c) Therapeutic range for prosthetic valves: 2.5-3.5
8) Platelets: normal 150,000-400,000/mm^3

e. Toxicology
   1) Alcohol: normal 0 mg/dL
   2) Dilantin: therapeutic 10-20 mcg/mL

2. Urine
   a. Glucose: normal negative
   b. Ketones: normal negative
   c. Specific gravity: normal 1.005-1.030
   d. Osmolality: normal 50-1200 mOsm/L
3. Cerebrospinal fluid analysis
   a. Properties
      1) Colorless, odorless; cloudy in bacterial meningitis
      2) Specific gravity: normal 1.007
      3) pH: normal 7.35
      4) Chlorides: normal 120-130 mEq/L
      5) Sodium: normal 140-142 mEq/L
      6) Glucose: normal 60% of serum glucose value; decreased in bacterial meningitis
   b. Protein: elevated in meningitis
      1) By lumbar puncture: normal 15-45 mg/dL
      2) By cisternal puncture: normal 10-25 mg/dL
      3) By ventricular puncture or catheter: normal 5-15 mg/dL
   c. Cells
      1) Leukocytes: normal 0-5/mm^3
      2) Erythrocytes: normal 0/mm^3
         a) NOTE: test tubes must be numbered to differentiate between traumatic puncture; if first test tube is bloody but others are clear, consider trauma; subarachnoid hemorrhage would cause all test tubes to be equally bloody
4. Other diagnostic studies (Table 6-16)

Intracranial Hypertension

Etiology

1. Mass lesion
   a. Hematoma
      1) Epidural
      2) Subdural
      3) Intracerebral
   b. Neoplasm
      1) Primary brain tumor
      2) Metastatic tumor
   c. Abscess
   d. Trauma: caused by local edema (e.g., contusion may act as a mass lesion)
2. Brain edema: most common cause of intracranial hypertension; may be localized or generalized
   a. Cytotoxic edema
      1) Intracellular swelling of neurons and glial cells
      2) Caused by any of the following:
         a) Hypoosmolality (e.g., low serum osmolality and sodium)
         b) Hypoxia (decreases ATP production, which impairs sodium-potassium pump)
         c) Cardiac arrest (cause of anoxic encephalopathy)
   b. Vasogenic edema
      1) Increase in extracellular fluid caused by breakdown of blood-brain barrier; increased vascular permeability and leakage of plasma protein
      2) Begins locally, becomes generalized
      3) Caused by any of the following:
         a) Trauma (e.g., contusion)
         b) Tumors
         c) Hemorrhage
         d) Abscesses
         e) Surgical trauma (e.g., craniotomy)
3. Cerebrovascular alterations
   a. Arterial vascular occlusions with cytotoxic and vasogenic edema
   b. Venous outflow obstruction: caused by decreased venous return from head
      1) Neck rotation, hyperextension, hyperflexion
      2) Tracheostomy ties or cervical collar
      3) Increased intrathoracic pressure
         a) Valsalva maneuver (e.g., coughing, vomiting, straining at stool)
         b) Positive pressure mechanical ventilation
         c) Positive end-expiratory pressure
   c. Increase in cerebral perfusion pressure (caused by hypertensive crisis)
   d. Vasodilation (caused by hypercapnia, hypoxia, hyperthermia, vasoactive drugs)
4. Increase in CSF volume (hydrocephalus)
   a. Increase in production of CSF (e.g., choroid plexus disease)
   b. Decrease in reabsorption of CSF
      1) Communicating hydrocephalus (e.g., subarachnoid hemorrhage, meningitis)
      2) Noncommunicating hydrocephalus (e.g., tumor, surgical, or traumatic edema, hemorrhage or infarction obstructing outflow of CSF)

Pathophysiology (Figure 6-24 on page 427)

1. Intracranial volumes
   a. Brain tissue: approximately 80-88%
      1) NOTE: Elderly patients and alcohol or drug abusers may have cerebral atrophy; traction on bridging vessels increases the risk of intracranial bleeding; hemorrhage or hematoma may be very large before symptomatic.
   b. Circulating blood: approximately 2-10%

Table 6-16 Neurologic Diagnostic Studies

Study	Purposes	Comments

Angiography	• Visualizes extracranial and intracranial vasculature
	• Identifies aneurysm, AV malformation, vasospasm, vascular tumors
	• Detects arterial occlusion and allows delivery of intraarterial therapy to restore blood flow
		• May cause local hematoma, vasospasm, vessel occlusion, allergic reaction to contrast media, transient or permanent neurologic dysfunction
		• Prior to test:
		  • Keep patient NPO for 4 hours and provide sedation prior to the study
		  • Check for allergy to iodine
		  • Evaluate renal function
		• After the test:
		  • Ensure hydration postprocedure (contrast medium used)
		  • Maintain bed rest for 8-12 hours
		  • Monitor arterial puncture point for hemorrhage or hematoma
		  • Monitor neurovascular status of affected limb
		  • Monitor for indications of systemic emboli
		  • Reevaluate renal function

Cisternogram	• Views CSF flow • Identifies hydrocephalus • Evaluates CSF leakage through a dural tear • Evaluates abnormality of structures at the base of the brain and upper cervical cord region	• Contraindicated in intracranial hypertension
Computerized tomography (CT); computerized axial tomography (CAT)	• Views intracranial structures: size, shape, location, shifts • Differentiates between tumors, hemorrhage, and infarction • Identifies hydrocephalus, brain edema, infectious processes, trauma, aneurysm, hematoma, AVM, brain atrophy, and subacute and old brain infarction • Evaluates arterial system if CT angiography studies performed	• Patient must be cooperative • Contrast media may be used; contrast media may be used after a noncontrast CT • Check for allergy to iodine or seafood prior to study • Patient will be NPO for 4-8 hours prior to the study • Sedation may be given • Monitor for signs of allergic reaction • Encourage fluids • Evaluate renal function when contrast media used
Digital subtraction angiography (DSA): brain; spine	• Visualizes the vasculature, especially carotid and larger cerebral arteries • Evaluates occlusive vascular disease • Identifies tumors, aneurysms, AVM, and vascular abnormalities	• May be done intravenously or intraarterially • If IV: less invasive with fewer complications than cerebral angiography • If intraarterial, care as for angiogram • Contrast media are used • Check for allergy to iodine or seafood prior to study • Patient will be NPO for 4-8 hours prior to the study • Monitor for signs of allergic reaction • Encourage fluids
Electroencephalography (EEG)	• Differentiates epilepsy from mass lesion • Detects focus of seizure activity • Evaluates drug intoxication • Evaluates electrical function of the brain which may be abnormal in the presence of cerebrovascular alterations • Localizes tumor, abscess, and other mass lesions • May be used in designation of brain death	• Stimulants, anticonvulsants, tranquilizers, and antidepressants may be withheld for 24-48 hours prior to the study • Hair shampooed before and after study

Continued

Table 6-16 Neurologic Diagnostic Studies—cont'd

Study	Purposes	Comments
Electromyography (EMG); nerve conduction velocity studies	• Detects muscle disease • Identifies peripheral neuropathies, nerve compression • Identifies nerve regeneration and muscle recovery	• Patient must be cooperative • Contraindicated in patients taking anticoagulants, with bleeding disorders, or with skin infection • May be uncomfortable for patient
Electronystagmography (ENG)	• Detects nystagmus, which may aid in identification of cerebellar or vestibular problem	
Evoked potential studies	• Evaluate brain's electrical potentials (responses) to external stimuli; evaluate sensory and somatosensory neurologic pathways • Identify neuromuscular disease, cerebrovascular disease, spinal cord injury, traumatic brain injury, peripheral nerve disease, and tumors • Determine prognosis in traumatic brain injury • Contribute to diagnosis of multiple sclerosis and brainstem injury	• Hair shampooed before and after study
Isotope ventriculography	• Visualizes CSF circulation system	• No CSF withdrawn • May cause meningeal irritation and aseptic meningitis
LP or cisternal puncture	• Obtains CSF for analysis • Measures CSF opening pressure (roughly equivalent to intracranial pressure for most patients if done recumbent and no blockage is present)	• Cisternal puncture is higher risk but may be used if scar tissue prevents lumbar puncture • Patient must be cooperative • Contraindicated in patients with intracranial hypertension because herniation may occur • Contraindicated in bleeding disorders and in patients receiving anticoagulants • Patient kept flat for 4-8 hours to prevent headache • May cause headache, low back pain, meningitis, abscess, CSF leak, or puncture of spinal cord
Magnetic resonance angiography (MRA)/ magnetic resonance imaging (MRI)	• As for CT • Visualizes tissue state (diffusion and perfusion) so that early ischemic changes are apparent (CT cannot visualize most early changes) • Identifies vascular lesions, tissue abnormalities, hemorrhage, infarction, epileptic foci, and multiple sclerosis • Identifies patency of large veins and venous sinuses • Identifies brainstem abnormalities • Identifies type, location, and extent of brain injury	• Patient must be cooperative • Contraindicated in patients with any implanted metallic device, including pacemakers • Tends to overestimate degree of stenosis
Magnetic resonance spectroscopy (also known as nuclear magnetic resonance [NMR] spectroscopy)	• Measures biochemical changes in the brain tissue • Detects abnormal changes as in brain tumors, epilepsy, stroke, and traumatic brain injury	• Patient must be cooperative • Contraindicated in patients with any implanted metallic device, including pacemakers

Table 6-16 Neurologic Diagnostic Studies—cont'd

Study	Purposes	Comments
Myelography	• Visualizes spinal subarachnoid space • Detects spinal cord lesions and cord or nerve root compression • Detects pressure on spinal nerve roots	• If done with oil-based iophendylate (Pantopaque), patient must lie flat for 4-8 hours after study • May cause headache, nerve root irritation, allergic reaction, or adhesive arachnoiditis • If done with water-soluble metrizamide (Amipaque), patient should have head of bed elevated • May cause headache, nausea, vomiting, back and neck ache, chest pain, seizures, hallucinations, speech disorders, dysrhythmias, or allergic reaction • Encourage fluid intake with either type of dye
Nerve conduction velocity studies	• Identifies peripheral neuropathies and nerve compression	• Needle electrodes are used
Oculoplethysmography (OPG)	• Indirectly measures ocular artery pressure • Reflects adequacy of cerebrovascular blood flow in the carotid artery	• Contraindicated in patients who have undergone eye surgery within the last 6 months, who have had lens implants or cataracts, or who have had retinal detachment • May cause conjunctival hemorrhage, corneal abrasions, or transient photophobia
Pneumoencephalography	• Visualizes ventricular system and subarachnoid space • Identifies intracranial tumors • Identifies brain atrophy	• Care as for LP • Contraindicated in patients with intracranial hypertension • May cause headache, nausea, vomiting, autonomic dysfunction, herniation, subdural hematoma, air embolus, or seizures • Patient kept flat for 12-24 hours after the study
Positron emission tomography (PET) or single photon emission-computerized tomography (SPECT)	• Evaluates oxygen and glucose metabolism • Measures cerebral blood flow, which may be altered by traumatic brain injury, seizure, ischemia, stroke, or neoplasm • Also used to evaluate dementia, depression, schizophrenia, and Alzheimer's disease	• Patient must be cooperative • Contraindicated in pregnant and breastfeeding patients
Radioisotope brain scan	• Identifies tumors, cerebrovascular disease, infarction, trauma, infectious processes, seizures	• Generally replaced by CT scan • Reassure patient that amount of radioactive material is minimal • Patient must be cooperative • Contraindicated in pregnant and breast-feeding patients
Regional cerebral blood flow (xenon [^{133}Xe] inhalation)	• Evaluates blood flow to the cerebral cortex • Identifies cerebrovascular disease • Detects regions of increased or decreased perfusion • Determines presence of collateral blood flow • Evaluates the effect of vasospasm on tissue perfusion	• Assure patient that amount of radioactive material is minimal • Contraindicated in pregnant and breast-feeding patients
Skull x-rays	• Detects skull fracture, facial fracture, tumor, bone erosion, cranial anomalies, air-fluid level in sinuses, abnormal intracranial calcification, and radiopaque foreign bodies	• Linear and basal fractures frequently missed by routine x-rays • Contraindicated in pregnant patients

Continued

Table 6-16 Neurologic Diagnostic Studies—cont'd

Study	Purposes	Comments
Somatosensory evoked potentials (SSEP)	• Evaluates neural pathways involving spinal cord, brainstem, thalamus, and cerebral cortex • Useful in diagnosis of multiple sclerosis, brain tumor, and spinal cord injury • Useful in determination of brain death	
Somnography	• Records EEG during sleep • Evaluates sleep and sleep disorders	
Spinal cord angiography	• Differentiates between spinal AVM, angioma, tumor, and ischemia	• As for angiogram • May cause thrombosis of spinal vessels and allergy to contrast agent
Spine x-rays	• Detects vertebral dislocation or fracture, degenerative disease, tumor, bone erosion, or calcification • Identifies structural spinal deficits and rules out associated cervical spine injuries	• Care must be taken to prevent fracture displacement and spinal cord injury • C1-C2 view best obtained via open mouth; C6-C7 best obtained with arms pulled down
Suboccipital puncture	• Obtains CSF for analysis • Measures CSF pressure • Rarely performed but may be useful when LP is contraindicated	• May cause trauma to the medulla
Transcranial Doppler	• Measures blood flow velocity through the cerebral arteries • Identifies vasospasm, emboli, vascular stenosis, and brain death	• Quality of findings and interpretation varies with user • Transtemporal window required (lacking in 14% of general population)
Ventriculography	• Obtains CSF for analysis • Measures CSF pressure • Is used especially when intracranial hypertension contraindicates LP	• May cause meningeal irritation, seizures, herniation, intracerebral or intraventricular hemorrhage

c. Cerebrospinal fluid: approximately 10%

2. Intracranial pressure: the pressure exerted by brain tissue, blood, and cerebrospinal fluid against the inside of the skull
   a. Measured as the pressure exerted by CSF within the ventricles of the brain
   b. Normal: 5-15 mm Hg
   c. Under normal circumstances, only slight fluctuation
3. Monro-Kellie hypothesis
   a. The cranium is an inexpansible vault.
   b. Inside the cranium is a closed system with three fluctuating volumes.
      1) Compensation is the ability of the cranium's contents to change or rearrange; compensation is more effective when volume increase is slower.
      2) If the volume of one of the constituents of the intracranial cavity increases, a reciprocal decrease in volume of one or both of the others will occur.
         a) Displacement of CSF from the cranium to the lumbar cistern
         b) Increased CSF reabsorption
         c) Compression of low-pressure venous system; blood is shunted to venous sinuses
   c. As successive units of any of the three volumes are added to the cranium, a critical point is reached where each additional unit of volume added increases ICP dramatically and herniation occurs.
      1) There is a volume-pressure relationship. (Figure 6-25)
      2) When the critical point is reached, herniation syndromes occur. (Figure 6-26 and Table 6-17)
4. Compliance
   a. The brain's ability to tolerate increases in volume without a corresponding increase in pressure.
   b. Compliance is poor if a small increase in volume causes a large increase in pressure
5. Cerebral perfusion pressure
   a. Pressure at which the brain tissue is perfused; used to estimate adequacy of cerebral blood flow (CBF)
   b. Calculated by subtracting ICP from MAP; MAP − ICP
   c. Normal CPP: 60-100 mm Hg; a CPP of greater than 60 mm Hg is considered a minimum desirable CPP in brain-injured patients
   d. Abnormal CPP

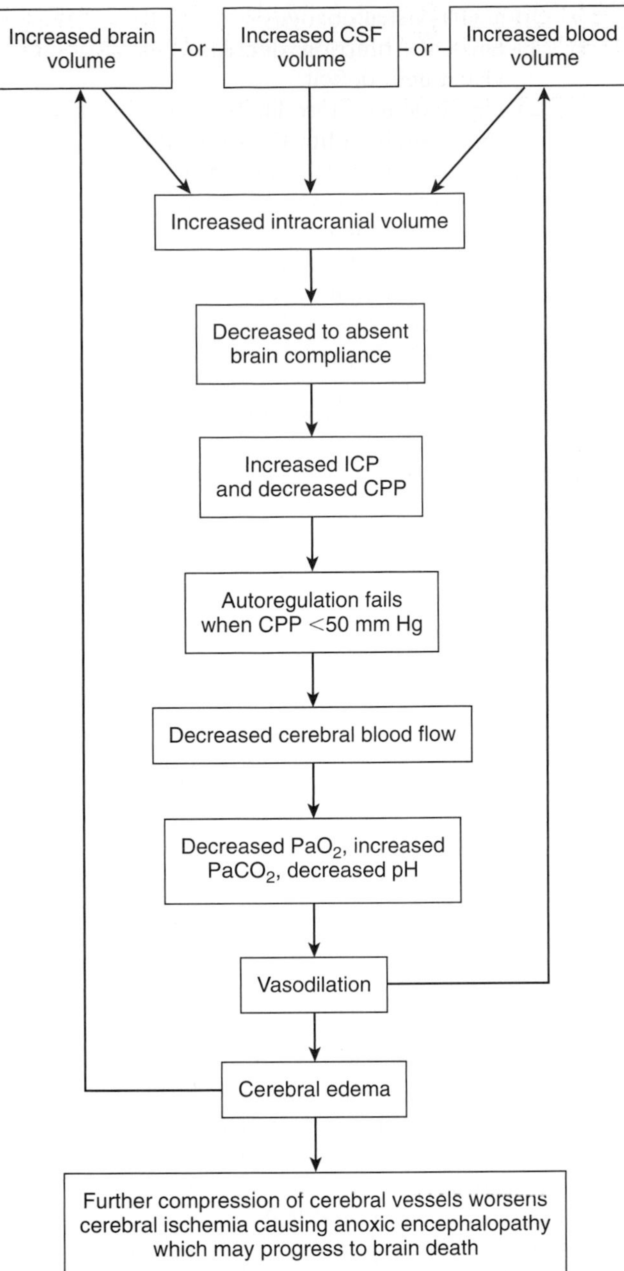

Figure 6-24 Summary of pathophysiology of intracranial hypertension. *CPP,* Cerebral perfusion pressure; *CSF,* cerebrospinal fluid; *ICP,* intracranial pressure; *$PaCO_2$,* partial pressure of carbon dioxide in arterial blood; *PaO_2,* partial pressure of oxygen in arterial blood.

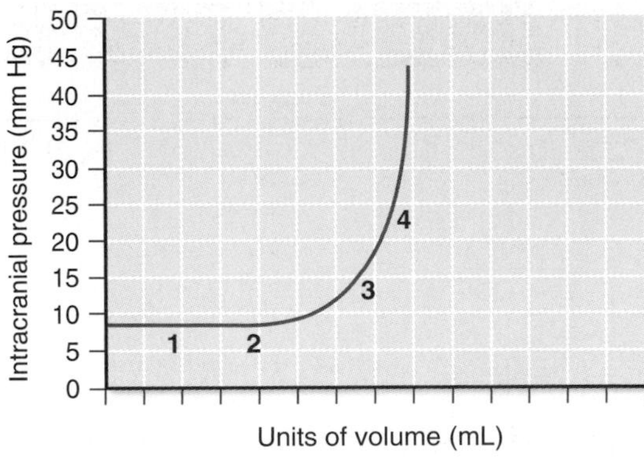

Figure 6-25 Intracranial pressure-volume curve. *1,* High compliance and low elastance. *2,* Lower compliance and higher elastance. *3,* High elastance and low compliance. *4,* Herniation. (See text for more complete description). (From Carlson, K. K. [Ed.]. [2009]. *Advanced critical care nursing.* St. Louis: Saunders.)

1) CPP greater than 150 mm Hg disrupts the blood-brain barrier and causes hyperperfusion and potentially brain edema.
2) CPP less than 50 mm Hg causes hypoperfusion and brain ischemia (although CPP of 70 mm Hg is required in most brain-injured patients and some require an even higher CPP to perfuse the brain).
3) CPP less than 40 mm Hg is associated with cerebral blood flow that is 25% of normal.
4) CPP less than 30 mm Hg causes irreversible ischemia.
5) As ICP approaches MAP, cerebral blood flow decreases; when they equalize, cerebral blood flow ceases and brain death is inevitable.

6. Autoregulation: the intrinsic ability of the cerebral blood vessels to dilate or constrict in response to changes in the brain's environment
   a. Enables the cerebral blood vessels to maintain cerebral blood flow in response to wide fluctuation in mean arterial pressure
   b. Autoregulation fails if CPP is less than 50 or greater than 150 mm Hg
7. Cerebral blood flow (CBF)
   a. Varies with changes in CPP and diameter of cerebrovascular bed
   b. Normal CBF: 50 mL/min/100 grams of brain
   c. Increased ICP and decreased CPP decreases CBF; the brain receives less oxygen and nutrients eventually causing neuronal death
8. Decompensation: brain loses its ability to compensate
   a. Pressure on cerebral vessels slows blood flow to the brain.
   b. Diminished circulation produces ischemia and an accumulation of carbon dioxide and lactic acid.
   c. Hypoxia and hypercapnia trigger vasodilation, which increases blood volume and brain edema.
   d. Brain edema increases ICP further.
   e. Compression of cerebral vessels occurs and causes further ischemia.
   f. Eventually cerebral circulation stops and brain death occurs.

Clinical Presentation

1. Stages of intracranial hypertension (Figure 6-27)
2. Change in level of consciousness
   a. Early: yawning, restlessness, confusion
   b. Late: diminishing level of consciousness, posturing
3. Cranial nerve changes

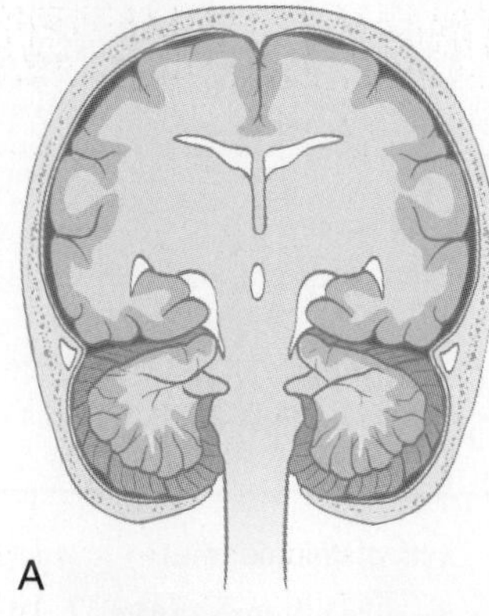

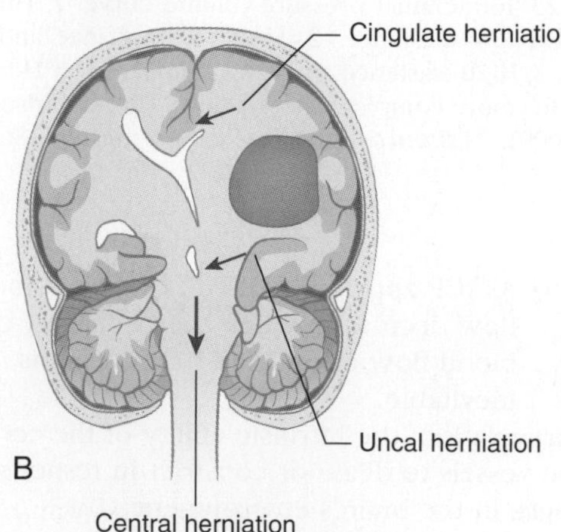

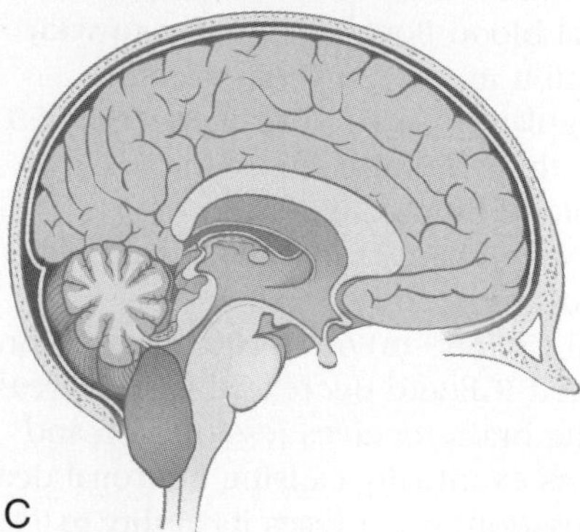

Figure 6-26 Herniation syndromes. **A,** Normal intracranial structures. **B,** Supratentorial herniation syndromes. **C,** Cerebellar tonsil herniation. (From McCance, K. L., & Huether, S. E. [2006]. *Pathophysiology: The biologic basis for disease in adults and children* [5th ed.]. St. Louis: Mosby.)

a. Oculomotor (III)
   1) Early
      a) Ipsilateral pupil changes
         i) Change in size, shape (oval)
         ii) Sluggish reaction to light
      b) Conjugate eye deviation
   2) Late
      a) Ipsilateral pupil changes
         i) Dilated, nonreactive-to-light pupil or pupils
         ii) Ptosis
         iii) Dysconjugate eye movement with brainstem lesions
b. Optic (II): visual changes
   1) Diplopia; blurring; decreased visual acuity; visual field deficit
   2) Papilledema: more likely to occur when ICP rises slowly rather than quickly
c. Trigeminal (V): impaired corneal reflex
d. Glossopharyngeal (IX) and vagus (X): impaired gag and swallowing

4. Motor changes: contralateral
   a. Due to compression or pressure on the corticospinal tracts
   b. Early: paresis, plegia
   c. Late: posturing
5. Vomiting: may occur especially with lesions below the tentorium
   a. Pressure on the vomiting center in the brainstem causes projectile vomiting without nausea.
6. Headache: increasing severity but inconsistent symptom
7. Seizures may occur.
8. Reflexes: decrease in or absence of reflexes (e.g., cough, gag, corneal reflexes)
9. Vital sign changes
   a. Cushing's triad
      1) Due to pressure on or ischemia of vasomotor center in brainstem
      2) Components
         a) Increased systolic BP
         b) Widening pulse pressure due to diastolic BP being normal or decreased along with increased systolic BP
         c) Bradycardia
   b. Respiratory pattern changes dependent on location of injury
   c. Temperature: Central hyperthermia may occur late in intracranial hypertension due to pressure on the thermoregulatory center in the hypothalamus.
10. ICP monitoring: elevated ICP
11. Diagnostic studies
   a. Lumbar puncture: contraindicated; may cause downward cerebellar herniation with medullary herniation and death
   b. CT scan: may show cause of intracranial hypertension or intracerebral shifts
   c. Cerebral angiography: may show cause of intracranial hypertension
   d. Skull x-ray: may show cause of intracranial hypertension and/or shift of pineal gland or sella turcica; rarely performed
   e. EEG: evaluates brain wave activity
   f. Evoked potentials: assesses brainstem integrity
   g. ECG
      1) May show prolonged QT interval
      2) Dysrhythmias: especially with subarachnoid hemorrhage

Collaborative Management

1. Monitor closely for clinical indications of intracranial hypertension; assist with insertion of

Table 6-17 Herniation Syndromes

Type of Herniation	Description	Symptomatology	Comments
Supratentorial			
Cingulate (or subfalcine) herniation	Expanding lesion of one hemisphere shifts laterally and forces the cingulate gyrus under the falx cerebri; compression of vessels causes brain edema, ischemia, and intracranial hypertension	• No specific clinical manifestations • May have altered LOC or plegia • Cheyne-Stokes ventilatory pattern may be seen	• Not life-threatening but a sign of brain decompensation • If condition not controlled, uncal or central herniation will occur
Uncal herniation	Expanding lesion in middle fossa or temporal lobe causes a lateral displacement which pushes the uncus of the temporal lobe over the edge of the tentorium; uncus may be lacerated by sharp edge of tentorium	• First symptom is unilateral (ipsilateral) pupil dilation with sluggish reaction to light → fixed, dilated pupils • Decreased LOC • Ventilatory pattern change • Contralateral hemiplegia progressing to posturing	• Most common herniation syndrome • Life-threatening when hemorrhage or brainstem compression occurs
Central (or transtentorial) herniation	Expanding lesions of the frontal, parietal, or occipital lobes or severe generalized edema cause downward displacement of the basal ganglia and diencephalon through the tentorial notch causing pressure on the midbrain	• First symptom is change in level of consciousness • Small, reactive pupils → fixed, dilated pupils • Ventilatory pattern changes → apnea • Decorticate posturing → flaccidity	• May be preceded by cingulate or uncal herniation • Life-threatening
Transcalvarial herniation	Extrusion of brain tissue through the cranium	• No specific clinical manifestations	• May occur through an opening from a skull fracture, craniotomy site, or burr hole • Risk of infection
Infratentorial			
Upward transtentorial herniation	Expanding mass lesion of cerebellum, brainstem, or fourth ventricle causes protrusion of the central area of the cerebellum and the midbrain upward through the tentorial notch	• First symptom is unilateral (ipsilateral) pupil dilation • Obstructive hydrocephalus occurs with rapid deterioration of neurologic status	• May be life-threatening
Downward cerebellar (or tonsillar) herniation	Expanding lesion of the cerebellum exerts downward pressure, sending cerebellar tonsils through the foramen magnum; compression and displacement of the medulla oblongata occurs	• Coma • Flaccid paralysis • Respiratory and cardiac arrest occur	• May be a complication of lumbar puncture when LP is performed in presence of high ICP • Causes death

ICP monitoring device if patient requires continuous monitoring.

2. Recognize factors that increase ICP (Box 6-1); prevent as many of these factors that you can; space activities that increase ICP that cannot be eliminated.
3. Prevent intracranial hypertension.
   a. Assess neurologic status frequently.
   b. Maintain adequate venous drainage from head.
      1) Assess patient's response to HOB elevation by using ICP, CO, BP and adjust accordingly; elevation of HOB to 30 degrees promotes venous drainage from the brain but may decrease cerebral blood flow by decreasing BP.
      2) Maintain head and neck in straight alignment to prevent compression of jugular veins.
      3) Prevent compression of jugular veins by tracheostomy ties, cervical collar; loosen if necessary.
   c. Maintain patent airway and ventilation.
      1) Endotracheal intubation
         a) Necessary if protective reflexes are absent

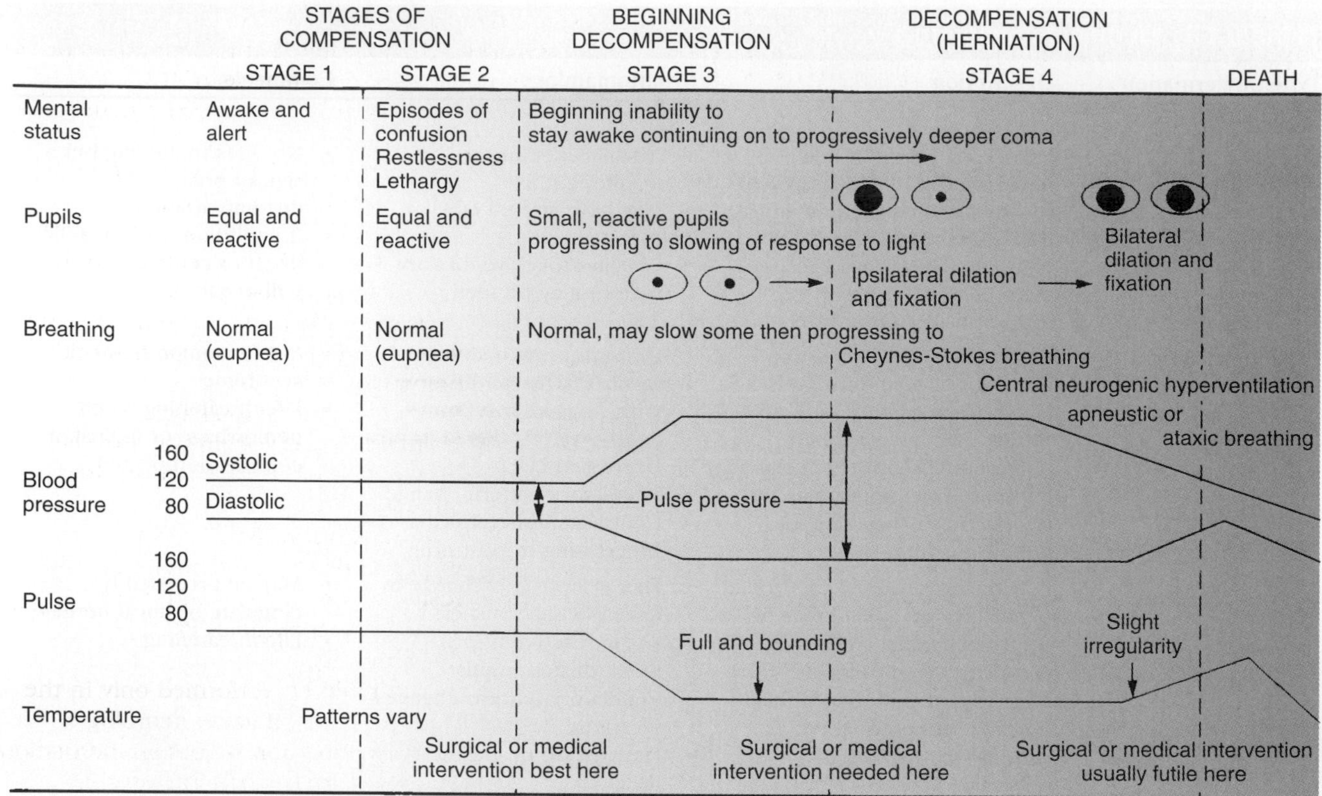

Figure 6-27 Clinical correlates of compensated and decompensated phases of intracranial hypertension. (From Beare, P. G., & Myers, J. L. [1994]. *Principles and practice of adult health nursing* [2nd ed.]. St Louis: Mosby.)

b) Indicated when GCS is less than 8 even in the absence of typical signs of acute respiratory failure

2) Mechanical ventilation may be necessary.
   a) Recognize that positive pressure mechanical ventilation will increase ICP; utilizing lower tidal volumes may minimize this effect.
   b) Recognize that positive end-expiratory pressure will increase ICP; utilizing only enough PEEP to maintain adequate PaO_2 may minimize this effect.

d. Prevent the increase in ICP caused by Valsalva maneuver.
   1) Instruct the patient to do the following:
      a) Exhale when turning in bed.
      b) Cough with mouth open if coughing is necessary.
      c) Avoid straining, bending, sneezing.
      d) Avoid hip flexion greater than 90 degrees.
   2) Discourage isometric exercise.
      a) Do not use footboard to prevent footdrop.
      b) Use high-top tennis shoes, on for 2 hours and off for 2 hours.
   3) Administer stool softeners as indicated.
   4) Treat nausea with antiemetics to prevent vomiting.
   5) Administer analgesics and/or sedatives prior to activities that may increase ICP.
   6) Prevent increase in ICP associated with suctioning.
      a) Suction only if necessary.
      b) Limit suctioning to 10 seconds.
      c) Limit suction to less than 120 mm Hg.
      d) Ensure that the catheter occludes no more than half the diameter of the endotracheal tube.
      e) Hyperoxygenate prior to and after suctioning.
      f) Lidocaine may be prescribed for IV use prior to suctioning to eliminate cough reflex.
         i) Dosage: 0.5-1.5 mg/kg
         ii) Disadvantage: may lower seizure threshold
      g) Do not suction via nose if there is evidence of head or facial trauma.

e. Monitor ICP during nursing care activities (e.g., turning, suctioning, enteral feedings); space activities to allow ICP to return to normal before performing another activity that may increase ICP.

f. Monitor ventilation and oxygenation; hypercapnia and/or hypoxemia may cause vasodilation and increase ICP.
   1) Arterial blood gases

Box 6-1 Causes of Intracranial Pressure Elevations

Ventilation and/or Oxygenation Problems

- Airway obstruction
- Hypercapnia
- Hypoxia
- Suctioning without hyperoxygenation
- Deep breathing

Position Changes

- Prone position
- Trendelenburg position
- Extreme hip flexion (greater than 90 degrees)

Decreased Venous Return from Head

- Neck flexion, hyperextension, or rotation
- Tight tracheostomy ties or cervical collar
- Increased intrathoracic pressure
- Positive pressure mechanical ventilation
- Positive end-expiratory pressure
- Valsalva maneuver
- Straining at stool
- Vomiting
- Coughing
- Suctioning
- Isometric exercise

Increased Metabolic Rate

- Hyperthermia
- Seizure activity
- Rapid eye movement (REM) sleep

Stress

- Disturbing conversation
- Noise
- Bright lights
- Pain or noxious stimuli

2) Pulse oximetry (SpO_2: oxygenation only)
3) Capnography ($PaCO_2$: ventilation only)

g. Maintain euvolemia.
   1) Hemodynamic monitoring may be necessary: Maintain PAOP 10-15 mm Hg.
   2) Administer intravenous fluids as prescribed: Avoid hypotonic fluids (e.g., D_5W) which may contribute to brain edema.

h. If CSF leakage is noted, do not pack nose or ears; apply mustache dressing under nose or 4 × 4-inch gauze over ear.

i. Reduce anxiety.
   1) Reorient patient frequently to person, place, date, and time.
   2) Explain procedures thoroughly.
   3) Do not conduct or allow emotionally disturbing conversations at bedside.
   4) Encourage family members to touch and talk to patient; let them know that many patients report an awareness during altered levels of consciousness.

j. Monitor ICP and calculate CPP; notify physician of significant changes or deteriorating trend.

4. Treat intracranial hypertension
   a. Providing therapy aimed at reducing volume of one of the three components of ICP
      1) CSF: drainage of CSF if intraventricular catheter in place
         a) Drainage is usually initiated when the ICP is greater than 20 mm Hg.
         b) Do not drain to ICP less than 15 mm Hg unless specifically instructed; rapid CSF drainage may cause the brain to pull away from the dura, rupturing bridging veins and possibly causing subdural hematoma.
         c) Record volume of drainage.
         d) Maintain closed system and asepsis during fluid drainage; high risk for infection
      2) Circulating blood volume
         a) Hyperventilation (with a manual resuscitation bag or mechanical ventilator) to maintain $PaCO_2$ 30-35 mm Hg
            i) Should be performed only in the presence of acute neurologic deterioration suggesting herniation because it works by causing alkalosis which constricts cerebral arteries reducing intracranial volume and pressure but also potentially reducing cerebral blood flow and causing brain ischemia; there is a delicate balance between vasoconstriction to decrease intracranial volume and pressure and vasoconstriction causing ischemia
            ii) Intended for short-term treatment only since renal compensation through excretion of sodium bicarbonate corrects pH within 2-3 days
            iii) SjO_2 monitoring is recommended to identify the $PaCO_2$ level that does not cause brain ischemia.
         b) Barbiturate-induced coma
            i) Actions
               (a) Decreases ICP by decreasing cerebral blood flow and metabolism
               (b) Decreases metabolic rate and oxygen consumption of the brain
               (c) May shunt blood from healthy brain tissue to ischemic areas
            ii) Preferred agent: pentobarbital (Nembutal)
               (a) Usually prescribed as 10 mg/kg IV over 30 minutes as a loading dose followed by 1 mg/kg/hr

(b) Maintain barbiturate level of 2.5-4.0 mg/dL
iii) Indications and expectations
(a) Indicated when ICP is greater than 40 mm Hg despite aggressive therapy
(b) Expect 10 mm Hg decrease in ICP within 10 minutes
(c) Discontinued when the ICP has been normal for at least 24-72 hours; patient should be on anticonvulsants prior to discontinuance as seizures may occur
iv) Considerations
(a) Monitor hepatic and renal function.
(b) Monitor cardiac status and daily weight; may decrease cardiac contractility.
(c) Must be intubated and mechanically ventilated.
(d) Must have ICP monitor; systemic arterial and pulmonary arterial pressure monitoring is recommended.
(e) Protect the corneas by instilling artificial tears and taping eyes shut or applying moisture chamber (i.e., plastic wrap taped in place over eyes).

3) Brain mass
a) Maintenance of euvolemia
i) Actions
(a) Maintains CO, MAP, and CPP
(b) Prevents hyperosmolality and increased blood viscosity which slows blood flow and may precipitate ischemia and occlusion
(c) Prevents brain edema caused by excess fluid administration
ii) Goals
(a) PAOP 10-15 mm Hg or CVP 5-10 mm Hg
(b) Serum osmolality less than 320 mmol/kg
(c) CPP greater than 60 mm Hg
iii) Considerations
(a) Isotonic crystalloids or colloids
(i) Colloids (e.g., dextran, albumin) frequently used but no evidence that they are superior to isotonic crystalloids and isotonic crystalloids are much more cost-effective
(b) Hypertonic saline may be utilized.
(c) Blood and/or blood products may be needed if there has been significant blood loss.
(d) Hypotonic solutions (e.g., D_5W) should be avoided since they reduce serum osmolality and contribute to brain edema.

b) Administration of diuretics
i) Osmotic diuretics (e.g., mannitol [Osmitrol])
(a) Actions
(i) Increases plasma osmolality which pulls fluid from brain tissue and decreases brain edema (this increase in intravascular volume is then eliminated by the kidney)
(ii) May decrease blood viscosity and increase CBF without raising ICP
(iii) May have a neuroprotective effect (under investigation)
(b) Dosage: usually prescribed as 0.25-1 g/kg IV; must be given with a 0.45-micron inline filter
(c) Onset and duration: starts to work within 15 minutes; lasts 2-6 hours; may be repeated every 1-4 hours
(d) Considerations
(i) Indwelling bladder catheter is recommended.
(ii) Monitor for clinical indications of fluid overload initially especially in patients with history of cardiovascular disease.
(iii) Monitor for fluid deficit.
(iv) May mask diabetes insipidus
(v) Monitor for electrolyte imbalance.
(vi) Monitor serum osmolality; should be less than 320 mmol/kg
(vii) Rebound intracranial hypertension may be seen ~8-12 hours after mannitol; furosemide given with mannitol to reduce the incidence of rebound; because of this undesirable rebound effect, continuous hypertonic saline

infusions are becoming standard of care for management of cerebral edema, with mannitol used for rescue dosing only

ii) Loop diuretics (e.g., furosemide [Lasix])

(a) Actions

(i) Reduces intracranial volume by reducing overall body fluid

(ii) Decreases CSF production (unknown mechanism)

(b) Dosage: usually prescribed as 0.5-1 mg/kg IV

iii) Replacement of circulating volume must be ensured to prevent hyperviscosity and dehydration

c) Surgical removal of brain mass: cerebral lobectomy may be performed as last resort (usually nondominant temporal lobe)

b. Prepare patient for surgery if indicated.

1) Débride open wounds and suture scalp laceration.

2) Elevate depressed skull fracture and repair dural tears.

3) Evacuate epidural or subdural hemorrhage or hematoma.

4) Control intracranial hemorrhage or hematoma.

5. Decrease metabolic requirements of the brain.

a. Administer prophylactic anticonvulsants as prescribed; usually no longer than 7 days

b. Maintain normothermia (less than 38° C); hypothermia (~33° C), although experimental, may be ordered to further lower metabolic and oxygen requirements.

1) Hyperthermia is aggressively treated as 1° C temperature elevation is associated with a 7% increase in metabolic rate and oxygen consumption.

2) Central fever is directly attributed to brain injury and reflects hypothalamic dysfunction.

a) Characterized by lack of sweating, absence of tachycardia, and may persist for days

b) Controlled best by external cooling but avoid shivering; use hypothermia blanket

i) Turn it off when the temperature reaches 38 ° C because the temperature of a neurologic patient will tend to drift downward after a hypothermia blanket is turned off.

ii) Do not allow the patient to shiver; small doses of meperidine (Demerol) or promethazine HCl (Phenergan) may be used to decrease shivering.

3) Peripheral fever is associated with infection.

a) Characterized by sweating and tachycardia

b) Controlled best by antipyretics (e.g., acetaminophen [Tylenol])

4) Large-bore central intravenous catheters may be placed for cooled solutions; less shivering is noted.

c. Administer sedatives, muscle paralytics, and/or barbiturates as prescribed; preferred agents are short-acting and/or reversible.

1) Analgesics and sedatives (e.g., morphine, propofol [Diprivan], midazolam [Versed])

a) Actions: reduces restlessness or agitation to decrease metabolic rate and oxygen consumption

b) Considerations

i) Monitor ventilatory status.

ii) May cause hypotension which will decrease CPP; fluid administration may be necessary to maintain preload

2) Muscle paralysis (e.g., pancuronium [Pavulon], atracurium besylate [Tracrium], vecuronium [Norcuron])

a) Actions

i) Reduces skeletal muscle activity, metabolic rate, and oxygen consumption

ii) Controls shivering and posturing, decreasing metabolic rate and oxygen consumption

b) Considerations

i) Must be mechanically ventilated

ii) Protect the corneas by instilling artificial tears and taping eyes shut.

iii) Always administer sedative with muscle paralytics.

3) Barbiturate-induced coma

d. Maintain calm, quiet environment.

1) Prevent loud noises, disturbing conversations.

2) Encourage family to touch the patient and speak to them encouragingly; a high percentage of patients remember things that were said or read to them while they were "unconscious."

6. Maintain MAP and CPP.

a. Assess for bleeding from chest, abdomen, pelvis, extremities.

b. Control scalp bleeding by applying pressure until sutured.

c. Administer IV fluids as prescribed.

d. Administer inotropes and/or vasopressors as prescribed to maintain MAP and CPP; maintain systolic BP ~140 mm Hg.

e. Calcium channel blockers (e.g., nimodipine [Nimotop]) and/or hypervolemic hemodilution may be used for vasospasm.

7. Monitor for complications.
   a. Permanent neurologic residual deficits
   b. Herniation
   c. Brain death

Encephalopathy

Definition

Global mental status dysfunction as a manifestation of a systemic or brain disorder

Etiology

1. Alterations in cerebral perfusion pressure such as anoxic or hypertensive encephalopathy (Figure 6-28)
2. Buildup of toxins such as in uremic or hepatic encephalopathy
3. Cellular changes that alter neurologic function such as hypoglycemia and Wernicke's encephalopathy
4. Metabolic imbalance such as hypothyroidism
5. Infection

Clinical Presentation: Varies with Etiology

1. Objective: varies
   a. Mild: memory loss, subtle personality changes
   b. Severe: dementia, loss of consciousness, seizures
2. Diagnostic: may clarify etiology

Collaborative Management

1. Maintain airway, oxygenation, and ventilation.
   a. Encourage deep breathing; if coughing is indicated (rhonchi are audible), instruct the patient to cough with mouth open.
   b. Administer oxygen to maintain SpO_2 of greater than or equal to 95% unless contraindicated.
   c. Assess swallow competency; have suction equipment available.
2. Resolve impairment in neurologic function if possible through treatment of cause.

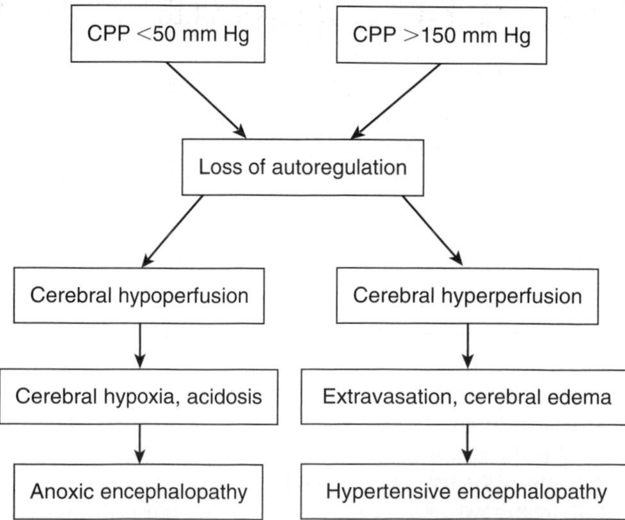

Figure 6-28 Effects of significant alterations in cerebral perfusion pressure. *CPP,* Cerebral perfusion pressure.

3. Maintain adequate hydration and electrolyte balance.
   a. Administer isotonic fluids as prescribed.
   b. Monitor closely for indications of overhydration or dehydration; evaluate urine output and urine specific gravity hourly.
4. Maintain nutritional status: Enteral nutritional support is preferred.
5. Prevent injury
   a. Administer prophylactic anticonvulsants as prescribed and use protective measures if seizure occurs
   b. Perform passive ROM and reposition the patient every 2 hours.
   c. Perform frequent skin assessment.
   d. Instill artificial tears every 2 hours to prevent corneal abrasions in patients who do not blink.
   e. Orient to time and place often; encourage family participation in reality orientation.

Craniotomy

Surgical Procedures

1. Craniotomy: opening of the cranium to allow access to the brain
   a. Supratentorial craniotomy is used to access the cerebral hemispheres and accomplish any of the following:
      1) Remove intracranial tumors, hematomas, abscesses, epileptic foci
      2) Clip or ligate aneurysm or arteriovenous (AV) malformations in the anterior circulation
      3) Place ventriculovenous, ventriculopleural, or ventriculoperitoneal shunt
      4) Débride fragments and necrotic tissue; elevate and realign bone fragments
   b. Infratentorial craniotomy is used to access the brainstem and cerebellum to allow removal of cerebellar tumors and hemorrhages, acoustic neuromas, tumors of the brainstem or cranial nerves, and abscesses.
   c. Transsphenoidal approach is frequently used to remove the pituitary gland; referred to as a *transsphenoidal hypophysectomy*
      1) A horizontal incision is made at the junction of the inner aspect of the upper lip and gingiva and extends laterally to the canine tooth on each side.
      2) The sella turcica is entered through the floor of the nose and the sphenoid sinus.
      3) Transphenoidal hypophysectomy is indicated for pituitary tumor or to control pain associated with metastatic cancer.
2. Craniectomy: removal of a portion of the cranium
3. Cranioplasty: repair of the cranium usually with a synthetic material
4. Burr holes: small holes drilled through the cranium to allow access to underlying structures; frequently used for any of the following:
   a. Evacuation of epidural or subdural hematoma

b. Insertion of intraventricular catheter for CSF drainage
c. Insertion of another form of ICP monitoring device (e.g., subarachnoid screw)

Preoperative Collaborative Management

1. Control pain and discomfort.
   a. Small doses of codeine or morphine may be prescribed.
   b. Care must be taken to avoid oversedation since it eliminates LOC, the most important assessment parameter.
2. Prepare patient for surgery.
   a. Anticonvulsants (e.g., phenytoin [Dilantin]) may be initiated preoperatively.
   b. Hair is washed with an antimicrobial shampoo the night before surgery; the operative area is usually shaved in the operating room (OR) or the OR holding area.
   c. Baseline neurologic status should be carefully recorded.
      1) Level of consciousness
      2) Glasgow coma score
      3) Communication deficits
      4) Cognitive deficits
      5) Motor deficits
      6) Sensory deficits
      7) Cranial nerve deficits
   d. Inform the patient and family what to expect after surgery.
      1) Equipment: IV catheter(s), oxygen therapy and possibly mechanical ventilation, indwelling bladder catheter, sequential compression stockings, possibly intraventricular catheter and ICP monitor
      2) Mild to moderate headache
      3) Photophobia
      4) Periorbital edema and bruising
      5) Head dressing and drain

Postoperative Collaborative Management

1. Prevent/monitor for clinical indications/treat intracranial hypertension
   a. Perform frequent neurologic assessments.
      1) Compare results with preoperative status.
      2) Check vision in patients having hypophysectomy.
   b. Monitor for clinical indications of intracranial hypertension (NOTE: This patient may have an intraventricular catheter in for monitoring ICP.)
   c. Teach patient to avoid causes of intracranial hypertension (Box 6-1).
   d. Prevent twisting of head or neck or flexion of neck to allow jugular vein drainage; support head, neck, shoulders when turning patient in bed.
   e. Control conditions that increase cerebral metabolic rate.
      1) Anticonvulsants for seizures
      2) Antipyretics, cooling blankets for hyperthermia
      3) Sedation as indicated for restlessness
      4) Muscle paralytics, barbiturates to decrease the oxygen requirements of the brain (ICP monitoring is required because the most important assessment parameter [LOC] is eliminated
   f. Administer treatments for intracranial hypertension as prescribed.
   g. Prevent/treat hypertension, hypotension to maintain CPP of 60-100 mm Hg
   h. Position patient appropriately.
      1) If supratentorial craniotomy
         a) Elevate head of bed 30 degrees.
         b) If large mass removed, do not allow the patient to lie on operative side
      2) If infratentorial craniotomy
         a) Position flat with small pillow under nape of neck.
         b) Do not allow on back for 48 hours.
      3) If transsphenoidal craniotomy (e.g., hypophysectomy): Elevate head of bed 30 degrees.
      4) If insertion of interventricular shunt: Position flat on nonoperative side.
      5) Other specific positioning may be prescribed by the surgeon.
2. Maintain airway, oxygenation, and ventilation
   a. Encourage deep breathing; if coughing is indicated (rhonchi are audible), instruct the patient to cough with mouth open.
   b. Administer oxygen to maintain SpO_2 of greater than or equal to 95% unless contraindicated.
   c. Assess swallow competency; have suction equipment available.
3. Maintain adequate hydration and electrolyte balance.
   a. Administer isotonic fluids as prescribed; avoid D_5W and other hypotonic solutions.
   b. Prevent overhydration, which can predispose to brain edema.
   c. Monitor closely for indications of overhydration or dehydration; evaluate urine output and urine specific gravity hourly.
   d. Assess head dressing hourly; notify surgeon if large amounts of drainage are noted.
4. Relieve headache.
   a. Inform patient to notify the nurse at the onset of headache; severe pain is not normal, notify physician
   b. Administer small doses of morphine or codeine avoiding oversedation; when the patient can take oral medications, acetaminophen with codeine is usually used.
   c. Decrease environmental stimuli.
   d. Apply cool compresses to decrease periorbital edema; dressing may be clipped if too tight (clip on side opposite surgical site).
5. Prevent injury.
   a. Institute seizure precautions.
      1) Have suction equipment available.

2) Have extra pillows available that can be placed between patient and side rails.
3) Assess onset, progression, and postictal period if seizure occurs.
4) Administer anticonvulsants as prescribed.

b. Perform passive ROM and reposition the patient every 2 hours.
c. Perform frequent skin assessment.
d. Instill artificial tears every 2 hours to prevent corneal abrasions in patients who do not blink; a moisture chamber may be created using plastic wrap.
e. Orient to time and place often; encourage family participation in reality orientation.
f. Apply restraints only if indicated for self-protection.

6. Prevent/monitor for infection.
   a. Administer prophylactic and/or therapeutic antibiotics as prescribed.
   b. Monitor head dressing, drains for purulent drainage; assess wound during aseptic dressing changes for redness, swelling, induration, and drainage.
   c. Do not put tubes (e.g., suction catheter, nasogastric tube) into nose if patient has transphenoidal approach; warn the patient not to blow or pick nose.
   d. Note drainage of CSF. (CSF leak increases risk of intracranial infection.)
      1) Assessment
         a) Rhinorrhea
         b) Otorrhea
         c) Excessive swallowing
      2) Management
         a) Mustache dressing for rhinorrhea
         b) 2 × 2-inch dressing over ear for otorrhea; sterile uribag may also be used
   e. Monitor for and control hyperthermia: treat temperatures of greater than 38° C with hypothermia blanket and/or acetaminophen.
7. Monitor for complications.
   a. Intracranial hypertension: Brain edema usually peaks in about 48-72 hours.
   b. Brain ischemia, infarction
   c. Cerebral hemorrhage
   d. CSF leak (NOTE: CSF leak is normal for up to 72 hours after transsphenoidal hypophysectomy.)
   e. CNS infection: encephalitis; meningitis
      1) Clinical indications of CNS infection: headache, photophobia, nuchal rigidity, positive Kernig's and Brudzinski's signs; fever
      2) Treatment: antibiotics
   f. Seizures
   g. Fluid and electrolyte imbalance
      1) Diabetes insipidus
         a) Pathophysiology
            i) Central or neurogenic DI: Decrease in production of ADH or brain edema causes blockage in the pathway from the hypothalamus (where ADH is produced) to the posterior pituitary (where ADH is stored and released).
            ii) Nephrogenic DI: decrease in the responsiveness of the renal tubule to ADH
         b) Clinical indications: thirst; polydipsia; polyuria (4-20 L/day); specific gravity of urine 1.005 or less; increased serum sodium; hyperosmolality
         c) Treatment: fluid replacement, vasopressin (ADH) for central DI; drugs to increase the responsiveness of the renal tube to ADH (e.g., chlorpropamide [Diabinese]) for nephrogenic DI
      2) Syndrome of inappropriate antidiuretic hormone (SIADH)
         a) Pathophysiology
            i) Increase in production or release of ADH, ectopic (e.g., tumor) source of ADH, or increase in responsiveness of the renal tubule to ADH
            ii) Increase in renal retention of water causes hyponatremia by dilution
         b) Clinical indications: decreased urine output; weight gain; confusion and lethargy; specific gravity of urine 1.035 or greater; decreased serum sodium (high potential for seizures)
         c) Treatment: fluid restriction; diuretics; hypertonic (3%) saline may be necessary if sodium level very low
      3) Cerebral salt wasting syndrome (CSW)
         a) Pathophysiology
            i) Poorly understood: Hypotheses include the following:
               (a) Increased activity of the sympathetic nervous system causing exaggerated renal pressure-natriuresis
               (b) Presence of circulating natriuretic factors (e.g., atrial natriuretic peptide)
            ii) Renal loss of sodium leads to hyponatremia.
         b) Clinical indications: hyponatremia, hypovolemia, high or normal serum osmolality, high urine sodium, osmolality, and specific gravity, increased BUN
            i) Frequently confused with syndrome of inappropriate antidiuretic hormone (SIADH) which would cause hypervolemia, low serum osmolality, and dilutional hyponatremia
         c) Treatment: fluid and sodium replacement, possibly requiring hypertonic (3% or 5%) saline

i) As opposed to SIADH which requires primarily fluid restriction and possibly sodium replacement

h. Hydrocephalus: frequently transient due to swelling

i. Deep vein thrombosis (DVT): Prevention methods include the following:
   1) Use sequential compression devices rather than graduated elastic stockings because these patients are at high risk for DVT; may be applied prior to surgery
   2) Low-dose heparin may be prescribed; low-molecular-weight heparin may be used.

j. Stress ulcer (frequently referred to as *Cushing's ulcer*): Prophylaxis with histamine$_2$ receptor antagonists or proton pump inhibitors is usually prescribed.

Traumatic Brain Injuries

Etiology

Blunt or penetrating trauma (risk is decreased by helmets, airbags, seatbelts, alcohol, drugs)

1. Motor vehicle crash
2. Falls
3. Violence: assault; gunshot or knife wound
4. Sports-related injuries (e.g., boxing, football)
5. Industrial accidents

Pathophysiology

See Figure 6-29.

Clinical Presentation

1. Classification of head injuries
   a. Mild: GCS 13-15
   b. Moderate: GSC 9-12
   c. Severe: GSC 3-8

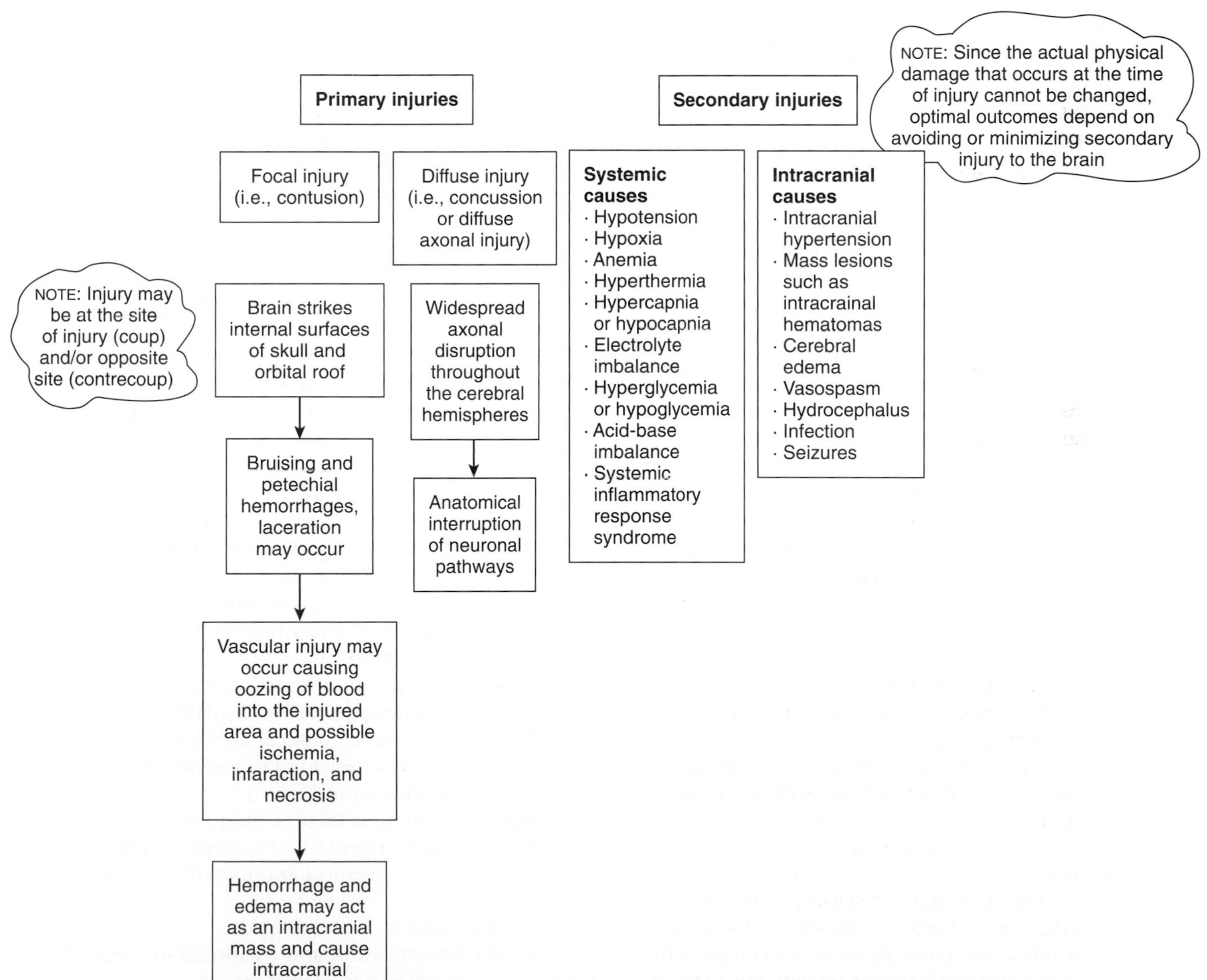

Figure 6-29 Traumatic brain injuries: pathophysiology of primary injuries and possible causes of secondary injury.

2. Concussion: may present with focal neurologic deficit or alteration in LOC that clears within 6-12 hours or less
   a. Subjective
      1) History of precipitating event
      2) Unconsciousness for 10-15 minutes
      3) Headache
      4) Scalp tenderness or pain at injury site
      5) Dizziness
      6) Visual changes
      7) Sluggishness
      8) Nausea/vomiting
      9) Memory loss
         a) Retrograde or antegrade amnesia may occur
         b) Posttraumatic amnesia, related to the events of the injury and events immediately preceding the injury, usually lasts less than 5 minutes
   b. Objective
      1) Confusion, restlessness, irritability
      2) Disorientation
3. Contusion: Signs vary depending on severity of trauma and area of brain involved; neurologic deficit persists less than 24 hours.
   a. Subjective
      1) History of precipitating event
      2) Memory loss
   b. Objective
      1) Change in LOC
      2) Motor or sensory dysfunction
      3) Cranial nerve dysfunction
      4) Focal neurologic signs (e.g., hemiparesis, hemiplegia may be seen)
      5) Seizures
      6) Clinical indications of intracranial hypertension may be seen
4. Diffuse axonal injury
   a. Subjective
      1) History of precipitating event
   b. Objective
      1) Loss of consciousness may last days to weeks and is usually followed by long periods of retrograde and posttraumatic amnesia.
      2) May have purposeful movements, withdrawal from pain, and restlessness
      3) Posturing (i.e., decorticate or decerebrate) may be present.
      4) Permanent residual deficits in memory and cognitive and intellectual functioning occur; permanent residual psychological or personality changes are common.
      5) Death rates are high and many of these patients may persist in a vegetative state; vegetative state is characterized by return of wakefulness (eyes open and sleep patterns observed) but without observable signs of cognition.
      6) Profound residual deficits
5. Diagnostic
   a. CT scan, MRI, magnetic resonance angiography (MRA), magnetic resonance spectroscopy (MRS)
      1) May show brain edema, areas of petechial hemorrhages with severe contusions, and hemispheric shift
      2) May detect presence of associated injuries such as carotid or vertebral dissection as may occur with acceleration/deceleration mechanism of injury
      3) May help predict functional recovery, degree of disability, and rehabilitation potential based upon measurement of chemicals in the brain
   b. EEG: may show brain wave abnormalities
   c. Somatosensory evoked potentials: may show prolongation of transmission of impulses through the brainstem to help predict whether there will be a return to consciousness

Collaborative Management

1. Perform a complete assessment for primary and secondary injuries
   a. Remember that an adult head injury patient is not hypotensive due to a blood loss from a closed head injury, therefore look for other causes of hypotension
   b. Remember that hypotension decreases CPP, increases mortality dramatically, and contributes to secondary brain injury
2. Maintain airway, ventilation, and oxygenation
   a. Assume that the patient has a spinal injury until radiologic clearance of spine: Do not tilt or hyperextend the head; use jaw-thrust technique to maintain open airway.
   b. Use oral or nasopharyngeal airway until lateral spine x-rays rule out fracture.
      1) Do not use nasopharyngeal airway or nasal suctioning if facial or skull fracture is present.
      2) Do not use oral airways in conscious patients since they stimulate the gag reflex.
   c. Assist with rapid sequence intubation if intubation is required.
   d. Administer oxygen as needed to maintain SpO_2 greater than or equal to 95% unless contraindicated.
   e. Prevent aspiration: Position patient on side and have suction equipment available.
3. Prevent/monitor for clinical indications of intracranial hypertension (see Intracranial Hypertension section).
4. Maintain CPP of at least 60 mm Hg; MAP challenge with intraparenchymal PbO_2 monitoring to assess cerebral autoregulation and individualize MAP and CCP goals
   a. Therapies to increase MAP
      1) Identification and treatment of cause of hypotension if present
      2) Fluid resuscitation: isotonic crystalloids, colloids, hypertonic saline, and blood products as prescribed

3) Vasopressors may be required in low systemic vascular resistance states (e.g., septic shock and neurogenic shock) or to raise MAP when ICP is elevated

b. Therapies to decrease elevated ICP (see Intracranial Hypertension section)

5. Employ therapies to maintain brain tissue oxygenation ($PbtO_2$) greater than 10-15 mm Hg, utilizing a specialized intraparenchymal monitor which accounts for all causes of brain tissue hypoxia
   a. Optimize oxygen-carrying capacity by maintaining hemoglobin/hematocrit at desired levels (typically hemoglobin of 7-10 mg/dL and hematocrit of 25-30%).
   b. Evaluate for and treat cerebral vasospasm with calcium channel blockers (e.g., nimodipine) as needed.
   c. Maintain body and brain euthermia to reduce oxygen consumption.
      1) Brain temperature probes are included in some intraparenchymal brain oxygen probe kits.
      2) Intravascular cooling may be utilized for maintenance of euthermia.
   d. Maintain PaO_2 greater than 90 mm Hg; evaluate for and treat acute lung injury, pneumothorax, or aspiration pneumonia as needed.
   e. Maintain upper-range normocapnia ($PaCO_2$ 40-45 mm Hg) if tolerated (i.e., may cause increased ICP); perform $PaCO_2$ challenge to assess CO_2 vasoreactivity and its effect on $PbtO_2$.
   f. Adjust ventilator settings as needed.
      1) Perform O_2 challenge to evaluate intraparenchymal $PbtO_2$ responsiveness.
      2) To decrease minute ventilation, allowing $PaCO_2$ to rise
         a) Decrease tidal volume.
         b) Decrease ventilation rate.
      3) To increase $PbtO_2$
         a) Increase FiO_2 considering guidelines to prevent oxygen toxicity.
         b) Increase PEEP.
            i) Identify optimum PEEP by evaluating a pressure-volume curve.
            ii) Avoid excessive PEEP since it may increase ICP.
         c) Increase inspiratory time to increase mean airway pressure; patient must be adequately sedated to prevent intolerance, agitation, and increased oxygen consumption.
         d) Increase tidal volume (minimum 4 mL/kg ideal body weight for height).
         e) Change ventilator modes to control pressure and volume (i.e., PRVC) but monitor closely for lung injury.
6. Prepare for surgery if indicated.
7. Prevent/monitor for complications.
   a. Vasogenic brain edema
   b. Neurogenic pulmonary edema
      1) Pathophysiology: thought to be due to massive sympathetic discharge
      2) Clinical presentation: pulmonary edema with normal PAOP
      3) Treatment
         a) Elevate head of bed 30 degrees, avoiding hip flexion.
         b) Administer codeine as prescribed for sedation.
         c) Administer osmotic diuretics (e.g., mannitol) and beta-blockers (e.g., propranolol) as prescribed.
         d) Utilize mechanical ventilation as necessary to maintain ventilation.
         e) Utilize oxygen and PEEP as necessary to maintain oxygenation.
            i) Weigh the benefits of PEEP (i.e., improves oxygenation by increasing the driving pressure of oxygen) against the risks (i.e., may increase ICP by reducing venous return).
   c. Sympathetic storm/dysautonomia
      1) Pathophysiology: an immediate sympathetic surge as an attempt to compensate for the effects of the injury
      2) Clinical presentation: hyperdynamic cardiac function with tachycardia, hypertension, hyperthermia, pupillary dilation, dysrhythmias, profuse sweating, hyperglycemia, agitation, muscle rigidity and flexor or extensor posturing
      3) Treatment: sedatives, opiates (e.g., morphine), beta-blockers (e.g., propranolol or esmolol), dopaminergics (e.g., bromocriptine), alpha agonists (e.g., clonidine), GABA-B agonist (e.g., baclofen), and/or anticonvulsant (e.g., gabapentin)
   d. Cerebral vasospasm
   e. Seizures
   f. Fluid and electrolyte imbalance: DI, SIADH, CSW (see Craniotomy section)
   g. Stress ulcers (frequently referred to as *Cushing's ulcers*)
   h. Postconcussion syndrome: persistent headache; inability to concentrate, memory problems, decreased problem-solving ability, irritability, emotional lability, depression, decreased libido, dizziness, tinnitus, diplopia, photophobia, decreased energy level, equilibrium disturbances
   i. Residual neurologic deficits
   j. Persistent coma

Skull Fractures

Etiology

1. Motor vehicle crash
2. Falls
3. Violence: assault, gunshot wounds, knife wounds

4. Sports-related accidents (e.g., boxing or football)
5. Industrial injuries

Pathophysiology (Figure 6-30)

1. Linear fractures (account for 80% of skull fractures)
   a. Fracture with no displacement of bone
   b. May interrupt major vascular channels
      1) Linear fractures of the temporal-parietal bones may tear the middle meningeal artery leading to epidural hematoma.
      2) Linear fractures of the occipital bone may tear the occipital artery leading to epidural hematoma.
2. Depressed
   a. Fracture that depresses outer table of skull
   b. May cause brain laceration
   c. May cause intracranial hematoma
3. Basal
   a. Fracture of base of skull
   b. May cause injury to one or more cranial nerves or cause tearing of the dura with CSF leak

Clinical Presentation

1. Linear
   a. Subjective
      1) History of precipitating event or condition
      2) Scalp tenderness
   b. Objective
      1) Swollen, ecchymotic area on scalp
      2) May have scalp laceration (NOTE: Because of the mobility of the scalp, the fracture may not lie directly beneath laceration.)
2. Depressed
   a. Subjective
      1) History of precipitating event or condition
      2) Headache
   b. Objective
      1) May have altered level of consciousness with focal neurologic deficits
      2) May have scalp laceration
         a) Open fracture: scalp laceration present
         b) Closed fracture: no scalp laceration present
      3) Hemiparesis, hemiplegia
      4) Seizures
      5) Depressed frontal fracture may cause cranial nerve I (olfactory) deficit (i.e., anosmia).
      6) Depressed temporal may cause cranial nerve VII (facial) or VIII (acoustic) deficits; may see ipsilateral facial paralysis (VII) or hearing or equilibrium problems (VIII).
3. Basal
   a. Subjective
      1) History of precipitating event or condition
   b. Anterior fossa
      1) May have rhinorrhea; usually lasts 2-3 days
      2) May have *raccoon eyes*; takes 3-4 hours after injury to develop
      3) May have injury to CNI (olfactory), causing anosmia
      4) May have facial fractures
   c. Middle fossa
      1) May have otorrhea or rhinorrhea
      2) May have CSF or blood behind the tympanic membrane if the tympanic membrane remains intact; may cause hearing deficit
      3) May have *Battle's sign*; takes 4-6 hours after injury to develop
      4) May have cranial nerve injuries
   d. Posterior fossa
      1) May have epidural hematoma which may result in signs of intracranial hypertension
      2) May have cerebellar, brainstem, or cranial nerve signs
         a) Visual changes
         b) Tinnitus
         c) Facial paralysis
         d) Conjugate eye deviation
4. Diagnostic
   a. Skull x-ray
      1) Linear or depressed skull fractures may be seen on plain films
      2) Basal skull fracture is difficult to confirm on x-ray; pneumocephalus, opacity of the mastoid or sphenoid sinus, or an air-fluid level in one of the sinuses may be seen.
   b. CT, MRI: may visualize depressed fractures

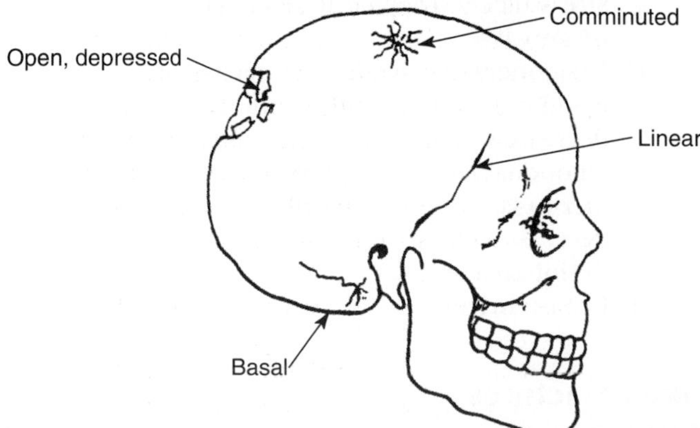

Figure 6-30 Types of skull fractures. (From Barker, E. [2008]. *Neuroscience nursing: A spectrum of care* [3rd ed.]. St. Louis: Mosby.)

Collaborative Management

1. Prevent/monitor for clinical indications/treat intracranial hypertension (see Intracranial Hypertension section)
2. Maintain airway, ventilation, and oxygenation
   a. Assume that the patient has a spinal injury until radiologic clearance of spine: Do not tilt or hyperextend the head; use jaw-thrust technique to maintain open airway.
   b. Use oral or nasopharyngeal airway until lateral spine x-rays rule out fracture; do not use nasopharyngeal airway or nasal suctioning if facial or skull fracture is present.

   c. Do not use oral airways in conscious patients because they stimulate the gag reflex.
   d. Assist with rapid sequence intubation if intubation is required.
   e. Administer oxygen as needed to maintain SpO_2 greater than or equal to 95% unless contraindicated.
   f. Prevent aspiration: Position patient on side and have suction equipment available.
3. Linear
   a. Monitor for clinical indications of intracranial hypertension or neurologic deficit.
   b. No specific treatment required in the absence of neurologic symptoms
4. Depressed
   a. Monitor for clinical indications of intracranial hypertension or neurologic deficit.
   b. Protect brain under cranial defect from injury; position patient away from cranial defect.
   c. Prevent/monitor for intracranial infection from open fracture.
      1) Ensure meticulous cleansing and débridement of associated scalp laceration.
      2) Surgical intervention is indicated if the depression of the skull is greater than the thickness of the skull (5-7 mm) and should be done emergently if scalp laceration or brain laceration is present
      3) Note indications of infection: fever; leukocytosis; redness, swelling, purulent drainage from wound
      4) Obtain culture if appropriate.
   d. Monitor for hemorrhage; removal of bone fragment from a venous sinus may result in hemorrhage; blood must be available
5. Basal
   a. Prevent CNS infection.
      1) Detect rhinorrhea/otorrhea; if present:
         a) Do not obstruct flow: Use mustache dressing.
         b) Elevate HOB 30 degrees.
      2) Avert further tearing of dura by discouraging sneezing, blowing nose, and the Valsalva maneuver; instruct patient to cough with mouth open and to exhale when turning rather than holding the breath.
      3) Do not use nasal O_2, nasogastric tube, nasopharyngeal tube, or nasotracheal tube.
6. Monitor for complications.
   a. Linear: epidural hematoma
   b. Depressed
      1) Laceration of brain tissue by brain fragments
      2) Intracerebral hemorrhage or contusion
      3) CNS infection (e.g., meningitis, encephalitis)
   c. Basal
      1) Intracerebral hemorrhage
      2) CNS infection (e.g., meningitis, abscess)
      3) Cranial nerve injury
      4) Carotid cavernous fistula
         a) Rare but serious complication
         b) Occurs when blood escapes from the carotid artery into the cavernous sinus
         c) Clinical indications include bruit and pulsation of orbit over affected eye, exophthalmos, headache, and visual disturbances.

Intracranial Hematomas

Etiology: Usually Trauma

1. Subdural hematoma (SDH) (15-30% of patients with head trauma and 50-70% of all hematomas)
   a. May occur spontaneously, particularly if patient has coagulation disorder or is taking anticoagulants
   b. Is prevalent in older patients with cerebral atrophy and alcoholics; may be bilateral
   c. May also be due to purulent effusion
2. Epidural hematoma (EDH) (5-8% of patients with head trauma and 20-30% of all hematomas): often associated with linear skull fractures that cross major vascular channels
3. Intracerebral hematoma (ICH) (2-20% of patients with head trauma)
   a. May occur as result of gunshot wound or stab wound, laceration of brain from a depressed skull fracture, severe acceleration-deceleration injury
   b. Intracerebral bleeding caused by aneurysm, AV malformation, vascular tumor, or rupture of a vessel due to hypertension is described as a *hemorrhagic stroke* and will be discussed in the section on Hemorrhagic Stroke

Pathophysiology (Figure 6-31)

1. Subdural hematoma
   a. Usually venous bleeding; arterial origin is rare
   b. Accumulates below dura mater
   c. Classification
      1) Acute SDH: signs/symptoms occur within 48 hours after injury
      2) Subacute SDH: signs/symptoms occur within 2 weeks after injury
      3) Chronic SDH: signs/symptoms may occur weeks to months after injury
         a) Fibroblasts accumulate around the hematoma and encapsulate it.
         b) Hemolysis of the clot liberates plasma proteins; this causes the encapsulated area to have a high osmotic pressure.
         c) This causes an influx of water and swelling of the mass.
2. Epidural hematoma
   a. Usually arterial bleeding; associated with tearing of arteries from skull fractures
      1) Linear fractures of the temporal-parietal bones may tear the middle meningeal artery leading to epidural hematoma.
      2) Linear fractures of the occipital bone may tear the occipital artery leading to epidural hematoma.

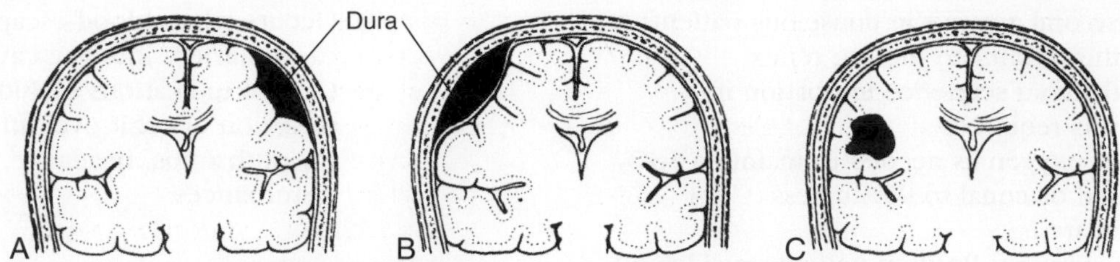

Figure 6-31 Types of hematomas. **A,** Subdural. **B,** Epidural. **C,** Intracerebral. (From Carlson, K. K. [Ed.]. [2009]. *Advanced critical care nursing.* St. Louis: Saunders.)

   b. May be due to venous bleeding; associated with fractures that cross major vascular channels such as the superior sagittal or transverse sinus (posterior fossa EDHs are usually of venous origin)
   c. Accumulates above the dura mater
3. Intracerebral hematoma: hematoma into brain mass itself: may be due to bleeding caused by missile injury (e.g., gunshot wound or knife) or severe acceleration-deceleration force that causes bleeding into deep cerebral tissues

Clinical Presentation

1. SDH
   a. Subjective
      1) History may include precipitating event or condition (in chronic SDH the patient may not be able to link to any particular event, either because they cannot remember or that there is no true precipitating event [spontaneous]).
      2) Headache
      3) Increasing irritability progressing to confusion progressing to decreased LOC
   b. Objective
      1) Decreased LOC
      2) Ipsilateral oculomotor paralysis
      3) Contralateral hemiparesis/hemiplegia
2. EDH
   a. Subjective
      1) History of precipitating event or condition
      2) History of short period of unconsciousness followed by lucid interval and then rapid deterioration; lucid interval may be absent if initial blow is significant
      3) Headache
   b. Objective
      1) Increasing irritability progressing to confusion progressing to decreased LOC
      2) Ipsilateral oculomotor paralysis
      3) Contralateral hemiparesis/hemiplegia
3. ICH
   a. Subjective
      1) History of precipitating event or condition
   b. Objective
      1) Varies with area of brain involved, size of hematoma, and rate of blood accumulation
      2) May or may not show clinical indications of intracranial hypertension
4. Diagnostic
   a. Skull and cervical spine x-rays: may reveal associated skull or spine fractures
   b. LP: contraindicated by intracranial hypertension
   c. CT scan: will show an area of increased density; may show midline shift
   d. MRI: shows hematoma
   e. Cerebral angiogram (rarely performed): may reveal avascular area with displacement or stretching of vessels

Collaborative Management

1. Detect/treat cranial, intracranial, and extracranial injuries
2. Maintain airway, ventilation, and oxygenation
   a. Assume that the patient has a spinal injury until radiologic clearance of spine: Do not tilt or hyperextend the head; use jaw-thrust technique to maintain open airway.
   b. Use oral or nasopharyngeal airway until lateral spine x-rays rule out fracture; do not use nasopharyngeal airway or nasal suctioning if facial or skull fracture is present.
   c. Do not use oral airways in conscious patients since they stimulate the gag reflex.
   d. Assist with rapid sequence intubation if intubation is required.
   e. Administer oxygen as needed to maintain SpO_2 greater than or equal to 95% unless contraindicated.
   f. Prevent aspiration: Position patient on side and have suction equipment available.
3. Prevent/monitor for clinical indications of intracranial hypertension (see Intracranial Hypertension section).
4. Prevent further bleeding; osmotic diuretics are generally not used since the tamponade effect of the hematoma helps to stop the bleeding.
5. Prepare patient for surgery.
   a. EDH and SDH
      1) Usually burr hole and clot evacuation, though small hematomas may be observed through serial CT scans to verify hematoma's gradual reabsorption
      2) Mortality increases dramatically if surgery is delayed.
   b. ICH
      1) Surgery is indicated if ICH is large or there is a deteriorating neurologic status.

2) Alternative treatment to surgery: stereotactic aspiration
   a) Stereotactic placement of a small catheter into the center of the hematoma
   b) Urokinase is injected and catheter sealed for 6 hours
   c) Application of gentle suction to aspirate any liquefied hematoma
   d) Repeat of cycle 8 times over 2 days
3) The FUNC score prediction tool (Rost et al., 2008) can be used following ICH to predict long-term functional independence to assist physicians, patients, and families in decision-making regarding care and inclusion in clinical trials; variables include the following:
   a) ICH volume
   b) Patient age
   c) ICH location
   d) GCS Score
   e) Pre-ICH cognitive impairment

6. Detect/treat postoperative rebleed and/or brain edema; monitor closely for clinical indications of intracranial hypertension or deterioration of neurologic status.
   a. HOB is usually elevated 20-30 degrees for acute and subacute subdural and epidural hematoma.
   b. Physician may request that HOB be flat on side after surgery for removal of chronic subdural hematoma.
7. Prevent seizure activity: Administer anticonvulsants prophylactically or therapeutically as prescribed.
8. Monitor for complications.
   a. Intracranial hypertension
   b. Hydrocephalus
   c. CNS infection
   d. Fluid and electrolyte imbalance: DI, SIADH, CSW (see Craniotomy section)
   e. SIADH
   f. Seizures

Hydrocephalus

Definition

Excessive accumulation of CSF within the ventricular spaces of the brain

1. Noncommunicating or intraventricular hydrocephalus: caused by obstruction within the ventricular system
2. Communicating or extraventricular: caused by impaired reabsorption of CSF
   a. Hydrocephalus ex vacuo: associated with cerebral atrophy
   b. Normal-pressure hydrocephalus: associated with arachnoid obstruction caused by adhesions and thickening of the arachnoid

Etiology

1. Noncommunicating
   a. Congenital abnormalities in the ventricular system
   b. Mass lesions (e.g., tumor)
   c. Scarring
   d. Subarachnoid hemorrhage
2. Communicating
   a. Subarachnoid hemorrhage
   b. Meningitis
   c. Mass causing compression of the subarachnoid space
   d. Head injury
   e. Craniotomy
   f. Congenital abnormalities of the subarachnoid space
   g. High venous pressure within the sagittal sinus (e.g., thrombosis, sinus occlusion, heart failure)

Pathophysiology

See Figure 6-32.

Clinical Presentation

1. Subjective
   a. History of unsteady, broad-based gait with a history of falling and/or declining memory and cognitive function in normal-pressure hydrocephalus
   b. Headache
   c. Blurred vision, diplopia
   d. Nausea
2. Objective
   a. Change in level of consciousness
   b. Inattentiveness
   c. Vomiting
   d. Ataxia
   e. Urinary incontinence
   f. May have clinical indications of intracranial hypertension

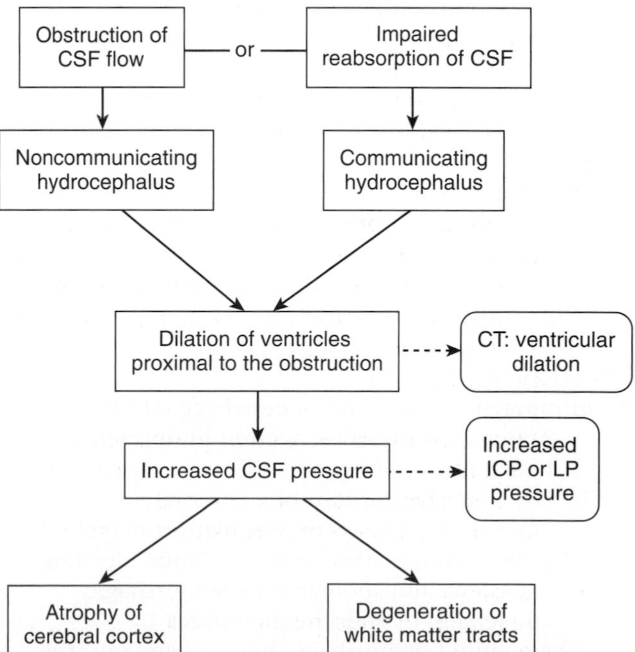

Figure 6-32 Pathophysiology of hydrocephalus. Dotted lines connect pathology to clinical presentation. *CSF,* Cerebrospinal fluid; *CT,* computed tomography; *ICP,* intracranial pressure; *LP,* lumbar puncture.

3. Diagnostic
   a. LP: shows increased pressure
   b. CT: shows increase in size of ventricles
   c. MRI: shows increase in size of ventricles
   d. Radioisotope cisternogram: useful in diagnosis of normal-pressure hydrocephalus

Collaborative Management

1. Maintain airway, ventilation, and oxygenation
   a. Oropharyngeal or nasopharyngeal airway as needed to hold tongue away from hypopharynx in obtunded patient
   b. Endotracheal intubation as needed in patients without airway protective reflexes; sedation is recommended prior to intubation
   c. Oxygen as needed to maintain SpO_2 greater than or equal to 95% unless contraindicated
   d. Mechanical ventilation as needed for hypoventilation, hypercapnia, and respiratory acidosis
   e. Prevention of aspiration
      1) Position with head of bed elevated 30 degrees.
      2) Assess swallow competency and have suction equipment available.
2. Prevent/treat intracranial hypertension.
   a. Treatment of cause
      1) Surgery for removal of mass lesion
      2) Ventricular bypass into the normal intracranial channel
   b. Measures to decrease CSF volume
      1) Ventriculostomy or lumbar drain
      2) Ventriculoperitoneal shunt
         a) Proximal tip in a lateral ventricle with distal tip placed in peritoneum
         b) Fluid from lateral ventricle is drained into the peritoneum
   c. Diuresis for normal-pressure hydrocephalus
3. Monitor for complications
   a. Intracranial hypertension
   b. Herniation

Hemorrhagic Stroke

Definition

Neurologic deficit caused by interruption of blood flow to the brain caused by vessel rupture

Etiology

1. Intraparenchymal brain hemorrhage (IPBH)
   a. Trauma: described in section on intracranial hematomas
   b. Hypertensive rupture of a cerebral vessel
   c. May also be caused by vascular intracerebral tumor, fibrinolytics, anticoagulants, bleeding disorders, and spontaneous hemorrhagic conversion of an ischemic infarct
2. Subarachnoid hemorrhage: hemorrhage into the subarachnoid space
   a. Cerebral aneurysm: weakened bulging area on an intracranial blood vessel; account for the majority of subarachnoid hemorrhage
      1) Most cerebral aneurysms are small (2-6 mm), saccular, and occur at bifurcations in circle of Willis
         a) Saccular (berry) aneurysms: usually congenital defects
         b) Fusiform aneurysms: from atherosclerosis
         c) Mycotic aneurysms: from necrotic vasculitis and septic emboli (rare)
         d) Traumatic aneurysms: from skull fracture disrupting vessel (very rare)
   b. AV malformation
      1) A tangle of abnormal arteries and veins: Arteries feed directly into veins without a capillary bed.
      2) Always congenital
      3) May occur in other circulatory systems including the spinal cord

Pathophysiology (Figure 6-33)

1. Aneurysm
   a. Two contributing factors
      1) Congenital weakness
      2) Stress (e.g., hypertension)
   b. The aneurysm may act as mass lesion if intact and large.
   c. Weakness of an artery and high pressure (90% of ruptured aneurysm associated with hypertension) lead to hemorrhage; hemorrhage most likely when aneurysm is 8-10 mm in size
2. AV malformation: congenital tangle of arteries and veins

Clinical Presentation

1. Subjective
   a. History
      1) Hypertension present in 90% of cases of ruptured aneurysm
      2) Most patients have had a "warning leak" days or weeks prior to bleed
         a) Headache
         b) Generalized, transient weakness
         c) Fatigue
         d) Ptosis, diplopia, blurred vision
   b. Sudden, severe headache
      1) Frequently described as "the worst headache of my life"
      2) Sudden: described as a "thunder clap" or "like being hit in the head"
      3) Localized progressing to generalized
      4) May radiate to neck and back
   c. Nausea and vomiting may be present if severe bleed
2. Objective
   a. Restlessness progressing to altered LOC
      1) Loss of consciousness is common in hemorrhage from aneurysm.
      2) Loss of consciousness is uncommon in hemorrhage from AVM.
   b. If hemorrhage into ventricles
      1) Nuchal rigidity

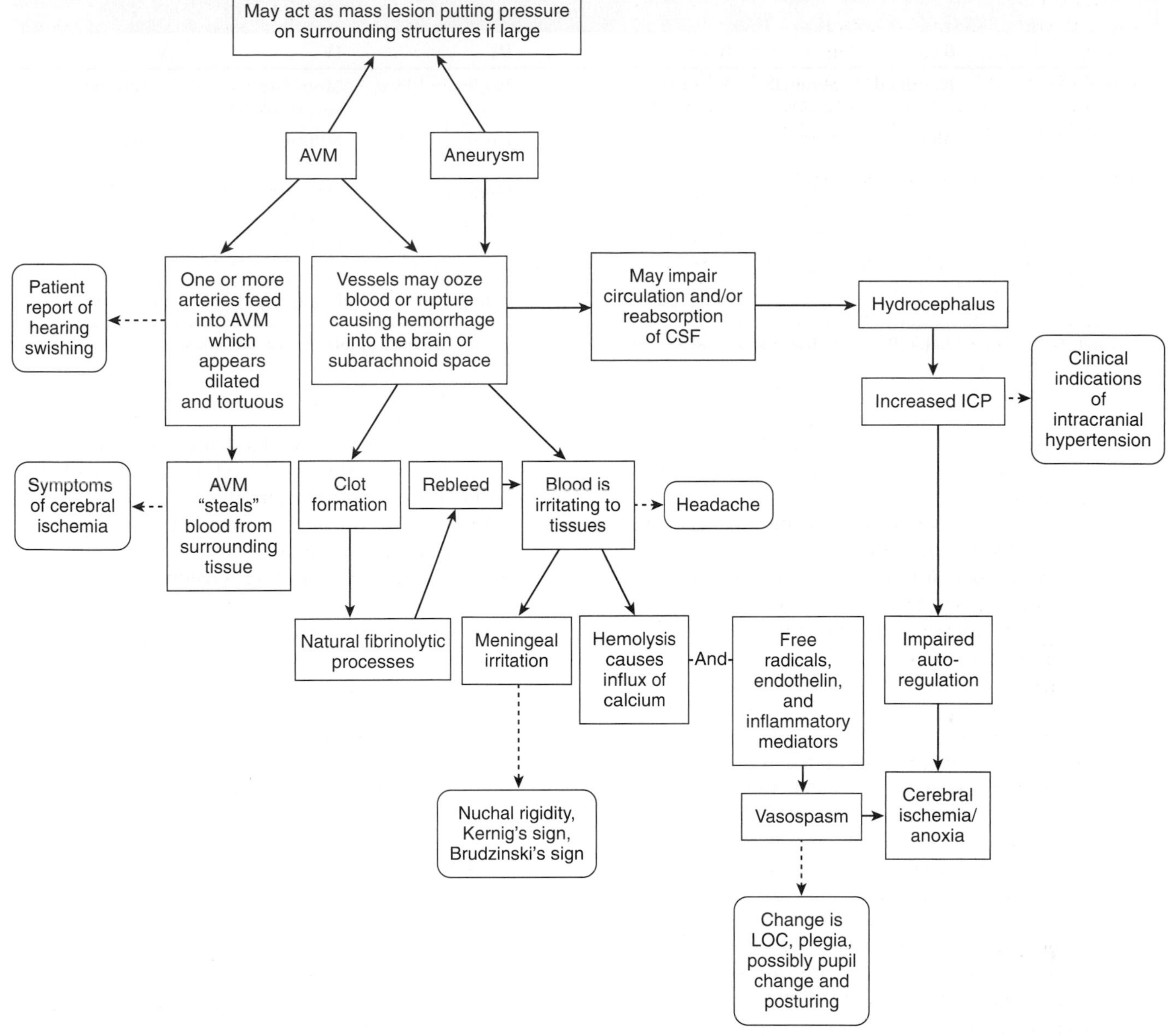

Figure 6-33 Pathophysiology of hemorrhagic stroke. Dotted lines connect pathology to clinical presentation. *AVM,* Arteriovenous malformation; *CSF,* cerebrospinal fluid; *ICP,* intracranial pressure; *LOC,* level of consciousness.

2) Photophobia
3) Kernig's sign, Brudzinski's sign
4) Hyperthermia

c. Neurologic deficit
d. Seizures
e. Site and size determine specific clinical presentation
f. Hunt and Hess aneurysm grading system (Table 6-18)

3. AVM specifically
   a. May have bruit and report a constant swishing sound in the head with each heartbeat
   b. Motor/sensory defects
   c. Aphasia
   d. Dizziness, syncope
4. Diagnostic
   a. Serum
      1) Hyponatremia may be present due to SIADH or cerebral salt wasting
      2) PT, aPTT may be abnormal
   b. ECG
      1) Changes that may occur with SAH
         a) Flattened, peaked, or inverted T wave
         b) Presence of U wave
         c) QT prolongation
      2) Dysrhythmias are common; torsade de pointes has been associated with SAH
   c. Echocardiography: may show decreased ejection fraction due to "stunned" myocardium; mechanism unknown
   d. LP: performed only if CT is nondiagnostic and there are no clinical indications of intracranial hypertension

Table 6-18 Hunt and Hess Aneurysm Grading System

Grade	0	I	II	III	IV	V
Description	No bleed	Minimal bleed	Mild bleed	Moderate bleed	Moderate → severe bleed	Severe bleed
LOC	Alert	Alert	Awake	Drowsy	Stupor	Coma; moribund appearance
Headache	None	Minimal	Mild → moderate	Moderate → severe	Moderate → severe	Moderate → severe
Nuchal rigidity	None	Slight	Yes	Yes	Yes	Yes
Neurologic deficit	None	No	Minimal (e.g., cranial nerve palsy)	Mild (e.g., hemiparesis)	Moderate (e.g., hemiplegia)	Severe (e.g., posturing)

From Hunt, W.E. & Hess, R.M. (1968). Surgical risks as related to time of intervention in the repair of intracranial aneurysms, *J Neurosug,* 28(14).

1) Reveals bloody CSF, elevated protein in acute SAH; it is important to number the test tubes
   a) If only test tube #1 is bloody: traumatic tap
   b) If all test tubes are bloody: bloody tap
2) Reveals xanthochromic (dark amber) CSF if hemorrhage occurred several days (more than 5 days) ago

e. Transcranial Doppler: aids in diagnosing vasospasm
f. CT: identifies extent of subarachnoid hemorrhage or intraparenchymal brain hemorrhage that may be suspicious of aneurysm; detects presence of hydrocephalus
g. MRI/MRA
   1) May reveal small aneurysms that are not visualized with CT
   2) May reveal ICH and intraventricular blood
   3) May show vasospasm
h. Cerebral angiogram: will illustrate size, shape, and location of aneurysm; allows direct evaluation for vasospasm

Collaborative Management

1. Maintain airway, ventilation, and oxygenation
   a. Maintain airway
      1) Oropharyngeal or nasopharyngeal airway may be needed to hold tongue away from hypopharynx in obtunded patient.
      2) Endotracheal intubation may be needed in patients without airway protective reflexes; sedation is recommended prior to intubation and administration of lidocaine may reduce the risk of increased ICP.
   b. Maintain oxygenation and ventilation.
      1) Administer oxygen as needed to maintain SpO_2 greater than or equal to 95% unless contraindicated.
      2) Initiate mechanical ventilation as needed for hypoventilation.
   c. Prevent aspiration.
      1) Position patient on side.
      2) Have suction equipment available.
2. Minimize potential for rebleed and promote stabilization of patient: Rebleed occurs most often within 10 days after hemorrhage.
   a. Maintain BP within 10% of prehemorrhage levels; hypotension is associated with hypoperfusion, and hypertension is associated with rebleeding
      1) Calcium channel blocker (e.g., nicardipine [Cardene], alpha- and beta-blocker (e.g., labetalol [Normodyne] or direct vasodilator (e.g., hydralazine [Apresoline]) for hypertension
      2) Vasopressors (e.g., phenylephrine [Neo-Synephrine], norepinephrine [Levophed]) for hypotension
   b. Decrease environmental stimuli (these interventions may be referred to as *aneurysm precautions*).
      1) Provide a quiet, dimly lit private room.
      2) Enforce bed rest with HOB elevated 15-30 degrees.
      3) Instruct patient regarding how to avoid Valsalva maneuver (e.g., cough with mouth open, exhale when turning in bed, stool softeners).
      4) Instruct visitors that the patient should not be upset in any way; limit number of visitors and duration of visits.
      5) Do not perform any rectal procedures (e.g., rectal temperature, enemas).
      6) Provide sedation (usually phenobarbital) if patient is restless.
      7) Treat fever with acetaminophen.
   c. Administer analgesics for headache but avoid oversedation that would impair assessment.
      1) Utilize short-acting narcotics (e.g., morphine, fentanyl, codeine).
      2) Avoid benzodiazepines.
   d. Prepare patient for surgery or interventional neuroradiology procedures.
      1) Aneurysm
         a) Indications
            i) Surgery to secure the aneurysm is indicated within 72 hours

b) Surgical
   i) Clipping: occlusion of the neck of the aneurysm with a ligature or metal clip; most common treatment especially if there is a well-defined neck
   ii) Wrapping or coating
      (a) Reinforcement of the sac with muscle, fibrin foam, or solidifying polymer
      (b) These procedures carry a higher risk of rebleeding, therefore complete obliteration is recommended.
   iii) Ligation: proximal ligation of a feeding vessel
   iv) Bypass grafts: Redirect blood flow to prevent feeding an aneurysm.

c) Endovascular procedures
   i) Detachable coils: made of soft platinum; the device molds itself into the inner diameter of the aneurysmal dilation to cause thrombosis; an average of five coils are need to occlude the aneurysm; a clot forms and evidentially the base of the aneurysm endothelializes and is cut off
   ii) Intravascular balloon placement: Silicone microballoon is placed into the aneurysm and detached.

2) AVM
   a) Surgical excision
   b) Stereotactic radiosurgery if AVM may not be safely excised
   c) Glue embolization: injection of glue into the arterial pedicle to cause thrombosis and block blood flow into the malformation
   d) Embolization of the AVM with Silastic beads
   e) Preoperative embolization followed by surgical excision

3) Intraparenchymal brain hemorrhage (IPBH)
   a) Surgical removal of the clot depends on the size and location of the clot, the patient's ICP, and neurologic status
      i) Massive hematoma (greater than 3 cm diameter) with brainstem compression or intracranial hypertension
      ii) Hydrocephalus
      iii) Surgical-accessible lesions

4) Provide postoperative management as described in Craniotomy section; monitor for clinical indications of intracranial hypertension or rebleeding.

3. Prevent/monitor for clinical indications/treat intracranial hypertension (see Intracranial Hypertension section)

4. Prevent/monitor for ischemia related to vasospasm following SAH due to aneurysm.
   a. Recognize risk factors that increase the risk of the occurrence and severity of vasospasm.
      1) Concomitant conditions
         a) Hyperglycemia: Controlling serum glucose may reduce the risk of vasospasm following SAH.
      2) CT: diffuse, thick blood in the subarachnoid space on CT scan especially if around the base of the brain
      3) Location: hemorrhage in one of the vessels of the circle of Willis
      4) Time frame: Vasospasm occurs anytime from the third day postbleed to 2-3 weeks after the initial bleed (peak incidence 5-12 days)
   b. Monitor for clinical indications of vasospasm
      1) Headache or worsening of headache
      2) Visual changes
      3) Change in LOC
      4) Confusion
      5) Pupil change
      6) Focal neurologic deficit (e.g., hemiparesis, aphasia)
      7) Seizures may occur
      8) Increase in ICP if being monitoring; blood may be visible in CSF if intraventricular catheter in place
      9) Transcranial Doppler
         a) Often performed daily after SAH or more often if indicated
         b) Note trends in flow velocity; intracranial blood flow velocities greater than 100-120 cm/second suggest vasospasm; greater than 200 cm/second suggest severe vasospasm
         c) Correlate with clinical assessment
      10) Angiography
         a) Definitive study for diagnosis of cerebral vasospasm
         b) Narrowing of arterial vessels may be seen on angiography before clinical indications of vasospasm are noted.
   c. Provide therapies for the prevention and treatment of cerebral vasospasm.
      1) Early clipping with flushing of excess blood and clots from the basal cisterns
      2) Calcium channel blockers to prevent and/or reduce vasospasm
         a) Nimodipine (Nimotop) is the preferred agent because it is lipid-soluble and therefore able to cross the blood-brain barrier
            i) Dosage: 60 mg orally every 4 hours for 14 days posthemorrhage
            ii) Adverse effects: hypotension; dose may be reduced to 30 mg every 2-4 hours
         b) Prolonged-release nicardipine implants may be placed parallel to the ruptured artery and adjacent to the clot.

c) Intrathecal nicardipine infusion may be administered via a lumbar drainage catheter.

3) Triple-H therapy (hypertension, hypervolemia, hemodilution)
 a) Goals: to increase CPP and CBF, and decrease risk of brain ischemia
 b) Components
  i) Hypertension
   (a) The most debated of the three; some physicians use only hypervolemia and hemodilution, especially prior to clipping
   (b) Goal
    (i) Maintain systolic BP approximately 60 mm Hg above baseline but not in excess of 160 mm Hg before the aneurysm has been clipped or otherwise secured.
    (ii) Maintain systolic BP of 160-200 mm Hg after clipping.
   (c) Vasopressors (e.g., phenylephrine [Neo-Synephrine], dopamine [Intropin]) may be needed if patient hypotensive; dobutamine (Dobutrex) may also be used to augment the cardiac output
  ii) Hypervolemia and hemodilution
   (a) Isotonic crystalloids and/or colloids (e.g., albumin)
   (b) Hypervolemia: Goal is to maintain a PAOP of 14-20 mm Hg and/or CVP 10-12 mm Hg
   (c) Hemodilution: Goal is to maintain a hematocrit of 30-33%; patients with hematocrit levels of less than 25% require blood transfusion to optimize cerebral oxygenation
 c) Usually maintained for 14 days after hemorrhage
 d) Controversies related to triple-H therapy
  i) Not every patient responds.
  ii) Significant costs
  iii) Potential complications: pulmonary edema, myocardial ischemia, coagulopathy, electrolyte imbalance, rebleeding

4) Transluminal cerebral balloon angioplasty
 a) Goal: widening of the stenotic segment with a balloon-tipped catheter
 b) Limitation: can only be used with larger, accessible vessels
 c) Complications
  i) Vessel rupture
  ii) Restenosis rarely occurs

5) Intraarterial injection of vasodilating agent (e.g., verapamil, nicardipine, nimodipine, milrinone, or papaverine)
 a) Goal: relief of spasm of vessels too distal for the use of angioplasty; most beneficial when used during angioplasty
 b) Complications: intracranial hypertension, brain ischemia

6) Magnesium: intravenous infusions may decrease cerebral ischemia and improve patient outcomes

7) Statins: may decrease vasospasm and the risk of mortality

5. Provide instruction and counseling regarding lifestyle modification and need for pharmacologic therapy.
 a. Nonpharmacologic therapies
  1) Weight normalization
  2) Cessation of tobacco use
  3) Limitation of alcohol consumption to 1-2 alcoholic beverages daily
  4) Regular aerobic exercise in moderation
  5) Complementary therapies: relaxation; imagery, biofeedback
  6) Stress reduction
  7) Yearly flu and pneumococcal vaccine
  8) Recognition of symptoms of recurrence and when to call the physician
 b. Pharmacologic agents
  1) Control of hypertension, hyperlipidemia, and diabetes mellitus

6. Monitor for complications
 a. Vasospasm (in aneurysms)
 b. Rebleeding
 c. Brain edema and intracranial hypertension
 d. Hydrocephalus: may require temporary diversion with intraventricular catheter or lumbar drain and more long-term management through placement of a ventriculoperitoneal shunt
 e. Fluid and electrolyte imbalance: DI, SIADH, CSW (see Craniotomy section)
 f. Seizures: Prophylactic anticonvulsants are frequently prescribed because the increase in BP, increase in metabolic rate and oxygen demand, and compromised ventilation and oxygenation during seizure activity could be devastating.
 g. Dysrhythmias (e.g., prolonged QT interval and torsades de pointes)
 h. Deep vein thrombosis and pulmonary embolism: Utilize sequential compression devices.

Ischemic Stroke

Definitions

1. Transient ischemic attack (TIA): episode of neurologic impairment attributed to focal cerebral ischemia (Box 6-2)

Box 6-2 Symptoms Occurring during Transient Ischemic Attacks

Anterior Circulation	Posterior Circulation
• Ipsilateral monocular visual defect (amaurosis fugax) or homonymous hemianopsia • Contralateral sensory or motor defects • Aphasia (if dominant hemisphere affected) • Ipsilateral headache • Seizure activity	• Bilateral visual defect; diplopia • Bilateral sensory or motor defects • Dysphagia • Occipital headache • Vertigo, syncope (drop attack), dizziness, ataxia

   a. Resolves within 24 hours (usually less than 1-2 hours)
   b. May be described as a zone of penumbra without central infarction
2. Ischemic stroke: sudden, severe disruption of the cerebral circulation with a subsequent loss of neurologic function caused by thrombus or embolus
3. Lacunar stroke: special subset of thrombotic stroke seen almost exclusively in hypertensive patients; small perforating vessel thrombosis

Etiology

1. Thrombosis
   a. Intracranial arteriosclerosis
   b. Extracranial (i.e., carotid) atherosclerosis
   c. Hypertension
   d. Hypercoagulability (e.g., polycythemia)
2. Embolism
   a. Mural thrombi
      1) Dysrhythmia (e.g., atrial fibrillation)
      2) Ventricular aneurysm
   b. Carotid artery atherosclerosis
   c. Bacterial endocarditis
   d. Valvular heart disease
   e. Prosthetic cardiac valves
   f. Deep vein thrombosis with patent foramen ovale
   g. Air or fat embolism (see Chapter 5)

Pathophysiology (Figure 6-34)

1. Risk factors include the following:
   a. Family history
   b. Hypertension
   c. Smoking
   d. Diabetes mellitus
   e. Valvular heart disease
   f. Coronary artery disease
   g. Heart failure
   h. Hyperlipidemia
   i. Obesity
   j. Sedentary lifestyle
   k. Drugs
      1) Alcohol, especially heavy episodic consumption
      2) Stimulants (e.g., cocaine, phenylpropanolamine)
      3) Oral contraceptives
   l. Dysrhythmias, especially atrial fibrillation
   m. Hypercoagulability

Clinical Presentation

1. Subjective
   a. May have history of any of the following:
      1) Transient ischemic attack (TIA)
      2) Hypertension
      3) Cardiovascular disease
      4) Arteriosclerosis
      5) DM
   b. Sudden onset of signs and symptoms
      1) Thrombotic stroke usually occurs at night and is often discovered on awakening; likely caused by decrease in cardiac output and blood pressure with less flow through an area of critical stenosis
      2) Embolic stroke is more likely to occur when the patient is active.
2. Objective
   a. Varies depending on area of vessel involved and extent of injury (Box 6-3)
3. Diagnostic
   a. Serum
      1) Lipids: may be elevated
      2) Glucose
         a) Hypoglycemia may mimic stroke.
         b) Hyperglycemia frequently seen in stroke
      3) Clotting profile: baseline desirable before fibrinolytics
   b. ECG: may show dysrhythmias as a possible cause of cerebral emboli; Holter monitor may identify dysrhythmia
   c. Echocardiography: may show intracardiac source for cerebral emboli (e.g., ventricular aneurysm, bacterial endocarditis)
   d. LP: may be done to differentiate hemorrhagic from thrombotic stroke if there are no signs of intracranial hypertension
   e. Doppler carotid studies: may show carotid artery stenosis
   f. Transcranial Doppler: may be used to localize vessel occlusions and experimentally to assist with clot lysis
   g. CT
      1) Normal early in ischemic stroke
      2) Identifies the location and characteristics of subacute and old infarctions, the presence or absence of gross hemorrhage, and the presence or absence of a mass lesion
      3) May show distortion or shift of ventricles
      4) CT performed 24 hours postfibrinolytic therapy to rule out intracranial hemorrhage
   h. MRI
      1) Shows presence of early ischemic changes when a CT still looks normal
      2) Identifies changes in the cranial or spinal structures

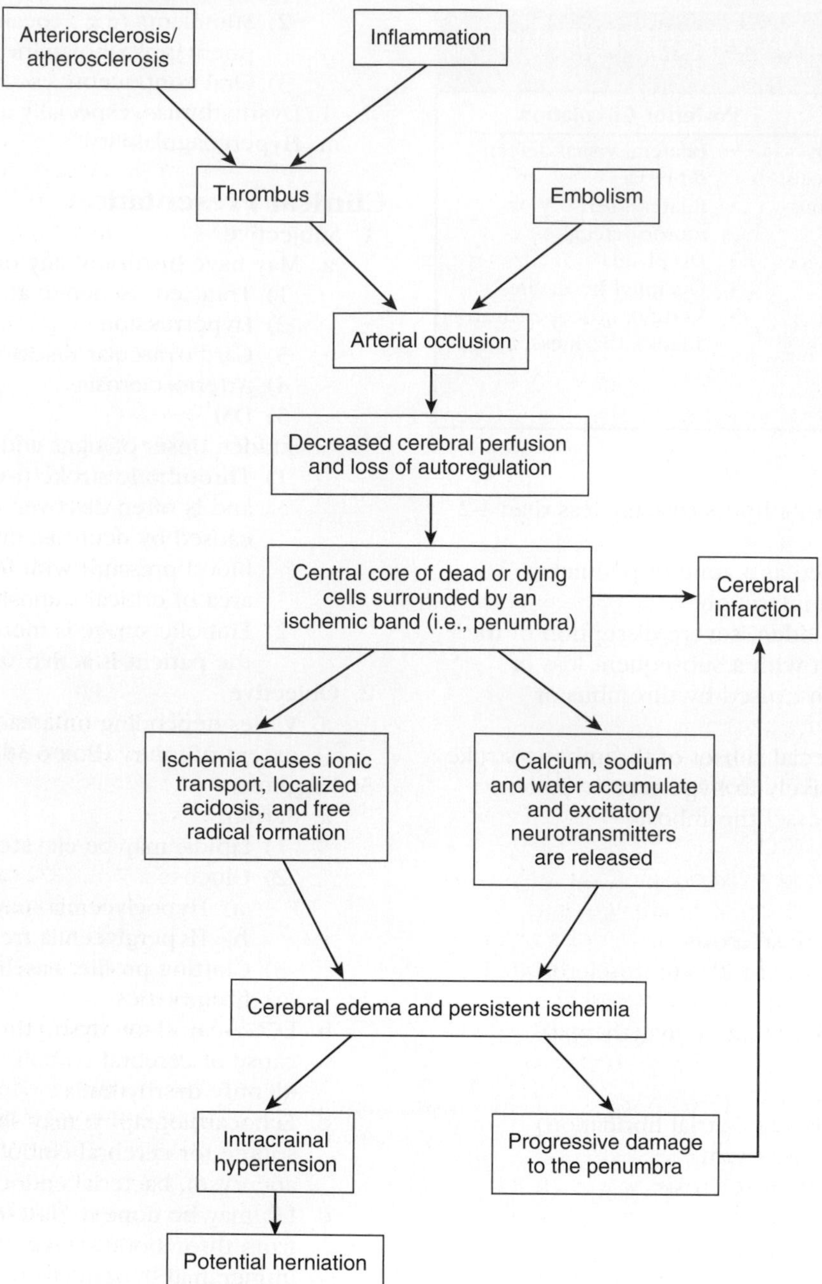

Figure 6-34 Pathophysiology of ischemic stroke.

Box 6-3 Clinical Indications Related to Vascular Occlusion

Anterior Cerebral Artery
- Impaired gait
- Contralateral paralysis of leg and foot
- Personality changes: flat affect; inappropriate emotional responses
- Mental impairment

Middle Cerebral Artery
- Hemiplegia of face and arm on contralateral side
- Contralateral sensory deficit
- Aphasia if dominant hemisphere affected
- Homonymous hemianopsia
- Apraxia, agnosia, neglect if nondominant hemisphere affected
- Dysarthria
- Dysphagia

Posterior Cerebral Artery
- Cortical blindness
- Perseveration (abnormal persistence of a response)
- Homonymous hemianopsia

Vertebral or Basilar Artery
- Weakness of tongue
- Ipsilateral facial numbness and weakness
- Dizziness
- Nystagmus
- Dysarthria
- Dysphagia
- Ataxia
- "Locked-in" syndrome (quadriplegia and mutism with intact consciousness)

i. Cerebral angiography: identifies occlusion, stenosis, aneurysms, and hemorrhage in arterial system

Collaborative Management

1. Maintain airway, ventilation, and oxygenation.
   a. Maintain airway.
      1) Oropharyngeal or nasopharyngeal airway may be needed to hold tongue away from hypopharynx in obtunded patient.
      2) Endotracheal intubation may be needed in patients without airway protective reflexes.
   b. Maintain oxygenation and ventilation.
      1) Administer oxygen as needed to maintain SpO_2 greater than or equal to 95% unless contraindicated.
      2) Turn patient frequently; 60-degree lateral rotation therapeutic bed is helpful to prevent pneumonia in these patients.
      3) Initiate mechanical ventilation as needed for acute respiratory failure.
   c. Prevent aspiration.
      1) Position patient on side.
      2) Have suction equipment available.
2. Detect changes in neurologic status and restore or maintain cerebral blood flow (Figure 6-35).
   a. Utilize the NIHSS (Table 6-9) to assess changes in neurologic status.
   b. Correct possible causes and contributing factors.
      1) Assist in electrical or pharmacologic conversion of atrial fibrillation or administer anticoagulants to prevent mural thrombi.
      2) Administer antihypertensives to control blood pressure only if BP greater than 220/120 mm Hg, cardiac ischemia, heart failure, or aortic dissection exist, fibrinolytic therapy is planned, or intracerebral hemorrhage is identified on CT
         a) Hypotension *must* be avoided since cerebral autoregulation is lost in the area of ischemia/infarction.
         b) Nicardipine (Cardene), labetalol (Normodyne), or hydralazine (Apresoline) may be used.
      3) Control hyperglycemia with intravenous insulin infusion.
   c. Administer fibrinolytics as prescribed.
      1) Goal: lysis of an occluding clot to restore blood flow to the compromised but potentially viable penumbra
      2) Seven Ds of stroke care (AHA)
         a) Detection of early indications and determination of time of onset
            i) Time of onset is either witnessed or the time that last known normal neurologic function was noted.
         b) Dispatch of emergency medical care
         c) Delivery of the patient to the nearest facility capable of implementing the most current stroke guidelines
         d) Door and rapid triage in the emergency department
         e) Data collected to aid in decision making
            i) Baseline CT and/or MRI to exclude intracranial hemorrhage and other risk factors for intracranial hemorrhage
            ii) History, physical examination, laboratory
         f) Decision made regarding whether the patient meets criteria for fibrinolytics and does not have contraindications (Box 6-4)
         g) Drug within 3-4.5 hours of the onset of symptoms
      3) Dosage and routes
         a) Intravenous alteplase (Activase)
            i) Total dose: 0.9 mg/kg with maximum dose of less than or equal to 90 mg
            ii) Bolus: 10% of this total dose over 1 minute
            iii) Infusion: remaining 90% of this total dose administered over 60 minutes
         b) Intraarterial
            i) Catheter is placed into the cerebral circulation under fluoroscopy
            ii) Dose of alteplase (Activase) approximately half of intravenous dose
      4) Management
         a) Monitor vital signs and neurologic status.
         b) Prior to fibrinolytic administration, maintain BP less than 185 mm Hg systolic and less than 110 mm Hg diastolic; labetalol (Normodyne), nicardipine (Cardene), hydralazine (Apresoline), or enalaprilat (Vasotec) are recommended.
         c) After fibrinolytic administration, maintain systolic BP less than 180 mm Hg and diastolic BP less than 105 mm Hg; postfibrinolytic therapy, BP should be managed with labetalol (Normodyne), nicardipine (Cardene), or nitroprusside (Nipride) if necessary.
         d) Do not administer anticoagulants or platelet aggregation inhibitors for 24 hours after intravenous fibrinolytic.
         e) Repeat CT at 24 hours postfibrinolytic.
         f) As in Table 3-13 (see page 166)
   d. Administer anticoagulants and platelet aggregation inhibitors as prescribed if fibrinolytics are contraindicated or after 24 hours post IV fibrinolytics.
      1) Anticoagulants (e.g., heparin) are especially important if emboli are of cardiac origin such as atrial fibrillation.

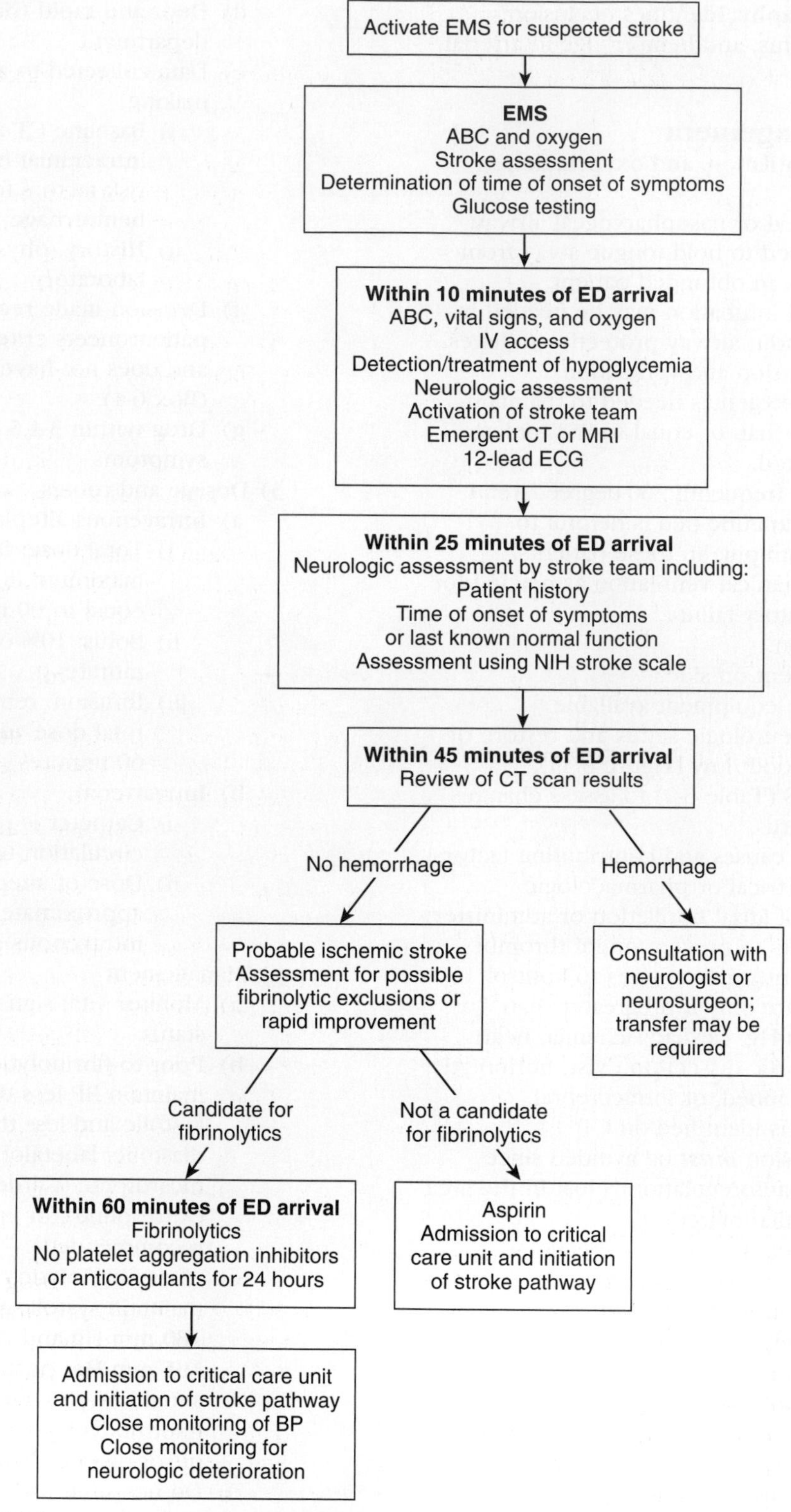

Figure 6-35 Suspected stroke algorithm. *ABC,* Airway, breathing, circulation; *BP,* blood pressure; *CT,* computed tomography; *ECG,* electrocardiogram; *EMS,* emergency management system; *IV,* intravenous; *MRI,* magnetic resonance imaging; *NIH,* National Institutes of Health. (Data from Jauch, E. C., Cucchiara, B., Adeoye, O., Meurer, W., Brice, J., Chan, Y. Y., et al. [2010]. Part 11: Adult stroke: 2010 American Heart Association Guidelines for Cardiopulmonary Resuscitation and Emergency Cardiovascular Care. *Circulation, 122*[18 Suppl 3], S818-828.).

Box 6-4 Inclusion and Exclusion Criteria for the Use of Fibrinolytics in Ischemic Stroke

Inclusion

Diagnosis of ischemic stroke causing measurable neurologic deficit

Onset of symptoms less than 3-4.5 hours prior to initiation of infusion

Age greater than or equal to 18 years

Exclusions If Within 3 Hours of Onset of Symptoms

Head trauma or previous stroke within previous 3 months

Suspicion of intracerebral hemorrhage by symptoms or CT or history of previous hemorrhagic stroke

Puncture of a noncompressible artery within the previous 7 days

Uncontrolled hypertension (i.e., systolic BP greater than 185 mm Hg or diastolic BP greater than 110 mm Hg)

Evidence of active bleeding on physical examination

Significant risk of bleeding (e.g., platelet count 100,000/mm^3, use of anticoagulants with aPTT greater than upper limit of normal, INR greater than 1.7, or PT greater than 15 seconds)

Serum glucose less than 50 mg/dL

CT evidence of multilobar infarction (i.e., hypodensity greater than one third of cerebral hemisphere)

Relative Exclusions If Within 3 Hours of Onset of Symptoms

Only minor neurologic deficit or rapidly resolving neurologic deficit

Seizure at onset with postictal neurologic deficit

Major surgery or serious trauma within 14 days

Recent (i.e., within 21 days) gastrointestinal or genitourinary hemorrhage

Recent (i.e., within 3 months) acute myocardial infarction

Additional Exclusions If Not Within 3 Hours But Within 4.5 Hours of Onset of Symptoms

Age greater than 80 years

Severe stroke (i.e., NIHSS greater than 25)

On anticoagulant therapy regardless of INR

History of both diabetes and prior ischemic stroke

Data from Jauch, E. C., Cucchiara, B., Adeoye, O., Meurer, W., Brice, J., Chan, Y. Y., et al. (2010). Part 11: Adult stroke: 2010 American Heart Association Guidelines for Cardiopulmonary Resuscitation and Emergency Cardiovascular Care. *Circulation, 122*(18 Suppl 3), S818-828.

a) Low-molecular-weight heparin subcutaneously may be used for DVT prophylaxis.

2) Platelet aggregation inhibitors
 a) Oral agents (e.g., ASA, Aggrenox, ticlopidine [Ticlid], clopidogrel [Plavix]) or IV agents abciximab [ReoPro], eptifibatide [Integrilin], tirofiban HCl [Aggrastat]) as prescribed
  i) IV agents being studied for primary use within 24 hours of stroke symptoms
 b) Especially important in patients with carotid, intracranial, or vertebrobasilar artery stenosis

c) Contraindicated for 24 hours after IV fibrinolytics

e. Prepare patient for surgical procedures as requested.
 1) Endarterectomy or carotid artery angioplasty with or without stenting for patients with signs of cerebrovascular insufficiency who have not had completed stroke (see Vascular Disease section of Chapter 3).
 2) Intraarterial mechanical embolectomy with or without fibrinolytic administration
 3) Craniotomy with evacuation of clot depending on size, location, and neurologic status
 4) Decompressive hemicraniectomy where there are severe cerebral edema, hemispheric shifting and potential herniation

3. Prevent/monitor for clinical indications/treat intracranial hypertension (see Intracranial Hypertension section) especially during the first 72 hours
4. Maintain fluid and electrolyte balance and nutritional status.
 a. Administer intravenous fluids as prescribed.
 b. Assess gag and swallow reflexes before PO fluids; routine use of a bedside dysphagia screening tool is recommended.
 c. Initiate early enteral feedings within 24-48 hours if unable to take food by mouth
5. Decrease metabolic requirements.
 a. Enforce bed rest initially.
 b. Administer minor tranquilizers as prescribed but do not oversedate.
 c. Administer stool softeners as prescribed.
 d. Treat hyperthermia with antipyretics, passive cooling (i.e., fans), and cooling blankets; hypothermia therapy may be initiated.
6. Assess patient's ability to communicate and establish means of communication; consult speech therapist as soon as possible in aphasic patients.
7. Protect patient from injury.
 a. Provide assistance during ambulation because patient may have postural imbalance related to hemiparesis/hemiplegia.
 b. Orient patient often and provide explanations of care because confusion and disorientation as well as memory deficits may occur concomitantly with aphasia.
 c. Administer prophylactic anticonvulsants as prescribed.
8. Prevent deformities, decubiti, and hazards of immobility.
 a. Reposition every 2 hours.
 b. Perform passive ROM exercises every 2 hours; assist with active ROM exercises when patient is able to assist.
9. Maximize independence in ADL; allow the patient to do whatever he or she can.
10. Provide emotional support and encourage participation in support groups.

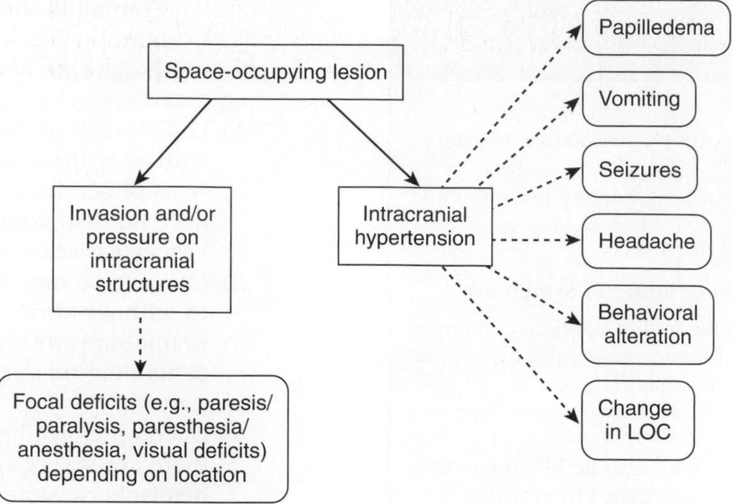

Figure 6-36 Pathophysiology of brain tumors. Dotted lines connect pathology to clinical presentation. *LOC,* Level of consciousness.

11. Provide instruction and counseling regarding lifestyle modification and need for pharmacologic therapy.
    a. Nonpharmacologic therapies
        1) Weight normalization
        2) Dietary modifications
            a) Low saturated fat
            b) Low (2-3 gram) sodium
            c) ADA diet for control of blood glucose for patient with DM
        3) Cessation of tobacco use
        4) Limitation of alcohol consumption to 1-2 alcoholic beverages daily
        5) Regular aerobic exercise in moderation
        6) Complementary therapies: relaxation; imagery, biofeedback
        7) Stress reduction
        8) Yearly flu and pneumococcal vaccine
        9) Recognition of symptoms of TIA or stroke and when to call the physician
    b. Pharmacologic agents
        1) Control of hypertension, hyperlipidemia, and diabetes mellitus
        2) Platelet aggregation inhibitors and/or anticoagulants
        3) Discontinuance of oral contraceptive agents in premenopausal females and hormone replacement therapy in postmenopausal females
12. Monitor for complications.
    a. Persistent neurologic trauma
    b. Brain edema
    c. Seizures: prophylactic anticonvulsants
    d. Fluid and electrolyte imbalance: DI, SIADH, CSW (see Craniotomy section)
    e. Spastic paralysis may cause contractures.
        1) Range of motion
        2) Splints
    f. Pneumonia
    g. Deep vein thrombosis, pulmonary embolism
        1) Subcutaneous LMWH or unfractionated heparin is usually used prophylactically.
        2) Sequential compression devices may also be used.
    h. Urinary tract infection, urosepsis
    i. Pressure ulcers

Brain Tumor

Etiology: Multifactorial or Unknown

1. Congenital
2. Hereditary factors

Pathophysiology (Figure 6-36)

1. Primary brain tumors are categorized by their cell type; metastatic brain tumors are of the cell type of the primary tumor (Table 6-19).

Clinical Presentation

1. Subjective
    a. Headache
        1) Occurs at night after retiring
        2) Present and worse on awakening
        3) May be relieved by midmorning
    b. Visual changes
2. Objective
    a. Seizures: new onset
    b. Personality changes
    c. Vomiting without preceding nausea
        1) More common in morning
    d. Papilledema
    e. Change in LOC
    f. Hormonal changes if pituitary involved
    g. Specific to affected area of brain (Table 6-20)
3. Diagnostic
    a. Hormone levels: may be abnormal if pituitary tumor
    b. Chest x-ray: may show primary tumor of lung
    c. Skull x-ray: may show shift of pineal gland
    d. EEG: aids in identification of seizure activity

Table 6-19 Types of Brain Tumors

Type	Comments
Gliomas • Astrocytomas (initially benign but prone to become malignant) • Oligodendrogliomas (usually benign but may become malignant) • Ependymomas (usually benign but may become malignant) • Medulloblastomas (highly malignant) • Glioblastoma multiforme (highly malignant)	• Most in cerebrum, but medulloblastoma in cerebellum and ependymomas in ventricular system • Most grow rapidly, but medulloblastoma is rapidly invasive • Most nonencapsulated; cannot be incised completely
Meningioma	• Benign, slow growing • Usually encapsulated; surgical cure possible • Recurrence possible
Pituitary adenoma	• Usually benign • Surgical approach usually successful
Acoustic neuroma	• Benign or low-grade malignancy • Arise from sheath of Schwann cells found on eighth cranial nerve • Will regrow if not completely excised • Surgical resection often difficult due to location
Metastatic tumor	• Malignant • Cancer cells spread to the brain via the circulatory system, usually from lung, breast, or prostate cancer • Surgical resection difficult and prognosis poor

e. Brain scan: identifies the tumor
f. Bone scan: may show bone cancer
g. CT: identifies the tumor
h. MRI: identifies the tumor and effect on surrounding tissue
i. Angiography: may show vascular shifts due to tumor or may show vascularity of tumor
j. Biopsy: classifies tumor cell type

Collaborative Management

1. Prevent/monitor for clinical indications/treat intracranial hypertension (see Intracranial Hypertension section); glucocorticoids are frequently used to reduce brain edema
2. Maintain airway, oxygenation, and ventilation.
   a. Maintain airway.
      1) Oropharyngeal or nasopharyngeal airway may be needed to hold tongue away from hypopharynx in obtunded patient.

Table 6-20 Clinical Manifestations of Tumors Specific to Affected Area of Brain

Area	Clinical Manifestations
Frontal lobe	• Personality changes • Inappropriate behavior: loss of social behavior • Inappropriate affect: quiet, flat • Inattentiveness, inability to concentrate • Emotional lability • Recent memory loss • Decreased intellectual ability • Motor changes: hemiparesis, hemiplegia • Seizure activity possible • If dominant hemisphere: expressive aphasia
Parietal	• Sensory changes: hyperesthesia, paresthesia, loss of two-point discrimination • Constructional apraxia • Loss of right-left discrimination • Homonymous hemianopsia • Seizure activity possible
Temporal	• Poor judgment • Irritability • Regressive behavior • Auditory disturbances • Olfactory, visual, and gustatory hallucinations • Psychomotor seizures • If dominant hemisphere: receptive aphasia
Occipital lobe	• Visual disturbances: visual field defects • Visual hallucinations • Seizure activity possible: visual aura
Pituitary or hypothalamus	• Visual disturbances • Hormone imbalance: hypopituitarism or hyperpituitarism • Temperature regulation problems • Changes in sleep patterns
Brainstem	• Dysphagia • Vomiting • Ataxia • Nystagmus • Vomiting: with or without nausea • Decreased corneal reflex • Ventilatory pattern changes
Cerebellum	• Ataxia • Nystagmus • Unsteady gait • Decreased coordination • Vomiting: with or without nausea • Intentional tremors • Seizure activity possible

      2) Endotracheal intubation may be needed in patients without airway protective reflexes.
   b. Maintain oxygenation and ventilation.
      1) Administer oxygen as needed to maintain SpO_2 greater than or equal to 95% unless contraindicated.

2) Initiate mechanical ventilation as needed for hypoventilation.
c. Prevent aspiration.
1) Position patient on side.
2) Have suction equipment available.
3. Prepare patient for surgery, radiation, and/or chemotherapy.
a. Surgery
1) Purposes of craniotomy for brain tumor
a) Debulk tumor to relieve pressure.
b) Resect and remove tumor (usually followed by radiation).
c) Insert shunt for hydrocephalus.
2) Postcraniotomy care (see Craniotomy section)
b. Radiation: after surgery for incompletely excised tumor or for nonsurgically accessible tumor
1) Whole-brain radiation therapy in high doses or superfractionated therapy
2) Brachytherapy or interstitial irradiation: placement of a radioactive source in contact with or implanted into the brain tumor
c. Radiosurgery: closed-skull destruction of an intracranial target with ionizing beams of radiation; an intracranial guiding device aids in focusing the beams of radiation
1) Bragg peak proton beam
2) Linear accelerator radiosurgery
3) Gamma knife therapy
d. Chemotherapy
1) Used after debulking in combination with radiotherapy, after irradiation, or for tumor recurrence
2) Antineoplastic agent determined by tumor type; more than one agent may be used
4. Monitor for complications
a. Fluid and electrolyte imbalance: DI, SIADH, CSW (see Craniotomy section)
b. Brain ischemia
c. Hydrocephalus
d. Brain edema
e. Seizures
f. Herniation

Status Epilepticus

Definitions

1. Seizure: sudden, paroxysmal episode of exaggerated activity or abnormal behavior caused by excessive discharge of cerebral neurons; Table 6-21 describes types of seizures.

Table 6-21 Types of Seizures

Type	Features	Duration
Generalized: Loss of Consciousness		
Absence (petit mal)	• Momentary loss of consciousness • Blank stare, cessation of activity • Eye blinking, lip smacking may occur • May lose muscle tone	Seconds
Tonic-clonic (grand mal)	• May be preceded by an aura and a cry from forced expiration • Loss of consciousness • Symmetrical tonic-clonic extremity movements • May experience apnea with cyanosis until tonic phase ends • May bite tongue, may be incontinent • Postictal fatigue, muscle soreness, confusion, lethargy, and/or headache	3-5 minutes
Myoclonic	• Short, abrupt muscle contractions of arms, legs, and torso • Contractions may be symmetrical or asymmetrical	Seconds
Clonic	• Muscle contraction and relaxation but slower than with myoclonic seizure	Several minutes
Tonic	• Abrupt increase in muscle tone of torso and face • Flexion of arms; extension of legs	Seconds
Atonic	• Abrupt loss of muscle tone • May cause falling and injuries related to fall	Seconds
Partial: Focal at Onset but May Evolve into a Generalized Seizure		
Simple partial	• Consciousness not impaired • Abnormal unilateral movement of arm, leg, or both • Patient may sense abnormal smell, sound, or sensation, such as numbness, tingling, or burning • Tachycardia or bradycardia, tachypnea, skin flushing, epigastric discomfort	Seconds to minutes
Complex partial	• Loss of consciousness but eyes may be open • Lip smacking, chewing, picking at clothing • Mumbling, speaking in repetitive phrases • Posturing or jerking movements • Postictal confusion, amnesia common	Minutes

2. Status epilepticus: seizure activity of 30 minutes or more duration caused by a single seizure or a series of seizures in which there is no return of consciousness between seizures
   a. Note that a more current definition is seizure activity lasting at least 10 minutes because treatment is generally initiated within 10 minutes preventing the continuation of seizure activity for 30 minutes.

Etiology

1. Preexisting history of seizure disorder
   a. Withdrawal from anticonvulsant medications
   b. Acute alcohol withdrawal
   c. Acute withdrawal from chronically used drugs that have sedative or depressant effects (e.g., barbiturates)
   d. Acute condition which lowers the seizure threshold
2. No preexisting history of seizure disorder
   a. Brain trauma
   b. Stroke: ischemic or hemorrhagic
   c. CNS infection: meningitis, encephalitis, abscess
   d. Brain tumors
   e. Encephalopathy: anoxic (e.g., post-cardiac arrest), hypertensive, or metabolic
      1) Hypoglycemia
      2) Hepatic failure
      3) Uremia
      4) Hyperosmolality
   f. Electrolyte imbalance
      1) Hyponatremia
      2) Hypocalcemia
      3) Hypomagnesemia
   g. Drug or alcohol withdrawal
   h. Drug toxicity: lidocaine, meperidine, theophylline, salicylates, cyclic antidepressants, cocaine
   i. Sepsis

Pathophysiology

See Figure 6-37.

Clinical Presentation

1. Subjective
   a. History may include precipitating event or condition
      1) History of epilepsy
      2) History of noncompliance in taking anticonvulsant drugs
      3) History of chronic drug or alcohol use
2. Objective
   a. Alteration in LOC
   b. Tonic and/or clonic body movements
   c. Incontinence of urine or stool
   d. Involuntary motor activities: lip smacking, swallowing, chewing
3. Diagnostic
   a. Evaluation of cause
      1) Blood urea nitrogen (BUN): increased in uremia, hyperosmolality
      2) Liver function studies: increased in hepatic failure
      3) Drug and alcohol levels

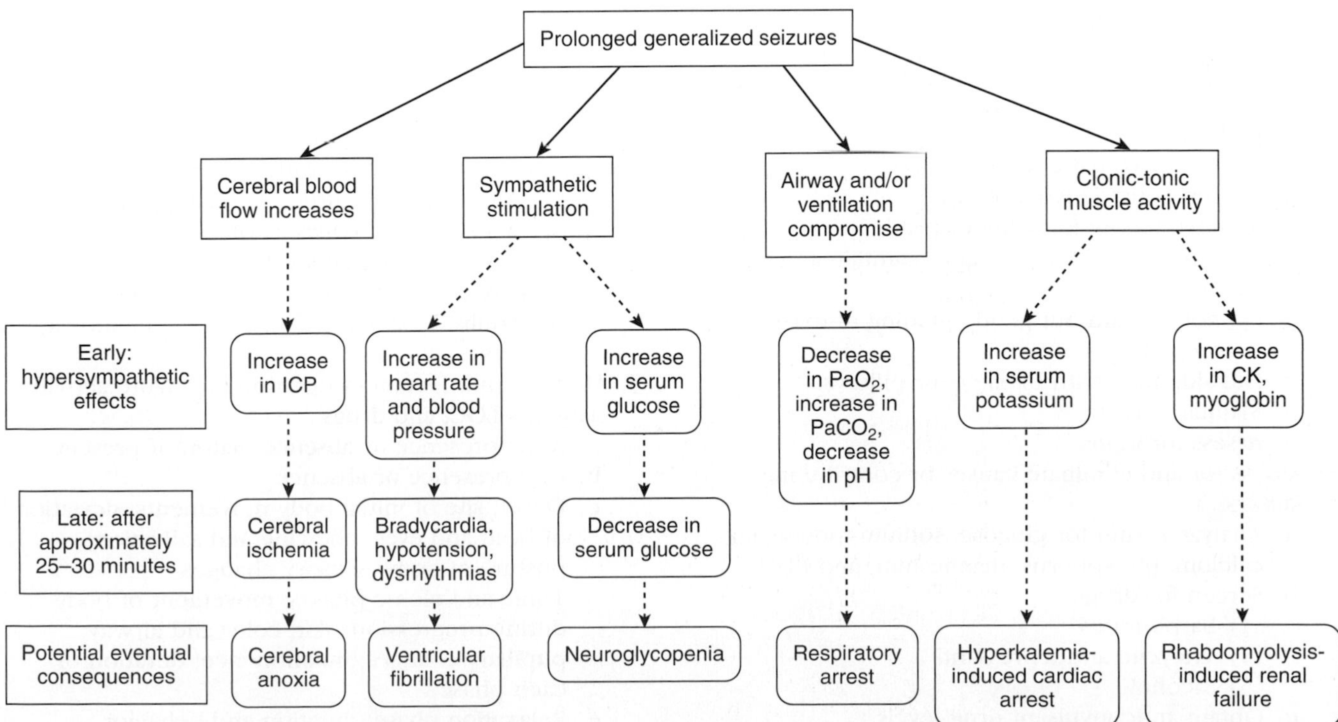

Figure 6-37 Pathophysiology of status epilepticus. Dotted lines connect pathology to clinical presentation. *CK,* Creatine kinase; *ICP,* intracranial pressure; *$PaCO_2$,* partial pressure of carbon dioxide in arterial blood; *PaO_2,* partial pressure of oxygen in arterial blood.

4) Anticonvulsant drug levels: subtherapeutic in noncompliance
b. Serum
1) Electrolytes: hyperkalemia
2) Glucose: increased early; decreased late
3) CK: increased
4) Lactic acid: increased
5) Arterial blood gases: may show hypercapnia, hypoxemia
c. Urine: may show myoglobinuria
d. Skull x-rays: may show cause
e. EEG: will show seizure activity
f. CT, MRI, MRA: may indicate pathologic conditions (e.g., mass lesions)
g. LP: may show meningitis as cause

Collaborative Management

1. Establish and maintain airway and adequate ventilation.
   a. Insert artificial airway if ventilation and oxygenation are inadequate.
      1) Utilize nasopharyngeal airway or nasotracheal intubation if mouth cannot be opened; do not try to force mouth open.
      2) Monitor ABGs and pulse oximetry.
   b. Maintain oxygenation and ventilation.
      1) Administer oxygen as needed to maintain SpO_2 greater than or equal to 95% unless contraindicated.
      2) Initiate mechanical ventilation as needed for hypoventilation.
   c. Prevent aspiration.
      1) Position on side: Do not just turn head to side; turn body on side.
      2) Have suction equipment available; suction as indicated.
2. Protect patient from injury and prevent complications during seizure.
   a. Call for help.
   b. Do not leave patient.
   c. Loosen constrictive clothing.
   d. Remove pillow from under head.
   e. Turn patient to the side and maintain an open airway.
   f. Do not restrain but gentle guiding of extremities is acceptable.
   g. Pad side rails with blankets or pillows.
   h. Maintain privacy.
   i. Assess for injury.
3. Assess for and eliminate causes or contributing factors.
   a. Analyze serum for glucose, sodium, potassium, calcium, phosphorus, magnesium, and BUN.
   b. Screen for drugs.
      1) Barbiturates
      2) Tricyclic antidepressants
      3) Alcohol
   c. Obtain anticonvulsant drug levels.
   d. Obtain blood cultures if patient is hyperthermic.
   e. Correct contributing factors that lower seizure threshold (e.g., hypoxemia, acid-base imbalance, electrolyte imbalance, hyperthermia, hypermetabolism).
4. Stop seizure activity.
   a. Initiate IV.
   b. Administer 100 mg thiamine and 50 mL of $D_{50}W$ if alcohol ingestion or hypoglycemia is suspected (thiamine is given with the dextrose to prevent Wernicke's encephalopathy especially if patient has chronic malnutrition).
   c. Administer benzodiazepine or other drugs if seizures persist after dextrose and thiamine (Table 6-22).
      1) Benzodiazepine to stop the seizure
         a) First choice: lorazepam (Ativan)
         b) Second choice: diazepam (Valium)
      2) Agents to prevent recurrence to be given after benzodiazepine
         a) Phenytoin (Dilantin)
         b) Fosphenytoin (Cerebyx)
         c) Phenobarbital
      3) Other agents for refractory status epilepticus
         a) Pentobarbital (Nembutal)
         b) Midazolam (Versed)
         c) Propofol (Diprivan)
         d) Levetiracetam (Keppra)
         e) Lacosamide (Vimpat)
         f) Rarely used intravenous agents: thiopental, valproic acid, etomidate, paraldehyde, lidocaine
         g) Rarely used inhalation anesthetics: halothane, isoflurane, nitrous oxide
      4) Monitor closely for hypotension; administer fluids as prescribed.
      5) Monitor for respiratory depression; ventilation with manual resuscitation bag and mask may be required; endotracheal intubation may be required
      6) Reduce the infusion rate as prescribed after at least 12 hours without seizures.
      7) Monitor serum drug concentrations and adjust drug dosages as prescribed to maintain optimal levels.
   d. Prepare patient for surgical procedures that may be required for removal of tumor, hematoma, or abscess.
5. Monitor and document duration of seizure activity, patient's LOC, and drugs.
   a. Aura: presence or absence; nature if present
   b. Cry: presence or absence
   c. Onset: site of initial body movements; deviation of head and eyes; chewing and salivation; posture of body; sensory changes
   d. Tonic and clonic phases: movement of body during progression; skin color and airway; pupillary changes; incontinence; duration of each phase
   e. Relaxation phase: duration and behavior
   f. Postictal phase: duration; ability to remember anything about the seizure; orientation; pupillary changes; headache; injuries

Table 6-22 Anticonvulsant Drugs

Drug	IV Dosage	Time to Stop Seizure/Duration of Anticonvulsant Effect	Adverse Effects
Lorazepam (Ativan)	0.1 mg/kg (not to exceed 8 mg/kg) at a rate no faster than 2 mg/min	6-10 minutes/12-24 hours	• Respiratory depression • Tachycardia • Hypotension • Dysrhythmias
Diazepam (Valium)	0.15-0.25 mg/kg at a rate of no faster than 5 mg/min	1-3 minutes/30 minutes	• Respiratory depression • Tachycardia • Hypotension • Dysrhythmias
Phenytoin sodium (Dilantin)	10-20 mg/kg at a rate no faster than 50 mg/min; must be mixed in saline	30 minutes/24 hours	• Hypotension • Dysrhythmias; blocks • Hepatitis • Nephritis • Blood dyscrasias
Fosphenytoin (Cerebyx)	15-20 mg/kg phenytoin equivalent (PE) at a rate no faster than 150 mg/min; may be administered intramuscularly	15 minutes/24 hours	• Hypotension (less risk than phenytoin) • Dysrhythmias (less risk than phenytoin) • Nephritis • Blood dyscrasias
Phenobarbital (Phenobarbital sodium, Luminal)	20 mg/kg at a rate no faster than 50 mg/min (not actively seizing) or 100 mg/min (actively seizing)	20-30 minutes/48 hours	• Respiratory depression • Hypotension • Angioedema • Thrombophlebitis
Levetiracetam (Keppra)	500-1500 mg over 15 minutes; must be diluted	15-30 minutes/6-30 hours	• Somnolence • Dizziness, vertigo • Vomiting, diarrhea • Irritability
Lacosamide (Vimpat)	200-400 mg over 30-60 minutes	1-4 hours/13 hours	• Dizziness • Ataxia • Diplopia • Cardiac rhythm and conduction abnormalities

   g. Duration: from aura to relaxation
   h. Drugs administered
6. Monitor and assess condition closely to prevent complications.
   a. Insert nasogastric tube to prevent vomiting and aspiration.
   b. Monitor cardiac rate and rhythm and BP.
   c. Have cardiovascular drugs available.
   d. Assess neurologic status frequently.
7. Provide reassurance and comfort during postictal period.
   a. Elevate HOB 30 degrees.
   b. Reassure and reorient patient as he or she awakens.
   c. Provide privacy and calm environment.
   d. Discretely clean patient if he or she was incontinent.
   e. Allow the patient to sleep.
8. Maintain fluid and electrolyte balance.
   a. Assess electrolytes, calcium, magnesium, and renal and hepatic function.
   b. Monitor for indications of myoglobinuria (e.g., cola-colored urine); administer treatment for myoglobinuria as prescribed (fluids and osmotic diuretics [e.g., mannitol]).
9. Monitor for complications.
   a. Injury during seizure
   b. Acute respiratory failure
   c. Aspiration
   d. Acid-base imbalance, electrolyte imbalance
      1) Respiratory or metabolic acidosis
      2) Hyperkalemia
   e. Hypoglycemia: Monitor serum glucose and administer parenteral dextrose as required.
   f. Hyperthermia: Treat body temperature greater than 40° C with antipyretics and/or hypothermia blanket.
   g. Renal failure related to myoglobinuria
      1) Monitor serum CK to detect rhabdomyolysis and note change in urine color (i.e., cola-colored) to detect myoglobinuria.
      2) Treat myoglobinuria with fluids, mannitol, and sodium bicarbonate as prescribed.
   h. Residual neurologic deficits

CNS Infections

Definitions

1. Meningitis: acute inflammation of the brain and spinal cord that may involve all meningeal membranes; may be bacterial, fungal, or viral

2. Encephalitis: acute inflammation of the parenchyma of the brain and meninges
3. Brain abscess: accumulation of pus within the brain tissue; surrounded by inflamed tissue

Etiology

1. Meningitis
   a. Bacterial
      1) Associated factors
         a) Otitis media
         b) Sinusitis, upper respiratory infection, or pneumonia
         c) Penetrating head injury
         d) Basal skull fracture
         e) Intracranial surgery
         f) ICP monitoring
         g) Septicemia, septic embolus
      2) Organisms
         a) *Haemophilus influenzae*
         b) *Neisseria meningitidis (meningococcal)*
         c) *Diplococcus pneumoniae (pneumococcal)*
         d) *Streptococcus pneumoniae*
         e) *Escherichia coli*
         f) *Enterobacter*
         g) *Klebsiella*
         h) *Pseudomonas*
         i) *Serratia*
         j) *Salmonella*
         k) Gonococcus
   b. Fungal
      1) Associated factors
         a) Immunosuppression
            i) AIDS
            ii) Histoplasmosis
            iii) After organ transplantation
            iv) Steroid therapy
            v) Cancer
         b) Contaminated needles or syringes from drug abuse
      2) Organisms
         a) Cryptococcosis
         b) Coccidioidomycosis
         c) Mucormycosis
         d) Candidiasis
         e) Aspergillosis
   c. Viral
      1) Associated factors
         a) Immunosuppression
      2) Organisms
         a) Coxsackievirus
         b) Echovirus
         c) Adenovirus
         d) Arbovirus
         e) Poliovirus
         f) Herpes simplex virus
         g) Myxovirus (e.g., influenza, mumps, measles)
         h) Western equine
   d. Parasitic
      1) *Plasmodium* (malaria)
      2) *Toxoplasma gondii*
2. Encephalitis (almost always viral)
   a. Associated factors
      1) Mosquito or tick bite (arbovirus)
      2) Recent viral infection
      3) Recent vaccination: measles, mumps, rubella
      4) Immunocompromise
   b. Organisms
      1) Arbovirus (e.g., West Nile virus, eastern equine encephalitis)
      2) Herpes simplex
      3) Rubella
      4) Rubeola
      5) Mumps
      6) Mononucleosis
3. Brain abscess
   a. Associated factors
      1) Middle-ear and mastoid infection
      2) Sinus infection
      3) Penetrating head injuries, skull fractures
      4) Compound fractures
      5) Osteomyelitis of the skull
      6) Neurosurgical or oral surgical procedures
      7) Metastatic abscess
   b. Organisms
      1) *Streptococci*
      2) *Staphylococci*
      3) *Pneumococci*

Pathophysiology

See Figure 6-38.

Clinical Presentation

1. Meningitis
   a. Subjective
      1) History of precipitating event or condition
      2) Headache that gets progressively worse
      3) Chills
      4) Nausea, vomiting
      5) Photophobia, pain when moving eyes
   b. Objective
      1) Infectious signs
         a) Fever
         b) Tachycardia
         c) Chills
         d) Skin rash: most likely with meningococcal meningitis
      2) Meningeal irritation
         a) Headache
         b) Nuchal rigidity
         c) Brudzinski's sign
         d) Kernig's sign
      3) Neurologic abnormalities
         a) Change in LOC
         b) Confusion, delirium
         c) Cranial nerve involvement (e.g., pupil changes)
         d) Focal neurologic signs
         e) Seizures
   c. Diagnostic
      1) Serum

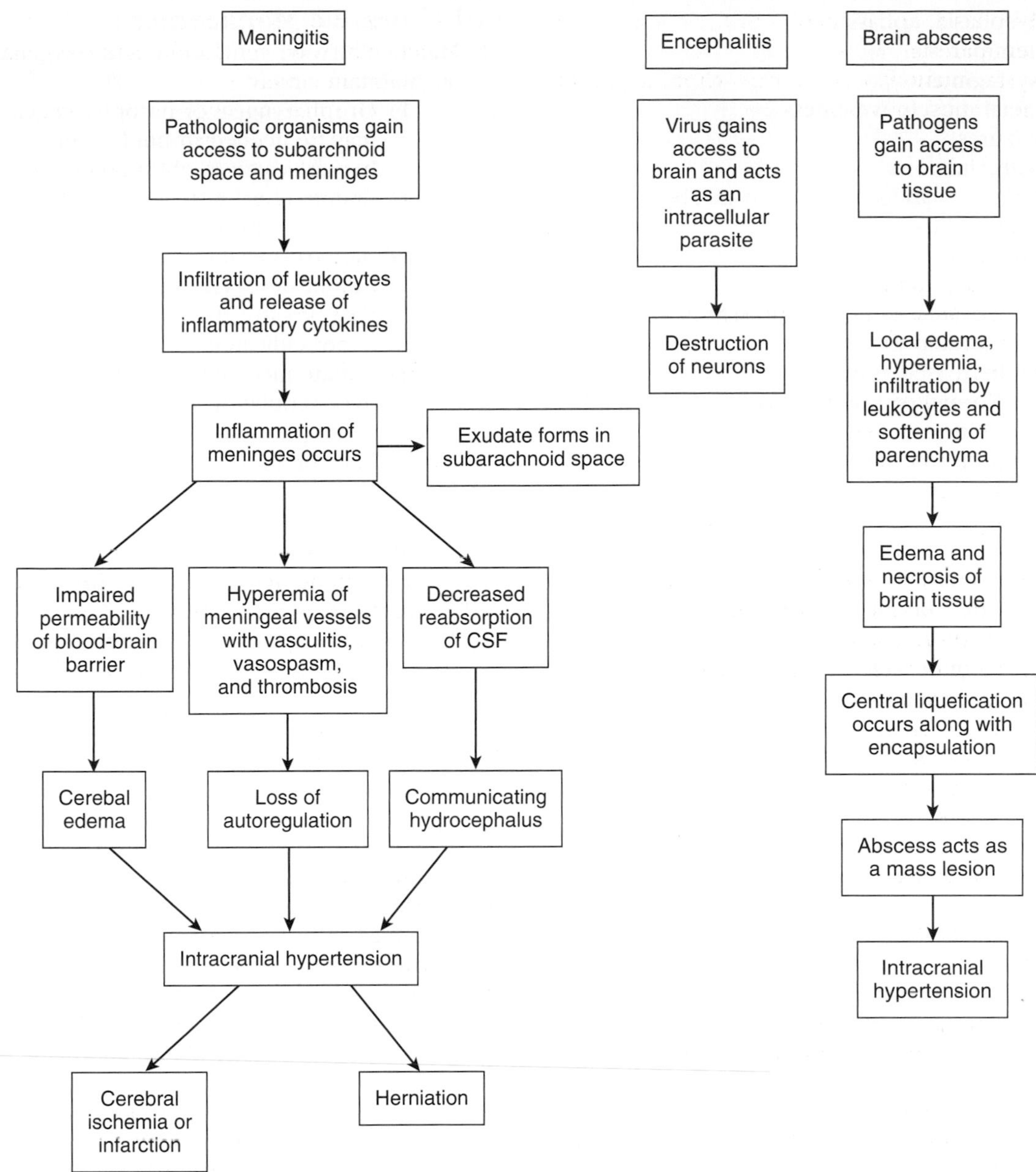

Figure 6-38 Pathophysiology of brain CNS infections. *CSF,* Cerebrospinal fluid.

a) Blood cultures: may be positive for causative organism
b) WBC: elevated

2) LP
a) Elevated CSF pressure (normal LP 80-180 mm/H_2O, measured at lumbar level, with patient in side-lying position)
b) Increased WBCs in CSF
c) Elevated protein in CSF in most cases
d) Decreased glucose content in CSF in bacterial meningitis (glucose in CSF is normally 60% of serum glucose)
e) CSF is cloudy in bacterial meningitis
f) Glucose content in CSF is normal and CSF is clear in viral meningitis.
g) Culture: may identify organism

3) CT: normal but CT scan of the head is frequently routinely obtained prior to the performance of an LP to identify occult intracranial abnormalities and avoid the risk of brainstem herniation secondary to the LP

2. Encephalitis
a. Subjective
1) History may include precipitating event or condition (e.g., mosquito or tick bite, contact with dead or sick bird).
2) Headache
3) Blurred vision, diplopia, photophobia
4) Weakness
5) Dysphagia
6) Gastrointestinal symptoms may occur.

b. Objective
1) Change in level of consciousness: lethargy, coma
2) Fever
3) Nuchal rigidity

4) Dysphasia, aphasia
5) Hemiparesis
6) Nystagmus
7) Facial muscle weakness
8) Seizures
9) Hallucinations
10) Parkinsonian-like rigidity in tick-borne viral encephalitis

c. Diagnostic
1) Lumbar puncture
a) Elevated or normal pressure
b) Elevated protein
c) Increased WBC
d) Normal or low glucose
e) Culture: may identify organism
2) Brain biopsy: required for diagnosis of herpes simplex encephalitis
3) EEG: may show seizure activity
4) CT: normal early in course; later low-density lesions may be seen
5) MRI: may be more definitive than CT scan
6) IgM antibody to West Nile virus for West Nile encephalitis in serum or CSF

3. Brain abscess
a. Subjective
1) History may include precipitating event or condition.
2) Headache: constant and severe; increased with straining
3) Malaise
4) Irritability
5) Chills
6) Nausea, vomiting
7) Muscle weakness
8) Symptoms vary according to location in the brain

b. Objective
1) Change in LOC
2) Confusion
3) Hemiplegia
4) Fever
5) Nuchal rigidity may be present
6) Dysphasia/aphasia
7) Seizures
8) Signs vary according to location of brain

c. Diagnostic
1) CT scan: may show localized changes in brain density
2) EEG: may show electrical silence at abscess location
3) Lumbar puncture
a) Increased pressure
b) Increased WBC
c) Elevated protein
d) Normal glucose
4) Brain biopsy: may identify organism
5) Brain scan: locates abscess greater than 1 cm in size
6) Angiogram: locate temporal lobe and cerebellar abscesses

Collaborative Management

1. Maintain airway, ventilation, and oxygenation.
a. Maintain airway.
1) Oropharyngeal or nasopharyngeal airway may be needed to hold tongue away from hypopharynx in obtunded patient.
2) Endotracheal intubation may be needed in patients without airway protective reflexes.
b. Maintain oxygenation and ventilation.
1) Administer oxygen as needed to maintain SpO_2 greater than or equal to 95% unless contraindicated.
2) Initiate mechanical ventilation as needed for hypoventilation.
c. Prevent aspiration.
1) Position patient on side.
2) Have suction equipment available.

2. Treat infection.
a. Administer antibiotics (need to be fat-soluble to cross blood-brain barrier) to treat bacterial infection as prescribed.
b. Administer antivirals to treat herpes simplex encephalitis as prescribed.
c. Prepare patient for surgical excision and drainage of brain abscess.

3. Prevent/monitor for clinical indications/treat intracranial hypertension (see Intracranial Hypertension section)
a. Steroids may be prescribed to decrease inflammation in bacterial meningitis: Dexamethasone (Decadron) is usually prescribed either before or with the first dose of antibiotics.

4. Maintain fluid and electrolyte balance.
a. Administer intravenous fluids as prescribed.
b. Monitor for overhydration and diabetes insipidus.

5. Control body temperature to less than 38° C.
a. Administer antipyretics.
b. Utilize hypothermia blanket.
c. Utilize meperidine (Demerol) as prescribed to control shivering (NOTE: though chlorpromazine (Thorazine) is sometimes used to prevent shivering, it lowers seizure threshold and should be avoided).

6. Prevent/monitor for/control seizures
a. Institute seizure precautions.
b. Administer anticonvulsant therapy as prescribed.

7. Treat headache with nonsedating analgesics (e.g., codeine).

8. Prevent transmission of disease.
a. Universal precautions are adequate for most patients with CNS infections.
b. Droplet precautions
1) *Haemophilus influenzae* and *Neisseria meningitidis* (meningococcal) may be transmitted by droplets generated during coughing, sneezing, talking, intubation, and bronchoscopy so droplet precautions should be initiated if there is a clinical suspicion of one of these pathogens.

2) These precautions should be continued for 24 hours after the start of effective antibiotic therapy until another organism is confirmed.

c. Antibiotic prophylaxis for close contacts is indicated for *Haemophilus influenzae* and *Neisseria meningitidis* (meningococcal).

d. Vaccination
   1) Vaccination for *Haemophilus influenzae* is now incorporated into the routine immunization schedule for children.
   2) Vaccination for 4 serogroups of meningococcus (i.e., quadrivalent meningococcal vaccine) is recommended for high-risk populations, including military recruits, persons traveling to an area with high risk of meningococcal disease, college students living in dormitories, and patients postsplenectomy
   3) Pneumococcal vaccine is thought to be about 50% effective in preventing pneumococcal meningitis.

9. Monitor for complications.
   a. Seizures: Prophylactic anticonvulsant may be prescribed.
   b. Disseminated intravascular coagulation (DIC)
   c. Fluid and electrolyte imbalance: DI, SIADH, CSW (see Craniotomy section)
   d. Brain edema and intracranial hypertension
   e. Subdural effusions
   f. Hydrocephalus
   g. Cranial nerve deficits
   h. Waterhouse-Friderichsen syndrome
      1) A major complication of meningococcal meningitis
      2) Overwhelming bacteremia with massive bilateral adrenal hemorrhage
      3) Causes acute adrenal crisis and potentially death
   i. Residual neurologic deficits (e.g., motor or cognitive deficits, memory loss, hearing or vision loss, seizure disorder)

Neuromuscular Disorders

Muscular Dystrophy

1. Definition: group of familial disorders that cause degeneration of skeletal muscle fibers; associated with progressive, symmetrical weakness and wasting of skeletal muscle groups
2. Etiology: genetic
3. Pathophysiology
   a. Degeneration of skeletal muscle fibers
   b. Replacement of muscle tissue with connective tissue and fat
   c. Number of muscle fibers is decreased and the remaining fibers are inflamed and may exhibit necrosis.
   d. Progressive weakness and muscle atrophy
4. Clinical presentation
   a. Subjective
      1) History of frequent falls
      2) Weakness
   b. Objective
      1) Muscle weakness and atrophy
      2) Lack of gross motor control
      3) Kyphoscoliosis is common
      4) Respiratory muscle weakness with tachypnea and decreased tidal volume
      5) Cardiac anomalies are common.
      6) Moderate developmental disability
      7) Smooth muscle dysfunction with megacolon, volvulus, and malabsorption syndromes
   c. Diagnostic: CK increased to approximately 10 × normal

Multiple Sclerosis

1. Definition: a progressive demyelinating disorder of the white matter of the brain and spinal cord; the optic and oculomotor cranial nerves and the spinal nerve tracts are most often affected while the peripheral nervous system is not affected
2. Etiology: genetic predisposition with environmental (e.g., viral) insult
3. Pathophysiology
   a. Possible precipitators include stress, fatigue, pregnancy, or respiratory tract infection
   b. Immune response results in recurrent inflammatory reaction leading to peripheral vasculitis
   c. Breakdown of blood-brain barrier with migration of B lymphocytes into the CNS
   d. B lymphocytes secrete immunoglobulin G antibodies
   e. Macrophages remove degenerating myelin causing scattered demyelination of the white matter of the brain and spinal cord
   f. Proliferation of neuroglial tissue (i.e., gliosis) in the white matter of the CNS
   g. This proliferation causes hard yellow plaques of scar tissue, which damages the axon fiber.
   h. Nerve transmission is disrupted.
   i. Remission results from health of demyelinated areas but symptoms become irreversible as the disease progresses.
4. Clinical presentation
   a. Clinical course
      1) Exacerbations and remissions
      2) May progress rapidly causing death or disability but most patients live productive lives with prolonged remissions
   b. Subjective
      1) Fatigue
      2) Sensory impairment (e.g., burning, pins and needles)
      3) Blurred vision, diplopia
      4) Urinary urgency
      5) Dysphagia
   c. Objectives
      1) Nystagmus
      2) Poor articulation

3) Weakness
4) Paralysis ranging from monoplegia to quadriplegia
5) Spasticity and hyperreflexia
6) Intentional tremor
7) Ataxia
8) Incontinence

d. Diagnostic
1) MRI: detects lesions and used to evaluate progression; most sensitive diagnostic test for multiple sclerosis
2) CT: lesions within the brain's white matter
3) CSF: elevated immunoglobulin G levels, normal WBC, and normal protein levels
4) EEG: frequently abnormal
5) Evoked potential studies and somatosensory evoked potentials (SSEP): slowed conduction

e. Specific syndromes
1) Corticospinal syndrome: symmetrical muscle weakness, spastic paralysis, and bowel and bladder incontinence
2) Brainstem syndrome: dysfunction of cranial nerves III through XII with nystagmus, dysarthria, facial nerve weakness, and paresthesia
3) Cerebellar syndrome: spastic gait, ataxia, intentional tremor, hypotonia
4) Cerebral syndrome: optic neuritis, impaired vision, intellectual deterioration

Amyotrophic Lateral Sclerosis (ALS)

1. Definition: chronic progressively debilitating disease that causes degeneration of the upper and lower motor neurons and muscular atrophy
2. Etiology: unknown but the following may be factors:
   a. Genetic
   b. Virus
   c. Nutritional deficiency
   d. Metabolic interference
   e. Autoimmune process
3. Pathophysiology
   a. Glutamine may be a factor; accumulates to toxic levels at the synapses
   b. Reduction of the number of motor neurons in cortex, brainstem, and spinal cord and degeneration of remaining motor neurons
   c. Progressive degeneration of axons with loss of myelin
   d. Nonfunctional scar tissue replaces normal neuronal tissue in the corticospinal tract in lateral column of spinal cord.
4. Clinical presentation
   a. Subjective
      1) Generalized muscle weakness
      2) Dyspnea if brainstem involved
   b. Objectives
      1) Muscle atrophy, fasciculations, weakness
      2) Paralysis especially forearms and hands
      3) Impaired speech, chewing, and swallowing with drooling and choking
   c. Diagnostic: primarily history and physical examination
      1) EMG: lower motor neuron denervation
      2) Muscle biopsy: lower motor degeneration

Guillain-Barré Syndrome

1. Definition: acquired acute inflammatory demyelinating axonal polyneuropathy affecting motor more than sensory nerves; also referred to as acute inflammatory demyelinating polyradiculopathy or acute demyelinating polyneuropathy
2. Etiology: autoimmune disease triggered by a preceding bacterial or viral illness; associated infection usually *Campylobacter jejuni*
   a. Predisposing factors include the following:
      1) Surgery
      2) Vaccination
      3) Viral illness
      4) Rabies
      5) Hodgkin's disease or other malignancy
      6) Lupus erythematosus
3. Pathophysiology
   a. Macrophages and lymphocytes destroy the myelin sheath of peripheral nerves
   b. Inflammation and swelling of axons
   c. Segmental demyelination of the peripheral nerves, both posterior (sensory) and anterior (motor) nerve roots
   d. Distance between nodes of Ranvier lengthens which impairs saltatory conduction along nerve roots
   e. Remyelination gradually transpires
   f. Autonomic nerve transmission may also be impaired
   g. Clinical course usually three phases
      1) Acute phase: from onset of symptoms to when no further deterioration develops; usually from 1 to 3 weeks
      2) Plateau phase: no change in symptoms; usually lasts up to 2 weeks
      3) Recovery phase: symptoms improve as remyelination occurs; usually lasts from months to years
4. Clinical presentation
   a. Subjective
      1) History of diarrhea or upper respiratory infection a few days or weeks before development of neurologic symptoms
      2) Numbness, pain, paresthesia, or paresis of the limbs
         a) Position and vibratory sensations are more affected than superficial sensation
         b) Paresthesias usually involving hands and feet
      3) Weakness and fatigue
   b. Objective
      1) Bilateral progressive paralysis beginning in legs and then progressing to arms, trunk, and face

a) Loss of deep tendon reflexes
b) Facial weakness due to involvement of CNVII
c) Bulbar (i.e., speech and swallowing) muscles may be involved resulting in difficulty chewing, swallowing, dysarthria, and cough if bulbar weakness
d) Usually plateaus or improves by fourth week
2) Respiratory muscle weakness may cause tachypnea, decreased tidal volume, impaired cough, and acute respiratory failure
3) Autonomic dysfunction may occur, manifested by tachycardia or bradycardia, hypotension or hypertension, ileus, urinary retention, and loss of or significant increase in perspiration

c. Diagnostic
1) CSF: high protein without cellular abnormality
2) EMG and nerve conduction velocity studies show impairment of nerve transmission
3) If acute respiratory failure: ABGs show decreased PaO_2, increased $PaCO_2$, decreased pH

Myasthenia Gravis

1. Definition: disorder of voluntary muscles caused by a defect in nerve impulse transmission at the neuromuscular junction
2. Etiology: acetylcholine receptor antibodies at the neuromuscular junction
   a. Genetic susceptibility
   b. Immunologic
   c. Lymphoid hyperplasia or tumor of thymus
3. Pathophysiology
4. Clinical presentation
   a. Clinical course: exacerbations and remissions
      1) Symptoms are milder on awakening and worsen as the day progresses.
      2) Short rest periods temporarily restore muscle function.
      3) Symptoms may be more severe during menses, emotional stress, infection, and exposure to sunlight or cold.
   b. Subjective
      1) May have history of other autoimmune diseases such as systemic lupus erythematosus, rheumatoid arthritis, polymyositis, or Graves' disease
      2) May have history of recurrent respiratory infection
      3) Exertional fatigue and weakness: worsens with activity and improves with rest
         a) Muscles of eyes, face, mouth, throat, and neck usually affected first: may complain of diplopia, choking, aspiration
   c. Objective
      1) Ptosis
      2) Impaired extraocular movement
      3) Facial droop, expressionless face
      4) Extreme muscle weakness
      5) Difficulty chewing and swallowing
      6) Drooping jaw
      7) Bobbing head
      8) Weight loss related to nutritional impairment
      9) Nasal, low-volume but high-pitched monotonous speech pattern
      10) May have difficulty maintaining head in erect position
      11) If acute respiratory failure: ABGs show decreased PaO_2 and SaO_2, increased $PaCO_2$, decreased pH
   d. Diagnostic
      1) Edrophonium chloride (Tensilon) test: strength increases significantly with administration of drug
      2) Repetitive single-fiber EMG: rapid fatigue of muscle fibers
      3) Nerve conduction studies: show slowed conduction
      4) Antibodies for AChR and MuSK: positive
      5) CT and MRI of mediastinum to detect presence of thymoma

Collaborative Management of Neuromuscular Disorders

1. Maintain airway, ventilation, and oxygenation.
   a. Utilize oropharyngeal or nasopharyngeal airway as needed to hold tongue away from hypopharynx in obtunded patient.
   b. Assist with endotracheal intubation as needed in patients without airway protective reflexes; sedation is recommended prior to intubation.
   c. Encourage deep breathing.
   d. Administer oxygen as needed to maintain SpO_2 greater than or equal to 95% unless contraindicated.
   e. Initiate mechanical ventilation as needed for hypoventilation.
   f. Prevent aspiration.
      1) Position with head of bed elevated 30 degrees.
      2) Assess swallow competency; have suction equipment available.
2. Promote comfort and treat pain.
   a. Gabapentin (Neurontin) or amitriptyline (Elavil) are frequently used for neuropathic pain.
   b. Reposition frequently.
3. Maintain adequate hydration and electrolyte balance.
   a. Administer isotonic fluids as prescribed.
   b. Monitor closely for indications of overhydration or dehydration; evaluate urine output and urine specific gravity hourly.
4. Maintain nutritional status.
   a. Enteral nutritional support may be required if dysphagia precludes oral feeding.
5. Prevent injury.
   a. Perform passive ROM and reposition the patient every 2 hours.

b. Obtain physical therapy consult.
c. Perform frequent skin assessment.
d. Instill artificial tears every 2 hours to prevent corneal abrasions in patients who do not blink; a moisture chamber may be created using plastic wrap.
e. Orient to time and place often; encourage family participation in reality orientation.

6. Administer pharmacologic agents and therapies specific to diagnosis.
   a. Specific to muscular dystrophy: none
   b. Specific to multiple sclerosis
      1) Corticosteroids and adrenocorticotropin hormone (ACTH)
      2) Interferon and/or glatiramer (Copaxone), an immunomodulator
      3) Baclofen (Lioresal) and tizanidine (Zanaflex): muscle relaxants
      4) Monitor for the following complications
         a) Injuries from falls
         b) Constipation
         c) Urinary tract infection
         d) Pneumonia
   c. Specific to ALS
      1) Riluzole (Rilutek), an antiglutamate
      2) Dantrolene (Dantrium) and baclofen (Lioresal): muscle relaxants
      3) Thyrotropin-releasing hormone
   d. Specific to Guillain-Barré
      1) Atropine for bradycardia or beta-blocker for tachycardia
      2) IV immune globulin
      3) Corticosteroids
      4) Plasmapheresis early: usually 3-5 plasma exchanges
      5) Anticoagulant (e.g., subcutaneous low-molecular-weight heparin) for DVT prophylaxis
      6) Monitor for the following complications.
         a) Autonomic dysfunction
         b) SIADH
   e. Specific to myasthenic gravis
      1) Anticholinesterase drugs such as pyridostigmine (Mestinon)
      2) Corticosteroids
      3) Immunosuppressants
      4) Azathioprine
      5) Cyclosporine
      6) Plasmapheresis
      7) Thymectomy
      8) Monitor for the following complications; which may cause respiratory arrest:
         a) Myasthenic crisis: severe muscle weakness causes quadriparesis or quadriplegia, dyspnea, decreased tidal volume and vital capacity, pronounced dysphagia; occurs 3-4 hours after medication
         b) Cholinergic crisis: severe muscle weakness as in myasthenic crisis that occurs 30-60 minutes after anticholinesterase medication (especially if dose increase); other symptoms include diarrhea, cramping, fasciculation, bradycardia, pupillary constriction, increased salivation, increased perspiration

LEARNING ACTIVITIES

CHAPTER 6

1. Complete the following crossword puzzle related to neurologic anatomy, physiology, and assessment.

ACROSS

2. The opening at the base of the skull where the brain connects to the spinal cord (2 words)
4. Difficulty with swallowing
14. Cerebrospinal fluid is produced in capillary networks called ___ plexuses
15. This type of aphasia is also referred to as motor
17. The intrinsic ability of the cranium's contents to change to prevent an increase in intracranial pressure
21. The part of the brain that coordinates muscle movement with sensory input
22. This branch of the autonomic nervous system is frequently referred to as "fight or flight"
23. This type of cell forms the blood-brain barrier
24. The protective coverings of the brain and spinal cord
26. The middle layer of the meninges is the _____ mater; blood vessels and cerebrospinal fluid are located here
29. A diagnostic study to evaluate the brain's electrical activity (abbrev)
30. A primary neurotransmitter for the sympathetic nervous system
31. Unpleasant sensation
33. The vascular structure that is invaluable for collateral circulation (3 words)
35. An unsteady or staggering gait
36. Another term for sympathetic
40. Double vision
41. MAP - ICP; normally 60-100 mm Hg (abbrev)
48. During this refractory period the nerve cannot be stimulated again
50. A pathologic reflex of grasping whatever is placed in the hand with failure to release on command
51. An abnormal sensitivity to light
52. The enzyme that breaks down acetylcholine
53. This cranial nerve controls lateral eye movement
54. The brain's ability to tolerate increases in volume without a corresponding increase in pressure
56. The intrinsic ability of the cerebral blood vessels to dilate or constrict to stable cerebral blood flow
59. This lobe controls vision
60. The cranial nerve that controls visual acuity
61. The nodes of _____ allow rapid conduction of impulses by saltatory conduction
62. SBP + (2 × DBP)] divided by 3; normally 70-105 mm Hg (abbrev)
63. The type of paralysis seen with lower motor neuron lesion
64. The sympathetic and parasympathetic nervous systems constitute the _____ nervous system
66. This cranial nerve controls swallowing
67. A check for arm weakness is to ask the patient to hold the arms even and observe for _____
68. Difficulty with articulation
70. The outermost layer of the meninges is the _____ mater
72. A chemical that acts as a bridge for transmission of impulses
76. These neurons are responsible for myelin formation in the CNS
78. _____'s sign is pain in the neck when the leg is extended; indicates meningeal irritation
79. The inability to understand or express verbal communication
83. These lobes control sensory function
84. Loss of half of the visual field
87. These nerve cells provide support, nourishment, and protection of the neurons
88. The loss of motor function
89. The type of paralysis seen with upper motor neuron lesion
93. This area of the midbrain is responsible for wakefulness (3 words)
95. Unidirectional conduction of an impulse from one neuron to the next
97. These cells are responsible for the transmission of nerve impulses
99. The brain must have a continuous supply of oxygen and _____

DOWN

1. The cranial nerve that controls sensation on the face
3. This is the predominant neurotransmitter for the parasympathetic nervous system
5. The respiratory centers are located in the _____
6. A loss of sensation
7. This pressure is the pressure exerted from the intracranial contents (abbrev)
8. In chronic _____ state the patient is unaware of self and surroundings
9. This test should never be performed if the patient has clinical indications of intracranial hypertension (abbrev)
10. This acts as a cushion for the brain and the spinal cord (abbrev)
11. ____'s triad is a late indication of intracranial hypertension
12. The scoring system used to standardize observation of responsiveness in neurologic patients
13. The inability to recognize objects through the special senses
14. Another term for parasympathetic
16. These neurons transmit impulses away from the spinal cord or brain
18. The cranial nerves, spinal nerves, and peripheral nerves constitute the _____ nervous system
19. The spinal _____ extends from the brainstem to L2
20. The component of the neuron that conducts impulses toward the cell body
25. This posturing is also referred to as abnormal extension
27. Slow movement
28. This type of aphasia is also referred to as sensory
32. This type of nerve cell is part of the reticuloendothelial system and is responsible for phagocytosis
34. This band of brain tissue connects the left and right cerebral hemispheres (2 words)
35. The component of the neuron that conducts impulses away from the cell body to other neurons or to end-organs
37. Contraction of a muscle and a jerk of the affected limb which is tested by tapping the tendon with a hammer (abbrev)
38. The cranial nerve that controls pupillary constriction
39. A synapse between the axon of one neuron and the cell body of another neuron would be referred to as _____
42. The normal response to stroking the sole of the foot is the _____ reflex
43. The fold of the dura that separates the cerebral hemispheres from the cerebellum
44. This portion of the brainstem controls cardiac and respiratory centers
45. Another word for body
46. This branch of the autonomic nervous system may be described as "steady state"
47. CSF leak from the nose
49. This bone divides the interior of the skill into 3 fossae: anterior, middle, and posterior
50. Four paired masses of gray matter in the deeper layers of each hemisphere are called the basal _____
55. This portion of the skull has 8 bones
57. Peripheral pain may be tested with pressure to the _____ (2 words)
58. The posterior portion of these lobes controls voluntary motor function

61. This is a test of balance to check for cerebellar dysfunction
65. Arching associated with brainstem injury
69. This spinal tract carries pain, temperature, light touch, pressure, and pain
71. This posturing is also referred to as abnormal flexion
73. This type of hydrocephalus is most likely to occur from trauma, including surgical trauma
74. CSF leak from the ears
75. The cranial nerve that allows you to smile
77. This area of the diencephalon is responsible for temperature regulation
80. The skin covering the cranium
81. This type of neuron has one axon and more than one dendrite
82. These nerve cells line the ventricles of the brain and aid in secretion of CSF
85. Neurons that transmit impulses to the spinal cord or brain
86. A lack of inflection while talking
90. The innermost layer of the meninges is the _____ mater
91. May be partial or generalized
92. The coating or sheath that speeds transmission along the axon
94. This lobe controls long-term memory
96. This nerve originates at C3, C4, and C5 and innervates the diaphragm
98. The most important assessment parameter in a patient with a neurologic condition (abbrev)

2. Match the area of the brain to the associated function.

___ 1. Anterior frontal lobe
___ 2. Posterior frontal lobe
___ 3. Parietal lobe
___ 4. Occipital lobe
___ 5. Temporal lobe
___ 6. Cerebellum
___ 7. Medulla
___ 8. Hypothalamus
___ 9. Wernicke's area
___ 10. Thalamus
___ 11. Limbic system
___ 12. Broca's area

a. Responsible for verbal expression
b. Regulates cardiac, vasomotor, and respiratory functions
c. Receives visual stimuli
d. Maintains equilibrium
e. Regulates endocrine and autonomic functions
f. Receives auditory stimuli
g. Receives sensory stimuli
h. Involved in emotional and sexual response
i. Responsible for language interpretation
j. Contains the motor strip which controls voluntary motor functions
k. Controls judgment, insight, and reasoning
l. Relays sensory and motor input to the cerebrum

3. Your patient has had a traumatic brain injury. His blood pressure is 80/50 mm Hg and his ICP is 20 mm Hg. Calculate his cerebral perfusion pressure. Should you be concerned? Why? ____

____

4. Identify the following physiologic alterations as being associated with either sympathetic or parasympathetic.

	Sympathetic	Parasympathetic
Bronchodilation		
Coronary artery dilation		
Hypersalivation		
Increased blood glucose		
Increased perspiration		
Increased intestinal motility		
Pupil constriction		
Tachycardia		

5. Think about the following ventilatory patterns and identify the site of lesion which would cause them.

Pattern	Site of Lesion
CNS hyperventilation	
Cheyne-Stokes	
Cluster (or Biot's)	
Ataxic	
Apneustic	

6. Name and identify how to assess the cranial nerves.

Cranial Nerve	Name	Method of Assessment
I		
II		
III		
IV		
V		
VI		
VII		
VIII		
IX		
X		
XI		
XII		

7. List 10 factors that can increase intracranial pressure that can and should be eliminated.

1. ______
2. ______
3. ______
4. ______
5. ______
6. ______
7. ______
8. ______
9. ______
10. ______

8. Identify 6 interventions that can decrease intracranial pressure and identify if they decrease brain mass, CSF, or blood.

Intervention	What Is Decreased?
1.	
2.	
3.	
4.	
5.	
6.	

9. Match the following sign or symptom associated with the neurologic condition.

___ 1. Brainstem lesion	a. Kernig's sign
___ 2. Chronic subdural hematoma	b. Fatigue and muscle weakness
___ 3. Subarachnoid hemorrhage	c. Ascending paralysis
___ 4. Status epilepticus	d. Change in LOC, pupillary changes, respiratory pattern changes, Cushing's triad
___ 5. Dural tear	e. Periorbital edema
___ 6. Postcraniotomy	f. Increased LP pressure, vomiting
___ 7. Upper motor neuron lesion	g. Rhinorrhea
___ 8. Meningeal irritation	h. Personality change
___ 9. Intracranial hypertension	i. "Worst headache of my life"
___ 10. Basal skull fracture	j. Myoglobinuria
___ 11. Guillain-Barré syndrome	k. Absence of doll's eyes (i.e., oculocephalic reflex)
___ 12. Myasthenia gravis	l. Babinski's reflex
___ 13. Hydrocephalus	m. Battle's sign

10. Your patient has had a hemorrhagic stroke. She has nuchal rigidity and decerebrate posturing. She does not vocalize at all and will not open her eyes even to pain. What is her Glasgow Coma Score? What grade bleed is this on the Hunt and Hess aneurysm grading scale? ______________________________

____

11. Identify the following factors as being associated with which complication of subarachnoid hemorrhage: vasospasm or rebleed.

	Vasospasm	Rebleed
Occurs either immediately after the bleed or between 7-10 days after the bleed		
Caused by calcium influx into the vessel		
Occurs any time after 3 days		
Treated by hypervolemic hemodilution and calcium channel blockers		
Caused by lysis of the protective clot		
Prevented by early clipping if the patient is stable enough		

12. List 5 ways that the use of fibrinolytics for ischemic stroke is different from fibrinolytics for myocardial infarction.

1. ______________________________

2. ______________________________

3. ______________________________

4. ______________________________

5. ______________________________

13. Describe CSF changes in the following conditions.

Bacterial meningitis	
Viral meningitis	
Subarachnoid hemorrhage	

14. List 5 observations to make and 5 interventions to perform during a seizure.

Observations to Make
Interventions

15. Match the neuromuscular disorder to the pathophysiology of the disorder.

___ 1. Amyotrophic lateral sclerosis
___ 2. Guillain-Barré
___ 3. Muscular dystrophy
___ 4. Multiple sclerosis
___ 5. Myasthenia gravis

a. Familial degeneration of skeletal muscle fibers
b. Acute inflammation and demyelination of motor more than sensory nerves
c. Immune-mediated inflammation and destruction of myelin with replacement with glial scar tissue
d. Autoimmune destruction of cholinergic receptors at the neuromuscular junction
e. Degeneration of motor neurons in the brainstem and spinal cord

16. Complete the following crossword puzzle dealing with neurologic conditions and treatment.

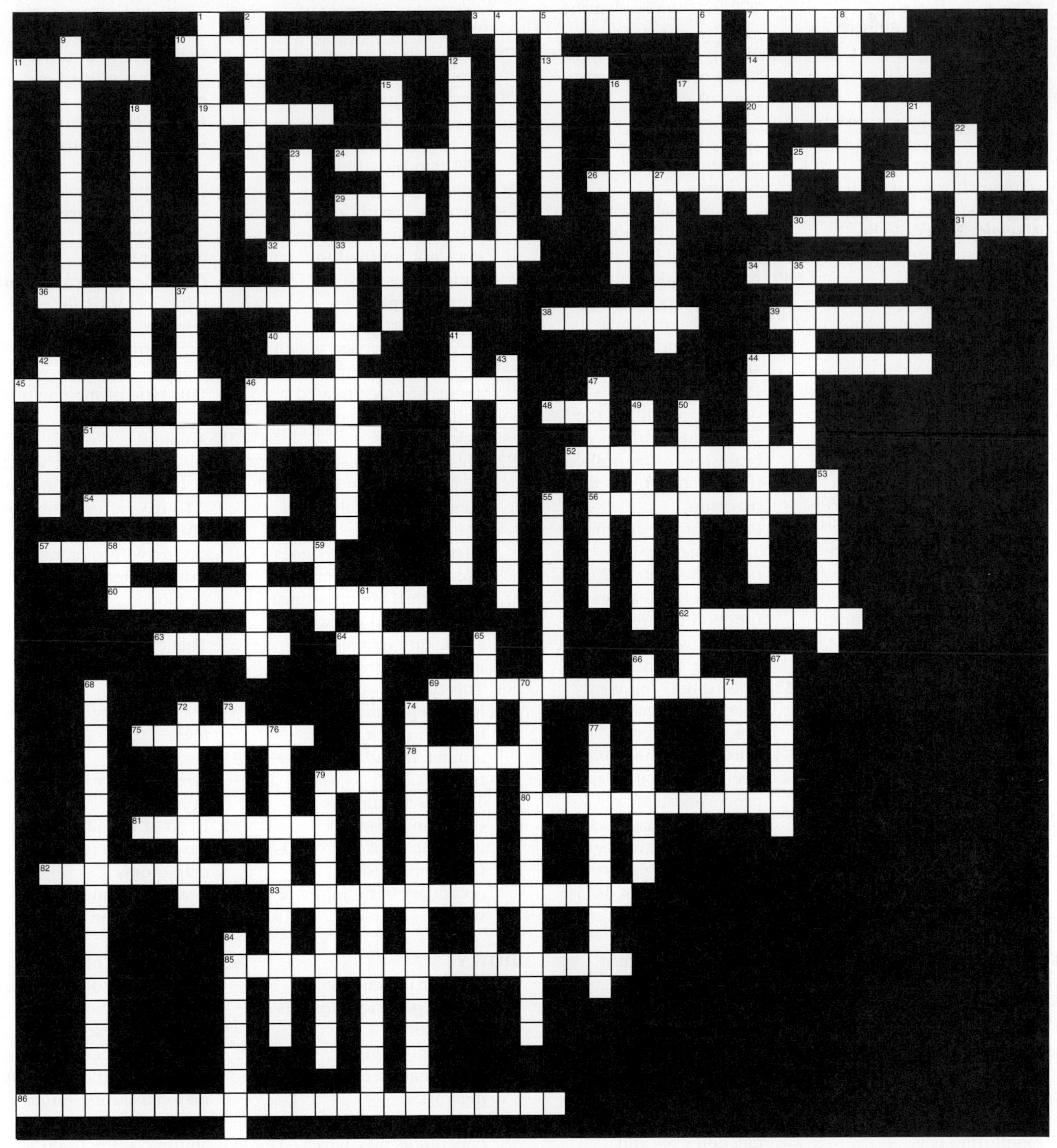

ACROSS

3. This type of crisis occurs after an increase in anticholinesterase dose
7. Elevation ____ in the CSF occurs in meningitis
10. This type of encephalopathy is caused by severe elevation of BP
11. This organ may be removed for myasthenia gravis
13. A severe injury to the brain that causes prolonged unconsciousness, brainstem dysfunction, and profound residual deficits (abbrev)
14. This test is used for myasthenia gravis; muscle weakness decreases when this drug is given
17. State of unconsciousness in which the patient cannot be awakened
19. This type of skull fracture of the temporal bone may tear the middle meningeal artery and cause epidural hematoma
20. The most common type of cerebral aneurysm
24. This type of encephalopathy is caused most often by out-of-hospital cardiac arrest
25. Focal cerebral ischemia that resolves within 24 hours (abbrev)
26. Diabetes _____ is a complication of head trauma or craniotomy that causes polyuria
28. The ____ in the CSF is reduced in bacterial meningitis
29. A _____ hole is drilled into the cranium to allow access for aspiration of a clot or to place an intracranial catheter for monitoring ICP
30. Skull fractures affecting this fossa may cause rhinorrhea and Battle's sign
31. A subjective sensation that often precedes a seizure
32. Rupture of a cerebral aneurysm is sometimes referred to as a _____ hemorrhage because the blood vessels are located in this space
34. Tight cervical collar or trach ties may increase ICP by compressing these veins
36. This type of drug is most likely to be used first to control seizures
38. Cerebrospinal fluid is produced in capillary networks called ___ plexuses
39. _____'s triad of vital sign changes is a late sign of intracranial hypertension
40. A side-to-side herniation
44. The primary symptom of hemorrhage from a cerebral aneurysm is sudden, severe _____
45. Herniation with a downward shift of the brain causing the brainstem to be pushed through the foramen magnum
46. Repair of the cranium
48. This degenerative neuromuscular disease selectively affects motor function (abbrev)
51. Process which occurs in multiple sclerosis
52. This drug is frequently used to prevent/treat vasospasm (generic)
54. This type of herniation occurs with bilateral processes such as cerebral edema; also called central herniation
56. This type of brain tumor is initially benign but is prone to become malignant
57. This neuromuscular condition causes ascending paralysis (2 words)
60. The enzyme that breaks down acetylcholine
62. Skull fracture affecting this fossa may cause raccoon eyes and otorrhea
63. When these muscles are affected in neuromuscular conditions, speech and swallowing difficulties result
64. The first sign of uncal herniation is a dilated, sluggish, or nonreactive ____
69. A treatment used in autoimmune disorders to remove antibodies
75. An abnormal weakness of an artery; most commonly occurs in the circle of Willis
78. Drooping of the eyelid; seen in myasthenia gravis
79. Autoregulation fails if the ___ is less than 50 mm Hg or greater than 150 mm Hg (abbrev)
80. Central _____ is associated with injury to the hypothalamus and does not respond to antipyretics such as acetaminophen
81. A complication of cerebral aneurysm which occurs most commonly in about 3-5 days; treated with calcium channel blockers
82. This hypothesis states that the cranium is an inexpansible vault and if one of the three intracranial volumes goes up, one of the other two intracranial volumes must go down or there will be a resultant increase in intracranial pressure
83. This type of hydrocephalus is most likely to occur from trauma, including surgical trauma
85. This dysrhythmia is a common cause of ischemic stroke (2 words)
86. Common cause of secondary brain injury (2 words)

DOWN

1. Monitor patients with status epilepticus for this indication of rhabdomyolysis
2. Inflammation of the meninges
4. Patients with status epilepticus may have ____ and require parenteral dextrose
5. This drug may be used to reduce the increase in ICP associated with suctioning (generic)
6. This type of cerebral edema is caused by hyponatremia, ischemia, or hypoxia
7. Patients with status epilepticus have elevated CK and ____
8. This type of hematoma is caused by an arterial bleed and causes rapid deterioration
9. Brainstem lesions may cause this type of eye movement
12. Generalized seizures involve these phases (2 words)
15. This type of stroke is caused by aneurysm or arteriovenous malformation
16. Care after traumatic brain injury is primarily directed toward preventing this type of injury
18. This type of meningitis is highly contagious
21. A complication of cerebral aneurysm which frequently occurs at about 7-10 days after the bleed
22. This type of rigidity occurs with meningeal irritation from infection or blood
23. Bruise on the brain
27. This type of stroke is caused by thrombus or embolism
33. Used to reduce peripheral fever
35. Excessive ____ at synapses may be a factor in ALS
37. Head of bed should be flat after this type of craniotomy
41. Uncal herniation causes dilation of the _____ pupil
42. This type of partial seizure is associated with loss of consciousness
43. Prolonged QT interval frequently seen in subarachnoid hemorrhage may cause this serious cardiac complication
44. Shifting of the brain within or out of the cranium
46. Stroke causes _____ paresis or plegia
47. A common complication of chronic degenerative neuromuscular conditions
49. This type of crisis occurs in a patient with myasthenia gravis especially in infection or trauma
50. This complication may occur after craniotomy,

traumatic brain injury, hemorrhagic stroke, or meningitis
53. An osmotic diuretic used for increased ICP
55. Speech impairment seen in myasthenia gravis
58. The first sign of tentorial herniation is a change in ____ (abbrev)
59. Early signs of multiple sclerosis primarily affect the _____ (plural)
61. The primary risk and cause of death in neuromuscular disorders (3 words)
65. This type of craniotomy is often used for removal of the pituitary gland
66. Opening of the cranium
67. This type of intracranial hematoma is caused by a venous bleed and causes symptoms that develop over several days
68. This study is frequently used to evaluate patients after subarachnoid hemorrhage for vasospasm (2 words)
70. This disease is the result of decreased effect of acetylcholine at the neuromuscular junction (2 words)
71. This electrolyte is affected by diabetes insipidus, syndrome of inappropriate ADH, and cerebral salt-wasting syndrome
72. This type of skull fracture may cause cranial nerve defects
73. Acute respiratory failure occurs in myasthenic _____
74. Used to reduce central fever (2 words)
76. Head of bed should be elevated after this type of craniotomy
77. A major risk factor for stroke
79. This type of hydrocephalus may be caused by subarachnoid hemorrhage or meningitis
84. This type of cerebral edema is caused by breakdown of the blood-brain barrier from trauma, tumor, abscess, hemorrhage

The Gastrointestinal System

CHAPTER 7

Selected Concepts in Anatomy and Physiology

General Information About the Gastrointestinal System

1. Functions of the gastrointestinal (GI) system
   a. Digestion and absorption of nutrients
   b. Elimination of waste material
   c. Detoxification and elimination of bacteria, viruses, chemical toxins, and drugs
2. Processes of the gastrointestinal system (Figure 7-1)
   a. Ingestion
   b. Digestion
   c. Absorption
   d. Elimination
3. Structures of the gastrointestinal system (Figure 7-2)
   a. Alimentary canal: from the mouth to the anus
      1) Oropharynx
      2) Esophagus
      3) Stomach
      4) Small intestine: divided into duodenum, jejunum, and ileum
      5) Large intestine: divided into cecum, ascending colon, transverse colon, descending colon, sigmoid colon, and rectum
   b. Accessory organs of digestion
      1) Liver
      2) Gallbladder
      3) Pancreas
4. Cell layers
   a. All areas of the gastrointestinal tract have the same cell layers (external to internal).
      1) Serosa: outermost layer that is frequently continuous with the peritoneum
      2) Muscularis
      3) Submucosa
      4) Mucosa: innermost layer that is exposed to dietary mucosa
5. Peritoneum
   a. The abdominal viscera are covered by the peritoneum.
      1) The parietal layer lines the abdominal cavity wall.
      2) The visceral layer covers the abdominal organs.
      3) The peritoneal cavity is a potential space between the parietal and visceral layers.
   b. There are two folds of the peritoneum.
      1) The mesentery contains blood and lymph vessels and attaches the small intestine and part of the large intestine to the posterior abdominal wall.
      2) The omentum contains fat and lymph nodes.
         a) Lesser omentum from lesser curvature of stomach and upper duodenum to the liver
         b) Greater omentum from stomach over the intestines

Alimentary Canal

1. Oropharynx
   a. Location: mouth to esophagus
   b. Description
      1) Oral cavity
         a) Lips
         b) Cheeks
         c) Palate
         d) Teeth
         e) Tongue
            i) Mucus glands
            ii) Serous glands
         f) Salivary glands
            i) Parotid glands (2)
            ii) Submandibular glands (2)
            iii) Sublingual glands (2)
      2) Muscles of mastication
      3) Pharynx
         a) Nasopharynx
         b) Oropharynx
         c) Laryngopharynx
   c. Secretions: saliva (Table 7-1)
      1) Stimulated by the thought, sight, smell, or taste of food
      2) Consists of:

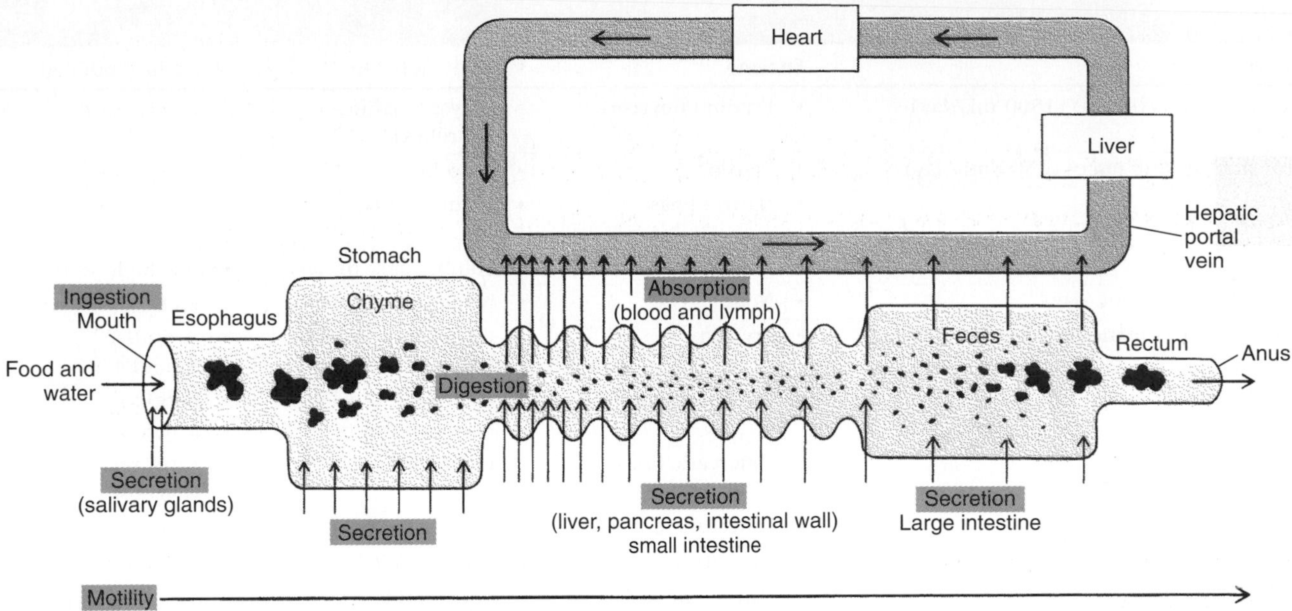

Figure 7-1 Summary of processes of the gastrointestinal system. (From Kinney, M.R., et al. [1998]. *AACN's clinical reference for critical care nursing* [4th ed.]. St. Louis: Mosby.)

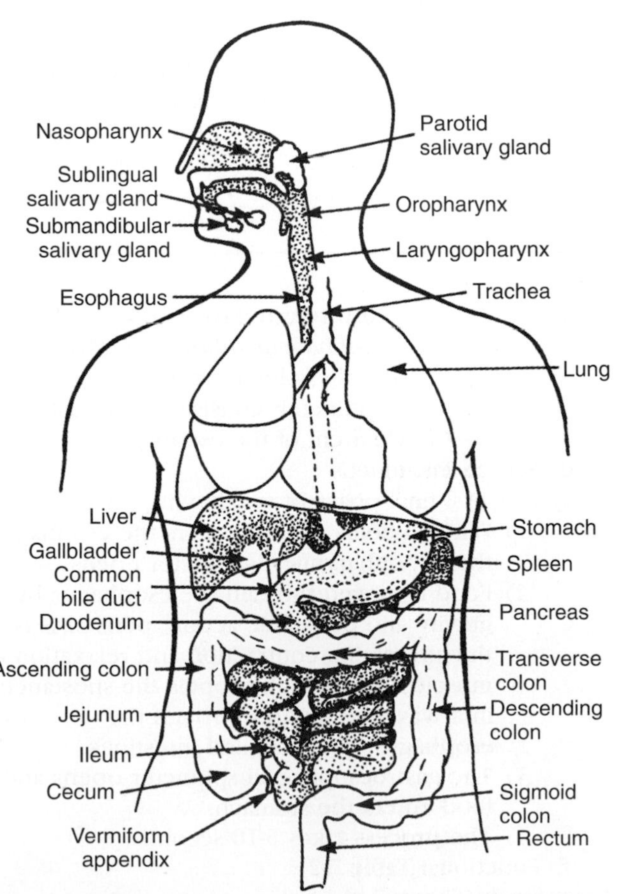

Figure 7-2 Structures of the gastrointestinal system. (From Kinney, M.R., et al. [1998]. *AACN's clinical reference for critical care nursing* [4th ed.]. St. Louis: Mosby.)

a) Ptyalin (amylase): begins the breakdown of polysaccharides (starches) to disaccharides

b) Mucus: provides lubricant

3) Volume: 1500 mL/day

d. Process

1) The teeth break up the food into smaller pieces to increase surface area for digestive enzymes to act.

2) The masseter muscles are innervated by cranial nerve V (trigeminal).

3) The tongue moves the food around in the mouth for better chewing and moves the food to the back of the throat to begin the process of swallowing.

4) Swallowing (deglutination) consists of three stages; only stage one occurs in the mouth.

a) Voluntary: The tongue forces the bolus of food into the pharynx.

b) Pharyngeal: The bolus of food passes from the pharynx to esophagus; the epiglottis closes to protect the larynx.

c) Esophageal: The bolus of food passes from the esophagus to the gastroesophageal sphincter.

e. Functions: Table 7-2

2. Esophagus

a. Location

1) Lies behind the trachea

2) Passes through the thoracic cavity and the diaphragm; passes through the diaphragm at the diaphragmatic hiatus

b. Description: hollow tube from the pharynx to the stomach; approximately 25 cm in length and 2 cm in diameter

Table 7-1 Digestive Enzymes

Source	Enzyme	What It Acts On	What Is Produced
Salivary glands (saliva) (1500 mL/day)	• Ptyalin (amylase)	• Polysaccharides (starches)	• Disaccharides
Stomach (gastric juice) (2500 mL/day)	• Pepsin	• Proteins	• Polypeptides
	• Gastric lipase	• Emulsified fats	• Fatty acids • Glycerol
	• Renin	• Soluble milk protein	• Insoluble form
Liver (bile) (500 mL/day)	• None	• Nonemulsified fats	• Emulsified fats
Pancreas (pancreatic juice) (1500 mL/day)	• Trypsin	• Denatured proteins • Polypeptides	• Peptides • Amino acids
	• Chymotrypsin	• Proteins • Polypeptides	• Peptides • Amino acids
	• Pancreatic lipase	• Emulsified fats	• Fatty acids • Glycerol
	• Pancreatic amylase	• Disaccharides	• Polysaccharides
	• Nucleases	• Nucleic acids	• Nucleotides
	• Carboxypeptidase	• Polypeptides	• Smaller polypeptides
Small intestine (1000 mL/day)	• Enterokinase	• Trypsinogen	• Trypsin
	• Aminopeptidase	• Polypeptides	• Smaller polypeptides
	• Dipeptidase	• Dipeptides	• Amino acids
	• Sucrase	• Sucrose	• Glucose • Fructose
	• Lactase	• Lactose	• Glucose • Galactose
	• Maltase	• Maltose	• Glucose
	• Nucleotidase	• Nucleotides	• Nucleosides • Phosphoric acid
	• Nucleosidase	• Nucleosides	• Purine • Pentose
	• Intestinal lipase	• Fat	• Glycerides • Fatty acids • Glycerol

c. Structure (Figure 7-3)
   1) Cell layers (external to internal)
      a) Does not have a serosa layer
      b) Muscularis
         i) Type of muscle
            (a) Upper one third: skeletal muscle
            (b) Lower two thirds: smooth muscle
         ii) Direction of muscle
            (a) Inner: circular
            (b) Outer: longitudinal
      c) Submucosa
      d) Mucosa: lined with mucous membrane, which secretes a protective mucoid substance
   2) Sphincters
      a) Hypopharyngeal
         i) Also referred to as the *upper esophageal sphincter* (UES)
         ii) Made of cricopharyngeal muscle
      b) Gastroesophageal
         i) Also referred to as the *lower esophageal sphincter* (LES)
         ii) A physiologic rather than anatomic sphincter: consists of the last 2-4 cm of the esophagus

d. Secretions: mucus

e. Process: final phase of swallowing (involuntary)
   1) When a bolus of food enters the esophagus, the hypopharyngeal sphincter opens.
   2) Food is moved through the esophagus by gravity and peristaltic action; peristalsis is the alternating contraction and relaxation of muscle fibers which propels the substance in a wavelike motion through the esophagus, stomach, and intestines.
   3) The gastroesophageal sphincter opens and food enters the stomach.
   4) The process takes 5-10 seconds.

f. Functions: Table 7-2

3. Stomach (Figure 7-4)
   a. Location: inferior to the diaphragm with approximately 80-85% of the organ to the left of midline

Table 7-2 Functions of the Components of the Gastrointestinal System

Component	Function
Oropharynx	• Salivation • Ingestion • Mastication • Lubrication and moistening of food • First, second stage of swallowing
Esophagus	• Third stage of swallowing • Lubrication of food • Provision of vent for increased gastric pressures
Stomach	• Secretion of gastric enzymes • Mixing of food with gastric enzymes • Reduction of osmolality of food • Absorption of water • Movement of food through the pylorus
Small intestine	• Receipt of chyme from the stomach and move chyme forward to facilitate proper absorption of proteins, carbohydrates, fats, electrolytes, vitamins, minerals, drugs, and water • Receipt of bile and pancreatic fluid to aid in digestion • Movement of chyme via peristalsis and segmentation • Bacteria in the small intestine help break down and digest protein and, to some degree, fat
Large intestine	• Secretion of mucus to lubricate and protect intestinal lining • Movement of chyme through colon to rectum and initiate urge to defecate • Storage of feces • Elimination of digestive wastes: defecation • Absorption of water and electrolytes • Synthesis of vitamins (folic acid, riboflavin, vitamin K, nicotinic acid) • Metabolism of blood urea to ammonia
Liver	• Secretion of bilirubin, bile salts, cholesterol, fatty acids, calcium, and other electrolytes into bile • Storage of amino acids, glucose, vitamins, minerals (copper, iron), and blood • Vitamins: riboflavin, nicotinic acid, pyridoxine, vitamins A, D, E, K, B_{12} • Conversion of complex sugars to simple sugars • Conversion of carbohydrates to fats • Conversion of stored glucose (glycogen) to glucose (process is called *glycogenolysis*) • Conversion of amino acids and fats to glucose (process is called *gluconeogenesis*) • Conversion of amino acids to fatty acids and triglycerides • Formation of phospholipids and cholesterol • Formation of lipoproteins from triglycerides and peptides • Conversion of amino acids to plasma proteins (e.g., albumin, fibrinogen, globulins) • Phagocytosis of old RBCs • Formation of clotting factors and heparin • Conversion of ammonia to urea • Conversion of creatine to creatinine • Conversion of vitamin D_3 to 25-hydroxycholecalciferol • Detoxification of bacteria • Biotransformation of drugs to active and/or inactive metabolites • Deactivation of certain hormones
Gallbladder	• Collection, concentration, and storage of bile • Passageway for bile from liver to intestine • Regulation of bile flow • Release of bile

Pancreas	• Exocrine function
	  • Secretion of pancreatic juice for digestion of carbohydrates, proteins, and fats
	  • Secretion of bicarbonate to neutralize chyme
	• Endocrine function
	  • Secretion of insulin and glucagon

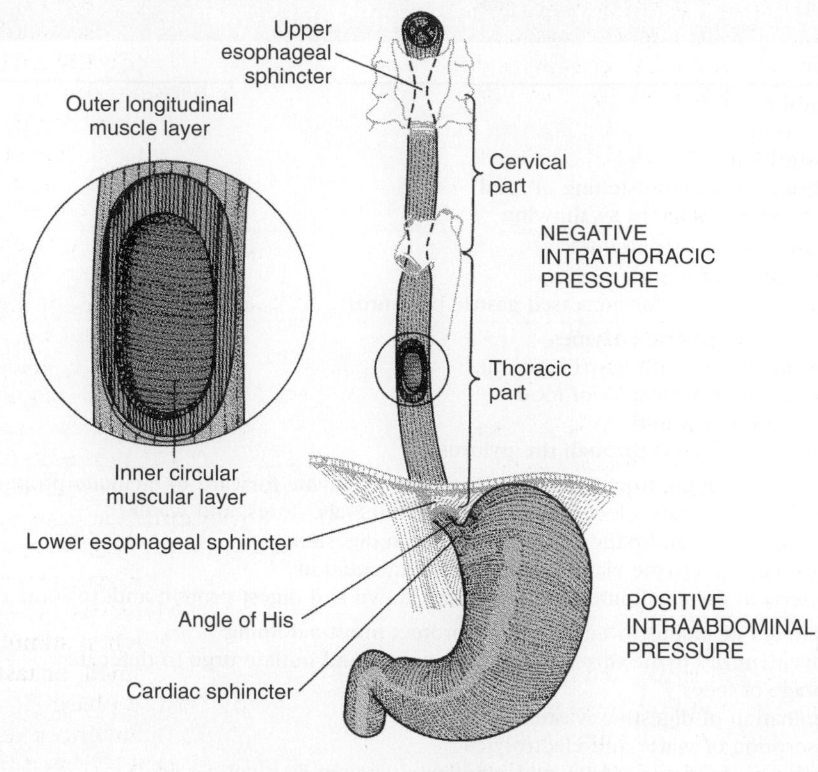

Figure 7-3 Anatomy of the esophagus. (From Beare, P. G., & Myers, J. L. [1994] *Principles and practice of adult health nursing* [2nd ed.]. St Louis: Mosby.)

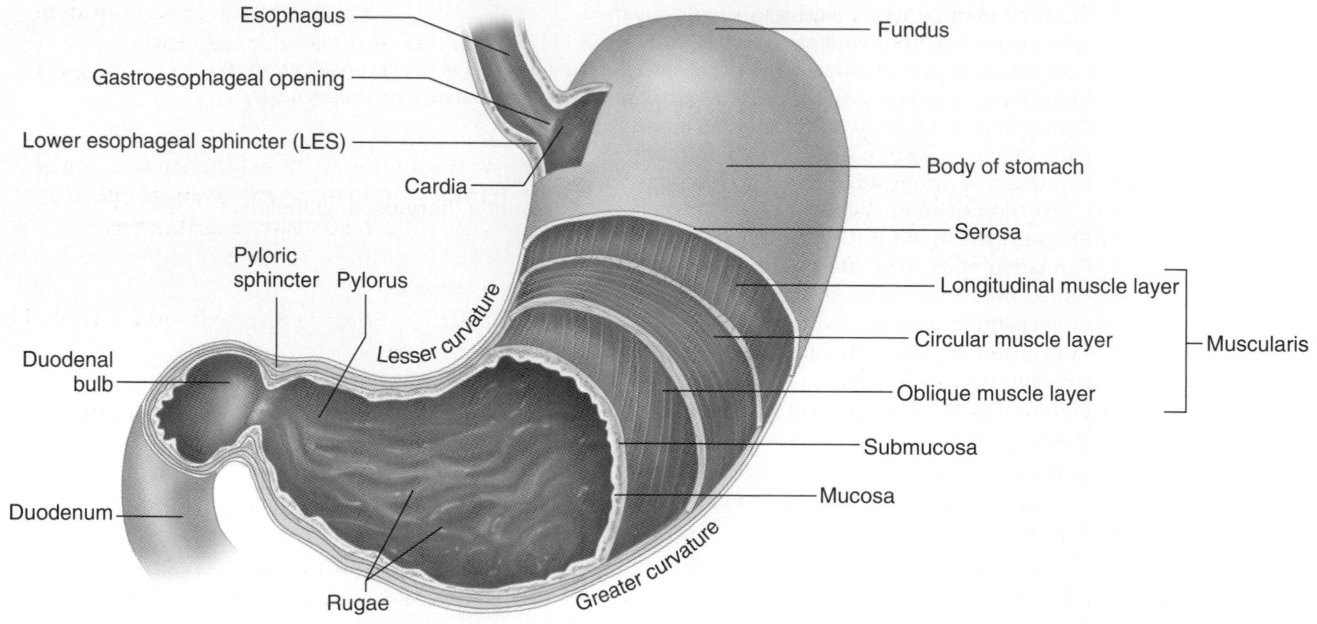

Figure 7-4 Anatomy of the stomach. (From Patton, K. T. & Thibodeau, G. A. [2013]. *Anatomy & physiology* [8th ed.]. St Louis: Mosby.)

b. Description
   1) Largest dilation of the GI tract
   2) Approximately 25-30 cm in length and 10-15 cm at maximal diameter
   3) Relatively little muscle tone, which permits increased distention

c. Structure
   1) Anatomical divisions
      a) Cardia: portion of stomach that immediately adjoins the esophagus
      b) Fundus: dome-shaped portion of stomach that extends left of the cardia

c) Greater curvature: lateral, convex side
d) Body: major area (belly) of stomach
e) Lesser curvature: medial, concave side
f) Antrum: lower portion close to pylorus
2) Sphincters
a) Cardiac: between esophagus and stomach
b) Pyloric: between stomach and duodenum
3) Layers of stomach wall (external to internal)
a) Serosa: continuous with the peritoneum
b) Muscularis
i) Outer: longitudinal muscle fibers
ii) Middle: circular muscle fibers
iii) Inner: transverse muscle fibers
c) Submucosa
i) Blood vessels
ii) Lymph vessels
iii) Connective tissue
iv) Fibrous tissues
d) Mucosa: contains rugae, which are thick folds on the interior of the stomach; rugae do all of the following:
i) Increase surface area for exposure
ii) Allow for distention
iii) Contain the openings of the gastric glands
e) Gastric glands
i) Cardiac glands: just distal to the gastroesophageal junction; secrete pepsinogen and mucus
ii) Oxyntic glands: fundic area
(a) Mucous neck cells secrete mucus.
(b) Chief cells secrete pepsinogen.
(c) Oxyntic (also referred to as *parietal*) cells secrete:
(i) Hydrochloric acid
(ii) Intrinsic factor
(d) Enterochromaffin (endocrine) cells secrete serotonin.
iii) Pyloric glands: antral area
(a) Gastrin secreted by G-cells
(b) Serotonin secreted by enterochromaffin cells

d. Secretions: Table 7-1
1) Description: Gastric secretions are clear and contain water, salts, enzymes, and hydrochloric acid.
2) Gastric secretions are stimulated when a bolus of food enters the upper portion of the stomach.
3) Gastric secretions contain the following
a) Hydrochloric acid
i) Stimulated by: histamine, acetylcholine, gastrin
ii) Functions
(a) Denature protein and break intermolecular bonds
(b) Activate a number of enzymes secreted by stomach
(c) Kill bacteria
b) Pepsinogen
i) Activated by hydrochloric acid to form pepsin
ii) Function: Pepsin catalyzes splitting of bonds between particular types of amino acids in protein chains.
c) Intrinsic factor: mucoprotein necessary for intestinal absorption of vitamin B_{12} in the ileum; deficiency of vitamin B_{12} causes pernicious anemia
d) Mucus: contributes to the maintenance of the gastric mucosal barrier
4) Control of gastric secretion
a) Cephalic phase
i) Mediated by parasympathetic nervous system (PNS)
ii) Release of hydrochloric acid (HCl) when stimulated by thought, sight, smell, or taste of food
b) Gastric phase
i) Enhances acid secretion
ii) Stimulated by distention of stomach and digestion products of food
c) Intestinal phase
i) Continuation of gastric acid secretion but in lesser amounts
ii) Stimulated by distention, hypertonic solution, acid, and fat within duodenum

e. Process
1) As food moves toward the pyloric sphincter at the distal end of the stomach, peristaltic waves increase in force and intensity.
2) The food bolus becomes a substance known as *chyme*.
3) Gastric motility is affected and controlled by various factors.
a) Affected by the following:
i) Quantity and pH of contents
ii) Degree of mixing
iii) Peristalsis
iv) Ability of the duodenum to accept the chyme
b) Controlled by the following:
i) Sympathetic and parasympathetic nervous systems
ii) Reflexes
iii) Gastric hormones
4) Chyme is pumped through the pyloric sphincter into the duodenum.
5) The stomach empties as chyme moves through the pyloric channel.
a) Rate of gastric emptying proportional to the volume of the stomach's contents
b) Regulation of gastric emptying affected by the following:

i) Consistency of the fluid chyme; liquids selectively move through the pylorus before solids
ii) Receptiveness of the duodenum
c) Factors inhibiting gastric emptying
i) Chyme with high lipid content
ii) High acidity in antrum
iii) Emotions: pain, anxiety, sadness, hostility
iv) Hormones: secretin and cholecystokinin
d) Food usually stays in the stomach 2-6 hours after ingestion.
f. Function: Table 7-2
4. Small intestine
a. Description
1) Length: 7 m; diameter: 2.5 cm
2) Extends from pylorus to ileocecal valve
b. Structure
1) Divisions
a) Duodenum: short segment only 30 cm long
b) Jejunum: the next two fifths after the duodenum; approximately 250 cm long
c) Ileum: the last three fifths after the duodenum; approximately 350 cm long
2) Layers of wall (external to internal)
a) Serosa: continuous with the peritoneum
b) Muscular
c) Submucosal
d) Mucosal
3) Sphincters
a) Pylorus: from stomach to duodenum
b) Ileocecal: controls flow of contents into large intestine and prevents reflux from the large intestine back into the ileum
4) Villi
a) Fingerlike projections of mucosa and submucosa prominent in duodenum and jejunum increase surface area.
b) Contain a single lymph vessel called a *lacteal* and a dense capillary bed to aid in absorption
c) Contain many different types of cells to absorb fat, CHO, or protein and/or secrete enzymes and mucus
i) Brunner's glands: cells that secrete mucus; primarily in duodenum
ii) Goblet cells: cells that secrete mucus
iii) Crypts of Lieberkühn: cells that produce watery mucus called *succus entericus*, a carrier substance for absorption of nutrients when the villi come in contact with the chyme
iv) Paneth's cells: uncertain function but may regulate intestinal flora
v) Peyer's patches
(a) Cells in mucosa and submucosa
(b) Lymphoid follicles that carry out antibody synthesis
c. Secretions
1) Stimulated by the presence of chyme in the duodenum and release of gastric hormones
2) Table 7-1
d. Process
1) Movement of chyme
a) During fasting and sleeping states: Muscle contraction moves from antrum to ileum to sweep the gut of contents.
b) During eating state
i) Concentric, segmenting contractions take place in the jejunum; help to mix secretions of the small intestines with the chyme particles
ii) Slow, propulsive contractions (peristalsis) slowly push the chyme in the direction of the large intestine.
iii) Continuous shortening and lengthening of the villi constantly stir the intestinal contents.
c) The movement of chyme from the small intestine to the large intestine regulated by gastroileal reflex; increased contractions in the ileum as the chyme nears the large intestine
d) Movement of chyme through small intestine approximately 3-10 hours
e. Function: Table 7-2
5. Large intestine
a. Description: length: 90-150 cm; diameter: 4-6 cm extending from ileum to anus
b. Structure
1) Divisions (Figure 7-5)
a) Cecum
b) Colon
i) Ascending colon
ii) Transverse colon
iii) Descending colon
iv) Sigmoid colon
c) Rectum
2) Flexures
a) Hepatic: bend at the liver; in the RUQ
b) Splenic: bend at the spleen; in the LUQ
3) Sphincters
a) Ileocecal: from small intestine to cecum
b) Anal: internal and external anal sphincters
4) Layers of large intestinal wall
a) Serosa: continuous with the peritoneum
b) Muscularis
c) Submucosa
d) Mucosa
c. Process
1) Movement of intestinal contents
a) Haustral shuttling
i) Periodic uncoordinated tonic contractions or segmentations of

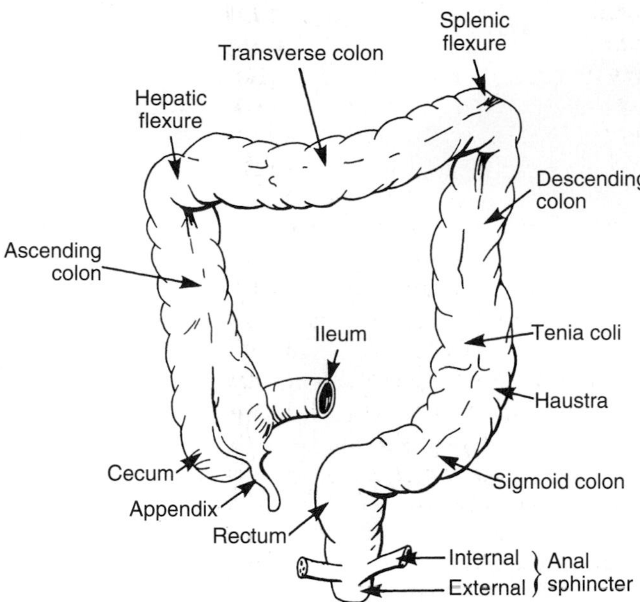

Figure 7-5 Anatomy of the large intestine. (From Kinney, M.R., et al. [1998]. *AACN's clinical reference for critical care nursing* [4th ed.]. St. Louis: Mosby.)

both the longitudinal and circular muscles

ii) Contents displaced short distances

iii) Weak peristaltic contractions that move the chyme through the large intestine

b) Phasic, random, nonpropulsive contractions

i) Last 30 seconds to 2 minutes

ii) Contents displaced short distances in both directions

iii) Mixes the stool material and helps in the absorption of liquid contents without advancement toward the anus

c) Spontaneous mass movements

i) Fecal contents are pushed forward by mass movements that typically occur only a few times each day.

ii) Mass movements are stimulated by gastrocolic reflexes initiated when food enters the duodenum from the stomach, especially after the first meal of the day.

iii) These movements move feces into the rectum.

iv) The defecation reflex occurs when feces enters the rectum; peristaltic waves in the rectum and relaxation of the internal and external anal sphincter occur.

v) Afferent impulses are transmitted to the sacral segment of the spinal cord, from which reflex impulses are transmitted back to the colon and rectum, initiating relaxation of the internal anal sphincter.

vi) Evacuation of the colon may be facilitated by Valsalva maneuver.

2) Factors that enhance colonic motility
   a) High-residue diet
   b) Hyperosmolality
   c) Fluids
   d) Irritation of colon (e.g., spicy foods)
   e) Irritant laxatives
3) Factors that inhibit colonic motility
   a) Low-residue diet
   b) Anticholinergic drugs
   c) Opiates
4) Movement of fecal contents through small intestine approximately 12 hours

d. Function: Table 7-2

Accessory Organs of Digestion (Figure 7-6)

1. Liver

a. Location: in RUQ, fitting snugly against right inferior diaphragm

b. Description
1) Largest organ in the body: 1.5 kg
2) Attached to the abdominal wall by the falciform ligament, which also divides the left and right lobes
3) Four main lobes
   a) Right: larger than left
   b) Left
   c) Caudate
   d) Quadrate
4) Covered by a thick capsule of connective tissue (called *Glisson's capsule*); contains blood vessels and lymphatics
5) Capsule covered by a layer of serosa continuous with the peritoneum

c. Structure
1) Lobes are divided into lobules.
2) Lobules are the functioning unit of the liver; there are over 1 million lobules.
   a) Hepatic cells (hepatocytes) are arranged in chains around a central vein.
   b) Blood flows through sinusoids, which separate the hepatic chains.
   c) The sinusoids receive oxygenated blood from branches of the hepatic artery and nutrient-rich blood from branches of the hepatic portal vein; the hepatic cells remove oxygen, nutrients, and toxins from the blood.
   d) Each lobule has its own hepatic artery, portal vein, and bile duct, collectively called the *portal triad.*
   e) The lobule is composed of branching plates of liver cells radiating from center to periphery.
   f) Kupffer cells, which are responsible for phagocytosis, line the sinusoids; Kupffer

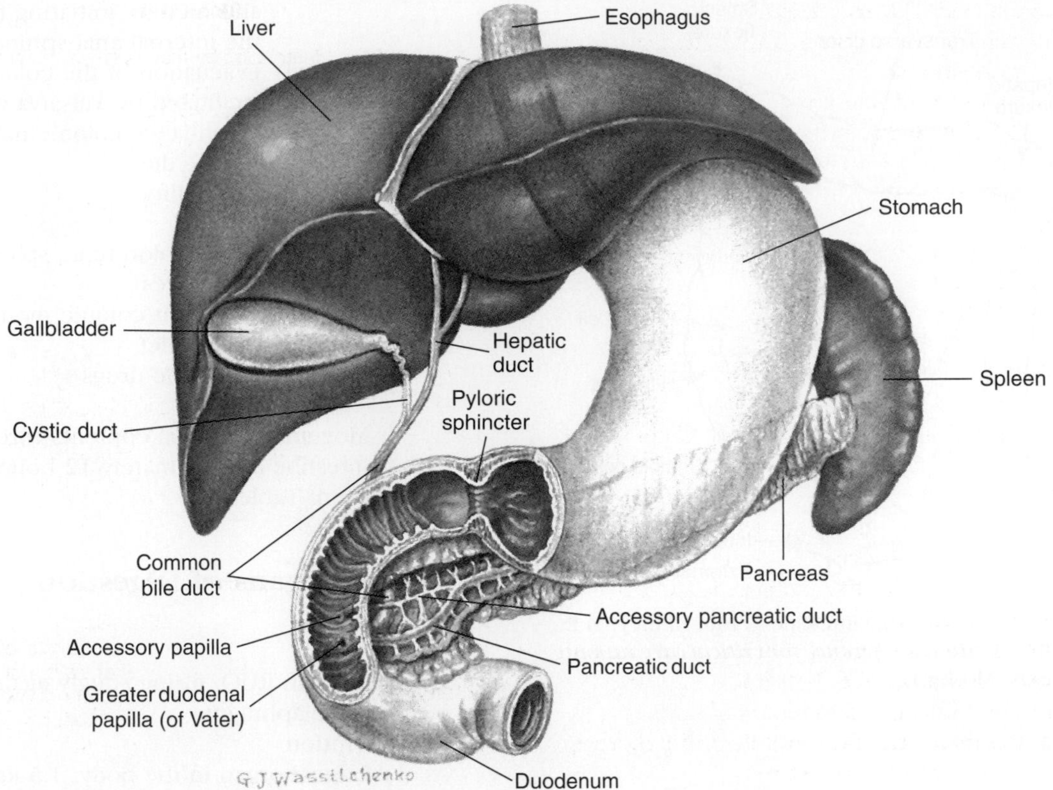

Figure 7-6 Accessory organs of the gastrointestinal system. (From Doughty, D. B., & Jackson, D. B. [1993]. *Gastrointestinal disorders: Mosby's clinical nursing series*. St Louis: Mosby.)

cells are a part of the reticuloendothelium system; they destroy old or defective red blood cells and remove bacteria and foreign particles from the blood.

g) Ducts
   i) Bile canaliculi are located between the hepatic cells and empty bile into the small bile ducts.
   ii) Small bile ducts join to form the right and left hepatic ducts.
   iii) Left and right hepatic ducts merge to form the common hepatic duct.
   iv) Cystic duct from the gallbladder joins the common hepatic duct to form the common bile duct. (Figure 7-7)
   v) The pancreatic duct joins the common bile duct and together they empty into the duodenum through the ampulla of Vater.
   vi) The sphincter of Oddi is a valve in the common bile duct, which regulates the passage of bile from the common bile duct into the duodenum.

d. Secretions: bile (described under Gallbladder)
e. Function: Table 7-2

2. Gallbladder
   a. Location

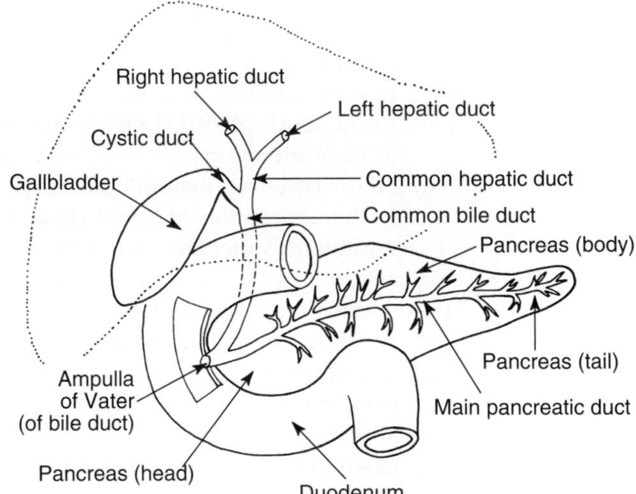

Figure 7-7 Ductal systems of the gastrointestinal tract. (From Kinney, M.R., et al. [1998]. *AACN's clinical reference for critical care nursing* [4th ed.]. St. Louis: Mosby.)

      1) Attached to undersurface of liver
      2) Connected to the upper portion of the duodenum by the common bile duct
   b. Description
      1) Saclike organ about 7-10 cm in length and 3 cm in diameter
      2) Storage capacity of 50-70 mL

3) Layers (exterior to interior)
   a) Serous layer: continuous with the peritoneum
   b) Smooth muscle layer
   c) Mucous membrane layer (has rugae which allow an increase in gallbladder size)

c. Structure
   1) There are four anatomical divisions of the gallbladder.
      a) Fundus: distal portion of the body that forms a blind sac
      b) Body: connects the fundus to the infundibulum
      c) Infundibulum: connects the body to the neck
      d) Neck: narrows into the cystic duct
   2) The cystic duct merges with the common hepatic duct to form the common bile duct, which joins with the pancreatic duct to form ampulla of Vater.
   3) The sphincter of Oddi is at the terminal end of the common bile duct, located at the entrance into the duodenum.
      a) Regulates the flow of bile and pancreatic juices into the intestine
      b) Inhibits the entry of bile into the pancreatic duct
      c) Prevents reflux of intestinal contents into the duct

d. Secretions
   1) Table 7-1
   2) Bile
      a) Bile is produced by the liver and stored in the gallbladder.
      b) The gallbladder contracts in response to the hormone cholecystokinin when food is present in the small intestine; release is stimulated when fatty food is present in the small intestine.
      c) The action of bile is to assist in the absorption of fats by emulsifying the fat and breaking down large fat droplets into small droplets.
      d) Bile is composed of the following:
         i) Water
         ii) Bile pigments
         iii) Bile salts
         iv) High concentration of cholesterol
         v) Some neutral fat, phospholipid, and inorganic salts
      e) The major bile pigment is bilirubin, a breakdown product of hemoglobin.
         i) Metabolism (Figure 7-8)
            (a) The heme portion of the hemoglobin molecule is converted to bilirubin by reticuloendothelial cells, released into the bloodstream, and binds to albumin as fat-soluble, unconjugated bilirubin (indirect).
            (b) In the liver, indirect bilirubin is bound to glucuronic acid to form water-soluble conjugated (direct) bilirubin, which is excreted into the hepatic ducts.

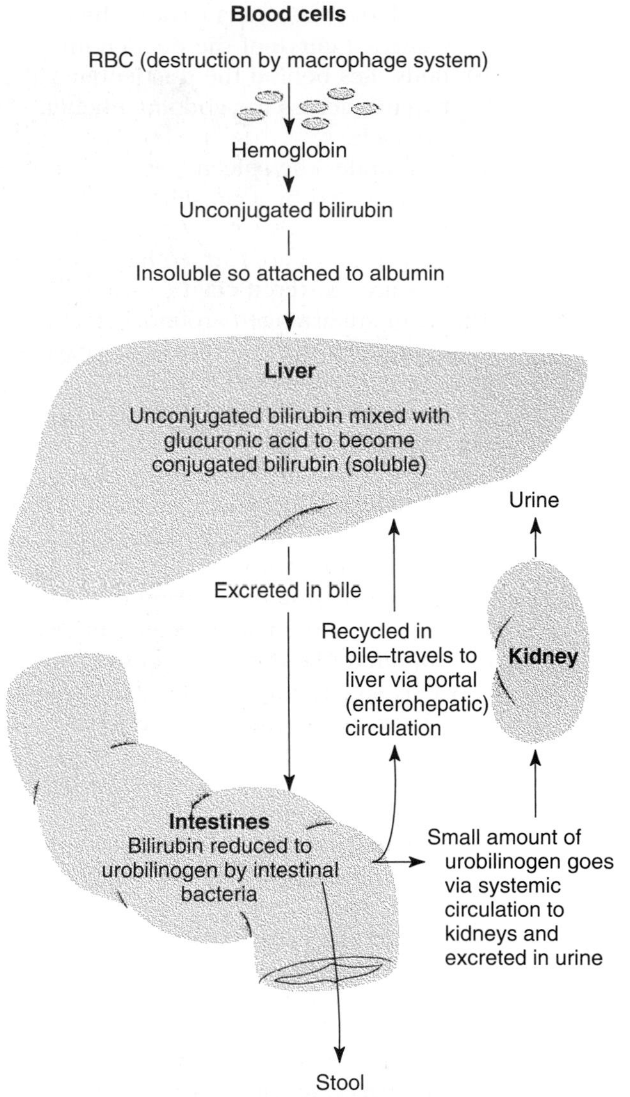

Figure 7-8 Bilirubin metabolism. (From Lewis, S. M., Heitkemper, M. M., & Dirksen, S. R. [2000]. *Medical-surgical nursing: Assessment and management of clinical problems* [5th ed.]. St. Louis: Mosby.)

e. Process
   1) Contraction of the gallbladder is stimulated by the hormone cholecystokinin.

f. Function: Table 7-2

3. Pancreas
   a. Location: lies in the posterior curvature of the stomach; lies behind duodenum and spleen (Figure 7-6)
   b. Description
      1) Length: 15-20 cm; diameter: 5 cm
      2) Anatomical divisions

a) Head: over the vena cava in the C-shaped curve of the duodenum
b) Body: lies behind the duodenum and extends across the abdomen behind stomach
c) Tail: under the spleen

3) Not surrounded by a capsule

c. Structure

1) Connected lobes are formed by lobules.
2) Lobules are clustered cells.
3) The acini are arranged around a small central lumen; they secrete their enzymes into the central lumen.
4) These central lumina are drained into ductules.
5) Ductules drain into intralobular ducts, which drain into interlobular ducts, which empty into the pancreatic duct (also called the *duct of Wirsung*).
6) The pancreatic duct runs from the tail to the head of the pancreas and unites with the common bile duct to form the ampulla of Vater, which empties into the duodenum.
7) Cells have exocrine and endocrine functions.
   a) Acinar cells have exocrine (through a duct) functions.
   b) Alpha and beta cells of the islets of Langerhans have endocrine (ductless) functions.
      i) Alpha cells secrete glucagon.
      ii) Beta cells secrete insulin.
      iii) Delta cells secrete somatostatin.

d. Secretions: Table 7-1

1) Pancreatic secretions are triggered by the presence of undigested food in the small intestine.
2) Acinar cells secrete a high concentration of sodium bicarbonate, water, sodium, potassium and digestive enzymes (lipase, amylase, trypsin, ribonuclease, deoxyribonuclease).
   a) Trypsinogen: secreted in inactive form; activated in contact with bile salts
   b) Chymotrypsinogen: secreted in inactive form; activated in contact with bile salts
3) Secretions are controlled by the following:
   a) Vagus nerve and parasympathetic nervous system
   b) Hormonal: secretin and cholecystokinin

e. Functions: Table 7-2

Gastrointestinal Hormones

See Table 7-3.

Blood Supply (Figure 7-9)

1. Arterial: aorta→aortic arch→thoracic arch→abdominal aorta→
   a. Celiac artery: The following branches of the celiac artery supply these specified organs:
      1) Left gastric: supplies stomach and esophagus
      2) Hepatic to right gastric: supplies stomach
      3) Gastroduodenal: supplies stomach and duodenum
      4) Cystic: supplies gallbladder

Table 7-3 Gastrointestinal Hormones

Hormone	Source	Stimulus for Release	Action
Gastrin	Gastric mucosa of the antrum of the stomach and the pylorus	Partially digested proteins in pylorus	• Stimulates release of gastric juices
Secretin	Duodenal mucosa	Partially digested proteins, fats, and acids in intestine	• Inhibits gastric motility and acid secretions • Pancreatic bicarbonate secretion
Cholecystokinin	Duodenal mucosa	Fats in duodenum	• Increases gallbladder contraction • Decreases stomach tone
Gastric inhibitory peptide	Small intestine mucosa	Fat and carbohydrate in duodenum	• Stimulates secretion of insulin • Decreases motor activity of the stomach • Slows emptying of gastric contents into the small intestine
Vasoactive intestinal peptide	Small intestine mucosa	Acid in the duodenum	• Stimulates intestinal juice • Inhibits gastric secretion
Enterogastrone	Small intestine mucosa	Partially digested proteins, fats, and acids in intestine	• Inhibits gastric secretion and motility • Relaxation of sphincter of Oddi and contraction of gallbladder
Villikinin	Small intestine mucosa	Chyme in intestine	• Stimulates movement of intestinal villi
Pancreozymin	Duodenal mucosa	Partially digested proteins, fats, and acids in duodenum	• Stimulates pancreatic juice

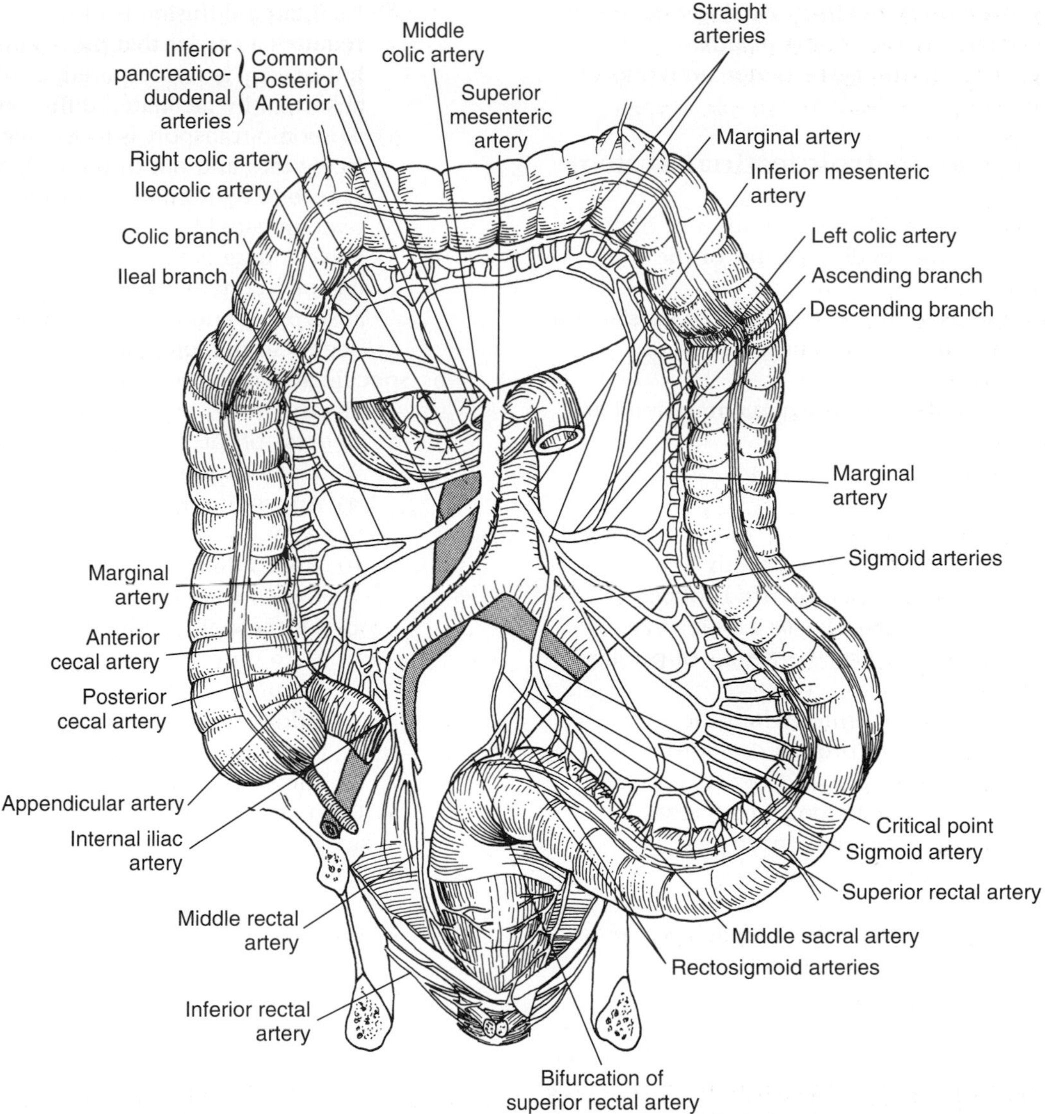

Figure 7-9 Arterial blood supply of the gastrointestinal system. (From Society of Gastroenterology Nurses and Associates SGNA [1993]. *Gastroenterology nursing: A core curriculum.* St Louis: Mosby.)

5) Splenic: supplies stomach, pancreas, and spleen

b. Superior mesenteric arteries supply the following:
   1) Jejunum
   2) Ileum
   3) Cecum
   4) Ascending colon
   5) Part of transverse colon

c. Inferior mesenteric arteries supply the following:
   1) Transverse, descending, and sigmoid colon
   2) Rectum

d. Hepatic artery and vein supply the liver.

2. Venous
   a. Portal vein collects and delivers blood from entire venous drainage of GI tract to liver; branches: gastric; splenic; superior mesenteric; inferior mesenteric
   b. Portal vein subdivides into liver sinusoids, which then unite with branches from hepatic artery to form hepatic vein, which empties into inferior vena cava.
   c. Partially metabolized digestive products are brought to liver sinusoids where hepatocytes complete the next stage of metabolism.

Nervous Innervation

1. Extrinsic
   a. Parasympathetic nervous system (PNS): increases the activity of the GI tract; innervated via the vagus nerve
   b. Sympathetic nervous system (SNS): decreases the activity of the GI tract; innervated via SNS fibers, which run parallel to the major blood vessels of the GI tract
2. Intrinsic
   a. Located inside the wall of GI tract

b. Consists of extensions from extrinsic nerves of the autonomic nervous system (ANS)
c. Form two major and three minor networks of plexuses

Functions of the Gastrointestinal System

1. Ingestion
   a. Ingestion begins with the sensation of hunger, controlled by the feeding center of the hypothalamus.
   b. Ingestion ends with the sensation of satisfaction provided by the satiety center also in the hypothalamus.
   c. Food and liquids enter the alimentary tract at the mouth.
2. Secretion: Table 7-1
3. Digestion
   a. Carbohydrates: 4 kcal/g
      1) Digestion begins in the mouth where polysaccharides (starch) are broken down to disaccharides (e.g., sucrose, lactose, maltose) by the action of ptyalin (amylase).
      2) The process continues when the disaccharides are broken down to monosaccharides (e.g., glucose, galactose, fructose) by the action of pancreatic amylase and intestinal enzymes (e.g., sucrase, lactase, maltase).
   b. Proteins: 4 kcal/g
      1) Digestion begins in the stomach where pepsin breaks down proteins into polypeptides.
      2) The process continues when the polypeptides are broken down into peptides and amino acids in the small intestine by the action of trypsin, chymotrypsin, carboxypeptides from the pancreas, and aminopeptidases and dipeptidase from the intestinal villi.
   c. Fats: 9 kcal/g
      1) Digestion of fats that are already emulsified (e.g., cream and butter) begins in the stomach by lipase.
      2) Digestion of nonemulsified fat occurs in the small intestine with emulsification of the fat by bile and pancreatic lipase.
      3) Fat is broken down into glycerol and fatty acids.
4. Absorption
   a. Basic absorption mechanisms
      1) Active transport requires an energy source (e.g., ATP) to move substances into and out of the cell; substances absorbed by active transport include proteins, glucose, sodium, and potassium.
      2) Passive diffusion is passive movement from an area of high solute concentration to an area of low solute concentration; substances absorbed by passive diffusion include free fatty acids and water.
      3) Facilitated diffusion is movement that requires a carrier that moves into the cell, but energy is not required; a substance absorbed by facilitated diffusion is fructose.
      4) Nonionic transport is movement of solutes freely into and out of the cell; substances absorbed by nonionic transport include unconjugated bile salts and drugs.
      5) Solvent drag is flow of water to higher osmotic concentration; it contributes to absorption and reduction in osmolality that occurs in the jejunum.
   b. Specific absorption in small intestine
      1) Electrolyte absorption: active transport from all areas of intestine
      2) Water absorption: small and large intestine
         a) Approximately 2 L of fluid is ingested daily.
         b) Approximately 7 L of fluid is secreted by the GI tract daily.
         c) Of these 9 L, 7500 mL are reabsorbed with only 1500 mL reaching the cecum.
         d) Additional fluid is reabsorbed in the large intestine, but only 200 mL is lost in the stool.
      3) CHO absorption
         a) Fructose by facilitated diffusion
         b) Glucose and galactose by active transport
      4) Protein absorption: amino acids absorbed by active transport in ileum and jejunum
      5) Fat absorption
         a) Micellar solubilization of fatty acid with bile salt to form micelle
         b) Diffusion of micelle into jejunal cell
         c) Delivery of fatty acids to circulation via lymphatic system
      6) Water-soluble vitamin absorption: all areas of small intestine by passive diffusion (absorption of vitamin B_{12} requires intrinsic factor)
      7) Fat-soluble vitamin absorption: absorbed in jejunum (bile salts required)
      8) Calcium absorption: mainly in duodenum (vitamin D required)
      9) Iron absorption: all areas of the intestine (especially in duodenum) by active transport; stored as protein-bound iron
5. Synthesis
   a. Bacteria in the large intestine produce vitamin K.
   b. Peyer's patches in the small intestine play a role in antibody synthesis.
6. Effect on fluid and electrolyte balance
   a. Gastric losses are acidic; increased gastric losses (e.g., nasogastric suction, vomiting) cause metabolic alkalosis, hypokalemia, hyponatremia, and hypovolemia.
   b. Intestinal losses are alkaline: Increased intestinal losses (e.g., biliary losses, pancreatic fistula, intestinal suction, diarrhea) cause metabolic

acidosis, hypokalemia, hyponatremia, and hypovolemia.

Assessment of the GI System

Interview

1. Chief complaint: why the patient is seeking help and duration of the problem
   a. Nonspecific problems/complaints
      1) Change in appetite
      2) Fatigue or weakness
      3) Unintentional weight loss or weight gain
      4) Fever and chills
   b. Abdominal pain: describe PQRST (Table 7-4)
      1) Provocation: relationship to food, drugs, activity, position, bowel movements, breathing, and stress
      2) Palliation

Table 7-4 Differentiation of Abdominal Pain

Condition	Description of Pain	Associated Signs/Symptoms
Abdominal aortic aneurysm	• Abdominal • Ripping or tearing • May radiate to back	• Pulsatile mass in abdomen • If ruptured, clinical indications of hypoperfusion and shock
Appendicitis	• Epigastric or periumbilical pain; later localizes to RLQ • Dull to sharp • May be referred to right shoulder • McBurney's sign: pain with palpation at McBurney's point (i.e., point at ⅓ the distance between the right anterior iliac crest and the umbilicus) • Rovsing's sign: pain in RLQ with palpation of LLQ indicates peritoneal irritation • Iliopsoas sign: abdominal pain caused by hyperextension of right hip	• Anorexia, nausea, vomiting • Fever • Diarrhea • Leukocytosis • Clinical indications of peritoneal irritation if ruptured
Cholecystitis	• Epigastric or RUQ • Cramping • May be referred to below right scapula • Murphy's sign: pain with deep breath while the nurse palpates under the right costal margin	• Nausea and vomiting especially after fatty foods • Abdominal tenderness in RUQ • Leukocytosis
Diverticulitis	• LUQ • Cramping • Tenderness over descending colon	• Vomiting, diarrhea • Fever, chills • Bloating
Gastritis	• Epigastric or slightly left of midline • May be described as indigestion	• Nausea and vomiting • May have hematemesis • Abdominal tenderness
Intestinal obstruction	• Epigastric or periumbilical • Sharp if small intestine; dull if large intestine	• Change in bowel habits • Melena or hematochezia • Hyperactive to hypoactive bowel sounds
Mesenteric ischemia	• Diffuse midabdominal • Severe	• Nausea and vomiting may occur • Diarrhea or constipation
Pancreatitis	• Epigastric or periumbilical LUQ • Boring; worsened by lying down • May be referred to back, left flank, or left shoulder	• Nausea and vomiting • Mild fever • Abdominal tenderness • May have Cullen's sign (i.e., bluish discoloration at umbilicus) indicating intraperitoneal bleeding or Grey Turner's sign (i.e., bluish discoloration at flanks) indicating retroperitoneal bleeding • May be jaundiced
Peptic ulcer	• Epigastric or RUQ • Gnawing or burning • May be referred to back	• Abdominal tenderness • Hematemesis (gastric) or melena (duodenal) • Clinical indications of peritoneal irritation if perforated
Strangulated hernia	• Localized • Severe • Generalized if bowel obstruction	• Distention if bowel obstruction

a) Ineffective or effective treatments
b) Alleviating factors (e.g., position)
3) Quality: sharp, dull, tearing, cramping, burning, gnawing, stabbing, aching, colicky
a) Visceral pain
i) Dull, poorly localized
ii) May be caused by organic lesions or functional disturbance within the GI tract
b) Somatic pain
i) Sharp, well localized
ii) May be caused by inflammation of abdominal organs which causes peritoneal irritation
c) Referred pain
i) Pain experienced at a distance from the disease process
ii) May be explained by the embryologic origins of the structures involved
4) Region: location
a) May be poorly localized
b) May be referred pain
i) Pain may be felt in a remote area that is supplied by the same nerve as the diseased or damaged organ.
ii) The pain is usually sharp and localized but not over area of injury.
5) Radiation
6) Severity: 0-10 scale
7) Timing: constant, intermittent; duration
c. Abdominal distention
1) Bloating (i.e., subjective feeling of abdominal fullness) versus distention (i.e., objective increase in abdominal girth)
2) Abdominal volume must be increased by at least 1 L for physical enlargement to occur.
d. Change in bowel elimination
1) Change in color of stools
a) Clay-colored stools indicate biliary obstruction.
b) Tarry stools (melena) indicate upper GI bleeding.
c) Bloody stools (hematochezia) indicate lower GI bleeding.
2) Change in consistency or shape of stools
a) Flattened on one side may indicate partial obstruction.
3) Change in frequency of stools
4) Excessive flatus
5) Use of laxative or enemas
6) Relationship to food, drugs, and alcohol
e. Nausea/vomiting
1) Onset and duration
2) Frequency
3) Character and color; presence of blood in vomitus (hematemesis)
4) Palliation
a) Ineffective or effective treatment
b) Alleviating factors
5) Timing
a) Time of day
b) Relationship to food, odors, drugs, alcohol, activity, bowel movements
6) Aggravating factors
7) Associated pain
f. Abdominal trauma
1) Gunshot entrance and exit wound
2) Knife wounds
3) Burns or abrasions
4) Ecchymotic areas associated with blunt trauma
g. Dentition problems
1) Caries
2) Gingivitis
3) Poor-fitting dentures
h. Odynophagia (i.e., painful swallowing)
i. Dysphagia (i.e., difficulty swallowing)
j. Dyspepsia (i.e., impaired digestion): may be manifested by indigestion, nausea, abdominal pain, bloating, belching, and/or early satiety
k. Eructation (i.e., belching)
l. Flatulence
m. Edema
n. Abnormal bruising or bleeding
o. Jaundice
p. Change in color of urine: dark brown or orange urine may indicate biliary obstruction
q. Pruritus
r. Fecal incontinence
s. Rectal bleeding
t. Anal discomfort or pressure
2. History of present illness: Use PQRST format.
3. Past medical history
a. Past illnesses
1) Jaundice
2) Anemia
3) Obesity: use of liquid diets, gastrointestinal bypass, gastric balloon, etc.
4) Eating disorders (e.g., bulimia, anorexia nervosa)
5) Substance abuse
a) Alcohol
b) Drug abuse
c) Chronic drug use of potentially hepatotoxic agents such as acetaminophen
6) Peptic ulcer disease
7) GI hemorrhage
8) Cholelithiasis
9) Hepatic disease
a) Cirrhosis
b) Hepatitis
c) History of blood transfusion
10) Pancreatitis
11) Cancer
12) Irritable bowel syndrome
13) Inflammatory bowel disease (e.g., ulcerative colitis, Crohn's disease, antibiotic-associated colitis, *Clostridium difficile* colitis)

        14) Diverticulitis
        15) Polyps
        16) Hemorrhoids
        17) Renal disease
        18) Cardiovascular disease
        19) Diabetes mellitus
        20) COPD (high incidence of peptic ulcer disease)
    b. Past injury: abdominal trauma
    c. Past surgical procedures
    d. Past diagnostic studies (e.g., endoscopy, x-rays, stool exam for occult blood)
    e. Food intolerances or allergies; type of reaction if allergy
4. Family history
    a. Eating disorders (e.g., obesity, anorexia nervosa, bulimia)
    b. Anemia
    c. Peptic ulcer disease
    d. Pancreatic disease (e.g. pancreatitis, pancreatic cancer)
    e. Diabetes mellitus
    f. Liver disease (e.g., cirrhosis, hepatitis)
    g. Malabsorption syndrome
    h. Inflammatory bowel disease (e.g., ulcerative colitis, Crohn's disease)
    i. Irritable bowel syndrome
    j. Alcoholism
    k. Cancer
5. Social history
    a. Relationship with spouse or significant other; family structure
    b. Occupation
    c. Educational level
    d. Stress level and usual coping mechanisms
    e. Recreational habits
    f. Exercise habits
    g. Dietary habits
        1) Appetite
        2) Usual foods
        3) Number and time of meals and snacks
        4) Fluid intake
        5) Food restrictions
            a) Intolerances
            b) Prescribed restrictions
            c) Religious restrictions
        6) Change in eating habits
    h. Usual bowel habits
    i. Caffeine intake
    j. Tobacco use: Record as pack-years (number of packs per day times the number of years of smoking).
    k. Alcohol use: Record as alcoholic beverages consumed per month, week, or day.
    l. Exposure to toxins or infectious disease
    m. Travel
6. Medication history
    a. Prescribed drugs, dose, frequency, time of last dose
    b. Nonprescribed drugs
        1) Over-the-counter drugs, including herbal drugs and remedies
        2) Substance abuse
    c. Patient understanding of drug actions and side effects
    d. Drugs causing potential problems for patients with gastrointestinal problems
        1) Antibiotics
        2) Aspirin
        3) Nonsteroidal antiinflammatory drugs (NSAIDs) (e.g., ketorolac [Toradol], ibuprofen [Motrin])
        4) Corticosteroids
        5) Acetaminophen (Tylenol)
        6) Many drugs have anorexia, nausea, or vomiting as side effects
        7) Many drugs are hepatotoxic (Box 7-1).
    e. Drugs frequently used for gastrointestinal problems
        1) Antacids, H_2 receptor antagonists, proton pump inhibitors
        2) Stool softeners
        3) Laxatives
        4) Cathartics
        5) Anticholinergics
        6) Corticosteroids
        7) Antidiarrheals
        8) Antiemetics
        9) Tranquilizers
        10) Sedatives
        11) Barbiturates

Vital Signs

1. Blood pressure: a. sitting, lying, standing, especially in hemorrhaging patient; b. systolic BP less than 100 mm Hg and HR greater than 100/min indicates at least a 20% reduction in blood volume
2. Heart rate
3. Respiratory rate
4. Temperature
5. Height
6. Weight
7. Body mass index (BMI): takes into account not just weight but also height to indicate body fat; goal for most people is a BMI of 18-25

Inspection

1. Landmarks (Figure 7-10)
    a. Xiphoid
    b. Costal margin
    c. Midline
    d. Umbilicus
    e. Anterior superior iliac crest
    f. Symphysis pubis
    g. The abdomen may be divided into:
        1) Four quadrants (Figure 7-11): Horizontal and vertical lines intersect at the umbilicus.
        2) Nine regions (Figure 7-12)
2. General survey
    a. Apparent health status
    b. Apparent age relative to chronological age
    c. Level of consciousness

Box 7-1 Hepatotoxic Agents

6-Mercaptopurine (Purinethol)
Acetaminophen (Tylenol)
Acetylsalicylic acid (ASA)
Allopurinol (Zyloprim)
Amiodarone (Cordarone)
Amitriptyline (Elavil)
Ampicillin (Polycillin)
Carbamazepine (Tegretol)
Carbon tetrachloride
Chlorambucil (Leukeran)
Chloramphenicol (Geopen)
Chlordiazepoxide (Librium)
Chlorpromazine (Thorazine)
Chlorpropamide (Diabinese)
Cimetidine (Tagamet)
Clindamycin (Cleocin)
Cyclosporine (Sandimmune)
Dantrolene (Dantrium)
Diazepam (Valium)
Doxepin (Sinequan)
Erythromycin estolate (Ilosone)
Ethanol
Ethrane
Ferrous sulfate
Fluothane
Haloperidol (Haldol)
Halothane
Hydrochlorothiazide (HydroDIURIL)
Imipramine (Tofranil)
Indomethacin (Indocin)
Isoniazid (Isoniazid)
Ketoconazole (Miconazole)
Meprobamate (Equanil)
Methotrexate (Methotrexate)
Methyldopa (Aldomet)
Monoamine oxidase (MAO) inhibitors
Nicotinic acid
Oral contraceptives
Oxacillin (Prostaphlin)
Penicillin (Pen Vee K)
Penthrane
Phenazopyridine (Pyridium)
Phenobarbital (Luminal)
Phenylbutazone (Butazolidin)
Phenytoin (Dilantin)
Probenecid (Benemid)
Prochlorperazine (Compazine)
Promethazine (Phenergan)
Propoxyphene (Darvon)
Propylthiouracil (PTU)
Quinidine
Rifampin (Rifadin)
Sulfonamides (Bactrim, Septra, Gantrisin)
Tetracyclines (Achromycin)
Tolbutamide (Orinase)
Trimethobenzamide (Tigan)
Tripelennamine (Pyribenzamine)

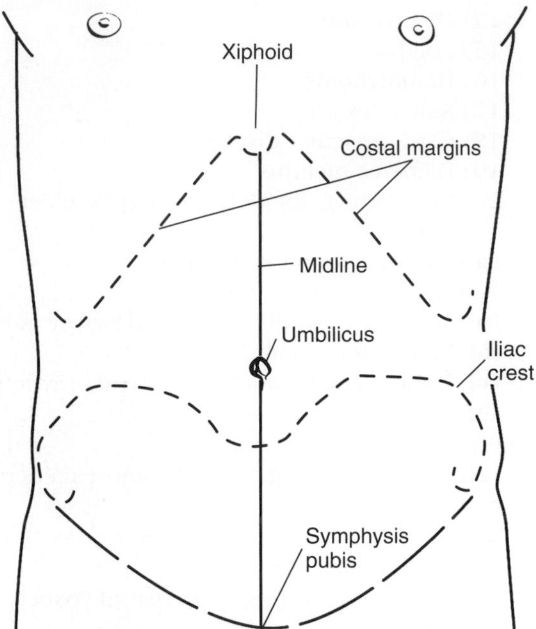

Figure 7-10 Landmarks of the abdomen.

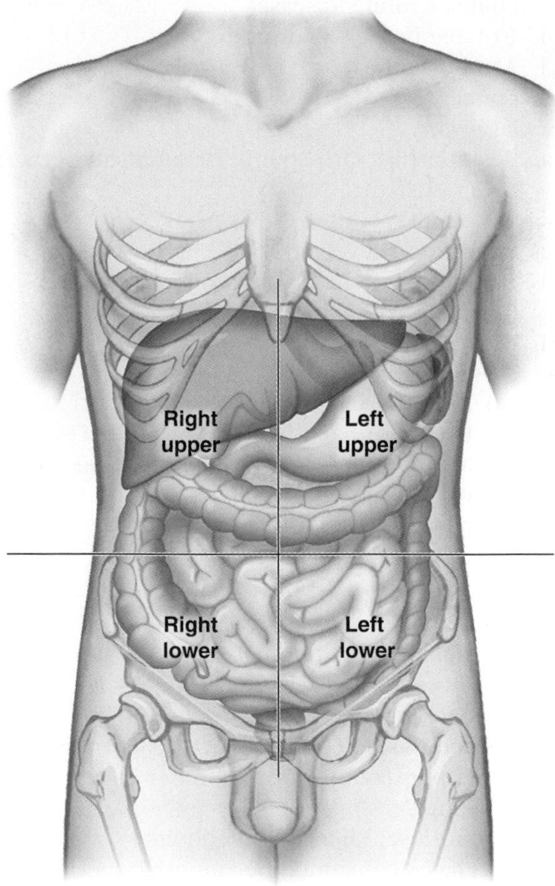

Figure 7-11 The abdomen divided into four quadrants: right upper quadrant (RUQ), left upper quadrant (LUQ), right lower quadrant (RLQ), and left lower quadrant (LLQ). (From Patton, K. T., & Thibodeau, G. A. [2013]. *Anatomy & physiology* [8th ed.]. St Louis: Mosby.)

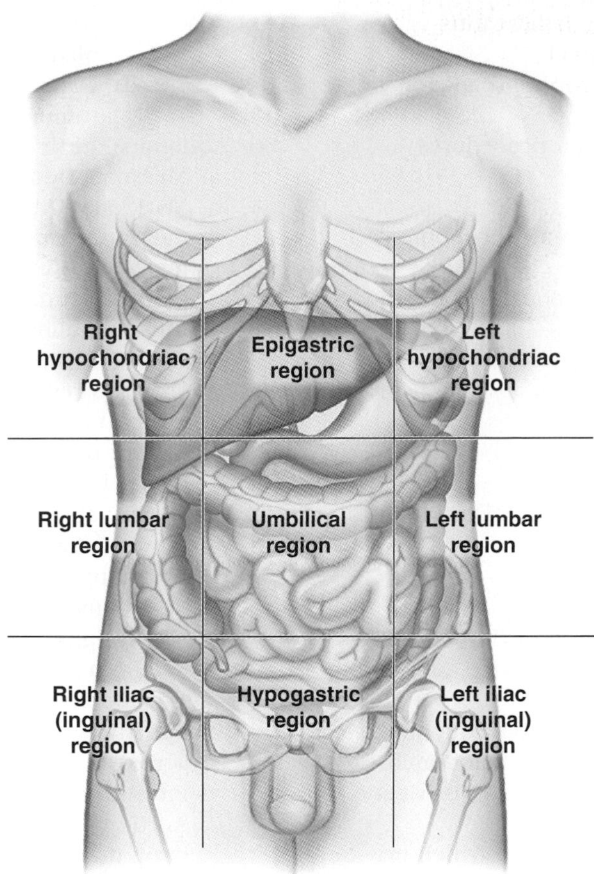

Figure 7-12 The abdomen divided into nine regions: epigastric, umbilical, hypogastric, right and left hypochondriac, right and left lumbar, and right and left iliac (inguinal). (From Patton, K. T., & Thibodeau, G. A. [2013]. *Anatomy & physiology* [8th ed.]. St Louis: Mosby.)

   d. Gross deformity
   e. Nutritional status
   f. Stature/posture
      1) Patient flexing his or her knees to relieve abdominal tension is frequently seen in peritonitis.
      2) Patient leaning forward to relieve abdominal pain is frequently seen in pancreatitis.
   g. Gait
3. Mouth
   a. Lips: color; texture; lesions; swelling; symmetry
   b. Gums: inflammation; retraction; hypertrophy; bleeding; lesions
   c. Teeth: caries; state of repair; occlusion; dentures: fit; gum ulceration caused by ill-fitting dentures
   d. Tongue: swelling; laceration; lesions; coating
   e. Mucosa: moisture; lesions; color
   f. Odor
      1) Fetor hepaticus: sweet fecal odor caused by hepatic failure
      2) Feculent breath: foul fecal odor caused by severe bowel obstruction
      3) Severe halitosis: foul odor may be caused by poor dental hygiene or neoplasms of esophagus or stomach
4. Skin
   a. Color: should be homogeneous over the entire abdomen
      1) Pallor: anemia
      2) Jaundice: occurs when bilirubin is greater than 3 mg/dL; associated with any of the following:
         a) Liver disease
         b) Biliary obstruction
         c) Excessive hemolysis
      3) Bluish: due to infiltration of the abdominal wall with blood
         a) Location
            i) Grey Turner's sign: ecchymosis to flanks indicative of retroperitoneal bleeding (e.g., from pancreas, duodenum, kidneys, vena cava, aorta)
            ii) Cullen's sign: ecchymosis around umbilicus indicative of intraperitoneal bleeding (e.g., liver or spleen)

b) Causes
i) Hemorrhagic pancreatitis
ii) Infarcted bowel
iii) Ruptured ectopic pregnancy

b. Lesions or discoloration
1) Scars: trauma or surgical procedures
2) Striae
a) Usually vertical
b) Initially pinkish or bluish, become silvery with time
c) May be caused by pregnancy, obesity, or ascites
d) Purplish striae may be caused by Cushing's syndrome
3) Rash
4) Ecchymosis
5) Abrasions
6) Spider angioma: may be associated with
a) Vitamin B_{12} deficiency
b) Liver disease
c) Pregnancy
7) Palmar erythema: seen in cirrhosis and hepatic failure

c. Shiny, edematous abdomen
1) Ascites: intraperitoneal fluid frequently associated with cirrhosis, intraabdominal malignancy (e.g., liver, ovarian), or right ventricular failure
2) Anasarca: entire body edema, which may be seen in end-stage heart failure or renal failure

d. Superficial vascularity
1) May be caused by obstruction of inferior vena cava or portal vein
2) Caput medusae: pronounced dilation of the periumbilical veins radiating from the umbilicus; seen in severe portal venous hypertension

e. Stoma: location; color; drainage; condition of peristomal skin

f. Draining wounds: location; drainage; condition of surrounding skin

g. Fistula: location; drainage; condition of surrounding skin

5. Contour of abdomen
a. Profile
1) Normal: flat from xiphoid process to pubic symphysis
2) Scaffold: concave abdomen seen in malnutrition
3) Distention or protuberance
a) Diffuse and symmetrical
i) Fat
ii) Flatus
iii) Fetus (i.e., pregnancy)
iv) Feces (i.e., obstruction)
v) Fluid (i.e., ascites)
vi) Fatal growths (i.e., malignancy)
vii) Fibroids
b) Distention in upper quadrants: gastric dilation; pancreatic cyst, malignancy
c) Distention in lower quadrants: pregnancy; uterine fibroid; distended bladder; ovarian tumor
d) Distention in one quadrant: hernia; tumor; cyst; obstruction; organomegaly

6. Abdominal girth
a. Measure abdominal girth at largest area.
b. Mark on either side of tape measure so that measurements are consistently at same location.
c. One-inch increase is equal to an increase in intraabdominal volume of 500-1000 mL.

7. Weakness of abdominal wall
a. Diastasis recti abdominis: abnormal separation of the two abdominal rectus muscles when the patient tenses abdominal muscles by raising his or her head from the bed
b. Hernia: abdominal, umbilical, or inguinal

8. Movement of abdomen
a. Breathing: normal
1) Women generally breathe thoracically when upright.
2) Both men and women generally breathe abdominally when supine.
b. Peristalsis: abnormal to see waves of peristalsis across the abdomen: generally associated with intestinal obstruction
c. Aortic pulsation: normally visible at the end of expiration in a supine patient especially if patient is thin; pulsatile swelling in the epigastrium suggests an abdominal aortic aneurysm or an epigastric solid tumor overlying the aorta

9. Umbilicus
a. Color
1) Bluish (Cullen's sign): due to infiltration of the abdominal wall with blood
2) Inflammation: may be seen with poor hygiene
b. Contour
1) Deeply inverted: obesity
2) Everted: pregnancy or ascites
3) Nodular (Sister Mary Joseph's nodule): may indicate intraabdominal carcinoma (especially stomach) with metastasis to the navel

Auscultation

1. Auscultation is done prior to percussion or palpation to prevent "stirring up" the abdomen; therefore, order for physical assessment of the abdomen is inspection, auscultation, percussion, palpation.
2. Preparation: may be helpful to put pillow under knees to relax abdominal muscles
3. Bowel sounds
a. Method
1) Use diaphragm with light pressure for 1 minute in each of the four abdominal quadrants.
2) Disconnect nasogastric suction.

   3) If bowel sounds are hypoactive, 5 minutes of auscultation without audible bowel sounds is required before documenting the absence of bowel sounds.
  b. Normal bowel sounds: bubbling or soft gurgling noises heard every 5-20 seconds in an irregular pattern; heard in all quadrants
   1) Return of bowel motility after surgery
    a) Small intestine: 4-24 hours
    b) Stomach: 2-4 days
    c) Colon: 3-7 days
   2) Feeding prior to return of bowel sounds after surgery is now considered safe.
   3) Bowel sounds are not considered an indication of feeding tolerance.
  c. Abnormal bowel sounds
   1) Very infrequent or absent bowel sounds
    a) Functional obstruction: paralytic ileus
    b) Advanced mechanical intestinal obstruction
   2) Loud, hyperactive (but normal pitched) bowel sounds: hyperperistalsis (e.g., diarrhea, catharsis caused by GI bleeding)
   3) High-pitched “rushing” bowel sounds: early mechanical small intestinal obstruction
   4) Low-pitched “rushing” bowel sounds: early mechanical large intestinal obstruction
4. Succussion splash: roll patient side to side while listening over left upper quadrant; indicative of pyloric obstruction
5. Vascular sounds
  a. Method: Use bell over specified areas.
  b. Bruits
   1) Listen over midline and renal and femoral arteries.
   2) If bruit is noted, check circulation to extremities; if decreased blood flow is noted, aneurysm should be suspected.
    a) Notify physician.
    b) Keep patient quiet.
    c) Do not palpate abdomen.
  c. Venous hum: hum of medium tone created by blood flow in a large, engorged vascular organ such as liver or spleen
6. Peritoneal friction rub: scratchy sound heard over inflamed spleen or neoplastic liver

Percussion

1. Percussion tones normally heard over abdomen
  a. Dull: liver, full sigmoid colon, full bladder
  b. Flat: bone
  c. Tympany: gastric bubble, bowel
2. Tests for ascites
  a. Fluid wave: Tap one side of the abdomen and feel for the wave to hit the hand on other side of abdomen; have a colleague or the patient place the ulnar surface of his or her hand at the abdomen's midline to stop skin transmission.
  b. Shifting dullness: Percuss dullness indicating fluid at flanks while patient supine, mark fluid level, turn patient on one side, and note shift of dullness line.
  c. Midline dullness: Dullness at midline with the patient leaning forward in a standing position indicates intraabdominal fluid.
3. Organ borders
  a. Liver (dullness between right lung resonance and bowel tympany)
   1) Normal span 6-12 cm in the right midclavicular line
   2) Enlarged and tender in RVF, hepatitis, mononucleosis
   3) May be large or small in cirrhosis
   4) Absence of liver dullness: may indicate free air in peritoneum from bowel perforation
  b. Spleen (dullness under left diaphragm): if percussible, should be less than 7 cm at the left midaxillary line
  c. Stomach (tympany under left costal margin)
  d. Bladder (dullness above symphysis pubis): percussible only if enlarged
  e. Intestine (tympany over abdomen): may percuss dullness over LLQ if sigmoid colon is full

Palpation

1. Method
  a. Warm hands.
  b. Examine each quadrant.
  c. Always palpate tender areas last.
  d. Carry on conversation with patient to keep him or her (and the abdominal muscles) relaxed, and place a pillow under the knees and a pillow under the head.
2. Light palpation: use fingertips to depress 1-2 cm; note the following:
  a. Temperature
  b. Moisture
  c. Superficial skin reflexes: movement of the umbilicus toward the quadrant that is stroked
  d. Voluntary guarding
   1) Patient may voluntarily splint abdominal muscles, especially when sensitive spot is touched; watch for nonverbal indicators of pain during palpation.
  e. Involuntary guarding or rigidity
   1) Diffuse rigidity suggests an infectious, neoplastic, or inflammatory process in the peritoneal cavity.
   2) Rigid, boardlike abdomen is associated with acute perforation of a viscus with spillage of air or GI contents into the peritoneal cavity.
  f. Tender areas
  g. Large masses
   1) If mass is pulsatile, refrain from additional abdominal palpation because this may be an abdominal aortic aneurysm.
   2) If mass is not pulsatile, describe the following:
    a) Size
    b) Location
    c) Consistency

d) Contour
e) Tenderness
f) Mobility
3. Deep palpation: Use one hand on top of the other to depress 4-5 cm.
a. Do not use deep palpation in the following situations:
1) Polycystic kidneys
2) After renal transplant
3) Malignant tumor: may cause seeding
4) Recent surgery
b. Note the following:
1) Direct tenderness
a) Associated with local inflammation of the abdominal wall, the peritoneum, or a viscus
2) Rebound (or indirect) tenderness (also referred to as *Blumberg's sign*)
a) Performed by pressing into the tender area and then letting go
b) If the pain is exacerbated when pressure is released, rebound tenderness is present and peritoneal inflammation is suspected.
c) Rebound tenderness is especially significant when it occurs at a site away from the area of direct tenderness.
3) Organ size
a) Liver edge: may be palpable
i) Ask patient to take a deep breath; move hand in and up to check for tenderness, smoothness of edge.
(a) Tenderness is frequently caused by hepatitis or engorgement caused by right ventricular failure.
(b) Hard, lumpy liver is associated with cancer or cirrhosis.
ii) A normal size liver may be palpable especially in patients with COPD due to hyperinflation of lungs; hepatomegaly exists only if liver span by percussion is greater than 12 cm.
b) Gallbladder: palpable only if enlarged with stones; if palpable, located under liver edge in right upper quadrant
4) Splenic tenderness
a) Palpate left side of abdomen with patient in lateral decubitus position.
b) Note any tenderness.
c) Spleen is palpable only if significantly enlarged (e.g., injury, leukemia, mononucleosis, portal hypertension).
5) Aortic pulsation: Check for lateral expansion, which may indicate an aneurysm.
4. Ballottement
a. Gentle repetitive bouncing of tissues against the hand
b. May be used to evaluate organ enlargement

Intraabdominal Pressure

1. Definitions
a. Intraabdominal pressure (IAP): the pressure within the abdominal cavity
1) Normal IAP is ~5-7 mm Hg
2) Variations in IAP
a) Position changes
b) Obesity
c) Breathing, mechanical ventilation, PEEP
b. Abdominal perfusion pressure: difference between the MAP and the IAP; greater than 60 mm Hg is desirable
c. Intraabdominal hypertension (IAH): sustained or repeated elevation of IAP greater than or equal to 12 mm Hg
1) Grade I: 12-15 mm Hg
2) Grade II: 16-20 mm Hg
3) Grade III: 21-25 mm Hg
4) Grade IV: greater than 25 mm Hg
d. Abdominal compartment syndrome (ACS): sustained ICP greater than 20 mm Hg that is associated with new organ dysfunction/failure
1) Primary: condition associated with injury or disease in the abdominal-pelvic region
2) Secondary: condition that does not originate from the abdominal-pelvic region
3) Recurrent: condition in which ACS redevelops after previous surgical or medical treatment of primary or secondary ACS
2. Methods of measurement
a. Assist with placement of an access for measuring IAP
1) Via a catheter (e.g., peritoneal dialysis catheter) inserted into peritoneal cavity and attached to a transducer
2) Via a catheter inserted into the sample port of an indwelling urinary catheter and attached to a transducer (Figure 7-13)
a) Accuracy of this method is affected by neurogenic bladder, abdominal packing, elevation of the head of the bed, pelvic fracture or hematoma, and intraperitoneal adhesions.
b. Attach a pressure monitoring system with the air-fluid interface of the transducer leveled to the midaxillary line at the iliac crest (Gallagher, 2010).
c. Place the patient in supine position.
d. After drainage of the bladder, remove air from the system and then instill 25 mL of isotonic sterile saline into the bladder.
e. Allow 30-60 seconds equilibration time after instillation of saline before measurement of pressure.
f. Measure the pressure at end-expiration.
3. Conditions associated with risk for intraabdominal hypertension and abdominal compartment syndrome include the following:
a. Conditions that cause an increase in intraabdominal volume

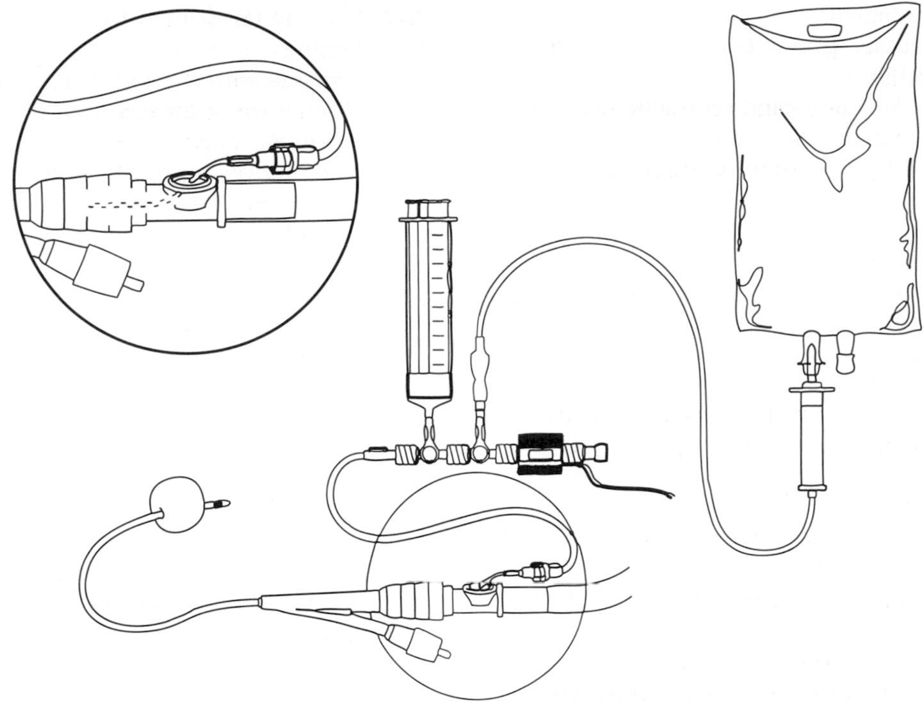

Figure 7-13 Measurement of intraabdominal pressure using an intravenous catheter into the specimen port of the urinary drainage tubing. (From Cheatham, M. L. [1999]. Intra-abdominal hypertension and abdominal compartment syndrome. *New Horizons,* 7[1], 96-115.)

1) Intraabdominal or retroperitoneal masses
2) Ascites or hemoperitoneum
3) Pneumoperitoneum (e.g., laparoscopic procedures)
4) Gastrointestinal tract dilation (e.g., gastroparesis, ileus, volvulus, intestinal obstruction)
5) Abdominal or pelvic trauma
    a) Pelvic fractures
    b) Intraperitoneal or retroperitoneal hemorrhage or hematoma
    c) Visceral edema due to ischemia and/or massive fluid resuscitation
6) Use of military antishock trousers (MAST) or pneumatic antishock garments (PASGs)

b. Conditions that decrease abdominal wall compliance
    1) Abdominal surgery
    2) Abdominal wall bleeding

c. Conditions that affect both intraabdominal volume and abdominal wall compliance
    1) Obesity
    2) Sepsis, severe sepsis, septic shock
    3) Acute pancreatitis
    4) Massive fluid resuscitation
    5) Major burns
    6) Liver or kidney transplantation

4. Clinical implications
    a. A critical level of IAH has not been established: an IAP of 25 mm Hg has been traditionally considered a critical value, although levels as low as 10 mm Hg may cause organ dysfunction.
    b. There is a volume-pressure curve: the abdominal wall can compensate for increases in intraabdominal volume up to a point, then any additional increase in intraabdominal volume results in a rapid increase in IAP and compromised organ perfusion.
    c. Pathophysiologic consequences of intraabdominal hypertension
        1) Cardiovascular
            a) Increased HR
            b) Increased CVP, PAP, PAOP
            c) Increased SVR
            d) Decreased CO/CI
            e) Decreased venous return from extremities
        2) Pulmonary
            a) Increased respiratory rate
            b) Decreased tidal volume, increased $PaCO_2$, decreased PaO_2, SaO_2
            c) Decreased compliance: increased intrathoracic pressure; increased peak inspiratory pressure
            d) Increased intraalveolar fluid
            e) Increased risk of compression atelectasis
        3) Neurologic
            a) Increased intracranial pressure (ICP)
            b) Decreased cerebral perfusion pressure (CPP)
        4) Renal
            a) Decreased glomerular filtration rate and urine output
            b) Urethral compression

5) Gastrointestinal
   a) Decreased portal, celiac, and mesenteric blood flow
      i) Severe mesenteric ischemia may occur and lead to multiple organ dysfunction syndrome (MODS).
   b) Increased intestinal permeability and bacterial translocation that increase risk of sepsis
   c) Increased risk of peptic ulcer
6) Immunology: release of proinflammatory cytokines that may lead to SIRS and MODS
7) Elevated serum lactate, metabolic acidosis

5. Treatment of intraabdominal hypertension and abdominal compartment syndrome
   a. Measure IAP at least every 2-4 hours in patients at risk for IAH; continuous monitoring is indicated for high-risk patients; titrate therapy to maintain IAP less than 15 mm Hg
   b. Optimize hydration status and avoid excessive fluids.
      1) Hypertonic crystalloids and/or colloids to allow expansion of vascular volume without excessive fluid volume
      2) Diuresis, dialysis, and/or ultrafiltration as indicated
      3) Hemodynamic monitoring is recommended to guide fluid administration
   c. Improve abdominal wall compliance.
      1) Head-of-bed elevation at 20 degrees between pressure readings
         a) Avoid prone positioning.
         b) Consider reverse Trendelenburg position.
      2) Encouragement to take deep breaths to prevent atelectasis and facilitate venous return to the heart
      3) Sedation and analgesia; neuromuscular blockade may be considered
      4) Removal of constrictive dressing, binders, eschar
   d. Decompress the GI tract as prescribed
      1) Gastric and/or rectal tube
      2) Prokinetic agents (e.g., metoclopramide, erythromycin)
      3) Slowing or discontinuance of enteral nutrition
      4) Enemas
      5) Colonoscopic decompression
   e. Evaluate and eliminate intraabdominal space-occupying lesions
      1) Abdominal ultrasound or CT scan
      2) Paracentesis if free fluid is cause
      3) Surgical evacuation of hematoma, mass lesion, etc.
   f. Optimize perfusion
      1) Goal-directed fluid resuscitation
      2) Maintenance of abdominal perfusion pressure greater than or equal to 60 mm Hg; fluids, inotropic agents, and/or vasopressors may be necessary
   g. Prepare the patient for decompression laparotomy as requested in symptomatic patients with IAP of greater than or equal to 25 mm Hg or greater than 15 with evidence of organ ischemia.
      1) Surgical approach is most commonly a full midline laparotomy from xiphoid to pubis.
         a) Less invasive procedures such as a subcutaneous linea alba fasciotomy may be used.
      2) Excess fluid, blood, and blood clots are removed.
      3) Recognize that reperfusion washes anaerobic metabolic byproducts from the viscera which may cause hypotension; fluids, mannitol, and sodium bicarbonate may be used prior to and during decompression surgery.
      4) The abdomen is left open after surgery for repair after swelling has subsided (usually within 5-7 days).
         a) Vacuum-assisted closure (VAC) may be used after surgery to continue to reduce edema.

Diagnostic Studies

1. Serum chemistries
   a. Sodium: normal 136-145 mEq/L; elevated in dehydration from severe diarrhea or intestinal obstruction
   b. Potassium: normal 3.5-5.5 mEq/L; decreased in GI losses from upper or lower GI tract
   c. Chloride: normal 96-106 mEq/L
      1) Elevated in dehydration
      2) Decreased in vomiting, diarrhea, or intestinal obstruction
   d. Calcium: normal 8.5-10.5 mg/dL; decreased in acute pancreatitis
   e. Phosphorus: normal 3-4.5 mg/dL
      1) Elevated in intestinal obstruction
      2) Decreased in malnutrition or malabsorption syndromes
   f. Magnesium: normal 1.5-2.2 mEq/L; decreased in chronic diarrhea
   g. Glucose: normal 70-115 mEq/L; elevated in diabetes mellitus, pancreatitis
   h. BUN: normal 5-20 mg/dL
   i. Creatinine: normal 0.7-1.5 mg/dL
   j. Gastrin: normal less than 200 nn/L; elevated in Zollinger-Ellison syndrome (gastrin-producing pancreatic tumor) or G-cell hyperplasia that may cause peptic ulcer disease
   k. Ammonia: byproduct of protein metabolism
      1) Normal 15-110 mOsm/dL
      2) Elevated in hepatic failure, renal failure, heart failure
   l. Iron: normal 50-150 mcg/dL
   m. Iron-binding capacity: 250-410 mcg/dL
   n. Lactate: negative
   o. Carcinoembryonic antigen (CEA): normal less than 2 ng/mL; elevated in cancer of the colon,

lung, pancreas, stomach, breast, head, neck, prostate

p. Bilirubin
   1) Total: normal 0.3-1.3 mg/dL; elevated in hepatic disease, biliary obstruction, or excessive hemolysis
   2) Direct (i.e., conjugated): normal 0.1-0.3 mg/dL; elevated in biliary obstruction
   3) Indirect (i.e., unconjugated): normal 0.1-1.0 mg/dL; elevated in hepatic disease or excessive hemolysis

q. Serum proteins
   1) Total protein: normal 6-8 g/dL
   2) Albumin: normal 3.5-5 g/dL; half-life is 19-20 days, so poor indicator of acute changes in nutritional status
   3) Prealbumin: normal 15-35 mg/dL; half-life is only 2-3 days, so indicates changes in nutritional status better than albumin
   4) Transferrin: normal 250-300 mg/dL; half-life is only 8-10 days, so indicates changes in nutritional status better than albumin
   5) Globulin: normal 1.5-3 g/dL
   6) Albumin/globulin ratio (A/G): normal 1.5/1 to 2.5/1; reverse in chronic hepatitis, chronic liver disease
   7) Fibrinogen: normal 0.1-0.4 g/dL

r. Serum lipids
   1) Cholesterol: normal 150-200 mg/dL
   2) Triglycerides: normal 40-150 mg/dL

s. Pepsinogen: normal 200-425 units/mL
   1) Elevated in hemoconcentration
   2) Decreased in malnutrition or hemorrhage

t. Enzymes
   1) Alkaline phosphatase: normal 30-85 IU/L; elevated in cirrhosis, rheumatoid arthritis, biliary obstruction, liver tumor, hyperparathyroidism
   2) Amylase: normal 56-190 IU/L; elevated in acute pancreatitis, pancreatic cancer, pancreatic pseudocysts, perforated peptic ulcer, mesenteric thrombosis, ectopic pregnancy, renal failure, mumps
   3) Lipase: normal up to 150 units/L; elevated in acute or chronic pancreatitis, duodenal ulcer, biliary obstruction, cirrhosis, hepatitis; stays elevated longer than amylase in pancreatitis
   4) Alanine aminotransferase (ALT): normal 5-36 units/mL
      a) Formerly called *SGPT*
      b) Elevated in hepatitis, cirrhosis, liver tumor, hepatotoxic drugs, cholestasis, infectious mononucleosis
   5) Aspartate aminotransferase (AST): normal 15-45 units/mL
      a) Formerly called *SGOT*
      b) Elevated in hepatitis, cirrhosis, acute pancreatitis, skeletal muscle disease or trauma, liver tumor
   6) Gamma-glutamyl transferase (GGT): normal 5-38 IU/L; elevated in hepatitis, cirrhosis, liver tumor, cholestasis, alcohol ingestion, myocardial infarction
   7) Lactate dehydrogenase (LDH): normal 90-200 IU/L; elevated in hepatitis, hemolytic anemia, pancreatitis, muscular dystrophy, pulmonary infarction, myocardial infarction, pernicious anemia, renal disease

u. Serology for viral hepatitis

2. Hematology
   a. Hematocrit: normal 40-52% for males; 35-47% for females
   b. Hemoglobin: normal 13-18 g/dL for males; 12-16 g/dL for females
   c. White blood cells (WBC): normal 3,500-11,000
      1) Differential: shift to left (increase in bands) indicates acute infection
   d. Erythrocyte sedimentation rate: normal up to 15 mm/hr for males; up to 20 mm/hr for females
3. Clotting profile: may be abnormal in liver disease
   a. Prothrombin time (PT): normal 12-15 seconds; therapeutic 1.5-2.5 times normal
   b. Activated partial thromboplastin time (aPTT): normal 25-38 seconds; therapeutic 1.5-2.5 times normal
   c. Activated clotting time (ACT): normal 70-120 seconds; therapeutic 150-190 seconds
   d. Thrombin time: normal 10-15 seconds
   e. Bleeding time: normal 1-9.5 minutes
   f. International normalized ratio (INR): normal less than 2
   g. Platelets: normal 150,000-400,000/mm^3
4. Urine
   a. Glucose: normal negative
   b. Ketones: normal negative
   c. Amylase: normal negative
   d. Bilirubin: normal negative
   e. Urobilinogen: normal 0.3-3.5 mg/dL
      1) Elevated in hepatocellular disease
      2) Decreased in complete biliary obstruction
   f. Specific gravity: 1.005-1.030
   g. Osmolality: 50-1200 mOsm/liter
5. Gastric contents
   a. Gastric analysis with a nasogastric tube
      1) Histamine or insulin is administered prior to collection of a sample of gastric contents.
      2) Gastric contents are analyzed for the presence of hydrochloric acid.
      3) Have antihistamine (e.g., diphenhydramine [Benadryl]) or 50% dextrose available.
   b. pH determination
      1) Method
         a) Flush nasogastric tube with 20 mL of tap water and then clear tube with air before aspirating.
         b) Do not use the same syringe used to give antacids or H_2 receptor antagonist to obtain the sample for pH testing.

2) Used for the following:
   a) To determine tube placement: stomach pH 1-3, intestine pH 6.5 or greater
   b) To determine effectiveness of H_2 receptor antagonist and/or antacid therapy: pH of 3.5-5 is desirable

6. Stool
   a. Fecal occult blood test: normal negative
   b. Ova, parasites, blood (OPB): normal negative; specimen must be warm
   c. Fecal fat: normal 5 g/24 hr
      1) Elevated in cystic fibrosis, Crohn's disease, biliary tract obstruction, pancreatic duct obstruction
      2) Specimen must be sent to laboratory in a wax-free container.
   d. Pus: normal none
   e. Urobilinogen: normal 0-4 mg/day
      1) Decreased in biliary obstruction
      2) Specimen must be sent to laboratory in a light-resistant container.
   f. Culture: normal intestinal flora
   g. Assay for clostridium difficile toxin A or B: positive is diarrhea is caused *c. difficile*, an opportunistic infection caused primarily by suppression of normal flora by antibiotic therapy
7. Other diagnostic studies (Table 7-5)

GI Drugs (Table 7-6)

Decrease Gastric Acidity and/or Protect Gastric Mucosa

1. Indications: prevention or treatment of peptic ulcer
2. Types of agents and specific actions
   a. Antacids
      1) Examples
         a) Aluminum-magnesium complex (Riopan)
         b) Magnesium hydroxide and aluminum hydroxide (Maalox, Mylanta)
         c) Calcium carbonate (TUMS)
      2) Actions
         a) Buffers gastric acid
         b) Increases pH to decrease the activity of pepsin
   b. Histamine (H_2) receptor antagonists
      1) Examples
         a) Cimetidine (Tagamet)
         b) Ranitidine (Zantac)
         c) Famotidine (Pepcid)
         d) Nizatidine (Axid)
      2) Action: blocks the action of histamine on parietal cells to inhibit volume and concentration of gastric secretions
   c. Proton pump inhibitors
      1) Examples
         a) Omeprazole (Prilosec)
         b) Lansoprazole (Prevacid)
         c) Pantoprazole sodium (Protonix)
      2) Action: inactivate hydrogen pump causing prevention of the formation of hydrochloric acid by parietal cells
   d. Mucosal protectant (prostaglandin E_1-analog)
      1) Example: misoprostol (Cytotec)
      2) Actions
         a) Enhances the body's normal gastric mucosal protective mechanisms
         b) Increases mucosal blood flow
         c) Decreases gastric acid secretion
   e. Mucosal protectant
      1) Example: sucralfate (Carafate)
      2) Actions
         a) Combines with gastric acid and forms an adhesive protective coating over an ulcer crater
         b) Adsorbs pepsin
3. Controversies of prophylaxis
   a. Costs of prophylaxis are considerable, and the number needed to treat to prevent even one case of GI bleeding is significant.
   b. Risks of changing the pH of the gastric secretions
      1) May impair digestion
      2) May impair absorption of drugs normally absorbed in the acid environment of the stomach
      3) May increase the risk of pneumonia: Bacteria that are normally killed in the acid medium of the stomach live, proliferate, and ascend the esophagus and are silently aspirated into the lungs.
   c. Who should probably definitely receive prophylaxis?
      1) Patients already exhibiting GI bleeding (though not technically prophylaxis at this point)
      2) Patients with a history of GI bleeding
      3) Patients with head injury
      4) Patients with burns

GI Hemorrhage

1. Octreotide acetate (Sandostatin)
   a. GI indications
      1) Severe diarrhea associated with carcinoid tumors or vasoactive intestinal peptide tumors
      2) GI bleeding (off-label)
      3) GI or pancreatic fistula (off-label)
      4) After partial pancreatectomy (Whipple procedure) (off-label)
   b. Actions
      1) Inhibits release of vasodilatory hormones to cause vasoconstriction of the viscera and decrease portal vein flow and portal hypertension
      2) Suppresses secretion of serotonin, gastroenteropancreatic peptides, and growth hormones
      3) Stimulates fluid and electrolyte absorption from GI tract and prolongs GI transmit time
2. Vasopressin
   a. GI indication: GI hemorrhage

Table 7-5 Gastrointestinal Diagnostic Studies

Study	Evaluates	Comments

Angiography: celiac or mesenteric	• Evaluates portal vasculature
	• Diagnoses source of gastrointestinal bleeding
	• Evaluates cirrhosis, portal hypertension, vascular damage resulting from trauma, intestinal ischemia, tumors
	• May be used to treat GI bleeding using vasopressin
		• Bowel preparation (e.g., cathartics) as prescribed
		• NPO for 8 hours prior to the study
		• Sedative is usually prescribed prior to the procedure
		• Contrast media used
		  • Check for allergy to iodine prior to the study
		  • Monitor for allergic reaction following procedure
		  • Ensure hydration following procedure
		Postprocedure
		• Keep extremity in which catheter was placed immobilized in a straight position for 6-12 hours
		• Monitor arterial puncture point for hemorrhage or hematoma
		• Monitor neurovascular status of affected limb
		• Monitor for indications of systemic emboli

Barium enema (also called lower GI series) NOTE: Meglumine diatrizoate (Gastrografin) may be used especially if bowel perforation is suspected	• Visualizes the movement, position, and filling of various segments of the colon after instillation of barium by enema • Diagnoses colorectal lesions, diverticulitis, inflammatory bowel disease, strictures, fistulas • Evaluates colon size, length, and patency	• Low-fiber diet for 1-3 days prior to the study • Bowel preparation with bowel irrigation (e.g., GoLYTELY) and cathartics • NPO for 8-12 hours prior to study • Cathartics must be given after study • Contraindicated if bowel perforation or obstruction exists
Barium swallow, upper GI series, and small bowel follow-through NOTE: Ordered according to which area or areas need to be evaluated (e.g., upper GI with small bowel follow-through means stomach, pylorus, duodenum; barium swallow with upper GI means esophagus, stomach, pylorus) NOTE: Meglumine diatrizoate (Gastrografin) may be used especially if bowel perforation is suspected	• Visualizes the position, shape, and activity of the esophagus, stomach, duodenum, and jejunum • Diagnoses esophageal lesions, varices, or esophageal motility disorders, hiatal hernia, gastric ulcers and tumors, small bowel obstruction, small bowel lesions, Crohn's disease • Evaluates gastric and small bowel motility	• Bowel preparation with bowel irrigation (e.g., GoLYTELY) and cathartics • NPO for 8-12 hours prior to study • Cathartics must be given after study • Contraindicated if bowel perforation or obstruction exists

Cholecystography (oral, intravenous, percutaneous transhepatic, or common bile duct)	• Assesses gallbladder function, patency of the biliary system, and presence of gallstones
	• Diagnoses extrahepatic or intrahepatic jaundice, biliary calculi, biliary obstruction, common bile duct injury
		• Percutaneous transhepatic cholangiography is contraindicated in patients with bleeding disorders
		• Fatty meal the day before the study, but the evening meal is fat free
		• Enema may be given the evening prior to the study
		• NPO 8-12 hours prior to the study
		• Contrast medium is administered orally the evening prior to the study, administered intravenously immediately prior to the study, injected percutaneously into the bile duct, or injected directly into the common bile duct during surgery
		  • Check for allergy to iodine prior to the study
		  • Monitor for allergic reaction following procedure
		  • Ensure hydration following procedure
		• Monitor for clinical indications of bile leakage, hemorrhage, or peritonitis after percutaneous transhepatic cholangiography

Continued

Table 7-5 Gastrointestinal Diagnostic Studies—cont'd

Study	Evaluates	Comments

Computed tomographic (CT) scan of abdomen	• Diagnoses tumors, pancreatic cancer or cysts, pancreatitis, biliary tract disorders, obstruction versus nonobstructive jaundice, cirrhosis, liver metastases, ascites, lymph node metastases, aneurysm
	• Evaluates vasculature and focal points found on nuclear scans
	• Used to direct biopsy of tumors or aspiration of abscess
		• No special preparation required
		• If contrast medium is used:
		  • Check for allergy to iodine prior to the study
		  • Monitor for allergic reaction postprocedure
		  • Ensure hydration postprocedure

Endoscopic retrograde cholangiopancreatography (ERCP)	• Diagnoses biliary stones, ductal stricture, ductal compression, neoplasms of the pancreas and biliary system • Evaluates patency of biliary and pancreatic ducts, jaundice, pancreatitis, cholecystitis, hepatitis	• Same as for esophagogastroduodenoscopy • Contraindicated if patient is uncooperative or if bilirubin is greater than 3.5 mg/dL • Monitor for clinical indications of pancreatitis (most common complication) after study • Monitor for clinical indications of sepsis
Endoscopy • Esophagogastro-duodenoscopy • Colonoscopy • Proctosigmoidoscopy	• Directly visualizes mucosa of areas of the GI tract • Esophagogastroduodenoscopy can be extended to visualize the pancreas and gallbladder • Esophagogastroduodenoscopy is used to diagnose esophagitis, esophageal ulcers, esophageal strictures, esophageal varices, hiatal hernia, gastritis, gastric ulcers, pyloric obstruction, pernicious anemia, foreign bodies, duodenal inflammation or ulcers and to evaluate esophageal or gastric motility, bleeding, lesions, status of surgical anastomoses • Esophagoscopy, gastroscopy may also be used therapeutically for sclerosis of varices • Proctosigmoidoscopy diagnoses rectosigmoid cancer, strictures, polyps, inflammatory processes, hemorrhoids and evaluates bleeding from rectosigmoid, surgical anastomoses • Colonoscopy diagnoses diverticular disease, obstruction, strictures, radiation injury, polyps, neoplasms, bleeding, ischemia • Colonoscopy or sigmoidoscopy may be used therapeutically for removal of polyps • Biopsies may be taken during any endoscopy	• Sedation may be prescribed, especially for colonoscopy • Bowel preparation with gastric irrigation (e.g., GoLYTELY) and cathartics required before lower GI endoscopy • NPO 4-8 hours prior to study • Keep NPO until gag reflex returns if sedation used • Monitor closely after procedure for clinical indications of perforation or hemorrhage

Table 7-5 Gastrointestinal Diagnostic Studies—cont'd

Study	Evaluates	Comments
Flat plate of abdomen (may also be referred to as *KUB*)	• Diagnoses perforated viscus, paralytic ileus, mechanical obstruction, intraabdominal mass • Evaluates the distribution of visceral gas (and identifies free air in the peritoneum indicative of bowel perforation) • Evaluates organ size	• No preparation required

Liver biopsy	• Obtains tissue specimen for microscopic evaluation
	• Diagnoses liver disease or malignancy
		• May be performed open or closed
		  • Open is done in surgery
		  • Closed biopsy may be done at bedside
		• Clotting profile is evaluated preprocedure
		  • Closed biopsy is contraindicated if platelet count is less than 100,000/mm^3
		• Patient must be cooperative because he or she must take a deep breath and hold for closed biopsy
		• Type and crossmatch for two units of blood preprocedure
		• NPO for 4-8 hours before study
		Postprocedure
		• Position patient on right side for 2 hours
		• Pressure dressing is applied, and the patient is on bed rest for 24 hours
		• Observe for:
		  • Hemorrhage: hypotension or dyspnea (subphrenic hematoma)
		  • Pneumothorax: dyspnea; chest pain; diminished breath sounds on right; hypoxemia
		  • Sepsis: fever; leukocytosis; rebound tenderness

Liver scan	• Diagnoses cirrhosis, hepatitis, tumors, abscesses, cysts, tuberculosis	• No preparation required
Magnetic resonance imaging (MRI)	• Evaluates liver, biliary tree, pancreas, spleen • Differentiation between cyst and solid mass • Diagnoses hepatic metastasis • Evaluates abscesses, fistulas, source of GI bleeding • Used for staging of colorectal cancer	• Cannot be used in patients with any implanted metallic device, including pacemakers • No special preparation required • Cannot be done on a patient being mechanically ventilated • Must be able to lie flat and still for ~30-60 minutes during the scan; sedation may be necessary
Paracentesis	• Analysis of fluid removed during peritoneal tap • Diagnoses intraperitoneal bleeding with diagnostic peritoneal lavage	• Monitor for peritoneal leakage after tap • Monitor for clinical indications of infection or peritonitis after tap
Percutaneous transhepatic cholangiography	• Diagnoses extrahepatic or intrahepatic jaundice, biliary calculi, bile duct obstruction, bile duct injury • Evaluates the patency of the biliary ductal system	• Contraindicated in uncorrected coagulopathy, allergy to iodine, severe ascites, cholangitis • Monitor closely for clinical indications of bleeding or peritonitis
Percutaneous transhepatic portography	• Diagnoses esophageal varices and visualizes portal venous circulation	• As for angiography

Continued

Table 7-5 Gastrointestinal Diagnostic Studies—cont'd

Study	Evaluates	Comments
Radionuclide imaging (hepatobiliary scintigraphy) • HIDA scan • PIPIDA scan	• Diagnoses hepatocellular disease, hepatic metastasis, biliary disease, lower GI bleeding, gastric reflux	• NPO 2 hours prior to study • Must be able to lie flat and still for 60 minutes during the scan
Schilling test	• Evaluates ileal absorption of vitamin B_{12} • Diagnoses pernicious anemia caused by intrinsic factor and inadequate ileal absorption of intrinsic factor-vitamin B_{12} complex	• IM vitamin B_{12} and oral radioactive B_{12} are given and 24-hour urine specimen is collected
Ultrasound of abdomen	• Evaluates the pancreas, biliary ducts, gallbladder, liver • Identifies tumor, abdominal abscesses, hepatocellular disease, splenomegaly, pancreatic or splenic cysts • Differentiates obstructive from nonobstructive jaundice	• All barium must have been cleared from the GI tract prior to ultrasonography • NPO for 8 hours prior to study • If for evaluation of gallbladder: fat-free meal the evening prior to study • Must be able to lie flat and still for 30 minutes during the procedure

b. Actions: constricts mesenteric arterioles and decreases portal circulation and pressure

Malnutrition

Definitions

1. Malnutrition: Dietary intake of essential nutrients is insufficient to meet the metabolic demands of the body.
   a. Macronutrients: carbohydrate (CHO); protein; fat
   b. Micronutrients: vitamins; minerals; water
2. Types of malnutrition
   a. Marasmus: gradual wasting of body fat and somatic muscle with preservation of visceral proteins as seen in prolonged starvation and chronic illness
   b. Kwashiorkor: visceral protein wasting with preservation of fat and somatic muscle as seen in poverty; the patient may appear well-nourished, overweight, or obese, and edema may be present
   c. Mixed marasmus and kwashiorkor: type most commonly seen in hospitalized patients and associated with the highest mortality and morbidity

Etiology

1. Decreased nutrient intake
   a. Recent weight loss
   b. Recent change in diet; fad or limited diet
   c. Eating disorder (e.g., obesity, bulimia, anorexia nervosa). NOTE: Obesity is not the same as overnourished, and many obese patients are protein malnourished.
   d. Anorexia
   e. Nausea
   f. Difficulty chewing or swallowing (e.g., stomatitis, dysphagia)
   g. Depression
   h. Alcoholism or drug addiction
   i. Social history of poverty, disability, living alone
   j. Loss of the sense of taste or smell
   k. Use of drugs known to alter dietary intake or food utilization (e.g., antacids, antibiotics, laxatives, antineoplastics)
2. Decreased absorption
   a. Diseases of the GI tract
   b. Malabsorptions (e.g., diarrhea, steatorrhea)
   c. Parasites
   d. Pernicious anemia
   e. Intestinal bypass or resection
   f. Drugs (e.g., antacids, cholestyramine, neomycin, alcohol)
3. Increased nutrient losses
   a. Recurrent vomiting, diarrhea
   b. GI disease such as peritonitis, inflammatory bowel disease
   c. Diabetes mellitus
   d. Hemorrhage
   e. Peritoneal dialysis or hemodialysis
4. Increased nutrient requirements
   a. Recent surgery or trauma
   b. Chronic illnesses such as malignancy or renal, liver, lung, or heart disease or diabetes mellitus
   c. Prolonged hypercatabolic state (e.g., multiple trauma, major surgery, sepsis, burns)
   d. Hyperthyroidism
   e. Hypoxia
5. Nosocomial malnutrition: related to mismanagement or inattention to nutritional requirements of hospitalized patients

Table 7-6 Selected GI Drugs

Drug	Administration	Adverse Effects	Nursing Implications
Octreotide acetate (Sandostatin)	For GI hemorrhage • SC:50-150 mcg bid or tid • IV injection (for GI bleeding): 25-50 mcg followed by IV infusion • IV infusion (for GI bleeding): 25-50 mcg/hr for 48 hours	• Crthostatic hypotension • Anorexia, nausea, vomiting, abdominal pain • Diarrhea, constipation, steatorrhea • Abdominal bloating, flatulence • Increase in liver enzymes • Anxiety • Dizziness • Drowsiness • Heartburn • Hypoglycemia or hyperglycemia • Rectal spasm	• Monitor HR, BP • Monitor for GI complaints and/or bleeding and serum glucose • Note contraindication: known hypersensitivity • Note that this drug is tolerated better than vasopressin for GI bleeding especially in patients with CAD • Note pain or burning at injection site • Do not administer if precipitation or discoloration occurs
Prototype PPI Pantoprazole sodium (Protonix)	• IV injection: 40 or 80 mg over 2 minutes; may also be diluted in 100 mL and infused over 15 minutes; followed by infusion • IV infusion: 8 mg/hr • PO: 40 mg twice daily	• Headache • Diarrhea, abdominal pain, flatulence • Rash • Hyperglycemia	• Monitor for GI complaints and/or bleeding and serum glucose • Note contraindications: known hypersensitivity
Prototype H_2 receptor antagonist Ranitidine (Zantac)	• PO: 150 mg once or twice daily or 300 mg at bedtime • IM: 50 mg every 6-8 hours • IV injection: 50 mg in 20 mL slowly every 6-8 hours or 50 mg in 100 mL over 15-20 minutes • IV infusion: mix 300 mg in 250 mL (1.2 mg/mL); usual dose 6.25-12.5 mg/hr	• Dizziness • Elevated liver enzymes, hepatotoxicity • Headache • Malaise	• Monitor HR, BP, liver enzymes, gastric pH • pH is maintained at 3.5 or greater • Note contraindications: known hypersensitivity • Use cautiously in liver disease, renal disease
Vasopressin (Pitressin)	For GI hemorrhage • IV infusion: mix 100 units/100 mL (1 IU/mL) and administer at 0.1-0.8 IU/min (concurrent nitroglycerin is recommended with doses higher than 0.4 IU/min) • Administer through central venous catheter	• Bradycardia • Hypertension • Fever • Water intoxication (SIADH), hyponatremia • Nausea, abdominal cramps • Tremor • Headache • Seizures • Coma • Constriction of cardiac arteries, resulting in chest pain and myocardial ischemia	• Monitor HR, BP, daily weight, serum sodium • Note contraindications: known hypersensitivity, nephritis • Use cautiously in coronary artery disease • Administer NTG as prescribed concurrently with IV vasopressin infusion to prevent potential complications related to cardiac ischemia • Prevent extravasation because necrosis may occur; treat with phentolamine (Regitine)

a. NPO status for diagnostic studies or postoperatively
b. Feedings not advanced
c. Wait and see
  1) If appetite improves
  2) If nausea, vomiting resolves
  3) If ileus resolves

Pathophysiology

1. Atrophy of mucosal cells in the small bowel can occur in as little as 72 hours without nutrient intake in individuals with even minor acute illness or injury; this cell atrophy is a major facilitator for bacterial translocation, a common cause of sepsis and MODS in critically ill patients.

2. Inadequate calories cause glycogenolysis and gluconeogenesis.
3. Stress of critical illness; stress hormones cortisol and glucagon have catabolic functions
   a. Hypermetabolism
   b. Glycogenolysis with increased glucose utilization
   c. Gluconeogenesis with increased protein and fatty acid utilization
   d. Insulin resistance
   e. Depletion of lean body tissue
4. Glycogenolysis, gluconeogenesis, and stress hormones all lead to hyperglycemia.
   a. Level of serum glucose is related to the degree of illness/injury.
   b. Hyperglycemia requires treatment with insulin to keep serum glucose within normal levels because hyperglycemia interferes with immune function.
5. Malnutrition causes immunodeficiency, poor wound healing, or eventually organ failure.

Clinical Presentation

1. Subjective
   a. Anorexia
   b. Diarrhea
   c. Weakness, fatigue, apathy
   d. Irritability
   e. Headache
2. Objective
   a. Dull, brittle, dry hair, hair loss
   b. Integumentary changes
      1) Pale, dry, flaky skin
      2) Poor skin turgor
      3) Poor wound healing
      4) Peripheral edema
      5) Transverse ridging of fingernails
   c. Oral changes
      1) Fissures at angles of lips (cheilosis)
      2) Hyperemic tongue; papillae may be hypertrophic or atrophic
      3) Gum and teeth problems: loss of teeth; dental caries; bleeding or receding gums
   d. Muscle wasting
   e. Ascites
   f. Hepatomegaly, splenomegaly
   g. Neurologic changes
      1) Altered mental status
      2) Loss of balance and coordination
   h. Weight loss
      1) Degrees of loss: 10% loss significant; 20% loss indicates malnutrition
      2) Loss of more than 1 kg/week associated with primarily protein loss
      3) Body mass index (BMI)
         a) Formula: Weight (kg)/Ht (m) × Ht (m)
         b) Optimal: 20-25
         c) Obesity: greater than 25
         d) Underweight: less than 20
   i. Diminished skinfold and arm circumference measurement (rarely used in critical care)
      1) Triceps skinfold
         a) Measurement of skinfold thickness with calipers
         b) Reflects measurement of the subcutaneous fat reserves of the body; normal 7.5-16.5 mm; less than 3 mm indicates severely depleted fat stores
      2) Midarm muscle circumference
         a) Measurement of middle of upper nondominant arm
         b) Reflects measurement of body's muscle stores
3. Diagnostics
   a. Visceral protein measurements
      1) Albumin: decreased
         a) Reflects changes in nutritional status slowly because half-life 10-20 days
            i) Normal: 3.5-5 g/dL
            ii) Mild depletion: 2.8-3.4 g/dL
            iii) Moderate depletion: 2.1-2.7 g/dL
            iv) Severe depletion: less than 2.1 g/dL
         b) May be secondary to liver disease, nephrotic syndrome, hypercatabolism
         c) May reflect overhydration
      2) Prealbumin: decreased
         a) More reliable than albumin for monitoring overall protein status in acute care setting; half-life 24 hours
      3) Transferrin: decreased; half-life 8-10 days
      4) Retinol-binding protein: decreased; half-life 10 hours; decreases with even minor stress; significance not fully understood
      5) Hemoglobin/hematocrit: may be decreased
      6) Tests for immunocompetence
         a) Total lymphocyte count (TLC): decreased
            i) Formula: TLC = WBC (in mm^3) × % of lymphocytes
               (a) Normal: 1500 to $2500/mm^3$
               (b) Mild depletion: less than $1500/mm^3$
               (c) Moderate depletion: less than $1200/mm^3$
               (d) Severe depletion: less than $800/mm^3$
            ii) May be decreased by stress, steroids, renal failure
            iii) May be increased by infection, leukemia, myeloma
         b) Cell-mediated immunity: skin tests for the following:
            i) *Candida albicans*
            ii) Mumps
            iii) Purified protein derivative (PPD) of tuberculin

b. Somatic (skeletal) protein measurements
   1) Midarm muscle circumference
   2) 24-hour urine specimen for creatinine
c. Nitrogen balance study may show negative nitrogen balance.
   1) Requires 24-hour dietary record to evaluate nitrogen intake and 24-hour urine collection to measure urine urea nitrogen and evaluate nitrogen loss
   2) Reliable only when renal function is normal

Collaborative Management

1. Prevent/detect negative nitrogen balance and malnutrition.
   a. Weigh daily at same time, and on same scale.
   b. Monitor diagnostic studies reflective of visceral protein stores (e.g., albumin, transferrin, prealbumin).
2. Ensure delivery of adequate and appropriate nutrients.
   a. Indication for nutritional support: when the patient is required to be NPO for greater than 5 days or if patient is unable to meet nutritional needs with oral feedings
      1) Note that 1 L of 5% dextrose provides only 170 kcal; while this provides fluids and delays gluconeogenesis for a short period of time, catabolism occurs after approximately 5 days at basal metabolic rate and earlier in a hypermetabolic patient.
   b. Nutritional support within 48 hours of injury or critical illness may lessen the hypercatabolic state; nutritional support does the following:
      1) Promotes anabolism to prevent negative nitrogen balance and loss of visceral and somatic protein stores
      2) Provides needed nutrients for cellular energy
      3) Supports healing and the immune system
      4) Enhances feeling of well-being
   c. Calculation of nutritional requirements
      1) Protein
         a) Basal protein requirement is 0.8 grams/kg/day.
         b) Most critically ill patients require approximately 1.5 g/kg/day.
         c) Patients with direct protein loss (e.g., crush injuries, burns, hemorrhage) require 2-3 g/kg/day.
         d) Note that too much protein is associated with azotemia.
      2) Calories: 25-80 kcal/kg/day; varies according to age, activity level, metabolic rate, nutritional status, severity of illness, and other factors
         a) Basal or minimal illness: 25 kcal/kg/day
         b) Moderate illness: 35 kcal/kg/day
         c) Sepsis or extensive trauma: 45 kcal/kg/day
         d) Burns: 80 kcal/kg/day
         e) Note that overfeeding is associated with electrolyte imbalance, especially hypophosphatemia.
      3) Fluids: 25-35 mL/kg/day with an additional 150 mL/day for each degree of body temperature above 37° C
   d. Distribution of nutrients to ensure adequate nonprotein calories to prevent the protein catabolism
      1) Protein: 15-20%
      2) CHO: 50-60%
      3) Fats: 20-30%
         a) Note that propofol (Diprivan) is delivered in a 10% lipid emulsion vehicle, and these fat calories need to be included in total calorie allotments; consult with the dietitian regarding the amount of propofol that the patient is receiving in a 24-hour period so that these fat calories are included in the nutritional support plan.
   e. Specialty supplements and effects
      1) Glutamine
         a) Nonessential neutral amino acid that plays an important role in maintaining normal intestinal structure and function; may be "conditionally" essential in critical illness
         b) Provision of glutamine to stressed patients is thought to support the integrity of the gut and decrease the rate of protein catabolism.
            i) Glutamine deficiency causes gut mucosal atrophy and eventually intestinal necrosis leading to bacterial translocation and sepsis.
            ii) Glutamine supplementation provides enterocytes their preferred energy source and prevents gut-induced SIRS.
         c) Use of glutamine in patients with intracranial pathology is questionable, especially if seizures are occurring, because glutamine is a predominant stimulatory neurotransmitter.
      2) Arginine
         a) Semiessential amino acid
         b) Provision of arginine is thought to do the following:
            i) Promote nitrogen retention
            ii) Improve protein turnover
            iii) Improve wound healing
            iv) Enhance immune function
            v) Aid in production of nitric oxide, a potent regulator of vascular tone and cardiac contractility
         c) Arginine supplementation reduces the risk of infection and sepsis and promotes wound healing.
      3) Nucleotides
         a) Have a role in energy transfer

b) Provision of nucleotides enhances natural killer (NK) cell activity and supports growth and function of metabolically active cells, such as lymphocytes and macrophages.

4) Branched-chain amino acids: leucine, isoleucine, valine
   a) Have beneficial effects on nitrogen balance in patients under stress
   b) These are especially helpful in patients with hepatic failure or encephalopathy, but temporary lowering of daily protein intake is likely to produce the same effect.
5) Medium-chain triglycerides (MCT)
   a) These are less irritating and more easily absorbed by the small bowel mucosa.
   b) They may be better than long-chain triglycerides (LCT) for patients with compromised GI function, SIRS, or sepsis.
6) Essential polyunsaturated fatty acids (PUFAs): omega-6 (e.g., linoleic acid) and omega-3 (e.g., α-linolenic acid) fatty acids: aid in efficient functioning of the immune system
7) Dipeptide/tripeptide formulas: may be used for patients with malabsorption (e.g., severe Crohn's disease, bowel edema, inflammation, or ischemia)

f. Administer nutritional support either enterally or parenterally (Figure 7-14).
g. Administer enteral nutritional support (Table 7-7) to patients with a functioning GI tract requiring nutritional support; remember "if the gut works, use it."
h. Administer parenteral nutritional support (Table 7-8 on page 514) to patients without a functioning GI tract requiring nutritional support; may also be used with oral or enteral nutrition to increase the amount of nutrients provided in hypermetabolic patients
i. Ensure a smooth transition from enteral or parenteral feedings to oral nutrition.
   1) Consult with the dietitian and the physician regarding plans for this transition.
      a) Parenteral to enteral feeding: TPN rate is cut in half when one half to one third of the patient's total caloric requirements are met by enteral feeding and discontinued when total caloric requirements are met by enteral feedings.
      b) Parenteral to oral diet
         i) Start with clear liquids and advance to full liquids while observing for aspiration.
         ii) Advance to solid food after 2-3 days of liquids and decrease TPN by one half if at least 500 kcal is consumed.
         iii) Discontinue nutritional support when the patient is able to tolerate sufficient oral nutrition for 2 to 3 days.
         iv) High-protein and high-calorie drinks, shakes, and puddings may be used as nutritional supplements to augment small, frequent meals.
      c) Enteral to oral diet
         i) Monitor oral intake and utilize nutritional supplements to boost caloric intake if needed.
         ii) Cyclic enteral feeding may be considered if calorie intake is consistently inadequate; usually administered at night
   2) Continue to monitor daily weight and food intake during transition times.

3. Provide frequent oral hygiene; teeth should be brushed before meals to avoid aspiration of harmful bacteria.
4. Prevent skin breakdown.
   a. Monitor for changes in edema.
   b. Keep skin clean and dry.
   c. Turn every 2 hours and use special mattresses as indicated.

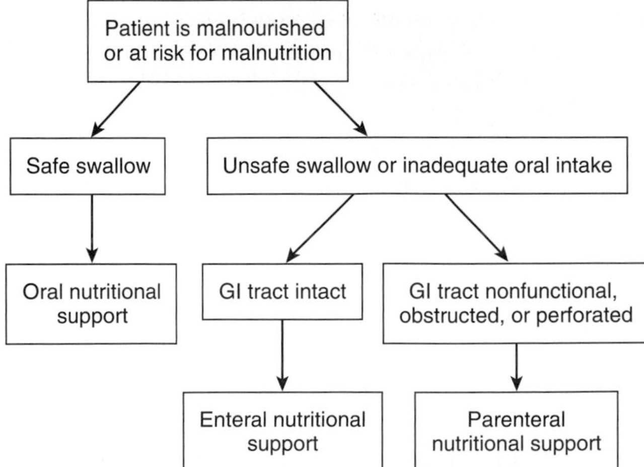

Figure 7-14 Nutritional support options. (Adapted from Manuel, A., & Maynard, N. D. [2009]. *Nutritional support*. Retrieved November 1, 2011, from *http://www.medscape.com/viewarticle/703713*)

Upper GI Hemorrhage

Definitions

1. Peptic ulcer: a sharply defined erosion in mucosa, which may involve the submucosa and muscular layers of the esophagus (~5%), stomach (~15%), or duodenum (~80%)
2. Esophageal varices: dilation of the submucosal esophageal veins
3. Mallory-Weiss tear: acute longitudinal tear of the esophagus caused by forceful retching
4. Gastritis: a generalized inflammation of the gastric mucosa

Text continued on p. 513

Table 7-7 Enteral Nutritional Support

Consideration	Comments
Indication	Patient has functioning GI tract but unable to consume adequate nutrients

Advantages	• Preferred route for patients with functional GI tract
	  • Maintenance of gut structure and absorptive ability
	  • Reduced incidence of sepsis by prevention of translocation of GI bacteria into blood or lymph
	  • Fewer complications than parenteral route
	  • Lower cost than parenteral route
	  • Early enteral

Disadvantages	• Decreased gastric and intestinal motility often accompanies critical illness and may lead to an inability to achieve adequate caloric intake as well as increase the risk of gastroesophageal reflux with resultant aspiration

Contraindications	• Absolute contraindications
	  • Diffuse peritonitis
	  • Intestinal obstruction
	    — Functional obstruction (e.g., paralytic ileus)
	    — Structural obstruction (e.g., tumor, volvulus, adhesion)
	  • Intestinal perforation
	• Relative contraindications
	  • Gastrointestinal ischemia
	  • Enterocutaneous fistula
	  • Severe acute pancreatitis especially if hemorrhagic
	• Severe malabsorption

Routes and choice of tubes	Routes
	• Gastric
	  • Advantages
	    — Maintains natural bactericidal quality of acid environment
	    — Provides some protection from stress ulceration
	  • Disadvantage: increases risk of aspiration especially in patients with gastric atony, which is common in critically ill patients
	    — Percutaneous endoscopic gastrostomy (PEG) may decrease this risk since the tube does not cause gastroesophageal sphincter incompetence
	• Intestinal
	  • Advantage: reduces risk of gastroesophageal regurgitation and microaspiration of gastric contents
	  • Disadvantage: placing tube is frequently difficult because critically ill patients frequently have delayed gastric motility; placement methods may include the following:
	    — Blind insertion
	      • Turn patient to right side and twist tube during advancement after gastric confirmation
	      • Air insufflation technique: instillation of 350-500 mL of air into the stomach
	      • Use of metoclopramide (Reglan)
	    — Fluoroscopic or endoscopic placement (e.g., percutaneous endoscopic jejunostomy [PEJ])
	    — Surgical (needle jejunostomy tube)
	Choice
	• Small-gauge tube that is placed below the gastroesophageal sphincter (such as percutaneous endoscopic gastrostomy [PEG]) tube or jejunostomy tube [including needle jejunostomy which may be done at the conclusion of a laparotomy] is preferred, especially in patients with potential for impaired gastric motility and high risk of aspiration (Bourgault et al., 2007)
	• Short-term (less than 6 weeks)
	  • Nasogastric or orogastric tube
	  • Nasointestinal or orointestinal tube (this may be advanced to the duodenum or jejunum)
	  • Needle jejunostomy
	• Long-term (greater than 6 weeks)
	  • Gastrostomy
	  • Jejunostomy

Continued

Table 7-7 Enteral Nutritional Support—cont'd

Consideration	Comments

Types of formulas	• Monomeric (also referred to as *elemental*) diets (e.g., Vivonex, Vivonex HN, Criticare HN, Vital HN, Travasorb NH, Impact, Stresstein) contain predigested nutrients: required when feeding is delivered distal to presence of digestive enzymes (distal jejunum); hyperosmolar
	• Polymeric formulas contain intact protein and require a functional GI system
	  • Intact protein and lactose-free enteral diets (e.g., Sustacal, Ensure, Enrich, Osmolite)
	  • Intact protein, lactose-free, high-density enteral diets (e.g., Magnacal, Isocal HCN, Sustacal HC, Ensure Plus, Ensure Plus HN)
	  • Blenderized meat-based enteral diets (e.g., Vitaneed, Compleat B)
	  • Specialized enteral diets
	    — Immune-boosting formulas (e.g., Immune-Aid, Impact, Perative, Replete): contain glutamine, arginine, and/or nucleotides
	    — Trauma (e.g., TraumaCal, Traum-Aid HBC, Vivonex TEN)
	    — Hepatic (e.g., Travasorb Hepatic, Hepatic-Aid): increased branched-chain amino acids
	    — Pulmonary (e.g., Pulmocare): higher proportion of fats, less CHO to reduce CO_2 production
	    — Renal (e.g., Travasorb Renal, Amin-Aid): essential amino acids
	    — Diabetic (e.g., Glucerna, Suplena)
	    — Fiber-containing formulas (e.g., Ensure with fiber, Jevity, Sustacal with fiber)
	• Modular
	  • CHO (e.g., Polycose, Nutrisource Modular System [carbohydrate])
	  • Protein (e.g., ProMod, Nutrisource Modular System [protein])
	  • Lipid-Medium Chain Triglycerides (e.g., MCT oil, Nutrisource Modular System [lipid])
	  • Lipid-Long Chain Triglycerides (e.g., Nutrisource Modular System [lipid LCT])
	• Note calorie concentration (most 1 kcal/mL but some critical care solutions have 2 kcal/mL and Pulmocare, which is higher in fat, has 1.5 kcal/mL)
	• Note osmolality (isotonic is 250-350 mOsm/L; hypertonicity contributes to dehydration and diarrhea)

Pattern of delivery	• Intermittent (cannot be used below the pylorus) • Continuous; provides more protection from stress ulcers • Cyclic: feeding may be discontinued for periods of time during the 24-hour period; infusion frequently initiated during nighttime hours

Monitor	• Position of the feeding tube
	  • X-ray is the only reliable method for confirming placement of enteral tubes; x-ray should be obtained to confirm desired placement prior to administering formula or medication by the tube for the first time
	  • Other nondefinitive methods include:
	  — pH of aspirate may be helpful but not definitive: pH of 1-3 in stomach without pH-altering drugs, 3-5 in stomach with pH-altering drugs, greater than 7 in small intestine
	  — Color of aspirate may be helpful but not definitive
	    • Stomach: green, cloudy, or colorless
	    • Intestine: yellow or brown
	    • Tracheobronchial: tan, white, pale yellow, or clear
	  — Auscultation over stomach when air is injected through the tube (air insufflation) is NOT recommended due to poor sensitivity
	• GI tolerance of enteral feeding
	  • Abdominal distention or complaints of discomfort or fullness
	  • Vomiting
	  • Excessive residual volumes
	• Intake and output totaled every 8-12 hours
	• Weight daily
	• Bedside glucose testing by fingerstick q 6 hours; serum glucose by laboratory daily
	• Electrolytes daily
	• BUN daily
	• Proteins, trace elements, liver function studies weekly

Table 7-7 Enteral Nutritional Support—cont'd

Consideration	Comments

General guidelines	• Start feedings within 24-48 hours of admission or when fully resuscitated and hemodynamically stable
	• Use an infusion pump for continuous infusion
	• Do not add blue food coloring (or methylene blue) to the enteral feeding; it is no longer recommended to add blue food coloring to enteral feedings for the following reasons:
	  • May result in generalized absorption of the dye from the GI tract; more likely in patients with multiple organ failure
	    — Discoloration of body fluids and tissues
	    — May cause fatal liver toxicity
	    — Causes questionable specificity because discoloration of tracheal secretions may have occurred by systemic route
	  • May result in infection due to contamination of the food coloring
	  • Interferes with occult blood testing
	  • Causes allergic reactions in some people due to presence of FD&C yellow No. 5
	  • Has relatively low sensitivity as an indication of aspiration
	• Keep HOB elevated 30 to 45 degrees during and 30-60 minutes after intermittent feeding and continuously for continuous feeding
	• Give formula full-strength but start at 25 mL/hr; increase rate by 25 mL/hr every 4 hours if tolerated until desired rate achieved
	• Check for residual volume every 4-6 hours or before next intermittent feeding; checking residuals is not recommended with small-lumen tubes because they tend to collapse and aspiration of gastric contents can cause clogging (Kenny & Goodman, 2010)
	  • If residual is greater than 200 mL (Kenny & Goodman, 2010)
	    — The aspirate should be reinstilled in the absence of abdominal pain or distention; flush with water after reinstillation of aspirate
	    — The feeding should be continued and rechecked in 1 hour
	      • If the residual is still greater than 200 mL, the infusion should be stopped for 4 hours and then rechecked
	        ○ If the residual is still greater than 200 mL, notify physician
	        ○ If the residual is less than 200 mL, restart feeding at 50% the original rate and monitor
	      • Note that frequent interruptions may compromise adequacy of nutritional support
	  • If large residual volumes continue to limit feeding and impair nutritional support, consider the following interventions:
	    — Place the patient on the right side for 20 minutes prior to recheck
	    — Consult with the physician regarding the use of a drug to increase gastric motility (e.g., metoclopramide [Reglan], erythromycin); erythromycin has the potential risk of bacterial resistance
	    — Advance the tube to below the pylorus (intestinal motility usually not affected by same factors as gastric motility)
	    — Consult with the dietitian regarding a more calorie-dense formula in order to reduce required volume
	    — Monitor and treat hyperglycemia to avoid gastroparesis
	• Use strict aseptic technique in administration of enteral feedings; discard feeding system after 24 hours if an open system or after 48 hours if a closed system
	• Administer free water in volume of 1 mL/kcal to prevent hyperosmolality

Complications of enteral alimentation	• Clogged feeding tube
	  • Recognize factors that increase risk of clogging the tube
	    — Calorie-dense formula
	    — Protein formulas
	    — Instillation of crushed medications
	    — Small-bore feeding tube
	    — Gravity drip
	  • Prevent clogging
	    — Use an infusion pump for continuous feedings and by flushing with water when indicated
	      • Flush with 30 mL of water before and after medication administration via tube
	      • Flush with 30 mL of water before and after intermittent feedings or every 4 hours with continuous feedings
	      • Flush with 30 mL of water after checking for residuals
	      • Flush with 30 mL of water every 4 hours
	    — Use liquid-form medications when possible
	  • Attempt to reestablish patency of a clogged tube by flushing with warm water (note that cranberry juice or cola has not been shown to be more effective than water); if warm water is not successful in unclogging the tube, a physician's order for pancreatic enzymes or pancreatic enzyme-sodium bicarbonate suspension may be requested (note that proper tube placement confirmation is crucial prior to using pancreatic enzymes); tube replacement may be required

Continued

Table 7-7 Enteral Nutritional Support—cont'd

Consideration	Comments

	• Tube displacement
	  • Tape tube securely and monitor for a change in external length
	  • Prevent vomiting with antiemetics
	• Nausea/vomiting
	  • Slow feeding
	  • Allow feeding to come to room temperature before infusion
	  • Reduce osmolality of the feeding by diluting with water
	  • Decrease amount of fat in feeding
	  • Administer lactose-free formula
	  • Consider the use of drugs to increase gastric motility (e.g., metoclopramide [Reglan], erythromycin)
	  • Consider the need to move the tube from the stomach into the duodenum
	• Endotracheal aspiration of tube feeding
	  • Elevate head of bed 30-45 degrees at all times if feeding is continuous; during and for 30-60 minutes after intermittent feeding
	  • Keep cuff inflated during feeding if patient is intubated or has tracheostomy
	  • Check for residual volumes every 4-6 hours if administering gastric feedings through a large-bore tube
	• Diarrhea
	  • Caused by decreased plasma colloidal oncotic pressure (COP) due to low serum proteins
	    — Maintain adequate nutritional support; diarrhea will resolve when plasma proteins are more normal
	    — Administer intravenous albumin as prescribed
	  • Bacterial contamination
	    — Wash hands before manipulation of equipment and use clean technique; wipe top of formula cans with an alcohol wipe
	    — Utilize a closed system if possible
	    — Change administration system daily or according to policy
	    — Do not allow solutions to hang at room temperature for more than 4 hours if an open system or 24 hours if a closed system
	    — Avoid antidiarrheals, which slow peristalsis and increase the risk of sepsis
	  • Hypertonicity
	    — Initiate enteral feedings at a slow rate and/or half strength; gradually increase rate and/or strength
	    — Use isotonic solutions if possible; dilute hyperosmolar feeding with free water
	  • Alteration in normal flora from antibiotics and proliferation of *clostridium difficile*
	    — Administer metronidazole (Flagyl) or vancomycin
	    — Encourage yogurt (with active cultures) or *lactobacillus acidophilus* to restore normal flora
	  • Also:
	    — Consider the addition of fiber (e.g., Jevity)
	    — Use only lactose-free formulas
	    — Consider discontinuance of causative medications (e.g., elixirs containing sorbitol or antacids)
	    — Administer pancreatic enzymes for pancreatic insufficiency
	• Constipation
	  • Add fiber
	  • Increase free water
	  • Increase activity if possible
	  • Administer laxative as prescribed
	• Dehydration
	  • Monitor daily weight and intake and output
	  • Administer free water as indicated
	• Electrolyte imbalance
	  • Treat cause (e.g., diarrhea)
	  • Monitor serum electrolytes
	  • Replace electrolytes as prescribed
	  • Consult with the physician and dietician regarding modification of formula
	• Hyperglycemia
	  • Monitor serum glucose every 6 hours
	  • Consult with physician and dietician regarding modification of formula
	  • Administer insulin as prescribed
	• Overfeeding
	  • Monitor renal and liver function studies
	  • Monitor for fluid overload, hyperglycemia, hyperlipidemia, electrolyte imbalance
	  • Consult with the physician and dietician regarding caloric and protein prescriptions

Table 7-7 Enteral Nutritional Support—cont'd

Consideration	Comments

	• Refeeding syndrome
	  • Start feedings slowly, especially in high-risk patients (e.g., NPO for several days, existing malnutrition, alcoholism, sepsis); may take 24-48 hours to get intake to recommended level of nutrition
	  • Monitor glucose, potassium, phosphorus; insulin, electrolyte replacement may be required
	• Inadequate feeding (Bourgault et al., 2007)
	  • Minimize interruptions
	  • Stop feedings immediately prior to minor procedures and then restart within 1 hour after procedures
	  • Stop feedings no more than 4 hours before major procedures

Etiology

1. Peptic ulcer
   a. *Helicobacter pylori:* a bacterial infection that has been identified as a common cause of recurrent ulcer disease
   b. Other predisposing factors
      1) Genetic predisposition
      2) Smoking
      3) Diet
         a) Coffee or tea
         b) Carbonated beverages
         c) Beer
      4) Drugs and therapies
         a) Antineoplastics
         b) Radiation therapy
         c) Drugs that alter the mucosal barrier
            i) Alcohol
            ii) NSAIDs (e.g., ASA, ibuprofen, indomethacin)
         d) Drugs that decrease gastric mucosal renewal: corticosteroid, phenylbutazone
         e) Drugs that increase acid stimulation
            i) Coffee (because of peptides, not caffeine)
            ii) Nicotine
            iii) Reserpine
         f) Hormones (e.g., estrogen)
      5) High physiologic stress situation
         a) COPD
         b) Multiple traumas
         c) Major surgery
         d) Myocardial infarction
         e) Hepatic failure
         f) Renal failure
         g) Burns: referred to as *Curling's ulcer*
         h) Neurologic trauma: referred to as *Cushing's ulcer*
            i) Cerebral trauma
            ii) Spinal cord injury
            iii) Neurosurgery
         i) Acute respiratory distress syndrome
         j) Mechanical ventilation for more than 5 days
         k) Coagulopathy
         l) Sepsis
         m) Shock
         n) Multiple organ dysfunction syndrome
2. Cirrhosis: portal hypertension
   a. Cirrhosis
      1) Alcoholic cirrhosis: most likely
      2) Viral or toxic hepatitis
      3) Chronic biliary obstruction
      4) Chronic right ventricular failure
   b. Portal vein thrombosis
   c. Hepatic venous outflow obstruction
   d. Congenital hepatic fibrosis
   e. Schistosomiasis: a parasitic infection
3. Mallory-Weiss tear: forceful retching and vomiting (e.g., alcoholism, particularly binge drinking, or bulimia)
4. Gastritis
   a. Dietary intolerances, especially milk intolerance
   b. Alcohol
   c. Drugs such as aspirin, steroids, NSAID
   d. Uremia
   e. Certain systemic diseases such as hepatitis
   f. Ingestion of strong acids or alkalis (referred to as corrosive gastritis)

Pathophysiology

See Figure 7-15 on page 517.

Clinical Presentation

1. Peptic ulcer
   a. Subjective
      1) History: epigastric pain, previous ulcer, previous GI bleeding, alcoholism, liver disease
      2) Epigastric pain
      3) Fatigue, weakness
      4) Thirst
      5) Anxiety
   b. Objective
      1) Bleeding
         a) Blood or coffee-grounds material appears in vomitus if gastric ulcer
         b) Black stools if duodenal
         c) If bleeding is gradual, faintness, fatigue, and pallor may be only indications
      2) Hyperactive bowel sounds

Table 7-8 Parenteral Nutritional Support

Considerations	Comments
Indications	• When the enteral route is contraindicated (see Table 7-7) • When the enteral route is ineffective (high caloric needs or shock)

Routes	• Central vein: referred to as *total parenteral nutrition* (TPN)
	  • Allows the administration of hypertonic glucose solutions because of rapid dilution by blood as the solution enters the great vessel
	  • Subclavian or internal jugular usually used; percutaneously inserted central catheter (PICC) may also be used
	• Peripheral vein: referred to as *peripheral parenteral nutrition* (PPN)
	  • Used for patients who cannot take in sufficient nutrition enterally for 5-7 days but are not hypermetabolic
	  • Not usually adequate to provide sufficient calories for critically ill patients because of osmolality (and therefore calorie) limitations

Type of catheter	• Short-term: peripheral or central venous catheter; multilumen catheter usually used to provide lumen for parenteral nutrition, lumen for blood and/or fluids, lumen for parenteral drugs • Long-term: Hickman, Broviac, or Groshong catheter; Infuse-a-Port; Port-a-Cath

Solution: 1 L of standard TPN formula (25% dextrose and 8.5% amino acids) provides ~1,000 kcal (1 kcal/mL)	• CHO: hypertonic dextrose
	  • Concentrations
	    — TPN: usually 25% but may be as high as 35% dextrose
	    — PPN: no more than 10% dextrose
	  • CHO and fats provide enough calories for maximal protein sparing effect
	  • Dextrose provides 3.4 cal/g
	• Protein: crystalline amino acids 2.5%-8.5%; includes essential and nonessential (note that no more than 5% amino acid solution via parenteral line [i.e., PPN]) amino acids and provides 4.3 cal/g
	  • Specialized formulas are available for specific diseases
	    — Hepatic failure (e.g., HepatAmine, Branch Amin): branched-chain amino acids
	    — Renal failure (e.g., RenAmin, NephrAmine): essential amino acids
	• Fats: oil-in-water emulsions composed of soybean oil or a combination of soybean oil and safflower oil that provide fatty acids as long-chain triglycerides
	  • 30-50% of nonprotein calories should be supplied by lipids not exceeding 2.5 g/kg/day
	    — Linoleic acid, the only essential fatty acid, should provide at least 4% of the total calorie intake to prevent deficiency of essential fatty acid
	    — Excessive amounts of lipids may have a detrimental effect on pulmonary function and the reticuloendothelial system
	  • Concentrations
	    — 10% lipids provide 1.1 kcal/mL
	    — 20% lipids provide 2 kcal/mL
	    — 30% lipids provide 3 kcal/mL
	  • Medium-chain triglycerides are immediately oxidized for fuel and may be preferred in SIRS and sepsis
	• Electrolytes: sodium chloride; potassium; calcium; magnesium; phosphate
	• Buffer: acetate or bicarbonate
	• Minerals: iron; zinc; copper; manganese; cobalt; iodine; chromium; selenium
	• Vitamins: multivitamins 1 ampule daily
	  • Vitamin K (10-20 mg) should be administered every week; may be given IM or subcutaneously or added to TPN solution as phytonadione (AquaMEPHYTON)
	  • Thiamine replacement should be considered, especially when chronic alcohol ingestion is known or suspected, to prevent Wernicke's encephalopathy
	• 3-in-1 admixture has everything in one infusion rather than lipid piggybacked in separately
	  • Advantages: lower cost with less equipment, waste, and nursing time
	  • Disadvantage: risk of solution instability; monitor closely for a cream-colored layer (also referred to as *creaming*) or a complete emulsion crack with a separation of the oil and water and return to pharmacy if separation noted

Table 7-8 Parenteral Nutritional Support—cont'd

Considerations	Comments
Possible additives	• Regular insulin (note that sliding scale insulin still must be administered as needed) • Heparin • H_2 receptor antagonists • Metoclopramide (Reglan) • NOTE: All additives should be added under laminar hood (in pharmacy department) rather than on nursing unit
Monitor	• Vital signs and infusion rate at least every 4 hours (depending on the acuity of the patient) • Intake and output totaled every 8-12 hours • Weight daily • Bedside glucose testing by fingerstick q 6 hours; serum glucose by laboratory daily • Electrolytes daily • BUN daily • CBC, proteins, trace elements, liver function studies, triglycerides, cholesterol, platelet count, prothrombin time weekly • Catheter site

General guidelines	• Utilize strict sterile technique during catheter insertion and management
	• Assess patient for central venous catheter insertion complications (pneumothorax, hemothorax, chylothorax, arterial puncture); request chest x-ray after insertion of central venous catheter; do not initiate fluids at a rate faster than KVO until chest x-ray confirms placement
	• Ensure a dedicated catheter or lumen of a multilumen catheter for TPN infusion
	  • Do not use a catheter or lumen that has been previously used for CVP measurements or for the prolonged administration of crystalloid solution or blood products
	  • Do not use the catheter (or lumen) for drawing blood samples or infusing any other fluids
	• Assess the solution prior to infusion
	  • Examine expiration date and discard any expired solutions
	  • Do not hang cloudy solutions
	  • Monitor closely for emulsion crack if hanging 3-in-1 solution (also called *total nutrient admixture* [TNA]); do not hang solution if a layer of fat is seen separated at top of bag
	• Initiate at 1200-2400 cal/day and increase to desired caloric intake as prescribed
	• Remove from refrigerator 30 minutes prior to infusing
	• Keep rate constant (volumetric pump required)
	• Utilize an inline filter; 0.22 micron if lipids are piggybacked in distal to filter; 1.2 micron if TNA used because smaller filter will not allow lipids to flow through
	• Change dressing every 48 hours or according to hospital policy or anytime that the dressing becomes soiled
	  • Gauze and tape or semipermeable transparent dressing (e.g., Op-Site, Tegaderm); note that semipermeable transparent dressing has been associated with a higher rate of catheter-related infection and sepsis than standard gauze and tape probably because of inadequate permeability and infrequency of dressing change; they should not be used in patients with oily skin or acne near catheter insertion site
	• Change tubing every 24-72 hours or according to hospital policy; lipid tubing (including TNA tubing) should be changed every 24 hours
	• Do not allow a bag to hang more than 24 hours

Continued

Table 7-8 Parental Nutritional Support—cont'd

Considerations	Comments

Complications	• Allergic reaction (especially to lipids)
	  • Note fever, chills, shivering, chest or back pain
	  • Stop infusion
	• Infection and sepsis
	  • Utilize meticulous aseptic technique with all aspects of catheter care; change dressing every 48 hours or whenever soiled; change tubing every 24-72 hours; minimize number of entries into the system
	  • Monitor for clinical indications of catheter-related sepsis: fever, leukocytosis, glucose intolerance, redness, swelling, tenderness, and purulent drainage at insertion site
	  • Obtain blood cultures (not through this catheter), remove catheter and culture tip
	• Hyperglycemia
	  • Monitor serum glucose levels
	  • Administer insulin therapy; usually administered as insulin drip if serum glucose greater than 500 mg/dL
	• Hyperosmolar nonketotic dehydration
	  • Monitor serum glucose levels
	  • Administer insulin therapy; usually administered as insulin drip if serum glucose greater than 500 mg/dL
	  • Administer 5% dextrose and hypotonic saline ($\frac{1}{4}$ or $\frac{1}{2}$) or D_5W (depending on patient's serum osmolality) to correct free water deficit
	  • Discontinue TPN until patient is stable as prescribed
	• Hypoglycemia
	  • Prevent interruption of TPN infusion (e.g., catheter occlusion or accidental removal)
	  • Use infusion pump (mandatory)
	  • Never discontinue TPN abruptly unless for HHS
	• Electrolyte imbalances: hyperchloremic metabolic acidosis; hyponatremia; hypokalemia; hypocalcemia; hypomagnesemia; hypophosphatemia
	  • Adjust TPN solution concentration and/or alteration of infusion rate as prescribed
	• Refeeding syndrome: fluid imbalance; hypokalemia; hypophosphatemia; hypoglycemia or hyperglycemia
	  • Monitor fluid, electrolyte, glucose levels especially during the first 24-48 hours after TPN initiated
	  • Adjust TPN solution concentration and/or alteration of infusion rate as prescribed
	• Increased CO_2 production
	  • Monitor closely for clinical indications of hypercapnia; request ABGs as indicated
	  • Decrease the percentage of calories supplied by CHO and increase percentage of calories supplied by fats if hypercapnia occurs or during weaning
	• Air embolism
	  • Prevent air embolus by the following:
	    — Ask the patient to hold his or her breath or perform Valsalva maneuver during catheter insertion, tubing changes, and catheter removal
	    — Purge all air from tubing before attachment to catheter
	    — Use air-eliminating filters on central line tubing
	    — Use Luer-Lok connections
	  • Note dyspnea, hypotension, churning murmur over precordium, confusion
	  • If clinical indications of air embolism do occur:
	    — Place patient in Trendelenburg position on left side
	    — Aspirate air with a syringe attached to the central venous catheter
	    — Administer oxygen
	• Subclavian thrombosis (rare)
	  • Monitor for swelling of involved arm, face, neck, erythema, fever
	  • Remove catheter
	  • Administer fibrinolytic or anticoagulation therapy as prescribed

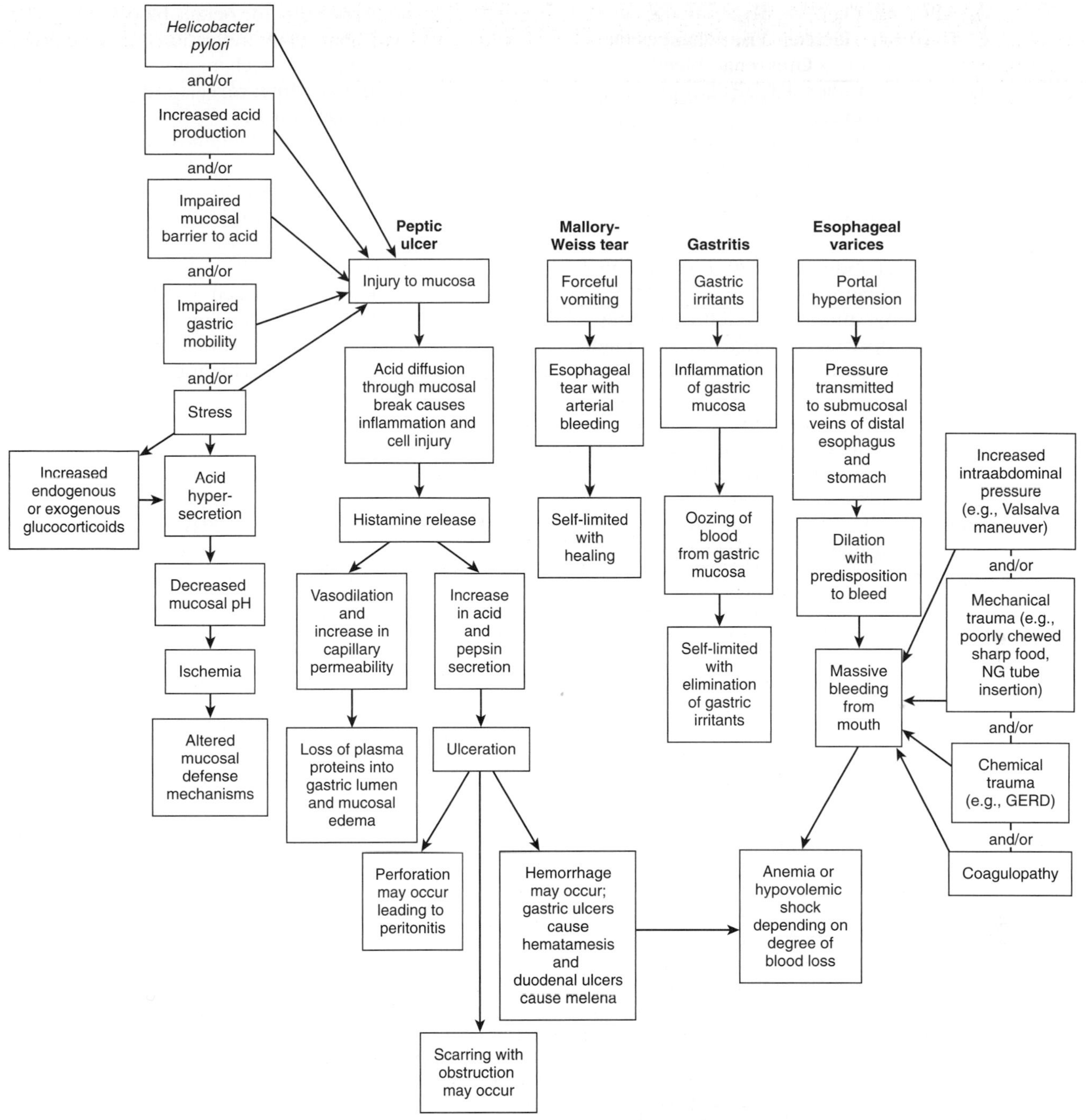

Figure 7-15 Pathophysiology of upper GI hemorrhage.

3) Patient may have signs of acute abdomen if ulcer perforates (Box 7-2); other terms for an acute abdomen include *surgical abdomen* or *hot belly*

c. Diagnostic

1) Serum

a) Gastrin level: may be elevated in gastric ulcer

b) Amylase: elevated if perforation causes penetration into the pancreas and causes acute pancreatitis

c) Total proteins, albumin, and transferrin may be decreased because many of these patients are malnourished.

Box 7-2 Clinical Indications of an Acute Abdomen

Abdominal pain
Abdominal distention
Rigid, boardlike abdomen
Rebound tenderness
Diminished or absent bowel sounds
Nausea, vomiting
Fever
Leukocytosis

- d) CBC: anemia
- e) Hgb, Hct: decreased but changes may take 4-6 hours after acute bleed
- f) Clotting studies: PT, aPTT prolonged if liver is affected

2) Gastric analysis: may show hyperacidity or blood in the gastric secretions
3) Stools for occult blood: positive
4) ECG: may show indications of ischemia (e.g., ST-T wave changes)
5) Flat plate of abdomen: may show free air under diaphragm indicating perforation
6) Gastroscopy: important in differentiating cause of upper GI bleeding; can determine ulcer presence, location, and stage of healing
7) Upper GI series: may show anatomic deformity created by ulcer crater; may show delayed gastric emptying if edema or scarring is present
8) Biopsy: may be done to rule out gastric cancer or malignant gastric ulcer
9) Angiography
   - a) Rarely performed
   - b) May reveal bleeding site or sites
   - c) May include the placement of a catheter for intraarterial administration of vasopressors (e.g., vasopressin)

2. Esophageal varices
   - a. Subjective
     1) History of precipitating causes (e.g., excessive, chronic alcohol intake)
     2) Report of sudden, painless hemorrhage orally
   - b. Objective
     1) Bright red blood gushing from mouth (average blood loss is 10 units)
     2) Jaundice
     3) Abdominal distention
     4) Hyperactive bowel sounds
     5) Melena
     6) Hepatomegaly
     7) Splenomegaly
     8) Clinical indications of hypoperfusion: tachycardia; tachypnea; hypotension; cool, clammy skin; decreased urine output; agitation; confusion
   - c. Diagnostic
     1) Serum
        - a) BUN: elevated
        - b) Bilirubin: may be elevated
        - c) Albumin: decreased because of liver disease
        - d) AST, ALT, LDH: elevated due to liver disease
        - e) Hematology: Hgb, Hct decreased
        - f) Clotting studies: PT, aPTT prolonged because of liver disease
        - g) Arterial blood gases: may reveal metabolic acidosis related to shock and hypoperfusion
     2) Stool: positive for occult blood
     3) ECG: may show indications of ischemia (e.g., ST-T wave changes)
     4) Barium swallow: reveals the presence of esophageal varices
     5) Esophagogastroduodenoscopy: reveals the presence of esophageal varices
     6) Percutaneous transhepatic portography: reveals esophageal varices and measures pressure in the portal circulation
     7) Angiography
        - a) Rarely performed
        - b) May reveal bleeding site or sites
        - c) May include the placement of a catheter for intraarterial administration of vasopressors (e.g., vasopressin)
3. Mallory-Weiss tear: hematemesis after forceful vomiting
4. Gastritis: coffee-grounds hematemesis

Collaborative Management

1. Ensure airway, oxygenation, and ventilation.
   - a. Position for optimal ventilation and to prevent aspiration.
     1) Elevate head of bed 30-45 degrees.
     2) Turn to left side.
   - b. Administer oxygen as necessary to maintain SpO_2 at 95% unless contraindicated; in patients with COPD, administer oxygen to achieve a SpO_2 of ~90%.
   - c. Ensure availability of oropharyngeal suctioning equipment at bedside.
   - d. Assist with endotracheal intubation as requested to reduce risk of aspiration.
     1) Prior to balloon tamponade for esophageal varices: recommended to prevent obstruction of airway in case of accidental dislodgement of the esophageal balloon
     2) Prior to endoscopy if indicated
2. Maintain hemodynamic stability.
   - a. Monitor blood loss and hemodynamic stability.
     1) Insert large-bore orogastric or nasogastric tube and perform gastric lavage.
        - a) Note that gastric lavage does not truly aid in clotting as previously believed and may actually dislodge clots; purposes of gastric lavage include the following:
          - i) Monitor bleeding
          - ii) Remove nitrogenous materials (blood) out of the gut so that they will not be converted to ammonia nitrogenous materials from the GI tract
          - iii) Allow visualization during endoscopy
        - b) Use room temperature saline for lavage; problems with the use of iced lavage
          - i) Less effective in cessation of bleeding
          - ii) Prolongation of clotting times
          - iii) Hypothermia

(a) Causing a shift of the oxyhemoglobin dissociation curve to the left, decreasing tissue delivery of oxygen
(b) Causing the patient to shiver, increasing oxygen consumption
2) Insert indwelling urinary catheter to evaluate hourly urine output.
3) Assist with insertion of arterial catheter and pulmonary artery catheter in patients with severe hemorrhage.

b. Replace circulating blood volume.
1) Insert at least two short (1¼-inch) large-gauge (16 or 18) peripheral intravenous catheters; blood is drawn for laboratory analysis and for type and crossmatch for two units of blood during the catheter insertion.
2) Administer crystalloids initially as prescribed; colloids may also be prescribed.
a) Maintain urine output of 0.5-1 mL/kg/hr.
b) Maintain PAOP of ~12-15 mm Hg.
c) Avoid lactated Ringer's (LR) in patients with liver disease.
3) Administer blood and blood products as prescribed.
a) Red packed cells should be given early if significant blood loss is suspected to prevent tissue hypoxia; indications include the following:
i) Persistent hemodynamic instability after 2 L of crystalloid
ii) Hematocrit less than 25%
iii) Clinical indications of hypoperfusion (see Table 2-2)
b) Fresh blood is preferred, especially in patients with liver disease, because it is lower in ammonia than banked blood.
c) After multiple transfusions, consideration should be given to replacement of clotting factors, platelets, and calcium.

c. Control bleeding
1) Administer octreotide acetate (Sandostatin) as prescribed (see Table 7-6).
2) Administer vasopressin intravenously as prescribed (see Table 7-6).
3) Assist with diagnostic/therapeutic endoscopy.
a) Diagnostic: to identify the specific cause of the bleeding
b) Therapeutic for peptic ulcer or Mallory-Weiss tear
i) Endoscopic thermal therapy uses heat to cauterize the bleeding vessel.
ii) Endoscopic injection therapy uses hypertonic saline, epinephrine, or dehydrated alcohol to cause localized vasoconstriction of the bleeding vessel.
c) Therapeutic for esophageal varices
i) Endoscopic injection therapy (i.e., sclerotherapy)
(a) Sclerosing agent (ethanolamine oleate [Ethamolin], morrhuate sodium [Scleromate], sodium tetradecyl [Sotradecol]) is injected into the varix and surrounding tissue; the sclerosing agent causes variceal inflammation, venous thrombosis, and eventually scar tissue; repeated injections may be necessary to completely decompress the bleeding varix and decrease the risk of recurrent hemorrhage.
(b) Varices are categorized as I-IV by their size; class III and IV are at high risk to bleed if not already bleeding.
(c) Monitor for complications of sclerotherapy.
(i) Retrosternal pain
(ii) Transient fever
(iii) Transient dysphagia
(iv) Local ulceration
(v) Pulmonary symptoms including diminished breath sounds
(vi) Bleeding
(vii) Stricture
(viii) Perforation
(ix) Sepsis
(d) Sclerosing is repeated in 4-7 days and every 6-8 months thereafter.
ii) Esophageal variceal ligation: Rubber bands or O-rings are placed on the target vessels at gastroesophageal junction.
4) Stop bleeding in esophageal varices through measures that lower venous pressure.
a) Administer beta-blockers (e.g., propranolol) as prescribed.
b) Assist in placement of a multiple-lumen tube for balloon tamponade (Figure 7-16 and Table 7-9) if bleeding cannot be controlled pharmacologically, endoscopically, or through use of transjugular intrahepatic portosystemic shunt (TIPS).

d. Correct coagulopathy; frequently significant in patients with esophageal varices and liver disease
1) Administer vitamin K as prescribed; recombinant clotting factors (e.g., rFVIIa) may be prescribed.

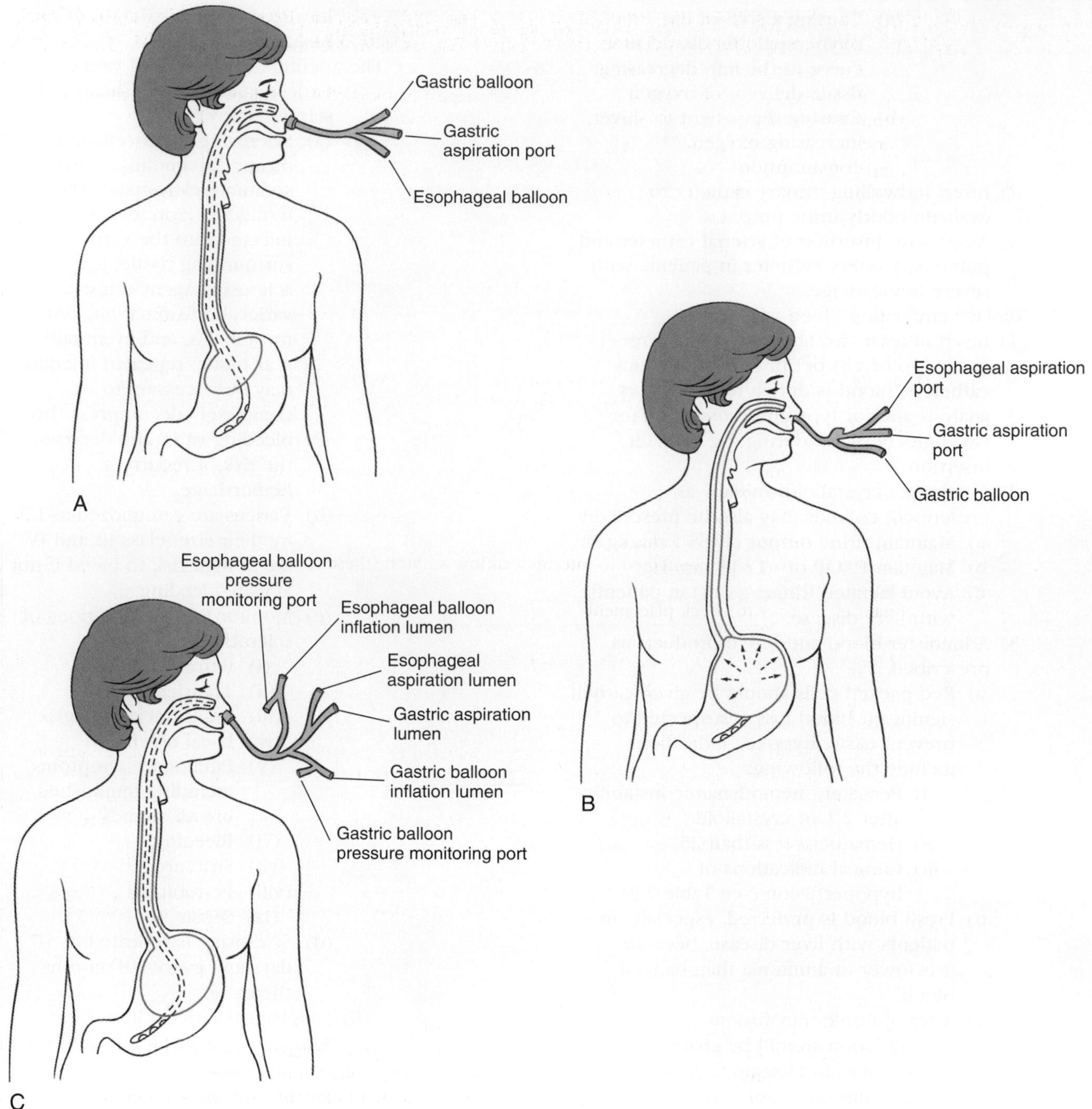

Figure 7-16 Esophageal tamponade tubes. **A,** Sengstaken-Blakemore tube. **B,** Linton tube. **C,** Minnesota tube. (From Urden, L., Stacy, K., & Lough, M. [2009]. *Critical care nursing: Diagnosis and management* [6th ed.]. St. Louis: Mosby.)

2) Monitor closely for bleeding.
3) Monitor clotting studies.
4) Avoid invasive procedures and injections.

3. Prepare patient for surgery if necessary to control bleeding.
   a. Peptic ulcer
      1) Indications for surgery
         a) Continuation of bleeding despite treatment
         b) Administration of greater than eight units of blood over 24 hours
         c) Hemorrhage to the point of hypotension or shock
         d) Rebleeding after homeostasis achieved
         e) Perforation with evidence of pneumoperitoneum
      2) Surgical interventions
         a) Oversewing of bleeding point
         b) Vagotomy: dividing the vagus nerve along the esophagus
            i) Decreases acid secretion in the stomach

Table 7-9 Balloon Tamponade for Esophageal Varices	
Action	• Applies pressure to esophageal and intragastric varices
Tubes	• Sengstaken-Blakemore (SB) tube (Figure 7-16): esophageal balloon; gastric balloon; gastric suction • Linton (L): gastric balloon; esophageal suction; gastric suction • Minnesota (M) tube: esophageal balloon; gastric balloon; esophageal suction; gastric suction
Lumens	• Gastric balloon: 200-500 mL for SB tube; 450-500 mL for M tube; 700-800 for L tube • Esophageal balloon: usually 20 mm Hg (25 cm H_2O) but may be as high as 30-40 mm Hg to control bleeding • Gastric suction: nonvented • Esophageal suction: nonvented

Insertion	• Generally done by physician but may be done by specifically trained nurse
	• Check balloon for leaks prior to insertion by inflating with air and putting in a basin of saline
	• Utilize viscous lidocaine or Cetacaine to anesthetize the nose and posterior pharynx
	• The catheter is advanced to ~50 cm mark
	• The gastric balloon is inflated to ~200-300 mL; the lumen is double-clamped to prevent leakage
	• The catheter is pulled back until resistance is met and then a nasal sponge is placed at the nose to keep the gastric balloon up against the gastroesophageal junction
	  • A football helmet with face mask may also be used
	    — If a helmet is used, check fit closely; skin breakdown is frequently caused by an ill-fitting helmet
	  • 0.5-1.0 kg weight may be hung over the end of the bed
	• The esophageal balloon is inflated to a pressure of 20-40 mm Hg until bleeding is controlled; the lumen is double-clamped to prevent leakage
	• The suction lumens are connected to intermittent low suction (these are nonvented)
	• Label all lumens
	• Obtain chest x-ray to check placement

Management	• Monitor and maintain airway
	  • Elevate head of bed to 45 degrees unless patient is unconscious; if patient is unconscious, elevate HOB 15 degrees on left side
	  • Have suction equipment available
	  • Intubation is desirable but not absolutely required
	  • Suction the oropharynx and nasopharynx often because the patient cannot swallow with the tube in
	    — Not as much of an issue with Minnesota tube because there is suction above the esophageal balloon
	    — A small nasogastric tube may be inserted into the nostril opposite the SB tube to drain secretions that collect above the esophageal balloon
	• Maintain pressures at prescribed levels
	  • Periodic deflation at specific intervals (e.g., every 4 hours) may be prescribed because the pressures required to control bleeding exceed the pressure of capillary filling, and ischemia or necrosis may occur
	    — Monitor closely for bleeding during any time of deflation
	• Have scissors at bedside to release pressure from esophageal balloon if it accidentally moves into the pharynx and acute respiratory distress occurs
	• Keep second tube in the room for replacement if necessary
	• Maintain traction on tube to keep gastric balloon pulled up against the gastroesophageal junction
	• Note amount of pressure/volume in each part of tube; maintain inflation of balloons
	• Ensure patency of the gastric suction lumen and keep connected to low intermittent suction to prevent aspiration or retention of blood in the gut which is likely to increase ammonia levels
	• Monitor closely for skin breakdown at mouth or nose; lubricate every 8 hours with water-soluble lubricant
	• Deflation of the esophageal balloon is usually done at 24 hours; deflation of the gastric balloon is usually done at 48 hours; monitor closely for recurrent bleeding when balloons are deflated

Complications	• Airway obstruction • Aspiration • Perforation of esophagus: sudden epigastric or substernal pain, respiratory distress, increased bleeding, shock • Dysrhythmias • Chest pain • Bronchopneumonia • Laceration, ulceration of stomach • Pressure necrosis of hypopharynx, esophagus, or upper stomach • Hiccoughs

ii) If ulcer is prepyloric, vagotomy should be performed to prevent obstruction.

c) Vagotomy and pyloroplasty

i) Pyloroplasty: surgical procedure in which the pylorus is cut and resutured to relax the muscle and widen the opening into the duodenum

d) Vagotomy and antrectomy

i) Antrectomy: surgical removal of the antrum to decrease acidity

(a) With gastroduodenal reconstruction (i.e., Billroth I) (Figure 7-17*A*)

(b) With gastrojejunal reconstruction (i.e., Billroth II) (Figure 7-17*B*)

e) Total gastrectomy: gastrectomy with anastomosis of esophagus to the duodenum or jejunum (Figure 7-17*C*)

i) Monitor for:

(a) Early dumping syndrome (hyperosmolality effect related to a hyperosmolar bolus of food being "dumped" into the duodenum because of absence of pyloric valve and normal, more gradual gastric emptying): occurs within 30 minutes after eating; dizziness, weakness; tachycardia; cool, clammy skin

(b) Late dumping syndrome (hyperinsulinism effect related to an increase in insulin production by the pancreas in response to a large bolus of food causing an increase in blood glucose): occurs 2 hours after meal; complaints of dizziness, weakness, restlessness; tachycardia; cool, clammy skin; malabsorption

(c) Pernicious anemia: related to removal of parietal cells that make intrinsic factor necessary for the absorption of vitamin B_{12} in the ileum

b. Esophageal varices

1) Indications for surgery

a) Continuation of bleeding despite treatment

b) Administration of greater than eight units of blood over 24 hours

c) Hemorrhage to the point of hypotension or shock

d) Rebleeding after homeostasis achieved

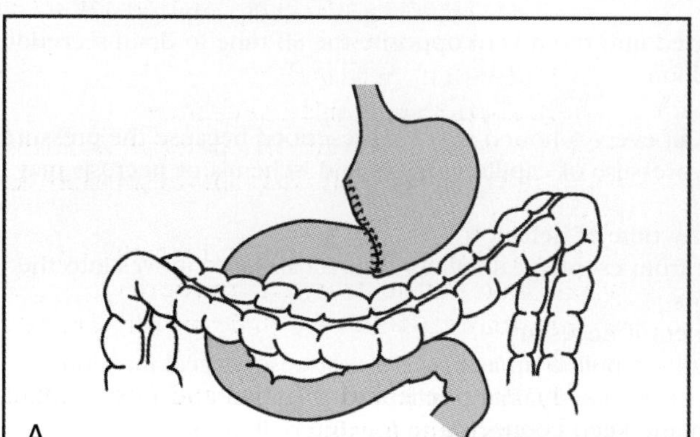

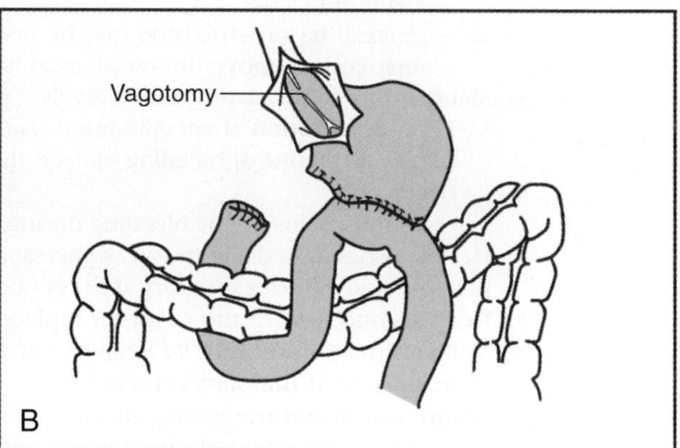

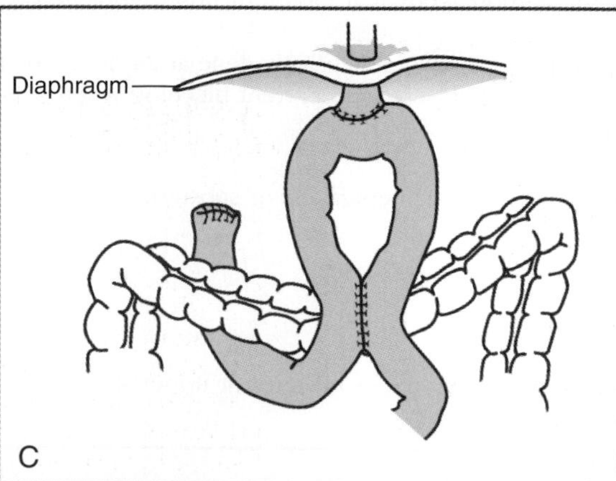

Figure 7-17 Gastric resection procedures. **A,** Billroth I. **B,** Billroth II. **C,** Total gastrectomy.

2) Portal-systemic shunt: portacaval, mesocaval, or splenorenal
   a) Lowers portal pressure by diverting blood flow
   b) Associated with a higher incidence of hepatic encephalopathy and avoided if possible
3) Transjugular intrahepatic portosystemic shunt (TIPS)
   a) Invasive angiographic method; less invasive than surgical shunt
   b) Shunts blood between the portal and systemic venous systems entirely within the liver; connection is made between the hepatic and portal veins and a stent is placed in the tract
   c) Complications: hemorrhage; renal failure; septic shock; shunt stenosis; hepatic encephalopathy

4. Prevent encephalopathy.
   a. Remove nitrogenous materials from the GI tract.
      1) Perform gastric lavage with room-temperature saline so that bacteria in GI tract cannot digest the globin (i.e., protein).
      2) Administer osmotic laxatives (e.g., lactulose) as prescribed.
      3) Administer enemas as ordered.
   b. Monitor patients with portacaval shunts closely for clinical indications of elevated ammonia levels (e.g., confusion, irritability, decreased attention span, apathy, slurring of speech).
5. Prevent further damage to the gastric mucosa caused by gastric irritants, hyperacidity, and/or impaired mucosal barrier.
   a. Discontinue any gastric irritants.
   b. Administer pharmacologic agents that decrease gastric acidity and/or protect gastric mucosa (see Table 7-6).
      1) Decrease gastric pH to 3.5-5 (normal pH of gastric secretions is 1-3).
         a) Antacids (e.g., aluminum-magnesium complex [Riopan], magnesium hydroxide and aluminum hydroxide [Maalox, Mylanta], calcium carbonate (TUMS)
         b) Histamine (H_2) receptor antagonist (e.g., ranitidine [Zantac], famotidine [Pepcid], nizatidine [Axid])
         c) Proton pump inhibitors (e.g., omeprazole [Prilosec], lansoprazole [Prevacid], esomeprazole [Nexium])
      2) Provide agents to improve the mucosal barrier to acid.
         a) Prostaglandin E_1-analog (e.g., misoprostol [Cytotec])
         b) Mucosal protectant (aluminum hydroxide, sulfated sucrose): (e.g., sucralfate [Carafate])
   c. Provide required nutritional support by enteral route if possible.
   d. Remove nasogastric or orogastric tube after lavage is completed (and enteral nutritional support is not required) because the gastric tube may increase acid production by stimulating gastric secretion.
   e. Administer drug therapy for *Helicobacter pylori;* any of the following combinations may be prescribed:
      1) Bismuth subsalicylate + metronidazole + tetracycline + H_2 receptor antagonist
      2) Omeprazole + clarithromycin
      3) Ranitidine bismuth citrate + clarithromycin
      4) Lansoprazole + amoxicillin + clarithromycin
      5) Lansoprazole + amoxicillin
6. Decrease anxiety.
   a. Maintain a calm and reassuring approach.
   b. Administer anxiolytics as prescribed and indicated; avoid hepatotoxic agents if the patient has liver disease.
   c. Keep the patient and family informed regarding patient status.
   d. Encourage discussion of fears and concerns.
   e. Assess for alcohol withdrawal syndrome (Box 7-3); if present:
      1) Administer CNS depressants (e.g., diazepam [Valium], chlordiazepoxide [Librium]) as prescribed.
         a) Most drugs used for this purpose, including diazepam (Valium) and chlordiazepoxide (Librium), have potential for liver toxicity; dosage is adjusted and liver function studies are monitored.
      2) Reorient frequently.
      3) Encourage family attendance.
7. Maintain fluid and electrolyte balance: Evaluate sodium, potassium, calcium, and magnesium and replace as prescribed.
8. Maintain nutritional status by administering appropriate nutrients when appropriate.
   a. Recommendations for patients with peptic ulcer
      1) Provide bland proteins and fats in small, frequent meals.

Box 7-3 Alcohol Withdrawal Syndrome

Early	Late
Mild tachycardia	Marked tachycardia
Mild hypertension	Marked hypertension
Nausea, vomiting	Hyperthermia
Diaphoresis	Dehydration
Pruritus	Delirium
Visual disturbances	Delusions
Time disorientation	Hallucinations
Tremors	Tonic-clonic seizures
Anxiety, agitation	
Sleep disturbances	

   2) Avoid stimulants of gastric secretions (e.g., coffee, tea, cola, spicy foods, alcohol).
   3) Progress to full diet as soon as possible.
  b. Recommendations for patients with esophageal varices
   1) Give clear liquids initially; progress diet as indicated.
   2) Avoid alcohol-containing mouthwash and drugs.
   3) Encourage thorough chewing of foods, especially hard, sharp foods like crackers as they may mechanically injure varices causing recurrence of bleeding.
9. Monitor for complications.
  a. Aspiration pneumonitis
  b. Recurrent bleeding, hemorrhage
  c. Perforation
  d. Peritonitis
  e. Penetration into surrounding tissues (e.g., acute pancreatitis)
  f. Gastric outlet syndrome related to ulcer inflammation and mucosal edema
  g. Obstruction due to ulcer scarring at the pylorus
  h. Myocardial infarction
  i. Cerebral infarction
  j. Disseminated intravascular coagulation (DIC)
  k. Sepsis
  l. Shock: hypovolemia or septic

Hepatic Failure/Encephalopathy

Definitions

1. Hepatic failure: inability of the liver to perform organ functions
  a. Acute liver failure (ALF) (previously referred to as *fulminant hepatic failure*): onset of coagulopathy (INR greater than or equal to 1.5) and any degree of encephalopathy within 25 weeks of the appearance of symptoms of liver failure in the absence of underlying liver disease (Larson, 2010)
2. Hepatic encephalopathy: neurologic failure as a result of hepatic failure

Etiology

1. Acute liver failure
  a. Hepatotoxic drugs (Box 7-1) (e.g., acetaminophen, halothane, methyldopa, isoniazid [INH], 3,4-methylenedioxy-methamphetamine [Ecstasy]) or toxins (*Amanita* mushrooms, carbon tetrachloride, sea anemone sting)
  b. Viruses
   1) Fulminant viral hepatitis (Table 7-10)
   2) Herpes simplex
   3) Herpes zoster
   4) Epstein-Barr
   5) Adenovirus
   6) Cytomegalovirus
  c. Ischemia (e.g., shock and multiple organ dysfunction syndrome [MODS])
  d. Trauma
  e. Reye's syndrome
  f. Budd-Chiari syndrome (i.e., hepatic vein obstruction)
  g. Acute fatty liver of pregnancy
  h. Acute hepatic vein occlusion
2. Chronic liver failure with an acute situation (e.g., peritonitis, GI hemorrhage, catabolism)
  a. Cirrhosis
  b. Wilson's disease
  c. Primary or metastatic tumors of the liver

Pathophysiology (Figure 7-18)

1. Cirrhosis
  a. Liver parenchymal cells are progressively destroyed and replaced with fibrotic tissue resulting in impaired hepatic function; three quarters of the liver can be destroyed before symptoms appear.
  b. Distortion, twisting, and constriction of central sections cause impedance of portal blood flow and portal hypertension.
2. Fulminant hepatitis: Liver cells fail to regenerate and necrosis occurs.

Clinical Presentation

1. Subjective
  a. History of precipitating event
  b. Irritability
  c. Personality change
  d. Disorientation
  e. Weakness, fatigue
  f. Anorexia, nausea, vomiting
  g. Right upper quadrant dull abdominal pain
  h. Abdominal fullness
  i. Change in bowel habits
  j. Weight loss
2. Objective
  a. General: emaciation, cachectic appearance
  b. Cardiovascular
   1) Tachycardia, dysrhythmias
   2) Bounding pulses
   3) Hypertension or hypotension
   4) Flushed skin
   5) Spider angioma on upper trunk, face, neck, arms
   6) Jugular venous distention
   7) Distended superficial vessels on abdomen (caput medusae)
  c. Pulmonary
   1) Tachypnea or hyperpnea
   2) Decreased respiratory excursion
  d. Neurologic
   1) Peripheral neuropathy
   2) Slow, slurred speech
   3) Asterixis
   4) Hyperactive reflexes
   5) Seizures
   6) Positive Babinski's reflex in encephalopathy
   7) Extreme lethargy or coma in encephalopathy

Table 7-10 Types of Viral Hepatitis

Type	Route	Incubation Period	Onset/Chronicity	Comments
A (HAV; infectious hepatitis, enteric hepatitis)	Fecal-oral	2-6 weeks	Acute onset Chronicity does not develop	• 99% resolves but 1% becomes fulminant • Treatment is supportive
B (HBV; serum hepatitis)	Parenteral Sexual Perinatal	4-24 weeks	Insidious onset Chronicity develops in less than 5%	• 1% becomes fulminant • 15-25% develop liver cancer • Treatment includes interferon alfa-2b (Intron A); antivirals such as lamivudine (Epivir) or famciclovir (Famvir) may also be prescribed
C (HCV; non-A, non-B hepatitis; posttransfusion hepatitis)	Parenteral Sexual Perinatal	2-20 weeks	Insidious onset Chronicity develops in 50-60%	• 20-50% develop cirrhosis • 20% develop liver cancer • 20% develop liver failure • Treatment includes interferon alfa-2b (Intron A) or peginterferon alpha-2b (Peg-Intron) and ribavirin (Virazole); may also include corticosteroids
D (HDV; delta virus)	Superinfection or coinfection in patient with chronic hepatitis B	4-24 weeks	Acute onset Chronicity common with superinfection	• Up to 30% become fulminant • Most have worsening active hepatitis • Treatment is as for hepatitis B
E (HEV; enteric non-A, non-B hepatitis)	Fecal-oral Perinatal	2-8 weeks	Acute onset Chronicity does not develop	• Generally benign and self-limiting; however, 10-20% mortality when it occurs during pregnancy
F (HFV)	Parenteral Sexual Perinatal			• Now considered a variant of hepatitis B
G (HGV)				• Very little known

e. Gastrointestinal
   1) Fetor hepaticus
   2) Ascites
   3) Hematemesis
   4) Hepatomegaly early; liver atrophy occurs later
   5) Splenomegaly
   6) Ascites
   7) Bowel sounds: diminished
   8) Clay-colored (pale) stools if biliary obstruction
   9) Steatorrhea (i.e., excessive fat in stool)
   10) Esophageal varices and/or hemorrhoids

f. Renal
   1) Oliguria
   2) Dark amber urine

g. Hematologic/Immunologic
   1) Abnormal bruising, bleeding
   2) Susceptibility to infection
   3) Poor wound healing

h. Integumentary
   1) Jaundice; usually noted in the sclera first
   2) Palmar erythema
   3) Petechiae
   4) Bruises
   5) Edema
   6) Pruritus
   7) Spider angioma

i. Endocrine changes
   1) Hypogonadism: testicular atrophy and reduced testosterone levels in men
   2) Gynecomastia in men
   3) Altered hair distribution

3. Diagnostic
   a. Serum
      1) Sodium: may be decreased or normal
      2) Potassium: may be decreased
      3) Calcium: may be decreased
      4) Magnesium: may be decreased
      5) BUN: may be elevated due to dehydration, hepatorenal syndrome, or GI bleeding
      6) Glucose: may be elevated or decreased

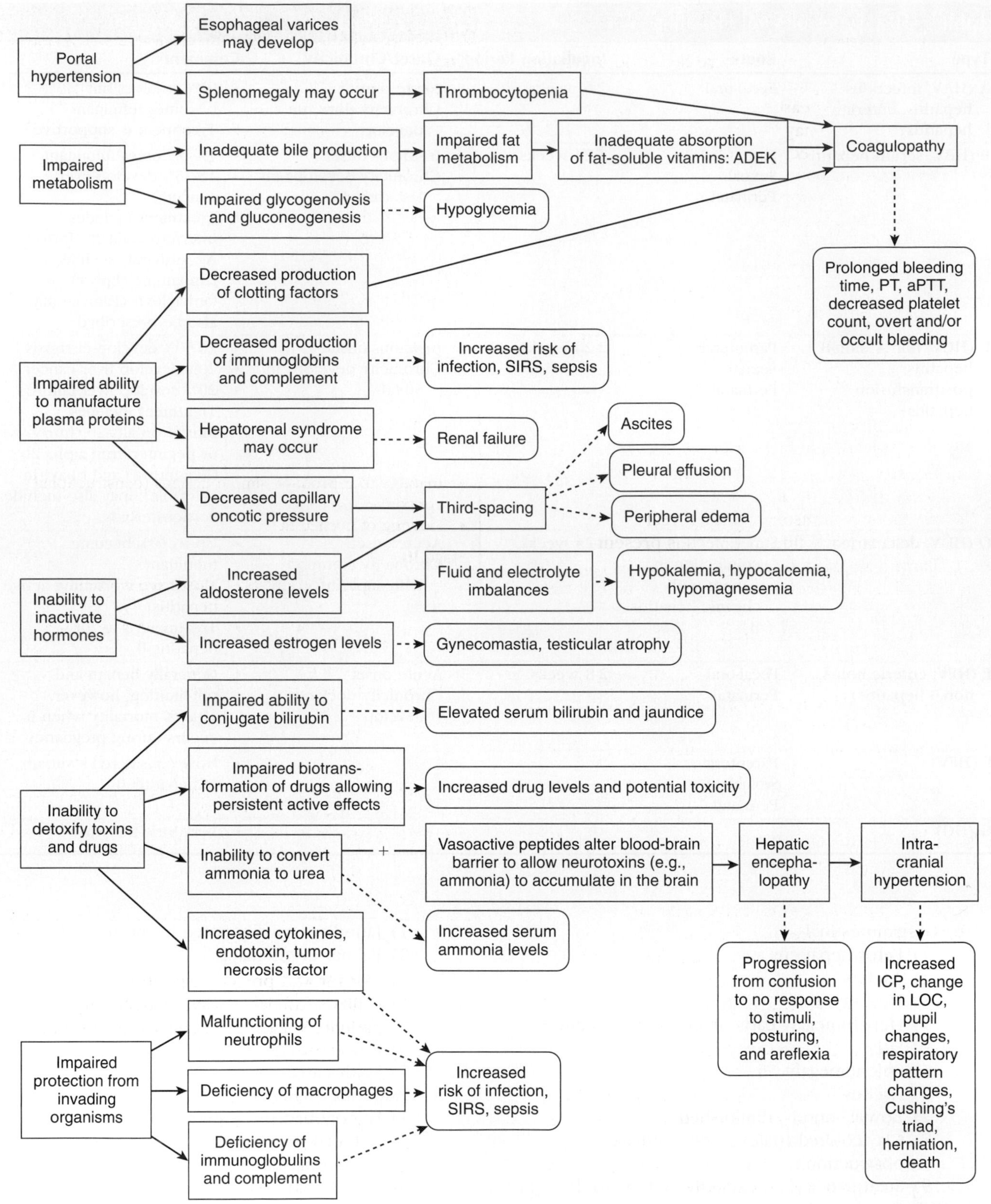

Figure 7-18 Pathophysiology of hepatic failure. Dotted lines connect pathology to clinical presentation.

7) Creatinine: may be elevated due to hepatorenal syndrome
8) Cholesterol: elevated
9) ALT, AST, LDH: elevated
   a) AST/ALT ratio greater than 1 suggests chronic liver failure or tumor.
   b) AST/ALT ratio less than 1 suggests hepatitis.
10) Alkaline phosphatase: elevated
11) Bilirubin: elevated
12) Ammonia: elevated in encephalopathy

13) Total protein, serum albumin, fibrinogen: decreased
14) Hgb, Hct: may be decreased if hemorrhage or hypersplenism
15) WBC: decreased; if normal or elevated, infection may be present
16) Platelets: decreased in splenomegaly
17) Arterial blood gases
 a) Respiratory alkalosis
 b) Hypoxemia may be seen

b. Urine
 1) Sodium: decreased
 2) Bilirubin: elevated in biliary obstruction
 3) Urobilinogen
  a) Elevated in hepatocellular disease
  b) Decreased in complete biliary obstruction

c. Chest x-ray: may show pleural effusion or atelectasis
d. Flat plate of abdomen: may reveal hepatosplenomegaly; abdominal haziness may be seen if ascites is present
e. Abdominal ultrasound: may reveal intraabdominal fluid if ascites is present
f. Barium swallow or esophagogastroduodenoscopy may be done to identify presence of esophageal varices.
g. Liver scan: may show diffuse changes of cirrhosis
h. Liver biopsy: may show fatty infiltration (early) or severe degeneration and scarring (advanced)
i. Endoscopic retrograde cholangiopancreatography: may identify biliary obstruction
j. Paracentesis: Cytologic examination may be done to rule out malignancy; ascites fluid has low specific gravity, low protein concentration, and cell counts.
k. EEG: shows abnormal and generalized slowing in patients with encephalopathy
l. Lumbar puncture: may be done to rule out neurologic cause of altered consciousness; CSF shows increase in glutamine

4. Stages of encephalopathy (Box 7-4)

Box 7-4 Stages of Encephalopathy

Stage I

- Mild confusion
- Decreased attention span
- Difficulty performing simple arithmetic computations (e.g., count backward from 100 by 7s)
- Decreased response time
- Forgetfulness
- Mood changes
- Slurred speech
- Personality changes
- Irritability
- Disruption in sleep-wake patterns
- EEG normal

Stage II

- Lethargy
- Confusion
- Apathy
- Aberrant behavior
- Tremor and asterixis (also referred to as *liver flap*)
- Inability to reproduce simple designs (constructional apraxia)
- Slowing of normal EEG

Stage III

- Somnolent with diminished responsiveness to verbal stimuli
- Severe confusion and incoherence following arousal
- Speech incomprehensible
- Tremor and asterixis
- Hyperactive deep tendon reflexes
- Hyperventilation
- EEG abnormal

Stage IV

- No response to stimuli or abnormal (e.g., decorticate or decerebrate) posturing to stimuli
- Areflexia except for pathologic reflexes
- Positive Babinski's reflex
- Fetor hepaticus
- EEG abnormal

Collaborative Management

1. Identify and treat cause of hepatic failure.
 a. Administer N-acetylcysteine (Mucomyst) for acetaminophen toxicity; must be administered within 24 hours of acetaminophen ingestion
 b. Administer antivirals (e.g., acyclovir, ganciclovir) as prescribed for viral causes; interferon may also be prescribed.
 c. Prevent further injury to the liver.
  1) Avoid hepatotoxic drugs.
  2) Avoid alcohol-containing mouthwash or medications.
 d. Monitor liver function studies.
2. Maintain airway, oxygenation, and ventilation.
 a. Elevate head of bed 30-45 degrees especially if ascites restricts diaphragmatic excursion.
 b. Monitor for and prevent aspiration.
  1) Utilize artificial airways as necessary in patients with altered consciousness and airway protective mechanisms (e.g., gag reflex).
  2) Intubation is usually required at stage III hepatic encephalopathy.
 c. Administer oxygen as necessary to maintain SpO_2 at 95% unless contraindicated; in patients with COPD, administer oxygen to achieve a SpO_2 of ~90%.
 d. Assist in management of ascites that cause decreased diaphragmatic excursion and ventilation difficulties.
  1) Monitor closely for clinical indications of atelectasis.
  2) Assist with paracentesis as necessary; patient may need paracentesis if extremely dyspneic.

3) Administer aldosterone antagonists (also referred to as *potassium-sparing diuretics*) (e.g., spironolactone [Aldactone]) as prescribed; loop diuretics may also be required as aldosterone antagonists tend to lose their effectiveness over time.
4) Restrict sodium to 500 mg/daily and restrict fluids to 1500 mL/day as prescribed; be alert to clinical indications of hypovolemia.
5) LeVeen or Denver shunt may be performed when patient is stable.
   a) Surgical procedures that shunt ascites fluid into the superior vena cava
   b) LeVeen shunt uses positive abdominal pressure caused by descent of the diaphragm during inspiration to open an intraperitoneal valve and shunt fluid from the peritoneum to the superior vena cava.
   c) Denver shunt adds a subcutaneous pump that can be compressed manually to irrigate the intraperitoneal tubing.

e. Control respiratory alkalosis associated with hyperammonemia.
   1) Avoid assist-control mode since it will perpetuate the problem.
   2) Utilize SIMV; muscle paralysis and sedation may be required to control $PaCO_2$ levels.

f. Monitor closely for ARDS.
   1) Monitor for clinical indications of respiratory distress and SpO_2.
   2) Utilize mechanical ventilation strategies to prevent ventilator-induced lung injury: V_T ~ 6 mL/kg.

3. Maintain adequate circulating volume and fluid and electrolyte balance.
   a. Monitor closely for indications of fluid and electrolyte imbalances.
      1) Monitor vital signs and hemodynamic parameters; invasive hemodynamic monitoring is usually indicated in stage III and IV hepatic encephalopathy.
      2) Weigh daily at same time on same scale.
      3) Measure abdominal girth daily for patients with ascites.
      4) Monitor serum osmolality, sodium, potassium, calcium, and magnesium.
   b. Maintain circulating blood volume.
      1) Administer colloids as prescribed to improve capillary oncotic pressure and reduce third-spacing; avoid protein-containing colloids (e.g., albumin) in hepatic encephalopathy.
      2) Administer crystalloids as prescribed; avoid lactated Ringer's solution because the liver is responsible for converting lactate to bicarbonate.
   c. Maintain vascular tone: Vasopressors may be necessary, especially in stage III or IV hepatic encephalopathy.
   d. Administer electrolyte replacement as prescribed.
   e. Monitor for hepatorenal syndrome.
      1) Observe urine output closely; note clinical indications of hepatorenal syndrome.
         a) Oliguria (less than 0.5 mL/kg/hr)
         b) Low urinary sodium
         c) Elevated BUN, serum creatinine
         d) Low serum sodium (i.e., dilutional hyponatremia)
         e) Moderately reduced GFR (less than 50 mL/min) as evaluated by 24-hour urine
      2) Administer diuretics as prescribed while monitoring closely for clinical indications of intravascular depletion and azotemia.
         a) Avoid thiazide diuretics.
         b) Utilize aldosterone antagonists (also frequently referred to as potassium-sparing diuretics) (e.g., spironolactone [Aldactone]) as prescribed.
         c) Utilize loop diuretics as prescribed; sometimes administered after albumin
            i) Albumin pulls fluid back into the intravascular space.
            ii) Furosemide (Lasix) then eliminates fluids by preventing reabsorption of sodium and water in the renal tubules.
      3) Prepare patient for hemodialysis or continuous renal replacement therapy (CRRT) as prescribed; unfortunately frequently unresponsive to treatment
         a) CRRT preferred because less likely to precipitate rapid osmolar shifts that can cause intracranial hypertension
   f. Administer H_2 receptor antagonists and/or antacids as prescribed to maintain pH 3.5-5 to reduce the risk of stress ulcer and GI hemorrhage.

4. Prevent and reduce elevated levels of toxins including ammonia.
   a. Stop nitrogen-containing drugs: ammonium chloride, urea
   b. Administer lactulose (combination of galactose and fructose) orally or via NG tube as prescribed.
      1) Acts as a chelating (bonds with) agent of ammonia by changing gut pH which results in ammonia excretion
      2) Changes gut flora to foster growth of nonammonia-forming bacteria
      3) Acts as an osmotic laxative; dose is usually adjusted for two semiformed stools/day
   c. Administer antibiotic to kill the bacteria that convert nitrogenous wastes to ammonia as prescribed.
      1) Rifaximin (Xifaxan) is a nonabsorbable antibiotic that is now preferred over neomycin.
      2) Neomycin has been traditionally used and may be prescribed by oral or NG tube; if used, monitor for auditory or renal toxicity.

d. Administer magnesium citrate orally and/or tap water enemas as prescribed to remove nitrogenous wastes from the GI tract.
e. Prevent constipation with fiber, stool softeners, enemas.
f. Assist with the use of liver support systems.
   1) Hemodialysis: blood circulated through a porous filter for rapid removal of fluid and solutes
   2) Continuous renal replacement therapy (CRRT): blood circulated through a porous filter for slow removal of fluid and solutes
   3) Hemoperfusion: hemodialysis or CRRT with a charcoal or resin exchange filter added
   4) Therapeutic plasma exchange: plasma removed and replaced by donor plasma
   5) Bioartificial liver support: Blood flows through a hollow fiber cartridge loaded with either cultured human or porcine hepatocytes.
   6) Extracorporeal liver perfusion: blood circulated through a human or animal liver in vitro

5. Prevent/assess for/treat intracranial hypertension and progression of hepatic encephalopathy.
   a. Perform frequent neurologic checks; invasive intracranial pressure monitoring may be utilized, especially in grade III and IV hepatic encephalopathy.
   b. Avoid hepatotoxic agents (see Box 7-1).
   c. Avoid sedatives and analgesics and/or reduce dosage if necessary; diphenhydramine (Benadryl) or oxazepam (Serax) may be used for restlessness because they can safely be eliminated.
   d. Provide adequate rest; maintain bed rest in hepatic encephalopathy.
   e. Avoid activities that increase ICP (see Intracranial Hypertension section of Chapter 6).
      1) Teach the patient to avoid Valsalva maneuver and other activities that increase intraabdominal or intrathoracic pressure.
      2) Maintain normal $PaCO_2$ and hypoxemia, which increase intracranial pressure.
   f. Institute seizure precautions.
   g. Administer hypertonic saline or mannitol (Osmitrol) and/or drainage of cerebrospinal fluid (if ICP catheter in place) as prescribed for cerebral edema.

6. Decrease portal hypertension.
   a. Administer beta-blockers as prescribed.
   b. Prepare the patient for a shunt as requested.
      1) Interventional radiologic procedure: TIPS (described in the GI Hemorrhage section)
      2) Surgical procedure (e.g., portacaval shunt): associated with higher incidence of hepatic encephalopathy than TIPS

7. Maintain normal serum glucose and nutritional status.
   a. Monitor serum glucose every 4-6 hours.
   b. Administer IV dextrose solution continuously; D_{10} may be required to prevent hypoglycemia.
   c. Increase dietary protein (0.6-1 g/kg/day) for patients with cirrhosis and hepatic failure, but restrict dietary protein (to less than 0.5 g/kg/day) in hepatic encephalopathy.
      1) Ensure that adequate CHO is provided to prevent muscle (protein) catabolism and muscle wasting (caloric requirements 35-40 kcal/kg/day).
      2) Add protein in 20-gram increments during recovery from encephalopathy.
   d. Use appropriate route for nutritional support.
      1) Oral: Administer antiemetics as prescribed prior to each meal and whenever indicated to prevent nausea (nausea is a significant impairment to oral nutritional intake in these patients).
      2) Enteral
         a) Necessary in patients with altered consciousness
         b) Elemental formulas (e.g., Vivonex) frequently used while maintaining protein restrictions if indicated (i.e., hepatic encephalopathy)
      3) Parenteral
         a) Branched-chain amino acid formulas may be used in encephalopathy; dextrose and lipids are needed to prevent the metabolism of parenteral amino acids or somatic protein (i.e., catabolism) for energy requirements.
   e. Administer vitamins and minerals.
      1) Fat-soluble (i.e., A, D, E, K) vitamins
      2) Thiamine and other B vitamins

8. Prevent and monitor for injury and infection.
   a. Prevent and monitor for skin breakdown.
      1) Alleviate pruritus
         a) Cornstarch baths
         b) Skin lubricating lotions
      2) Place hands in cotton gloves at night to prevent scratching during sleep.
      3) Administer cholestyramine (Questran) as prescribed to reduce bile pigment accumulation in skin.
   b. Prevent and monitor for bleeding.
      1) Avoid aspirin and NSAIDs
      2) Avoid invasive procedures, including injections, if possible.
      3) Administer vitamin K, fresh frozen plasma, and platelets as prescribed.
      4) Administer aminocaproic acid (Amicar) as prescribed.
   c. Monitor closely for clinical indications of infection and sepsis.
      1) Administer microbials as prescribed: antibiotics and antifungals.

9. Assess for clinical indications of alcohol withdrawal syndrome (see Box 7-3).

a. Administer sedatives as prescribed: most of these agents, including chlordiazepoxide (Librium) and diazepam (Valium), are hepatotoxic so doses are adjusted and liver enzymes are monitored.
b. Avoid alcohol-containing mouthwash or medications.

10. Participate in consideration of long-term treatment of hepatic failure.
    a. Early evaluation of candidacy for liver transplantation
11. Monitor for complications.
    a. Malnutrition resulting in immunosuppression, poor wound healing, and edema
    b. Coagulopathy
    c. Hemorrhage may be due to:
        1) Esophageal varices
        2) Coagulopathy
        3) Disseminated intravascular coagulation (DIC)
    d. Hypoglycemia
    e. Electrolyte imbalance
    f. Acute respiratory failure related to intrapulmonary shunt or noncardiac pulmonary edema
    g. Pancreatitis
    h. Infection, sepsis
    i. Acute renal failure related to hepatorenal syndrome, acute tubular necrosis, or hypovolemia
    j. Seizures
    k. Cerebral edema

Acute Pancreatitis

Definition

Acute inflammation of the pancreas; forms include the following:

1. Mild acute pancreatitis (previously referred to as interstitial pancreatitis)
    a. Edematous pancreas with little necrosis damage
    b. Hypovolemia may occur as a result of fluid leak into the peritoneal cavity
    c. Usually resolves within approximately 7 days
2. Severe acute pancreatitis (previously referred to as *necrotizing pancreatitis*)
    a. Extensive necrosis of pancreas and peripancreatic tissue and fat
    b. Erosion into blood vessels with hemorrhage
    c. SIRS frequently occurs.
    d. High incidence of complications and death

Etiology

1. Obstruction of common bile duct
    a. Cholelithiasis
    b. Postendoscopic retrograde cholangiopancreatography (ERCP)
2. Alcoholism
    a. Chronic alcohol intake leads to secretory and structural changes in the pancreas contributing to duct obstruction.
    b. Alcohol increases the amount of trypsinogen.
3. Hypertriglyceridemia
4. Drugs
    a. Thiazide diuretics
    b. Furosemide
    c. Estrogen
    d. Procainamide
    e. Tetracycline
    f. Sulfonamides
    g. Corticosteroids
    h. Azathioprine (Imuran)
    i. Opiates
5. Peptic ulcer with perforation
6. Cancer, especially tumors of pancreas or lung
7. Injury to pancreas
    a. Trauma
    b. Surgical
        1) Gastric
        2) Biliary
        3) Duodenal
    c. Iatrogenic
8. Radiation injury
9. Pregnancy: third trimester; ectopic pregnancy
10. Ovarian cyst
11. Hyperparathyroidism or other causes of hypercalcemia
12. Lupus erythematosus
13. Infections
    a. Mumps
    b. Coxsackievirus B
    c. *Mycoplasma*
    d. Infectious mononucleosis
    e. Viral hepatitis
    f. Human immunodeficiency virus (HIV)
    g. Intestinal parasites (e.g., *Ascaris*)
14. Ischemia (e.g., shock and multiple organ dysfunction syndrome)
15. Postcardiopulmonary bypass
16. Infection, sepsis
17. Hereditary factors
18. Idiopathic (20% of cases)

Pathophysiology

See Figure 7-19.

Clinical Presentation

1. Subjective
    a. Abdominal pain
        1) Precipitation: may occur after a heavy, especially if fatty, meal or a drinking binge
        2) Palliation: may be eased by leaning forward or by assuming fetal position
        3) Quality: "boring"
        4) Region: diffuse in epigastrium but may be left upper quadrant
        5) Radiation: to back or flanks
        6) Severity: moderate to very severe
        7) Timing: sudden onset; constant
    b. Associated symptoms
        1) Abdominal tenderness, guarding

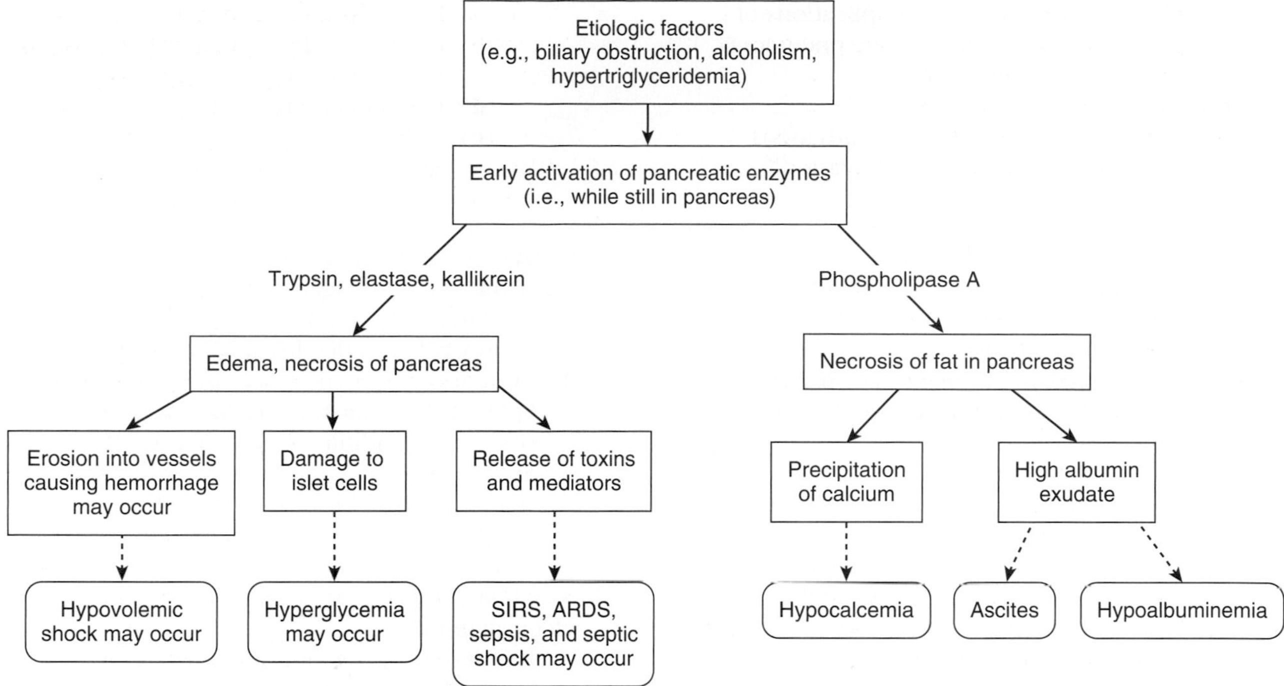

Figure 7-19 Pathophysiology of pancreatitis. Dotted lines connect pathology to clinical presentation.

2) Nausea, vomiting, retching
3) Dyspepsia
4) Flatulence, diarrhea
5) Weight loss
6) Weakness

2. Objective
   a. Tachycardia
   b. Hypotension may be seen due to decreased circulating volume due to effusion or hemorrhagic; may be decreased due to septic shock
   c. Fever: usually low-grade (e.g., 37.8-39° C)
   d. Jaundice if biliary obstruction
   e. Vomiting
   f. Hematemesis
   g. Grey Turner's sign or Cullen's sign may be seen with hemorrhage
   h. Abdominal distention
   i. Bowel sounds: decreased or absent
   j. Indications of peritoneal irritation: involuntary guarding during palpation of the abdomen, rebound tenderness
   k. Epigastric mass may be palpable especially if pseudocyst
   l. Ascites may be present.
   m. Steatorrhea (bulky, pale, foul-smelling, floating)
   n. Breath sounds changes: may be diminished due to atelectasis, pleural effusion, or ARDS; crackles may also be heard
   o. Chvostek's or Trousseau's signs may be positive in hypocalcemia
3. Diagnostic
   a. Serum
      1) Potassium: decreased
      2) Calcium: decreased
      3) Magnesium: decreased
      4) Glucose: elevated if endocrine function of the pancreas is compromised
      5) Triglycerides: may be elevated
      6) Amylase: usually elevated to greater than three times normal
         a) Peaks at 4-24 hours after onset of symptoms; usually returns to normal within 4 days
         b) May not be elevated when pancreatitis is due to hypertriglyceridemia
      7) Lipase: elevated
         a) Stays elevated longer than amylase
         b) More specific than amylase
      8) Albumin: decreased
      9) BUN: may be elevated due to hypovolemia
      10) AST, ALT, LDH, alkaline phosphatase, bilirubin: elevated in liver or biliary disease
      11) Hct: decreased with hemorrhage; elevated with hemoconcentration due to third-spacing
      12) WBC: usually elevated with shift to the left
      13) Arterial blood gases
         a) Metabolic acidosis
         b) Respiratory complications may cause respiratory acidosis and hypoxemia.
   b. Urine: amylase usually elevated
   c. Stool: increase in fecal fat
   d. ECG: may suggest MI (e.g., ST-T wave elevations)
   e. Chest x-ray
      1) May show bilateral or only left pleural effusion, elevated left hemidiaphragm, left atelectasis

2) May show pulmonary complications of pancreatitis (e.g., atelectasis, pneumonia, ARDS, pleural effusion)

f. Flat plate of abdomen
   1) May show cause (e.g., cholelithiasis)
   2) May show ileus and bowel dilation
   3) May show calcified pancreatic stones

g. Upper GI
   1) May show delayed gastric emptying
   2) May show enlargement of duodenum
   3) May show presence of dilated loop of smooth bowel adjacent to the pancreas

h. Abdominal ultrasound: may show pancreatic swelling, edema, gallstones, pseudocyst, or peripancreatic fluid collections

i. CT scan with contrast
   1) May show enlargement, edema, or necrosis of the pancreas
   2) May show complications of pancreatitis (e.g., pancreatic pseudocyst or abscess)
   3) Balthazar and Ranson's system for grading pancreatitis by CT findings
      a) Grade A: Normal pancreas
      b) Grade B: Focal or diffuse enlargement of pancreas
      c) Grade C: Mild peripancreatic inflammatory changes
      d) Grade D: Fluid collection in a single location
      e) Grade E: Multiple fluid collections or gas within the pancreas or peripancreatic inflammation

j. MRI: shows inflammatory changes within the pancreas

k. Endoscopic retrograde cholangiopancreatography (ERCP)
   1) Contraindicated in acute pancreatitis; used more often in chronic pancreatitis
   2) Identifies ductal changes or calculi

l. HIDA scan: may identify hepatocellular disease from biliary obstruction as cause of pancreatitis

m. Peritoneal lavage: positive for blood in hemorrhagic pancreatitis

4. Ranson's prognostic criteria
   a. Scoring
      1) Each of the following criteria increases the severity (and mortality) in pancreatitis.
         a) Only 1-2 criteria: mild pancreatitis; mortality approximately 1%
         b) More than 6 criteria: severe pancreatitis; predicted mortality greater than 60%
   b. Criteria
      1) At the time of admission or diagnosis
         a) Age over 55 years
         b) WBC over 16,000/mm^3
         c) Serum glucose greater than 200 mg/dL
         d) Serum lactate dehydrogenase (LDH) greater than 350 units/L
         e) Serum aspartate aminotransferase (AST) greater than 250 units/L
      2) After 48 hours
         a) Hct drop greater than 10%
         b) Increase in BUN greater than 5 mg/dL
         c) Calcium less than 8 mg/dL
         d) Base deficit greater than 4 mEq/L
         e) Estimated fluid sequestration greater than 6 L
         f) PaO_2 less than 60 mm Hg

Collaborative Management

1. Maintain airway, oxygenation, and ventilation.
   a. Elevate head of bed 30-45 degrees, especially if ascites restricts diaphragmatic excursion.
   b. Administer oxygen as necessary to maintain SpO_2 at 95% unless contraindicated; in patients with COPD, administer oxygen to achieve a SpO_2 of ~90%.
   c. Monitor SpO_2 closely and evaluate work of breathing in detection of development of atelectasis and/or ARDS.
2. Maintain adequate circulating volume and fluid and electrolyte balance.
   a. Administer crystalloids and colloids as prescribed to restore circulating blood volume.
   b. Monitor sodium, calcium, potassium, magnesium, and phosphate.
      1) Administer calcium replacement orally or intravenously as prescribed.
      2) Administer potassium replacement as prescribed.
      3) Restrict sodium to 500 mg/daily for patients with ascites.
   c. Measure abdominal girth daily in patients with ascites.
   d. Weigh daily at same time on same scale.
3. Decrease release of and destruction by pancreatic enzymes.
   a. Assist with treatment of cause.
      1) Alcohol cessation if alcohol related
      2) Cholecystectomy after resolution of pancreatitis if caused by cholelithiasis
      3) Discontinuance of offending drug if drug induced
      4) Statins, niacin, fibrates, or omega-3 fatty acids if related to hypertriglyceridemia
   b. Maintain NPO status during acute phase and with any recurrence of pain.
   c. Insert nasogastric tube to decompress the stomach and decrease risk of vomiting until ileus is resolved.
   d. Administer drugs as prescribed to decrease secretion of pancreatic enzymes (see Table 7-6).
      1) Octreotide acetate (Sandostatin) IV or subcutaneously
      2) $Histamine_2$ receptor antagonists IV
   e. Keep environment free of food odors.
   f. Perform mouth care with water or normal saline only; do not use alcohol-containing or flavored mouthwash or toothpaste.
4. Prevent and treat pain and discomfort.
   a. Maintain bed rest; encourage knee flexing while in supine position to relax abdominal muscles.

b. Maintain quiet environment, comfortable temperature, and dim lighting.
c. Administer analgesics.
   1) Opiates (e.g., morphine, hydromorphone) preferably administered via patient-controlled analgesia (PCA)
      a) NOTE: Though meperidine (Demerol) for years has been considered the analgesic of choice in acute pancreatitis, recent studies show no significant difference between morphine and meperidine in the degree of spasm of the sphincter of Oddi.
   2) Neurolytic block of the celiac plexus for severe persistent pain
d. Utilize nonpharmacologic pain relief methods (e.g., imagery, distraction).
e. Treat nausea with prescribed antiemetics.
f. Ensure adequate sleep and rest.

5. Administer appropriate nutritional support considering restrictions.
   a. Administer nutritional support during acute phase of illness.
      1) Parenteral nutrition initially
      2) Enteral nutrition below the duodenum after ileus is resolved
         a) Though enteral feeding has traditionally been thought to be contraindicated in acute pancreatitis, recent studies indicate that enteral feeding may be safely administered if the tube is below the ligament of Treitz (e.g., jejunostomy tube)
         b) Advantages over parenteral nutrition include the following:
            i) Maintains immune responsiveness and gut integrity
            ii) Reduces risk of bacterial translocation
            iii) Fewer complications
   b. Clear liquids or elemental diet (e.g., Vivonex) may be used after inflammation subsides (pain subsides, serum amylase normal) progressing to low fat, full liquids and eventually progressing to a regular diet.
   c. Avoid alcohol and food high in fat.
   d. Administer fat-soluble vitamins, thiamine, and folic acid as prescribed.
   e. Monitor serum glucose levels closely and administer glucose or insulin as indicated.
6. Prevent and monitor for infection.
   a. Prophylactic antibiotics as prescribed
      1) Antibiotics are prescribed that effectively penetrate the pancreatic tissue and provide good coverage against gram-negative enteric and anaerobic organisms (e.g., imipenem/cilastatin [Primaxin], ofloxacin [Floxin], metronidazole [Flagyl]).
      2) If no improvement after 1 week, CT-guided aspiration may be performed; bacteria in aspirate suggest infected pancreatic necrosis and indicate the need for surgery.
   b. Monitor for clinical indications of abscess formation (e.g., increase in abdominal pain, vomiting, fever, leukocytosis).
7. Prepare patient for surgical measures for relief of pancreatitis if necessary (during acute phase, surgery is performed only if absolutely necessary).
   a. Cholecystectomy if bile reflux is the cause of pancreatitis
   b. Drainage and removal of abscess or pseudocysts
   c. Pancreatic resection/total pancreatectomy
      1) Used if pancreas and/or other organs are necrotic
      2) After surgical débridement of necrotic tissue, the abdomen may be left open and packed or closed with drains in place.
      3) Total pancreatectomy; results in diabetes and other metabolic difficulties
         a) Islet cell autotransplantation is sometimes performed.
         b) Segmental pancreatic autotransplantation is sometimes performed: part of viable pancreatic tissue reimplanted following total pancreatectomy
8. Maintain normal serum glucose levels.
   a. Monitor serum glucose levels closely.
   b. Administer insulin as indicated and prescribed.
   c. Maintain constant infusion of TPN solution or enteral feedings.
9. Assess for clinical indications of alcohol withdrawal syndrome (see Box 7-3).
   a. If present, administer sedatives as prescribed; most of these agents, including chlordiazepoxide (Librium) and diazepam (Valium), are hepatotoxic; doses are adjusted and liver enzymes are monitored.
   b. Avoid alcohol-containing mouthwash or medications.
10. Monitor for complications.
   a. Hypoglycemia or hyperglycemia
   b. Hypocalcemia
   c. Pseudocysts
      1) Caused by collection of inflammatory debris, pancreatic secretions, and necrotic tissue in the pancreatic tissue; may cause compression of portal vein or bile duct or rupture and peritonitis and sepsis
      2) Clinical presentation includes pain or ache in the abdomen, a feeling of bloating, or poor digestion of food.
      3) Complications related to the pseudocyst include infection of the pseudocyst with a pancreatic abscess, bleeding into the pseudocyst, or intestinal obstruction of the intestine by the pseudocyst.
      4) Collaborative management includes nothing for small cysts or drainage by surgical, endoscopic, or percutaneous approach for larger cysts.

d. Pancreatic abscess
   1) Caused by accumulation of pus in or near the pancreas
   2) Clinical presentation includes fever, palpable mass, abdominal tenderness, nausea, vomiting, and leukocytosis.
   3) Collaborative management includes surgery for drainage.
e. Pancreatic fistula
   1) Caused by a communication between the pancreas and the skin
   2) Clinical presentation includes drainage of extremely alkaline pancreatic secretions onto the skin and severe excoriation.
   3) Collaborative management includes fluid and electrolyte replacement; octreotide acetate (Sandostatin) may be used.
f. Hypovolemic shock
   1) Caused by exudate of protein-rich fluid into retroperitoneal space or by erosion into the vascular bed and hemorrhage
   2) Clinical presentation includes tachycardia, hypotension, oliguria, and other indications of hypoperfusion.
   3) Collaborative management includes volume resuscitation, including crystalloids, colloids, blood administration for hemorrhagic pancreatitis
g. Systemic inflammatory response syndrome (SIRS)
h. Pleural effusion
i. Acute respiratory distress syndrome
j. GI bleeding
k. Disseminated intravascular coagulation (DIC)
l. Sepsis
m. Acute renal failure
n. Perforation

Intestinal Infarction/ Obstruction/Perforation

Definitions

1. Intestinal infarction: necrosis of the intestinal wall resulting from ischemia
2. Intestinal obstruction: failure of the intestinal contents to progress forward through the lumen of the bowel; may be partial or complete
   a. Mechanism
      1) Functional obstruction: caused by loss of peristalsis; usually referred to as paralytic ileus
      2) Structural (i.e., mechanical) obstruction: caused by factors that occlude the bowel lumen
   b. Severity
      1) Simple: luminal obstruction without compromise of blood supply
      2) Strangulated: luminal obstruction with compromise of blood supply
   c. Extent: partial versus complete
   d. Location: proximal versus distal
3. Intestinal perforation: penetration of the lumen of the intestine with resultant spillage of intestinal contents into the peritoneal cavity

Etiology

1. Infarction
   a. Arteriosclerosis
   b. Vasculitis
   c. Mural thrombus, emboli: post-MI; atrial fibrillation; ventricular aneurysm; endocarditis
   d. Hypercoagulability (e.g., polycythemia, postsplenectomy)
   e. Surgical procedures involving aortic clamping (e.g., abdominal aortic aneurysm repair)
   f. Vasopressors
      1) Endogenous due to sympathetic nervous system stimulation (e.g., shock)
      2) Exogenous (e.g., norepinephrine, high dose dopamine)
   g. Strangulated intestinal obstruction
   h. Intraabdominal infection
   i. Cirrhosis
2. Obstruction
   a. Functional (i.e., paralytic ileus): most common type of intestinal obstruction
      1) Abdominal surgery
      2) Hypokalemia
      3) Intestinal distention
      4) Peritonitis
      5) Intestinal ischemia
      6) Severe trauma
      7) Spinal cord injury
      8) Ureteral distention
      9) Pneumonia
      10) Pleuritis
      11) Subphrenic abscess
      12) Pancreatitis
      13) Acute cholecystitis
      14) Pelvic abscess
      15) Narcotics (e.g., morphine)
      16) Sepsis
   b. Structural (i.e., mechanical)
      1) Small bowel: Most obstructions occur in the small bowel, especially at the ileum.
         a) Postoperative adhesions: most common
         b) Incarcerated hernia
         c) Volvulus
         d) Foreign body
         e) Neoplasm
         f) Crohn's disease
      2) Large bowel: most often the sigmoid colon
         a) Neoplasm: most common
         b) Stricture
         c) Intussusception
         d) Diverticulitis
         e) Fecal or barium impaction
3. Perforation
   a. Peptic ulcer
   b. Bowel obstruction
   c. Appendicitis, diverticulitis
   d. Penetrating wound

Pathophysiology

See Figure 7-20.

Clinical Presentation

1. Infarction
   a. Subjective
      1) May have history of precipitating event
      2) Anorexia
      3) Pallor
      4) Abdominal pain
         a) Severe cramping, periumbilical or nonspecific diffuse
         b) Abdominal pain related to mesenteric ischemia may be referred to as *abdominal angina*
      5) Abdominal tenderness
      6) Urgency to have a bowel movement
   b. Objective
      1) Tachycardia
      2) Hypotension
      3) Tachypnea
      4) Fever
      5) Clinical indications of dehydration
      6) Vomiting: persistent, may be bloody
      7) Abdominal distention
      8) Abdominal guarding and rigidity
      9) Urgent and bloody diarrhea
      10) Hypoactive or absent bowel sounds
      11) Weight loss
   c. Diagnostic
      1) Serum
         a) BUN: elevated due to dehydration
         b) Alkaline phosphatase: elevated
         c) Amylase: elevated

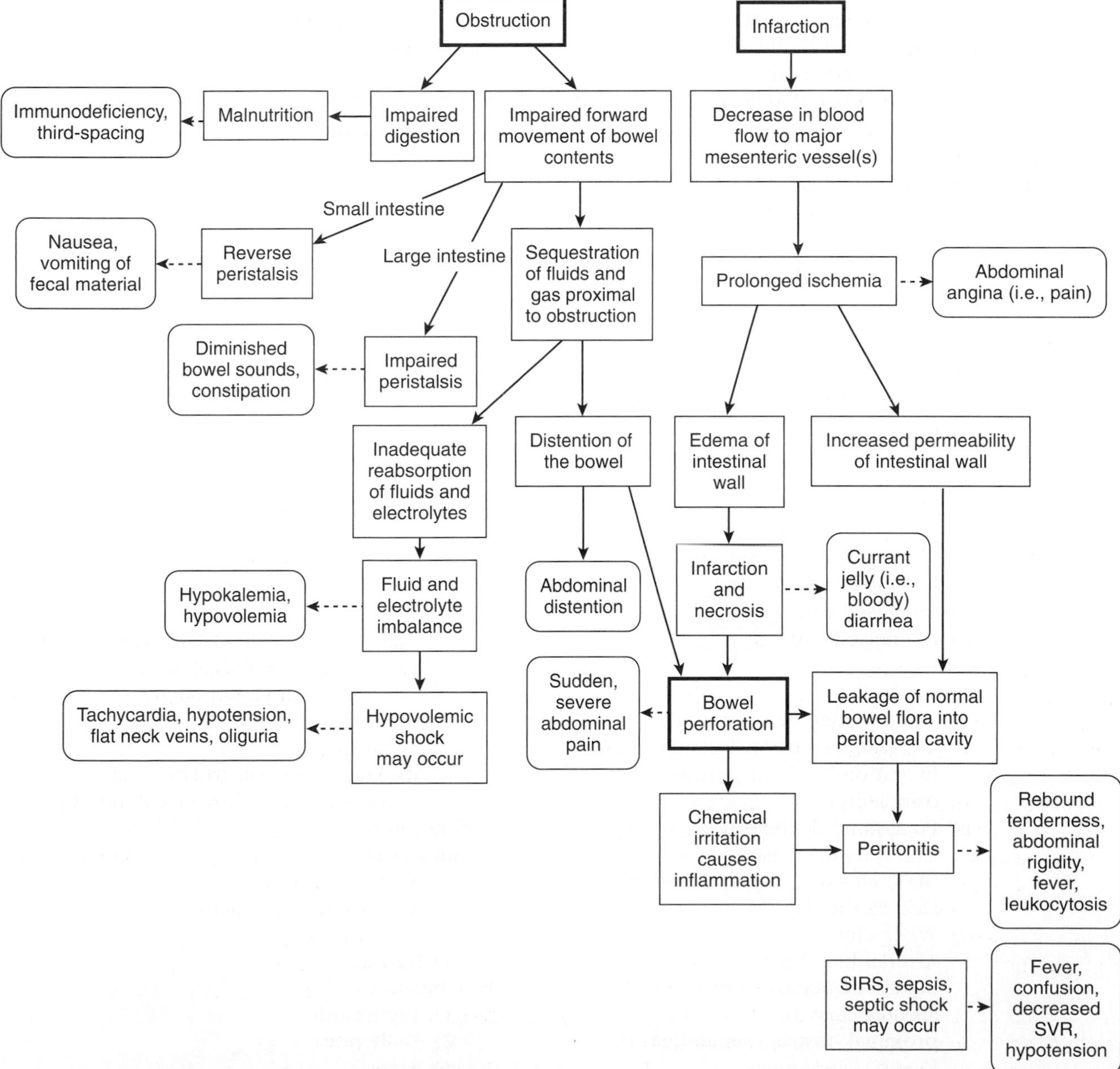

Figure 7-20 Pathophysiology of intestinal obstruction/infarction/perforation. Dotted lines connect pathology to clinical presentation.

d) Hematocrit: elevated
e) WBC: elevated
f) Arterial blood gases: metabolic acidosis
2) Stool: guaiac positive
3) Angiography: shows occlusion of the arterial supply
4) Sigmoidoscopy: shows dusky, ischemic bowel

2. Obstruction
   a. Small bowel
      1) Subjective
         a) May have history of precipitating event
         b) Abdominal pain
            i) Pain that is colicky and of shorter duration with bilious vomiting may be more proximal; pain that is progressive and lasting for several days with abdominal distention may be more distal.
            ii) Steady, severe, localized pain may indicate strangulation.
         c) Changes in bowel habits
            i) Early or partial bowel obstruction: normal stools or diarrhea
            ii) Late or complete obstruction: constipation or absence of stools
      2) Objective
         a) Vomiting early: may be projectile and/or fecal
            i) Clear gastric fluid: obstruction at the pylorus
            ii) Gastric contents and bile
               (a) Obstruction in the proximal small intestine
               (b) Paralytic ileus
            iii) Brown fecal: obstruction in the distal small intestine
         b) Abdominal distention
         c) Clinical indications of dehydration
         d) Bowel sounds: high-pitched
            i) Increased early
            ii) Decreased late
      3) Diagnostic
         a) Serum
            i) Sodium: may be decreased, increased, or normal depending on hydration level and serum osmolality
            ii) Potassium: decreased
            iii) Chloride: decreased
            iv) BUN: elevated due to dehydration
            v) Hct: elevated
            vi) WBC: elevated
            vii) Arterial blood gases: usually metabolic acidosis but metabolic alkalosis may be seen with proximal obstruction and gastric losses
         b) Upper GI: may show point of obstruction
         c) Flat plate of abdomen: shows dilated loops of gas-filled bowel
         d) CT: aids in differentiation of cause and location of obstruction
         e) MRI: aids in differentiation of cause and location of obstruction
   b. Large bowel
      1) Subjective
         a) May have history of precipitating event
         b) Dull pain
         c) Change in bowel habits: thin, ribbonlike stools progressing to constipation to absence of stools with watery discharge
         d) Decrease in flatus
      2) Objective
         a) Vomiting late
         b) Abdominal distention
         c) Bowel sounds: low-pitched
            i) Increased early
            ii) Decreased late
         d) Melena may occur if large bowel obstruction is caused by ulcerative colitis, cancer, or diverticulitis.
      3) Diagnostic
         a) Serum
            i) Sodium: may be decreased, increased, or normal depending on hydration level and serum osmolality
            ii) Potassium: decreased
            iii) Chloride: decreased
            iv) BUN: elevated due to dehydration
            v) CEA: elevated if due to cancer
            vi) Hematocrit: may be elevated due to dehydration or decreased due to hemorrhage; large intestinal tumor frequently causes slow bleeding
            vii) WBC: elevated
            viii) Arterial blood gases: metabolic acidosis
         b) Stools: may be positive for occult blood in large bowel obstruction due to ulcerative colitis, cancer, or diverticulitis
         c) Flat plate of abdomen: shows dilated loops of gas-filled bowel
         d) Barium enema: may show point of obstruction
         e) Endoscopy: obstruction may be visible on sigmoidoscopy or colonoscopy

3. Perforation
   a. Subjective
      1) Abdominal pain
      2) Abdominal tenderness
      3) Anorexia
      4) Nausea
   b. Objective
      1) Tachycardia
      2) Tachypnea
      3) Fever
      4) Vomiting
      5) Rigid, "boardlike" abdomen

6) Rebound tenderness
7) Absence of liver dullness due to free air in peritoneum
8) Bowel sounds: diminished or absent

c. Diagnostic
1) Serum: WBC elevated
2) Flat plate of abdomen: free air in peritoneum may be seen
3) Upper GI: contraindicated

Collaborative Management

1. Maintain airway, oxygenation, and ventilation.
a. Elevate head of bed 30-45 degrees.
b. Administer oxygen as necessary to maintain SpO_2 at 95% unless contraindicated; in patients with COPD, administer oxygen to achieve a SpO_2 of ~90%.
2. Maintain adequate circulating volume and fluid and electrolyte balance.
a. Assess fluid status.
1) Daily weight at same time on same scale.
2) Hemodynamic monitoring may be necessary during fluid resuscitation.
b. Administer crystalloids and colloids as prescribed to restore circulating blood volume.
c. Administer blood and blood products as needed; whole blood or packed cells should be given early if significant bleeding is suspected; after multiple transfusions, consideration should be given to replacement of clotting factors, platelets, and calcium.
d. Monitor sodium, calcium, potassium, and phosphate; administer electrolyte replacement as indicated.
e. Discontinue vasopressors if cause of ischemia.
3. Prevent and treat pain and discomfort.
a. Maintain bed rest.
b. Maintain quiet environment, comfortable temperature, and dim lighting.
c. Administer analgesics (e.g., morphine) (NOTE: Analgesics are sometimes withheld until the diagnosis is made).
d. Encourage knee flexing while in supine position to relax abdominal muscles.
e. Utilize nonpharmacologic pain relief methods (e.g., imagery, distraction, music).
f. Treat nausea with prescribed antiemetics.
g. Perform mouth care after emesis.
4. Prevent perforation of bowel if obstruction present.
a. Discontinue all oral intake.
b. Insert a nasogastric tube or orogastric tube as prescribed to decompress the stomach, prevent vomiting, and reduce the risk of aspiration.
c. Administer drugs as prescribed to enhance GI motility in partial intestinal obstruction.
1) Erythromycin
2) Metoclopramide HCl (Reglan)
3) Octreotide (Sandostatin)
d. Insert a rectal tube as prescribed to reduce trapped air in complete large bowel obstruction.
e. Prepare patient for therapeutic colonoscopy as requested.
1) Air insufflation for intussusception
2) Cecal dilation or endoscopic balloon duodenal dilation for small bowel obstruction
f. Assist with palliative procedures to enhance quality of life in patients with terminal disease associated with bowel obstruction.
1) Insertion of distal gastric or jejunal tubes
2) Colonic dilation
3) Insertion of intestinal stents
5. Prepare the patient for surgery as requested: Surgery is indicated for vascular obstruction, complete bowel obstruction, and bowel perforation; a strangulated obstruction is a surgical emergency.
a. Bowel preparation with cathartics, enemas, and sterilization prior to surgery
1) Nonabsorbable aminoglycoside (e.g., neomycin) usually is used for bowel sterilization.
2) Do not give cathartics or enemas for patients who are completely obstructed.
b. Procedures
1) Infarction
a) Exploratory laparotomy and embolectomy and/or arterial reconstruction with resection of irreparably damaged bowel
2) Obstruction
a) Correction of cause
i) Laparoscopic adhesiolysis: for obstruction caused by adhesion
ii) Herniorrhaphy: for reduction of hernia
iii) Reduction of volvulus or intussusception
b) Bowel resection: may require temporary or permanent bowel diversion with colostomy
i) Right hemicolectomy: for tumors in the cecum and ascending colon
ii) Left hemicolectomy: for tumors of the descending and sigmoid colon; prepare patient for the possibility of colostomy (temporary or permanent) in cases of left-sided obstruction
iii) Transverse colectomy: for tumors of the middle or left transverse colon
iv) Low anterior resection: for proximal and midrectal tumors
v) Abdominoperineal resection: for malignant lesions of the lower sigmoid colon, rectum, and anus; requires permanent colostomy
3) Perforation
a) Repair of perforation may require bowel resection; a temporary bowel diversion

may be performed to allow the anastomosis to heal.
    b) Antibiotic lavage may be done during surgery.
  c. Answer the patient's questions about the planned procedures.
  d. Prepare the patient for adjuvant therapy if required for colon cancer.
    1) Chemoembolization: the infusion of a concentrated dose of an antineoplastic agent into the hepatic artery to embolize the agent
    2) Radiation therapy
    3) Brachytherapy: the placement of radioactive seeds in the area where the tumor was removed
    4) Chemotherapy: the administration of an antineoplastic agent before, during, or after surgery
    5) Cryosurgery: the freezing of liver metastasis
6. Prevent/monitor for infection.
  a. Administer antibiotics as prescribed.
  b. Reduce leakage of intestinal bacteria and risk of peritonitis and sepsis if perforation has occurred.
    1) Keep the patient immobilized to reduce the chemical irritation to the peritoneum.
    2) Antibiotics are given preoperatively.
    3) Antibiotic lavage may be done during surgery.
    4) Antibiotics are given postoperatively.
  c. Monitor closely for clinical indications of infection and sepsis.
    1) Measure temperature every 4 hours.
    2) Assess HR and BP hourly.
    3) Note changes in mental status.
    4) Note changes in color and character of wound drainage.
    5) Monitor changes in WBC.
  d. Clean around drains aseptically and protect skin around drains postoperatively.
7. Administer appropriate nutritional support considering restrictions.
  a. Administer nutritional support parenterally in the acute phase.
  b. Provide oral feedings and advance diet when condition and postoperative paralytic ileus have resolved.
  c. Administer vitamin and mineral supplements as prescribed.
8. Monitor for complications.
  a. Fluid and electrolyte imbalance
  b. Hemorrhage
  c. Sepsis
  d. Peritonitis
  e. Respiratory distress secondary to abdominal distention
  f. Shock: hypovolemic or septic
  g. Abscess
  h. Perforation

Abdominal Trauma

Definition

Trauma that occurs between the nipple line to midthigh

Etiology

1. Penetrating trauma (e.g., motor vehicle collision; assault; sharp instruments [e.g., knife; gunshot wound; impalement])
2. Blunt trauma (e.g., motor vehicle collision; assault; fall; sport injury)
3. Iatrogenic trauma
  a. Peritoneal tap
  b. Endoscopy
  c. Biopsy
  d. Cardiopulmonary resuscitation

Pathophysiology

1. Seldom a single-organ injury
2. High-velocity penetrating trauma
  a. Extensive destruction of contact tissue
  b. Severe associated blast effect on the surrounding tissues
  c. Liver most often affected by penetrating trauma
3. Blunt trauma
  a. Due to direct injury, crushing force between two objects, acceleration/deceleration, shearing, twisting
  b. Pressure injury
  c. Spleen most often affected by blunt trauma; pancreas is frequently injured with spleen.

Clinical Presentation

1. Subjective
  a. Abdominal pain: may be poorly localized or referred
    1) Kehr's sign: left shoulder pain indicative of splenic rupture caused by blood below diaphragm that irritates the phrenic nerve
    2) Rovsing's sign: pain in RLQ with palpation of LLQ indicates peritoneal irritation
  b. Abdominal tenderness
2. Objective
  a. Seat belt sign: ecchymosis across the lower abdomen caused by seat belt
  b. Hematoma: Note location.
    1) Hematoma in flank area may be seen in renal injury.
  c. Entrance and exit wounds
  d. Grey Turner's or Cullen's sign: may be seen
  e. Coopernail's sign (ecchymosis of scrotum or labia): indicative of fractured pelvis
  f. Rigid abdomen: may indicate intraabdominal bleeding
  g. Ballance's sign (i.e., resonance over right flank with patient on left side): indicative of ruptured spleen
  h. Diminished femoral pulses: may be seen in vascular injury
  i. Loss of liver dullness: indicates perforation with free air in peritoneum

j. Clinical indications of hypoperfusion or shock (see Table 2-2)
k. Clinical indications of perforation (e.g., severe abdominal pain, fever, nausea, vomiting)
l. Clinical indications of peritonitis (e.g., involuntary guarding, abdominal rigidity, rebound tenderness)
m. Specifics related to organ injured (Table 7-11)

3. Diagnostic
   a. Serum
      1) Glucose: elevated due to stress
      2) Amylase: may be elevated if injury to pancreas or bowel
      3) ALT, AST, and LDH: may be elevated if liver injury
      4) Hgb, Hct: decreased with hemorrhage
      5) WBC: may be elevated if infection is present or if spleen is ruptured
      6) Platelets: elevated if spleen is injured
      7) PT, aPTT: may be prolonged
      8) Drug and alcohol screens: may be positive
   b. Urine
      1) May show hematuria if renal trauma
      2) May show myoglobinuria if crush injury has occurred
   c. Stool: may be positive for occult blood
   d. Chest x-ray: used to rule out concurrent thoracic injury; identify free air under diaphragm
   e. Flat plate of abdomen: may show free air in peritoneum if stomach or bowel is perforated
   f. IVP: if hematuria is present to look for renal trauma
   g. Angiography: may show vascular injury
   h. CT scan or MRI: to identify areas of injury
   i. Focused abdominal sonography for trauma (FAST)
      1) Use: detects fluid or blood in the pericardium, abdomen, or pelvis and allows visualization of the spleen and liver
         a) While cannot reliably identify injury to intraabdominal organs (requires CT), can accurately predict the need for laparotomy in trauma patients; very good sensitivity and excellent specificity
      2) Advantages over diagnostic peritoneal lavage (DPL)
         a) More rapid: generally completed in less than 5 minutes
         b) Requires no preparation
         c) Noninvasive
         d) No contraindications
   j. Diagnostic peritoneal lavage (DPL): may be done to assess for intraabdominal bleeding, though FAST is usually the preferred screening study
      1) Assist with placement of peritoneal catheter; if gross blood is obtained with catheter insertion, immediate exploratory laparotomy is indicated.
      2) Instill 1 L of normal saline over 15-20 minutes.
      3) Move the patient side to side after fluid instillation to distribute the lavage fluid.
      4) Drain.
      5) Send for analysis.
         a) Considered positive if lavage fluid is grossly bloody or contains the following:
            i) RBC greater than 100,000/mm^3
            ii) WBC greater than 500/mm^3
            iii) Amylase greater than 175 units/dL
            iv) Bile, bacteria, intestinal content
         b) Considered positive if newsprint cannot be read through the lavage fluid (i.e., newsprint sign)
         c) Major limitation of peritoneal lavage is that it does not detect diaphragmatic or retroperitoneal injuries
   k. Specifics related to organ injured (Table 7-11)

Collaborative Management

1. Maintain airway, oxygenation, and ventilation.
   a. Stabilize the cervical spine.
   b. Elevate head of bed 30-45 degrees to allow for optimal diaphragmatic excursion.
   c. Administer oxygen as necessary to maintain SpO_2 at 95% unless contraindicated; in patients with COPD, administer oxygen to achieve a SpO_2 of 90% by pulse oximetry.
   d. Place oropharyngeal or nasopharyngeal airway in patients with altered consciousness; assist with endotracheal intubation if required.
2. Detect bleeding and maintain adequate circulating volume.
   a. Detect bleeding by performing head-to-toe assessment and assisting with peritoneal lavage; peritoneal lavage is especially important in an unconscious patient because subjective report of tenderness or pain is absent.
   b. Insert indwelling urinary catheter to evaluate hourly urine output unless contraindicated; contraindications include the following:
      1) Blood around the urinary meatus
      2) Perineal or scrotal hematoma
      3) Displacement of the prostate gland noted during rectal exam by physician
   c. Assist with insertion of arterial catheter and pulmonary artery catheter in patient with hemodynamic instability.
   d. Insert two short (1¼-inch) large-gauge (16-18) peripheral intravenous catheters; draw blood samples for laboratory analysis and type and crossmatch for blood.
   e. Administer intravenous fluids to restore circulating blood volume.
      1) Crystalloids
      2) Colloids
      3) Blood and blood products
         a) Whole blood or packed cells should be given early if significant bleeding is suspected.

Table 7-11 Clinical Indications of Organ Injury

Organ	Suspect Injury to This Organ if	Clinical Indications of Injury	Complications
Liver	• Seat belt sign • Local sign of injury (RUQ) • Lower right rib fracture • Blunt or penetrating trauma • Acceleration/deceleration MVC • Presence of other abdominal injuries	• RUQ pain, tenderness, and guarding • Referred pain to right shoulder • Increase in abdominal girth and rigidity • Increased pain on inspiration • Clinical indications of shock • Leukocytosis • Elevated ALT, AST, LDH • Decreased Hgb and Hct • Abnormal clotting studies • Chest x-ray: elevated diaphragm on right side • Injury evident on FAST • Positive peritoneal lavage if performed	• Shock • Infection, sepsis • Subdiaphragmatic abscess • Clotting abnormalities • Atelectasis, pneumonia, ARDS • Hepatic failure
Spleen	• Seat belt sign • Local sign of injury (LUQ) • Lower left rib fractures • Left pneumothorax • Blunt or penetrating trauma to abdomen • Acceleration/ deceleration MVC • Presence of other abdominal injuries	• LUQ pain, tenderness, and guarding • Increased abdominal girth and rigidity • Kehr's sign • Ballance's sign • Increased pain on inspiration • Clinical indications of shock • Decreased Hgb and Hct • Injury evident on FAST • Positive peritoneal lavage • Shock	• Shock • Atelectasis, pneumonia, ARDS • Infection, sepsis especially if splenectomy performed • Subdiaphragmatic abscess
Pancreas	• Seat belt sign • Presence of other abdominal injuries • MVC • Blunt or penetrating trauma to abdomen	• Epigastric, back, or shoulder pain • Abdominal tenderness and guarding • Increased abdominal girth • Diminished bowel sounds • Clinical indications of shock • Hyperglycemia or hypoglycemia • Elevated serum lipase • Leukocytosis • Positive peritoneal lavage for amylase but unreliable because the pancreas is located retroperitoneally	• Shock • Diabetes • Pancreatitis • Pancreatic abscess or pseudocyst • Pancreatic fistula • Atelectasis, pneumonia, ARDS
Stomach	• Penetrating trauma to abdomen • Presence of other abdominal injuries	• Epigastric or LUQ pain and tenderness • Hematemesis or bloody aspirate from NG tube • Rebound tenderness • Clinical indications of shock • Leukocytosis • Positive peritoneal lavage • Free air on flat plate of abdomen	• Atelectasis, pneumonia, ARDS • Gastric fistula
Intestine	• Seat belt sign • Presence of other abdominal injuries • Blunt trauma with deceleration • Penetrating injury	• Local sign of injury (e.g., ecchymosis, abrasion) • Nausea, vomiting • Abdominal pain: may be referred or rebound • Absent bowel sounds • Leukocytosis • Positive peritoneal lavage for blood and fecal matter • Free air on flat plate of abdomen • Positive fecal occult blood test	• Ileus • Peritonitis, sepsis • Abscess • Intestinal ischemia, infarction, obstruction, perforation • Fistula
Abdominal vessels	• Other abdominal injuries • Blunt or penetrating abdominal injury • Sudden deceleration in MVC or fall	• Clinical indications of shock • Abdominal distention and guarding • Increased abdominal girth and rigidity • Abdominal bruit • Diminished femoral pulses if aorta or iliac injury • Mottled lower extremities • Cullen's sign • Decreased Hgb and Hct • Shock	• Shock • Mesenteric ischemia or infarction • Infection, sepsis

b) Consideration should be given to replacement of clotting factors, platelets, and calcium after multiple transfusions.
f. Control bleeding.
1) Pressure can be applied to overt bleeding site.
2) Prepare patient for exploratory laparotomy as indicated.
a) Penetrating injury invading the peritoneum
b) Clinical indications of perforation (e.g., acute abdomen)
c) Free air in peritoneum on x-ray
d) Shock
e) GI hemorrhage
f) Massive hematuria
g) Evisceration
h) Positive peritoneal lavage
i) Surgical indications on CT scan or angiography

3. Prevent and treat pain and discomfort.
   a. Maintain bed rest.
   b. Maintain quiet environment, comfortable temperature, and dim lighting.
   c. Administer analgesics (e.g., morphine); may be contraindicated until diagnoses are made
   d. Encourage knee flexing while in supine position to relax abdominal muscles in patients with peritoneal irritation.
   e. Utilize nonpharmacologic pain relief methods (e.g., imagery, distraction, music).
4. Maintain fluid and electrolyte balance.
   a. Monitor sodium, calcium, potassium, magnesium, and phosphate.
   b. Administer electrolyte replacement as indicated.
5. Decompress GI tract.
   a. Insert nasogastric tube; use orogastric tube in patients with midface fractures.
   b. Monitor nasogastric output for color, amount, and odor of drainage.
   c. Cover any eviscerated organs with saline-soaked pads.
6. Administer appropriate nutritional support considering restrictions.
   a. Administer nutritional support parenterally acutely.
   b. Provide oral feeding and advance diet when condition is surgically resolved.
   c. Administer vitamin and mineral supplements.
7. Prevent/monitor for infection.
   a. Observe for signs of peritonitis (e.g., fever, peritonitis, leukocytosis).
   b. Monitor abdominal girth.
   c. Administer antibiotics as prescribed; antibiotic lavage may be performed during exploratory laparotomy if bowel perforation has occurred.
   d. Maintain asepsis of wounds and drains.
   e. Monitor bowel sounds.
   f. Evaluate tetanus immunization status and administer tetanus toxoid if indicated for penetrating trauma, abrasion, cuts, etc.
8. Monitor for complications.
   a. Obstruction
   b. Perforation
   c. Peritonitis
   d. Pancreatitis
   e. Infection, abscess, sepsis
   f. Hemorrhage
      1) Retroperitoneal
      2) Intraperitoneal
   g. Shock: hypovolemic or septic
   h. DIC
   i. Atelectasis, pneumonia, ARDS
   j. Organ failure
   k. Abdominal compartment syndrome

GI Surgery

Procedures Frequently Requiring Critical Care

See Table 7-12 and Figures 7-21 through 7-25.

Postoperative Management for GI Surgeries

1. Maintain airway, oxygenation, and ventilation.
   a. Monitor airway patency and utilize artificial airways as indicated; many of these patients will still be intubated and receiving mechanical ventilation.
   b. Monitor SpO_2 and administer oxygen to maintain SpO_2 at 95% until contraindicated.
   c. Position the patient with head of bed elevated to 30 to 40 degrees unless contraindicated; side-lying position is frequently more comfortable for patients who have had rectal or perineal procedures.
   d. Utilize short-term breathing trials to evaluate the patient's ability to maintain spontaneous breathing so that weaning and extubation can be accomplished as soon as possible.
   e. Encourage deep breathing and incentive spirometry.
   f. Maintain hydration, encourage leg exercises, and ambulate as soon as possible to prevent DVT and pulmonary embolism.
2. Prevent/monitor for fluid volume deficit and/or electrolyte imbalance.
   a. Monitor vital signs, hemodynamics, urine output, daily weights, and laboratory values.
      1) Utilize CVP or PA catheter when in place to evaluate fluid status.
      2) Evaluate electrolyte values as indicated.
      3) Monitor hemoglobin and hematocrit as indicated.
      4) Weigh daily.
   b. Administer fluids as prescribed: crystalloids and colloids.
   c. Monitor drains if in place for change in amount or character of drainage.
   d. Expect mobilization of third-spaced fluids and increase in urine output on second or third

Table 7-12 GI Surgical Procedures Frequently Requiring Critical Care

Surgical Procedure	Description	Indication
Billroth I (also referred to as *gastroduodenostomy*) (Figure 7-17)	• Resection of the antrum of the stomach and anastomosis of the remainder of the stomach to the duodenum	• Ulcer or malignancy
Billroth II (also referred to as *gastrojejunostomy*) (Figure 7-17)	• Resection of the antrum of the stomach and anastomosis of the remainder of the stomach to the jejunum leaving the duodenal stump and accompanied by a vagotomy	• Ulcer or malignancy
Complete gastrectomy (Figure 7-17)	• Removal of the stomach with anastomosis of the esophagus to the jejunum leaving the duodenal stump	• Ulcer or malignancy
Whipple procedure (also referred to as *radical pancreaticoduodenectomy*) (Figure 7-21)	• Removal of the lower stomach and duodenum with anastomosis of the remaining stomach to the jejunum with partial or total pancreatectomy and a possible splenectomy	• Cancer of the pancreas • May also be performed for resection of necrotic tissue as a result of pancreatitis
Esophagogastrectomy (Figure 7-22)	• Removal of all or a portion of the esophagus, possibly with a portion of the stomach, with anastomosis to the remaining portion of the stomach	• Cancer of the lower and middle third of the thoracic esophagus • Corrosive esophagitis
Esophagoenterostomy (may also be referred to as *esophagogastrectomy with a colon interposition*) (Figure 7-23)	• Removal of all or a portion of the esophagus along with replacement with a segment of the colon	• Cancer of the esophagus • Corrosive esophagitis
Colon resection with end-to-end anastomosis; may include colostomy	• Removal of a portion of the colon; may include formation of a colostomy • Temporary colostomy may be developed to temporarily divert bowel contents to allow for healing of the anastomosis • May be performed laparoscopically	• Tumor, bleeding, inflammation, necrosis, or trauma of the large intestine
Total colectomy and ileostomy	• Removal of the entire large intestine and the formation of a stoma from the end of the ileum • May also include surgical formation of a continent ileostomy (i.e., Kock pouch) or ileoanal reservoir	• Ulcerative colitis
Abdominoperineal resection	• Removal of the anus, rectum, and sigmoid colon with creation of a permanent colostomy	• Malignancy of the rectum
Restrictive Procedures for Morbid Obesity		
Vertical banded gastroplasty (VBG)	• Partitioning of the stomach near the gastroesophageal junction to create a small gastric pouch and outlet • Less commonly performed today due to lack of sustained weight loss	• Morbid obesity (e.g., BMI greater than 40 kg/m^2 or BMI of greater than 35 kg/m^2 with serious medical problems)
Gastric banding (Figure 7-24)	• Placement of a prosthetic device around the gastric cardia to limit oral intake • May be done laparoscopically	• Morbid obesity (e.g., BMI greater than 40 kg/m^2 or BMI of greater than 35 kg/m^2 with serious medical problems)
Malabsorptive Procedures for Morbid Obesity		
Intestinal bypass	• Formation of an anastomosis between the upper small intestine and the lower small intestine or large intestine • Less commonly performed today due to high complication rate	• Morbid obesity (e.g., BMI greater than 40 kg/m^2 or BMI of greater than 35 kg/m^2 with serious medical problems)
Roux-Y gastric bypass (RYGB) (Figure 7-25)	• Combines gastric restriction and malabsorption; in addition to creating a gastric pouch, the small bowel is resected so that the upper jejunum is connected to the pouch and the lower jejunum is anastomosed to the biliopancreatic limb; digestive juices do not come into the small bowel until the lower jejunum, so absorption is decreased • Usually performed via laparoscopic technique	• Morbid obesity (e.g., BMI greater than 40 kg/m^2 or BMI of greater than 35 kg/m^2 with serious medical problems)

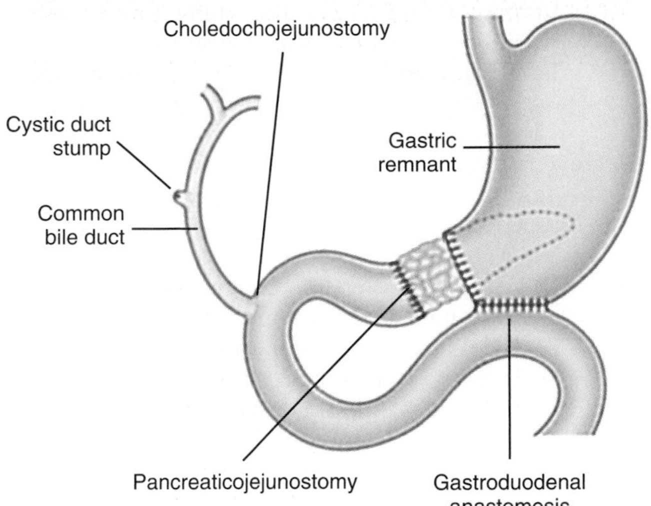

Figure 7-21 Whipple procedure (also referred to as *radical pancreaticoduodenectomy)*. (From Lewis, S. M., et al. [2011]. *Medical-surgical nursing: Assessment and management of clinical problems* [8th ed.]. St. Louis: Mosby.)

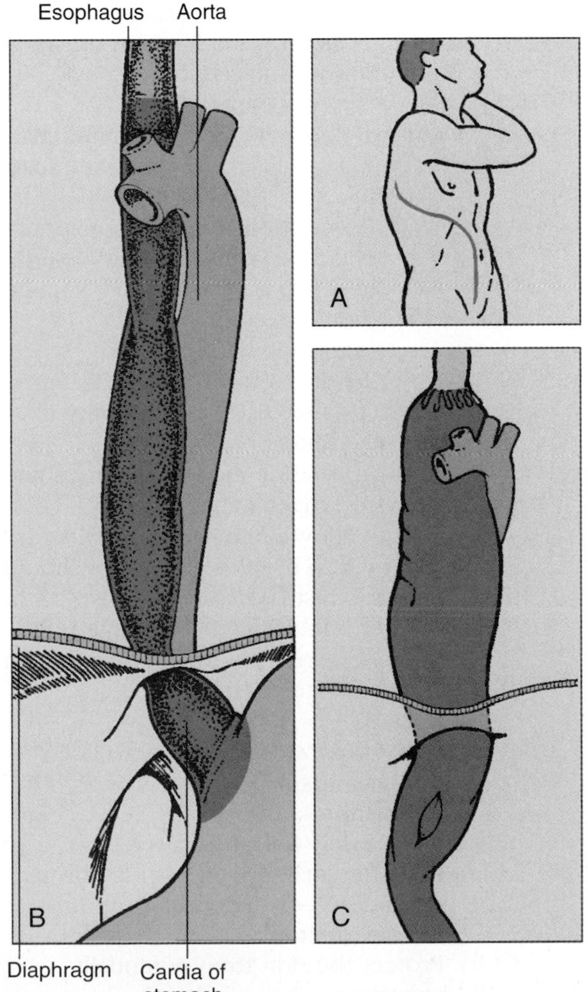

Figure 7-22 Esophagogastrectomy. **A,** Incision. **B,** Shaded portion to be resected. **C,** Completed reconstruction. (From Beare, P. G., & Myers, J. L. [1998]. *Adult health nursing* [3rd ed.]. St. Louis: Mosby.)

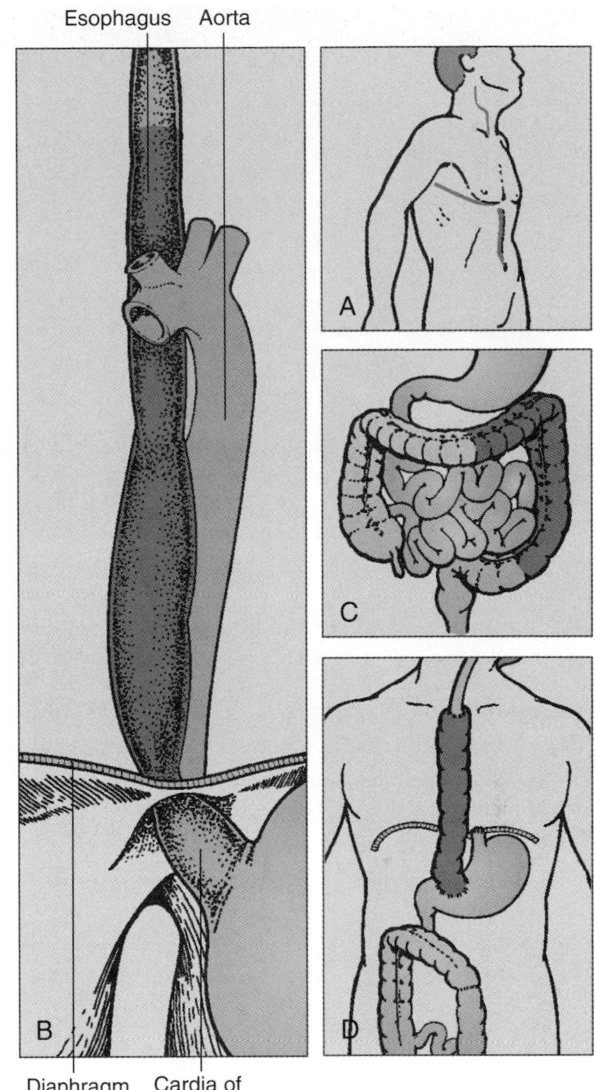

Figure 7-23 Esophagoenterostomy. **A,** Incision. **B,** Shaded portion to be resected. **C,** Portion of colon to be used. D, Completed reconstruction. (From Beare, P. G., & Myers, J. L. [1998]. *Adult health nursing* [3rd ed.]. St. Louis: Mosby.)

postoperative day; monitor for changes in electrolyte levels.

e. Monitor for petechiae, ecchymosis, changes in clotting profile, and frank bleeding that may indicate a coagulopathy, such as DIC.

3. Prevent and/or treat pain.
   a. Administer narcotics (e.g., morphine, hydromorphone, fentanyl) by patient-controlled analgesia as prescribed; epidural analgesia may be utilized.
   b. Administer NSAIDs as prescribed to augment the analgesic effect of narcotics by acting as antiprostaglandins.
      1) Initially ketorolac (Toradol)
      2) Oral agents (e.g., ibuprofen [Motrin], naproxen [Naprosyn, Anaprox]) when able to take drugs by mouth
   c. Utilize noninvasive pain control measures.

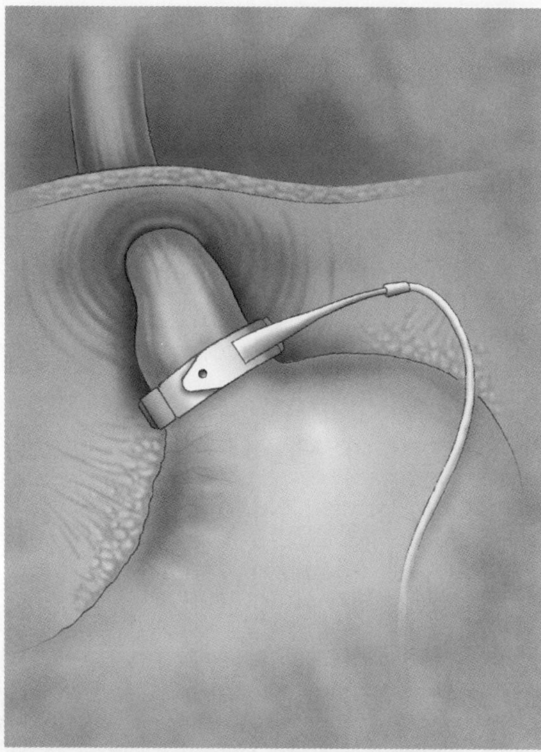

Figure 7-24 Example of gastric banding. (From American Association of Operating Room Nurses. [2004]. AORN bariatric surgery guideline. *AORN Journal, 79*[5], 1026-1052.)

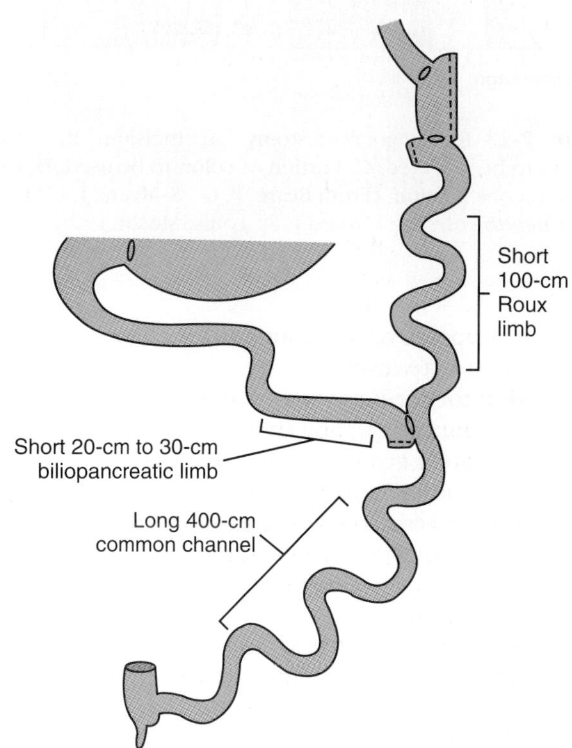

Figure 7-25 Example of gastric bypass: Roux-en-Y proximal gastric bypass. (From American Association of Operating Room Nurses. [2004]. AORN bariatric surgery guideline. *AORN Journal, 79*[5], 1026-1052.)

d. Teach the patient how to splint the incision during coughing; teach the family how to assist.
e. Administer antiemetics for nausea; provide mouth care after each episode of vomiting and assess positioning of nasogastric tube if still in place.

4. Prevent/monitor for infection.
   a. Monitor closely for clinical indications of infection.
      1) Evaluate temperature at least every 4 hours.
      2) Assess color, character, and odor of drainage from incision line, drains, tubes.
      3) Assess for clinical indications of peritonitis (e.g., abdominal pain, abdominal distention, rigid, boardlike abdomen, rebound tenderness, diminished or absent bowel sounds, nausea, vomiting, fever, leukocytosis) caused by anastomosis leak.
      4) Monitor for clinical indications of intraabdominal abscess (e.g., abdominal pain, fever, leukocytosis).
   b. Administer antibiotics prophylactically and therapeutically as prescribed.
   c. Provide incision and drain care aseptically.
      1) Protect the skin from excoriation by changing incisional dressing and dressings around drains as indicated.
      2) Change packing as prescribed.
         a) Some patients may have wounds that are left open and packed with saline-soaked dressings.
            i) Do not utilize packing soaked with Betadine (iodine); known effects of Betadine on open wounds include the following:
               (a) Toxic to fibroblasts
               (b) Decreases epithelialization
               (c) Increases susceptibility to infection
               (d) Iodine may be absorbed and cause nephrotoxicity.
         b) Do not allow dressings to become dry (i.e., wet to dry); the dressings should be still moist (i.e., wet to moist) at the time of removal and replacement to prevent disruption of granulating tissue.
      3) Irrigate the wound with saline as prescribed.
         a) Do not utilize hydrogen peroxide because it is damaging to new epithelium.
      4) Monitor closely for a fistula tract.
         a) Look for small openings along or near the incision or drain site; output is usually green or yellow.
         b) Protect the skin from potentially excoriating drainage by placing a wound drainage bag over the fistula; also allows measurement of fluid loss and collection of sample for electrolyte analysis to guide fluid and electrolyte replacement

d. Monitor serum glucose and administer insulin to keep serum glucose within normal limits.
e. Assess approximation of wound edges for indications of possible dehiscence or evisceration.

5. Reduce acidity of gastric secretions.
   a. Maintain NPO status while gastric suction is required.
   b. Administer antacids, H_2 receptor antagonists, and/or proton pump inhibitors as prescribed.
   c. Administer octreotide acetate (Sandostatin) as prescribed to suppress secretion of pancreatic peptides post-Whipple.
6. Maintain GI integrity.
   a. Monitor and maintain NG tube until return of bowel sounds.
      1) Ensure proper tube placement; do not manipulate a tube placed during surgery without consulting surgeon.
   b. Monitor closely for indications of anastomosis leak.
   c. Monitor for return of bowel sounds, flatus, BM.
   d. Assess and provide bowel diversion care as indicated (bowel resection with formation of a temporary or permanent bowel diversion).
      1) Maintain intactness of bowel diversion appliance.
      2) Keep peristomal skin clean and dry.
      3) Report any change in the drainage from the ileostomy/colostomy.
         a) Ileostomy: watery, excoriating, and continuous
         b) Ascending colostomy: watery or semisolid, excoriating, and continuous
         c) Transverse colostomy: pastelike or semisolid and occurs at unpredictable intervals; may be 3-5 days postoperative before any drainage
         d) Descending or sigmoid colostomy: formed stools that may be at predictable intervals (e.g., after breakfast) especially with irrigation routine; may be 3-5 days postoperative before any drainage
      4) Assess color of stoma and report any indications of ischemia.
         a) Stomal color should be the same color as the oral mucosa and it should be moist; report darkening such as burgundy or black.
      5) Report any stomal prolapse or retraction.
7. Maintain or improve nutritional status.
   a. Assess nutritional status: weight; BUN; serum albumin; total protein; Hgb and Hct
   b. Administer TPN initially as prescribed and progress diet as prescribed: usually small, frequent meals are indicated.
   c. Administer enteral feedings as prescribed; a jejunostomy tube may be placed for nutritional support.
   d. Monitor for diarrhea.
   e. Administer oral pancreatic enzymes (Creon, Pancrease, Viokase, Cotazym) with each meal as prescribed post-Whipple.
8. Provide size-sensitive care for patients with obesity.
   a. Ensure that appropriate bariatric equipment is available.
      1) Avoid derogatory terms such as "big boy bed."
   b. Recognize and discuss prejudice based on size and weight.
   c. Provide privacy and dignity.
      1) Weigh the patient in private.
      2) Close doors and curtains when examining the patient.
      3) Maintain confidentiality.
9. Assist with adjustment to diagnosis of cancer if malignancy present.
   a. Provide accurate information and clarification about the diagnosis, prognosis, and treatment plan when information is requested.
   b. Be realistic but do not eliminate hope.
   c. Give patient and family members time to discuss their feelings and concerns; encourage expression of goals for treatment.
   d. Refer patient and family to support groups or for counseling as indicated.
   e. Prepare the patient and family for additional treatments for malignancy if indicated such as the following:
      1) Radiation therapy
      2) Antineoplastic drug therapy
10. Monitor for complications.
    a. General
       1) Anastomosis leak
       2) Atelectasis, pneumonia, ARDS
       3) DVT, pulmonary embolism
       4) Infection, sepsis
       5) Prolonged ileus
       6) GI bleeding
       7) Stenosis or stricture
       8) Fistula
       9) Organ failure
          a) Cardiac
          b) Hepatic
          c) Pulmonary
          d) Renal
    b. Specific to gastric resections
       1) Dumping syndromes
          a) Early: hyperosmolality causing hypovolemic effect
          b) Late: hypoglycemia caused by hyperinsulinemic response
       2) Pernicious anemia
       3) Diarrhea
       4) Chronic gastritis
    c. Specific to Whipple procedure
       1) Delayed gastric emptying
       2) Pancreatic fistula
       3) Intraabdominal abscess
       4) Hemorrhage: usually due to injury to portal vein or vena cava
       5) Wound infection

6) Diabetes
7) Pancreatic exocrine insufficiency
8) Pancreatitis
9) Marginal ulceration

d. Specific to esophagogastrectomy
1) Esophageal stenosis or anastomotic stricture
2) Chylothorax
3) Myocardial ischemia
4) Dysrhythmias

e. Specific to restrictive procedures for morbid obesity
1) Pulmonary embolism
2) Stomal outlet stenosis
3) Severe gastroesophageal reflux
4) Erosive esophagitis
5) Band erosion
6) Herniation of the stomach upward inside the band
7) Band migration
8) Regaining of weight

f. Specific to malabsorptive procedures for morbid obesity
1) Pulmonary embolism
2) Gastric pouch outlet stricture
3) Jejunojejunostomy obstruction
4) Dumping syndrome
5) Prolonged nausea and vomiting
6) Cholelithiasis
7) Anemia
8) Vitamin (A, D, E, K, B_{12}) and mineral (calcium, folic acid, iron) deficiencies
9) Electrolyte imbalance
10) Lactose intolerance
11) Anemia
12) Offensive, foul-smelling soft bowel movements and flatus

11. Provide instruction to the patient and family regarding wound care, pharmacologic agents prescribed for home use, and signs/symptoms to report to the physician.

LEARNING ACTIVITIES

CHAPTER 7

1. Complete the following crossword puzzle related to gastrointestinal anatomy and physiology.

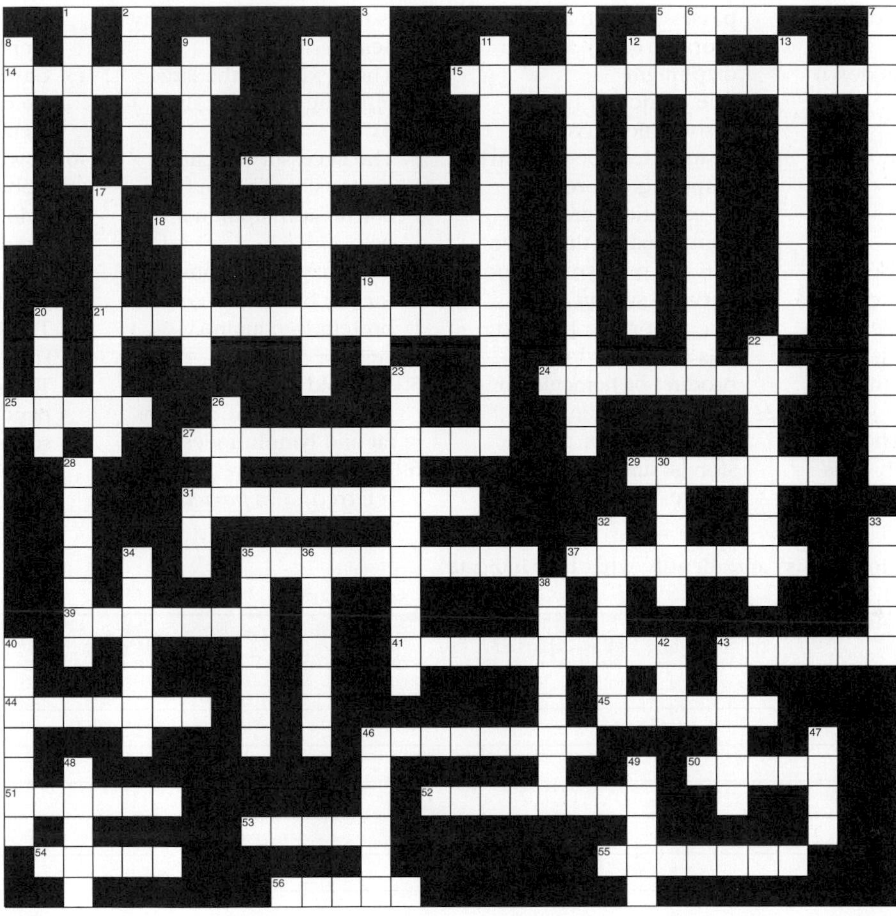

ACROSS

5. Sphincter of _____ is a valve in the common bile duct that regulates passage of bile
14. The accessory organ with both endocrine and exocrine functions
15. The process of converting fat and protein to glucose
16. The nutrient source that is broken down into amino acids
18. The nutrient source that is broken down into glucose, fructose, and galactose
21. Sphincter that is also referred to as the *upper esophageal sphincter*
24. This factor is necessary for the intestinal absorption of vitamin B_{12}
25. This substance is important in maintaining protection of the gastric mucosa from the effects of acid
27. The alternate contraction and relaxation of muscle fibers which propels food and chyme through the GI tract
29. The hormone responsible for the secretion of hydrochloric acid
31. Absorption of this type of vitamins requires the presence of bile salts; examples are ADEK (two words)
35. The first portion of the alimentary canal
37. The phase of gastric secretion that is stimulated by the thought, sight, smell, or taste of food
39. Enzyme in saliva that begins the breakdown of polysaccharides to disaccharides
41. This structure protects the airway by closing during swallowing
43. These cells are in the pancreas and responsible for exocrine function
44. Absorption of this mineral requires vitamin D
45. This duct comes from the gallbladder and joins the common hepatic duct to form the common bile duct
46. Intestinal losses are ____ so excess losses cause metabolic acidosis
50. Fingerlike projections of mucosa and submucosa in the duodenum and jejunum that increase surface area
51. The oral secretion stimulated by the thought, sight, smell, or taste of food
52. The vitamin that plays a chief role in the metabolic breakdown of glucose to yield energy in body tissue
53. _____'s patches are lymphoid follicles in the intestines
54. Thick folds on the interior of the stomach that increase surface area
55. The largest dilation of the GI tract

56. Viscous, semifluid stomach contents that move through the pylorus into the small intestine

DOWN

1. Dome-shaped portion of the stomach that extends left of the cardia
2. The upper portion of the stomach
3. Enzyme that breaks down lipid
4. The hormone that stimulates contraction of the gallbladder
6. Another term for swallowing
7. Sphincter that is also referred to as the *lower esophageal sphincter*
8. The flexure of the large intestine that is in the LUQ
9. Another term for chewing
10. The gastric acid which is stimulated by gastrin
11. The process of breaking down stored carbohydrate
12. The membrane which covers the abdominal viscera
13. Activated by hydrochloric acid to form pepsin
17. The hollow tube that passes through the thoracic cavity and the diaphragm
19. The branch of the autonomic nervous system that speeds gastric emptying (abbrev)
20. GI secretions are controlled by this nerve and the parasympathetic nervous system
22. The major bile pigment; this is a breakdown product of hemoglobin
23. The accessory organ responsible for the storage and release of bile
26. These cells in the pancreas secrete insulin
28. One of these lymph vessels is located in each villi
30. These cells in the pancreas secrete glucagon
31. The nutrient source that is broken down into fatty acids
32. The flexure of the large intestine that is in the RUQ
33. The accessory organ responsible for the conversion of ammonia to urea
34. The enzyme responsible for the breakdown of protein into amino acids
35. The fold of the peritoneum that contains fat and lymph nodes
36. These glands are also referred to as *parietal cells*; they secrete hydrochloric acid and intrinsic factor
38. Shortest segment of the small intestine
40. Enzyme that breaks down lactose
42. This branch of the autonomic nervous system slows gastric emptying (abbrev)
43. Gastric losses are ___ so excess losses cause metabolic alkalosis
46. Lower portion of the stomach, close to the pylorus
47. Fluid produced by the liver and stored in the gallbladder
48. The last section of the small intestine
49. These cells in the pancreas secrete somatostatin

2. Describe the following "signs" and identify what they indicate.

Sign	Description	Indicates
Ballance's		
Grey Turner's		
Cullen's		
Coopernail's		
Kehr's		
Chvostek's		
Trousseau's		

3. List three general causes of jaundice.

a. ______

b. ______

c. ______

4. Why is serum prealbumin a better assessment tool than albumin to evaluate improvement from nutritional support?

______

______

5. Calculate the caloric intake for a patient receiving total parenteral nutrition (TPN) with daily intake of 42 grams of protein, 250 grams of carbohydrate, and 140 grams of fat.

______

______

6. List four interventions for any patient with acute hemorrhage (regardless of location).
a. ______
b. ______
c. ______
d. ______

7. List five possible reasons for upper GI hemorrhage.
a. ______
b. ______
c. ______
d. ______
e. ______

8. List five methods to control bleeding in esophageal varices.
a. ______
b. ______
c. ______
d. ______
e. ______

9. List four classifications of drugs that are used to prevent ulcers and an example of each one.

Type	Example

10. Match the following clinical manifestations of hepatic failure with the pathophysiologic change (answers may be used more than once).

___ 1. Splenic engorgement
___ 2. Stretching of the liver capsule
___ 3. Decrease in the metabolism of testosterone
___ 4. Decrease in metabolism of aldosterone
___ 5. Decrease in production of plasma proteins
___ 6. Decrease in metabolism of estrogen
___ 7. Decreased production of clotting factors
___ 8. Decrease in conjugation and excretion of bilirubin

a. Petechiae, purpura, bleeding
b. Jaundice
c. Third-spacing
d. Testicular atrophy
e. Gynecomastia
f. Anemia, leukopenia, thrombocytopenia
g. Abdominal tenderness

11. List one type of diuretic that is indicated and one type of diuretic that is contraindicated for ascites in hepatic failure.

Indicated	Contraindicated

12. List five common causes of paralytic ileus.
a. ______
b. ______
c. ______
d. ______
e. ______

13. List five classic indications of an "acute abdomen" seen in intestinal perforation.

a. ______________________

b. ______________________

c. ______________________

d. ______________________

e. ______________________

14. Complete the following table. You may include more than one condition for each but include only conditions discussed in this chapter.

Clinical Finding	Condition
Elevated lipase, amylase	
Sudden, painless hematemesis	
Decreased protein	
Rebound tenderness	
Jaundice	
Hypocalcemia	
Bleeding tendencies	
Elevated ammonia	
Bloody diarrhea	
Hyperbilirubinemia	
Fetor hepaticus	
High-pitched rushing bowel sounds	
Succussion splash	
Management	**Condition**
Irrigate NG tube until clear	
Neomycin and lactulose	
Sclerosis during endoscopy	
Aldosterone antagonist diuretics	
NPO status	
Sengstaken-Blakemore tube	
Volume and blood replacement	
Billroth I or II	

15. Complete the following crossword puzzle related to gastrointestinal assessment, conditions, and treatments.

ACROSS

7. _____'s ulcer is a stress ulcer associated with cerebral trauma
8. Vomiting blood
9. A luminal intestinal obstruction with compromise of blood supply
11. The form of fluid replacement that is indicated for acute hemorrhage
14. Term for difficulty swallowing
16. Hepatitis B is sometimes referred to as _____ hepatitis
17. Hypertension of this circulation system is seen in cirrhosis
20. Generalized, massive edema
23. A drug used in GI hemorrhage to suppress gastrin (generic)
25. A syndrome of renal failure associated with hepatic failure
26. Conditionally essential amino acid that enhances the immune system and promotes wound healing
29. This osmotic diuretic may be used for cerebral edema in hepatic encephalopathy
30. Procedure now preferred over intestinal bypass for weight reduction for patients with morbid obesity (abbrev.)
32. A common description of the appearance of the stool seen with mesenteric infarction (2 words)
33. The term for tarry stools
35. _____ tenderness indicates that pain is more severe on release than with pressure
36. Electrolyte imbalance seen in acute pancreatitis
38. The type of drug frequently prescribed for patients with ascites
40. The location of pain in acute pancreatitis
41. This antibiotic may be used to stimulate peristalsis
43. This type of pain is sharp and well localized
45. This type of pain is experienced at a distance from the disease process
47. Intraabdominal _____ is when the intraabdominal pressure is above normal
50. Conditionally essential amino acid that aids in maintaining the integrity of the gut to prevent bacterial translocation
54. _____'s sign is caused by phrenic nerve irritation by subphrenic blood
55. This treatment for esophageal varices is performed during endoscopy
57. A complication of vasopressin therapy which causes water intoxication (abbrev.)
59. This drug is used for acetaminophen toxicity; must be administered within 24 hours of acetaminophen ingestion (generic)
62. A deficiency of this vitamin is commonly seen in alcoholism
63. This type of anemia is caused by a deficiency of intrinsic factor
66. Screening echo used in abdominal trauma (abbrev.)
69. Exploratory _____ may be necessary to localize organ injury and/or hemorrhage in trauma patients
71. Elevated _____ levels cause neurologic changes in patients with hepatic encephalopathy
74. Conversion of fat or protein to glucose
77. An osmotic laxative frequently used in hepatic encephalopathy (generic)
78. The route of nutritional support used in functional or structural obstruction
80. A common cause of acute pancreatitis
82. H_2 receptor antagonist (generic)
84. Serum _____ is elevated in acute pancreatitis
88. A drug that acts as mucosal barrier used to protect the gastric mucosa (generic)
89. This type of pain is dull and poorly localized
91. These must be kept at the bedside for a patient with balloon tamponade
93. This condition is manifested by coffee-grounds gastric aspirate
94. One controversy regarding the use of drugs which alter the pH of the gastric secretions is the increased incidence of _____
95. This procedure divides the vagus nerve along the esophagus to decrease acid secretion in the stomach
96. _____'s sign is indicative of splenic rupture
97. Spore-producing bacterium that is a common cause of diarrhea in critically ill patients (2 words)

DOWN

1. This type of ulcer causes an erosion in the mucosa of the esophagus, stomach, or duodenum
2. This drug may be used for GI hemorrhage but may cause myocardial or mesenteric ischemia (generic)
3. This condition may be caused by ulcer, appendicitis, diverticulitis, or intestinal obstruction; causes peritonitis
4. A stent is placed between the hepatic and portal veins in this procedure performed in patients with esophageal varices (abbrev)
5. The plasma protein most significant in maintaining capillary oncotic pressure
6. A gastric feeding tube that is endoscopically placed (abbrev)
7. _____'s is a stress ulcer associated with burns
9. This diuretic is frequently used for fluid retention in hepatic failure; blocks aldosterone (generic)
10. Type of parenteral catheter
12. Serum ____ is elevated in acute pancreatitis and is more specific than serum amylase
13. Analgesic of choice in pancreatitis is _____ or hydromorphone
15. Another term for bright red blood per rectum
18. An abnormal accumulation of fluid in the peritoneal cavity
19. The preferred method of nutritional support; should be used unless contraindications exist
21. This antibiotic was traditionally used in hepatic encephalopathy to kill intestinal bacteria that convert nitrogenous wastes to ammonia (generic)
22. Occurs as a result of a disruption in the integrity of the GI tract; causes an acute abdomen
24. May be caused by biliary obstruction, liver disease, or excessive hemolysis
27. Functional obstruction of the bowel
28. Small bowel obstruction causes reverse peristalsis and vomiting that is ___
31. Term for belching
34. This type of enteral formula is required if feeding is delivered distal to the jejunum
37. *Clostridium difficile* is usually initially treated with _____ (generic)
38. Term for impaired digestion
39. A complication of hernia that may cause bowel ischemia or infarction
42. This tube has four lumens and may be used for balloon tamponade in patients with esophageal varices
44. Hepatitis A and E are sometimes referred to as _____ hepatitis
46. This syndrome may occur after gastric resection; may be classified as early or late
48. Collection of inflammatory debris, pancreatic secretions, and necrotic tissue in the pancreas
49. A "maneuver" that facilitates evacuation of the colon
51. This test may cause pancreatitis (abbrev)
52. IV proton pump inhibitor (brand name)
53. A serious pulmonary complication of acute pancreatitis (abbrev)

56. A drug commonly used for suicide gesture that is a major cause of hepatic failure in adolescents (generic)
58. This macronutrient is restricted in hepatic encephalopathy
60. Abnormal function of the brain; may be caused by elevated ammonia levels
61. Abdominal pain experienced with mesenteric ischemia is frequently described as abdominal _____
64. Esophageal _____ causes sudden, painless hemorrhage by mouth; caused by portal hypertension
65. _____ tear is caused by forceful retching and vomiting (2 words)
67. Loud, hyperactive bowel sounds
68. The gentle repetitive bouncing of tissues against the hand; used to evaluate organ enlargement
70. A flapping tremor seen in hepatic encephalopathy
72. Intestinal perforation causes an _____ abdomen and requires surgical intervention
73. *Helicobacter* _____ is a bacteria associated with peptic ulcer
75. This tube has three lumens and may be used for balloon tamponade in patients with esophageal varices (2 words)
76. Bowel diversity that is most likely to cause skin erosion if excellent containment not achieved
79. _____'s procedure is also called a pancreatoduodenectomy
81. A nonabsorbable antibiotic that is now preferred over neomycin to kill intestinal bacteria that act on nitrogenous wastes to produce ammonia (brand)
83. Inflammation of the liver
85. Enteral feeding administration may be intermittent, continuous, or _____
86. _____'s sign is a bluish discoloration around the umbilicus; indicative of intraabdominal bleeding
87. _____'s sign is a bluish tint to the flanks that is indicative of retroperitoneal bleeding (2 words)
90. A type of shunt that is used for ascites
92. An obstruction here is manifested by vomiting and a succussion splash

The Renal System

Selected Concepts in Anatomy and Physiology

General Information

1. Functions of the renal system
   a. Regulation of homeostasis and the body's internal environment
      1) Regulation of extracellular fluid volume
      2) Regulation of extracellular fluid osmolality
      3) Regulation of electrolyte balance
      4) Excretion of metabolic wastes
      5) Regulation of acid-base balance (in conjunction with the pulmonary system)
   b. Production and release of hormones
      1) Regulation of blood pressure influenced by aldosterone and antidiuretic hormone (ADH)
      2) Stimulation of RBC production via erythropoietin
      3) Synthesis and release of prostaglandins
   c. Participation in activation of vitamin D
2. Components of the renal system (Figure 8-1)
   a. Two kidneys
   b. Two ureters
   c. Urinary bladder
   d. Urethra

Functional Anatomy

1. General characteristics of the kidney
   a. Location of kidney
      1) Posterior abdominal wall behind peritoneum
      2) Opposite last thoracic and first three lumbar vertebrae on each side of spine
      3) Right kidney slightly lower than left as a result of liver location
   b. Size, shape, weight of the kidney
      1) Size: approximately 10 × 5 × 2.5 cm or approximately fist-sized
      2) Shape: beanlike with convex lateral border, convex and concave medial border; long axis approximately vertical
      3) Weight: 120-170 grams per kidney
2. Extrarenal structures
   a. Renal capsule
      1) Thin, smooth layer of fibrous membrane that surrounds each kidney
      2) Acts as a protective layer
      3) Prevents kidney swelling
      4) Contains pain receptors
   b. Perirenal fat and renal fascia
      1) Support and protect the kidney
      2) Hold kidney in place
   c. Adrenal gland (also referred to as the *suprarenal gland*): rests on top of each kidney
   d. Hilum
      1) Concave notch of medial aspect of kidney
      2) Entry site for renal artery and nerves
      3) Exit site for renal vein and ureter
   e. Ureters
      1) Fibromuscular tubes located behind peritoneum; extend from kidney to posterior part of bladder floor
      2) Ureter walls composed of smooth muscle with mucosa lining and fibrous outer coat
      3) Collect urine from the renal pelvis and propel it to the bladder by peristaltic waves
      4) Ureters enter the superior, posterior bladder at an oblique angle; this angle and the peristaltic action of the ureters prevent reflux of urine
   f. Bladder
      1) Located behind symphysis pubis, below peritoneum
      2) Collapsible bag of smooth muscle
      3) Acts as a reservoir for urine until sufficient amount accumulates for elimination; expels urine from body by way of urethra
         a) Adults void approximately 5-9 times/day
         b) Volume of each voiding usually 100-300 mL but may be as much as 1 L
   g. Urethra
      1) Located behind symphysis pubis, anterior to the vagina in females; extends through the prostate gland and penis in males
      2) Acts as passageway for expulsion of urine from the urinary bladder to the urinary meatus, where it is expelled from the body

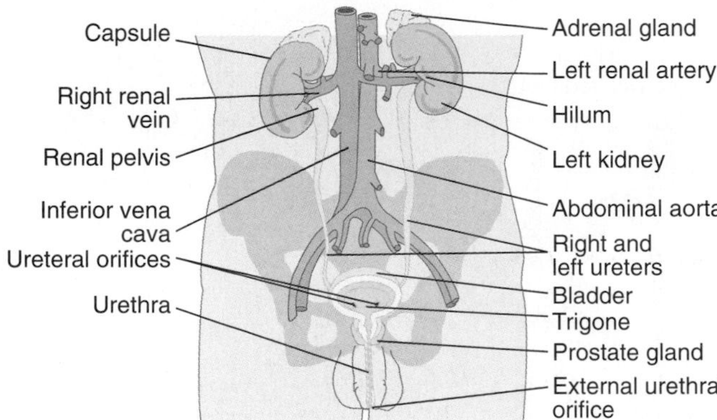

Figure 8-1 The kidneys and other structures of the urinary tract. (From Montague, S. E., Watson, R., & Herbert, R. [2005]. *Physiology for nursing practice* [3rd ed.]. Oxford: Bailliére Tindall.)

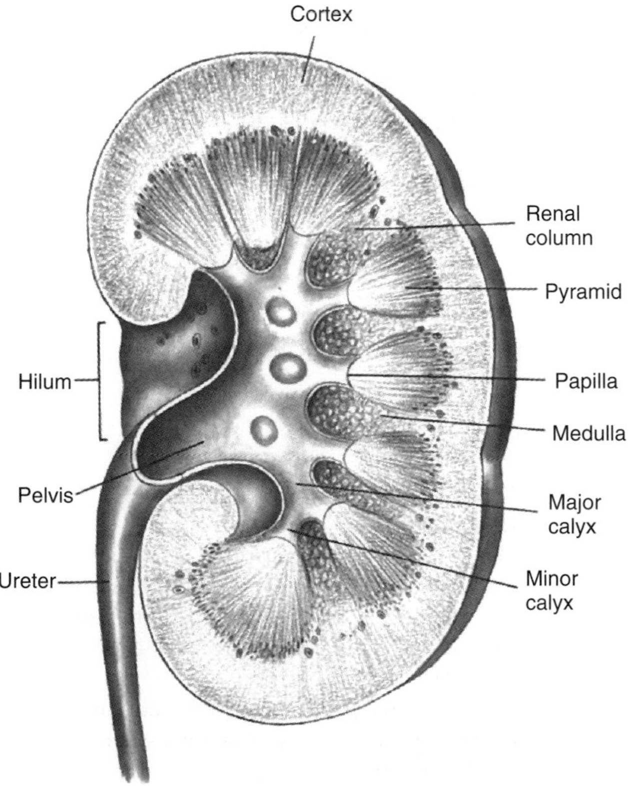

Figure 8-2 Cross-section of the kidney. (From Thompson, J. M., McFarland, G. K., Hirsch, J. E., & Tucker, S. M. [2002]. *Mosby's clinical nursing* [5th ed.]. St Louis: Mosby.)

3. Renal structures (Figure 8-2)
   a. Renal parenchyma
      1) Cortex
         a) Approximately 1 cm wide, reddish-brown and granular appearance
         b) Metabolically active portion of kidney where aerobic metabolism occurs and ammonia and glucose are formed
         c) Site of glomerulus, proximal and distal tubules
      2) Medulla
         a) Approximately 5 cm wide, darker than cortex and striated
         b) Comprised of 6-10 pyramids formed by collecting tubules and ducts
            i) Pyramids are triangular wedges of medullary tissue and are composed of collecting tubules.
            ii) Columns are inward extensions of cortical tissue between the pyramids; much of the kidney's blood vessels and nerves are in these columns.
            iii) Renal lobe is comprised of a pyramid and surrounding cortical tissue.
         c) Site of deepest part of Henle's loop
   b. Renal sinus: spacious cavity filled with adipose tissue, the renal pelvis, minor and major calyces, and the origin of the ureter
      1) Calyces
         a) Calyces are cuplike structures that drain the papillae.
         b) Eight to 12 minor calyces open into two to three major calyces that form the renal pelvis.
      2) Renal pelvis
         a) Papillae are at the apices of the renal pyramids; collecting tubules drain into minor calyces at papillae.
         b) Renal pelvis is like a small funnel tapering into the ureter; formed by the union of several calyces
         c) Urine flows from collecting duct to renal pelvis and into the ureter.
   c. Nephron: microscopic functional unit of kidney (Figure 8-3)
      1) Approximately 1 million in each kidney
      2) Able to compensate for significant degree of nephron destruction by:
         a) Filtering a greater solute (dissolved substances) load
         b) Hypertrophy of remaining functional nephrons
      3) Types of nephrons
         a) Cortical (85% of nephrons are cortical nephrons)
            i) The glomerulus is located in outer cortex.
            ii) Cortical nephrons contain short loops of Henle that dip into the outer edge of the medulla.
         b) Juxtamedullary (15% of nephrons are juxtamedullary nephrons)
            i) The glomerulus is located in inner cortex.
            ii) Juxtamedullary nephrons contain long loops of Henle that penetrate deep into medulla.
            iii) These nephrons are important in the kidney's ability to concentrate the urine.

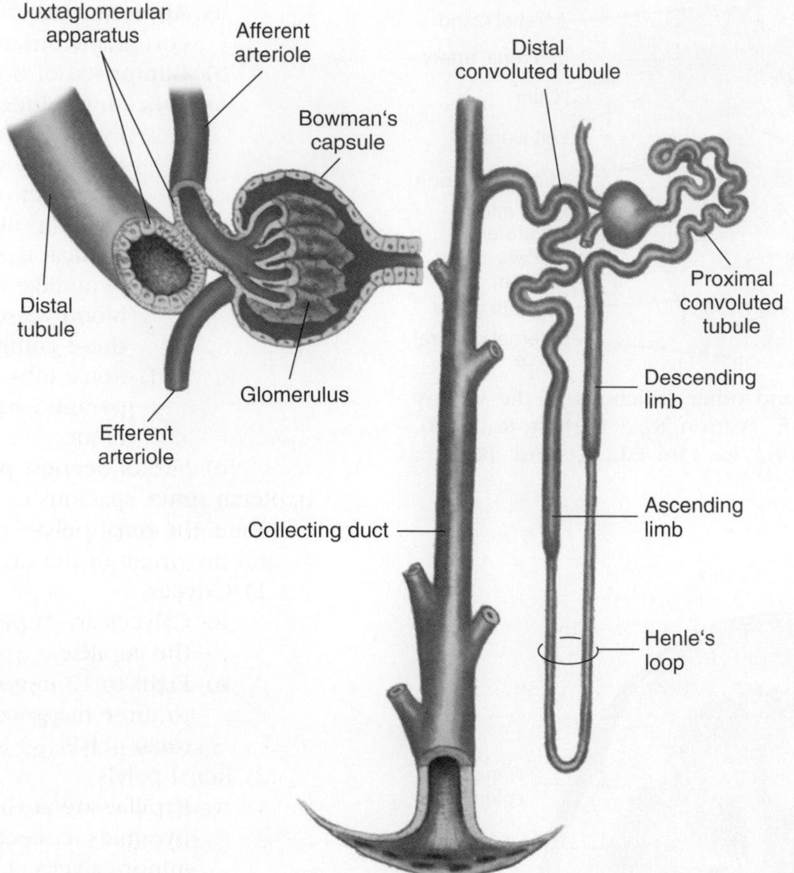

Figure 8-3 Components of the nephron. (From Urden, L. D., Stacy, K. M., & Lough, M. E. [2010]. *Critical care nursing: Diagnosis and management* [6th ed.]. St. Louis: Mosby.)

4) Functional segments
   a) Renal corpuscle: consists of Bowman's capsule and glomerulus
      i) The glomerulus is a cluster of tightly coiled capillaries that produces an ultrafiltrate; a portion of this ultrafiltrate eventually becomes urine.
      ii) Bowman's capsule is the funnel-shaped upper end of the proximal tubule.
   b) Renal tubules
      i) Segmentally divided into proximal convoluted tubule, loop of Henle, distal convoluted tubule
      ii) Responsible for reabsorption and secretion, which alter the volume and composition of the ultrafiltration to form the final urine volume and composition
   c) Collecting duct
      i) Several nephrons converge into a collecting duct.
      ii) The collecting duct relays the urine from the tubules to the minor calyx.

d. Renal vasculature
   1) Pathway of blood supply
      a) Renal arteries branch from the aorta.
      b) The renal arteries branch into interlobar arteries → arcuate arteries → interlobular arteries
      c) The interlobular arteries become the afferent arteriole that forms the glomerulus.
      d) The efferent arteriole leads out of the glomerulus and forms the peritubular capillary network.
      e) The efferent arteriole from the juxtamedullary nephron forms a different capillary network called the *vasa recta*.
         i) The vasa recta is a complex of long straight capillary loops that run parallel to the ascending and descending loop of Henle.
         ii) The vasa recta plays an important role in concentrating interstitial fluid found in the medulla.
         iii) Blood flow through the vasa recta is sluggish.

f) The peritubular capillary network leads to the interlobular vein that leads to the arcuate vein.
g) The arcuate vein leads to the interlobar vein that leads to the renal vein.
h) The renal vein empties into the inferior vena cava.

2) Renal blood flow
a) The kidneys receive 20-25% of the cardiac output, or approximately 1200 mL/min (600 mL/min for each kidney).
b) Autoregulation maintains constancy in glomerular filtration rate (GFR).
i) Systemic arterial pressure between 80-180 mm Hg prevents large changes in GFR because of the ability of the afferent arteriole to constrict or dilate.
(a) Increases in MAP cause constriction of the afferent arteriole that prevents the increased arterial pressure from raising the pressure in the glomerulus.
(b) Decreases in MAP cause dilation of the afferent arteriole, so more blood is allowed to flow into the glomerulus.
ii) Autoregulation fails at MAP of 60 mm Hg or less.

3) Juxtaglomerular apparatus consists of the macula densa and the juxtaglomerular cells.
a) The macula densa is a part of the distal tubule that lies close to the afferent and efferent arterioles.
b) Juxtaglomerular cells produce and store the enzyme renin that is secreted in response to hypotension.

e. Lymphatics
1) There is an abundant supply of lymphatics to the kidney.
2) Lymphatics from the kidney drain into thoracic duct.

f. Nervous innervation
1) The autonomic nervous system (ANS) supplies the primary innervation of the kidney and the urinary tract.
2) The renal plexus is formed by the superior splanchnic and inferior splanchnic nerves and enters the kidney at the hilum; the bladder, ureters, and urethra are supplied by the inferior mesenteric plexus, the hypogastric plexus, and the pubic nerve from the sacral region.
3) Both the sympathetic nervous system (SNS) and the parasympathetic nervous system (PNS) innervate the kidney but the SNS has the prominent effect on the kidney; SNS fiber endings are found in the afferent and efferent arterioles and in all sections of the tubule; effects on the kidney include the following:
a) Low level: increased sodium reabsorption within the proximal tubule
b) Moderate level: constriction of afferent and efferent arterioles decreases renal blood flow and glomerular filtration rate
c) High level: predominant effect of afferent arteriole constriction; extreme reduction in renal blood flow and potential cessation of glomerular filtration rate

Physiology

1. Formation of urine involves three processes: filtration, reabsorption, and secretion (Figure 8-4); major functions of each portion of the nephron (Figure 8-5)
a. Glomerular filtration: the pressure of the blood within the glomerular capillaries causes blood to be filtered into Bowman's capsule, where it begins to pass down to the tubule
1) Filtration is the transfer of water and dissolved substances through a permeable membrane from a region of high pressure to low pressure
2) Filtration depends on hydrostatic pressure that may be affected by the following:
a) Diminished renal perfusion from hypovolemia
b) Occlusion of the glomeruli from diabetic neuropathy

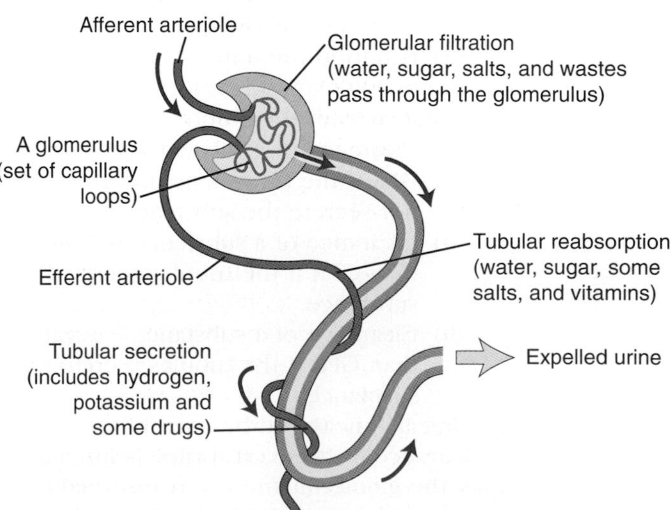

Figure 8-4 Processes of filtration, secretion, and reabsorption in the formation of urine. (From Leonard, P.C. [2005]. *Building a medical vocabulary with Spanish translations* [6th ed.]. St. Louis: Saunders.)

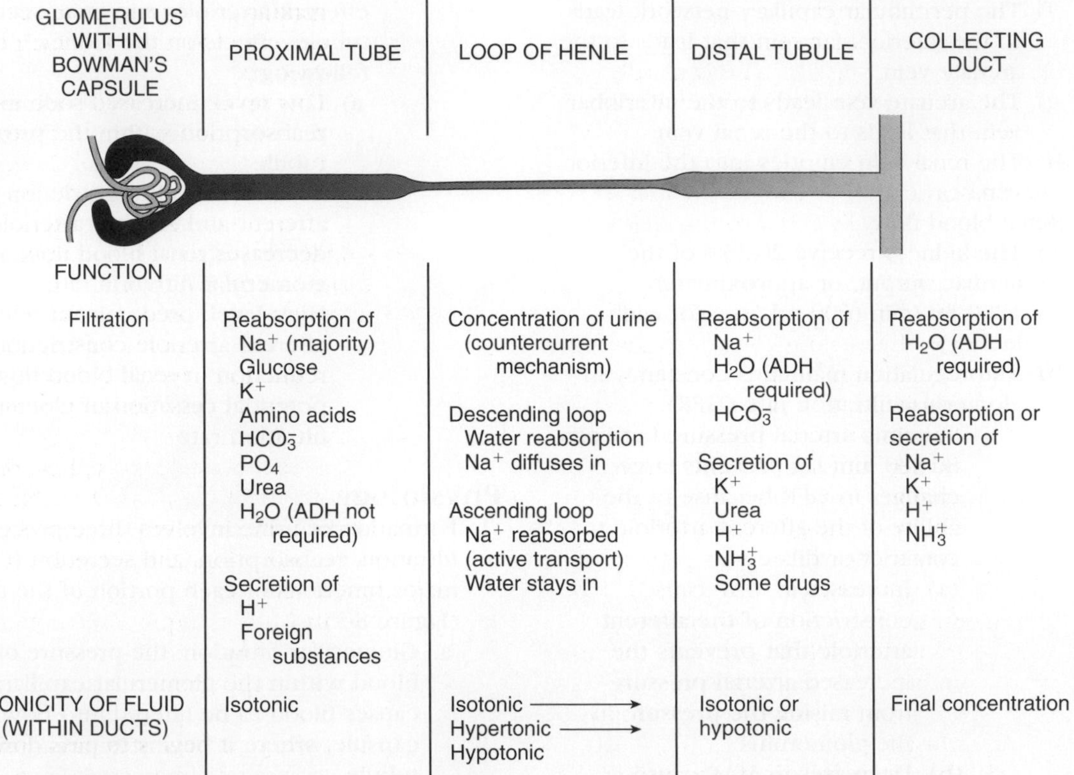

GLOMERULUS WITHIN BOWMAN'S CAPSULE
PROXIMAL TUBE
LOOP OF HENLE
DISTAL TUBULE
COLLECTING DUCT
FUNCTION
Filtration
Reabsorption of Na^+ (majority) Glucose K^+ Amino acids HCO_3^- PO_4 Urea H_2O (ADH not required)
Secretion of H^+ Foreign substances
Concentration of urine (countercurrent mechanism)
Descending loop Water reabsorption Na^+ diffuses in
Ascending loop Na^+ reabsorbed (active transport) Water stays in
Reabsorption of Na^+ H_2O (ADH required) HCO_3^-
Secretion of K^+ Urea H^+ NH_3^+ Some drugs
Reabsorption of H_2O (ADH required)
Reabsorption or secretion of Na^+ K^+ H^+ NH_3^+
TONICITY OF FLUID (WITHIN DUCTS)
Isotonic
Isotonic
Hypertonic
Hypotonic
Isotonic or hypotonic
Final concentration

Figure 8-5 Major functions of each portion of the nephron. (From Sole, M. L., Klein, D. G., & Moseley, M. J. [2005]. *Introduction to critical care nursing* [4th ed.]. Philadelphia: Saunders.)

c) Alteration in the plasma protein concentration from hypoproteinemia
d) Alterations in the basement membrane from an autoimmune disorder
e) Arteriolar constriction from SNS stimulation or vasopressors

3) Glomerular filtration rate (GFR)
   a) Dependent upon the following:
      i) Permeability of the capillary walls
      ii) Vascular pressure
      iii) Filtration pressure
   b) Clearance: complete removal of a substance from the blood
      i) Clearance of a substance equals GFR if the tubules neither reabsorb nor secrete the substance.
      ii) Clearance of a substance is less than GFR if the tubules secrete the substance.
      iii) Clearance of a substance is greater than GFR if the tubules secrete the substance.
   c) Clinically measured by creatinine clearance because creatinine is filtered by the glomeruli and not reabsorbed by the tubules
      i) Formula for GFR =

$$\frac{Ux \times v}{Px}$$

where: **x** = substance freely filtered through glomerulus and not secreted or absorbed by tubules (e.g., creatinine); **P** = plasma concentration of **x** (e.g., creatinine); **v** = urine flow rate/min; **U** = urine concentration of **x** (e.g., creatinine)

      ii) Creatinine clearance is a calculation of GFR by comparing serum creatinine with the amount of creatinine excreted in the urine over a 24-hour period
      iii) GFR must be maintained at a constant rate, and autoregulation ensures this constant rate; systemic mean arterial pressure must be maintained between 80-180 mm Hg to maintain regulation.

4) The glomerular membrane is a porous but semipermeable membrane.
   a) Glomerular filtrate (also called *ultrafiltrate*) is similar in composition to blood except that it lacks blood cells, platelets, and large plasma proteins; water, sodium, glucose, potassium, chloride, phosphate, urea, uric acid, creatinine, ammonia, phenol, calcium,

and magnesium pass through the glomerular membrane.

b) Glomerular filtrate volume is usually 120 mL/min, but 99% of this will be reabsorbed in the renal tubule.

b. Reabsorption: passage of a substance that the body needs from the lumen of the tubules through the tubular cells and into the capillaries
   1) Processes
      a) Active transport
         i) The force used when the cell membranes must move molecules "uphill" against a concentration gradient
         ii) Requires the use of energy and a carrier substance; the substance combines with a "carrier" and diffuses through the tubular membrane where they reenter the bloodstream
         iii) Substances moved by active transport include glucose, protein, amino acids, and phosphate.
      b) Passive transport: processes of osmosis and diffusion
         i) Diffusion: the passive movement of solute from an area of higher concentration to an area of lower concentration; urea and electrolytes are moved by diffusion
         ii) Osmosis: the passive movement of water from an area of lower solute concentration to an area of higher solute concentration
   2) Maximal tubular transport capacity: maximum amount of a substance that can be completely reabsorbed in 1 minute and reflects the renal threshold of a substance; if this threshold is exceeded, the substance appears in the urine (e.g., glucosuria)

c. Tubular secretion: passage of a substance not needed by the body from the capillaries through the tubular cells into the lumen of the tubule

d. Countercurrent mechanism utilizes the juxtamedullary nephrons with their long loops of Henle and occurs within the renal medullary interstitium.
   1) Countercurrent multiplication is the mechanism that enables the body to excrete urine with an osmolality higher than the osmolality of serum.
      a) Sodium chloride is transported out of the filtrate as it moves up the ascending limb of the loop of Henle, but water is not able to follow because this limb is impermeable to water.
      b) Some of sodium chloride enters the peritubular capillaries and is removed from the kidney, but some reenters the descending limb of the loop of Henle, making the filtrate more concentrated than the blood from which it was derived.
      c) This process increases the osmotic pressure in the capillaries and tubules of the papillary region of the kidney until it is four times stronger than that of the blood in the afferent arteriole.
   2) Countercurrent exchange is the maintenance component of the countercurrent mechanism.
      a) The vasa recta minimize the loss of solute from the interstitium by passive diffusion, maintaining the osmotic gradient necessary for the countercurrent multiplication process.

e. A total of 99% of the glomerular filtrate is reabsorbed from the tubules (especially the proximal limb); the remaining 1% is excreted as urine output.
   1) Normal urine output is approximately 1500 mL/day.
   2) Urine composition
      a) Water
      b) Nitrogenous wastes: urea, uric acid, creatinine, ammonia
      c) Ions: potassium, sodium, calcium, chloride, bicarbonate, hydrogen, phosphate, sulfate
      d) Hormones and their breakdown products
      e) Vitamins: particularly water-soluble B vitamins and Vitamin C
      f) Toxins
      g) Drugs
   3) Abnormal constituents: glucose, albumin, RBCs, calculi, casts, pigments

2. Excretion of metabolic waste products
   a. Urea
      1) Protein (either ingested or borrowed from protein stores) is broken down into amino acids and nitrogenous wastes.
      2) Urea nitrogen is the end product of protein metabolism; it circulates in the bloodstream and is excreted in the urine.
      3) Blood urea nitrogen varies with protein intake and hydration status so blood urea nitrogen (BUN) provides an unreliable evaluation of renal function.
   b. Creatinine
      1) Creatinine is a waste product of muscle metabolism.
      2) The normal kidney excretes creatinine at a rate equal to the kidney's blood flow or GFR.
      3) Serum creatinine is a better test for evaluation of renal function than BUN; urine creatinine clearance, which provides a comparison of serum creatinine and 24-hour urine creatinine, is an even better evaluation of renal function.

3. Renal regulation of acid-base balance (for more on acid-base balance, see Chapter 4)
   a. Tubular excretion of H^+ ions in exchange for sodium reabsorption
   b. Bicarbonate reabsorption into the circulation or excretion into the urine
   c. Excretion of H^+ ions in the urine as: NH_4Cl; H_2PO_4; H_20
   d. Renal response to acidosis
      1) Increased hydrogen ion secretion
      2) Increased bicarbonate reabsorption
      3) Production of ammonia to accommodate hydrogen ion excretion
   e. Renal response to alkalosis
      1) Decreased hydrogen ion secretion
      2) Increased bicarbonate excretion
      3) Decreased production of ammonia
4. Fluid balance
   a. Body fluids are dilute solutions of water and solutes.
   b. Measurement methods
      1) Milliliter (mL): the unit of measure for fluid volume
      2) Milliequivalent (mEq): the unit of measure for chemical combining activity of an electrolyte
      3) Milliosmoles (mOsm): the unit of measure for osmotic pressure based on the number of dissolved particles in solution
         a) Osmolality and osmolarity: frequently used interchangeably, though most calculations of body fluids are based on osmolality
            i) Osmolality: number of osmoles per kilogram of solution; expressed as mOsm/kg
               (a) Blood
                  (i) Normal: 280-295 mOsm/kg
                  (ii) Main constituent: sodium
               (b) Urine
                  (i) Normal: 50-1200 mOsm/kg H_2O
                  (ii) Main constituents: urea and sodium
            ii) Osmolarity: number of osmoles per liter of solution
               (a) Isotonic: the tonicity of body fluids; osmolarity of 280-295 mOsm/L
               (b) Hypotonic: lower tonicity than body fluids
               (c) Hypertonic: higher tonicity than body fluids
   c. The human body is mostly water
      1) Volume
         a) Adult males: 60% of total body weight in adult males is water.
         b) Adult females: slightly less water at 55% of total body weight due to higher percentage of body fat
         c) Older adults: less water at 45-55% of total body weight
         d) Obesity: body water decreases with increasing body fat
      2) Distribution (Figure 8-6A)
         a) Intracellular
            i) Fluid contained within the cells
            ii) Accounts for 40% of total body weight
         b) Extracellular

Intracellular
(40% body wt)
25 liters
40% of body weight
Intravascular
(5% body wt)
5 liters
5% of body wt
Interstitial
(15% body wt)
10 liters
15% of body weight
A

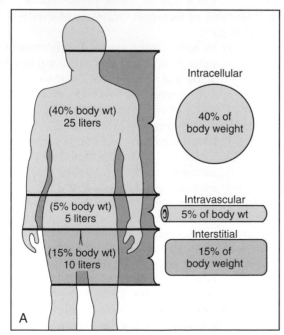

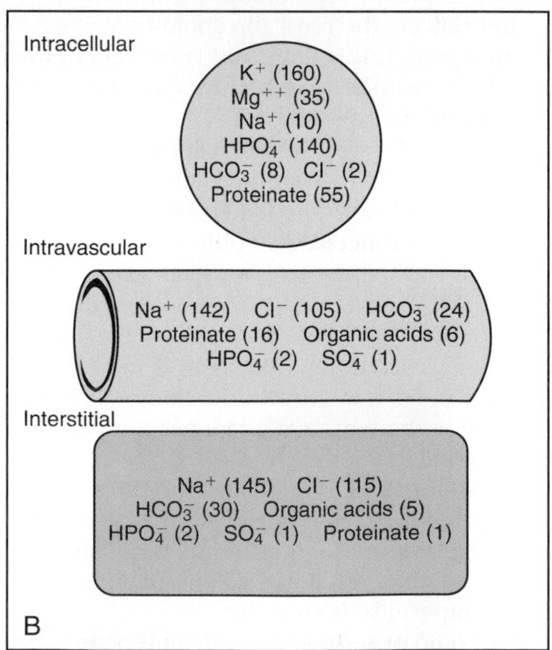

Figure 8-6 A, Distribution of body fluids. **B,** Electrolytes by fluid compartment. (From Urden, L. D., Stacy, K. M., & Lough, M. E. [2010]. *Critical care nursing: Diagnosis and management* [6th ed.]. St. Louis: Mosby.)

i) Fluid outside the cells
ii) Accounts for 20% of total body weight
iii) Distribution
(a) Interstitial
(i) Fluid surrounding the cells
(ii) Accounts for 15% of total body weight
(b) Intravascular
(i) Fluid contained within the blood vessels
(ii) Accounts for approximately 4% of total body weight
(c) Transcellular
(i) Fluid contained within specialized cavities of the body (e.g., cerebrospinal, pericardial, pleural, synovial, intraocular, digestive fluids)
(ii) Accounts for approximately 1% of total body weight

d. Homeostasis is the state of internal equilibrium within the body; fluid, electrolyte, and acid-base are in balance.
1) Water and solutes are in constant movement and are exchanged continuously.
a) Most of the membranes of the body are semipermeable; allowing free movement of water and many nonelectrolytes and selective movement of electrolytes according to concentration gradients.
b) Movement of fluids, electrolytes, and other solutes occurs by the following processes:
i) Diffusion: Solutes move from an area of higher solute concentration to an area of lower solute concentration.
ii) Osmosis: Solutions move from an area of lower solute concentration to an area of higher solute concentration.
iii) Active transport: use of an energy source to move solutes from an area of lower solute concentration to an area of higher solution concentration
iv) Filtration: use of the pushing pressure of hydrostatic pressure to move water and selective solutes through a semipermeable membrane
c) Movement into and out of the cell occurs by diffusion, osmosis, and active transport.
i) Hydrostatic pressures push
(a) Capillary hydrostatic pressure pushes fluid out of capillary and into interstitium.
(b) Interstitial hydrostatic pressure pushes fluid out of interstitium and into the capillary.
ii) Colloidal oncotic pressures pull
(a) Capillary colloidal oncotic pressure pulls and holds fluid in the capillary.
(b) Interstitial colloidal oncotic pressure pulls and holds fluid in the interstitium.
iii) Starling's law of the capillaries describes the movement of fluid into and out of the capillaries (for more on capillary dynamics, see Chapter 2)
(a) Pressure differences at the venous and arterial ends of the capillaries influence the direction and rate of water and solute movement.
(b) Pressures pushing fluid out of the capillary dominate at the arterial end; pressures pushing fluid back into the capillary dominate at the venous end.
d) Pathology
i) Third-spacing: fluid accumulation in any space that is not intravascular or intracellular (e.g., interstitial edema, ascites, pleural effusion, pericardial effusion)
(a) HF: Peripheral edema is caused by venous congestion and excessive hydrostatic pressure at the venous end.
(b) Malnutrition: Decrease in plasma proteins decrease capillary colloidal oncotic pressure and allow excessive fluid to leak out of the capillary.
(c) Fluid resuscitation with hypotonic solutions (e.g., D_5W): Fluids with osmolality less than serum cause movement of fluid out of the vascular bed into the interstitium.
2) Normal functioning of cells requires constancy of the body's compartments; imbalances disrupt homeostasis.

e. Water exchanges occur continuously.
1) Loss of water: total ~2400 mL/24 hr
a) Lungs (400 mL)
b) Skin (400 mL)
c) Kidneys (1500 mL)
d) Intestines (100 mL)

e) Losses are increased by any of the following:
i) Increased respiratory rate
ii) Fever
iii) Hot, dry environment
iv) Injury to the skin (e.g., burns)

2) Gains of water: total ~2400 mL/24 hr
a) Liquids (1500 mL)
b) Food (500 mL)
c) Oxidation of food and body tissues (400 mL)

f. Body fluid is regulated by the following mechanisms:
1) Thirst
a) Thirst mechanism is located in the anterior hypothalamus; osmoreceptor cells sense changes in serum osmolality and initiate impulses to produce the thirst sensation and the release of ADH.
b) The mechanism is stimulated by any of the following:
i) Intracellular dehydration
ii) Hypertonic body fluids
iii) Extracellular fluid loss
iv) Hypotension or decreased cardiac output
v) Angiotensin
vi) Dry mouth
c) The effect of thirst is the conscious desire to drink fluids (NOTE: Thirst is unreliable in the elderly or confused).

2) Antidiuretic hormone
a) ADH is produced by the hypothalamus, stored in and released by the posterior pituitary gland; release may be altered by intracranial processes (e.g., head injury, tumors, craniotomy) and extracranial processes (e.g., mechanical ventilation, tuberculosis).
b) ADH is stimulated by any of the following:
i) Hyperosmolality of extracellular fluid
ii) Decrease in extracellular fluid volume
iii) Hyperthermia
c) Effects of ADH include the following:
i) Acts on distal and collecting tubules, causing more water to be pulled from the tubule back into the blood
ii) Increases total volume of body fluid by decreasing urine volume

3) Renin-angiotensin-aldosterone (RAA) system (see Figure 2-22 on page 32)
a) RAA system is stimulated by any of the following:
i) Decreased blood pressure stimulating stretch receptors in juxtaglomerular cells
ii) Sympathetic nervous system stimulation
iii) Hyponatremia, hyperkalemia
iv) Increased adrenocorticotropin hormone (ACTH) levels
b) Effects of the RAA system include the following:
i) Angiotensin II causes vasoconstriction and secretion of aldosterone, a mineralocorticoid produced by the adrenal cortex.
ii) Aldosterone stimulates the renal tubules to reabsorb more sodium and water, which causes sodium retention, water retention, and decreased urine volume.
iii) Vasoconstriction and sodium and water retention increase blood pressure, which decreases renin secretion.

4) Atrial natriuretic peptide (ANP)
a) ANP is a hormonelike substance that is synthesized and stored by specialized atrial muscle cells.
b) ANP secretion is stimulated by the following:
i) Volume expansion
ii) Elevated cardiac filling pressures
c) Effects of ANP include the following:
i) Increased excretion of sodium and water by the kidney
ii) Decreased synthesis of renin and decreased release of aldosterone

5) Countercurrent mechanism of kidney: mechanism for concentration and dilution of urine

5. Electrolyte balance
a. Solutes are substances dissolved in a solution and may be electrolytes or nonelectrolytes.
1) Nonelectrolytes (e.g., glucose, proteins, lipids, oxygen, carbon dioxide, urea, creatinine, bilirubin) are solutes without an electrical charge; they stay intact in solution.
2) Electrolytes are solutes that dissociate into positive or negative ions when in solution and will generate an electrical charge when in solution.
a) Electrical charge
i) Cations are positive-charged ions
(a) Major intracellular cation is potassium (K^+)
(b) Major extracellular cation is sodium (Na^+)
(c) Other cations: Ca^{++}; Mg^{++}; H^+
ii) Anions are negative-charged electrolytes.
(a) Major intracellular anion is chloride (Cl^-)
(b) Major extracellular anion is phosphate (PO_4^{3-})
(c) Other anions: HCO_3^-

iii) In each fluid compartment, the various cations and anions balance each other to achieve electrical neutrality; there is no net charge within a fluid compartment (Figure 8-6*B*).

b. Renal regulation of electrolytes
   1) Excretion and/or retention of electrolytes
   2) Filter and reabsorb about half of unbound serum calcium and activate vitamin D_3, a compound that promotes intestinal calcium absorption
   3) Regulates phosphorus excretion

c. Summary of electrolyte normal values, roles, regulation, and food sources (Table 8-1)

6. Renal role in regulation of blood pressure
   a. Juxtaglomerular apparatus is a combination of specialized cells located near the glomerulus at the junction of the afferent and efferent arterioles; juxtaglomerular cells contain granules of inactive renin.
   b. Renin-angiotensin-aldosterone system as depicted in Figure 2-22
7. Red blood cell (RBC) synthesis and maturation
   a. Erythropoietin secretion
      1) Stimulates production of RBCs in bone marrow
      2) Prolongs life of RBC
   b. Postulated methods of erythropoietin synthesis and stimulus for secretion

Table 8-1 Electrolyte Summary

Electrolyte	Functions	Regulation and Factors Affecting Serum Level	Food Sources
Sodium: normal 136-145 mEq/L	• Maintains extracellular osmolality and volume • Maintains active transport mechanism in conjunction with potassium • Influences the kidney's regulation of the body's water and electrolyte status • Promotes the irritability of nerve tissue and the conduction of nerve impulses • Facilitates muscle contraction • Aids in some enzyme activities • Combines with bicarbonate and chloride to help regulate acid-base balance	• Aldosterone: causes sodium and water retention • Glomerular filtration rate: sodium excretion is increased when GFR is high; decreased when GFR is low • "Third factor": promotes sodium excretion by inhibiting sodium reabsorption; suppression of this factor ensures sodium reabsorption • Increase in sodium concentration stimulates water retention by ADH release diluting sodium back to normal level • Some excretion through skin in perspiration	• Bouillon • Celery • Cheeses • Dried fruits • Frozen, canned, or packaged foods • Monosodium glutamate (MSG) • Mustard • Olives • Pickles • Preserved meat • Salad dressings and prepared sauces • Sauerkraut • Snack foods • Soy sauce
Potassium: normal 3.5-5.0 mEq/L	• Promotes transmission of nerve impulses • Maintains intracellular osmolality • Activates several enzymatic reactions • Helps regulate acid-base balance • Influences kidney function and structure • Promotes myocardial, skeletal, and smooth muscle contractility	• Aldosterone: increase in intracellular potassium or decrease in serum sodium causes aldosterone release and potassium excretion • GFR: potassium excretion is directly related to GFR in a normal kidney • Obligatory loss: the kidneys are unable to conserve potassium; it may be flushed out by diuresis even in the presence of a body deficit; 40-50 mEq lost each day • Renal failure: if kidneys fail to excrete potassium normally from the body (e.g., renal failure), toxic levels can occur • pH: potassium shifts into the cell in alkalosis (causing hypokalemia) and out of the cell in acidosis (causing hyperkalemia)	• Apricots • Artichokes • Avocado • Banana • Cantaloupe • Carrots • Cauliflower • Chocolate • Dried beans, peas • Dried fruit • Mushrooms • Nuts • Oranges, orange juice • Peanuts • Potatoes • Prune juice • Pumpkin • Spinach • Sweet potatoes • Swiss chard • Tomatoes, tomato juice, tomato sauce

Continued

Table 8-1 Electrolyte Summary—cont'd

Electrolyte	Functions	Regulation and Factors Affecting Serum Level	Food Sources
Calcium: normal 8.5-10.5 mg/dL or 4.5-5.8 mEq/L (NOTE: Calcium is affected by albumin levels; to correct calcium, add 0.8 mg/dL for each 1 g/dL decrease in albumin)	• Hardens and strengthens bones and teeth • Aids in blood coagulation • Transmits neuromuscular impulses • Maintains cellular permeability • Serves essential role in cardiac contractility	• PTH: stimulated by a decrease in serum calcium; promotes calcium transfer from bone to plasma and aids in renal and intestinal absorption • Phosphorus: inhibits calcium absorption; calcium and phosphorus have an inverse relationship; if calcium goes up, phosphorus goes down and vice versa • Vitamin D: necessary for GI absorption; promotes calcium absorption • Calcitonin: aids transfer of calcium from plasma to bone which directly lowers serum calcium • Albumin: 50% of serum calcium is bound to serum albumin; therefore a decrease in serum albumin will lower the total calcium level but not the ionized calcium level and the patient will not have symptoms of hypocalcemia • pH: alkalosis increases binding between albumin and calcium so that the patient will exhibit symptoms of hypocalcemia, though total body calcium is normal; acidosis decreases binding between albumin and calcium so that the patient may exhibit symptoms of hypercalcemia • Corticosteroids: contribute to demineralization of the bone and calcium loss; large doses decrease calcium absorption in GI tract • Diuretic effect: calcium is lost, along with potassium and magnesium, in patients on diuretics	• Brazil nuts • Broccoli • Cheese • Collard, mustard, turnip greens • Cottage cheese • Eggnog • Ice cream • Milk and cream • Milk chocolate • Molasses • Oat flakes • Rhubarb • Seafood, especially sardines with bones • Sesame seeds • Soy flour • Spinach • Yogurt
Phosphorus: normal 3.0-4.5 mg/dL	• Aids in structure of cellular membrane • Essential for glucose metabolism in red cells; produces 2,3-diphosphoglyceric acid (2,3-DPG) as an end product • Regulates the delivery of oxygen to the tissues; 2,3-DPG encourages unloading between hemoglobin and oxygen • Essential for ATP or high-energy phosphate formation • May be connected with DNA, RNA, genetic coding • Helps maintain bone hardness • Aids in enzyme regulation (ATPase) • Used by kidney to buffer hydrogen ions (PO_4)	• PTH: inhibits renal reabsorption of phosphates; calcium and phosphorus have an inverse relationship; if calcium goes up, phosphorus goes down and vice versa • Alterations in GFR affect phosphate excretion; increased GFR decreases reabsorption of phosphorus; decreased GFR increases reabsorption of phosphorus	• Dried beans and peas • Eggs and egg products • Fish, poultry • Meats, especially organ meats • Milk and milk products • Nuts • Seeds • Whole grains

Table 8-1 Electrolyte Summary—cont'd

Electrolyte	Functions	Regulation and Factors Affecting Serum Level	Food Sources
Magnesium: normal 1.5-2.5 mEq/L	• Aids in neuromuscular transmission • Aids in cardiac contractility • Activates enzymes for cellular metabolism of CHO and proteins • Aids in maintaining the active transport mechanism at the cellular level • Aids in the transmission of hereditary information to offspring	• Not completely understood • Factors that influence calcium and potassium balance also affect magnesium • Deficiencies of these electrolytes usually occur together (e.g., diuretics cause the loss of all three) • Availability of sodium: sodium is necessary for the absorption of magnesium • Diuretics: cause the loss of excessive magnesium • PTH: affects magnesium reabsorption as it does calcium	• Bananas • Chocolate • Coconut • Grapefruit • Green, leafy vegetables • Legumes • Milk • Molasses • Nuts and seeds • Oranges • Refined sugar • Seafood • Soy flour • Wheat bran
Chloride: normal 96-106 mEq/L	• Maintains serum osmolality (along with sodium) • Combines with major cations to form important compounds (e.g., NaCl, HCl, KCl, CaCl) • Helps maintain acid-base balance through HCl production	• Indirectly affected by aldosterone • Changes almost always linked to sodium • pH: acidosis causes bicarbonate to be reabsorbed while chloride is excreted; alkalosis causes bicarbonate to be excreted while chloride is reabsorbed	• Bananas • Celery • Cheese • Dates • Eggs • Fish • Milk • Spinach • Table salt • Turkey

1) Normal kidneys either produce erythropoietin or synthesize an enzyme that catalyzes its formation.
2) Stimulation for formation is believed to be decreased PaO_2 in renal blood.

c. Interference in this process causes anemia in patients with chronic renal failure.

8. Prostaglandin synthesis
   a. Process occurs primarily in the medulla.
   b. Types of prostaglandins are as follows:
      1) Vasodilators: PGE_2, PGD_2, PGI_2
      2) Vasoconstrictors: PGA_2
   c. Release is stimulated by vasoactive substances (e.g., angiotensin, norepinephrine, bradykinins).
   d. Effects of prostaglandins include the following:
      1) Modulate the vasoconstrictive effects of angiotensin and norepinephrine; interference with this process may be one factor contributing to hypertension in patients with renal failure
      2) Increase renal blood flow, which results in arterial vasodilation, inhibition of the distal tubule's response to ADH, and promotion of sodium and water excretion
9. Renal role in bone mineralization
   a. Vitamin D is metabolized by the kidney from an inactive form to an active metabolite called *1,25-dihydroxycholecalciferol,* necessary for the absorption of calcium and phosphorus from the intestine.
   b. Interference in this process causes osteodystrophy in patients with chronic renal failure.

Assessment of Fluid, Electrolyte, and Renal Status

Interview

1. Chief complaint: common symptoms of fluid, electrolyte, or renal conditions
   a. Flank or costovertebral angle pain
      1) Unilateral or bilateral
      2) Constant or intermittent
      3) Aggravated by costovertebral angle percussion
      4) Dull ache to stabbing or throbbing pain
      5) Relieved only by analgesics or treatment of underlying disease
      6) Accompanying findings: hematuria; pyuria; change in urine volume
      7) Possible causes: renal calculi; bladder cancer; bacterial cystitis; acute glomerulonephritis; obstructive uropathy; perirenal abscess; polycystic kidney disease; acute pyelonephritis; renal infarction; renal cancer; renal trauma; renal vein thrombosis; acute pancreatitis
   b. Changes in pattern of urination
      1) Frequency: frequent voiding
      2) Nocturia: getting up at night to void (more than twice)

3) Dysuria: painful urination
4) Urgency: a feeling of the need to void immediately
5) Hesitancy: difficulty starting the flow of urine
6) Change in stream
7) Retention: incomplete emptying of the bladder
8) Incontinence: inability to control urination
9) Enuresis: incontinence of urine in bed at night

c. Change in urine output: increased or decreased amount
d. Change in appearance of urine
   1) Dilute: clear to light yellow
   2) Concentrated: dark, amber
   3) Pyuria: cloudy
   4) Hematuria: pink to red
   5) Bilirubinemia: orange to brown
   6) Myoglobinuria: tea- or cola-colored
   7) Hemoglobinuria: wine-colored
e. Neurologic
   1) Visual changes: may be associated with uremia, fluid overload, or electrolyte imbalance
   2) Paresthesias: may be associated with hypocalcemia
   3) Headaches: may be associated with fluid overload or uremia
   4) Seizures: may be associated with uremia, electrolyte imbalances, fluid overload
   5) Decreased ability to concentrate: may be associated with uremia, electrolyte imbalance, or fluid overload
   6) Apathy: may be associated with uremia
f. Cardiovascular
   1) Palpitations: may be seen with dysrhythmias in electrolyte imbalance
   2) Chest pain: may be seen with uremia or electrolyte imbalance
   3) Edema: may be associated with uremia, fluid overload, or hypoproteinemia
g. Pulmonary
   1) Dyspnea: may be seen in patients with renal failure as a result of left ventricular failure or pleural effusion
   2) Hemoptysis: seen in Goodpasture's syndrome
h. Gastrointestinal
   1) Halitosis: foul odor to breath; urinelike odor to breath may be associated with uremia; metallic taste in mouth
   2) Anorexia: may be associated with uremia
   3) Nausea or vomiting: may be associated with uremia, electrolyte imbalance, or fluid overload
   4) Constipation or diarrhea: may be related to fluid imbalance
i. Musculoskeletal
   1) Joint pain: may be associated with uremia, fluid imbalance, electrolyte imbalance
   2) Muscle weakness: may be associated with electrolyte imbalance
   3) Muscle pain or cramps: may be associated with uremia or electrolyte imbalance
j. Dermatologic
   1) Pruritus: may be associated with uremia
   2) Bruising: may be associated with uremia
   3) Delayed healing: may be associated with uremia
k. Sexual
   1) Impotence: may be related to uremia
   2) Diminished libido: may be related to uremia
   3) Infertility: may be related to uremia
l. Other general symptoms
   1) Fatigue: may be associated with uremia
   2) Fever: may be associated with infection or dehydration
   3) Thirst: may be associated with fluid imbalance
   4) Change in body weight: may be associated with uremia or fluid imbalance

2. History of present illness
   a. PQRST
   b. Accompanying symptoms
3. Past medical history
   a. Renal/urinary tract
      1) Urinary tract infection
      2) Calculi
      3) Renal insufficiency/failure
         a) Dialysis
         b) Renal transplantation
      4) Surgical procedures
   b. Cardiovascular
      1) Hypertension
      2) Arteriosclerosis/atherosclerosis
      3) Heart failure
      4) Bacterial endocarditis
   c. Pulmonary: tuberculosis
   d. Endocrine/metabolic
      1) Diabetes mellitus
      2) Gout
   e. Immunologic/hematologic
      1) Connective tissue disorders
         a) Lupus erythematosus
         b) Scleroderma
      2) Goodpasture's syndrome: hemoptysis with glomerulonephritis
      3) Hemophilia
      4) Disseminated intravascular coagulation
      5) Sickle cell disease
      6) Malignancy
      7) Blood transfusion
   f. Gynecologic: toxemia of pregnancy
   g. Infection
      1) Recent beta-hemolytic streptococcal infection
      2) Urinary tract infection (UTI)
4. Family history
   a. Renal
      1) Inherited glomerulonephritis
      2) Polycystic disease

3) Inherited nephritis (Alport's syndrome)
4) Amyloidosis
5) Malignancy

b. Cardiovascular
1) Hypertension
2) Coronary artery disease

c. Immunologic/hematologic
1) Hemophilia
2) Sickle cell disease

d. Endocrine: diabetes mellitus

5. Social history
a. Occupational exposure to toxins: lead, mercury, pesticides, methanol, radiation, carbon tetrachloride, phenol
b. Exercise habits: strenuous exercise in an unconditioned person may cause rhabdomyolysis
c. Fluid intake: type of fluids
d. Smoking: increased incidence of bladder cancer
e. Use of saccharin: increased incidence of bladder cancer

6. Medication history
a. Potentially nephrotoxic agents
1) Antimicrobials
a) Aminoglycosides
b) Cephalosporins
c) Sulfonamides
d) Amphotericin B
e) Bacitracin
f) Rifampin
2) Nonsteroidal antiinflammatory agents (e.g., ibuprofen, indomethacin, aspirin)
3) ACE inhibitors (e.g., captopril, enalapril)
4) Antineoplastics (e.g., cisplatin, methotrexate)
5) Analgesics containing phenacetin
6) Cyclosporin A
7) Methanol, ethylene glycol
8) Carbon tetrachloride
9) Contrast media
10) Heavy metals (e.g., lead, arsenic, mercury, uranium)
11) Insecticides and fungicides
12) Phencyclidine (PCP) and other street drugs

b. Diuretics
c. Antihypertensives
d. Anticoagulants
e. Electrolyte replacement therapy
f. Immunosuppressives
1) Corticosteroids
2) Azathioprine (Imuran)
3) Cyclophosphamide (Cytoxan)

Vital Signs

1. Blood pressure
a. Increased: seen in fluid overload, renal disease, hypertension
b. Decreased: must be fluid loss of 15-25% before systolic blood pressure falls
c. Postural drop (tilt positive): decrease of 15 mm Hg in systolic pressure when patient sits or stands may be earlier change of hypovolemia

2. Pulse
a. Increased: seen in SNS stimulation as may be seen in fluid overload or dehydration; response blunted or eliminated by beta-blockers
b. Postural: increases of pulse by 20 beats/min when the patient sits or stands may be earlier change of hypovolemia

3. Respiratory rate and rhythm
a. Tachypnea: seen in SNS stimulation as may be seen in fluid overload or dehydration
b. Kussmaul's: rapid, deep, gasping breaths seen in metabolic acidosis

4. Temperature: hyperthermia may be seen in dehydration

5. Weight changes
a. Change of 1 lb is equal to 500 mL; change of 1 kg is equal to 1 L
b. Evaluate weight before and after hemodialysis; evaluate weight after drainage of dialysate in patients on peritoneal dialysis
c. Weight loss resulting from generalized debilitation may be seen in renal failure.

Inspection and Palpation

1. Skin
a. Color
1) Yellowish-gray color is seen in renal failure.
2) Pallor may indicate anemia.
3) Petechiae or bruising may be seen in renal failure as a result of platelet dysfunction.

b. Skin texture
1) Rough, dry skin is seen in renal failure.
2) Uremic frost, a filmy coating over the skin, is seen in untreated uremia.

c. Lesions: Scratch marks may be seen as a result of pruritus in renal failure.

d. Skin turgor
1) Recoil should be immediate; decrease in skin turgor indicates interstitial dehydration but is not an early sign.
2) Evaluation of skin turgor to determine hydration status is not reliable in elderly patients because of poor elasticity.

e. Edema
1) Late change of overhydration because patient may gain 3-4 kg before edema is noticeable
2) Location
a) Edema related to renal disease is frequently facial initially.
b) Anasarca (generalized, massive edema and does not pit) may be seen in end-stage renal disease.

2. Mouth
a. Halitosis: uremic fetor (urinelike odor to the breath) noted in renal failure
b. Mucous membranes: Stickiness of the oral mucous membranes and tongue is the preferred

indicator of dehydration in the elderly; use a tongue blade to evaluate stickiness.

3. Eyes
   a. Periorbital edema seen in nephrotic syndrome and other forms of renal disease
   b. Cataract formation common in renal failure
4. Ears: nerve deafness common in renal failure
5. Neurologic status
   a. Change in level of consciousness may indicate azotemia or electrolyte imbalance
   b. Confusion may be indicative of uremia
   c. Seizures may indicate hyponatremia, cerebral edema
   d. Neuromuscular irritability and changes in muscle strength may reflect electrolyte imbalance.
6. Cardiovascular
   a. Dysrhythmias are common in electrolyte imbalance.
   b. Jugular venous distention (see Figure 2-30 in Chapter 2 for illustration)
      1) To evaluate JVD
         a) Place patient at a 45-degree angle.
         b) Identify the angle of Louis: raised notch that is created where the manubrium and the body of the sternum join; also called *manubriosternal junction* or *sternal angle.*
         c) Measure height of neck vein distention.
         d) Normal height of neck vein distention is 1-2 cm above the angle of Louis; neck vein distention of greater than 2 cm above the angle of Louis may be indicative of hypervolemia.
7. Abdomen
   a. Generalized edema and/or ascites: may be seen in renal failure
   b. Kidney
      1) The kidney may be palpated by "capture" technique; put one hand under the patient below the costal margin and the other hand on the abdomen below the costal margin; ask the patient to take a deep breath and move hands together to try to "capture" the kidney.
      2) The lower pole of a normal right kidney may be palpable because it is lower than the right (pushed down by the liver).
      3) A normal left kidney is not palpable.
      4) If kidney is palpable, evaluate the following:
         a) Size: Normal size is 10 × 5 × 2.5 cm or about the size of a fist.
            i) Increased size may be seen in acute renal disease, polycystic disease, obstructive uropathy, pyelonephritis, renal abscess or tumor.
            ii) Decreased size may be seen in advanced chronic renal failure.
         b) Discomfort: Pain or discomfort during palpation may indicate infection, calculi, tumor, hydronephrosis, or glomerulonephritis.
   c. Bladder
      1) The bladder is palpable in suprapubic area only when full.
      2) If palpable, the bladder should be felt as a smooth, round, firm organ that is sensitive to palpation.
8. Extremities
   a. Asterixis: a hand-flapping tremor induced by extending the arm and dorsiflexing the wrist; indicative of increased ammonia levels; seen in renal failure and hepatic encephalopathy
   b. Vascular access (e.g., fistula, AV graft, shunt): thrill over access indicates patency

Percussion

1. Thorax: Flatness at lung bases may indicate pleural effusion, which is frequently seen in renal failure.
2. Abdomen
   a. Elicitation of a fluid wave: indicative of ascites, which is frequently seen in end-stage renal failure
   b. Costovertebral angle (CVA): Tap over costovertebral angle with ulnar surface of hand.
      1) CVA tenderness may be seen in pyelonephritis, renal calculi, renal abscess or tumor, glomerulonephritis, or intermittent hydronephrosis.
      2) Bruising over CVA may indicate renal trauma.
   c. Bladder
      1) The bladder is percussible in suprapubic area only when it contains at least 150 mL.
      2) Dullness is audible above the symphysis pubis if the bladder is full of urine.
      3) Pain during percussion may indicate cystitis.

Auscultation

1. Vascular sounds
   a. Renal bruit: may be audible to the left or right of midline in periumbilical region in renal vascular disease or renal vascular trauma
   b. Vascular access (e.g., fistula, AV graft, shunt): Bruit over access indicates patency.
2. Heart sounds
   a. Rate and rhythm: Dysrhythmias may be seen in electrolyte imbalance.
   b. S_3: indicates heart failure
   c. Flow murmur: Mitral regurgitation murmur (systolic murmur heard best at apex with diaphragm) may be heard with fluid overload.
   d. Pericardial friction rub: may indicate pericarditis, a common complication of renal failure
3. Breath sounds: Crackles may indicate fluid overload, heard initially at bases.
4. Bowel sounds: Changes may indicate electrolyte imbalance.
   a. Hypoactive bowel sounds in hypokalemia
   b. Hyperactive bowel sounds in hyperkalemia

Urine Output

1. Important indicator of GFR
2. Decreased with diminished cardiac output or dehydration
3. Increased in overhydration
4. Volume parameters
   a. Normal output = 1500 mL/24 hr or at least 0.5 mL/kg/hr
   b. Polyuria: greater than 2500 mL/24 hr
   c. Oliguria: 100-400 mL/24 hr
   d. Anuria: 0-100 mL/24 hr

Bladder Volume by Portable Ultrasound Bladder Scanner

1. Uses
   a. Differentiate between an empty bladder and urinary retention, thereby avoiding unnecessary catheterization.
   b. Evaluate residual urine in the bladder after voiding.
2. Technology
   a. Portable ultrasound bladder scanner automatically computes the bladder volume based on cross-sectional images of the bladder.
   b. Components
      1) Instrument box with screen for digital display of bladder volume
      2) Handheld ultrasound transducer
3. Methodology
   a. Indicate patient gender.
   b. Wash the transducer tip and apply ultrasound gel.
   c. Position the tip of the transducer above the symphysis pubis and toward the bladder.
   d. Press the transducer button and hold until the machine beeps, indicating that scanning is complete.
   e. May be repeated once or twice more to evaluate consistency, which would indicate a reliable reading
   f. Wash gel from patient's abdomen and transducer tip.
4. Implication: Catheterization is generally indicated if bladder volume is greater than 300 mL.

Hemodynamic Monitoring

1. Right atrial pressure (RAP) (from proximal port of pulmonary artery catheter) or central venous pressure (CVP) (from catheter in superior vena cava): normal 2-6 mm Hg
   a. Increased in hypervolemia
   b. Decreased in hypovolemia
2. Pulmonary artery wedge pressure (PAOP): normal 8-12 mm Hg
   a. Increased in hypervolemia
   b. Decreased in hypovolemia

Diagnostic Studies

1. Serum
   a. Osmolality: normal 280-295 mOsm/kg
      1) Measures particles exerting osmotic pull per unit of water
      2) May be calculated:

$$(\text{Na} \times 2) + (\text{BUN}/2.6) + (\text{Serum glucose}/18)$$

      3) Reflects total body hydration
         a) Increased in dehydration
         b) Decreased with fluid overload
   b. Blood urea nitrogen (BUN): normal 5-20 mg/dL
      1) Reflects difference between rate of urea synthesis and its excretion by the kidneys
         a) Formed in the liver through enzymatic breakdown of protein
         b) Not as accurate an indicator of renal failure as is creatinine because BUN levels fluctuate greatly with protein intake but creatinine levels are relatively unchanged by protein intake and hydration level
      2) Abnormal values
         a) Increased with decreased renal blood flow or urine production, dehydration, some neoplasms, and certain antibiotics; increased BUN is also referred to as *uremia*
         b) Decreased in pregnancy, overhydration, severe liver disease, malnutrition
      3) BUN : creatinine ratio: normally ~10 : 1
         a) When BUN is elevated disproportionately to the creatinine (e.g., BUN:creatinine ratio 20 : 1), consider an extrarenal cause such as one of the following:
            i) Volume depletion (i.e., prerenal)
               (a) Insufficient fluid intake
               (b) Excessive fluid loss
                  (i) Diuresis
                  (ii) Vomiting
            ii) Poor renal perfusion
               (a) Shock
               (b) Sepsis
               (c) Decreased cardiac output
               (d) Renovascular disease
            iii) Protein catabolism
               (a) Starvation
               (b) Blood in the GI tract
               (c) Corticosteroids
         b) When BUN and creatinine are both elevated while maintaining the normal 10 : 1 ratio, consider a renal cause such as acute or chronic renal failure.
         c) When BUN:creatinine is lower than normal
            i) Decreased protein intake
            ii) Liver dysfunction
   c. Creatinine: normal 0.7-1.5 mg/dL
      1) Nonprotein end product of muscle metabolism
         a) More accurate than BUN in evaluating renal function because creatinine is

normally filtered by the glomerulus and not reabsorbed by the tubule.
   b) Unaffected by diet and fluid intake
  2) Abnormal values
   a) Increased
    i) A twice-normal (~3 mg/dL) creatinine level suggests 50% nephron loss
    ii) Greater than 10 mg/dL indicates end-stage renal disease with less than 10% of nephrons still functioning
   b) Decreased: muscular dystrophy

d. Electrolytes
  1) Sodium: normal 136-145 mEq/L
  2) Potassium: normal 3.5-5.5 mEq/L
  3) Chloride: normal 96-106 mEq/L
  4) Calcium: normal 8.5-10.5 mg/dL
  5) Phosphorus: normal 3.0-4.5 mg/dL
  6) Magnesium: normal 1.5-2.2 mEq/L

e. Anion gap: a calculated parameter (Table 8-2)
  1) Calculated by subtracting the anions from the cations
   a) (Sodium + Potassium) − (Chloride + Carbon dioxide content or bicarbonate)
   b) Normal: 5-15
  2) Helpful in determination of cause of metabolic acidosis
   a) A normal anion gap indicates that the reason for the metabolic acidosis is bicarbonate loss.
   b) An elevated anion gap indicates that the reason for the metabolic acidosis is an acid gain (e.g., lactic acid, ketoacid, toxins).

f. Glucose: normal 70-110 mEq/L

g. Arterial blood gases
  1) pH: normal 7.35-7.45
  2) $PaCO_2$: normal 35-45 mm Hg
  3) HCO_3: normal 22-26 mEq/L
  4) PaO_2: normal 80-100 mm Hg

h. Hematology
  1) Hematocrit: normal 40-52% for males; 35-47% for females
   a) Measures portion of blood volume occupied by RBCs
   b) Increased in dehydration or polycythemia
   c) Decreased with low RBCs or with normal hemoglobin and water overload
  2) Hemoglobin: normal 13-18 g/dL for males; 12-16 g/dL for females
  3) White blood cells (WBC): 3500-11,000/mm^3

i. Clotting profile
  1) Prothrombin time (PT): normal 12-15 seconds
  2) Partial thromboplastin time (PTT): normal 25-38 seconds
  3) Thrombin time: normal 10-15 seconds
  4) Bleeding time: normal 1-9.5 minutes
  5) Platelets: normal 150,000-400,000/mm^3

Table 8-2 Anion Gap

Considerations	Comments
Calculation of anion gap	(Na + K) − (Cl + [HCO_3 or CO_2 content])
Normal value	5-15
Causes of metabolic acidosis with normal anion gap: bicarbonate loss	Intestinal loss of bicarbonate • Diarrhea • Pancreatic fistula • Ureterosigmoidostomy Renal loss of bicarbonate • Carbonic anhydrase inhibitors (e.g., acetazolamide [Diamox]) • Aldosterone antagonists (also referred to as *potassium-sparing diuretics*) (e.g., triamterene [Dyrenium], spironolactone [Aldactone]) • Renal tubular acidosis • Adrenal insufficiency • Primary hypoaldosteronism Excessive gain of chloride • Large quantities of normal saline • Ammonium chloride • Arginine hydrochloride
Causes of metabolic acidosis with increased anion gap: metabolic acid gain	Renal failure Lactic acidosis • Shock • Hypoxemia/hypoxia • Severe anemia • Status epilepticus • Cyanide poisoning Ketoacidosis • Diabetic ketoacidosis • Starvation • Alcohol Drugs and toxins • Salicylates • Methanol • Ethylene glycol • Paraldehyde • High-dose carbenicillin Rhabdomyolysis

j. Serum proteins
  1) Total protein: normal 6-8 g/dL
  2) Albumin: normal 3.5-4.5 g/dL

k. Serum lipids
  1) Cholesterol: 150-200 mg/dL
  2) Triglycerides: 40-150 mg/dL

2. Urine
 a. Visual examination: clear, yellow
 b. Glucose: normal negative; glycosuria occurs when renal threshold for glucose is exceeded; renal threshold is variable and patient-specific, so there is no accurate method to predict serum glucose

c. Ketones: normal negative; ketonuria is seen in catabolism (e.g., starvation or diabetic ketoacidosis)
d. Protein: normal 0-8 mg/dL
   1) Proteinuria may occur after ingestion of a high-protein meal or can accompany renal changes of pregnancy.
   2) Consistent proteinuria suggests compromise of the glomerular membrane (e.g., nephrotic syndrome, glomerulonephritis).
e. Myoglobin: normal negative or less than 20 ng/mL; myoglobinuria indicates muscle breakdown
f. Hemoglobin: normal negative; hemoglobinuria indicates free hemoglobin in the urine such as occurs in hemolytic blood transfusion reaction, hemolytic or sickle cell anemia, fresh-water drowning, burns, disseminated intravascular coagulation (DIC)
g. Bilirubin: normal negative; urobilinogen indicates biliary obstruction or liver disease
h. Specific gravity: 1.005-1.030
   1) Increased with any condition causing hypoperfusion of kidneys leading to oliguria (e.g., shock, severe dehydration, proteinuria, glycosuria, contrast media)
   2) Decreased in diabetes insipidus, overhydration, and when renal tubules lose their ability to reabsorb water and concentrate urine as in early pyelonephritis
i. Osmolality: 50-1200 mOsm/kg
   1) Measures number of particles per unit of water in urine
   2) Depends upon the circulating titer of ADH and the rate of urinary solute excretion; should be 1.5 times that of serum osmolality
   3) Increased in fluid volume deficit due to retention of fluid by the body
   4) Decreased in fluid volume excess due to fluid being excreted by the kidney
j. Creatinine clearance
   1) Estimate of GFR
   2) Urine specimen for 24-hour period and a serum creatinine required
   3) Normal: 85-135 mL/min
k. Culture and sensitivity: normal no bacteria present; if bacteria are present, appropriate antibiotic therapy is identified
l. pH: normal 4-8 with average of 6
   1) Increased urinary acidity indicates that the body is retaining bicarbonate.
   2) Decreased urinary acidity (more alkaline) indicates that the kidney is retaining sodium and acids.
      a) Alkaline urine may be associated with urinary tract infection.
      b) Alkaline urine and serum acidosis are associated with renal tubular acidosis.
m. Spot urine electrolytes
   1) Evaluates the kidney's ability to conserve sodium and concentrate urine
   2) Measures sodium, potassium, and chloride concentrations in the urine
      a) Sodium: normal 40-220 mEq/L
      b) Potassium: normal 25-120 mEq/L
      c) Chloride: normal 110-250 mEq/L
n. Sediment
   1) Casts: precipitation from the kidney that takes the shape of the tubule where it was formed; normally none or occasional hyaline casts
      a) Hyaline casts: small amounts normal, but large amounts indicative of significant proteinuria
      b) Erythrocyte casts: indicative of glomerulonephritis or vasculitis
      c) Leukocyte casts: indicative of infectious process
      d) Granular casts: indicative of acute tubular necrosis, interstitial nephritis, acute or chronic glomerulonephritis, chronic renal failure
      e) Fatty casts: indicative of lipoid nephrosis or nephrotic syndrome
      f) Renal tubular casts: indicative of acute kidney injury
   2) Bacteria: abnormal in catheterized specimen
   3) Erythrocytes: small numbers normal; large numbers indicative of glomerulonephritis, interstitial nephritis, malignancy, infection, calculi, cystitis, or trauma
   4) Leukocytes: small numbers normal; large numbers indicative of infection, interstitial nephritis
   5) Renal epithelial cells: indicative of acute tubular necrosis, glomerulonephritis, interstitial nephritis
   6) Crystals: indicative of stone formation
   7) Eosinophils: indicative of allergic reaction in kidney

3. Other diagnostic studies (Table 8-3)

Drugs Affecting the Renal System

Diuretics

1. Action: excretion of fluid and sodium
2. Indications
   a. Hypertension
   b. Heart failure
   c. Edema
      1) Pulmonary (usually a loop diuretic)
      2) Cerebral (usually mannitol)
      3) Peripheral
   d. Drug toxicity (forced diuresis) (usually mannitol)
   e. Renal pigments (e.g. hemoglobinuria, myoglobinuria) (usually mannitol)
3. Types of diuretics and specific actions
   a. Thiazide diuretics
      1) Examples
         a) Hydrochlorothiazide (HydroDIURIL)
         b) Chlorthalidone (Hygroton, Thalitone)
         c) Chlorothiazide (Diuril)

Table 8-3 Renal Diagnostic Studies

Study	Purposes	Comments
Computerized tomographic (CT) scan	• Provides a view of kidneys, retroperitoneal space, bladder, prostate • Evaluates kidney size • Evaluates the kidney for tumors, abscesses, and obstruction	• No special preparation required • Can be safely used in patients with renal failure • Contrast medium may be used
Cystometrogram	• Evaluates the pressure exerted against the wall of the bladder to evaluate bladder tone	• No special preparation required • Urinary catheter inserted and saline instilled into bladder Postprocedure • Monitor for clinical indications of urinary tract infection
Cystoscopy	• Visualizes bladder and urethra for identification of pathology	Preprocedure • NPO after midnight if general anesthesia is to be used • Administer sedative if prescribed • No special preparation required Postprocedure • Pink-tinged urine is normal but gross hematuria is abnormal; monitor urine output • Encourage fluids

Intravenous pyelogram (IVP)	• Evaluates position, size, shape, and location of kidneys
	• Provides visualization of internal kidney (parenchyma, calyces, pelvis)
	• Evaluates filling of renal pelvis
	• Outlines ureters and bladder
	• Identifies presence of cysts and tumors
	• Identifies obstruction, congenital abnormality
		• Also called *excretory urogram*
		• Contraindicated in renal insufficiency, multiple myeloma, pregnancy, congestive heart failure, sickle cell disease
		• Bowel preparation (e.g., cathartics as prescribed)
		• NPO for 8 hours prior to the test
		• Contrast media used
		  • Check for allergy to iodine prior to the study
		  • Monitor for allergic reaction postprocedure
		  • Ensure hydration postprocedure

Kidneys, ureters, and bladder (KUB)	• Outlines kidneys, ureters, and bladder • Evaluates size, shape, and position of kidneys • Identifies location of calculi	• Also called *flat plate of abdomen* • Bowel preparation (e.g., cathartics may be prescribed if to be followed by IVP)
Magnetic resonance imaging (MRI)	• Differentiation between cyst and solid mass • Identifies infarction, trauma, obstruction	• More specific than renal ultrasonography or CT scan because it shows subtle density changes • Cannot be used in patients with any implanted metallic device, including pacemakers • No special preparation required

Nephrotomogram	• Evaluates segments of the kidney at different levels
	• Differentiates cysts from solid masses
		• Bowel preparation (e.g., cathartics as prescribed)
		• NPO for 8 hours prior to the test
		• Contrast media used
		  • Check for allergy to iodine prior to the study
		  • Monitor for allergic reaction postprocedure
		  • Ensure hydration postprocedure

Table 8-3 Renal Diagnostic Studies—cont'd

Study	Purposes	Comments

Renal angiography	• Evaluates renal vasculature
	• Identifies renal artery stenosis
	• Identifies cysts, tumors, infarction, trauma
		• Bowel preparation (e.g., cathartics) as prescribed
		• NPO for 8 hours prior to the test
		• Sedative is usually prescribed prior to the procedure
		• Contrast media used
		  • Check for allergy to iodine prior to the study
		  • Monitor for allergic reaction postprocedure
		  • Ensure hydration postprocedure
		Postprocedure
		• Keep extremity in which catheter was placed immobilized in a straight position for 6-12 hours
		• Monitor arterial puncture point for hemorrhage or hematoma
		• Monitor neurovascular status of affected limb
		• Monitor for indications of systemic emboli

Renal biopsy	• Obtains tissue specimen for microscopic evaluation	• May be performed open or closed • Clotting profile is evaluated preprocedure • Type and crossmatch for two units of blood preprocedure • Usually not performed if patient has only one functioning kidney (unless being done to evaluate possible transplant rejection) • Closed biopsy contraindicated in bleeding abnormalities, polycystic disease, hydronephrosis, neoplasm, urinary tract infection, and uncooperative patient Postprocedure • Pressure dressing is applied, and the patient is on bed rest for 24 hours • Observe for hematuria, flank pain, or hypotension
Renal radionuclide scan (renogram)	• Evaluates position, size, shape, and location of kidneys • Identifies obstruction, abscesses, cysts, tumors • Evaluates renal perfusion • Evaluates glomerular filtration, tubular function, and excretion • Assesses status of renal transplant	• Assure patient that the amount of radioactive material is minimal • Do not schedule within 24 hours after IVP • Ask patient to void prior to scan • Encourage fluids after the procedure

Retrograde pyelogram	• Evaluates position, size, shape, and location of kidneys
	• Outlines ureters and bladder
	• Identifies presence of cysts and tumors
	• Identifies obstruction
		• Does not require the kidney to excrete dye so may be used in patients with renal insufficiency
		• Bowel preparation (e.g., cathartics as prescribed)
		• NPO for 8 hours prior to the test
		• Contrast media used
		  • Check for allergy to iodine prior to the study
		  • Monitor for allergic reaction postprocedure
		  • Ensure hydration postprocedure
		• Monitor patient for clinical indications of urinary tract infection or sepsis

Ultrasonography	• Evaluates fluid versus solid mass • Identifies obstructions • Identifies cysts, abscesses, tumors, polycystic kidney disease • Identifies hemorrhage • Identifies urinary tract obstruction and leaks	• No special preparation required • Can be safely used in patients with renal failure • Contrast media may be used
Voiding cystourethrography	• Identifies abnormalities of lower urinary tract to determine presence of reflux and residual urine	• No special preparation required • Encourage fluids postprocedure

d) Polythiazide (Renese)
e) Indapamide (Lozol)
f) Metolazone (Mykrox, Zaroxolyn)

2) Actions
a) Inhibit sodium reabsorption in the ascending loop of Henle and the early distal tubule
b) Decrease water reabsorption

3) Potential adverse effects
a) Hyponatremia
b) Hypokalemia
c) Hypercalcemia
d) Hypomagnesemia
e) Hypovolemia
f) Hyperglycemia
g) Hyperuricemia
h) Increased BUN
i) Hepatitis
j) Anemia, thrombocytopenia, neutropenia

b. Loop diuretics: used most often in critical care because of their potency

1) Examples
a) Furosemide (Lasix)
b) Ethacrynic acid (Edecrin)
c) Bumetanide (Bumex)
d) Torsemide (Demadex)

2) Actions
a) Inhibit sodium reabsorption in the ascending loop of Henle
b) Decrease water reabsorption

3) Potential adverse effects
a) Hyponatremia
b) Hypokalemia
c) Hypocalcemia
d) Hypomagnesemia
e) Hypochloremic alkalosis
f) Hypovolemia
g) Hyperglycemia
h) Hyperuricemia
i) Increased BUN
j) Hearing loss
k) Thrombocytopenia, agranulocytosis, leukopenia, anemia

c. Osmotic diuretics

1) Example: mannitol (Osmitrol)

2) Actions
a) Expand intravascular volume and increase GFR
b) Increase osmolality of the tubular fluid leading to decreased absorption of sodium and water

3) Potential adverse effects
a) Hyponatremia
b) Hypokalemia
c) Hypocalcemia
d) Hypomagnesemia
e) Initial intravascular hypervolemia followed by hypovolemia
f) Increased intravascular volume may cause pulmonary edema in patients with poor cardiac function.
g) Hyperglycemia
h) Hyperuricemia
i) Increased BUN
j) Confusion

4) Aldosterone antagonists (frequently referred to as *potassium-sparing diuretics*)
a) Examples
i) Spironolactone (Aldactone)
ii) Triamterene (Dyrenium)
iii) Amiloride (Midamor)
b) Actions
i) Act as an aldosterone antagonist
ii) Block sodium and potassium exchange mechanism in the distal tubule, causing loss of sodium and water and retention of potassium
c) Potential adverse effects
i) Hyponatremia
ii) Hyperkalemia
iii) Hypocalcemia
iv) Hypomagnesemia
v) Hypovolemia
vi) Hyperchloremic metabolic acidosis

5) Carbonic anhydrase inhibitors
a) Examples: acetazolamide (Diamox)
b) Actions
i) Block the action of carbonic anhydrase in the proximal tubule, preventing bicarbonate and sodium reabsorption
ii) Cause increased water loss and a decrease in serum pH; may be used to treat metabolic alkalosis
c) Potential adverse effects
i) Hyponatremia
ii) Hypokalemia
iii) Hypocalcemia
iv) Hypomagnesemia
v) Hypovolemia
vi) Hyperchloremic metabolic acidosis
vii) Thrombocytopenia, agranulocytosis, leukopenia, anemia

d. Selected diuretics (Table 8-4)

Dopaminergic Stimulators

1. Dopamine infused at low doses is thought to be specific to dopaminergic receptors.
   a. Results are often unpredictable, and it can cause several alpha- and beta-induced side effects (Abay, Reyes, Everts, & Wisser, 2007).
   b. Diuretic effect is thought to be caused primarily by the inotropic effect of $beta_1$ stimulation.
2. Fenoldopam mesylate (Corlopam)
   a. Actions
      1) Dilates arterial system, decreasing afterload
      2) Stimulates dopamine D1 receptors in the kidneys, causing diuresis
   b. Indications
      1) Hypertension

Table 8-4 Selected Diuretics

Drug	Administration	Adverse Effects	Nursing Implications

Furosemide (Lasix)	• PO: 20-80 mg daily
	• IV injection: 20-120 mg; administer at rate not to exceed 10 mg/min; if initial dose is ineffective, the next dose is usually double the original dose
	• IV infusion: mix 250 mg in 250 mL (1 mg/mL); usual dose is 0.1-0.75 mg/kg/hr; not to exceed 4 mg/min
	• Maximum: 1 g/day
	• Do not mix with acidic solutions
	Other loop diuretics
	• Torsemide (Demadex): 5-20 mg daily PO or IV (over 2 minutes); may be titrated to desired effect but single dose should not exceed 200 mg
	• Bumetanide (Bumex): 0.5-1.0 mg IV; may be repeated at 2- to 3-hour intervals
		• Hypotension
		• Hypovolemia
		• Nausea, vomiting, abdominal pain
		• Rash
		• Electrolyte imbalance: hypocalcemia, hypokalemia, hypomagnesemia, hyponatremia
		• Acid-base imbalance: hypochloremic alkalosis
		• Increased uric acid and BUN
		• Renal failure
		• Hyperglycemia
		• Photosensitivity
		• Thrombocytopenia, agranulocytosis, leukopenia, neutropenia, anemia
		• Transient deafness (with rapid IV injection)
			• Monitor HR, BP, urine output, serum electrolytes, BUN, creatinine, uric acid, CBC, daily weights
			  • Monitor patients also on digitalis for clinical indications of digitalis toxicity
			  • Monitor serum glucose in patients with diabetes mellitus
			  • Monitor for clinical indications of gout
			• Note contraindications: known hypersensitivity to sulfonamides, anuria, hypovolemia, electrolyte depletion
			• Sulfonamide-sensitive patients may have allergic reaction to these drugs (furosemide, bumetanide, torsemide) because they are all sulfa derivatives
			• Use cautiously in diabetes mellitus, dehydration, severe renal disease, gout, hepatic disease
			• Do not administer if solution is yellow or if precipitate is present
			• Teach patient about potassium-rich foods

Mannitol (Osmitrol)	• IV infusion: 1-2 g/kg over 30-60 minutes; average dose 50-100 grams • Use inline filter when administering mannitol	• Tachycardia • Nausea, vomiting • Fluid and electrolyte imbalance • Pulmonary edema • Thirst • Phlebitis • Seizures • Rebound cerebral edema 8-12 hours after diuresis	• Monitor BP, HR, urine output, serum osmolality, serum electrolytes, BUN, uric acid, daily weights • Note contraindications: known hypersensitivity, active intracranial bleeding, anuria, severe dehydration • Use cautiously in severe renal failure, HF, dehydration • Check bottle or ampule for crystallization: discard and replace • Monitor closely for rebound effect: return of clinical indications of intracranial hypertension 8-12 hours after mannitol

2) Renal protection when patient is receiving nephrotoxic dyes

c. Selected dopaminergic stimulator (Table 8-5)

Fluid and Electrolyte Imbalances

Hypovolemia

1. Etiology
   a. Insufficient intake
   b. Inadequate replacement following excess fluid loss
   c. Excessive fluid losses
      1) Hemorrhage
      2) GI losses
         a) Nasogastric or intestinal suction
         b) Vomiting
         c) Diarrhea
         d) Fistula
      3) Renal losses
         a) Diuretics
         b) Aldosterone insufficiency (i.e., Addison's disease)
         c) Diuretic phase of acute kidney injury
         d) Osmotic diuresis due to hyperglycemia
      4) Increased insensible losses
         a) Diaphoresis
         b) Tachypnea
      5) Draining wounds

Table 8-5 Selected Dopaminergic Stimulator

Drug	Administration	Adverse Effects	Nursing Implications
Fenoldopam mesylate (Corlopam)	• IV infusion: mix 10 mg in 250 mL (40 mcg/mL); usual dose is 0.03-0.3 mcg/kg/min • Maximum: 1.7 mcg/kg/min	• Tachycardia, hypotension • Ventricular dysrhythmias • Dizziness • Anxiety • Headache • Flushing • Nausea, vomiting, abdominal pain • Hypokalemia • Increased intraocular pressure • Increased intracranial pressure	• Monitor HR, BP, urine output, neurologic status • Note contraindications: known hypersensitivity to fenoldopam or sulfite, intracranial hypertension • Use caution in patients with glaucoma or ocular hypertension and in patients on other drugs which may cause hypotension (e.g., beta-blockers)

d. Intravascular to extravascular shift (also called third-spacing)
   1) Ascites
   2) Intestinal obstruction
   3) Peritonitis
   4) Burns
2. Clinical presentation
   a. Subjective
      1) Weakness
      2) Anorexia, nausea, vomiting, constipation
      3) Thirst
      4) Syncope
   b. Objective
      1) Tachycardia
      2) Orthostatic hypotension
      3) Low-grade fever
      4) Flushed skin (fluid loss) or cool, clammy skin (blood loss)
      5) Flat jugular veins even when patient in flat position
      6) Dry, sticky tongue and mucous membranes
      7) Poor skin turgor
      8) Lethargy, disorientation, coma
      9) Oliguria
      10) Weight loss greater than 5% of body weight
      11) Hemodynamic changes: decreased CVP, PAOP, CO; increased SVR
   c. Diagnostic
      1) Hematocrit and serum osmolality increased if fluid lost; hematocrit decreased if blood lost
      2) Urine specific gravity greater than 1.03 if ADH osmoreceptor mechanism is intact
      3) BUN increased with normal creatinine (i.e., prerenal)
3. Collaborative management
   a. Monitor urine output, I & O, daily weight, and laboratory studies.
   b. Treat the cause.
      1) Antiemetics for vomiting
      2) Antidiarrheals for diarrhea
      3) Control of hemorrhage: local pressure, prepare patient for surgery
      4) Antibiotics for infection
   c. Replace fluids carefully to prevent hypervolemia.
      1) Oral fluids for mild deficits
      2) Parenteral fluids for moderate or severe deficits; replace fluids lost with similar fluids (e.g., blood for hemorrhage, normal saline with electrolytes for excessive diuresis, etc.)
      3) Close monitoring for clinical indications of fluid overload (e.g., S_3, crackles)
   d. Provide frequent oral and skin care.

Water Loss Syndromes

Serum osmolality greater than 295 mOsm/kg (may be referred to as hyperosmolar [or hypovolemic] hypernatremia)

1. Etiology: water loss in excess of sodium loss
   a. Inadequate water intake
   b. Hypertonic fluids or enteral feedings
   c. Diabetes insipidus
   d. Diabetes mellitus
   e. Excess TPN
   f. Watery diarrhea
2. Clinical presentation
   a. Subjective
      1) Weakness
      2) Thirst
      3) Syncope
   b. Objective
      1) Tachycardia
      2) Hypotension
      3) Low-grade fever
      4) Flushed skin
      5) Dry, sticky tongue and mucous membranes
      6) Poor skin turgor
      7) Thirst
      8) Mental irritability, confusion
      9) Oliguria to anuria (except diabetes insipidus)
   c. Diagnostic
      1) Hematocrit and serum osmolality increased
      2) Serum sodium increased (concentration effect)
3. Collaborative management
   a. Monitor urine output, I & O, daily weight, and laboratory studies.

b. Treat the cause.
    1) Vasopressin for central diabetes insipidus; chlorpropamide (Diabinese) for nephrogenic diabetes insipidus
    2) Insulin for diabetes mellitus and hyperglycemia
    3) Antidiarrheals for diarrhea
    4) Antiemetics for nausea and vomiting
c. Provide appropriate volume replacement and normalize serum osmolality: administer water in excess of sodium (e.g., D_5W or ½NS).
d. Maintain adequate urine output with adequate volume replacement.
e. Provide frequent oral and skin care.

Hypervolemia

1. Etiology
    a. Excessive intake of fluid
        1) Excess oral or parenteral fluids
        2) Excess use of saline enemas
    b. Retention of sodium and water
        1) Steroid therapy
        2) Heart failure
        3) Liver disease (e.g., cirrhosis)
        4) Stress response via ADH secretion, renin-angiotensin-aldosterone system
        5) Nephrotic syndrome
        6) Acute or chronic renal failure
    c. Interstitial to intravascular shift
        1) Remobilization of fluids after treatment of burns
        2) Administration of hypertonic or hyperosmolar solutions (e.g., 3% saline, albumin)
2. Clinical presentation
    a. Subjective
        1) Dyspnea
        2) Headache
    b. Objective
        1) Tachycardia
        2) Increased blood pressure
        3) Jugular venous distention
        4) Tachypnea, dyspnea, crackles
        5) Peripheral edema
        6) Ascites
        7) Increased urine output
        8) Muscle weakness
        9) Confusion, apathy, lethargy, coma
        10) Hemodynamic changes: increased CVP and PAOP
        11) Weight gain greater than 5% of body weight
        12) Clinical indications of pulmonary or cerebral edema
    c. Diagnostic
        1) Hematocrit and serum osmolality decreased
        2) BUN decreased
        3) Urine specific gravity less than 1.01 if ADH osmoreceptor mechanism is intact
        4) Chest x-ray may show pulmonary vascular congestion
3. Collaborative management
    a. Monitor urine output, I & O, daily weight, and laboratory studies.
    b. Prevent hypervolemia by closely monitoring IV fluids; volumetric or controller pumps must be used for patients predisposed to hypervolemia.
    c. Decrease excess volume.
        1) Restriction of fluids and/or sodium
        2) Diuretics as prescribed
        3) Hemodialysis or continuous renal replacement therapy (CRRT) may be utilized, especially if renal insufficiency is present.
    d. Provide frequent oral and skin care.

Water Excess Syndromes

May be referred to as *hypo-osmolar* (or *hypervolemic*) *hyponatremia*

1. Etiology: water gain in excess of sodium gain
    a. Replacement of isotonic body fluids with hypotonic solution (e.g., D_5W)
    b. Excess use of tap water enemas
    c. Psychogenic polydipsia
    d. GI or GU irrigation with hypotonic fluids (e.g., tap water or distilled water)
    e. Excessive ice chips
    f. Syndrome of inappropriate antidiuretic hormone (SIADH)
    g. Administration of oral hypoglycemic agents and tricyclic antidepressants
2. Clinical presentation
    a. Subjective
        1) Anorexia, nausea, vomiting
        2) Abdominal and muscle cramps
        3) Headache
        4) Weakness
    b. Objective
        1) Edema
        2) Lethargy
        3) Muscle twitching, seizures
        4) Confusion
    c. Diagnostic
        1) Serum osmolality less than 280 mOsm/kg
        2) Serum sodium decreased (dilution effect)
        3) Hematocrit decreased
3. Collaborative management
    a. Monitor urine output, I & O, daily weight, and laboratory studies.
    b. Decrease water and normalize osmolality.
        1) Restrict fluids.
        2) Administer diuretics as prescribed.
        3) Administer hypertonic (3%) saline as prescribed for severe hyponatremia.
            a) Usually administered no more rapidly than 100 mL/hr and no more than 400 mL/24 hr
            b) Monitor closely for clinical indications of fluid overload because it pulls fluid into the vascular space.
        4) Initiate CRRT as prescribed.
        5) Administer demeclocycline or lithium as prescribed for nephrogenic SIADH.
    c. Provide frequent oral and skin care.

d. Monitor for clinical indications of cerebral or pulmonary edema; institute seizure precautions.

Hyponatremia

1. Etiology: both sodium and water decreased
   a. Decreased sodium intake
      1) Sodium-restricted diet
      2) Alcoholism
   b. Increased sodium excretion
      1) Skin losses
         a) Diaphoresis
         b) Burns
      2) GI losses
         a) GI suctioning
         b) Vomiting
         c) Diarrhea
         d) Draining wound or fistula
         e) Laxative abuse
      3) Renal losses
         a) Diuretics: thiazide, loop
         b) Adrenal insufficiency
         c) Cerebral salt-wasting syndrome
      4) Adrenal insufficiency (i.e., Addison's disease)
2. Clinical presentation
   a. Subjective
      1) Anorexia, nausea, vomiting, abdominal cramps
      2) Apprehension
      3) Headache
      4) Weakness, fatigue
   b. Objective
      1) Tachycardia
      2) Postural hypotension
      3) Diarrhea
      4) Weight loss
      5) Decreased skin turgor
      6) "Fingerprinting" over sternum
      7) Personality changes
      8) Mental confusion, disorientation
      9) Lethargy progressing to coma
      10) Muscle cramps, muscle twitching, increased deep tendon reflexes (DTRs)
      11) Tremors, seizures
      12) Oliguria
   c. Diagnostic
      1) Serum sodium less than 136 mEq/L with normal serum osmolality
3. Collaborative management
   a. Monitor urine output, I & O, daily weight, and laboratory studies.
   b. Restore normal serum electrolyte levels.
      1) Increased dietary sodium for mild deficiency
      2) Parenteral sodium for moderate or severe deficiency
         a) Normal saline as prescribed
         b) Hypertonic (3%) saline as prescribed for severe hyponatremia
            i) Usually administered no more rapidly than 1-2 mL/kg/hr and no more than 400 mL/24 hr
            ii) Monitor closely for clinical indications of fluid overload because it pulls fluid into the vascular space.
      3) Potassium replacement may also be needed.
   c. Monitor for neurologic changes; institute seizure precautions.
   d. Provide frequent oral and skin care.

Hypernatremia

1. Etiology: Both sodium and water are increased.
   a. Excess salt (sodium chloride) consumption
   b. Excess/rapid administration of normal saline or hypertonic saline solution
   c. Administration of sodium bicarbonate, sodium polystyrene sulfonate (Kayexalate)
   d. Heart failure
   e. Renal failure
   f. Cirrhosis
   g. Steroid therapy
   h. Cushing's syndrome
   i. Primary hyperaldosteronism
   j. Salt water near-drowning, ingestion of salt water
2. Clinical presentation
   a. Subjective
      1) Thirst
      2) Muscle weakness and/or cramps
   b. Objective
      1) Tachycardia
      2) Hypertension
      3) Low-grade fever
      4) Edema
      5) Dry, sticky tongue and mucous membranes
      6) Flushed, dry skin
      7) Muscle rigidity, twitching
      8) Increased deep tendon reflexes (DTRs)
      9) CNS irritability: restlessness, agitation
      10) Mental confusion, disorientation
      11) Tremors, seizures
      12) Oliguria
      13) Weight gain
   c. Diagnostic
      1) Serum sodium greater than 145 mEq/L with normal serum osmolality
3. Collaborative management
   a. Monitor urine output, I & O, daily weight, and laboratory studies.
   b. Treat the cause.
   c. Restore normal serum electrolyte levels.
      1) Sodium restriction
         a) Mild restriction: 3-4 g/day; commonly referred to as a *"no added salt" diet*
         b) Moderate restriction: 2 g/day; consumption of only foods specifically "low sodium"
         c) Severe restriction: 500 mg/day; only low-sodium foods with avoidance of shellfish and limitation of dairy and meat
      2) Diuretics as prescribed
   d. Provide frequent oral and skin care.

e. Monitor for change in neurologic status; institute seizure precautions.

Hypokalemia

1. Etiology
   a. Poor potassium intake
      1) Starvation
      2) Alcoholism
      3) Administration of potassium-deficient parenteral fluids or nutrition
      4) Use of low-potassium dialysate
   b. Increased GI losses
      1) GI surgery
      2) Gastric or intestinal suction
      3) Vomiting
      4) Fistula
      5) Diarrhea
      6) Chronic malabsorption syndrome
      7) Laxative abuse
      8) Intestinal bypass surgery
   c. Increased renal losses
      1) Polyuria
      2) Renal tubular acidosis
      3) Sodium restriction
      4) Hypomagnesemia
      5) Hyperaldosteronism
      6) Licorice excess: increases aldosterone effect
      7) Heart failure
      8) Steroid therapy or Cushing's syndrome
      9) Cirrhosis
      10) Stress via renin-angiotensin-aldosterone system and release of corticosteroids
      11) Burns (as fluid shifts back into intravascular space 48-72 hours after fluid resuscitation)
      12) Drugs
         a) Diuretics: thiazide; loop
         b) Certain antimicrobials: aminoglycosides, amphotericin B, carbenicillin, penicillin
         c) Corticosteroids
   d. Skin losses
      1) Diaphoresis
   e. Extracellular to intracellular shift
      1) Alkalosis
      2) Insulin
      3) Treatment of diabetic ketoacidosis
      4) Refeeding syndrome
2. Clinical presentation
   a. Subjective
      1) Anorexia, nausea, vomiting
      2) Malaise, fatigue
      3) Dizziness
      4) Muscle cramps
   b. Objective
      1) Orthostatic hypotension
      2) Decreased GI motility and bowel sounds, paralytic ileus, constipation, abdominal distention
      3) Muscle weakness, possibly flaccid paralysis
      4) Decreased DTR
      5) Irritability, mental confusion, drowsiness to coma
      6) Respiratory muscle weakness causing shallow ventilation, dyspnea progressing to respiratory paralysis and respiratory arrest
      7) Polyuria, polydipsia, inability to concentrate urine
      8) Enhanced digitalis effect
      9) Decreased cardiac output, dysrhythmias, and cardiac arrest may occur.
   c. Diagnostic
      1) Serum potassium less than 3.5 mEq/L
      2) ECG changes
         a) Flat T waves and prominent U waves
         b) Depressed ST segment
         c) Prolonged QT and PR intervals
         d) Dysrhythmias (e.g., PVCs, ventricular tachycardia, ventricular fibrillation, torsades de pointes)
3. Collaborative management
   a. Monitor urine output, I & O, daily weight, and laboratory studies.
   b. Treat the cause.
      1) Correct alkalosis.
      2) Correct hypomagnesemia and/or hypocalcemia; hypokalemia that is refractory to treatment is frequently accompanied by hypomagnesemia and/or hypocalcemia.
      3) Discontinue causative drug if possible.
   c. Restore normal serum electrolyte levels.
      1) Increase dietary potassium for mild hyperkalemia; encourage use of potassium chloride salt substitute.
      2) Administer potassium supplements orally.
      3) Administer potassium parenterally for severe hypokalemia.
         a) Safety
            i) Never administer potassium IV push.
            ii) Always use an infusion pump.
            iii) Do not add to a preexisting infusion; if potassium is to be added to maintenance fluids, a new solution should be mixed to avoid uneven distribution of the potassium.
         b) Potassium "runs" IV as prescribed usually via minibag (usual safe maximum 10 mEq/100 mL over 1 hour but may be administered at 20 mEq/hr if serum potassium is less than 2.5 mEq/L)
            i) Concentration no greater than 10 mEq/100 mL if given via peripheral catheter or 20 mEq/100 mL if given via a central venous catheter
            ii) Administration in normal saline unless contraindicated; dextrose may stimulate insulin secretion and intracellular shift of potassium
            iii) NOTE: It takes 100-200 mEq of potassium to increase serum potassium by 1 mEq/L.

iv) Close monitoring of ECG when administering high concentrations of potassium
d. Monitor for clinical indications of digitalis toxicity if patient receiving digitalis preparation.
e. Teach patient about adequate potassium replacement if receiving diuretics; potassium-sparing diuretics may be used.

Hyperkalemia

1. Etiology
   a. Increased potassium intake
      1) Excessive administration/ingestion of potassium: oral or parenteral
      2) Excessive or too rapid potassium replacement
      3) Excessive use of KCl salt substitute
      4) Transfusion of banked blood; the longer the blood has been stored, the higher the extracellular potassium content
      5) Cardioplegic solution
      6) Drugs that contain potassium, such as potassium penicillin and potassium phosphate enemas
   b. Decreased potassium excretion
      1) Acute and chronic renal disease
      2) Adrenal insufficiency (i.e., Addison's disease)
      3) Drugs
         a) Potassium-sparing diuretics
         b) Angiotensin-converting enzyme (ACE) inhibitors or angiotensin receptor blockers
         c) Nonsteroidal antiinflammatory drugs
         d) Cyclosporine
   c. Cellular disruption with leak of intracellular potassium
      1) Crush injuries
      2) Rhabdomyolysis
      3) Hemolysis (e.g., blood transfusion reaction, fresh water near-drowning)
      4) Early burns
      5) Trauma
      6) Catabolism
      7) Lysis of tumor cells from chemotherapy
   d. Intracellular to extracellular shift
      1) Acidosis
      2) Insulin deficiency
      3) Malignant hyperthermia
      4) Drugs
         a) Massive digitalis overdosage
         b) Muscle paralyzing agents (e.g., succinylcholine)
   e. Pseudohyperkalemia
      1) Hemolyzed blood sample
      2) Sample drawn above an IV infusion containing potassium
      3) Traumatic venipuncture
      4) Delay in analysis of sample
2. Clinical presentation
   a. Subjective
      1) Nausea, vomiting, abdominal cramping, diarrhea
      2) Numbness, paresthesia of extremities
      3) Weakness, fatigue
   b. Objective
      1) Initially tachycardia progressing to bradycardia and cardiac arrest
      2) Decreased contractility, decreased cardiac output, hypotension
      3) Abdominal distention
      4) Hyperactive bowel sounds
      5) Muscle weakness progressing to flaccid paralysis
      6) Increased DTRs initially progressing to decreased to absent DTRs
      7) Respiratory muscle weakness may cause hypopnea, respiratory distress
      8) Lethargy, apathy, mental confusion
      9) Oliguria
   c. Diagnostic
      1) Serum potassium greater than 5 mEq/L
         a) Mild: 5-6 mEq/L
         b) Moderate: 6-7 mEq/L
         c) Severe: greater than 7 mEq/L
      2) ECG changes
         a) 5.5-6 mEq/L: tall, narrow, peaked T waves, shortened QT interval
         b) 6-7 mEq/L: wide QRS complexes, prolonged PR intervals
         c) 7-7.5: flattened to absent P waves, further widening of QRS complexes
         d) 8 or greater: fusion of QRS complexes and T waves, idioventricular rhythm, asystole
3. Collaborative management
   a. Monitor urine output, I & O, daily weight, and laboratory studies.
      1) Check BUN and creatinine levels for data about renal function.
   b. Treat the cause.
      1) Dialysis for renal failure
      2) Treatment of acidosis
      3) Insulin therapy for hyperglycemia
      4) Discontinuance of any causative drug if possible
         a) Potassium-sparing diuretics
         b) ACE inhibitors or angiotensin receptor blockers (ARBs)
         c) Nonsteroidal antiinflammatory drugs
   c. Restore normal serum electrolyte levels
      1) Potassium restriction
         a) Ensure that IV solution or TPN contain no potassium.
         b) Check medications for potassium content.
      2) Diuretics as prescribed: usually 40-80 mg furosemide (Lasix)
      3) Emergency treatment if potassium is greater than 6.5 mEq/L or dysrhythmias are present; however, patients with chronic renal failure may tolerate high levels of

potassium and not be symptomatic until 7 mEq/L or greater
   a) Dextrose and insulin as prescribed; this moves potassium back into the cell and the effect lasts about 4-6 hours; sodium polystyrene sulfonate (Kayexalate) should be given during this time
      i) Usual dosage is 50 mL of 50% dextrose and 10 units of insulin.
      ii) Monitor for increased or decreased serum glucose.
   b) Sodium polystyrene sulfonate (Kayexalate), an exchange resin, as prescribed; exchanges sodium for potassium and moves potassium out of the body via the GI tract
      i) Oral or by retention enema
         (a) Usual dose is 15-50 grams in 50-100 mL of 20% sorbitol orally
         (b) 50 grams in 200 mL of dextrose as retention enema
      ii) Sorbitol, an osmotic laxative, produces a cathartic effect only when given orally, and may contribute to intestinal necrosis when given by enema
   c) Nebulized albuterol as prescribed
      i) Usual dose is 10-20 mg nebulized over 15 minutes
      ii) Adverse effect: tachycardia
   d) Bicarbonate as prescribed to correct acidosis
      i) Usual dose 50 mEq IV over 5 minutes
      ii) This effect lasts 1-2 hours.
      iii) Adverse effects: hypernatremia, hyperosmolality
   e) Continuous renal replacement therapy (e.g., continuous venous-venous hemodialysis) if prescribed
d. Monitor for/prevent cardiac effects of hyperkalemia.
   1) Intravenous calcium as prescribed
      a) Usual dose 5-10 mL of 10% calcium chloride over 2-5 minutes
      b) Blocks the neuromuscular and cardiac effects
      c) Contraindicated if patient is receiving digitalis

Hypocalcemia

1. Etiology
   a. Decreased calcium intake or absorption
      1) Chronic insufficient dietary calcium intake
      2) Hypoparathyroidism
         a) Injury to parathyroid gland(s) during thyroidectomy
      3) Hypomagnesemia
      4) Acute and chronic renal failure
      5) Vitamin D deficiency or resistance
      6) Liver disease
      7) Postgastrectomy
      8) Chronic malabsorption syndrome
      9) Alcoholism
      10) Cushing's syndrome
      11) Steroid therapy
   b. Increased calcium excretion
      1) Diuretic therapy: loop, osmotic, potassium-sparing, carbonic anhydrase inhibitors
      2) Chronic diarrhea
      3) Hyperphosphatemia
      4) Diuretic phase of acute kidney injury
   c. Increased calcium binding, decreased ionized calcium
      1) Citrated blood administration
      2) Alkalosis
      3) Acute pancreatitis
      4) Drugs (e.g., aminoglycosides, cimetidine, heparin, theophylline)
2. Clinical presentation
   a. Subjective
      1) Abdominal cramps, biliary colic
      2) Muscle cramps
      3) Paresthesia of fingertips, circumoral area
   b. Objective
      1) Chvostek's sign: facial twitching in response to tapping on the facial nerve
      2) Trousseau's sign: carpal spasm after 3 minutes of inflation of a blood pressure cuff to a level above systolic pressure
      3) Muscle tremors
      4) Increased deep tendon reflexes (DTRs), carpopedal spasm
      5) Irritability, confusion, psychosis
      6) Memory loss
      7) Laryngospasm, stridor
      8) Tetany (characterized by cramps, twitching of the muscles, sharp flexion of the wrist and ankle joints, seizures)
      9) Seizures
      10) Decreased contractility, cardiac output
      11) Oliguria, anuria if renal calculi obstructive
      12) Bruising, bleeding
   c. Diagnostic
      1) Serum calcium less than 8.5 mg/dL (less than 4.5 mEq/L)
         a) If albumin is decreased, corrected total calcium can be calculated: measured total calcium + 0.8 × (4.0 − albumin)
         b) Hypocalcemia is present if serum ionized calcium is less than 4.1 mg/dL
      2) ECG changes
         a) Prolonged QT interval
         b) Dysrhythmias (e.g., torsades de pointes)
      3) Serum phosphate decreased
3. Collaborative management
   a. Monitor airway patency and ventilation; cricothyroidotomy may be necessary for severe laryngospasm.
   b. Monitor urine output, I & O, daily weight, and laboratory studies.

c. Treat the cause.
  1) Phosphate-binding antacids as prescribed for hyperphosphatemia
  2) Calcium administration, phosphate restriction, and phosphate-binding agents for renal failure
d. Restore normal serum electrolyte levels.
  1) High-calcium, low-phosphorus diet
  2) Oral calcium with vitamin D supplements as prescribed for mild hypocalcemia
  3) Calcium gluconate or calcium chloride IV as prescribed
    a) 10 mL of calcium gluconate contains 4.5 mEq of calcium; 10 mL of calcium chloride contains 13.6 mEq of calcium.
      i) Calcium chloride produces higher ionized calcium; however, calcium gluconate is frequently preferred because it is less irritating to tissues.
    b) Administration through central venous catheter if possible; if administered through a peripheral catheter, prevent extravasation which may cause necrosis and sloughing
    c) Slow administration: Dilute in 100 mL of D_5W and administer over 10-30 minutes.
    d) Close monitoring of BP and cardiac rhythm during calcium administration
  4) Magnesium as prescribed (hypocalcemia unresponsive to treatment may indicate concurrent hypomagnesemia)
e. Monitor for/prevent neurologic complications; institute seizure precautions.

Hypercalcemia

1. Etiology
  a. Increased calcium intake
    1) Excessive intake of calcium supplements or calcium antacids
    2) Milk-alkali syndrome related to milk and antacid intake
  b. Increased calcium absorption: hypophosphatemia
  c. Increased mobilization of calcium from bone
    1) Hyperparathyroidism
    2) Vitamin D excess
    3) Immobility
    4) Osteolytic lesions
    5) Malignancy especially breast, lung, lymphoma, multiple myeloma
    6) Paget's disease
    7) Leukemia
    8) Granulomatous disease (e.g., sarcoidosis, TB, histoplasmosis)
    9) Thyrotoxicosis
  d. Decreased calcium excretion
    1) Thiazide diuretics
    2) Adrenal insufficiency (i.e., Addison's disease)
    3) Renal tubular acidosis
    4) Hyperparathyroidism
    5) Oliguric phase of acute kidney injury
  e. Increased ionized calcium: acidosis
2. Clinical presentation
  a. Subjective
    1) Thirst
    2) Anorexia, nausea, vomiting, abdominal pain
    3) Malaise, fatigue, weakness
    4) Bone and/or flank pain; pathologic fractures may occur
    5) Depression
  b. Objective
    1) Decreased bowel sounds, constipation, paralytic ileus
    2) Neuromuscular weakness to flaccidity; decreased deep tendon reflexes (DTRs)
    3) Agitation, confusion, lethargy, stupor, coma
    4) Subtle personality changes progressing to psychosis
    5) Renal calculi
    6) Polyuria, polydipsia
    7) Azotemia
    8) Enhanced digitalis effect
  c. Diagnostic
    1) Serum calcium greater than 10.5 mg/dL (greater than 5.8 mEq/L)
    2) Serum phosphate decreased
    3) ECG changes: shortened QT interval, dysrhythmias and/or blocks
    4) X-ray: osteoporosis
3. Collaborative management
  a. Monitor urine output, I & O, daily weight, and laboratory studies.
  b. Treat the cause.
    1) Discontinuance of causative drugs
    2) Surgery, radiation, antineoplastics for malignancy
    3) Partial parathyroidectomy for hyperparathyroidism
  c. Restore normal serum electrolyte levels.
    1) Decrease calcium absorption.
      a) Low-calcium, high-phosphorus diet
      b) Corticosteroids
    2) Increase calcium excretion.
      a) Oral or parenteral fluids as prescribed; usually isotonic saline at 100-200 mL/hr
      b) Any of the following as prescribed:
        i) Loop diuretics (e.g., furosemide [Lasix])
        ii) Calcitonin
        iii) Phosphorus
        iv) EDTA (disodium salt)
      c) Dialysis may be utilized.
    3) Decrease bone resorption of calcium.
      a) Weight-bearing activities
      b) Any of the following as prescribed:
        i) Etidronate (Didronel)
        ii) Pamidronate (Aredia)
        iii) Gallium nitrate
        iv) Corticosteroids

v) Plicamycin (formerly known as *mithramycin*) (Mithracin)
vi) Inorganic phosphate

d. Monitor for/prevent cardiac effects of hypercalcemia: calcium channel blockers as prescribed.
e. Prevent renal calculi while correcting hypercalcemia: Agents for acidification of urine may be used because acidification of urine increases solubility of calcium.
f. Monitor for clinical indications of digitalis toxicity.

Hypophosphatemia

1. Etiology
   a. Inadequate intake of phosphorus
      1) Malnutrition
      2) Alcoholism
      3) Severe, prolonged vomiting
      4) Prolonged low-phosphorus or phosphate-free IV therapy or total parenteral nutrition therapy
   b. Decreased GI absorption or increased intestinal loss
      1) Excessive use of phosphate-binding gels such as aluminum hydroxide (Amphojel)
      2) Prolonged vomiting, gastric suction, sucralfate (Carafate)
      3) Chronic diarrhea
      4) Chronic malabsorption syndrome
      5) Vitamin D deficiency
   c. Increased renal excretion of phosphorus
      1) Thiazide diuretics
      2) Hypomagnesemia
      3) Hypokalemia
      4) Hyperglycemia
      5) Hyperparathyroidism
      6) Fanconi's syndrome
   d. Extracellular to intracellular shifts
      1) Parenteral glucose or insulin administration
      2) Alkalosis
      3) Large amounts of carbohydrate (refeeding syndrome)
      4) Treatment of diabetic ketoacidosis
      5) Beta-adrenergic drugs (e.g., albuterol [Proventil])
2. Clinical presentation
   a. Subjective
      1) Anorexia, nausea, vomiting
      2) Malaise, fatigue
      3) Paresthesia
      4) Bone pain
      5) Chest pain
   b. Objective
      1) Tachycardia, hypotension
      2) Tremors
      3) Muscle weakness
      4) Nystagmus, anisocoria
      5) Incoordination, ataxia
      6) Confusion, lethargy, coma
      7) Seizures
      8) Memory loss
      9) Respiratory muscle weakness and decreased respiratory excursion
      10) Heart failure: dyspnea, crackles
      11) Weight loss
      12) Hemolytic anemia
      13) Platelet dysfunction: petechiae, bleeding
      14) Immunosuppression
   c. Diagnostic
      1) Serum phosphate less than 3 mg/dL
      2) Increased serum and urine calcium
      3) ECG: dysrhythmias
      4) X-ray: skeletal abnormalities
3. Collaborative management
   a. Monitor urine output, I & O, daily weight, and laboratory studies.
   b. Treat the cause.
      1) Discontinuance of phosphate-binding gels
      2) Correction of hypercalcemia if cause of hypophosphatemia
   c. Restore normal serum electrolyte levels.
      1) High-phosphorus, low-calcium diet
      2) Oral phosphate supplements (e.g., Neutra-Phos [sodium and potassium phosphate], Phospho-Soda [sodium phosphate], K-Phos [potassium phosphate]) as ordered and monitor for signs of hypocalcemia when giving supplements
      3) Parenteral sodium phosphate or potassium phosphate IV as ordered and monitor for signs of hypocalcemia
         a) Usual dose
            i) If phosphate less than 1 mg/dL without adverse effects: usual dose is 0.6 mg/kg/hr.
            ii) If phosphate less than 2 mg/dL with adverse effects: usual dose is 0.9 mg/kg/hr.
         b) Utilization of central venous catheter if possible
         c) Intravenous phosphate is contraindicated in hypercalcemia.
   d. Monitor for cardiovascular, pulmonary, and neurologic effects of hypophosphatemia.

Hyperphosphatemia

1. Etiology
   a. Increased phosphorus intake
      1) Cathartic abuse with phosphate-containing laxatives and enemas
      2) Excessive vitamin D
      3) Transfusion of stored blood
      4) Acute elemental phosphorus poisoning
   b. Decreased phosphorus excretion
      1) Acute or chronic renal failure
      2) Hypoparathyroidism
   c. Intracellular to extracellular shifts
      1) Acidosis
      2) Malignant hyperthermia
      3) Severe hypothermia
   d. Cellular destruction

1) Neoplastic disease treated with chemotherapy
2) Catabolism
3) Rhabdomyolysis
2. Clinical presentation
a. As for hypocalcemia
b. Diagnostic: serum phosphate greater than 4.5 mg/dL
3. Collaborative management
a. Monitor airway patency; cricothyroidotomy may be necessary for severe laryngospasm.
b. Monitor urine output, I & O, daily weight, and laboratory studies.
c. Treat the cause.
1) Correction of hypocalcemia
2) Dialysis if renal failure is cause
3) Saline diuresis and urinary alkalization if tumor lysis syndrome or rhabdomyolysis
d. Restore normal serum electrolyte levels.
1) Low-phosphorus, high-calcium diet
2) Sucralfate (Carafate) or aluminum antacids to bind with phosphate in the GI tract as prescribed
3) Glucose and insulin as prescribed to shift phosphate into the cell (transient effect only)
e. Monitor for/prevent neurologic complications; institute seizure precautions.

Hypomagnesemia

1. Etiology
a. Decreased magnesium intake or absorption
1) Protein-calorie malnutrition
2) Starvation
3) Alcoholism
4) Prolonged low-magnesium or magnesium-free IV therapy or total parenteral nutrition therapy
b. Impaired absorption
1) Alcoholism
2) Intestinal malabsorption syndrome
3) Acute pancreatitis
c. Increased magnesium loss
1) Drugs
a) Diuretics
b) Antimicrobials: aminoglycosides, pentamidine, amphotericin B
c) Ethanol
d) Cisplatin
e) Cyclosporin A
2) Diuretic phase of acute kidney injury
3) Vomiting, gastric suction, fistula
4) Chronic diarrhea (e.g., ulcerative colitis; laxative abuse)
5) Hypoparathyroidism
6) Hyperaldosteronism
7) Steroids
8) Diabetic ketoacidosis
9) Heart failure
d. Increased magnesium binding: citrated blood administration
e. Extracellular to intracellular shift
1) Refeeding syndrome
2) Amino acid solutions
3) Insulin; treatment of DKA
4) Acute myocardial infarction
2. Clinical presentation
a. Subjective
1) Anorexia, nausea, vomiting, abdominal distention
2) Paresthesia of fingertips, circumoral area
3) Muscle cramps
4) Syncope
b. Objective
1) Tachycardia, hypotension
2) Chvostek's and Trousseau's signs
3) Tremors, increased DTRs, carpopedal spasm
4) Ataxia, nystagmus
5) Laryngospasm, stridor
6) Tetany
7) Seizures
8) Insomnia
9) Confusion, psychosis
10) Memory loss
11) Decreased contractility, cardiac output
12) Increased digitalis effect
c. Diagnostic
1) Serum magnesium less than 1.5 mEq/L
a) May have concurrent hypocalcemia, hypokalemia, and hypophosphatemia
2) ECG changes
a) Prolonged QT interval
b) Dysrhythmias especially torsades de pointes
3. Collaborative management
a. Monitor airway patency; cricothyroidotomy may be necessary for severe laryngospasm.
b. Monitor urine output, I & O, daily weight, and laboratory studies.
c. Treat the cause.
1) Nutritional support for malnutrition
2) Use of potassium-sparing diuretics if diuretics are needed since they spare magnesium
d. Restore normal serum electrolyte levels.
1) High magnesium diet
2) Oral magnesium supplements in the form of magnesium antacids as prescribed
3) Magnesium sulfate IV as prescribed
a) Usually administered slowly so that magnesium will be absorbed
i) 1-2 grams diluted in 100 mL and administered over 1 hour unless critical level, then 4-gram dose should be given over 2 hours
ii) 1-2 grams may be diluted in 10 mL and administered over 5-20 minutes for when life-threatening dysrhythmias (e.g., torsades de pointes) occur

        4) Calcium replacement as prescribed; most patients with hypomagnesemia are also hypocalcemic
    e. Monitor for/prevent neurologic complications; institute seizure precautions.
    f. Monitor for clinical indications of digitalis toxicity for patients on digitalis preparations.

Hypermagnesemia

1. Etiology
    a. Increased magnesium intake
        1) Magnesium antacids
        2) Magnesium sulfate IV
        3) Magnesium-containing antacids, laxatives, enemas
    b. Decreased magnesium excretion
        1) Acute/chronic renal failure
        2) Hyperparathyroidism
        3) Hypoaldosteronism
        4) Hypothyroidism
    c. Intracellular to extracellular shift
        1) Untreated ketoacidosis
        2) Burns
        3) Rhabdomyolysis
    d. Pseudohypermagnesemia: sample hemolysis
2. Clinical presentation
    a. Subjective
        1) Weakness, fatigue
        2) Nausea, vomiting
        3) Somnolence
        4) Diplopia
    b. Objective
        1) Bradycardia, hypotension
        2) Facial flushing
        3) Muscle weakness progressing to paralysis
        4) Decreased DTRs: Loss of patellar reflex occurs at levels greater than 8 mEq/L.
        5) Respiratory muscle weakness may cause hypoventilation and dyspnea.
        6) Respiratory muscle paralysis and apnea may occur with levels greater than 10 mEq/L.
        7) Confusion, somnolence, lethargy, coma
        8) Cardiopulmonary arrest
    c. Diagnostic
        1) Serum magnesium greater than 2.5 mEq/L
        2) ECG: prolonged PR, QRS, QT; bradycardias and blocks
3. Collaborative management
    a. Monitor and maintain airway and ventilation; intubation and mechanical ventilation may be necessary.
    b. Monitor urine output, I & O, daily weight, and laboratory studies.
    c. Treat the cause.
        1) Discontinuance of magnesium-containing antacids or laxatives, IV magnesium
    d. Restore normal serum electrolyte levels.
        1) Low-magnesium diet
        2) Diuresis
            a) NS or ½NS and furosemide (1 mg/kg) as prescribed if normal renal function
            b) Monitor for hypocalcemia, hypokalemia
        3) Dialysis if renal failure is cause of hypermagnesemia
        4) Dextrose and insulin may promote movement of magnesium into the cells (transient effect only).
    e. Monitor for/prevent neuromuscular, pulmonary, and cardiovascular complications.
        1) Intravenous calcium as prescribed
            a) Usual dose 5-10 mL of 10% calcium chloride over 2-5 minutes
            b) Blocks the neuromuscular and cardiac effects
            c) Contraindicated if patient is receiving digitalis

Acute Kidney Injury (AKI)

Formerly referred to as *acute renal failure*

Definition

Sudden decline in kidney function that causes fluid, electrolyte, and acid-base imbalance caused by decreased GFR and impaired clearance of small solutes

Etiology

1. Prerenal: disrupted blood flow to the kidney
    a. Decreased intravascular volume
        1) Hemorrhage
        2) GI losses: vomiting, diarrhea
        3) Renal losses: osmotic diuresis, diuretics, diabetes insipidus
        4) Skin losses: perspiration, burns, necrotizing fasciitis
        5) Volume shifts: peritonitis, ileus, pancreatitis
    b. Decreased cardiac output
        1) Myocardial infarction
        2) Heart failure
        3) Cardiomyopathy
        4) Cardiac tamponade
        5) Dysrhythmias
        6) Pulmonary embolism
    c. Vasodilation
        1) Sepsis
        2) Anaphylaxis
        3) Vasodilators
    d. Renovascular changes
        1) Renal artery atherosclerosis or thrombosis
        2) Sepsis
        3) Hepatorenal syndrome
        4) Abdominal aortic aneurysm
        5) Vasopressors
2. Intrinsic: damage to the renal tissue
    a. Cortical
        1) Glomerulonephritis
            a) Acute poststreptococcal
            b) Systemic lupus erythematosus
            c) Goodpasture's syndrome
            d) Bacterial endocarditis
        2) Vasculitis
            a) Periarteritis

            - b) Hypersensitivity angioedema
            - c) Pregnancy
        - 3) Interstitial nephritis
            - a) Acute pyelonephritis
            - b) Allergic nephritis
            - c) Severe hypercalcemia
            - d) Uric acid nephropathy
            - e) Myeloma of the kidney
            - f) Malignant hypertension
    - b. Medullary (i.e., acute tubular necrosis)
        - 1) Nephrotoxic agents
            - a) Antimicrobials
                - i) Aminoglycosides
                - ii) Cephalosporins
                - iii) Tetracyclines
                - iv) Penicillins
            - b) Antifungal: amphotericin B
            - c) Antineoplastics (e.g., cisplatin, methotrexate)
            - d) Nonsteroidal antiinflammatory drugs
            - e) Contrast dyes
            - f) Heavy metals (e.g., lead, arsenic, mercury, uranium)
            - g) Pesticides, fungicides
            - h) Chemicals (e.g., ethylene glycol, carbon tetrachloride)
            - i) Multiple myeloma
            - j) Heavy pigments
                - i) Rhabdomyolysis leading to myoglobinuria
                - ii) Hemolysis leading to hemoglobinuria
        - 2) Prolonged ischemic injury
            - a) MAP less than 60 mm Hg for 40 minutes or more
            - b) Aortic cross-clamping
            - c) Bilateral emboli to both kidneys, causing renal infarction
            - d) Vasoconstriction
            - e) Vasopressors (e.g., norepinephrine [Levophed], high-dose dopamine)
        - 3) Any of the causes of prerenal failure that are prolonged
- 3. Postrenal: disrupted urine flow
    - a. Mechanical
        - 1) Ureteral obstruction (e.g., strictures, calculi, neoplasm)
        - 2) Urethral obstruction (e.g., prostatic hypertrophy)
        - 3) Edema
    - b. Functional
        - 1) Neurogenic bladder (e.g., diabetic neuropathy, spinal cord injury)
        - 2) Ganglionic blocking agents

Pathophysiology

See Figure 8-7.

Clinical Presentation

1. Subjective
    - a. Flank pain may be present.
    - b. Uremic syndrome
        - 1) Irritability
        - 2) Insomnia
        - 3) Inability to concentrate
        - 4) Anorexia, nausea, vomiting
        - 5) Metallic taste
        - 6) Fatigue, weakness
        - 7) Anxiety
    - c. Dyspnea if pulmonary edema is present
    - d. Headache
    - e. Pruritus
    - f. Decreased libido
    - g. Weight loss or weight gain
2. Objective
    - a. Genitourinary
        - 1) Decrease in urine volume
            - a) Nonoliguria: dilute urine output greater than 400 mL/24 hr
            - b) Oliguria: urine output less than 400 mL/24 hr
            - c) Anuria: urine output less than 100 mL/24 hr
                - i) Rare but may be seen in complete obstruction (postrenal)
        - 2) Altered excretion of drugs; toxic drug levels
        - 3) Bladder distention may be noted with postrenal failure.
    - b. Neurologic
        - 1) Change in behavior
        - 2) Confusion
        - 3) Change in level of consciousness
        - 4) Focal neurologic deficits
        - 5) Tremors, twitching, increased DTR
        - 6) Asterixis
        - 7) Seizures
    - c. Gastrointestinal
        - 1) Bleeding gums
        - 2) Uremic breath
        - 3) Abdominal distention
        - 4) Malnutrition
        - 5) GI bleeding, melena
        - 6) Constipation or diarrhea
        - 7) May have paralytic ileus
    - d. Respiratory
        - 1) Deep, rapid breathing (i.e., Kussmaul's respirations)
        - 2) Pulmonary edema
            - a) Bilateral crackles
        - 3) Hemoptysis may be seen along with acute kidney injury in Goodpasture's syndrome
    - e. Cardiovascular
        - 1) Tachycardia
        - 2) Dysrhythmias
        - 3) Uremic pericarditis
            - a) Pericardial friction rub
        - 4) Hypertension
        - 5) Vascular access
            - a) Bruit
            - b) Thrill
            - c) Neurovascular assessment of limb
    - f. Musculoskeletal
        - 1) Impaired mobility

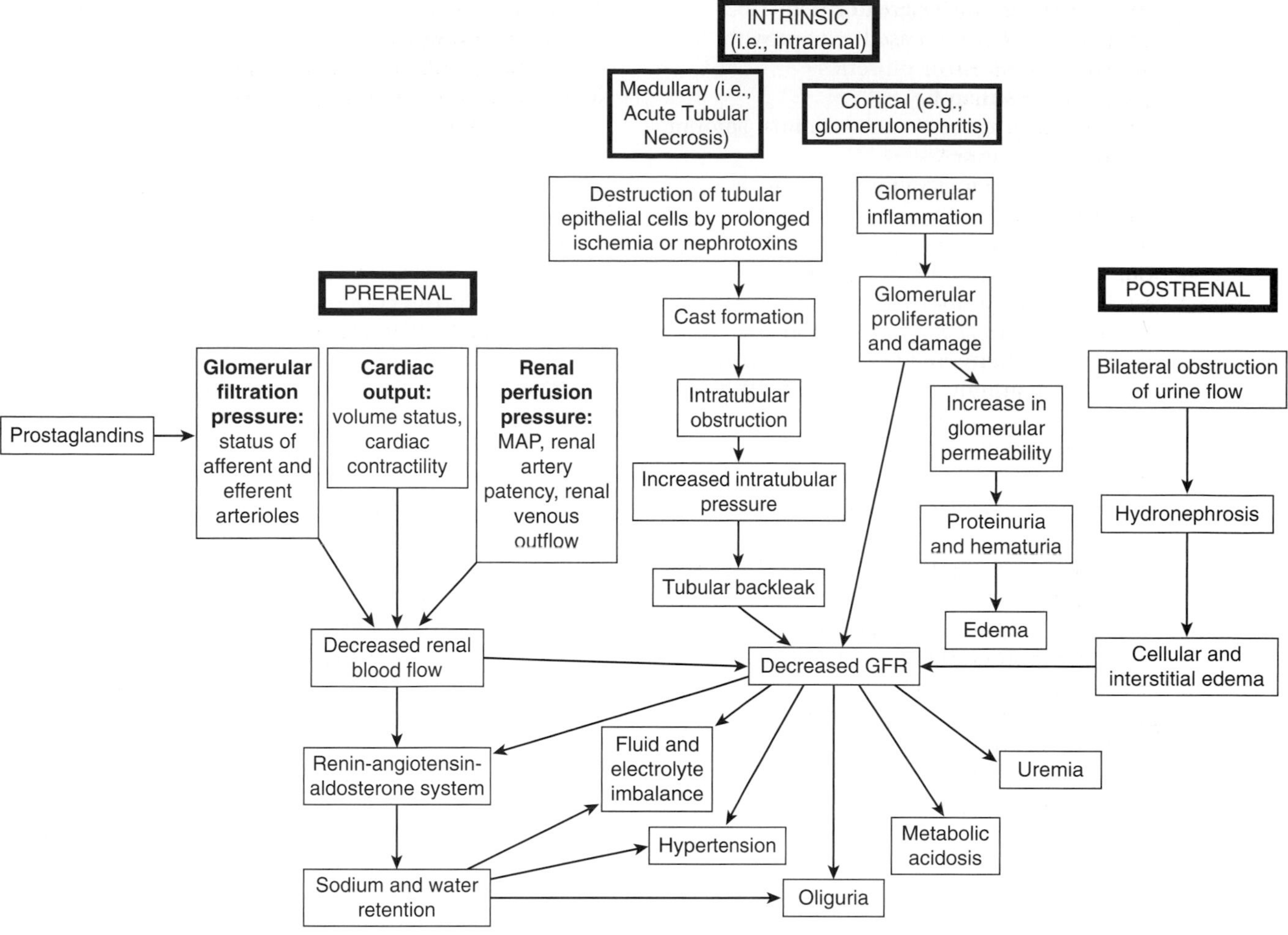

Figure 8-7 Pathophysiology of acute kidney injury.

2) Muscle weakness
g. Integument
1) Dry skin
2) Pruritus
3) Edema
4) Bruising
5) Pallor
6) Uremic frost (end-stage)
h. Hematologic/immunologic
1) Increased susceptibility to infection, sepsis
2) Petechiae, bruising, bleeding
3. Diagnostic
a. Blood
1) Elevated BUN, creatinine
2) Hyperkalemia
3) Hyperphosphatemia
4) Hypocalcemia
5) Hypermagnesemia
6) Sodium level is dependent on water balance.
a) Normal or dilutional hyponatremia
7) Hyperuricemia
8) Arterial blood gases: metabolic acidosis with increased anion gap
9) Hematology
a) Hematocrit, hemoglobin usually decreased; may be increased in prerenal failure due to dehydration
b) Platelets: decreased
10) Clotting profile: Bleeding time may be increased.
b. Urine
1) Varies; dependent on type of acute kidney injury
2) Decreased creatinine clearance
c. Radiologic
1) KUB, renal ultrasonography, or computed tomography may indicate cause of postrenal failure.
2) Chest x-ray may show:
a) Pericardial effusion
b) Pleural effusion
c) Pulmonary edema
d. Renal biopsy: most definitive diagnostic test especially for glomerulonephritis
4. Diagnostics by type of acute kidney injury
a. Prerenal
1) Oliguria
2) Urinary sodium less than 20 mEq/L
3) Increased BUN with BUN:creatinine ratio greater than 10:1 (usually 20:1)

4) Urine specific gravity greater than 1.02
5) Urine osmolality increased except with metabolic acidosis or diuretics
6) Urine pH less than 6
7) No protein in urine or only minimal amount of protein in urine
8) Sediment in urine: hyaline casts, finely granular casts

b. Intrinsic
1) Cortical
a) Urine output may be normal (nonoliguria), oliguria, or polyuria.
b) Urine sodium greater than 20 mEq/L
c) BUN:creatinine increased with 10:1 ratio
d) Urine specific gravity varies
e) Urine pH greater than 6
f) Moderate to heavy proteinuria
g) Sediment in urine: RBCs, WBCs, casts
2) Medullary
a) Urine output may be normal (nonoliguria), oliguria, or polyuria.
b) Urine sodium greater than 20 mEq/L
c) Urine specific gravity 1.010
d) BUN:creatinine increased with 10:1 ratio
e) Urine specific gravity 1.01-1.015
f) Urine pH greater than 6
g) Minimal to moderate proteinuria
h) Sediment in urine: tubular epithelial cells, tubular casts, rare RBCs

c. Postrenal
1) Oliguria with partial obstruction; anuria with complete obstruction
2) Urine sodium 20-40 mEq/L
3) BUN:creatinine increased with 10:1 ratio
4) Urine specific gravity 1.01-1.015
5) Urine pH greater than 6
6) Sediment in urine: RBCs, WBCs, calculi, uric acid crystals, hyaline casts
7) KUB, IVP may show obstruction and/or ureteral dilatation
8) May have positive culture for bacteria

5. RIFLE classification system (Table 8-6): correlates with outcomes
6. Stages of acute renal injury (Table 8-7)

NOTE: Some patients (especially when acute renal injury is related to nephrotoxins) go through only three phases: onset, nonoliguric, recovery.

Collaborative Management

1. Prevent/treat the cause.
a. Administer acetylcysteine (Mucomyst) and/or fenoldopam (Corlopam) as prescribed along with adequate hydration to prevent dye-related acute tubular necrosis.
b. Administer fluids, diuretics (usually mannitol), and sodium bicarbonate as prescribed for rhabdomyolysis with myoglobinuria.
c. Monitor serum creatinine when using nephrotoxic agents (e.g., aminoglycosides, amphotericin B, vancomycin).
d. Prevent/treat abdominal hypertension and abdominal compartment syndrome.
e. Support renal perfusion and improve glomerular filtration rate through appropriate treatment.
1) Volume to improve preload in patients with hypovolemia as evidenced by decreased RAP, PAOP
2) Inotropes to improve contractility in patients with decreased contractility as evidenced by decreased RVSWI, LVSWI
3) Vasopressors to increase afterload in patients with massive vasodilation as evidenced by decreased SVR
4) Low-dose dopamine has shown no evidence of benefit when used in patients with acute oliguric renal failure and can predispose the patient to bowel ischemia through splanchnic vasoconstriction and is no longer recommended for the management of acute oliguric renal failure.
5) Fenoldopam (Corlopam), a dopaminergic stimulator, may be prescribed to increase renal blood flow.
6) Diuretic trial as prescribed if patient is not anuric

Table 8-6 Rifle Classification System for Degrees of Acute Kidney Injury

Grades of Severity	Serum Creatinine	Glomerular Filtration Rate	Urine Output
Risk	1.5 × normal	Decreased by greater than 25%	Less than 0.5 mL/kg for 6 hours
Injury	2 × normal	Decreased by greater than 50%	Less than 0.5 mL/kg for 12 hours
Failure	3 × normal or greater than mg/dL	Decreased by greater than 75%	Less than 0.5 mL/kg for 24 hours or anuria for 12 hours
Loss	Complete loss of renal function for greater than 4 weeks		
End-stage kidney disease	Complete loss of renal function with need for renal replacement therapy for greater than 3 months		

Adapted from Bellomo, R., Ronco, C., Kellum, J. A., Mehta, R. L., & Palevsky, P. (2004). Acute renal failure—definition, outcome measures, animal models, fluid therapy and information technology needs: the Second International Consensus Conference of the Acute Dialysis Quality Initiative (ADQI) Group. *Crit Care, 8*(4), R204-212.

Table 8-7 Stages of Acute Kidney Injury

	Onset	Oliguric-Anuric	Diuretic	Recovery
Definition	Period of time from the precipitating event to the beginning of oliguria or anuria	Period of time when urine output is less than 400 mL/24 hr	Period of time between urine output of greater than 400 mL/24 hr until when laboratory values stabilize	Period of time between when the laboratory values stabilize until they are normal
Duration	Hours to days	1-2 weeks	1-2 weeks	3-12 months
BUN/creatinine	Normal or slight increase	Increased	Begins to decrease	Almost normal
Urine output	Decreased; about 20% of normal	Less than 400 mL/24 hr; about 5% of normal	May exceed 3 L/24 hr; about 150-200% of normal	Back to 100% of normal
Mortality	5%	50-60%	25%	10-15%
Other characteristics		• Metabolic acidosis • Water gain with dilutional hyponatremia • Hyperkalemia • Hypocalcemia • Hyperphosphatemia • Hypermagnesemia • Azotemia	• Metabolic acidosis • Sodium may be normal or decreased • Hyperkalemia continues	• Uremia, acid-base imbalances, and electrolyte imbalances gradually resolve

NOTE: Some patients (especially when acute kidney injury is related to nephrotoxins) go through only three phases: onset, nonoliguric, and recovery.

a) Controversial because diuretics in acute renal injury may increase mortality (Mehta, Pascual, Soroko, & Chertow, 2002).

b) Agents

i) Loop diuretics (e.g., furosemide [Lasix], bumetanide [Bumex])

ii) Osmotic diuretics (e.g., mannitol [Osmitrol])

(a) Frequently used for rhabdomyolysis

(b) Contraindicated in HF, pulmonary edema

f. Administer immunosuppressants and initiate plasmapheresis for immune-mediated causes of acute renal injury (e.g., Goodpasture's syndrome).

2. Maintain fluid, electrolyte, and acid-base balance.

a. Fluid

1) Monitor for clinical indications of fluid overload.

2) Maintain sodium and water restriction and encourage the patient to remain within prescribed restrictions.

a) Restrict fluid: 24-hour restriction usually determined by adding 500 mL (for insensible loss) to the previous day's urine output

b) Space fluid allowances over the entire 24-hour period.

c) Treat thirst by offering ice chips (must be included as intake), wet washcloths, misting the mouth, and providing mouth care.

d) Restrict sodium (usually 1-2 g/day).

b. Potassium

1) Monitor for clinical indications of hyperkalemia.

2) Maintain potassium restriction (usually 40 mEq/day); do not allow salt substitute (KCl) on dietary trays.

c. Phosphorus

1) Monitor for clinical indications of hyperphosphatemia.

2) Maintain phosphorus restrictions.

3) Administer phosphate-binding agents (e.g., Basaljel, Amphojel).

a) These aluminum-containing phosphate-binding agents may contribute to dialysis encephalopathy due to accumulation of aluminum; calcium carbonate (Caltrate) or calcium acetate (PhosLo) may be prescribed instead.

4) Treat hypocalcemia with calcium administration; increasing calcium will decrease phosphorus.

d. Magnesium

1) Monitor for clinical indications of hypermagnesemia.

2) Maintain dietary magnesium restrictions.

3) Do not administer magnesium-containing medications (e.g., Maalox, magnesium sulfate, magnesium citrate).

e. Monitor arterial blood gases for acid-base imbalance.

1) Initiate dialysis to eliminate nitrogenous wastes as prescribed for metabolic acidosis.

2) Administer sodium bicarbonate or Carbicarb as prescribed.
   a) Generally used only for severe metabolic acidosis (pH less than 7.1)
   b) Monitor for hypernatremia.
   c) Monitor for hypocalcemia caused by increased binding between albumin and calcium and decrease in ionized calcium.

3. Diminish the accumulation of nitrogenous wastes.
   a. Maintain protein restriction; usually 0.6 g/kg/day initially but may be as high as 1-1.5 g/kg/day if on hemodialysis or continuous renal replacement therapy (CRRT); 1.5-2 g/kg/day if on peritoneal dialysis
   b. Provide protein foods of high biological value (i.e., contain all essential amino acids).
   c. Provide adequate caloric intake to prevent catabolism and utilization of dietary protein for energy needs: usually greater than or equal to 35-40 kcal/kg/day.
   d. Initiate dialysis as indicated and prescribed.
      1) Indications for dialysis in the patient with acute kidney injury generally include the following:
         a) Volume overload (especially with pulmonary edema)
         b) Uncontrollable hyperkalemia
         c) Uncontrollable hyperphosphatemia
         d) Uncontrollable acidosis
         e) Symptomatic uremia (e.g., neurologic changes)
         f) Pericarditis
         g) Seizures or coma
         h) BUN 80-100 mg/dL or greater but may be initiated at BUN greater than 50-60 mg/dL
         i) Serum creatinine 10 mg/dL or greater
      2) Contraindications for dialysis
         a) Hemodynamic instability: Continuous renal replacement therapy (CRRT) may be used in these situations.
         b) Inability to tolerate anticoagulation
         c) Lack of vascular access
      3) Maintenance of patency and prevention of infection of vascular access (if present)
         a) Palpate shunt, fistula, AV graft for thrill; auscultate for bruit; note change in bright red color in tubing in shunt; palpate pulses and check capillary refill distal to access.
         b) Do not allow venipuncture, IV cannulation, injections, blood pressure measurements in limb with shunt, fistula, or AV graft.
         c) Monitor for constrictive clothing or dressing in limb with shunt, fistula, or AV graft.
         d) Monitor for bleeding; use pressure dressing to stop bleeding; bulldog clamps (always kept clamped to dressing) are used on shunt tubing to stop bleeding.
         e) Note any redness, induration, or purulent drainage around access; culture any purulent drainage; change dressing as for central venous catheter.
         f) Instruct patient not to disturb scabs at puncture sites at fistula or AV graft for hemodialysis.
      4) Maintenance of patency and prevention of infection of peritoneal access
         a) Note any redness, induration, or purulent drainage around access; culture any purulent drainage.
         b) Provide aseptic catheter care.
            i) Wash with antibacterial soap.
            ii) Dress with light gauze dressing.
            iii) Aseptic catheter manipulation
         c) Culture peritoneal dialysate outflow fluid periodically or as indicated.

4. Prevent further damage to the kidney by nephrotoxic agents.
   a. Note that dosages of drugs eliminated by the kidney are decreased and the interval between doses is increased.
   b. Monitor peak/trough serum drug levels when appropriate (e.g., aminoglycosides).
   c. Monitor urine creatinine clearance when patient is receiving nephrotoxic agents.
   d. Prevent contrast dye-related nephrotoxicity.
      1) Increase oral and/or parenteral fluids.
      2) Administer acetylcysteine (Mucomyst) as prescribed.
         a) Acts as an oxygen free radical scavenger
         b) Usual dose is 600 mg orally every 12 hours the day before and the day of the radiologic procedure that requires contrast.
      3) Administer fenoldopam (Corlopam) as prescribed.
         a) Acts as a dopaminergic stimulator to improve renal blood flow
         b) Usual dose is an intravenous infusion of 0.05 to 0.1 mcg/kg/min for 60-90 minutes before the injection of the contrast material and continued for 4 hours after the injection if no adverse reactions occur.
   e. Monitor for changes in urine color that may indicate the presence of heavy pigments that may cause acute tubular necrosis.
      1) Myoglobinuria: tea or cola colored
      2) Hemoglobinuria: wine colored

5. Provide adequate nutrition while maintaining dietary restrictions.
   a. Provide high biological protein within protein restriction.
   b. Provide enough calories to prevent catabolism of somatic protein stores.
   c. Increase dietary calcium.

d. Decrease dietary sodium, potassium, and phosphorus.
6. Prevent fluid volume deficit during the diuretic phase.
   a. Monitor for clinical indication of fluid volume deficit.
   b. Volume may be replaced hourly during this phase by replacing the last hour's urine output during the following hour.
7. Prevent infection: Initiate dialysis as prescribed when BUN level greater than 80-100 mg/dL because BUN values above this level are associated with increased risk of infection.
8. Prevent injury: Initiate dialysis as prescribed when BUN level greater than 80-100 mg/dL because BUN values above this level are associated with neurologic changes.
9. Monitor for and treat anemia and platelet dysfunction.
   a. Monitor hemoglobin, hematocrit, and RBCs.
   b. Treat anemia as prescribed.
      1) Folic acid, iron, vitamin B_{12}
      2) Recombinant erythropoietin (Epogen)
         a) Cannot be used with CRRT as it is dialyzed
      3) Packed RBCs: only prescribed if the patient is symptomatic of anemia (e.g., dyspnea, chest pain, syncope, hypotension)
   c. Monitor for clinical indications of platelet dysfunction (e.g., petechiae, ecchymosis, bleeding).
   d. Administer desmopressin (DDAVP) as prescribed for platelet dysfunction.
10. Promote comfort.
   a. Administer antipyretics as prescribed.
   b. Utilize emollient or cornstarch baths.
11. Monitor for complications.
   a. Renal: Chronic renal failure will develop in 25-30% of patients with acute kidney injury.
   b. Cardiovascular
      1) Dysrhythmias
      2) Hypertension
      3) Pericarditis, cardiac tamponade
      4) Pulmonary edema
   c. Neurologic
      1) Coma
      2) Seizures
   d. Metabolic
      1) Electrolyte imbalances
         a) Hyperkalemia
         b) Hyperphosphatemia
         c) Hypermagnesemia
         d) Hypocalcemia
      2) Acid-base imbalance: metabolic acidosis
   e. Gastrointestinal
      1) Peptic ulcer disease
      2) GI hemorrhage
   f. Hematologic
      1) Anemia
      2) Uremic coagulopathies
   g. Infection
      1) Increased susceptibility to pneumonias
      2) Septicemias
      3) Urinary tract and wound infections
   h. Miscellaneous: drug toxicity

Chronic Kidney Disease

Definition

1. Progressive and irreversible destruction of kidney structures
2. Stages (Table 8-8)

Etiology

1. Diabetes mellitus
2. Hypertension
3. Glomerulonephritis
4. Polycystic kidney disease
5. Irreversible acute kidney injury

Pathophysiology

See Figure 8-8.

Collaborative Management

1. As for acute kidney injury
2. Maintain ventilation, oxygenation, and circulation.
   a. Assessment for clinical indications of pericarditis, heart failure, hypertension and assistance with treatment.
   b. Assessment for clinical indications of life-threatening fluid, electrolyte, and/or acid-base imbalance and assistance with treatment
      1) Hypervolemia
      2) Hyperkalemia
      3) Hypermagnesemia
      4) Metabolic acidosis
3. Initiate and maintain renal replacement therapy.
4. Maintain safety.
   a. Adjustment of drug dosages
   b. Monitoring for delirium and uremic encephalopathy
   c. Mobility assistance to prevent fracture
   d. Avoidance of invasive procedures and monitoring for bleeding
5. Provide patient and family education.
   a. Dietary restrictions
   b. Prevention of complications
   c. Participation in care and decision-making

Renal Replacement Therapy

Dialysis

1. Definition: separation of solutes by differential diffusion through a semipermeable membrane that is placed between the two solutions (Figure 8-9)
2. Purposes
   a. Eliminate excess body fluids
   b. Maintain or restore electrolyte balance
   c. Maintain or restore acid-base balance
   d. Eliminate nitrogenous wastes and toxins from the blood

Table 8-8 Stages of Chronic Kidney Disease

Stage	Severity	GFR (mL/min)	Progression	Symptoms	Intervention
1	Kidney damage but normal or increased GFR	Greater than 90	None apparent	Usually none but may be hypertensive	Screening for risk factors
2	Kidney damage with mild decrease in GFR	60-89	Increasing PTH Early bone disease Increasing BUN and creatinine	Subtle • Hypertension	Screening/reduction of risk factors
3	Moderate: decreased GFR	30-59	Anemia Increasing BUN and creatinine	Mild • Anemia • Hypertension	Treatment and prevention of progression
4	Severe: decreased GFR	15-29	Increased triglycerides Metabolic acidosis Electrolyte imbalance Increasing BUN and creatinine	Moderate • Anemia • Hypertension • Hyperphosphatemia • Hyperkalemia • Edema	Treatment of complications and preparation for renal replacement therapy
5	End-stage kidney disease	Less than 15	Uremia requiring dialysis for survival	Severe • Anemia • Hypertension • Hyperphosphatemia • Hyperkalemia • Edema	Renal replacement therapy; possible renal transplant

Adapted from National Kidney Foundation. (2002). *KDOQI clinical practice guidelines for chronic kidney disease: Evaluation, classification, and stratification.* Retrieved January 2, 2012, from *http://www.kidney.org/professionals/KDOQI/guidelines_ckd/p4_class_g1.htm.*

3. Indications
   a. Acute or chronic renal failure
      1) Symptomatic uremia
      2) Uremic pericarditis
   b. Severe water intoxication
   c. Severe electrolyte imbalance
   d. Drug intoxication (drug must be dialyzable [e.g., alcohol, salicylates, lithium, barbiturates, some poisons])
   e. Hepatic encephalopathy/coma
4. Components
   a. Dialysate: solution of water, electrolytes (sodium, chloride, magnesium, bicarbonate), nonelectrolytes (glucose), buffer (acetate, lactate, or bicarbonate)
      1) Electrolyte concentration in the dialysate is adjusted to the patient's needs.
   b. Semipermeable membrane: peritoneum, extracorporeal membrane
   c. Patient's blood in contact with the membrane
5. Principles (Figure 8-10)
   a. Osmosis: A hypertonic solution is used as the dialysate to move water across the semipermeable membrane.
   b. Diffusion: The dialysate solution contains a concentration of selected solutes lower than the blood so that these solutes will move across the semipermeable membrane and into the dialysate solution.
   c. Filtration: In some forms of dialysis, there is a pressure difference between the sides of the semipermeable membrane with the highest pressure on the forward side of the membrane to act as a hydrostatic force pushing against the membrane to provide a filtration effect.
   d. Convection (in continuous renal replacement therapy [CRRT]): the transfer of solutes and solutions simultaneously moving across the semipermeable membrane
6. Variables affecting efficiency
   a. Size and number of the pores in the semipermeable membrane
   b. Surface area of the semipermeable membrane
   c. Thickness of the semipermeable membrane
   d. Size of the solute molecules
   e. Concentration of solutes in the blood
   f. Osmotic concentration
   g. Pressure gradients
   h. Temperature of the solution
   i. Rate of blood flow
7. Comparison of various types of dialysis (Table 8-9)
   a. Choice of right dialysis option
      1) Intermittent hemodialysis: therapy of choice for hemodynamically stable patients in hospital setting
      2) Peritoneal dialysis: suited for hemodynamically stable patients with intact peritoneum but has low efficiency
      3) Continuous renal replacement therapy (CRRT): suitable for critically ill or hemodynamically unstable patients and has a higher efficiency than peritoneal dialysis
8. Collaborative management
   a. Peritoneal dialysis
      1) Preparation

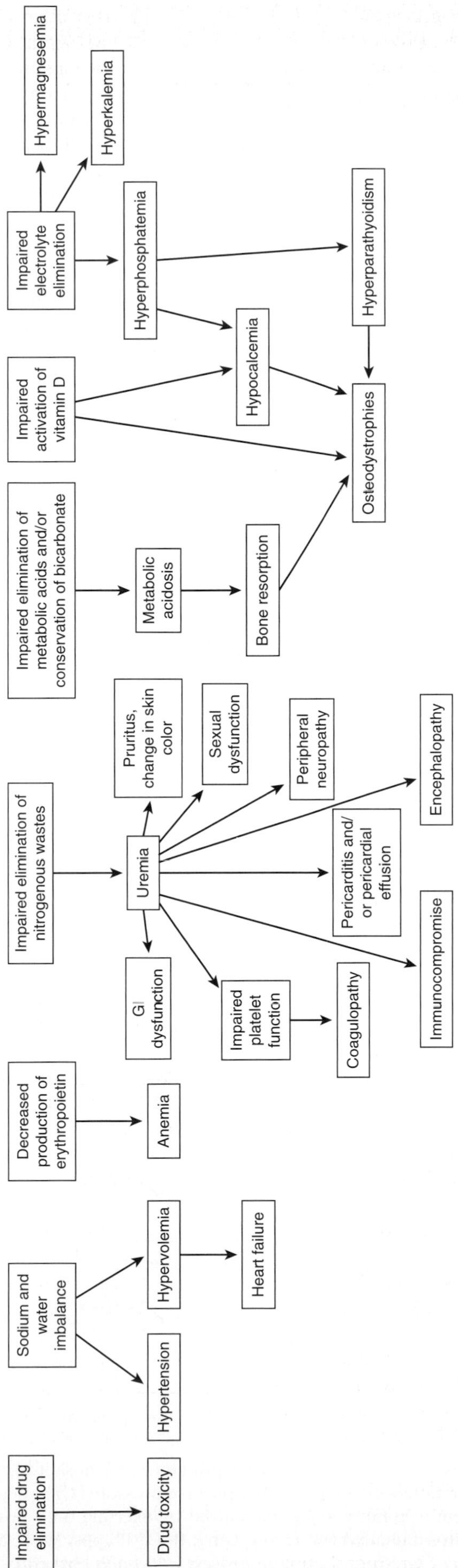

Figure 8-8 Pathophysiology of chronic kidney disease.

a) Prepare patient for insertion of peritoneal catheter. (Figure 8-11*A*)
   i) Explain procedure to patient.
   ii) Ask patient to void or insert urinary catheter prior to abdominal puncture.

b) Weigh patient before treatment and daily after draining dialysate.

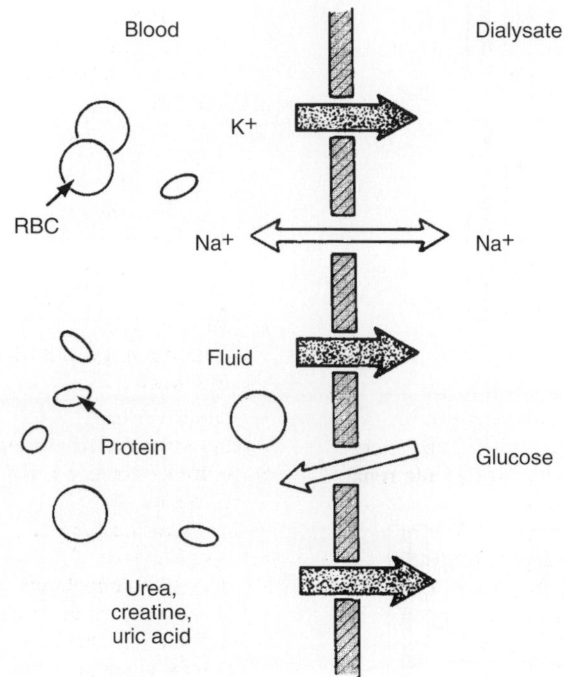

Figure 8-9 Osmosis and diffusion in dialysis. Net movement of major particles and fluid is illustrated. (From Long, B. C., Phipps, W. J., & Cassmeyer, V. L. [1993]. *Medical-surgical nursing: A nursing process approach* [3rd ed.]. St Louis: Mosby.)

2) Procedure (Figure 8-11*B*)
   a) Warm dialysate to body temperature.
   b) Ensure that prescribed medications have been added to dialysate: heparin; potassium chloride; antibiotics; lidocaine; etc.
   c) Instill 1-3 L of dialysate (usually 2 L) (inflow phase); this volume is usually infused at a rate of 2 L in 10-20 minutes.
   d) Allow to dwell in intraperitoneal space for 20-30 minutes (NOTE: if first exchange, do not allow dialysate to dwell; drain immediately to ensure catheter patency and placement)
   e) Drain and measure dialysate (outflow phase).
   f) Assess appearance of dialysate.
      i) Normal: clear, pale yellow or straw-colored
      ii) Cloudy: Suspect infection; culture and sensitivity is indicated.
      iii) Bloody: if occurs after the first four exchanges, suspect intraabdominal bleeding or coagulopathy
      iv) Amber: Suspect bladder perforation.
      v) Brownish: Suspect bowel perforation.
   g) If the amount drained is less than the amount instilled
      i) Turn patient side to side.
      ii) Apply gentle pressure to the abdomen.

3) Keep meticulous cumulative intake and output records (e.g., if drain is 300 mL less than the amount instilled [+300 mL] during one exchange but the next exchange yields

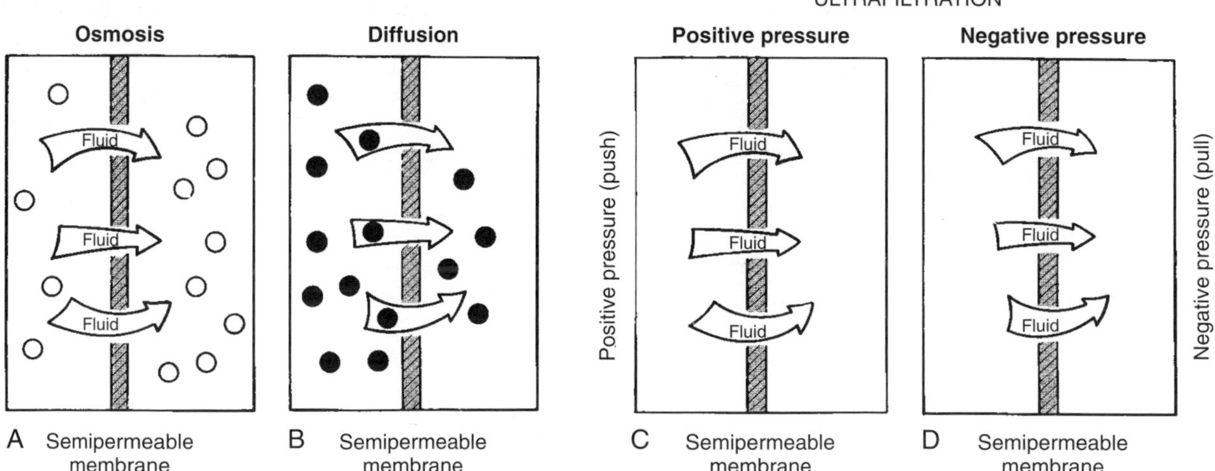

Figure 8-10 Dialysis is based on the following principles: Osmosis **(A)**, diffusion **(B)**, and ultrafiltration. Ultrafiltration occurs when either positive pressure **(C)** or negative pressure **(D)** is placed on the system. Ultrafiltration is maximized by exerting both positive and negative pressure on the system simultaneously. (From Long, B. C., Phipps, W. J., & Cassmeyer, V. L. [1993]. *Medical-surgical nursing: A nursing process approach* [3rd ed.]. St Louis: Mosby.)

Table 8-9 Types of Dialysis

	Hemodialysis	Intermittent Peritoneal Dialysis	CRRT Therapies
Principles	• Osmosis • Diffusion • Filtration	• Osmosis • Diffusion • Filtration	• Osmosis • Diffusion • Filtration • Convection

Treatment requirements	• Membrane: extracorporeal membrane or high coefficient membrane
	• Blood pump
	• Dialyzer
	• Dialysate
	• Vascular access
	• Anticoagulation
		• Membrane: peritoneum
		• Dialysate: 1.5%, 2.5%, 4.25%
		• Access: peritoneal catheter
			• Vascular access:
			  • CAVH and CAVHD are rarely done because they require arterial and venous access
			  • SCUF, CVVH, CVVHD, and CVVHDF require venovenous access
			• Blood pump
			• High-coefficient membrane hemofilter
			• Therapy fluid: predilution, postdilution, or dialysate

Specific indications	• Need for rapid treatment • Hemodynamically stable patient • Fluid overload unresponsive to diuretics • Electrolyte imbalance • Acute or chronic renal failure • Drug overdose or poison intoxication with dialyzable agent • Pulmonary edema refractory to diuretics	• Fluid overload • Electrolyte imbalance • Acute or chronic renal failure • Drug overdose or poison intoxication with dialyzable agent • Intact peritoneum • Inability to anticoagulate • Hemodynamic instability	• Fluid overload unresponsive to diuretics • Acute or chronic renal failure in hemodynamically unstable patient • Electrolyte imbalance • Drug overdose or poison intoxication with dialyzable agent • Inability to tolerate hemodialysis • May also be used in heart failure, sepsis, lactic acidosis, rhabdomyolysis, multiple organ dysfunction syndrome (MODS), hepatic failure
Contraindications	• Hemodynamic instability • Hypovolemia • Inadequate vascular access • Coagulopathy	• Rapid treatment required • Acute peritonitis • Recent abdominal surgery • Known abdominal adhesions • Abdominal trauma • Intraperitoneal hematoma • Recent vascular anastomosis of abdominal vessels • Respiratory distress • Sepsis • Extreme obesity • Coagulopathy	• Rapid treatment required • Systolic blood pressure less than 60 mm Hg for CAVH, CAVHD • Lack of venovenous access for SCUF, CVVH, CVVHD • Coagulopathy: relative; may increase risk during vascular access placement

Continued

Table 8-9 Types of Dialysis—cont'd

	Hemodialysis	Intermittent Peritoneal Dialysis	CRRT Therapies
Advantages	• Rapid and efficient; only 3-4 hours per session (usually 3 times weekly) unless overdose treatment, which may require 8-16 hours • Very efficient for small molecules; corrects biochemical disturbances quickly for time on therapy	• Equipment is easily and readily assembled • Fairly simple; requiring less staff and patient education • Relatively inexpensive • Minimal danger of acute electrolyte imbalance or hemorrhage • Dialysate can be individualized easily • Anticoagulation not required	• Removes solutes gradually • Decreased risk of hemodynamic instability • Provides flexibility in fluid administration • Allows adequate nutritional intake • Requires only minimal anticoagulation • Requires less staff education because it requires only catheter access instead of fistula or autograft • Can be used for physiologically unstable patients
Disadvantages	• Complex procedure requiring extensive staff training • Equipment expensive • Machine availability may be limited • Requires anticoagulation • Vascular access necessary	• Relatively slow to alter biochemical imbalances, usually requiring 36 hours for therapeutic effect • May cause protein loss • May be difficult to gain and maintain peritoneal access	• Patient must be in bed during entire treatment if femoral line in place or if unstable • May require anticoagulation • Vascular access necessary • Increased nursing care requirements • Complicates dosing of certain drugs such as antibiotics and agents which are dialyzable

Complications	• Access complications: bleeding, clotting, infection
	• Acute fluid and electrolyte imbalances
	• Hemorrhage
	• Hypovolemia
	• Air embolus
	• Disequilibrium syndrome caused by too rapid removal of waste products
	• Allergic reaction to membrane
	• Hepatitis
	• Dialysis encephalopathy (related to accumulation of aluminum from water used to prepare dialysate)
	• Infection
	• Dysrhythmias
		• Access complications: infection, dialysate leak, bleeding, and peritonitis
		• Too rapid fluid removal causing the following:
		• Hypovolemia
		• Hypernatremia
		• Hypervolemia caused by dialysate retention
		• Hypokalemia caused by potassium-free dialysate usage
		• Alkalosis caused by alkaline dialysate usage
		• Disequilibrium syndrome caused by too rapid a removal of waste products
		• Hyperglycemia caused by high glucose concentration of dialysate
		• Protein loss
		• Respiratory distress
			• Hypotension
			• Hypothermia
			• Hypovolemia or hypervolemia if too rapid or too slow fluid removal
			• Electrolyte imbalance of potassium, calcium, magnesium, and phosphate, depending on therapy
			• Acid-base imbalances
			• Access complications: bleeding, clotting, infection
			• Depletion syndrome: loss of vitamins and amino acids
			• Hemorrhage related to the following:
			  • Anticoagulation
			  • Disruption of filter or tubing
			• Infection
			• Air embolism

BP, Blood pressure; *CRRT*, continuous renal replacement therapy; *CVVH*, continuous venovenous hemofiltration; *CVVHD*, continuous venovenous hemodialysis; *CVVHDF*, continuous venovenous hemodiafiltration; *SCUF*, slow continuous ultrafiltration therapy.

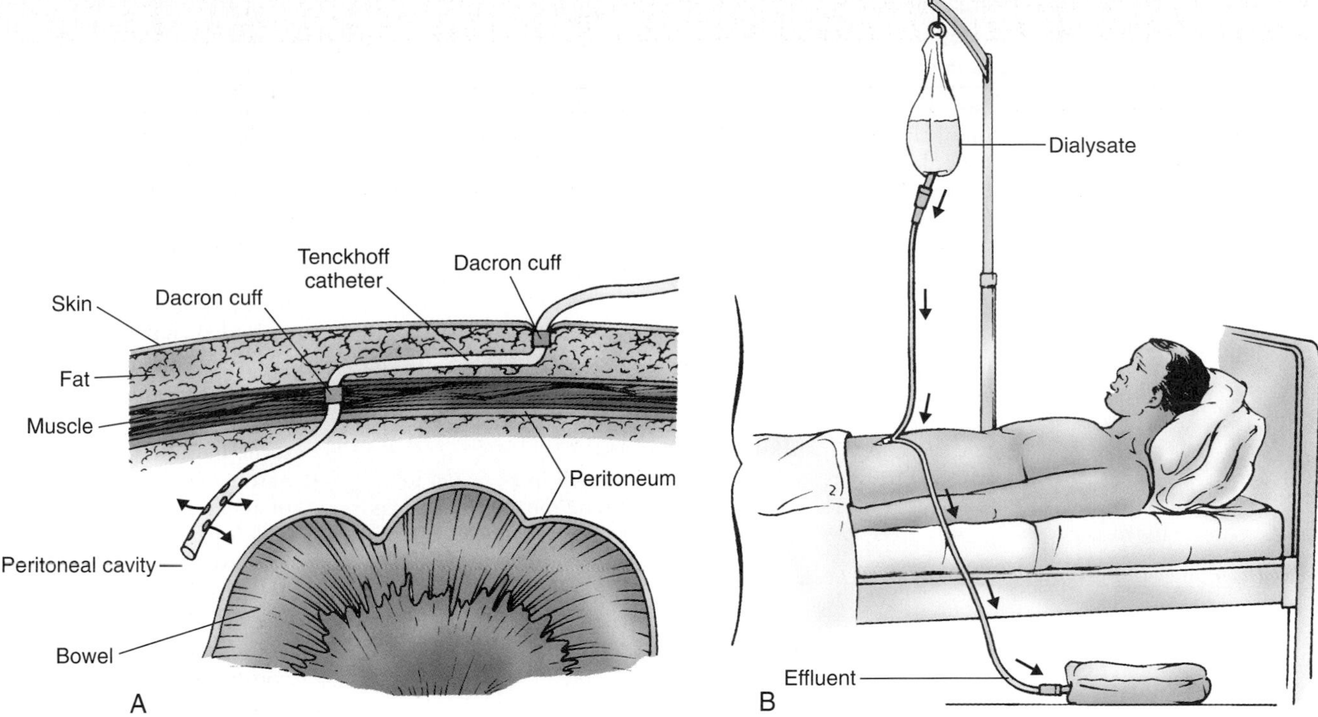

Figure 8-11 Manual peritoneal dialysis via an implanted Tenckhoff catheter. **A,** Catheter position in peritoneal cavity. **B,** Manual peritoneal dialysis process. (From Ignatavicius, D. D., & Workman, M. L. [2006]. *Medical-surgical nursing: Critical thinking for collaborative care* [5th ed.]. Philadelphia: Saunders.)

a drain volume of 400 mL more than the amount instilled [−400 mL], the cumulative volume is −100 mL).

4) Monitor for hypotension and respiratory distress, especially during inflow phase.
5) Monitor vital signs during outflow phase.
6) Monitor blood glucose levels in all patients; hyperglycemia is likely to occur in diabetic patients or when 4.25% dialysate is used.
7) Provide peritoneal catheter exit site care.

b. Hemodialysis
  1) Preparation
    a) Patient must have vascular access. (Table 8-10 and Figures 8-12 and 8-13)
    b) Weigh patient prior to hemodialysis.
    c) Do not administer drugs that may cause hypotension prior to hemodialysis.
      i) Antihypertensives
      ii) Antiemetics
      iii) Narcotics
      iv) Beta-blockers
      v) Calcium channel blockers
    d) Do not administer dialyzable drugs immediately prior to hemodialysis.
  2) Procedure (usually performed by specially trained hemodialysis nurse rather than critical care staff) (Figure 8-14)
    a) Vascular access is cannulated and/or connected to the dialyzer.
    b) Anticoagulation is maintained.
    c) Blood chemistries are monitored throughout the treatment.
    d) Vital signs are monitored frequently for evaluation of hemodynamic stability and tolerance.
    e) Hematocrit is monitored for changes that may indicate too rapid removal of fluid.
    f) Monitor the vascular access and the hemofilter for indications of clotting.

c. Selected complications
  1) Disequilibrium syndrome
    a) Caused by toxins (e.g., urea being rapidly removed from the blood but not as rapidly removed from the cerebrospinal fluid)
    b) The higher concentration of toxins in the brain cells may cause a shift of fluid into brain cells and cerebral edema.
    c) Clinical indications may include nausea, vomiting, headache, hallucinations, and seizures.

Table 8-10 Forms of Vascular Accesses for Dialysis

Access	Advantages	Disadvantages	Management
Double-lumen vascular catheter (Figure 8-12) inserted into subclavian, jugular, or femoral vein	• Easy insertion • Immediate use • High flow rates are achieved • No venipuncture required for access	• Externally located • Can be easily dislodged • Prone to infection and thrombosis • Femoral catheters are associated with a higher incidence of infection	• Monitor site daily and provide site care • Restrict use of this catheter to dialysis only • Administer heparin into catheter if prescribed • A fibrinolytic may be used to reestablish patency of an occluded catheter
Fistula (Figure 8-13*A*)	• Located internally • Greater longevity • Lower clotting and infection rates than external devices • No danger of disconnect	• Requires 4-6 weeks to mature prior to use • Requires venipuncture for access • May result in ischemia to affected limb (referred to as "vascular steal syndrome") • May thrombose	• Do not use limb for BP or venipuncture • Listen for bruit, feel for thrill: indicate patency • Assess neurovascular status of affected limb frequently • Teach patient exercises to increase blood flow in fistula (e.g., squeezing a ball) • Warn patient not to wear constrictive clothing
AV graft (Figure 8-13*B*)	• As for fistula • May be used for patients with vessels inadequate for fistula formation • Can be used earlier than traditional fistula	• As for fistula • Infection is more serious than with traditional fistula due to risk of disintegration and hemorrhage • May cause aneurysm formation	• As for fistula • Rotating puncture sites and applying pressure on needle removal aids in prevention of aneurysm and pseudoaneurysm

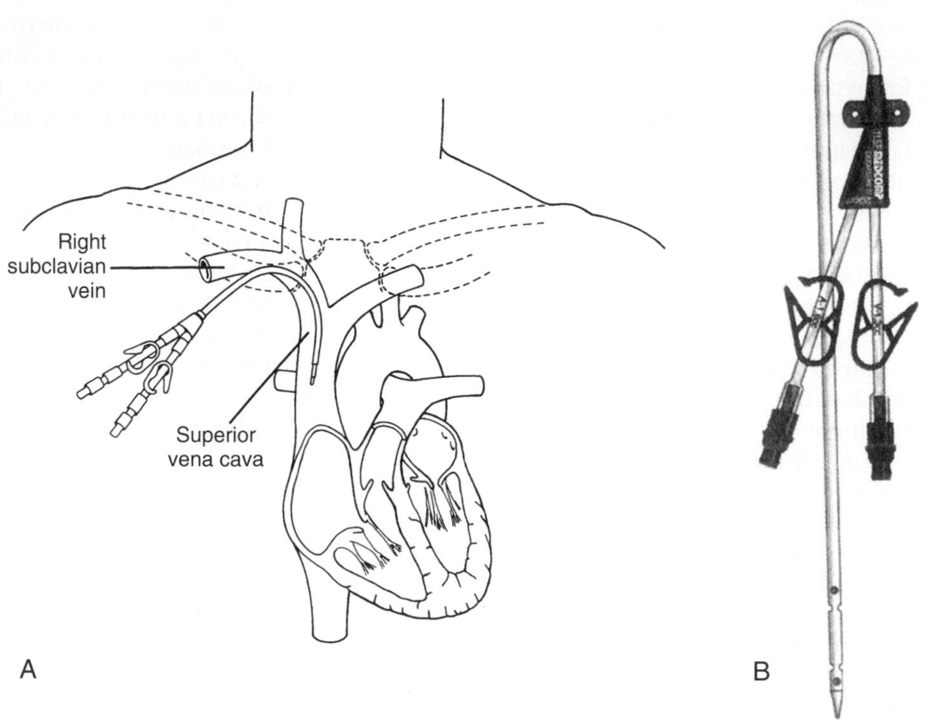

Figure 8-12 A, Temporary vascular access using subclavian dual-lumen venous catheter. **B,** Dual-lumen temporary catheter. (Courtesy MEDCOMP Corporation, Harleysville, PA.)

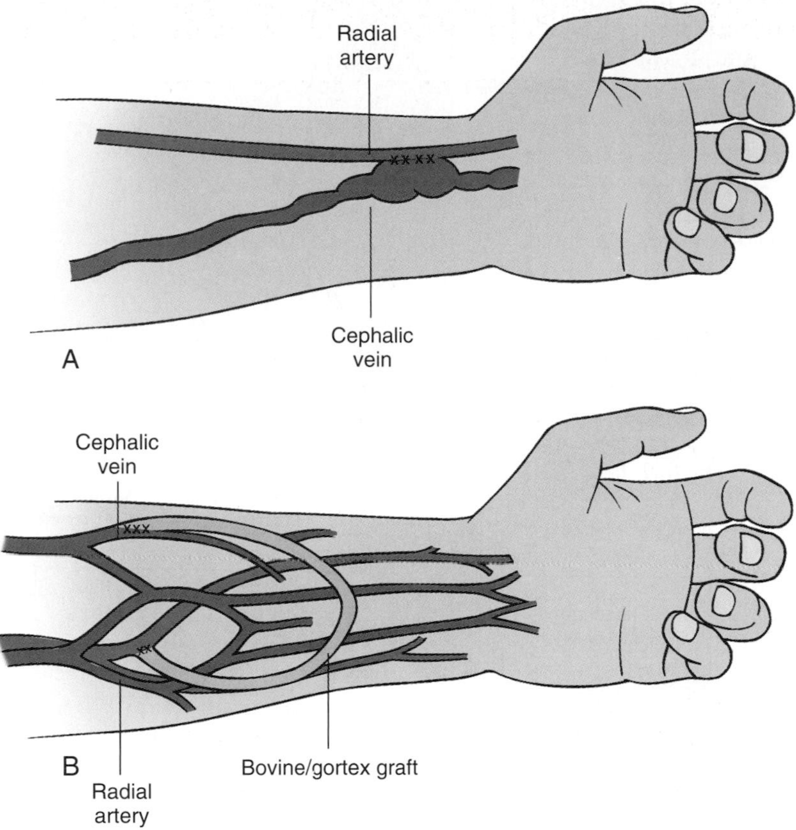

Figure 8-13 Permanent vascular accesses. **A,** A-V fistula. **B,** A-V graft. (From Urden, L. D., Stacy, K. M., & Lough, M. E. [2010]. *Critical care nursing: Diagnosis and management* [6th ed.]. St. Louis: Mosby.)

d) Collaborative management
   i) Use a smaller dialyzer.
   ii) Reduce blood pump speed.
   iii) Shorten dialysis time and dialyze more frequently.
   iv) Administer diazepam and phenytoin as prescribed for seizures.
2) Muscle cramps
   a) Caused by rapid water removal and sodium shifts
   b) Collaborative management
      i) Administer quinine as prescribed prior to dialysis.
      ii) Hypertonic saline during dialysis may also be prescribed.

d. Continuous renal replacement therapy (CRRT) (Table 8-11 and Figure 8-15)
   1) Preparation
      a) Patient must have vascular access.
      b) Heparin, citrate, and other combinations are placed in the port and need to be removed prior to initiation of treatment.
   2) Procedure
      a) Prepare hemofilter with dialysate solution.
      b) Connect vascular access to hemofilter.
      c) Initiate appropriate therapy and fluid as ordered.
      d) Set ultrafiltration rate to allow for appropriate removal of fluid and solutes as prescribed without causing or worsening hemodynamic instability.
      e) Fluid replacement if calculated according to the ultrafiltration rate.
      f) Change the filter set when unable to maintain prescribed rate or if filter clots and flow is stopped.

Renal Transplant

Renal replacement therapy for patients with chronic kidney disease

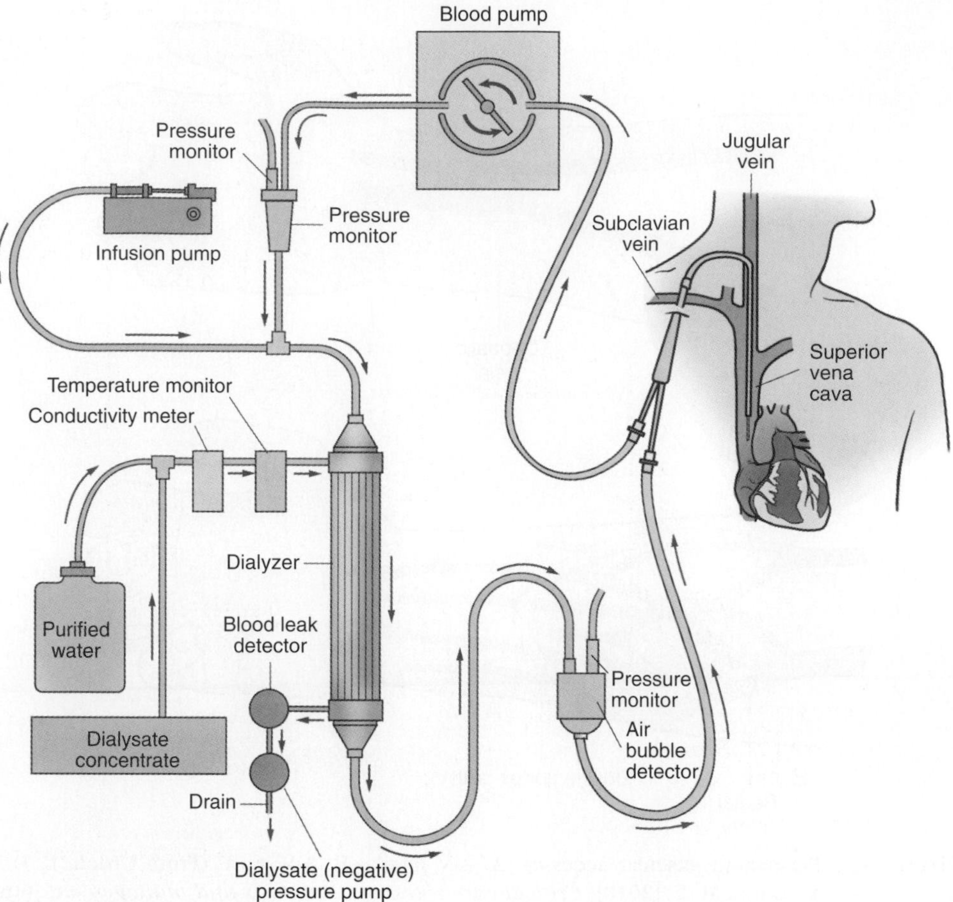

Figure 8-14 Components of a hemodialysis system. (From Urden, L. D., Stacy, K. M., & Lough, M. E. [2010]. *Critical care nursing: Diagnosis and management* [6th ed.]. St. Louis: Mosby.)

Table 8-11 Continuous Renal Replacement Therapy

Type	Ultrafiltration Rate	Function	Nursing Considerations
SCUF (slow, continuous ultrafiltration)	100-300 mL/hr	• Fluid removal	• Anticoagulation may be required
CVVH (continuous venovenous hemofiltration)	35 mL/kg/hr	• Fluid removal • Small- to moderate-sized solute removal by convection	• Fluid predilution or replacement required
CVVHD (continuous venovenous hemodialysis)	35 mL/kg/hr	• Fluid removal • Maximal solute removal by diffusion	• Dialysate solution is required
CVVHDF (continuous venovenous hemodiafiltration); not available on all equipment	Ultrafiltration is limited by amount of fluid predilution/postdilution or dialysate fluid infused	• Maximal fluid and solute removal by convection and diffusion	• Fluid replacement required • Dialysate solution required

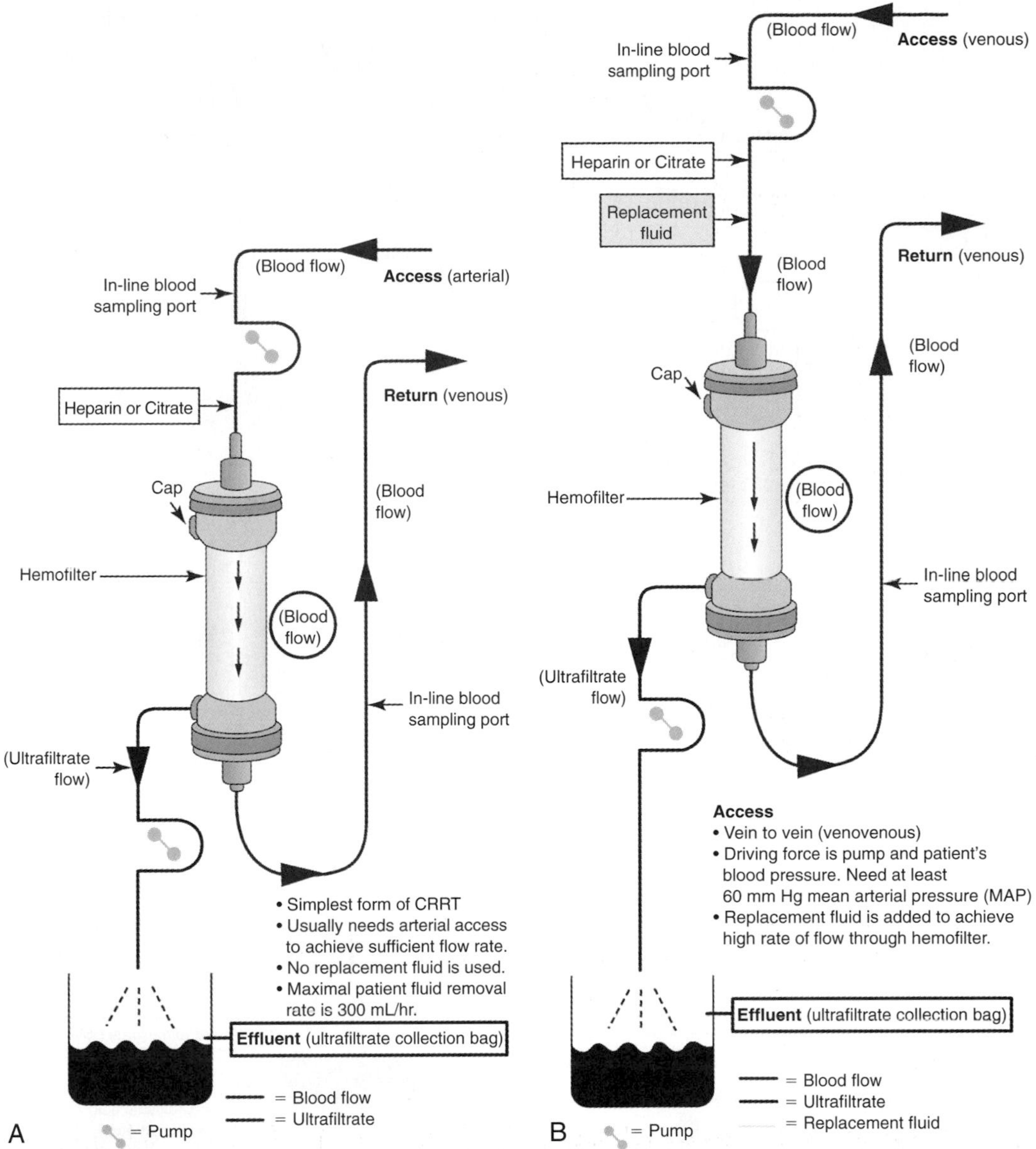

Figure 8-15 Continuous renal replacement therapy (CRRT) systems. **A,** Slow, continuous ultrafiltration (SCUF). **B,** Continuous venovenous hemofiltration (CVVH).

Continued

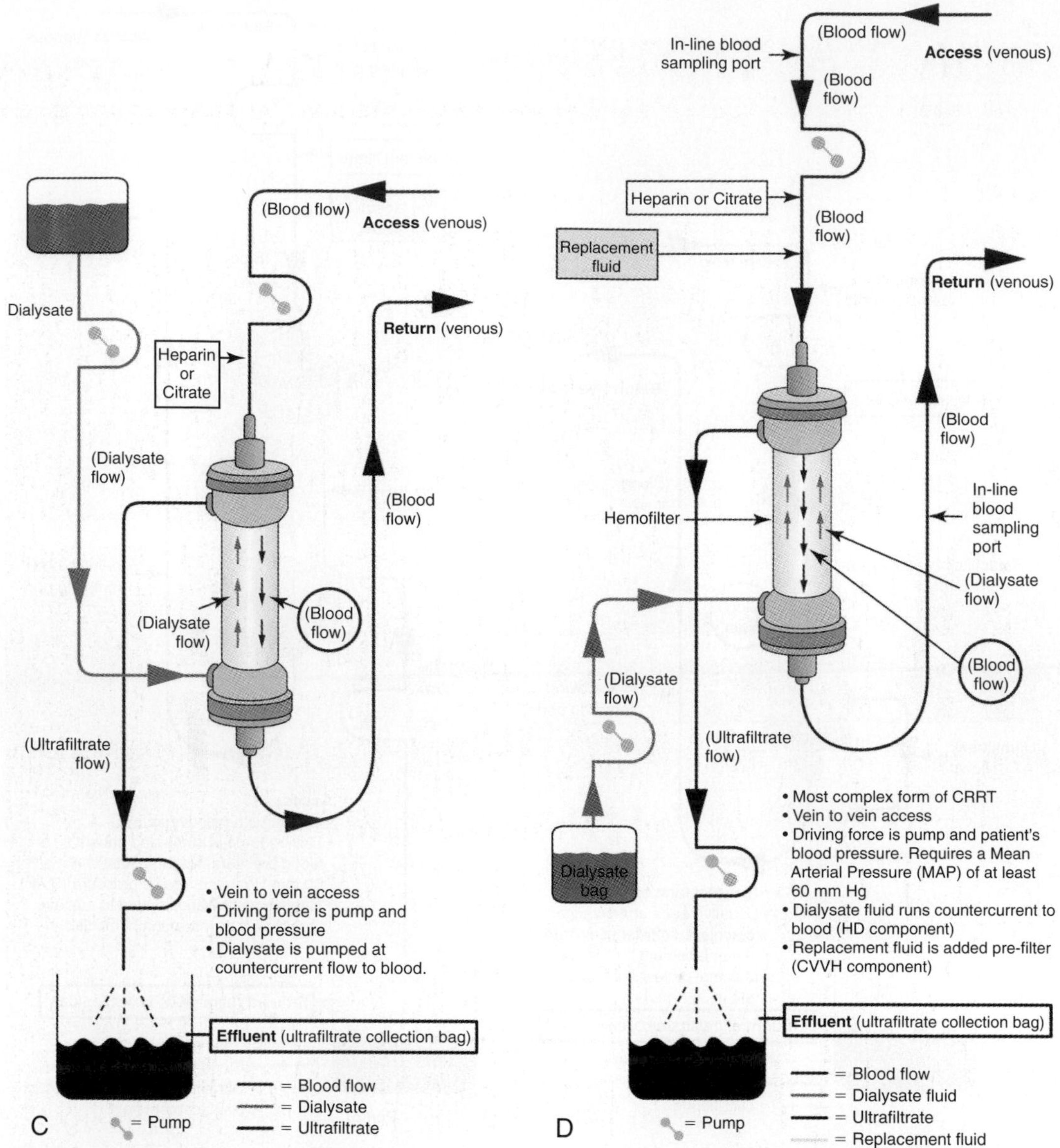

Figure 8-15, cont'd C, Continuous venovenous hemofiltration dialysis (CVVHD). **D,** Continuous venovenous hemodiafiltration (CVVHDF). (From Urden, L. D., Stacy, K. M., & Lough, M. E. [2010]. *Critical care nursing: Diagnosis and management* [6th ed.]. St. Louis: Mosby.)

LEARNING ACTIVITIES

CHAPTER 8

1. Complete the following crossword puzzle related to renal anatomy and physiology.

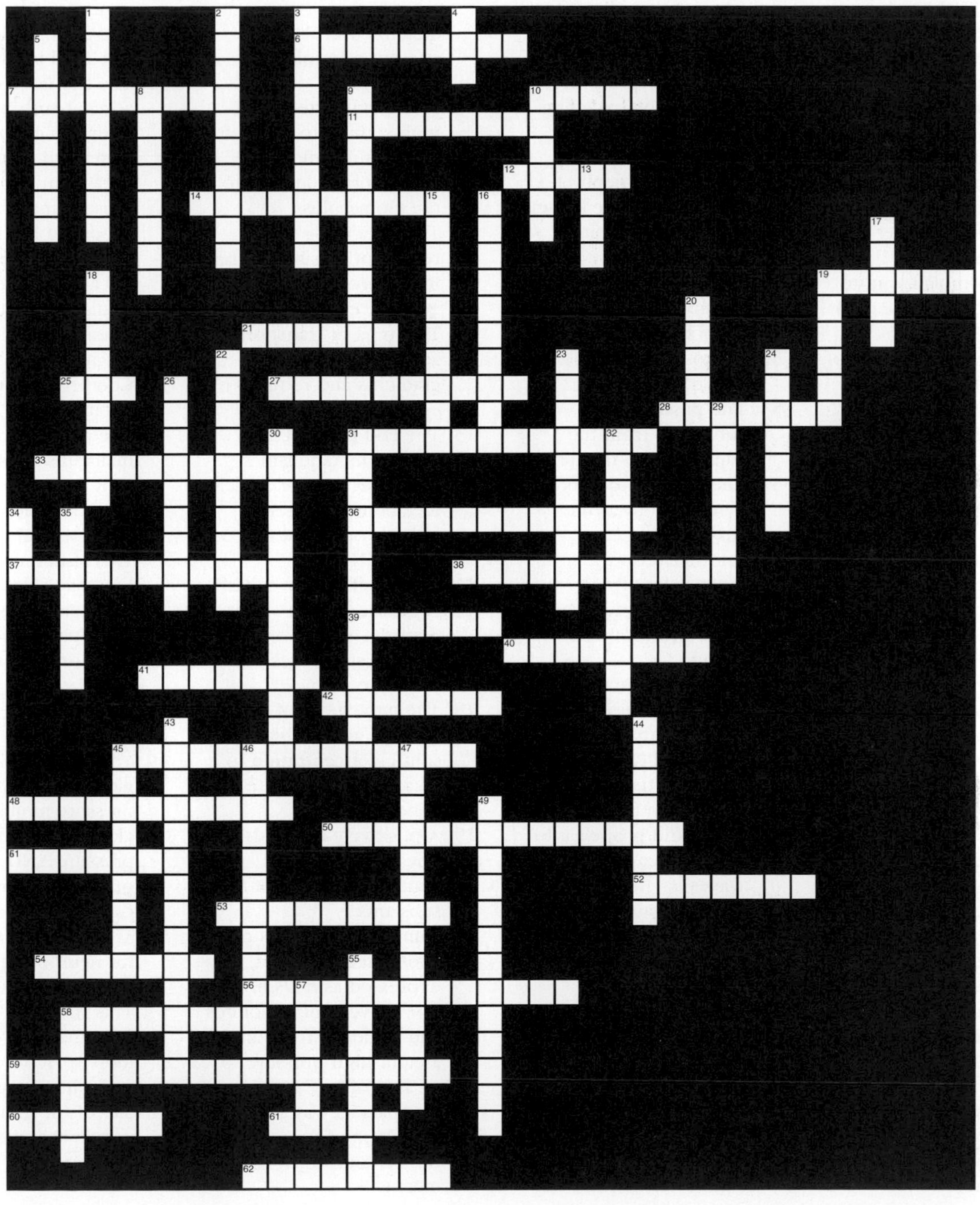

ACROSS

6. Indicates that the fluid has an osmolality less than body fluids; e.g., ½ NS
7. An estimate of a known substance in the plasma compared with the amount in the urine
10. A negatively charged ion
11. Indicates that the fluid has approximately the same osmolality as body fluids; e.g., normal saline
12. Cavity filled with adipose tissue, minor and major calyces, renal pelvis, and origin of the ureter
14. Indicates that the fluid has an osmolality more than body fluids: e.g., 3% saline
19. The inward extension of cortical tissue between the pyramids
21. A small funnel tapering into the ureter
25. This lab value reflects protein metabolism and is normally 10 times the creatinine value (abbrev)
27. The type of fluid loss (or gains) that cannot be measured
28. Urea is the result of the breakdown of this macronutrient
31. The fluid between cells
33. This substance is made by the kidney and modulates the vasoconstrictive effects of angiotensin and norepinephrine
36. The movement of substances from the tubule back into the capillaries
37. This pressure is a pushing pressure
38. The state of internal equilibrium within the body
39. The primary extracellular cation; reabsorbed primarily in the proximal convoluted tubule
40. The concentration of this ion determines pH
41. Vitamin D is necessary for the absorption of this mineral
42. This organ is a collapsible bag of smooth muscle
45. A complex physiologic process that allows for concentration of urine
48. The kidney aids in acid-base regulation primarily by excreting and retaining this extracellular anion
50. This type of nephron is important in the kidney's ability to concentrate urine
51. The thin layer of fibrous membrane that surrounds each kidney
52. Microscopic functional unit of the kidney
53. The passage of a substance from the capillary into the tubule
54. The endocrine gland that is referred to as the *suprarenal gland*
56. Another term for glomerular filtrate
58. This type of nephron has a short loop of Henle
59. This hormone is secreted in response to atrial stretch; causes excretion of sodium (2 words)
60. This structure collects urine from the renal pelvis and propels it to the bladder by peristaltic waves
61. This substance is secreted by the juxtaglomerular apparatus in response to low perfusion
62. Triangular wedges of medullary tissue; composed of collecting tubules

DOWN

1. The primary intracellular cation; reabsorbed primarily in the collecting duct
2. This area of the kidney includes the renal cortex and medulla
3. This electrolyte is crucial for cellular energy
4. This branch of the autonomic nervous system controls the afferent arterioles (abbrev)
5. This electrolyte works with sodium to maintain body fluid osmolality
8. This arteriole leads into the glomerulus
9. These increase the reabsorptive surface area in the proximal convoluted tubule
10. This type of transport is against concentration gradients and requires energy
13. The end product of protein metabolism
15. Waste product of muscle metabolism; better indicator of renal function than BUN
16. Cluster of tightly coiled capillaries in the nephron
17. Cuplike structures that drain the papillae
18. The movement of solutes from an area of high solute concentration to an area of low solute concentration
19. A positively charged ion
20. The human body is composed mostly of this substance
22. Number of osmoles per kilogram of solution; expressed as mOsm/kg
23. The movement of solutes and solutions from an area of high pressure to an area of low pressure
24. The passageway for expulsion of urine from the bladder to the urinary meatus
26. The capillary network that runs parallel to the ascending and descending loop of Henle (2 words)
29. The movement of solution from an area of low solute concentration to an area of high solute concentration
30. The fluid inside cells
31. The fluid inside vessels
32. The hormone of the adrenal cortex that causes retention of sodium and water and excretion of potassium
34. This hormone is produced in the hypothalamus and released by the posterior pituitary; it causes water retention in the renal tubule
35. Comprised of 6-10 pyramids
43. The process that maintains constancy in GFR
44. This arteriole leads out of the glomerulus
45. This structure consists of Bowman's capsule and the glomerulus
46. The fluid outside cells
47. The hormone that stimulates the release of RBCs from the bone marrow
49. This pressure is the glomerular hydrostatic pressure minus glomerular osmotic pressure AND hydrostatic pressure in Bowman's capsule (2 words)
55. This electrolyte is crucial for neuromuscular transmission
57. This structure includes proximal convoluted, loop of Henle, and distal convoluted segments
58. Site of the glomerulus, proximal and distal tubules

2. Number the structures below according to the order of their involvement in urine formation.
___Ureters
___Glomerulus
___Loop of Henle
___Proximal convoluted tubule
___Bladder
___Bowman's capsule
___Collecting ducts
___Distal convoluted tubule
___Urethra

3. Complete the following statements related to the movement of solutes and solutions.
Water moves by the process of __________.
Electrolytes move by the process of __________.
The sodium-potassium pump is an example of __________.
The use of a pushing pressure, such as hydrostatic pressure, is called __________.

4. A 72-year-old woman is brought to the emergency department from a long-term care facility. She had recently been started on enteral feedings. She has had a change in level of consciousness. Her sodium level is 150 mEq/L, her BUN is 80 mg/dL, and her serum glucose is 1000 mg/dL. Calculate her serum osmolality and identify what this serum osmolality indicates. What is the most likely cause of this abnormal serum osmolality? ______________________________

____

5. Identify the electrolyte or electrolytes that the statement describes.
a. Serum levels of this electrolyte go up in acidosis and down in alkalosis______________________________
b. These three electrolytes frequently go down together. ______________________________
____
c. Serum levels of this electrolyte go down in hypoalbuminemia.______________________________
d. These two electrolytes have an inverse relationship: When one goes down, the other goes up. ______________
____
e. These two electrolytes are frequently deficient in malnourished patients. ______________________________
____
f. Loss of either of these electrolytes causes hydrogen ions to move into the cell resulting in metabolic alkalosis. __________
____

6. Specify whether the following causes of metabolic acidosis would have a normal anion gap or an increased anion gap.

Condition	Normal Anion Gap	Increased Anion Gap
Shock		
Renal failure		
Diarrhea		
Diabetic ketoacidosis		
Salicylate overdose		
Renal tubular acidosis		
Rhabdomyolysis		
Carbonic anhydrase inhibitors		
Ethylene glycol poisoning		

7. Identify three major reasons for the BUN to be elevated in a patient with a normal creatinine.
a. ______________________________
b. ______________________________
c. ______________________________

8. Identify whether these signs and symptoms are indicative of electrolyte deficit or excess.

Sign/Symptom	Excess (Hyper)	Deficit (Hypo)
Sodium		
Weight gain		
Abdominal cramps		
Flushed, dry skin		
Postural hypotension		
Headache		
Hypertension		
Potassium		
Flat T waves, prominent U waves		
Decreased GI motility, paralytic ileus		
Intestinal colic, diarrhea		
Muscle cramps → flaccid paralysis		
Decreased cardiac contractility		
Tall, peaked T waves, widened QRS complex		
Calcium		
Tetany		
Decreased deep tendon reflexes		
Neuromuscular weakness, flaccidity		
Seizures		
Bone or flank pain		
Laryngospasm		
Phosphorus		
Tetany		
Fatigue		
Chest pain		
Dyspnea		
Increased deep tendon reflexes		
Abdominal cramps		
Magnesium		
Decreased deep tendon reflexes		
Anorexia, nausea, vomiting		
Cardiopulmonary arrest		
Lethargy		
Dysrhythmias, especially torsades de pointe		
Facial flushing		

9. Identify three electrolyte imbalances that enhance the digitalis effect and increase the chance of digitalis toxicity.
   a. ______
   b. ______
   c. ______

10. Identify the fluid, electrolyte, or acid-base imbalances to which these patients would be predisposed:
    a. A patient receiving regular doses of furosemide.
       1. ______
       2. ______
       3. ______
       4. ______
       5. ______
       6. ______

b. A patient with persistent vomiting.
   1. ______
   2. ______
   3. ______
   4. ______

c. A patient with acute kidney injury (oliguric phase).
   1. ______
   2. ______
   3. ______
   4. ______
   5. ______
   6. ______
   7. ______

d. A patient with diabetic ketoacidosis (before treatment).
   1. ______
   2. ______
   3. ______
   4. ______

e. A patient receiving multiple units of banked blood.
   1. ______
   2. ______
   3. ______

11. List three indications for dialysis in a patient with acute kidney injury.
   a. ______
   b. ______
   c. ______

12. Categorize the following causes of acute kidney injury as prerenal, intrarenal, or postrenal.

Condition	Prerenal	Intrarenal	Postrenal
Acute pyelonephritis			
Benign prostatic hypertrophy			
Contrast dyes			
Diuretics			
Aminoglycosides			
Glomerulonephritis			
Goodpasture's syndrome			
Hemorrhage			
Hepatorenal syndrome			
Hypersensitivity reactions			
Intraabdominal tumor			
Malignant hypertension			
Neurogenic bladder			
Prolonged hypotension			
Renal calculi			
Rhabdomyolysis with myoglobinuria			
Septic shock			

13. Identify the following characteristics as occurring during the oliguric or diuretic phase of acute kidney injury or both.

Characteristic	Oliguric Phase	Diuretic Phase	Both
Elevated BUN			
Hyperkalemia			
Metabolic acidosis			
Volume deficit			
Volume excess			

14. Complete the following crossword puzzle related to renal assessment, conditions, and treatments.

ACROSS

3. Urea is the result of the breakdown of this macronutrient
5. This type of diuretic may cause hyperkalemia, especially if the patient has renal insufficiency; e.g., spironolactone (2 words)
7. This condition occurs in renal failure and is caused by a deficiency of erythropoietin
8. A very serious complication of hyponatremia
9. A thiazide diuretic (generic)
15. This fluid/electrolyte imbalance is caused by inadequate fluid intake, inadequate fluid replacement, excessive fluid losses, or fluid shifts
17. An acute inflammation of the kidney associated with beta-hemolytic streptococcal infection
18. A long-term vascular access consisting of an internal artery-vein anastomosis
19. The separation of solutes by differential diffusion through a semipermeable membrane that is placed between two solutions
21. This electrolyte imbalance occurs in renal failure and contributes to hypocalcemia
23. Type of intrarenal failure that is caused by infectious processes
24. A renal replacement therapy that may be used in patients who cannot tolerate hemodialysis (abbrev)
26. This form of potassium may be used in DKA for ⅓-½ of potassium needed (2 words)
29. This type of candy may cause hypokalemia by increasing aldosterone effect
31. High levels of this electrolyte may cause respiratory paralysis and cardiopulmonary arrest
32. This lethal dysrhythmia is associated with hypokalemia, hypocalcemia, and hypomagnesemia (3 words)
35. This is a cause of hypoproteinemia in renal failure
37. The electrolyte imbalance primarily associated with refeeding syndrome
41. A dopaminergic agent that increases renal flow (generic)
43. Drugs used to prevent organ rejection in a posttransplant patient cause _____
44. The hand-flapping tremor seen in uremia
45. A potentially permanent renal replacement therapy for patients with chronic renal failure
46. This plasma protein has the most significant effect on intravascular oncotic pressure
47. May be used to correct metabolic acidosis if pH less than 7 or for hyperkalemia caused by acidosis (2 words)
48. This type of edema is frequently associated with nephrotic syndrome
49. This electrolyte imbalance is common in acute pancreatitis
51. This muscle paralytic agent, frequently used for intubation, may cause hyperkalemia
52. To move the kidney down to palpable range, the patient is asked to take a deep _____
54. Administration of blood can cause hypocalcemia because the ____ binds with calcium
56. This categorization of acute kidney injury is caused by disrupted urine flow; nephrolithiasis is an example of a cause of this type of renal failure
58. Calcium may be administered for hypocalcemia, hyperkalemia, and _____
59. This sign is carpal spasm after 3 minutes of inflation of a blood pressure cuff to a level above systolic pressure; indicates hypocalcemia
61. Precipitation from the kidney that takes the shape of the tubule where it was formed
62. A type of antibiotic that is associated with acute tubular necrosis
63. Excessive use of ____ can cause hypermagnesemia (plural)
64. Administration of ___, especially if old, can cause hyperkalemia
65. An aldosterone antagonist (also referred to as a *potassium-sparing diuretic*) (generic)
67. The most important intervention for a patient with prerenal failure is to ensure adequate intravascular ____
68. Presence of this protein in the urine is the result of the breakdown of skeletal muscle; may cause renal failure
70. The condition characterized by the breakdown of skeletal muscle; leads to myoglobinuria and may cause renal failure
73. Tenderness over this "angle" may indicate pyelonephritis
77. High levels of this electrolyte occur in renal failure; low levels occur in malnutrition
78. This postoperative complication is frequently associated with hypokalemia (2 words)
80. A carbonic anhydrase inhibitor frequently used to treat metabolic alkalosis (abbrev.)
82. Common form of CRRT (abbrev.)
85. The most common type of acute kidney injury in critically ill patients (abbrev.)
86. This is palpable over a fistula
88. Electrolyte imbalance that can occur with immobility and bone malignancy
89. This acid-base imbalance causes the shift of potassium from intracellular to extracellular
90. This type of dialysis is contraindicated if the patient has recent abdominal trauma or surgery
92. This type of renal syndrome is associated with loss of large amounts of protein, resultant edema, hyperlipidemia, and lipiduria
93. Use of this form of dialysis is frequently prohibited in critically ill patients due to hemodynamic instability
94. This phase of acute kidney injury is heralded by a dramatic increase in urine output

DOWN

1. This may result from hypocalcemia and cause compromise of the airway
2. A psychiatric disorder that causes hemodilutional hyponatremia (2 words)
3. The categorization of acute kidney injury that is caused by disrupted blood flow to the kidney
4. Serum levels of calcium and phosphorus are ____
6. A loop diuretic (generic)
10. Frequently used for diagnostic studies, this can cause acute tubular necrosis, especially if the patient is not adequately hydrated
11. Syndrome characterized by basement membrane damage and manifested by renal failure and hemoptysis
12. Treatment of ___ is always important in treating fluid and electrolyte imbalances
13. Solution of glucose and electrolytes used on one side of the semipermeable membrane to pull fluid and electrolytes
14. Significant changes in serum levels of this electrolyte cause T wave change and dysrhythmias
16. This type of renal syndrome is associated with loss of large amounts of protein, resultant edema, hyperlipidemia, and lipiduria

20. This complication of thyroidectomy may cause severe hypocalcemia
22. This is audible over a fistula
25. Dietary modification for patients with renal failure would include ____ of fluid, sodium, potassium, and phosphorus
27. This categorization of acute kidney injury is caused by damage to renal tissue
28. Presence of this protein in the urine is the result of massive hemolysis; may cause renal failure
30. A common cause of hypomagnesemia and hypophosphatemia
33. This disease is an endocrine disorder which causes hyponatremia and hyperkalemia due to deficiency of aldosterone
34. Very low urine ____ is a manifestation of diabetes insipidus as a possible cause of hypovolemia and hypernatremia (2 words)
36. An obvious manifestation of hypervolemia, right ventricular failure, or tension pneumothorax
38. This IV fluid is administered slowly and cautiously for severe hyponatremia (2 words)
39. ___ with dextrose is used for hyperkalemia with life-threatening dysrhythmias
40. ADH disorders cause gain or loss of ____, causing either hemoconcentration (DI) or hemodilution (SIADH)
42. This type of intrarenal failure is caused by nephrotoxic agents or prolonged ischemic injury
49. The electrolyte imbalance that occurs with crush injury, renal failure, and hemolysis
50. This drug by inhalation may be used for severe hyperkalemia
53. Loop diuretics such as furosemide work at the loop of _____
55. The hormone that stimulates the release of RBCs from the bone marrow
57. A condition characterized by cramps, seizures, twitching of the muscles, and sharp flexion of the wrist and ankle joints; associated with hypocalcemia
60. Increased levels of urea in the blood
66. An oxygen free scavenger which may be used after contrast dyes, especially if the patient has an elevated creatinine
69. Glomerulonephritis requires renal ____ for definitive diagnosis
71. This acid-base imbalance causes the shift of potassium from extracellular to intracellular
72. Emergent dialysis is indicated for a patient with hyperkalemia caused by ____ (2 words)
74. This sign is facial twitching in response to tapping on the facial nerve; indicates hypocalcemia
75. Dietary modifications for patients with renal failure include adequate ___ to avoid catabolism (which would increase BUN)
76. The amount of time that dialysate solution remains in the peritoneal cavity is referred to as the _____ time
79. An ion exchange agent used to decrease serum potassium (brand)
81. An osmotic diuretic (generic)
83. A cause of intrarenal failure that causes ischemia to the renal tubules
84. Pain in this area is frequently associated with renal conditions
87. This fluid/electrolyte imbalance is caused by excessive fluid intake, retention of sodium and water, or interstitial to intravascular shift
91. Levels of this electrolyte are greatly affected by water balance

The Endocrine System

Selected Concepts in Anatomy and Physiology

Functions

The endocrine system regulates secretion of hormones that alter metabolic body functions including all of the following:

1. Chemical reactions and transport of chemicals across cell membranes
2. Growth and development
3. Metabolism
4. Fluid and electrolyte balance
5. Acid-base balance
6. Adaptation
7. Reproduction

Components

1. Glands or glandular tissue that synthesize, store, and secrete hormones
   a. An endocrine gland is ductless but highly vascular.
   b. The location of endocrine glands is depicted in Figure 9-1.
2. Hormones
   a. Definition: complex chemical substances produced in one part or organ of the body that initiate or regulate the activity of an organ or a group of cells in another part of the body
      1) Hormones are released by endocrine glands in response to specific signals (e.g., low target gland hormone levels, low serum calcium, sympathetic nervous system innervation).
      2) Hormones are released directly into the bloodstream to be distributed throughout the body and to the target gland or target organ to initiate a response.
   b. Types include the following:
      1) Single amino acids (e.g., epinephrine, dopamine, thyroid hormones)
      2) Proteins (e.g., growth hormone, follicle-stimulating hormone)
      3) Steroids (e.g., androgens, aldosterone, cortisol)
   c. Endocrine glands and hormones significant in the care of critically ill patients are summarized in Table 9-1; hormones also are secreted by the following organs, although these organs are not normally considered part of the endocrine system.
      1) Gastrointestinal tract (e.g., gastrin, cholecystokinin, somatostatin, gastric inhibitory peptide, secretin, vasoactive intestinal peptide)
      2) Heart (e.g., atrial natriuretic hormone)
      3) Kidney (e.g., erythropoietin, renin, calcitriol)
3. Receptor cells: located in an organ or a group of cells in another part of the body

Process of Hormone Synthesis, Secretion, Effect, and Suppression

See Figure 9-2.

Regulation of Hormones

1. The hypothalamus regulates the secretion of hormones through secretion of releasing factors.
2. The pituitary gland is stimulated by these releasing factors from the hypothalamus to secrete stimulating factors.
3. The target gland is then stimulated to secrete the hormone.
4. The hormone binds with receptors in the target cells.
5. Regulation
   a. Self-regulation based on the concentration of the hormone present in the circulation; may also be influenced by electrolyte levels, metabolites, osmolality, fluid status, and other hormones
   b. Negative feedback: most common
      1) High hormone levels inhibit the release of the releasing factor from the hypothalamus or stimulating factor from the pituitary gland or secretion of the hormone from the gland.

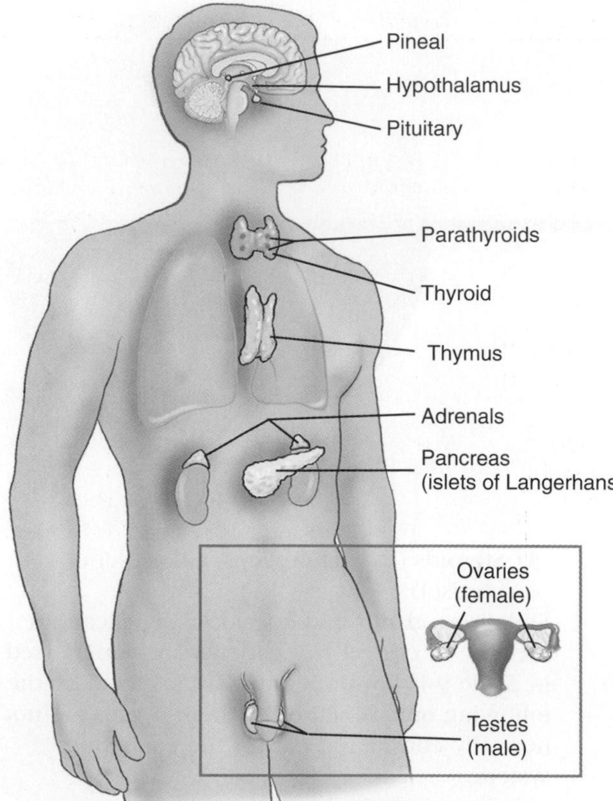

Figure 9-1 Location of endocrine glands. (From Shiland, B. J. [2010]. *Mastering healthcare terminology* [3rd ed.]. St. Louis: Mosby.)

c. Positive feedback: less common
   1) A hormone stimulates continued secretion until a specific level is reached.

d. Neural regulation as a result of stimulation of sympathetic division of autonomic nervous system; when stress is removed, SNS is no longer stimulated and epinephrine release is reduced

Endocrine Dysfunction

1. Classification
   a. Based on level of hormone activity
      1) Hyperfunction: increased hormonal activity
      2) Hypofunction: decreased hormonal activity
   b. Based on location of dysfunctional gland or response
      1) Primary disorders: disorder of the target gland (e.g., adrenal or thyroid gland)
      2) Secondary disorder: disorder of the stimulating gland (e.g., pituitary)
      3) Tertiary disorder: disorder of the hypothalamus
   c. Based on acuity
      1) Acute: beginning abruptly with marked intensity
      2) Chronic: developing slowly and persisting for a long period of time, often for the remainder of the lifetime of the individual
2. Causes of endocrine dysfunction
   a. Dysfunction of a particular gland
   b. Altered secretion of the stimulating hormones for that gland
   c. Altered response to the hormone itself at the target cell

Assessment of the Endocrine System

Interview

1. Chief complaint: why is the patient seeking help and the duration of the problem; because hormones affect every body tissue, numerous symptoms may indicate endocrine dysfunction
   a. General
      1) Easy fatigability, lethargy
      2) Sleep disorders
      3) Cold or heat intolerance
      4) Weight loss or gain, or rapid fluctuations in weight
      5) Increase in size of head, hands, or feet
   b. Dermatologic
      1) Pruritus
      2) Hair loss
      3) Changes in hair distribution
      4) Changes in quality of hair
      5) Changes in skin color or pigmentation
      6) Striae
      7) Changes in skin moisture
   c. Eyes: visual changes
   d. Neck
      1) Jugular neck vein distention
      2) Enlargement or nodules
   e. Cardiovascular
      1) Palpitations
      2) Syncope
   f. Pulmonary: dyspnea
   g. Neurologic
      1) Voice changes
      2) Tremors
      3) Nervousness
      4) Visual changes
      5) Loss of the sense of smell
      6) Headache
      7) Sensory changes
      8) Memory loss
      9) Personality changes
      10) Confusion, agitation
      11) Delusions, paranoia, depression
      12) Muscle twitching
      13) Seizures
   h. Gastrointestinal
      1) Change in appetite
      2) Nausea, vomiting
      3) Abdominal pain
      4) Constipation or diarrhea
      5) Incontinence
      6) Polyphagia
      7) Polydipsia
   i. Genitourinary
      1) Polyuria, oliguria, nocturia

Table 9-1	Endocrine Glands and Hormones Significant in the Care of Critically Ill Adults				
Hormone	**Actions**	**Releasing Factors**	**Target**	**Hypersecretion**	**Hyposecretion**
Hypothalamus: Controls the release of pituitary hormones					
Pituitary (Hypophysis)					
Anterior Pituitary (Adenohypophysis)					
Growth hormone (somatotropin)	• Stimulates protein anabolism • Mobilizes fatty acids • Conserves carbohydrates • Stimulates growth of bone, muscle, and cartilage	Growth hormone-releasing hormone (GRH) from hypothalamus in response to exercise, starvation, decreased amino acid levels, stress, hypoglycemia	All body cells capable of growth, especially muscle, bone, and cartilage cells	Giantism in children; acromegaly in adults	Dwarfism in children; possible decrease in organ weight in adults
Adrenocorticotropic hormone	• Stimulates growth and function of adrenal gland • Controls production and release of glucocorticoid hormones • Stimulates mineralocorticoid production • Stimulates androgen production	Corticotropin-releasing hormone (CRH) from hypothalamus in response to hypoglycemia, decrease in cortisol levels, hypoxia, trauma, surgery, physical and/or psychological stress	Cells of adrenal cortex	Cushing's disease	Adrenal insufficiency (chronic) and/or adrenal crisis (acute)
Thyroid-stimulating hormone (thyrotropin)	• Increases size and growth of thyroid cells • Increases synthesis of thyroid hormones • Releases stored thyroid hormones	Thyrotropin-releasing hormone (TRH) from the hypothalamus in response to cold temperature or a decrease in thyroid hormone levels	Cells of the thyroid gland	Hyperthyroidism	Hypothyroidism
Posterior Pituitary (Neurohypophysis)					
Antidiuretic hormone (vasopressin)	• Increases water reabsorption (inhibits diuresis) by kidney tubules and collecting ducts • Vasoconstriction of arterioles • Abdominal cramping	Increase in serum osmolality; hypernatremia; hypovolemia; hypoxia; hypotension; pain; trauma; stress; nausea; pharmacologic agents	Distal renal tubules and collecting ducts; smooth muscle of arterioles and GI tract	Syndrome of inappropriate antidiuretic hormone (SIADH)	Diabetes insipidus
Thyroid Gland					
Triiodothyronine (T_3) and thyroxine (T_4) NOTE: T_3 is more biologically active	• Stimulates metabolic rate • Increases protein synthesis • Increases carbohydrate and fat metabolism • Increases bone growth • Increases oxygen consumption • Increases metabolism and clearance of drugs	Thyroid-stimulating hormone (TSH) from anterior pituitary; thyrotropin-releasing hormone (TRH) from hypothalamus; cold temperature	Most body cells	Hyperthyroidism (chronic); thyroid storm or crisis (acute)	Hypothyroidism (chronic); myxedema coma (acute)

Continued

Table 9-1 Endocrine Glands and Hormones Significant in the Care of Critically Ill Adults—cont'd

Hormone	Actions	Releasing Factors	Target	Hypersecretion	Hyposecretion
Thyrocalcitonin (calcitonin)	• Reduces plasma calcium levels by inhibiting bone lysis and decreasing calcium resorption by the kidney	Increase in serum calcium, magnesium, or glucagon	Bone cells, kidney cells	Not significant	Not significant
Parathyroid Gland					
Parathyroid hormone (parathormone)	• Increases serum calcium by accelerating bone breakdown with release of calcium into the blood, increasing calcium reabsorption from intestine, and decreasing kidney tubule reabsorption of calcium • Decreases blood phosphate levels by increasing phosphate loss in urine • Increases reabsorption of magnesium by the renal tubules	Low serum calcium or magnesium or high serum phosphate level; catecholamines; cortisol	Bone cells, cells of GI tract and kidney	Hypercalcemia and hypophosphatemia; osteoporosis and possibly renal calculi; decreased neuromuscular irritability and muscle weakness	Hypocalcemia and hyperphosphatemia; neuromuscular irritability and tetany
Adrenal Cortex					
Glucocorticoids (i.e., cortisol)	• Increases blood glucose by stimulating gluconeogenesis in the liver • Inhibits glucose utilization by the cell • Inhibits protein anabolism • Promotes fatty acid mobilization • Inhibits inflammatory response	CRH from hypothalamus; ACTH from anterior pituitary	Most body cells	Cushing's syndrome	Addison's disease (chronic); adrenal crisis (acute)
Mineralocorticoids (i.e., aldosterone)	• Increases sodium and water reabsorption and potassium excretion	ACTH from anterior pituitary (minor effect); primary stimulus is renin-angiotensin system; decrease in serum sodium; increase in serum potassium	Distal and collecting tubules of kidney; sweat glands; salivary glands; intestines	Hyperaldosteronism	Addison's disease (chronic); adrenal crisis (acute)

Table 9-1 Endocrine Glands and Hormones Significant in the Care of Critically Ill Adults—cont'd

Hormone	Actions	Releasing Factors	Target	Hypersecretion	Hyposecretion
Adrenal Medulla					
Catecholamines (i.e. epinephrine, norepinephrine)	• Dilates pupils • Increases heart rate and contractility • Dilation of blood vessels to heart, brain, and skeletal muscle • Constriction of blood vessels to nonessential organs (i.e., skin, kidney, GI tract) • Bronchodilation • Increases in respiratory rate and depth • Increases in perspiration, peristalsis, and secretion in GI tract • Increases in blood sugar	Sympathetic nervous system innervation: insulin; histamine; anxiety; fear; pain; trauma; exercise; temperature extremes; hypoxia; hypotension; hypovolemia; excess thyroid hormone	Most body cells, vascular beds, smooth muscle	Exaggeration or prolongation of normal effects; may be caused by adrenal medulla tumor called *pheochromocytoma*	May have decrease in stress response or no noticeable effect
Pancreas					
Glucagon (from alpha cells)	• Stimulates glycogenolysis and gluconeogenesis to increase blood glucose • Inhibits glycolysis • Increases lipolysis	Decrease in blood glucose; elevated blood amino acid; catecholamines; exercise; starvation	Most body cells, especially liver cells	Hyperglycemia	Hypoglycemia
Insulin (from beta cells)	• Enables glucose to move into the cell • Aids in muscle and tissue oxidation of glucose • Enhances storage of glycogen • Increases protein synthesis • Inhibits lipolysis	Increase in blood glucose; gastrin; increase in growth hormone; ACTH; glucagon	Most body cells, especially liver cells	Hypoglycemia	Hyperglycemia (diabetes mellitus)

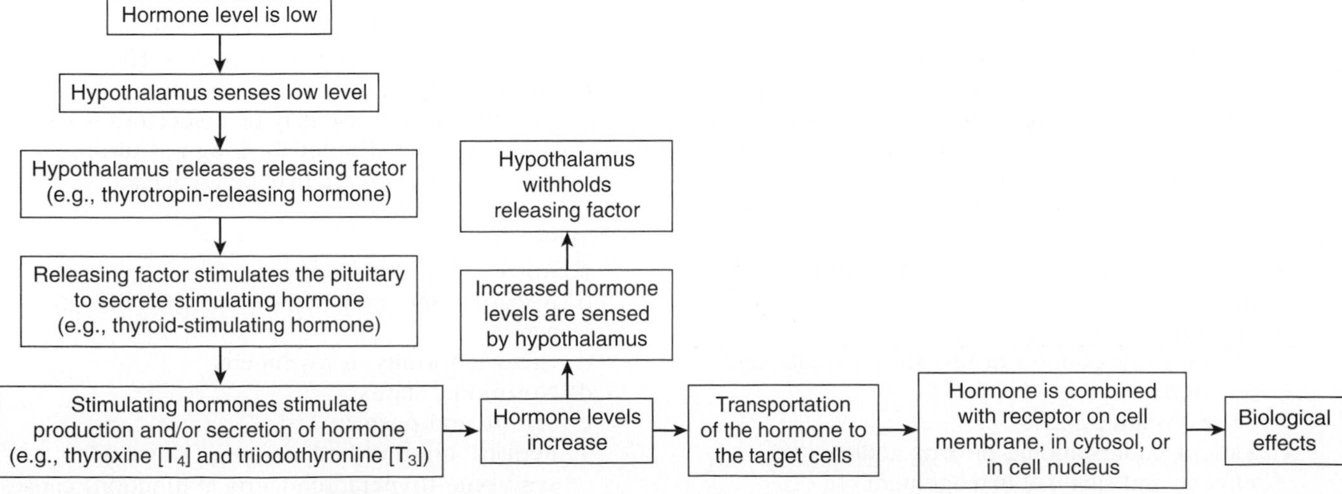

Figure 9-2 Process of hormone secretion, effect, and suppression.

2) Incontinence
3) Decreased libido
4) Menstrual irregularities

j. Musculoskeletal
1) Muscle or joint pain or aching
2) Muscle weakness
3) Muscle cramping
4) Muscle wasting
5) Twitching
6) Fractures

2. History of present illness: Use PQRST format (provocation, palliation, quality, quantity, region, radiation, severity, timing).
3. Past medical history: past illnesses or pathologic conditions that may result in endocrine dysfunction
   a. Trauma
   b. Ischemia or infarction
   c. Neoplasm
   d. Inflammation, infection
   e. Autoimmune conditions
   f. Acquired immunodeficiency syndrome (AIDS)
   g. Irradiation, antineoplastic drugs
   h. Surgical removal of an endocrine gland
   i. Interruption of prescribed pharmaceutical agent for treatment of a preexisting chronic endocrine dysfunction
4. Family history
   a. Diabetes mellitus
   b. Cardiovascular disease
   c. Cerebrovascular disease
   d. Cancer
5. Social history
   a. Relationship with spouse or significant other; family structure
   b. Occupation
   c. Educational level
   d. Stress level and usual coping mechanisms
   e. Recreational habits
   f. Exercise habits
   g. Dietary habits
      1) Usual diet
      2) Compliance with prescribed limitations
   h. Fluid intake
   i. Caffeine intake
   j. Tobacco use: recorded as pack-years (number of packs per day times the number of years the patient has been smoking)
   k. Alcohol use: recorded as alcoholic beverages consumed per month, week, or day
   l. Toxin exposure
   m. Travel
6. Medication history
   a. Prescribed drug, dose, frequency, and time of last dose
   b. Nonprescribed drugs
      1) Over-the-counter drugs, supplements, and herbs
      2) Substance abuse
   c. Patient understanding of drug actions, side effects, and sick day management
   d. Pharmacologic agents used to treat chronic endocrine dysfunction
      1) Hormone replacement
      2) Hormone suppressive agents
      3) Agents that trigger release of hormone or potentiate the effect of the hormone
      4) Vitamins or minerals necessary for body synthesis of hormones
   e. Evaluation of patient's compliance with prescribed therapy
   f. Pharmacologic agents that may alter endocrine function by either stimulating or inhibiting hormone release or interfering with hormone action at the target tissue; pharmacologic agents that may cause endocrine dysfunction are listed under Etiology for each endocrine condition

Inspection and Palpation

1. Vital signs
   a. BP: lying, sitting, standing; orthostatic BP changes due to hypovolemia may be seen in diabetes insipidus or diabetes mellitus
   b. Heart rate
      1) Bradycardia is frequently seen in hypothyroidism.
      2) Tachycardia may be associated with hyperthyroidism, infection (which may be a cause of DKA or HHS), hypovolemia (which may occur in DKA, HHS, or DI), and hypervolemia (which may occur in SIADH).
   c. Respiratory rate
      1) Bradypnea is frequently seen in hypothyroidism.
      2) Tachypnea may be associated with hyperthyroidism, infection (which may be a cause of DKA or HHS), hypovolemia (which may occur in DKA, HHS, or DI), and hypervolemia (which may occur in SIADH).
   d. Temperature
      1) Hypothermia may be associated with hypothyroidism.
      2) Hyperthermia may be associated with hyperthyroidism, with extreme hyperthermia during thyroid crisis.
      3) Hyperthermia may also indicate infection that may be a cause of DKA or HHS.
   e. Height and weight
      1) Weight increase may be associated with hypothyroidism or Cushing's syndrome.
      2) Weight decrease may be associated with hyperthyroidism.
2. General survey
   a. Apparent health status
   b. Apparent age (consistency with chronologic age)
   c. Gross deformity or asymmetry
   d. Nutritional status
   e. Stature and posture
   f. Redistribution of body fat (e.g., Cushing's syndrome [hyperadrenocortical function] causes

redistribution of fat with "buffalo hump," "moon face," and thick trunk with thin arms and legs)
   g. Gynecomastia in males: may be related to hypogonadism, hyperthyroidism, Cushing's syndrome
   h. Mobility
   i. Level of consciousness: Changes seen in cerebral function may occur.
   j. Presence of MedicAlert bracelet indicating chronic endocrine condition or steroid dependency
3. Head and neck
   a. Eyes
      1) Eyeballs
         a) Protruding eyeballs (exophthalmos): frequently seen in hyperthyroidism; lid lag frequently seen in patients with exophthalmos
         b) Sunken: may be seen in hypothyroidism or dehydration
      2) Strabismus: may be seen with hyperthyroidism
   b. Facial or periorbital edema: frequently seen in Cushing's syndrome; may also be seen in hypothyroidism
   c. Changes in visual acuity and visual fields: may be related to pituitary tumor
   d. Facial bone structure: facial changes including protruding forehead and prominent jaw seen in acromegaly
   e. Thyroid gland (the only endocrine gland that can be palpated)
      1) Enlargement or palpable mass or nodule
      2) Tenderness
      3) Presence of thrill
4. Skin and appendages
   a. Skin color changes
      1) Addison's disease causes characteristic "bronzing" of the skin.
      2) Gray-brown pigmentation around neck and axillae may be seen in Cushing's syndrome.
      3) Yellowish skin discoloration may be seen in hypothyroidism.
   b. Skin temperature: changes frequently seen in thyroid conditions
   c. Skin moisture and turgor
      1) Warm, moist, paper-thin skin may be seen in hyperthyroidism.
      2) Dry, scaly skin may be seen in hypothyroidism.
      3) Decreased skin turgor may be seen in dehydration, which may be seen in DI, DKA, and HHS.
   d. Skin lesions: acne; spider angiomas
   e. Mucous membranes: Note moisture.
   f. Scars (especially in neck area, which may indicate prior thyroid surgery)
   g. Bruising: Increased bruising may be seen in Cushing's syndrome.
   h. Striae: Purplish striae on abdomen may be seen in Cushing's syndrome.
   i. Hair changes
      1) Alopecia: may be seen in hyperthyroidism, hypothyroidism, and hypopituitarism
      2) Coarse hair: frequently seen in hypothyroidism
      3) Thin, silky hair: frequently seen in hyperthyroidism
      4) Increased body or facial hair: may be seen in acromegaly or Cushing's disease
   j. Brittle nails: frequently seen in hypothyroidism
   k. Enlargement and protrusion of tongue: may be seen in hypothyroidism or acromegaly
5. Cardiovascular
   a. Point of maximal impulse (PMI) displacement: may indicate cardiomegaly, which may be seen in hypothyroidism
   b. Heave: may be associated with heart failure, which may be seen in hyperthyroidism
   c. Peripheral pulses: increased or decreased quality
6. Pulmonary
   a. Odor of breath: acetone (fruity) breath noted in DKA
   b. Respiratory rate, depth, and rhythm
      1) Kussmaul's pattern associated with metabolic acidosis such as diabetic ketoacidosis
7. Neurologic
   a. Level of consciousness or mental status changes: may be related to intracranial mass (e.g., pituitary tumor), cerebral edema, or dehydration (e.g., ADH disorders)
   b. Pupil size, shape, and reactivity: Changes may be related to intracranial mass (e.g., pituitary tumor) or cerebral edema.
   c. Motor tone and strength
   d. Sensation
   e. Tremors
8. Gastrointestinal: abdominal mass or organ enlargement
9. Genitourinary: Suprarenal mass may indicate adrenal tumor (e.g., pheochromocytoma).

Percussion

1. Neurologic: Changes in deep tendon reflexes (increased or decreased) may be related to serum sodium changes seen in DI or SIADH.

Auscultation

1. Head and neck: thyroid gland bruits
2. Cardiovascular: heart sound changes
   a. S_3: indicative of HF, which may be seen in patients with hyperthyroidism
   b. Systolic murmur: frequently heard in high cardiac output states (e.g., hyperthyroidism)
3. Pulmonary
   a. Crackles noted with fluid overload and pulmonary edema
   b. Stridor noted in hypocalcemia associated with hypoparathyroidism
4. Gastrointestinal: bowel sound changes (hyperactive or hypoactive)

Diagnostic Studies

1. Serum
   a. Sodium: normal 136-145 mEq/L
   b. Potassium: normal 3.5-5 mEq/L
   c. Chloride: normal 96-106 mEq/L
   d. Calcium: normal 8.5-10.5 mg/dL
   e. Ionized calcium: normal 4.5-5.6 mg/dL
   f. Phosphorus: normal 3-4.5 mg/dL
   g. Magnesium: normal 1.5-2.2 mEq/L
   h. Glucose: normal 70-110 mg/dL
   i. Glycosylated hemoglobin: 4-7%
   j. Osmolality: normal 280-295 mOsm/kg
   k. BUN: normal 5-20 mg/dL
   l. Creatinine: normal 0.7-1.5 mg/dL
   m. Ketones: negative
   n. Thyroid-stimulating hormone (TSH): normal 2-10 mU/mL
   o. T_3: normal 0.2-0.3 mcg/dL
   p. T_4: normal 6-12 mcg/dL
   q. Antithyroglobulin antibody: normal less than 1:100; used in differential diagnosis of thyroid disease
   r. Radioactive iodine uptake test: normal 8-35%; increased in hyperthyroidism, iodine deficiency
   s. ACTH: normal 15-100 pg/mL in AM, less than 50 pg/mL in PM
   t. Cortisol: normal 6-28 mcg/dL at 8 AM, 2-12 mcg/dL at 4 PM
   u. ADH: normal 1-5 pg/mL
   v. Provocation tests: assess the endocrine gland's ability to respond to stimulus
      1) Assess the endocrine gland's reserve capacity
      2) Confirm hypo- or hyperfunction of the endocrine gland
   w. Arterial blood gases
      1) pH: normal 7.35-7.45
      2) $PaCO_2$: normal 35-45 mm Hg
      3) HCO_3: normal 22-26 mM
      4) PaO_2: normal 80-100 mm Hg
      5) SaO_2: normal 95-100%
   x. Hematocrit: normal 40-52% for males; 35-47% for females
   y. Hemoglobin: normal 13-18 g/dL for males, 12-16 g/dL for females
   z. White blood cells (WBC): normal 3500-11,000/mm^3
2. Urine
   a. Glucose: normal negative
   b. Ketones: normal negative
   c. Specific gravity: 1.005-1.03
   d. Osmolality: 50-1200 mOsm/kg
   e. 17-hydroxycorticosteroids: normal 4.5-10 mg/24 hr for males, 2.5-10 mg/24 hr for females
   f. 17-ketosteroids: normal 8-15 mg/24 hr for males, 6-12 mg/24 hr for females
3. Radiologic studies
   a. Skull series
   b. Chest x-ray
   c. Flat plate of abdomen (KUB)
   d. CT (computerized tomography) scan of head or abdomen
   e. Magnetic resonance imaging (MRI) of head or abdomen
   f. Pancreatic scan
   g. Thyroid scan
   h. Thyroid ultrasound
   i. Fine-needle aspiration biopsy of thyroid gland
   j. Adrenal angiography
   k. Brain scan
4. Other studies
   a. Electrocardiogram
   b. Electroencephalogram

Endocrine Pharmacology

Antidiuretic Hormone

1. Actions
   a. Increases water reabsorption in the renal tubule
   b. Reduces portal venous pressure through vasoconstriction
   c. Causes contraction of coronary, splanchnic, GI, pancreatic, skin, and muscular vascular beds
2. Indications
   a. Cardiac arrest (see Chapter 3)
   b. Gastrointestinal hemorrhage (see Chapter 7)
   c. Vasogenic forms of shock (i.e., septic) (see Chapter 11)
   d. Diabetes insipidus
3. Forms of ADH for DI (Table 9-2)
4. Side effects to monitor for: hypertension, chest pain, water intoxication, abdominal cramping

Insulin

1. Actions
   a. Stimulates cellular transport of glucose, amino acids, nucleotides, and potassium
      1) Glucose is converted to glycogen.
      2) Amino acids are used to build proteins.
      3) Fatty acids are incorporated into triglycerides.
   b. Promotes cell growth and division
2. Indication: hyperglycemia
3. Insulin preparations (Table 9-3)

Glucagon

1. Action: promotes the breakdown of glycogen, reduces glycogen synthesis, and stimulates biosynthesis of glucose to increase serum glucose level
2. Indication: hypoglycemia, beta-blocker intoxication with severe bradycardia
3. Administration: 0.5-1 mg IM, SC, or IV
4. Comments
   a. IV glucose is preferred in patients with severe hypoglycemia.
   b. Adequate glycogen stores are required so is ineffective if hypoglycemia is due to starvation
   c. Consciousness is expected within 20 minutes if used in patients who are unconscious due to

Table 9-2 Forms of Antidiuretic Hormone Replacement

Drug	Route	Comments
Synthetic ADH		
Vasopressin (Pitressin synthetic)	• IV, IM, SC: 5-10 units two to four times/day	• Short duration (2-8 hours)
ADH Analogs		
Desmopressin (DDAVP [1,deamino-8-D-arginine vasopressin], Stimate, Minirin)	• Nasal: 10-60 mcg every 12 hours (one to four sprays when 0.1 mg/mL) • IV, IM, or SC: 2-5 mcg two times/day • Oral: 100-300 mcg two to three times/day	• Relatively long duration (8-24 hours) with few side effects • May cause nasal congestion if given intranasally • Administer IV DDAVP via central vein catheter
Lysine vasopressin (DIAPID)	• Nasal: one to two sprays two to four times/day	• Shorter duration (4-6 hours) than DDAVP

Table 9-3 Characteristics of Insulin Preparations

Generic Name	Brand Name	Onset (min)	Peak (hr)	Duration (hr)
Short Duration/Rapid Acting				
Insulin lispro (SC)	Humalog	15-30	0.5-2.5	3-6.5
Insulin aspart	NovoLog	10-20	1-3	3-5
Insulin glulisine	Apidra	10-15	1-1.5	3-5
Short Duration/Slower Acting				
Human regular (IV)	Humulin R	Immediate	0.25-0.5	1-2
Human regular (SC)	Humulin R, Novolin R	30-60	1-5	6-10
Human regular (SC)	Exubera	15-30	0.5-1.5	6.6
Intermediate Duration				
Human NPH (SC)	Humulin N, Novolin N	60-120	6-14	16-24
Insulin detemir	Levemir	—	6-8	12-24*
Long Duration				
Insulin glargine	Lantus	70	No discernible peak	24

*Duration is dose dependent: At 0.2 unit/kg, duration is 12 hours, but at 2.5 units/kg, duration is 20-24 hours.
Adapted from Lehne, R. (2009). *Pharmacology for nursing care* (7th ed.). St. Louis: Saunders.

hypoglycemia; should be followed by oral carbohydrates and protein

Diabetes Insipidus (DI)

Definition

Clinical condition characterized by impaired renal conservation of water, resulting in polyuria, low urine specific gravity, dehydration, and hypernatremia; caused either by deficiency of ADH or decreased renal responsiveness to ADH

Etiology

1. Neurogenic (or central) DI: defect in synthesis or release of antidiuretic hormone (ADH) due to defect in hypothalamus, pituitary stalk, or posterior pituitary
   a. Primary: familiar, congenital, idiopathic
   b. Secondary
      1) Intracranial tumors: especially hypothalamic or pituitary; may be primary or metastatic tumor
      2) Extracranial neoplasm: leukemia; breast cancer
      3) CNS trauma: especially basal skull fracture
      4) Craniotomy
         a) Transient: Edema postcraniotomy causes obstruction of stalk between hypothalamus and posterior pituitary.
         b) Permanent: Hypophysectomy requires lifelong replacement of ADH.
      5) Intracerebral aneurysm, hemorrhage
      6) CNS infections (e.g., meningitis, encephalitis)
      7) Radiation
      8) Cerebral hypoxia and/or anoxic brain syndrome

Box 9-1 Drugs Affecting the Action of ADH

Drugs that Decrease the Amount or Action of ADH (May Cause DI)	Drugs that Increase the Amount or Effect of ADH (Some May Be Used to Treat DI)
• Alpha-adrenergic agents (e.g., norepinephrine) • Amphotericin B • Caffeine • Chlorpromazine (Thorazine) • Colchicine • Demeclocycline (Declomycin), a tetracycline derivative • Ethanol alcohol • Lithium • Phenytoin (Dilantin) • Reserpine (Serpasil) • Vinblastine	• Beta-adrenergic agents (e.g., isoproterenol) • Acetaminophen • Anticonvulsants: carbamazepine (Tegretol) • Antihyperlipidemics: clofibrate (Atromid-S) • Barbiturates • Cytotoxic agents: vincristine (Oncovin); cyclophosphamide (Cytoxan) • General anesthetics • Narcotics: morphine, meperidine • Nicotine • Oral hypoglycemics: chlorpropamide (Diabinese) • Thiazide diuretics: hydrochlorothiazide (HydroDIURIL) • Tricyclic antidepressants: amitriptyline (Elavil)

9) Granulomatous diseases (e.g., sarcoidosis, tuberculosis)
10) Drugs that inhibit the secretion of ADH (Box 9-1)
  a) Ethanol
  b) Phenytoin (Dilantin)
  c) Chlorpromazine (Thorazine)
  d) Reserpine (Serpasil)

2. Nephrogenic DI: defect in renal tubular response to ADH; usually less severe than neurogenic DI
   a. Congenital
   b. Renal disease
      1) Renal insufficiency
      2) Pyelonephritis
      3) Renal transplant
      4) Polycystic kidneys
      5) Metabolic diseases affecting the kidneys
         a) Amyloidosis
         b) Sarcoidosis
         c) Multiple myeloma
   c. Drugs that block the effect of ADH on the renal tubules (Box 9-1)
      1) Lithium
      2) Demeclocycline (Declomycin), a tetracycline derivative
      3) Alpha-adrenergic agents (e.g., norepinephrine)
      4) Caffeine
      5) Amphotericin B
      6) Colchicine
      7) Vinblastine
   d. Result of electrolyte imbalance
      1) Severe hypokalemia
      2) Hypercalcemia
3. Psychogenic DI
   a. Due to psychiatric disturbances with psychogenic polydipsia
   b. Also referred to as compulsive water drinking
4. Dipsogenic DI: due to an abnormality in the CNS thirst mechanism

Pathophysiology (Figure 9-3)

1. Deficiency of ADH or inadequate renal tubule response to ADH leading to inadequate antidiuresis
2. Diuresis of large volumes of hypotonic urine
3. Dehydration and hypernatremia
4. Potential shock and/or neurologic effects
5. Permanent versus temporary
   a. Permanent DI follows hypophysectomy (removal of pituitary gland).
   b. Temporary DI usually resolves within 3-5 days but may be up to 8 days.

Clinical Presentation

1. History of precipitating event: usually occurs within 24 hours of precipitating event but clinical indications may not occur for 1-3 days due to utilization of stored ADH
2. Subjective
   a. Thirst, especially for cold liquids
   b. Fatigue, weakness
3. Objective
   a. Polyuria: 5-15 L/24 hr; suspect DI if urine output is greater than 200 mL/hr for 2 consecutive hours
   b. Clinical indications of dehydration and volume depletion
      1) Weight loss
      2) Poor skin turgor
      3) Dry mucous membranes
      4) Sunken eyeballs
      5) Postural hypotension, tachycardia
      6) Decrease in CVP, RAP, and/or PAOP
   c. Neurologic signs resulting from hyperosmolality and hypernatremia
      1) Restlessness, confusion; irritability
      2) Seizures
      3) Lethargy, coma
4. Diagnostic
   a. Serum
      1) Sodium: elevated, greater than 145 mEq/L (hyperosmolar hypernatremia caused by water loss)
      2) BUN: elevated
      3) Increased serum osmolality: elevated, greater than 295 mOsm/kg
      4) Hct: elevated
      5) Serum ADH level: decreased (less than 1 pg/mL)
   b. Urine
      1) Specific gravity: decreased; less than 1.005

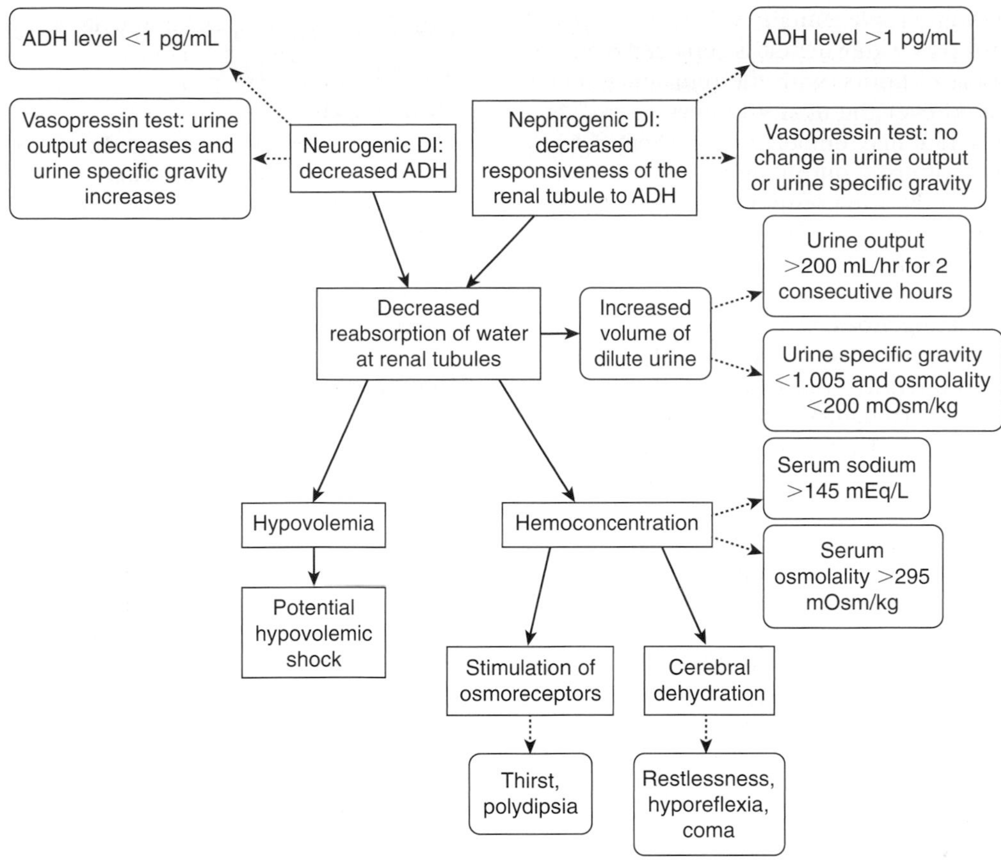

Figure 9-3 Pathophysiology of diabetes insipidus. Dotted lines connect pathology to clinical presentation. *ADH,* Antidiuretic hormone; *DI,* diabetes insipidus.

2) Osmolality: less than serum osmolality; less than 200 mOsm/kg

c. Water deprivation test may be performed. (NOTE: Because of the risks of dehydration, this test usually is not performed on a critically ill patient.)
   1) Prestudy weight, serum, urine osmolality, and urine specific gravity are measured.
   2) Fluid intake is withheld.
   3) Measurements are repeated hourly until one of the following occurs:
      a) Negative results: urine specific gravity exceeds 1.02; urine osmolality exceeds 800 mOsm/kg
      b) Positive results: 5% of body weight is lost or urine specific gravity does not increase after 3 consecutive hours
   4) Discontinue if hypotension, tachycardia, or lethargy occur.
   5) Inability to concentrate urine when fluid deprived suggests diabetes insipidus, and a vasopressin test should be performed

d. Vasopressin test
   1) Exogenous ADH (usually 5 units of aqueous vasopressin) is administered subcutaneously; urine specimens are collected every 30 minutes for 2 hours and evaluated for quantity and osmolality.
      a) If neurogenic DI: Urine output decreases and urine osmolality increases by more than 9%.
      b) If nephrogenic DI: No response to ADH will be seen.

Collaborative Management

1. Detect clinical indications of DI in high-risk patients.
   a. Monitor urine output hourly; measure urine specific gravity if indicated by an increase in urine output.
   b. Monitor weight daily and estimate fluid loss (1 kg = 1 L).
   c. Monitor serum sodium levels.
   d. Note or calculate serum osmolality.
   e. Monitor for clinical indications of hypovolemia and hypoperfusion.
   f. Monitor closely for changes in neurologic status.
2. Correct fluid deficit.
   a. Type of volume replacement
      1) Normal saline until intravascular volume is replaced (even if the patient is hypernatremic)
      2) Hypotonic solutions, such as 0.45% sodium chloride solution or D_5W, depending on degree of hyperosmolality once intravascular volume is restored

   b. Rate of volume replacement
      1) Half of free-water deficit is replaced over the first 24 hours, with the remaining deficit replaced over the next 48 hours.
      2) Hourly rate may initially be determined by volume of urine output and insensible losses (e.g., hourly urine output plus 50 mL/hr).
   c. Close monitoring for electrolyte losses and replace accordingly
3. Treat the cause.
   a. Administer exogenous ADH replacement as prescribed for neurogenic DI (see Table 9-2).
   b. Assist in preoperative preparation and postoperative management after hypophysectomy if pituitary tumor is the cause; usually done by transsphenoidal approach
      1) Incision is made in the gingiva above the maxilla, and then the pituitary gland is removed through the sphenoid.
      2) Antibiotic-impregnated nasal packing is usually maintained for 48-72 hours.
      3) CSF leak may be seen during first 72 hours; mustache dressing is used to collect CSF.
      4) Close monitoring of neurologic status, fluid and electrolyte balance, and urine output.
   c. Administer ADH potentiator as prescribed for nephrogenic DI (see Box 9-1).
      1) Chlorpropamide (Diabinese) used most often
         a) Stimulates the release of ADH from the pituitary gland and enhances its effect at the renal tubule
         b) Monitor for clinical indications of hypoglycemia.
      2) Thiazide diuretics (e.g., hydrochlorothiazide) and sodium restriction may also be used.
         a) Causes mild sodium depletion that enhances water reabsorption
         b) May be combined with indomethacin (Indocin) or amiloride (Midamor)
   d. Administer pharmacologic agents as prescribed for obsessive-compulsive behavior (e.g., serotonin reuptake inhibitors, tricyclic antidepressants, or monoamine oxidase inhibitors) or psychogenic polydipsia.
4. Correct electrolyte imbalance.
   a. Potassium replacement usually required
   b. Close monitoring of sodium; IV fluid with less sodium and more water (e.g., $D_5 \frac{1}{2}$ NS) if patient is hypernatremic or isotonic as serum sodium returns to normal
5. Maintain patient safety.
   a. Safe environment: side rails up; call light within reach
   b. Seizure precautions
   c. Frequent reorientation
6. Monitor for complications.
   a. Coma
   b. Hypovolemic shock
   c. Thromboembolism

Syndrome of Inappropriate Antidiuretic Hormone (SIADH)

Definition

1. Clinical condition characterized by impaired renal excretion of water, resulting in oliguria, high urine specific gravity, water intoxication, and hyponatremia
2. Caused either by excess of ADH or an ADH-like substance or an increased renal responsiveness to ADH

Etiology

1. Neurogenic SIADH: increased production and/or release of ADH
   a. Pituitary tumor
   b. CNS trauma
   c. Stroke: thrombotic or hemorrhagic
   d. Intracranial hematoma
   e. CNS infection: encephalitis, meningitis
   f. CNS hemorrhage
   g. Guillain-Barré syndrome
   h. Cerebral infarction or atrophy
   i. Nonmalignant pulmonary disease
      1) Tuberculosis
      2) Pneumonia
      3) Lung abscess
      4) Chronic obstructive pulmonary disease
      5) Positive pressure ventilation
2. Ectopic SIADH: production of a substance indistinguishable from ADH by tissue
   a. Oat-cell (small cell) cancer of the lung
   b. Duodenal cancer
   c. Pancreatic cancer
   d. Prostatic cancer
   e. Leukemia
   f. Lymphoma: Hodgkin's and non-Hodgkin's
   g. Thymoma
   h. Lymphosarcoma
3. Nephrogenic SIADH: pharmacologic agents that increase ADH secretion or ADH effect (see Box 9-1)
   a. General anesthetics
   b. Narcotics: morphine, meperidine
   c. Barbiturates
   d. Thiazide diuretics: hydrochlorothiazide (HydroDIURIL)
   e. Tricyclic antidepressants: amitriptyline (Elavil)
   f. Oral hypoglycemics: chlorpropamide (Diabinese)
   g. Acetaminophen
   h. Cytotoxic agents: vincristine (Oncovin); cyclophosphamide (Cytoxan)
   i. Nicotine
   j. Anticonvulsants: carbamazepine (Tegretol)
   k. Beta-adrenergic agents (e.g., isoproterenol)
   l. Antihyperlipidemics: clofibrate (Atromid-S)

Pathophysiology (Figure 9-4)

1. Increased secretion of ADH or an ADH-like substance or increased renal responsiveness to ADH
2. Failure of negative feedback system: ADH secretion continues in spite of low serum osmolality.

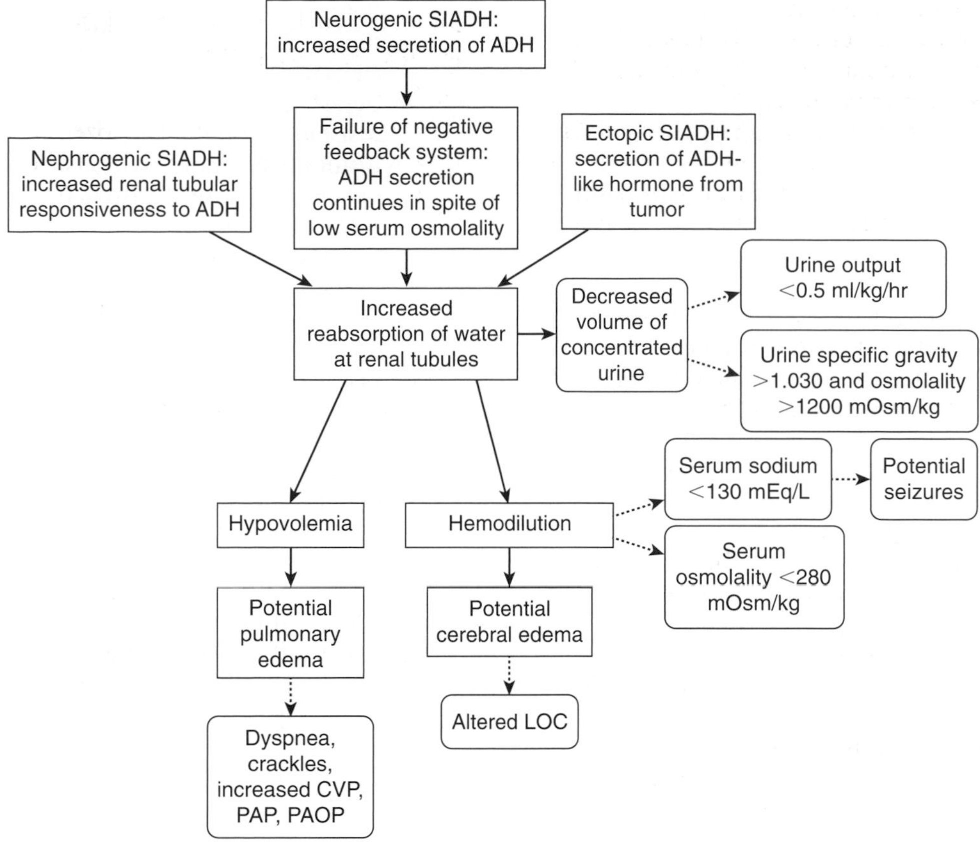

Figure 9-4 Pathophysiology of syndrome of inappropriate antidiuretic hormone (*SIADH*). Dotted lines connect pathology to clinical presentation. *ADH,* Antidiuretic hormone; *CVP,* central venous pressure; *LOC,* level of consciousness; *PAOP,* pulmonary artery occlusive pressure; *PAP,* pulmonary artery pressure.

3. Renal reabsorption of water increases.
4. Water intoxication
5. Hyponatremia, hypoosmolality
6. Potential cerebral edema and seizures

Clinical Presentation

1. Subjective
    a. Anorexia
    b. Nausea
    c. Dyspnea may be reported if pulmonary edema develops.
    d. Headache
    e. Inability to concentrate
    f. Muscle weakness and/or cramps
2. Objective
    a. Oliguria (less than 0.5 mL/kg/hr)
    b. Signs of fluid overload
        1) Tachypnea
        2) Hypertension
        3) Weight gain without edema
        4) Fever
        5) Jugular venous distention (JVD)
        6) Breath sound changes: crackles
        7) Increased CVP, PA, PAOP
    c. GI
        1) Vomiting
        2) Diarrhea
        3) Diminished bowel sounds
    d. Neurologic
        1) Personality changes
        2) Altered level of consciousness: confusion, lethargy → coma
        3) Decreased deep tendon reflexes
        4) Seizures related to hyponatremia
3. Diagnostic
    a. Serum
        1) Sodium: decreased; frequently less than 120 mEq/L (hypoosmolar hyponatremia caused by water retention)
        2) Potassium: may be decreased
        3) Calcium: may be decreased
        4) BUN: decreased
        5) Osmolality: decreased; less than 280 mOsm/L
        6) Plasma ADH: greater than 5 pg/mL
    b. Urine
        1) Specific gravity: elevated; greater than 1.03
        2) Osmolality: elevated; frequently greater than 1200 mOsm/L
    c. Water load test (NOTE: Because of the risks of fluid overload, this test usually is not performed in a critically ill patient)
        1) Patient is given an oral or IV fluid load (usually 20 mL/kg)
        2) Urine is collected over the next 5-6 hours.
            a) Normal (negative): excretion of 80% of amount of fluid administered

b) Positive: excretion of less than 40% of amount of fluid administered

Collaborative Management

1. Detect clinical indications of SIADH in high-risk patients.
   a. Monitor urine output hourly; measure urine specific gravity if indicated by a decrease in urine output.
   b. Monitor weight daily (1 kg = 1 liter).
   c. Monitor serum sodium levels.
   d. Note or calculate serum osmolality.
   e. Monitor for clinical indications of hypervolemia, pulmonary edema, and intracranial hypertension.
2. Treat the cause.
   a. Surgical intervention to remove malignant lesion if it is causative agent
   b. Demeclocycline (Declomycin), phenytoin (Dilantin), or lithium may be used to inhibit the action of ADH on the renal tubules, especially with ectopic ADH.
   c. Discontinuance of causative drugs if possible
3. Correct fluid volume excess.
   a. Fluid restriction based on amounts lost in urine and insensible losses; usually restricted to 1000 mL/day
   b. Diuretics to promote water excretion: usually furosemide (Lasix) or mannitol (Osmitrol)
4. Correct electrolyte imbalance.
   a. Dietary sodium should be encouraged.
   b. Hypertonic (3%) saline (usually 250-500 mL over several hours at rate of 1-2 mL/kg/hr) for serum sodium greater than 115 mEq/L or if patient is having seizures
      1) Hypertonic saline is usually discontinued when the serum sodium is 125 mEq/L.
      2) Monitor closely for clinical indications of pulmonary edema during and after hypertonic saline infusion.
   c. Potassium replacement may be needed.
5. Provide for patient safety.
   a. Safe environment: side rails up; call light within reach
   b. Seizure precautions
   c. Frequent reorientation
6. Monitor for complications.
   a. Intracranial hypertension
   b. Seizures
   c. Coma

Diabetic Ketoacidosis (DKA)

Definitions

1. Diabetes mellitus: a group of metabolic diseases characterized by hyperglycemia (confirmed fasting serum glucose of greater than or equal to 126 mg/dL) that results from defects in insulin secretion, insulin action, or both
   a. Type 1 diabetes is characterized by beta cell destruction, usually leading to absolute insulin deficiency; previously known as juvenile onset, type I, insulin-dependent diabetes mellitus (IDDM)
   b. Type 2 diabetes is characterized by insulin resistance and a relative (rather than absolute) insulin deficiency; previously known as age-onset, type II, non–insulin-dependent diabetes mellitus (NIDDM).
2. Hyperglycemic crises
   a. Diabetic ketoacidosis: hyperglycemic crisis associated with metabolic acidosis and elevated serum ketones; the most serious metabolic disturbance of type 1 diabetes mellitus
   b. Hyperglycemic hyperosmolar nonketotic condition: hyperglycemic crisis associated with the absence of ketone formation; most serious metabolic disturbance in type 2 diabetes mellitus

Etiology

1. Undiagnosed type 1 DM: 20% of patients with DKA
2. Causes in known type 1 DM
   a. Illness or infection
   b. Omission of exogenous insulin
   c. Trauma
   d. Surgery
   e. Noncompliance: too many calories
3. Causes in patients with or without diabetes
   a. Cushing's syndrome
   b. Hyperthyroidism
   c. Pancreatitis
   d. Pregnancy
   e. Drugs
      1) Glucocorticoids (e.g., prednisone)
      2) Thiazide diuretics (e.g., hydrochlorothiazide)
      3) Phenytoin (Dilantin)
      4) Sympathomimetics (e.g., epinephrine)
      5) Diazoxide (Hyperstat)

Pathophysiology

See Figure 9-5.

Clinical Presentation

1. Subjective
   a. Nausea
   b. Abdominal pain
   c. Polyphagia initially; may progress to anorexia with acidosis
   d. Weakness, fatigue
   e. Polydipsia
   f. Weight loss
   g. Headache
   h. Visual disturbances
2. Objective
   a. General
      1) Flushed, warm, dry skin
      2) Poor skin turgor
      3) Sunken eyeballs
      4) Hypothermia or hyperthermia
   b. Cardiovascular
      1) Tachycardia

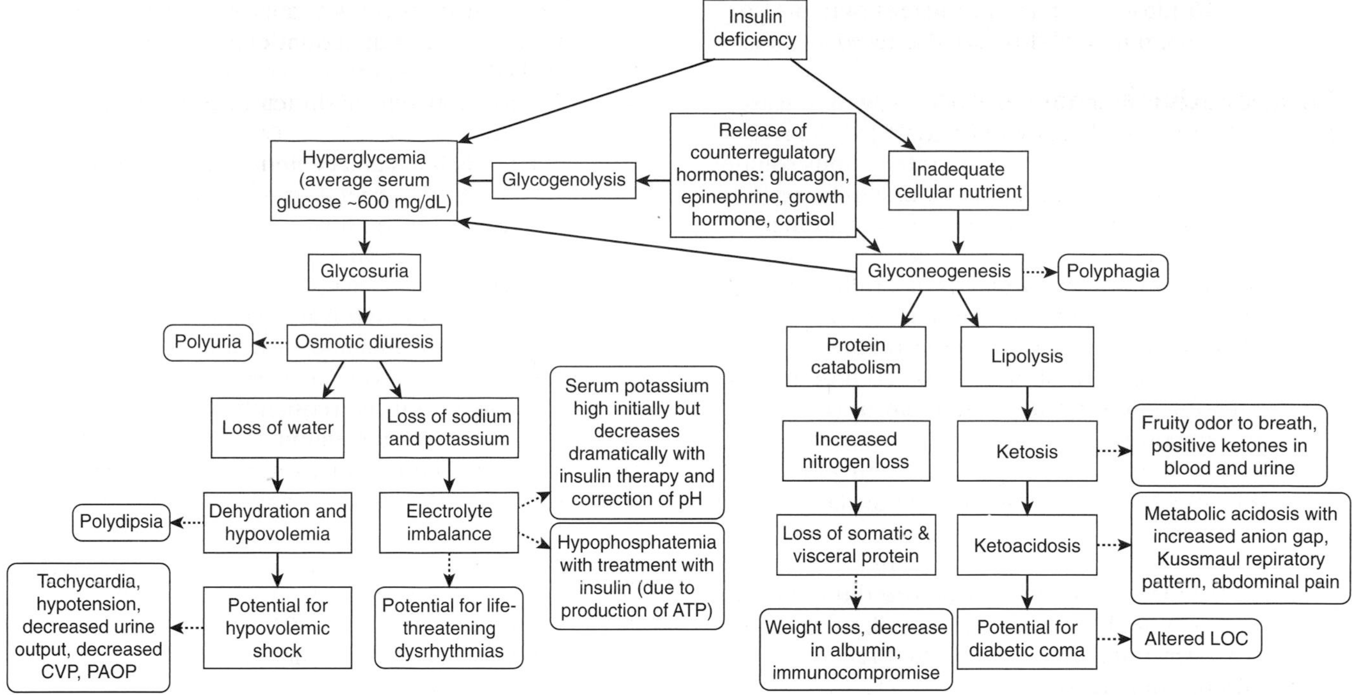

Figure 9-5 Pathophysiology of diabetic ketoacidosis (DKA). Dotted lines connect pathology to clinical presentation. *ATP,* Adenosine triphosphate; *CVP,* central venous pressure; *LOC,* level of consciousness; *PAOP,* pulmonary artery occlusive pressure.

2) Pulse may have decreased quality: 1+/3+
3) Orthostatic hypotension
4) Decreased CVP, PAP, PAOP, CO

c. Pulmonary
1) Kussmaul's ventilatory pattern
2) Acetone (fruity) odor to breath

d. Neurologic
1) Diminished deep tendon reflexes
2) Lethargy progressing to coma

e. Gastrointestinal
1) Vomiting
2) Hypoactive bowel sounds

f. Renal
1) Polyuria early
2) Oliguria late

3. Diagnostic
a. Laboratory
1) Serum
a) Glucose: elevated 300-800 mg/dL; average 600 mg/dL
b) Sodium: normal, elevated, or decreased depending on hydration status
c) Potassium
i) Elevated initially
ii) Decreased to normal or low as pH and dehydration are corrected
iii) Total body potassium is low.
d) Anion gap: elevated; greater than 15
i) Formula: $(Na^+ + K^+) - (Cl^- + HCO_3^-)$
ii) Normal: 5-15
iii) Increase in anion gap indicates an increase in metabolic acid (e.g., ketoacids).
e) Calcium: may be decreased
f) Phosphorus: normal initially but decreases with treatment with insulin and fluids
g) Magnesium: elevated initially and then decreased
h) Ketones: elevated; greater than 3 mOsm/kg
i) BUN and creatinine elevated with BUN:creatinine ratio greater than 10:1
j) Serum osmolality: elevated; usually 295-330 mOsm/kg
k) Lipids: may be elevated
l) Arterial blood gases: metabolic acidosis frequently with some degree of respiratory compensation
i) pH less than 7.3
ii) HCO_3 less than 15
iii) $PaCO_2$ less than 35 mm Hg
m) Hematocrit: elevated
n) WBC: elevated; unreliable indication of infection in DKA
2) Urine: positive for glucose and ketones

b. Electrocardiogram
1) May show changes associated with potassium levels
2) Sinus tachycardia is frequently seen.

Collaborative Management

1. Maintain oxygenation, ventilation, and circulation.
a. Oxygen by nasal cannula to maintain SpO_2 at least 95% unless contraindicated
b. Airway: intubation may be required if consciousness impaired
c. Correction of fluid volume deficit

1) Monitor for clinical and laboratory indications of dehydration, hypovolemia, and hypoperfusion.
2) Establish intravenous access with at least one large-gauge catheter.
3) Administer appropriate intravenous solution.
   a) Normal saline for the first 1-2 L or until the patient is hemodynamically stable; then normal (0.9%) saline if serum sodium is normal or if serum osmolality is less than 320 mOsm/kg; half-normal (0.45%) saline if hypernatremic or serum osmolality is less than 320 mOsm/kg
   b) Colloids such as albumin or plasma protein fraction may be needed, especially if the patient is hypotensive.
   c) Dextrose 5% is added (e.g., D_5NS or D_5½NS) when serum glucose reaches 250-300 mg/dL.
   d) Dextrose 10% may be used if serum glucose falls to 150 mg/dL or less.
4) Administer intravenous fluid replacement at appropriate rate.
   a) First hour: 10-30 mL/kg
   b) After first hour: 500-1000 mL/hr depending on cardiovascular status, volume deficit, and urine output
   c) Total volume deficit: usually 4-8 L

2. Normalize serum glucose level gradually.
   a. Monitor serum glucose every hour initially.
      1) Goal of insulin therapy is to decrease serum glucose by 50-100 mg/dL each hour.
      2) Rapid correction of serum glucose is associated with hypoglycemia, hypokalemia, and cerebral edema.
   b. Administer IV regular insulin injection as prescribed: usually 10-20 units (or 0.15 units/kg) followed by infusion.
   c. Initiate IV regular insulin infusion as prescribed: usually 5-10 units/hr (or 0.1 unit/kg/hr).
      1) Insulin is mixed in normal saline, and the IV tubing is flushed with 50 mL of insulin solution to saturate binding sites on the IV tubing before administration.
      2) Insulin infusion is usually decreased to 3-5 units/hr when serum glucose is less than 250 mg/dL and usually discontinued 1-2 hours after subcutaneous insulin is started.
   d. Administer subcutaneous regular insulin as prescribed: usually administered by sliding scale when serum glucose is less than 250 mg/dL, pH is greater than 7.2, and bicarbonate is greater than 18.

3. Correct electrolyte imbalance.
   a. Monitor for clinical, laboratory, and ECG indications of hyperkalemia (initially) and hypokalemia, hypophosphatemia, and hypomagnesemia (with insulin therapy).
   b. Replace potassium as prescribed.
      1) Potassium levels are monitored every 1-2 hours initially.
      2) Usually total body potassium is severely depleted, but serum levels show normal level or hyperkalemia due to an intracellular to extracellular shift because acidosis is present.
      3) Potassium replacement is started when potassium level is at upper limit of normal; usually in the form of KCl but a portion may be given in the form of KPO_4, depending on phosphorus levels
      4) Refractory hypokalemia suggests hypocalcemia and/or hypomagnesemia.
   c. Replace phosphorus as prescribed.
      1) Phosphorus is frequently low, especially with insulin therapy; replacement is indicated especially if patient is anemic, has HF, pneumonia, or any other cause of hypoxia (hypophosphatemia shifts the oxyhemoglobin curve to the left and impairs tissue oxygenation) or if the serum phosphate level is less than 1 mg/dL.
      2) One half to two thirds of potassium is replaced with KCl, and one third to one half of potassium is replaced with KPO_4.
      3) To prevent hypocalcemia, phosphate administration should not exceed 1.5 mEq/kg/24 hr.
   d. Replace magnesium as prescribed.
      1) Magnesium is frequently low.
      2) Usually replaced as 1-2 grams of 10% solution if renal function is adequate
   e. Monitor sodium and replace as prescribed.

4. Correct acid-base imbalance.
   a. Provide adequate rehydration and insulin therapy.
   b. Administer sodium bicarbonate as prescribed (NOTE: Sodium bicarbonate is only recommended for severe acidosis [pH 7 or less] and should be discontinued as soon as pH is 7.2.)
   c. Monitor for hyperchloremic acidosis caused by NaCl and KCl administration.

5. Ensure patient safety.
   a. Prevent aspiration due to paralytic ileus commonly seen in DKA.
      1) Keep head of bed elevated 30 degrees.
      2) Insert nasogastric tube as indicated.
   b. Maintain seizure precautions.
   c. Monitor serum glucose and electrolytes carefully.

6. Identify and treat cause.
   a. Assess for source of infection: Obtain cultures and administer antibiotics as prescribed.
   b. Assess knowledge level related to self-care; be alert to possible drug therapy errors, noncompliance with diet, and drug interactions.

7. Monitor for complications.
   a. Cardiovascular
      1) Hypovolemic shock
      2) Dysrhythmias
      3) Thromboembolism

4) Myocardial infarction
5) Pulmonary edema
b. Neurologic
1) Cerebral edema
2) Seizures
3) Coma
c. Pulmonary
1) ARDS
2) Pulmonary embolism
d. Endocrine: hypoglycemia
e. Renal
1) Acute renal failure
2) Electrolyte imbalances: potassium, sodium,; phosphorus, magnesium
f. Sepsis
8. Provide instruction and counseling regarding lifestyle modification and need for pharmacologic therapy.
a. Nonpharmacologic therapies
1) Monitoring and normalization of body weight
2) Dietary modifications
a) Low saturated fat
b) ADA diet for control of serum glucose
3) Cessation of tobacco use
4) Avoidance of alcohol
5) Regular aerobic exercise in moderation
6) Complementary therapies: relaxation; imagery, biofeedback
7) Stress reduction
8) Yearly flu and pneumococcal vaccine
9) Recognition of symptoms of hyperglycemia and hypoglycemia and when to call the physician
10) Measurement of body weight
b. Pharmacologic agents
1) Insulin therapy including sick day management
2) Control of hypertension, hyperlipidemia, and thyroid disorders

Hyperglycemic Hyperosmolar State (HHS)

Definition

Hyperglycemic crisis associated with the absence of ketone formation; most common severe metabolic disturbance in type 2 diabetes mellitus

Etiology

Usually seen in patients over 50 years old with glucose intolerance or type 2 diabetes mellitus; frequently iatrogenic

1. Noncompliance with diet or drug therapy in a patient with known type 2 DM
2. Acute illness
3. Trauma
4. Surgery
5. Infection
6. Pancreatitis
7. Burns
8. Hepatitis
9. Cushing's syndrome
10. Hyperthyroidism
11. Renal disease
a. Peritoneal dialysis
b. Hemodialysis
12. Hypertonic nutrition: enteral or parenteral
13. Alcohol
14. Drugs
a. Glucocorticoids (e.g., prednisone)
b. Thiazide diuretics (e.g., hydrochlorothiazide)
c. Loop diuretics (e.g., furosemide [Lasix])
d. Phenytoin (Dilantin)
e. Diazoxide (Hyperstat)
f. Immunosuppressive drugs
g. Beta-blockers (e.g., propranolol [Inderal])
h. Chlorpromazine (Thorazine)
i. Cimetidine (Tagamet)
j. Calcium channel blockers
k. Mannitol
l. Sympathomimetic drugs (e.g., epinephrine)
m. Thyroid preparations

Pathophysiology

See Figure 9-6.

Clinical Presentation

1. Subjective: weakness, fatigue
2. Objective
a. General
1) Weight loss
2) Flushed, warm, dry skin
3) Poor skin turgor
4) Polydipsia
5) Fever common
b. Cardiovascular
1) Tachycardia
2) Orthostatic hypotension
3) Decreased CVP, RAP, PAOP, CO/CI
c. Pulmonary: tachypnea
d. Neurologic
1) Sensory deficits: paresthesia
2) Motor deficits: paresis, plegia
3) Aphasia
4) Decreased deep tendon reflexes
5) Seizures
6) Lethargy progressing to coma
e. Renal
1) Polyuria early
2) Oliguria late
3. Diagnostic
a. Serum
1) Glucose 600-2000 mg/dL; average 1100 mg/dL
2) Sodium: normal or elevated
3) Potassium: decreased
4) Calcium: may be decreased
5) Phosphorus: decreased
6) Magnesium: decreased
7) Ketones: normal or only mildly elevated
8) BUN and creatinine: elevated with BUN : creatinine ratio greater than 10 : 1

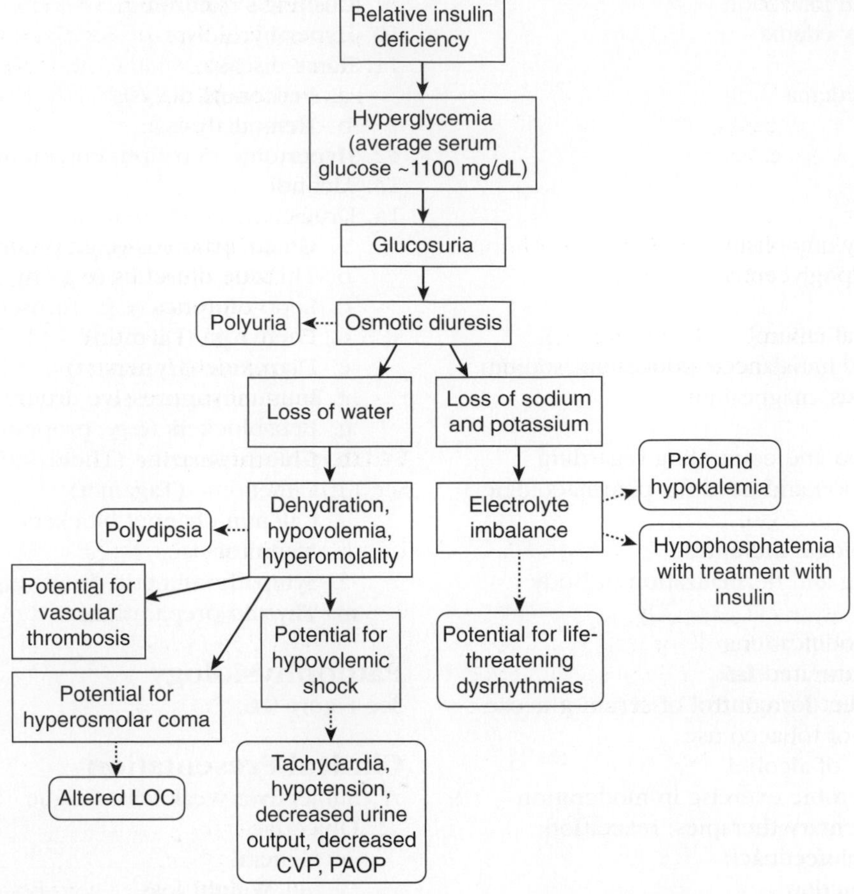

Figure 9-6 Pathophysiology of hyperglycemic hyperosmolar state (HHS). Dotted lines connect pathology to clinical presentation. *CVP,* Central venous pressure; *LOC,* level of consciousness; *PAOP,* pulmonary artery occlusive pressure.

9) Serum osmolality: elevated; usually greater than 330; may be as high as 450 mOsm/kg
10) Arterial blood gases
    a) Normal pH or only mildly acidotic
        i) Acidosis, if present, is lactic acidosis related to hypoperfusion instead of ketoacidosis
11) Hematocrit: elevated
12) WBC: elevated

b. Urine
    1) Glucose: positive
    2) Ketones: negative or trace
c. Electrocardiogram
    1) May show changes associated with potassium levels
    2) May show sinus tachycardia

Collaborative Management

1. Maintain oxygenation, ventilation, and circulation (as for DKA).
    a. Intravenous fluid replacement at appropriate rate: as for DKA except that total volume deficit is more significant (i.e., usually 8-15 L)
2. Normalize serum glucose level gradually (as for DKA).
    a. Even though HHS causes higher serum glucose levels, smaller amounts of insulin are needed to normalize serum glucose.
    b. IV insulin infusion usually discontinued when subcutaneous insulin is initiated; note that there is usually no overlap required in HHS
3. Correct electrolyte imbalance (as for DKA).
    a. Monitor for clinical, laboratory, and ECG indications of hypokalemia, hypophosphatemia, and hypomagnesemia (with insulin therapy).
4. Ensure patient safety (as for DKA).
5. Identify and treat cause.
    a. Assess for source of infection: Obtain cultures and administer antibiotics as prescribed.
    b. Monitor serum glucose in patients on enteral and parenteral nutrition, glucocorticoids, dialysis, and diuretics.
    c. Assess knowledge level related to self-care; be alert to possible drug therapy errors, noncompliance with diet, and drug interactions.
6. Monitor for complications.
    a. Cardiovascular
        1) Hypovolemic shock
        2) Dysrhythmias
        3) Thromboembolism
        4) Myocardial infarction
        5) Pulmonary edema
    b. Neurologic
        1) Intracranial hypertension
        2) Cerebral edema

3) Cerebral infarction
4) Coma
c. Pulmonary
1) ARDS
2) Pulmonary embolism
d. Endocrine: hypoglycemia
e. Renal
1) Acute renal failure
2) Electrolyte imbalances: potassium, sodium, phosphorus, and magnesium
f. Sepsis
7. Provide instruction and counseling regarding lifestyle modification and need for pharmacologic therapy (as for DKA).

Hypoglycemia

Definition

Less than normal serum glucose level.

1. Any serum glucose level of less than 70 mg/dL is hypoglycemia.
2. Symptomatic hypoglycemia generally occurs at a serum glucose level of 50 mg/dL or less, but symptoms may occur if a sudden decrease in serum glucose occurs even though the level is not less than 50 mg/dL.

Etiology

1. Insufficient nutrient intake
   a. Missed or delayed meal
   b. Nausea, vomiting
   c. Interrupted tube feedings or parenteral nutrition
2. Excessive insulin dose
   a. Poor visual acuity causing dose inaccuracy
   b. Change from pork or beef insulin to human insulin (Humulin)
   c. Injection in area of improved absorption
3. Drugs
   a. Sulfonylurea (e.g., glyburide, glipizide, glimepiride) therapy
      1) Renal insufficiency potentiates effects.
      2) Hepatic insufficiency delays metabolism and excretion and impairs gluconeogenesis and glycogenolysis.
      3) Potentiated by salicylates, sulfonamides, phenylbutazone, alpha-glucosidase inhibitors (e.g., acarbose [Precose], miglitol [Glyset])
   b. Ethanol
   c. Quinidine
   d. Disopyramide
   e. Alpha-blockers
   f. Salicylates
   g. Haloperidol
   h. Trimethoprim-sulfamethoxazole
4. Inadequate production of glucose
   a. Strenuous physical exercise or stress with inadequate adjustment of food intake and/or insulin dosage
   b. Excessive alcohol intake ingested without adequate food intake
   c. Glucagon deficiency
5. Postgastrectomy
6. Pancreatic islet cell necrosis: may occur with pentamidine therapy for *Pneumocystis carinii* infection; causes an acute increase in insulin release
7. Adrenal insufficiency
8. Severe liver disease
9. Pregnancy
10. Tumors
   a. Non–beta-cell tumors
      1) Malignant: sarcoma, mesothelioma, hepatomas, lymphoma, leukemia, adrenal carcinoma
      2) Benign: carcinoid and carcinoidlike tumors, pheochromocytoma
   b. Beta-cell tumors (i.e., insulinomas)

Pathophysiology

See Figure 9-7.

Clinical Presentation

1. Subjective
   a. Adrenergic (sympathetic) stimulation indicators
      1) Palpitations
      2) Anxiety
      3) Nausea
      4) Weakness
   b. Neuroglycopenic indicators
      1) Hunger
      2) Anxiety
      3) Paresthesia
      4) Blurred vision, diplopia
      5) Headache
      6) Irritability, difficulty with concentration
      7) Fatigue
2. Objective
   a. Adrenergic (sympathetic) stimulation indicators
      1) Diaphoresis
      2) Pallor, cool skin
      3) Tremors
      4) Piloerection
      5) Tachycardia, tachypnea
   b. Neuroglycopenic indicators
      1) Vasomotor changes: hypotension
      2) Slurred speech
      3) Agitation
      4) Confusion
      5) Staggering gait
      6) Sensory changes: paresthesias
      7) Motor changes: paresis, hemiplegia, paraplegia
      8) Seizures
      9) Coma
   c. Nocturnal hypoglycemia
      1) Restless sleep
      2) Nightmares
      3) Early morning headache
3. Diagnostic
   a. Serum glucose: 50 mg/dL or less
      1) 20 to 40 mg/dL is associated with seizures
      2) Less than 20 mg/dL is associated with coma
   b. Electrocardiogram: Sinus tachycardia is seen.
   c. BUN, creatinine, liver function studies

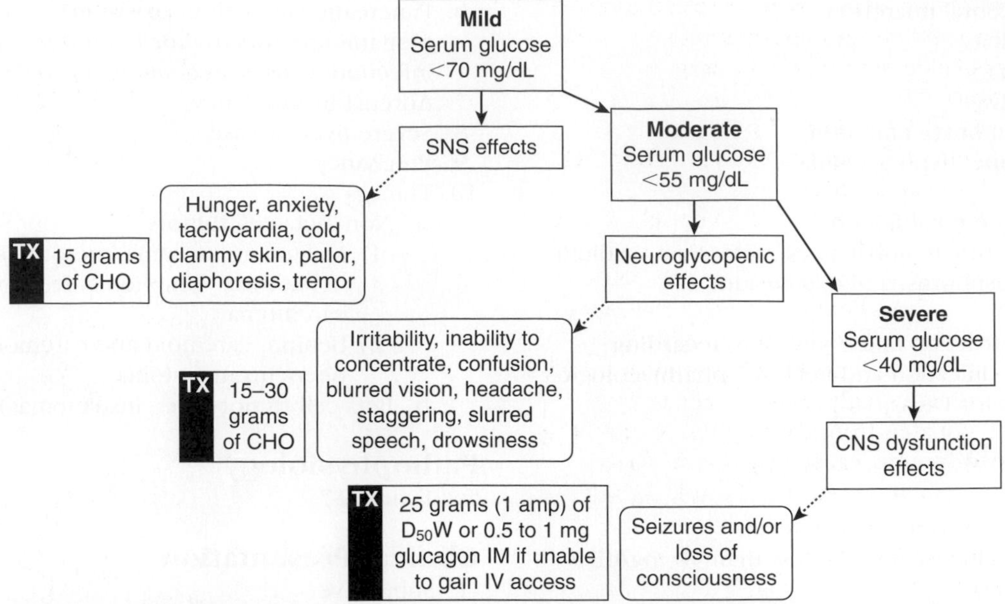

Figure 9-7 Pathophysiology of hypoglycemia. Dotted lines connect pathology to clinical presentation. *CHO,* Carbohydrate; *CNS,* central nervous system; *IM,* intramuscular; *IV,* intravenous; *SNS,* sympathetic nervous system; *TX,* treatment.

Box 9-2 Foods Providing 15 Grams of Carbohydrates for Treatment of Hypoglycemia

3 (5 g) glucose tablets
6 oz of apple or orange juice
6 oz of nondiet cola or other carbonated beverage
8 oz of skim or 1% milk
25 mL of $D_{50}W$ if patient is unable to take calories orally
4 cubes or 2 packets of sugar

d. Drug screen for possible drug cause may be indicated.

Collaborative Management

1. Restore normal serum glucose level.
   a. Measure serum glucose level immediately when clinical indications of hypoglycemia occur.
   b. Administer 15 grams (60 calories) of carbohydrates for conscious patients; for examples, see Box 9-2.
      1) Glucose tablets or gel is **required** if the patient has been receiving an alpha-glucosidase inhibitor (e.g., acarbose [Precose], miglitol [Glyset]) because these agents block the conversion of carbohydrates to glucose.
   c. Administer parenteral glucose if patient is unconscious.
      1) $D_{50}W$ injection: usually 50 mL (25 grams) over 3-5 minutes
         a) Thiamine 100 mg IV recommended prior to dextrose administration, especially in alcoholics to prevent Wernicke's encephalopathy
         b) $D_{10}W$ or D_5W infusion to follow as prescribed
      2) Glucagon 0.5 to 1 mg IM may be given to unconscious patients if unable to gain IV access
   d. Provide longer-acting carbohydrate source (milk, cheese, crackers) or regularly scheduled meal to avoid recurrence.
   e. Reassess serum glucose 15 minutes after treatment and every 15 minutes until serum glucose is within normal range; an additional 50 mL of $D_{50}W$ may be required for refractory hypoglycemia.
2. Prevent injury.
   a. Maintain airway if patient is unconscious.
   b. Monitor closely for seizures; maintain seizure precautions.
3. Identify and treat cause of hypoglycemia.
   a. Assess serum glucose by laboratory or bedside glucose-monitoring device as indicated.
   b. Anticipate times when the patient is most likely to exhibit hypoglycemia.
      1) Be aware of peak times for administered insulin therapy (Table 9-3).
      2) Be aware of missed or late meals or snacks that predispose the patient to hypoglycemia.
      3) Be aware of excessive exertion that may predispose the patient to hypoglycemia.
      4) Note any drugs that the patient is receiving that may potentiate insulin.
      5) Be aware (and make patient and family aware) that beta-blockers block the SNS (early) symptoms of hypoglycemia; serum glucose testing should be done more frequently in patients on beta-blockers.

c. Assess knowledge level related to self-care; be alert to possible drug therapy errors, noncompliance with diet, and drug interactions.
d. Assist with additional diagnostic studies if hypoglycemia is experienced by a patient who is not a known diabetic.
e. Consider Somogyi phenomenon (insulin-induced posthypoglycemic hyperglycemia) as cause of early morning hyperglycemia (Figure 9-8)
   1) The result of counterregulatory hormone secretion in response to hypoglycemia
   2) Results in early morning hyperglycemia after nighttime hypoglycemia; needs to be differentiated from dawn phenomenon (i.e., hyperglycemia caused by nocturnal elevations in growth hormone)
   3) Best documented by 3 AM serum glucose
   4) Treated by a decrease in insulin dose and/or bedtime snack
f. Administer hydrocortisone as prescribed if adrenal insufficiency is suspected.

4. Monitor for complications.
   a. Myocardial ischemia or infarction
   b. Seizures
   c. Coma
   d. Irreversible neurologic damage
5. Provide instruction and counseling regarding lifestyle modification and need for pharmacologic therapy.
   a. Importance of not skipping meals
   b. Recognition of symptoms of hyperglycemia and hypoglycemia and when to call the physician
   c. Insulin and/or oral hypoglycemic agents, including sick day management
   d. Control of hypertension, hyperlipidemia, and thyroid disorders

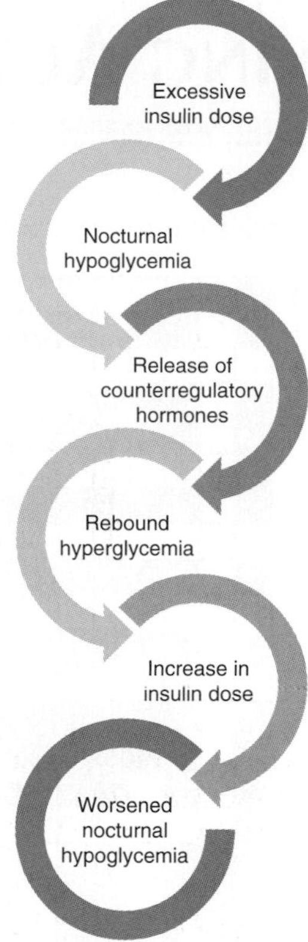

Figure 9-8 Somogyi effect.

LEARNING ACTIVITIES

CHAPTER 9

1. Complete the following crossword puzzle.

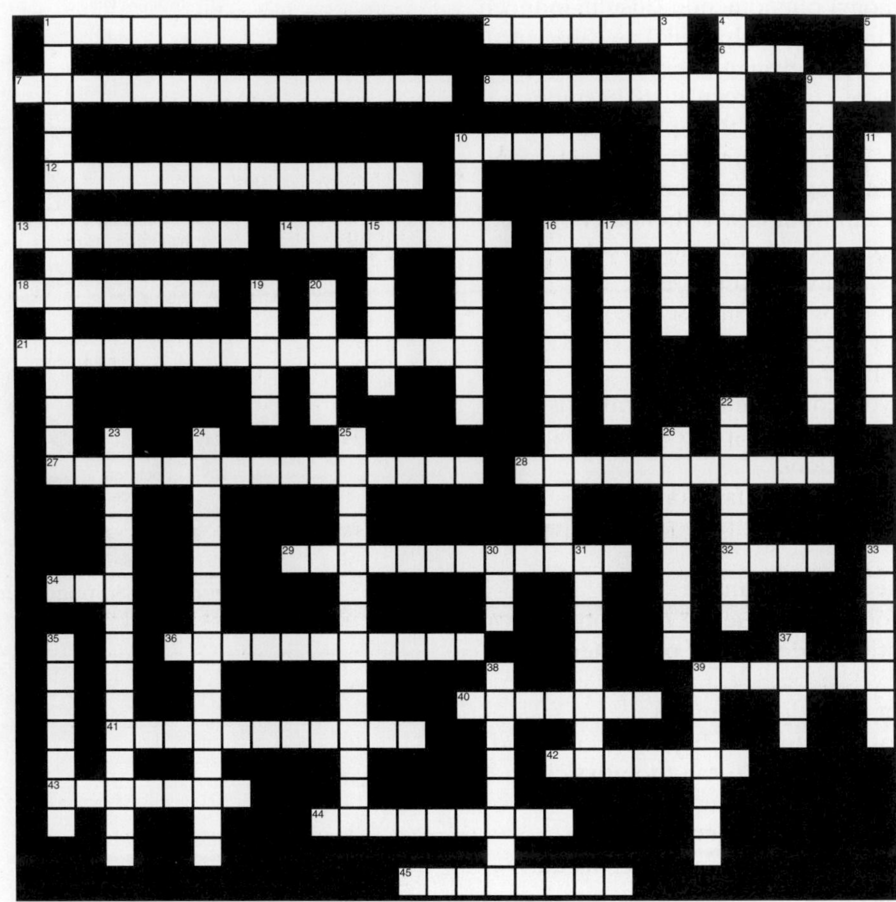

ACROSS

1. This organ produces glucagon and insulin
2. This area of the adrenal gland produces epinephrine and norepinephrine
6. This hormone is produced by the hypothalamus and stored in and released by the posterior pituitary (abbrev)
7. These hypoglycemic effects are caused by low brain glucose
8. This type of diabetes is caused by ADH deficiency
9. This hyperglycemic crisis occurs in type 2 diabetes mellitus or in patients with glucose intolerance (abbrev)
10. DKA causes an increase in this "gap"
12. This is most likely the result of insulin deficiency but also may be caused by stress, steroids, or insulin resistance
13. This hormone is considered a stress hormone and is produced by the adrenal cortex
14. This hormone triggers glycogenolysis and gluconeogenesis
16. In DI and HHS the serum becomes _____
18. Hyperglycemia caused by counterregulatory hormones released in response to hypoglycemia
21. This electrolyte imbalance occurs with insulin therapy in DKA because glucose moves into the cell and increased amounts of ATP are produced
27. Another term for the anterior pituitary
28. This type of DI is caused by decreased responsiveness of the renal tubule to ADH
29. The treatment for hypoglycemia in a conscious patient is 15 g of ____
32. This hormone is produced by the anterior pituitary gland that causes the production and release of hormones from the adrenal cortex (abbrev)
34. This hormone is produced by the anterior pituitary that stimulates the thyroid gland (abbrev)
36. This type of drug blocks the early symptoms of hypoglycemia
39. This endocrine gland is located on top of the kidney
40. _____'s syndrome is caused by an excess of hormones from the adrenal cortex
41. This electrolyte imbalance is noted in DKA as the acidosis is corrected and in HHS
42. This occurs in DKA but not in HHS
43. This hormone enables glucose to move into the cell

44. This type of endocrine disorder is caused by a problem with the pituitary gland
45. This type of diabetes is caused by insulin deficiency

DOWN

1. This benign tumor of the adrenal medulla causes labile hypertension
3. This hormone is secreted by the adrenal cortex and causes the retention of sodium and water
4. This is another name for ADH
5. The initial symptoms of hypoglycemia are caused by stimulation of the ___ (abbrev)
9. A serum glucose less than normal
10. This disorder is caused by excessive secretion of growth hormone in an adult
11. This type of DI results from a deficiency in the secretion of ADH from the posterior pituitary
15. The hormones from this area of the adrenal gland can be remembered as sugar (cortisol), salt (aldosterone), and sex (androgen)
16. This electrolyte imbalance is noted in DKA due to acidosis causing the shift of potassium from intracellular to extracellular
17. This type of endocrine disorder is caused by a problem in the target gland
19. These cells produce glucagon
20. This form of vasopressin replacement is used nasally in patients with permanent DI (abbrev)
22. This type of regulation controls the release or retention of hormones
23. Another term for the posterior pituitary
24. A complication in HHS caused by severe dehydration
25. This oral hypoglycemic agent potentiates the action of ADH on the renal tubules; may be used for nephrogenic DI (generic)
26. The change in urine output that occurs in DI, DKA, and HHS
30. This hyperglycemic crisis occurs in type 1 DM (abbrev)
31. This is given with glucose for hypoglycemia in patients with substance abuse to prevent Wernicke's encephalopathy
33. Insulin manufactured using recombinant DNA technology so nonantigenic (trade)
35. This endocrine gland is located in the neck and produces hormones that control metabolic rate
37. These cells produce insulin
38. _____'s respirations are seen in DKA due to the metabolic acidosis
39. _____'s disease is caused by a deficiency of hormones from the adrenal gland

2. Identify whether these factors increase or decrease ADH release or action.

Lithium	
Alcohol	
Chlorpropamide (Diabinese)	
Positive pressure ventilation	
Chlorpromazine (Thorazine)	
Phenytoin (Dilantin)	
Hydrochlorothiazide (HydroDIURIL)	
Anesthetic agents	
Demeclocycline (Declomycin)	
Beta stimulants	
Morphine sulfate	

3. Identify whether these factors are increased or decreased in DI and SIADH.

	DI	SIADH
Serum ADH		
Urine output		
Urine specific gravity		
Urine osmolality		
Serum osmolality		
Serum sodium		
Right atrial/pulmonary artery occlusive pressures		

4. A 45-year-old man was admitted to the surgical intensive care unit yesterday after a craniotomy. Today his urine output has increased dramatically over the last couple of hours. His urine output has been 600 mL over the last 2 hours, and the urine is very dilute with a specific gravity of 1.004. Calculate his serum osmolality and identify the likely cause of the following laboratory values.

Serum sodium	158 mEq/L
Serum potassium	3.8 mEq/L
Serum glucose	110 mg/dL
BUN	32 mg/dL
Serum creatinine	1 mg/dL
Hematocrit	45%
Urine osmolality	195 mOsm/kg

____

____

5. Complete this table.

	DKA	HHS
Type of diabetes mellitus		
Onset		
Typical serum glucose range		
Presence of ketosis		
pH		
Anion gap		
Respiratory pattern		
Breath odor		
Serum osmolality		
Serum sodium		
Serum potassium		
BUN		
Average fluid deficit		

6. Identify the following clinical indications as DKA, HHS, or both.

Serum glucose greater than 300 mg/dL	
Kussmaul's respirations	
pH less than 7.3	
Positive serum and urine ketones	
Abdominal pain	
Dehydration	
Lethargy → coma	
Serum glucose greater than 600 mg/dL	

7. Identify the following clinical indications as DKA, hypoglycemia, or both.

Headache	
Serum glucose more than 300 mg/dL	
Abdominal pain	
Cold, clammy skin	
Nervousness, tremors	
Polyuria	
Lethargy → coma	
Seizures → coma	
Glycosuria	
Tachycardia	
Agitation, difficulty with concentration	
Weakness, fatigue	
Fruity breath	
Serum glucose less than 50 mg/dL	

8. Match the following endocrine conditions with appropriate pharmacologic therapy. More than one therapy may be listed for each condition.

___ 1. Neurogenic DI
___ 2. Nephrogenic DI
___ 3. DKA
___ 4. HHS
___ 5. Hypoglycemia
___ 6. SIADH

a. 50% dextrose
b. Chlorpropamide (Diabinese)
c. Parenteral fluids
d. Insulin
e. Thiazide diuretics
f. Vasopressin
g. Loop diuretics
h. Potassium
i. 3% saline

The Hematologic and Immunologic Systems

Selected Concepts in Anatomy and Physiology

Purposes of the Hematologic and Immunologic Systems

1. Hematologic
   a. Provides the medium for transportation of oxygen, carbon dioxide, and nutrients to the tissues
   b. Maintains hemostasis
   c. Maintains internal environment, including participation in regulation of temperature and acid-base balance
2. Immunologic
   a. Protects the body's internal milieu against invading organisms and the development, growth, and dissemination of abnormal cells
   b. Maintains homeostasis by removing damaged cells from the circulation

Bone Marrow

1. Adults have 30-50 mL of bone marrow per kg of body weight
2. Most functioning bone marrow in adults is located in flat bones (vertebrae, skull, pelvic and shoulder girdles, clavicle, ribs, sternum) and proximal epiphysis of long bones.
3. The functions of the bone marrow include:
   a. Production of the following:
      1) Erythrocytes (red blood cells)
      2) Leukocytes (white blood cells), including granulocytes (i.e., neutrophils, eosinophils, basophils), agranulocytes (i.e., monocytes), and lymphocytes
      3) Thrombocytes (platelets)
   b. Recognition and removal of senescent cells
   c. Participation in cellular and humoral immunity

Spleen

1. White pulp: primarily supports humoral immunity; performs the following functions:
   a. Production of lymphocytes
   b. Stimulation of B cell activity to produce immunoglobulins; therefore, splenectomized patients have a greatly increased risk of sepsis with encapsulated microorganisms
   c. Storage site for splenic reticuloendothelial tissue and immunoglobulins
2. Red pulp: contains reticuloendothelial tissue; performs the following functions:
   a. Storage and release of RBCs into the circulation
      1) Caused by contraction of smooth muscle in the capsule surrounding the spleen and in invaginations of the capsule, called *trabeculae*
      2) When stimulated by the SNS, as much as 100 mL of concentrated RBCs can be released into the circulation, raising the hematocrit by 1-2%.
   b. Filtering and destruction (by the process of phagocytosis) of damaged or old erythrocytes (referred to as *culling*)
      1) Removes particles from intact RBCs without destroying them (referred to as *pitting*)
      2) Catabolizes hemoglobin released from RBCs that have been destroyed by the spleen; iron returned to the bone marrow for reuse
   c. Filtering and trapping foreign material, including bacteria and viruses
   d. Storage and release of platelets; destruction of damaged or senescent platelets

Liver

Performs the following functions:

1. Filtering of blood as it comes from the gastrointestinal tract
   a. Removal of foreign material, including microorganisms, damaged or old RBCs, and other degradation products by the Kupffer cells lining the sinusoidal beds of the liver
   b. Destruction of RBCs produces bilirubin, which the liver converts to bile, necessary for fat digestion.
2. Elimination of immune complexes (e.g., antigen-antibody complexes) from the blood

3. Detoxification of toxic substances that enter the blood
4. Manufacture of some clotting factors (i.e., vitamin K-dependent factors II, VII, IX, X) and antithrombin
5. Storage of blood (e.g., in heart failure, the liver becomes engorged with blood)

Lymphatic System

1. Lymph: pale yellow fluid that transports lymphocytes
   a. Composition
      1) Contains lymphocytes, granulocytes, enzymes, and antibodies
      2) Deficient in platelets and fibrinogen, so it coagulates very slowly
   b. Function: return of proteins and fat from GI tract, excess interstitial fluid, and certain hormones to the blood
2. Lymph circulation
   a. Lymphatic capillaries are somewhat larger than blood capillaries and irregular in diameter.
   b. Lymphatic vessels are formed by lymphatic capillaries.
   c. Lymph ducts drain into subclavian veins.
      1) The right lymphatic duct collects lymph from the right side of the head, neck, and thorax and from the right arm, right lung, right side of heart, and right upper surface of the diaphragm.
      2) The thoracic duct collects lymph from all other parts of the body.
   d. Lymph nodes are small, bean-shaped organs located along lymph vessels.
      1) Spongy and multichanneled on inside
      2) Sites of B and T cell lymphocyte production and maturation prior to distribution
      3) Functions
         a) Lymph nodes filter and allow WBCs to phagocytose bacteria and foreign material carried by lymph.
         b) Granulocytes, macrophages, and lymphocytes pass through the lymph node to return to the blood.
      4) Enlargement of lymph nodes
         a) This occurs with inflammation, infection, or malignancy.
         b) Enlargement of superficial nodes can be palpated; enlarged deep nodes can only be visualized on x-ray or computed tomography.
   e. Additional lymphoid tissue synthesizes immunoglobulins A (IgA) and E (IgE) and is located in the submucosa of the respiratory, intestinal, or genitourinary tracts.
      1) Mucosa-associated lymphoid tissues (MALT): clusters of T and B lymphocytes, macrophages, and phagocytes dispersed in the mucosal linings of the respiratory, gastrointestinal, and genitourinary tracts
      2) Gut-associated lymphoid tissue (GALT): Peyer's patches in the intestinal tract
3. Thymus
   a. Location: anterosuperior mediastinum below the thyroid gland; each lobe packed with lymphocytes
   b. Function
      1) Site of maturation and distribution of T lymphocytes
      2) Secretes a hormone, thymosin, which is thought to stimulate immune function
4. Glial cells
   a. Location: white matter of the brain
   b. Function: lymphocyte-rich tissue that functions to destroy foreign matter that crosses the blood-brain barrier

Blood

1. Plasma comprises 55% of total blood volume
   a. Composed of serum and plasma proteins, including prealbumin, albumin, serum globulins, fibrinogen, prothrombin, and plasminogen
   b. Hematocrit expresses the percentage of red blood cells in the total blood volume; affected by the fluid component of the blood
      1) Increased Hct may indicate polycythemia or hemoconcentration.
      2) Decreased Hct may indicate anemia or hemodilution.
2. All blood cells originate from pluripotential stem cells that differentiate into myeloid and lymphoid lineage cells.
   a. Erythroid stem cells (pronormoblasts) develop into reticulocytes and finally into erythrocytes.
   b. Myeloid stem cells (myeloblasts or monoblasts) develop into granulocytes and monocytes.
   c. Lymphoid stem cells (lymphoblasts) develop into B and T lymphocytes.
   d. Thrombocytic stem cells (megakaryoblasts) develop into thrombocytes.
3. Erythrocytes are also referred to as *red blood cells* or *RBC.*
   a. Structure
      1) Erythrocytes are nonnucleated round biconcave cells.
      2) The inner part of RBCs (referred to as *stoma*) is the location of hemoglobin attachment and contains the antigens that determine ABO and Rh blood type.
   b. Function of RBCs
      1) Transport oxygen from lungs to tissues
      2) Participate in maintenance of acid-base balance
      3) Provide insulation and weight to the blood
      4) Are highly permeable to hydrogen, chloride, and bicarbonate ions and water
   c. Types of RBCs
      1) Reticulocytes: immature RBCs
         a) Useful in assessing erythrocyte production; elevated reticulocyte count (i.e., greater than 25% of total RBC count) means that production of new RBCs is greater

b) Mature in 1-4 days after release and function like normal RBCs but may have a shortened life span
c) May be released after sudden blood loss, such as hemorrhage; repeated challenges to this compensatory mechanism lead to exhaustion of reserve reticulocytes
2) Erythrocytes: mature RBCs
a) Life span is approximately 120 days.
b) The spleen acts as RBC reservoir; contains 1-2% of circulating RBCs.

d. Erythropoiesis
1) Regulation
a) Determined by relationship of cellular oxygen requirement and general metabolic activity
i) Increased muscle mass causes higher RBC levels.
ii) Androgens increase RBC production while estrogens decrease them.
b) Bone marrow stimulated to make more RBCs by the hormone erythropoietin; erythropoietin secreted by the kidney in response to hypoxemia
2) Nutritional requirements for RBC and hemoglobin production
a) Iron and iron precursors such as ferritin
b) Vitamin B_{12}
c) Folic acid
d) Essential elements: zinc, selenium, and copper
3) Process
a) Stem cell
b) Erythroblast (has a nucleus)
c) Expulsion of nucleus
d) Erythrocyte
4) Hemoglobin synthesis
a) Synthesis takes place in bone marrow.
b) Hemoglobin consists of four globin chains and four heme groups per hemoglobin molecule; each hemoglobin molecule has two different types of globin (e.g., normal adult hemoglobin [referred to as HbA]), two alpha chains and two beta chains
c) The heme portion of hemoglobin molecules contains iron: more than two thirds of the body's iron is contained in hemoglobin and myoglobin.
i) Oxygen binds to the heme protein within the erythrocyte.
ii) The binding affinity of oxygen to hemoglobin is dependent upon acid-base balance, temperature, and levels of 2,3-DPG.
(a) Alkalosis, hypothermia, and decreased levels of 2,3-DPG cause the oxyhemoglobin dissociation curve to shift to the left, increasing the affinity between oxygen and hemoglobin; this facilitates the pickup of oxygen at the lung but impairs drop-off of oxygen at the tissues.
(b) Acidosis, hyperthermia, and increased levels of 2,3-DPG cause the oxyhemoglobin dissociation curve to shift to the right, decreasing the affinity between oxygen and hemoglobin; this impairs the pickup of oxygen at the lung but facilitates drop-off of oxygen at the tissues.

e. Destruction (hemolysis) of erythrocytes
1) Destruction of old and immature RBCs occurs in the liver and spleen.
2) Destruction of immature RBCs occurs primarily because they are misshapen or damaged.
3) Presenescent RBCs are removed from the circulation by the spleen, liver, or bone marrow for any of the following reasons:
a) RBC membrane abnormalities
b) Hemoglobin abnormalities
c) Abnormal metabolic functions
d) Physical trauma to the RBC
e) Antibodies
f) Infectious agents and toxins
4) Hgb and iron are returned to the bone marrow for reuse.
a) Heme is bound to haptoglobin for recirculation.
b) Iron is bound to transferrin for recirculation.
5) Erythrocyte destruction increases bilirubin production; bilirubin is transported to the liver attached to albumin.
a) Indirect bilirubin is unconjugated; this is before the liver has converted it to a water-soluble substance; indirect bilirubin becomes elevated in hemolytic states that overwhelm the liver's ability to conjugate or in liver disease when the liver is unable to adequately conjugate
b) Direct bilirubin is conjugated: this is after the liver has converted it to a water-soluble substance that will be excreted into the bile; direct bilirubin becomes elevated in biliary obstruction
c) Bilirubin is excreted via the gastrointestinal tract or as urobilinogen in the urine.

4. Leukocytes: phagocytic and immunologic systems
a. Cytokines: protein hormones synthesized by the various leukocytes
1) Act as chemical mediators of immunity and inflammation
2) Important in regulation of normal immune and inflammatory responses

Table 10-1	**Definitions of Selected Leukocyte Activities**
Opsonization	The process by which opsonins render bacteria more susceptible to phagocytosis by leukocytes; an opsonin is an antibody or complement split product that, when attached to foreign material, microorganism, or antigen, enhances phagocytosis of the substances by leukocytes and other macrophages
Chemotaxis (Figure 10-1)	The movement toward (positive) or away from (negative) a chemical stimulus; movement of neutrophils and monocytes toward an invading microorganism
Margination (Figure 10-1)	The process of the white blood cell sticking to the wall of the capillary
Diapedesis (Figure 10-1)	The passage of white blood cells through the walls of the vessels that contain them without damage to the vessels
Phagocytosis	The process by which certain cells engulf and destroy microorganisms and cellular debris; involves invagination, engulfment, internalization and formation of phagocyte vacuole, digestion of phagocytosed material by lysosomes and oxygen-derived radicals, and release of digested microbial products
Lysis	The destruction or dissolution of a cell through the action of a specific agent

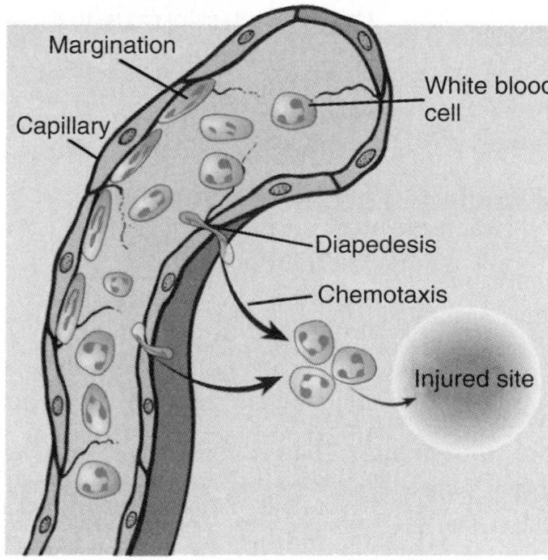

Figure 10-1 Illustration of margination, diapedesis, and chemotaxis. (From Lewis, S. M., et al. [2007]. *Medical-surgical nursing: Assessment and management of clinical problems* [7th ed.]. St. Louis: Mosby.)

3) Are causative factors in systemic inflammatory response syndrome (SIRS) (see Chapter 11)
4) Types of cytokines
   a) Monokines are synthesized by mononuclear phagocytes.
   b) Lymphokines are synthesized by lymphocytes.
   c) Macrophages secrete nonspecific cytokines such as tumor necrosis factor, interleukins, and interferons.

b. Granulocytes: active phagocytes
   1) Neutrophils (also known as *polymorphonuclear leukocytes [PMNs]*); largest component of granulocytes and the circulating WBC mass (40-80%)
      a) Function
         i) Neutrophils leave the blood vessel, migrate through the tissues, and search for microorganisms or damaged or old body cells; they then engulf, kill, and digest them through the process of phagocytosis. (Table 10-1 and Figure 10-1 describe some selected cellular processes of leukocytes, including phagocytosis.)
            (a) Neutrophils are the most actively phagocytic of granulocytes.
            (b) Neutrophils are attracted to inflammation and bacterial microorganisms.
            (c) After phagocytosis, the neutrophil dies.
            (d) Pus is the end product of neutrophil death.
            (e) Neutrophils exhibit a burst of oxygen consumption during phagocytosis known as a *respiratory burst*; this produces superoxide, hydrogen peroxide, and hydroxyl radicals; these oxygen-derived radicals normally function in destruction of microorganisms but may be injurious to normal body tissue.
         ii) Neutrophils contain cytoplasmic granules that include lysosomal enzymes, which aid in killing the microorganism.
      b) Life span after maturation: half-life 4-10 hours
      c) Maturity
         i) Bands are immature neutrophils.
            (a) Phagocytic
            (b) Increase in bands seen in acute bacterial infection; frequently referred to as a *shift to the left*
         ii) Segmented neutrophils (referred to as *segs*) are mature neutrophils.
            (a) Phagocytic

(b) Increase in mature segmented neutrophils seen in inflammation, liver disease, and pernicious anemia; frequently referred to as a *shift to the right*

d) Recruitment
   i) Movement into the tissues is stimulated by microorganisms or antigen-antibody reactions.
   ii) The bone marrow speeds maturation and release when more neutrophils are needed for phagocytosis.

e) Destruction: lost from the blood via the GI tract, pulmonary or oral secretions, and urine and into the tissues

2) Eosinophils: comprise 0-5% of WBC mass
   a) Functions
      i) Ingest immune complexes (antigen-antibody complexes) and inactive mediators of allergic response
      ii) Some phagocytic activity
      iii) Probably most important during parasitic infections and allergic reactions; especially important in helminth infections because these parasitic worms are too large to be phagocytized and eosinophils secrete chemicals that destroy the surface of the helminth
      iv) Also elevated in pulmonary and dermatologic inflammation and infection
   b) Life span after maturation: half-life in circulation approximately 30 minutes; in tissues 12 days
   c) Tissue eosinophils are present in large numbers on mucosal surfaces of the respiratory and gastrointestinal systems and the skin because these locations are common entry points for foreign material.

3) Basophils: comprise 0-2% of WBC mass
   a) Function
      i) Like mast cells, basophils contain heparin and histamine which are released as they degranulate during acute local or systemic allergic reactions; mast cells stay in the tissue, and basophils stay in the circulatory system; if a basophil leaves the circulatory system to stay in the tissue, it becomes a mast cell.
      ii) Basophils do not participate in phagocytic activity.
   b) Life span after maturation: unknown

c. Agranulocytes
   1) Mononuclear phagocytes
      a) Monocytes: comprise 3-8% of WBC mass
         i) Function
            (a) Some phagocytic activity
            (b) Differentiate into macrophages as they migrate into the tissues
         ii) Life span after maturation: circulating half-life 8-10 hours
      b) Macrophages (not measured in WBC count due to their location)
         i) Function
            (a) Greater phagocytic ability than PMNs or monocytes; especially involved in removal of damaged or senescent cells, cellular debris, and mutant or cancer cells
            (b) Produce the cytokine interleukin-1 (IL-1), which increases proliferation of T cells, stimulates the growth and development of B lymphocytes, causes fever, and stimulates the release of prostaglandin
            (c) Produce the cytokine alpha interferon which is important in the body's defense against viruses and tumors
            (d) Also produce IL-6, IL-8, and tumor necrosis factor (TNF)
         ii) Fixed or mobile
            (a) Fixed (or tissue) macrophages: stay in one organ and phagocytize live and dead debris
               (i) Lung: alveolar macrophages
               (ii) Brain: microglia
               (iii) Liver: Kupffer cells
               (iv) Bone: osteoclast
               (v) Peritoneum: peritoneal macrophages
               (vi) Kidney: mesangial cells
               (vii) Spleen: splenic mononuclear cells
            (b) Mobile macrophages: found primarily at sites of inflammation and in peritoneal, pleural, and synovial spaces; migrate through the circulatory system as monocytes
         iii) Life span: months or years
   2) Lymphocytes: comprise 10-40% of WBC mass
      a) T cells: comprise approximately 70-80% of lymphocytes
         i) Develop in the bone marrow; mature and differentiate in the thymus and the lymph node
         ii) Function: cellular immunity

iii) Types of T cells
   (a) Helper T cells (also referred to as *CD4 T lymphocytes, T4 lymphocytes, or* T_H) detect foreign cells and produce lymphokines to stimulate the production or activation of other cells to fight infection; lymphokines are soluble proteins which function as chemical communicators to transmit instructions to macrophages, lymphocytes, and tissue cells.
   (b) Cytotoxic T cells (also referred to as *killer cells or* T_C) emit chemicals which dissolve the foreign cell's membrane to kill the cell before the invader can use it as a base for multiplication.
   (c) Suppressor T cells (also referred to as *CD8 T lymphocytes, T8 lymphocytes,* or T_S) modulate the overall immune system by signaling B cells and T cells to slow down or stop their activity.
   (d) Memory T cells circulate in blood and lymph after the initial infection to allow ready response to subsequent invasion by the same organism.
   (e) Helper T cells typically carry the CD4 surface molecule; suppressor and cytotoxic T cells typically carry the CD8 surface molecule; normally there are twice as many CD4 cells as CD8 cells.

b) B cells: comprise approximately 10-20% of lymphocytes
   i) Develop and mature in the bone marrow (bursa); migrate to lymph nodes and lymphoid tissue for differentiation and antibody production or plasma cell differentiation
   ii) Function: production of immunoglobulins (humoral immunity)
      (a) Once activated, B cells become plasma cells.
         (i) Recognize specific foreign material
         (ii) Develop specific immunoglobulins to that antigen
      (b) Memory B cells circulate in blood and lymph after the initial infection to allow ready response to subsequent invasion by the same organism.

c) Natural killer (NK) cells (also referred to *as null cells*): comprise approximately 10% of lymphocytes
   i) Large granular cytotoxic lymphocytes that are neither T cells nor B cells (no surface marker exists on these lymphocytes)
   ii) Function
      (a) Kill nonspecifically and do not need prior exposure for activation
      (b) Involved in surveillance against tumors, some parasites, and viruses

Inflammation

1. Sequential physiologic response the body makes to injuries, immunologic processes, or foreign substances in the body; may be acute or chronic
   a. Occurs at sites of tissue damage irrespective of etiology
   b. May be local only or can become systemic; systemic response is now referred to as SIRS (discussion of SIRS and multiple organ dysfunction syndrome (MODS) is in Chapter 11)
2. Process
   a. Stage I: vascular stage
      1) Phases
         a) Phase 1: immediate but temporary vasoconstriction caused by trauma to vascular smooth muscle
         b) Phase 2
            i) Warmth, redness, swelling, pain, and loss of function are the five classic symptoms of the inflammatory response.
            ii) Injured tissues and cells secrete chemical mediators (Table 10-2); predominant effect is vasodilation and increase in capillary permeability, causing warmth, redness, and swelling.
               (a) Healing is enhanced by the increase in mobilization of nutrients to the area.
               (b) Tissue injury is decreased by diluting toxins or microorganisms that enter the area.
               (c) Pain is caused by tissue stretching and release of histamine and prostaglandin.
               (d) Loss of function is caused by tissue swelling and pain.
      2) The major leukocyte in this stage of inflammation is the tissue macrophage.

Table 10-2 Chemical Mediators of the Inflammatory Process

Chemical Mediator	Actions
Bradykinin	• Causes vasodilation • Increases capillary permeability • Enhances chemotaxis • Causes pain • Converts plasminogen to plasmin • Produces smooth muscle contraction (e.g., bronchospasm)
Collagenase	• Degrades clots
Complement cascade	• Triggers neutrophil aggregation • Increases capillary permeability • Activates mast cells and basophils
Elastase	• Degrades clots
Endorphin	• Causes vasodilation • Produces analgesia
Fibrinolysin	• Digests fibrin
Histamine	• Causes vasodilation • Increases capillary permeability • Increases heart rate and contractility • Produces bronchospasm • Increases secretion of mucus and gastric acid • Inhibits T cells
Interleukin-1 (IL-1)	• Stimulates protein catabolism • Causes fever • Activates lymphocytes • Stimulates fibroblasts
Interleukin-2 (IL-2)	• Activates B lymphocytes to make antibodies • Activates macrophages
Leukotriene	• Causes vasoconstriction • Increases capillary permeability • Produces smooth muscle contraction (e.g., bronchospasm)
Lipase	• Degrades fat
Plasminogen	• Degrades clots when activated to plasmin
Prostacyclin	• Causes vasodilation • Inhibits platelet aggregation • Increases capillary permeability
Prostaglandin (PGD_2, PGF_{2a})	• Vasoconstriction • Bronchoconstriction
Prostaglandin (PGE_2, PGI_2)	• Causes vasodilation • Produces smooth muscle relaxation (e.g., bronchodilation) • Promotes platelet aggregation • Increases capillary permeability • Activates lysosomal enzymes • Potentiates leukotrienes • Causes pain
Serotonin	• Causes vasodilation • Increases capillary permeability • Causes pulmonary vasoconstriction • Produces smooth muscle contraction (e.g., bronchospasm)
Thromboxane	• Causes vasoconstriction and endothelial damage • Causes pulmonary vasoconstriction • Acts as a potent platelet aggregator
Tumor necrosis factor (TNF)	• Causes necrosis of bacteria or tissue • Stimulates muscle catabolism • Induces fever

a) Response is immediate because the tissue macrophage is already in the tissue.
b) Granulocyte colony-stimulating factor (G-CSF) is secreted by the macrophage to stimulate the bone marrow to speed up the maturation and release of leukocytes.
c) Cytokines secreted by the macrophage attract neutrophils to the area of injury or invasion.

b. Stage II: cellular stage
   1) Major leukocyte in this stage of inflammation is the neutrophil, which attacks and destroys foreign material and removes necrotic tissue.
   2) Thromboxane (procoagulant) and prostacyclins (anticoagulants) act to wall off the site of injury and are part of the inflammatory process
c. Stage III: tissue repair and replacement
   1) Initiated at the time of injury
   2) Regeneration: replacement of lost cells with the same type of cells
   3) Repair: replacement of lost cells with connective tissue cells to form scar tissue; some loss of function occurs with the degree of loss dependent on the percentage of previously functional tissue replaced by scar tissue

Immunity

1. Definition: the protection of the body against pathogenic organisms or other foreign material; dependent on ability to recognize self from nonself
   a. Self is determined genetically; it is anything synthesized by a person's own particular DNA code.
   b. Nonself describes anything that is different in its chromosome structure and evokes a response from the immune system; antigens are chemical substances (almost always protein) that are viewed by the body as foreign (nonself).
      1) Nonself proteins may be normally pathogenic and warrant an immunologic response (e.g., foreign microbes).
      2) Nonself antigens/proteins that are not pathogenic but precipitate an immunologic response include allergens such as animal dander and plant pollens; the response is called a hypersensitivity reaction.
      3) When the body perceives an existing body cell as foreign due to surface markers or cellular changes and mounts a response against it, the response is called an autoimmune reaction.
2. Lines of defense
   a. First: skin and mucous membranes, acid secretions and enzymes, natural immunoglobulins
   b. Second: macrophages and neutrophils
   c. Third: cellular and humoral immunity
3. Innate immunity: body's inherent immune mechanisms; present at birth; do not require prior exposure to antigen for activation
   a. Anatomical: skin and mucous membranes
   b. Chemical
      1) Acid secretions in stomach, vagina, and mouth
      2) Digestive enzymes in the GI tract
      3) Tears and perspiration
      4) Lysosomes
      5) Natural immunoglobulins
      6) Cytokines
      7) Pyrogen (produced by granulocytes to cause an increase in body temperature)
   c. Cellular
      1) Normal bacterial flora: GI tract, vagina, and respiratory tract
      2) Tissue macrophages
      3) Leukocytes and mobile macrophages
      4) Inflammatory process
4. Acquired immunity: immunity developed by the body through the creation of antibodies and formation of T and B memory cells in response to exposure to foreign material (antigen)
   a. Types
      1) Passive acquired immunity: produced by the injection of antibodies or sensitized lymphocytes
      2) Active acquired immunity: produced by natural exposure to an antigen (e.g., infection) or administration of live attenuated vaccines (e.g., influenza "FluMist") that trigger a direct response from the body
   b. Cell-mediated immunity
      1) Particularly effective against viruses, parasites, some fungi, and bacteria harbored inside of cells; responsible for delayed hypersensitivity, transplant rejection, and malignancy surveillance and possibly destruction
      2) Primarily mediated by T cells
      3) Induced and regulated primarily through the production and activity of cytokines
      4) Process
         a) The macrophage is the first cell to detect most antigens.
         b) The macrophage processes the antigen and "presents" it to both T and B cells.
         c) T cells recognize the antigen as foreign when it is on the macrophage cell membrane.
         d) The antigen binds with an antigen receptor on the surface of the T cell, sensitizing the T cell.
         e) Sensitized T cells secrete lymphokines, which regulate and coordinate the immune response to combat foreign cells, protect the body against mutant or cancer cells, and destroy foreign tissue;

IL-8 is secreted by the macrophage and stimulates T cell division.

f) T cells are programmed to recognize the body's own tissue (self) from nonself (antigenic); autoimmune diseases are caused when the immune system cannot recognize self and the body is damaged by the immune system.

g) Natural killer cells also contribute to cellular immunity, especially in relation to cancer cell surveillance.

c. Humoral-mediated immunity

1) Primarily effective against bacteria and viruses

2) Primarily mediated by B cells

3) Process (Figure 10-2)

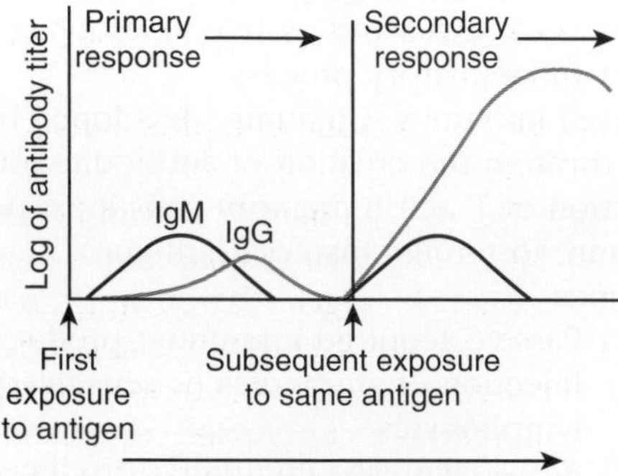

Figure 10-2 Primary and secondary immune responses. The introduction of antigen induces a response dominated by two classes of immunoglobulins, IgM and IgG. IgM predominates in the primary response, with some IgG appearing later. After the host's immune system is primed, another challenge with the same antigen induces the secondary response, in which some IgM and large amounts of IgG are produced. (From Lewis, S.M. et al. [2011]. *Medical-surgical nursing: Assessment and management of clinical problems* [8th ed.]. St. Louis: Mosby.)

a) Once activated, B cells become plasma cells and recognize specific foreign cells or antigens.

b) Plasma cells make antibodies (also called *immunoglobulins*) (Table 10-3).

i) Immunoglobulins (antibodies) are serum proteins that bind to specific antigens; they begin the process that causes lysis or phagocytosis of an offending antigen.

ii) One end of the immunoglobulin (Ig) molecule has a constant fragment with a fixed sequence of amino acids that is constant within the category of the immunoglobulin (e.g., IgG, IgM).

iii) The other end of the Ig has an antigen-binding fragment with an amino acid sequence specific to the antigen for which it was formed.

c) The first exposure to an antigen is followed by a latent phase in which no antibody levels are detected.

d) Primary response follows as serum antibody levels rise rapidly; maximal antibody response takes 3-5 days.

e) Levels plateau and finally decline.

f) Subsequent exposure to the antigen results in more rapid production of antibodies to that antigen and higher concentrations of the antibody; this is the basis for immunizations and the consequence of increasing severity of allergic reactions.

g) Inflammation occurs because antigen-antibody complexes (referred to as

Table 10-3 Immunoglobulins (Igs)

Ig	Actions	Comments
IgG	• Coats microorganisms (primarily bacteria and viruses) to enhance phagocytosis • Activates complement system	• Most abundant immunoglobulin (75-80% of total) • Present in intravascular and extravascular spaces • Crosses the placental barrier and provides natural immunity
IgA	• Protects epithelial surfaces against antigen adhesion and invasion • Protects against entry via the respiratory tract, GU, GI tracts • Activates complement system	• Present in many body secretions (e.g., saliva, tears, sweat, mucus, breast milk) • 10-15% of total
IgM	• Kills bacteria in bloodstream • Activates complement system	• First responder to bacterial or viral invasion • Present mostly in intravascular space • 5-10% of total immunoglobulins
IgD	• Not well understood • May activate B cells	• 1% of total immunoglobulins
IgE	• Attaches to mast cells and basophils and causes them to release their contents (e.g., histamine) in response to contact with specific antigens	• Present in serum, interstitial space, exocrine secretions and on basophils and mast cells • Very small (0.002) percentage of total immunoglobulins

immune complexes) attract white blood cells.
4) Immune complexes activate the complement cascade.
   a) Complement is a group of blood proteins: there are more than 20 of these proteins, but 11 are considered the primary complement elements.
      i) These are labeled C1 to C9, with C1 having three subunits (C1q, C1r, C1s).
      ii) C1 is primarily synthesized by the intestinal epithelium.
      iii) C2 and C4 are produced by macrophages.
      iv) C3, C6, and C9 are synthesized by the liver.
      v) C5 and C8 are synthesized by the spleen.
   b) When activated, they function as mediators to enhance various aspects of inflammatory response; they also do the following:
      i) Attract and stimulate PMNs
      ii) Kill microorganisms by punching holes in their cell membranes, allowing intracellular fluid to leak out; mononuclear phagocytes and monocytes then clear the debris from the bloodstream
      iii) Agglutinate the bacteria
      iv) Activate basophils and mast cells
      v) Complement deficiencies may be congenital or acquired and result in unusual infections and abnormal hypersensitivity reactions.
   c) They may be activated with or without previous exposure to the antigen.
      i) Anaphylactoid reaction: no previous exposure to the antigen; no true antigen-antibody interaction
      ii) Anaphylactic reaction: previous exposure to the antigen; involves antigen-antibody interaction (A more detailed description of anaphylactoid and anaphylactic reactions is in Chapter 11.)

d. Hypersensitivity (allergic) reactions
   1) Type I: immediate hypersensitivity reactions ranging from mild reaction with localized response to a severe systemic reaction referred to as *anaphylaxis*
      a) Reaction occurs within minutes (usually 5-20) of exposure to even a miniscule amount of the antigen.
      b) Caused by IgE specific to the antigen; the antigen binds to one end of IgE; IgE is bound to a mast cell or basophil; when the antigen attaches, the mast cell or basophil degranulates and histamine is released; slow-reacting substance of anaphylaxis (SRS-A) and eosinophil chemotactic factor of anaphylaxis (ECF-A) are also released; eosinophils are recruited to the site
      c) Example: anaphylactic reaction to a penicillin, insect venom, foods, or pollen
   2) Type II: cytotoxic hypersensitivity
      a) Reaction is usually within minutes to days.
      b) Caused by the combination of IgG, IgM, or IgA antibody and antigenic receptors on membranes of cells; complement cascade is activated; natural killer cells are involved in destruction of the immune complex and the cell to which it is attached and macrophages may phagocytize the immune complexes
      c) Example: mismatched blood transfusion reaction
   3) Type III: immune complex-mediated reaction
      a) Reaction is usually within hours.
      b) Caused by large quantities of antigen-antibody (IgG, IgM, or IgA) complexes that cannot be quickly and efficiently cleared by the reticuloendothelial system; complement cascade is activated; neutrophils are activated at the site of deposition; inflammatory process is stimulated and mediators are released
      c) Example: vasculitis and renal damage caused by immune complexes
   4) Type IV: delayed or cell-mediated hypersensitivity
      a) Reaction is within one or more days.
      b) Cause is poorly understood but is presumed to be cells that require time to migrate to the site; probably caused by previously sensitized lymphocytes and lymphokines that activate the inflammatory response at the site
      c) Example: skin testing for tuberculosis, contact dermatitis, and latex allergy

Hemostasis

1. Definition: the termination of bleeding by a complex process that involves integrated interactions among blood vessels, platelets, clotting factors, and the fibrinolytic system
2. Hemostatic mechanisms
   a. Vascular response
      1) Disruption of vascular integrity causes a sympathetic nervous system (SNS) response resulting in vasospasm and blood vessel constriction in the injured vessel.
      2) Thromboxane A_2, endothelin, the alpha-adrenergic system, and serotonin are thought to mediate this response.
   b. Platelet aggregation (thrombocytes)

1) Thrombocytes (platelets)
   a) Produced in bone marrow
   b) Life span is 9-12 days.
   c) Thrombopoiesis
      i) Thrombopoietin (a hormonelike erythropoietin for RBCs) is postulated to stimulate the production and release of thrombocytes.
      ii) Iron is needed for thrombopoiesis.
   d) Thrombocytes stored in and destroyed by the spleen
2) Process
   a) Endothelial damage exposes the basement membrane of the subendothelial collagen.
   b) Damaged tissues release chemicals (e.g., thromboplastin) to activate platelets.
   c) Activated platelets swell and develop hairlike projections.
   d) Swelling increases the surface area of the platelets for platelet adhesion and makes platelets more likely to aggregate.
   e) Granules and components necessary for the clotting process are released from the platelets; adenosine diphosphate (ADP) released by degranulation of the platelets enhances adhesiveness and aggregation.
      i) Adhesiveness: stickiness that aids in ability to stick to vessel walls occurs.
         (a) Enhanced by circulating von Willebrand factor (vWF), collagen, and endothelial collagen–specific glycoprotein Ia/IIb surface receptors.
         (b) Additional glycoprotein receptors, such as IIb, IIIa, IV, and V, progress this reaction to aggregation.
      ii) Aggregation: process of platelets adhering or clumping together to form the "platelet plug"
   f) Activated platelets become adhesive and aggregate.
   g) Platelet aggregation becomes large enough to form a platelet plug (sometimes referred to as *a white clot*) that seals the damaged blood vessel.
      i) This platelet plug lasts 2-5 hours and dissolves as fibrin clots replace the platelets.
   h) During aggregation of the platelets, platelet factor III (PFIII), an important contributor in the intrinsic pathway, is released.
   i) Platelets contain factor XIII (fibrin-stabilizing factor), essential in the formation of a stable fibrin clot.
3) Platelet function is affected by qualitative and quantitative factors.
   a) Qualitative changes
      i) Drugs that decrease the ability of the platelets to aggregate
         (a) Alcohol
         (b) Aspirin (ASA)
         (c) Ticlopidine (Ticlid)
         (d) Clopidogrel (Plavix)
         (e) GP IIb/IIIa platelet receptor blockers (e.g., abciximab [ReoPro], eptifibatide [Integrilin], tirofiban HCl [Aggrastat])
         (f) Nonsteroidal antiinflammatory agents (e.g., phenylbutazone [Butazolidin], ibuprofen [Motrin])
         (g) Quinidine
         (h) Dextran 40 (i.e., low-molecular-weight dextran)
         (i) Heparin
         (j) Aminoglycosides (e.g., gentamicin)
         (k) Loop diuretics (e.g., furosemide) and thiazides (e.g., hydrochlorothiazide)
         (l) Catecholamines (e.g., epinephrine, norepinephrine, dopamine)
         (m) Phenothiazines
         (n) Herbs such as ginkgo biloba, Chinese ginseng, chamomile, ginger
         (o) Vitamin E
      ii) Disorders that alter platelet quality
         (a) Catecholamine release
         (b) Diabetes mellitus
         (c) Hepatic cirrhosis
         (d) Hyperthermia/hypothermia
         (e) Malignant lymphomas
         (f) Sarcoidosis
         (g) Scleroderma
         (h) Systemic lupus erythematosus (SLE)
         (i) Thyrotoxicosis
   b) Quantitative changes
      i) Thrombocytopenia
         (a) Significance
            (i) Mild thrombocytopenia: platelet counts greater than 50,000/mm^3 but less than normal; surgery can generally be tolerated
            (ii) Moderate thrombocytopenia: platelet counts 20,000-30,000/mm^3; spontaneous bleeding may occur but

considered unlikely unless vascular injury occurs
- (iii) Severe thrombocytopenia: platelet counts less than 10,000/mm^3; spontaneous intracranial hemorrhages likely, high risk of bleeding without provocation

(b) Causes
- (i) Decreased production (e.g., bone marrow depression, vitamin B_{12} or folic acid deficiency, viral illness, estrogen, metabolic hormones [e.g., thyroxine, cortisol])
- (ii) Increased destruction (e.g., idiopathic thrombocytopenic purpura [ITP], disseminated intravascular coagulation [DIC], heat stroke, hypertension, artificial heart valves, large bore intravenous catheters [e.g., intra-aortic balloon pump], sepsis)
- (iii) Hypersplenism (e.g., portal hypertension)
- (iv) Heparin-induced thrombocytopenia (HIT)
- (v) Dilutional thrombocytopenia: caused by large volumes of fluids that do not contain platelets

ii) Thrombocytosis
- (a) Significance: may cause excessive thrombosis or bleeding, depending on the quality of the platelets
- (b) Causes
  - (i) Malignancy
  - (ii) Granulomatous disease
  - (iii) Polycythemia vera
  - (iv) Leukemia
  - (v) Postsplenectomy
  - (vi) Rheumatoid arthritis
  - (vii) Trauma
  - (viii) Vitamin E deficiency

c. Coagulation
1) Dependent upon presence of clotting factors, active ionized calcium, and functioning of the pathways
2) Blood coagulation factors (Table 10-4)
   - a) Consist of proteins, lipoproteins, and calcium, which is critical in the intrinsic, extrinsic and common pathways
   - b) Circulate as inactive; activated in a cascade fashion
3) Clotting pathways (Figure 10-3)
   - a) Pathways are cascades in which one action is dependent upon a preceding action or interaction.
   - b) A fibrin clot may be produced through activation of either the intrinsic or extrinsic pathway, although the factor VII-initiated extrinsic pathway is a more potent and significant initiator of clotting.
     - i) Intrinsic pathway
       - (a) Initiated by damage to red blood cells or platelets
       - (b) Time from activation through intrinsic pathway and common pathway to a clot: 2-6 minutes
       - (c) Tested by aPTT or factor Xa level
     - ii) Extrinsic pathway
       - (a) Initiated by injured tissue and subsequent release of tissue thromboplastin
       - (b) Time from activation through extrinsic pathway and common pathway to a clot: as short as 15-20 seconds
       - (c) Tested by PT
   - c) Common pathway
     - i) Platelet factor III and tissue thromboplastin combine to become a prothrombin activator.
     - ii) Prothrombin is converted to thrombin.
     - iii) Fibrinogen is converted to fibrin.
     - iv) Fibrin clot is formed.
     - v) Pathway is tested by aPTT, factor Xa levels, PT, fibrinogen level, and thrombin time.
   - d) Other prothrombotic mechanisms
     - i) Inflammation triggers thromboxane.
     - ii) Cancer procoagulants, such as cancer procoagulant (CP), or heat shock proteins (HSPs) enhance coagulability.

d. Anticoagulant mechanisms in normal system
1) Fibrinolytic system (Figure 10-4)
   - a) Activated clotting factors are cleared by the reticuloendothelial system.
   - b) Clot-lysing activities maintain blood in fluid state.
     - i) Process of clot breakdown takes approximately 7-10 days.

Table 10-4 Blood Coagulation Factors

Factor	Name(s)	Comments
I	Fibrinogen	• Synthesized in liver • Precursor to fibrin (Ia)
Ia	Fibrin	• Activated fibrinogen (I) becomes fibrin (Ia)
II	Prothrombin	• Synthesized in liver • Vitamin K dependent • Precursor to thrombin (IIa)
IIa	Thrombin	• Activated prothrombin becomes thrombin
III	Tissue thromboplastin Tissue factor	• First factor of extrinsic pathway
IV	Calcium	• Acts as an enzyme cofactor for most of the activation steps in intrinsic, extrinsic, and common pathways
V	Proaccelerin Labile factor Ac globulin	• Synthesized in liver • Combines with Xa and phospholipid to accelerate conversion of prothrombin (II) to thrombin (IIa)
VI	There is no designated factor VI	
VII	Proconvertin Stable factor	• Synthesized in liver • Vitamin K dependent • Part of extrinsic pathway • Complexes with tissue thromboplastin (III) to activate X
VIII	Antihemophiliac factor A	• Part of intrinsic pathway • Complexes with IXa and platelet phospholipid to activate X
IX	Plasma thromboplastin component Christmas factor Antihemophiliac factor B	• Synthesized in liver • Vitamin K dependent • Associated with factors VIII, XI, and XII in the intrinsic pathway
X	Stuart-Prower factor	• Synthesized in liver • Vitamin K dependent • Part of intrinsic and extrinsic pathways • Complexes with V and phospholipid to accelerate prothrombin (II) conversion
XI	Plasma thromboplastin antecedent	• May be synthesized in liver • May be vitamin K dependent • Part of intrinsic pathway • Associated with factors VIII, IX, and XII in the intrinsic pathway
XII	Hageman factor Contact factor	• First factor in intrinsic factor • Indirectly activates plasmin and complement cascades
XIII	Fibrin-stabilizing factor Fibrinase Laki-Lorand factor	• May be synthesized in liver • Activated by thrombin (IIa) • Produces a stronger, insoluble clot; stabilizes clot formation

Note: "a" after the factor indicates an activated factor.

ii) Blood (intrinsic pathway) or tissue (extrinsic pathway) plasminogen activators activate plasminogen to plasmin; therefore, once a clot is developed, steps are initiated to eliminate it.

iii) Plasmin works to lyse fibrin clots producing fibrin degradation products (FDPs) (also referred to as *fibrin split products [FSPs*]; FDPs have anticoagulant properties, and increased amounts of FDPs enhance potential for patients to bleed.

iv) Fibrinolytics speed up this process by either directly providing tissue plasminogen activator (e.g., alteplase [Activase], reteplase [Retavase]), tenecteplase (TNKase) or by triggering the process by adding a complex to cause the activation of the fibrinolytic system (streptokinase [Streptase]).

c) Controls of fibrinolysis

i) Plasminogen activator inhibitor type 1 (PAI-1) inactivates tissue plasminogen activator.

ii) Alpha$_2$-antiplasmin is an inhibitor of plasmin.

iii) Antithrombin is a serum protease that degrades specific coagulation factors IXa, Xa, and XIIa.

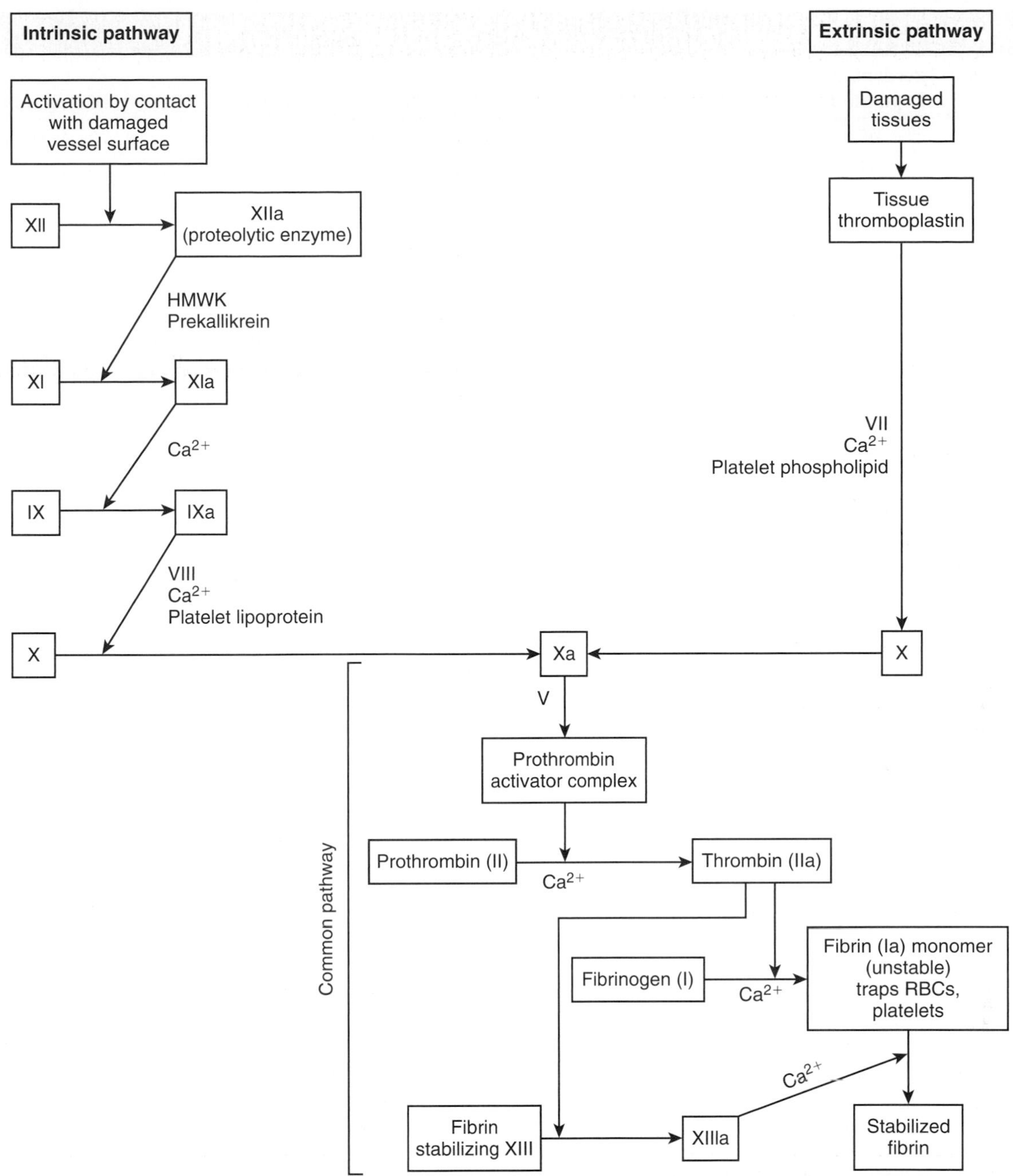

Figure 10-3 The clotting pathways: intrinsic, extrinsic, and common. (From Lewis, S.M. et al. [2011]. *Medical-surgical nursing: Assessment and management of clinical problems* [8th ed.]. St. Louis: Mosby.)

2) Antithrombin system
   a) Defends against excessive clotting
   b) Release of antithrombin III from mast cells
   c) Neutralizes the clotting capability of thrombin
   d) Extrinsic infusion of antithrombin III can provide anticoagulant effects.

e. Regulators of coagulation
   1) Calcium is required for activation of factors.
   2) Tissue factor pathway inhibitor (TFPI) inhibits excessive tissue factor activity.
   3) Protein C and thrombomodulin enhance degradation; absence leads to thrombophilia and excess clotting.
   4) Antithrombin III (ATIII) degradation is affected by intrinsic or extrinsic administration of heparins.
   5) Plasmin cleaved by tissue plasminogen activator (tPa)
   6) Prostacyclin (PGI_2) released by damaged endothelium or extrinsic administration inhibits platelet aggregation.

Table 10-5 ABO Blood Groups

Patient's ABO Group	Percentage of Population	Antigen on RBC	Antibodies in Plasma	Compatible RBCs	Compatible Plasma
O	47%	None	Anti-A, Anti-B	O	O, A, B, AB
A	41%	A	Anti-B	O, A	A, AB
B	9%	B	Anti-A	O, B	B, AB
AB	3%	A and B	None	O, A, B, AB	AB

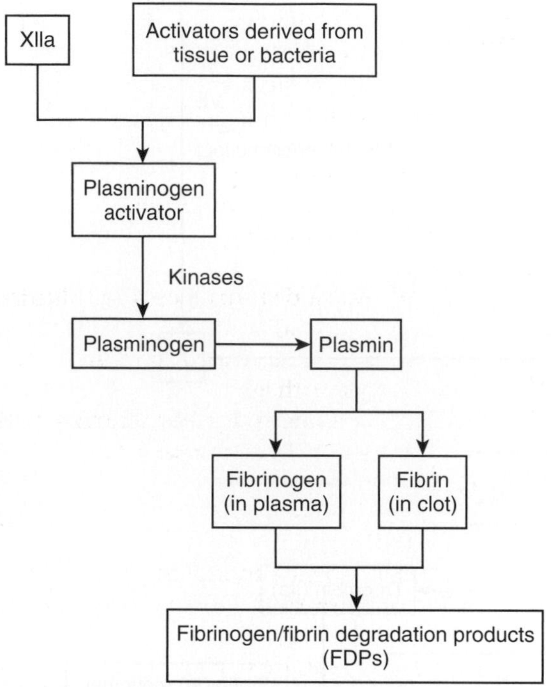

Figure 10-4 The fibrinolytic process. (From Lewis, S. M., et al. [2011]. *Medical-surgical nursing: Assessment and management of clinical problems* [8th ed.]. St. Louis: Mosby.)

Blood Groups

1. Three systems describe the most important antigens on red blood cells, tissues, and other cells.
   a. ABO system (Table 10-5)
      1) This system is concerned with antigens on the RBC that are designated A and B; the presence of these antigens is genetically controlled.
      2) Blood type is named for the antigen that is present on the RBC.
      3) Antibodies are present in the plasma for the antigen or antigens that are not present (e.g., B antibodies are found in group A blood because B antigens are absent).
         a) Blood that contains both A and B antigens is termed *type AB blood*.
         b) Blood that contains neither A nor B antigens is termed *type O blood*.
      4) Agglutination that occurs in mismatched blood is the basis for typing and crossmatching.
         a) Blood typing detects the major antigens: A, B, and Rh.
         b) Crossmatching detects the presence of major or minor RBC antigens in donor blood that can lead to reactions for a specific recipient.
   b. Rh system (Table 10-6)
      1) This system is concerned with a series of six common types of Rh antigens, each called an Rh factor.
      2) Each person has one of each of three pairs so they have three of these Rh factors designated c, C, d, D, e, and E.
      3) Only C, D, and E are antigenic enough to cause significant development of anti-Rh antibodies (and therefore to potentially cause blood transfusion reaction if nonmatched blood is administered).
      4) If C, D, or E antigens are present, the person is Rh+; if none of these three antigens is present, the person is Rh−; most (85%) of Americans are Rh+.
      5) Rh antibodies do not develop spontaneously; they only occur after exposure to Rh antigen (e.g., second exposure to non-Rh-matched blood or Rh− mothers pregnant with the second Rh+ fetus if anti-Rh globin [Rho-gam] was not given); delayed transfusion reactions can occur even after the first exposure to Rh+ blood and cause a mild transfusion reaction.
   c. Other red cell antigens
      1) Cold agglutinins
         a) These are antibodies that cause erythrocytes to coagulate when blood plasma temperature is below normal body temperature.
         b) Banked blood must be warmed to normal body temperature (37° C) before

Table 10-6 Rh Compatibility

Patient's Rh Type	RBC Rh Type for Transfusion	Plasma Rh Type for Transfusion
Positive	Positive or negative	Positive or negative
Negative	Negative	Positive or negative

giving the blood to a patient who has cold agglutinins.
c) Cold agglutinins more commonly occur in non-Caucasians, elderly patients, patients with autoimmune disease, or after viral infection; may be a temporary or permanent condition
2) Coombs' test: used to determine presence of hemolyzing antibodies
a) Direct: detects antibodies attached to red cells
b) Indirect: detects antibodies in serum
3) Other RBC antigens include Kell (third most common), Duffy, and Kidd.

d. Uncrossmatched type O negative packed red blood cells may be used safely in exsanguinating patient.
1) Whole blood is avoided to decrease the risk of reaction caused by anti-A and anti-B antibodies in type O plasma.
2) Blood antigen-antibody complexes may complicate later crossmatching and may cause future blood transfusion reaction to own blood type unless it is O negative.
3) Type-specific blood may be preferable, and type matching takes only 5-15 minutes.

e. Human leukocyte antigen (HLA)
1) Concerned with a group of antigenic substances found on many cell types (including WBCs and platelets but not on erythrocytes)
2) Detected serologically by cytotoxicity assays; HLA-A, HLA-B, HLA-C are found on all nucleated cells, but HLA-D and HLA-DR antigens are only located on B lymphocytes, monocytes, epidermal, and endothelial cells.
3) Very important in organ and tissue transplantation histocompatibility

Assessment of the Hematologic and Immunologic Systems

Interview

1. Chief complaint: why the patient is seeking help and duration of the problem
a. Symptoms which may be related to hematologic or immunologic conditions
1) General
a) Fatigue
b) Weakness
c) Chills
d) Fever
e) Weight loss
f) Night sweats
g) Apathy
h) Lethargy
i) Malaise
j) Abnormal bleeding, bruising, or swelling
k) Chronic or recurrent infections
l) Poor wound healing
m) Enlarged and/or tender lymph nodes
2) Specific
a) Skin
i) Dry, coarse skin
ii) Bruising or bleeding
(a) Mucosal bleeding: oral, gastrointestinal, urogenital
(b) Prolonged bleeding
(c) Petechiae
(d) Bruising easily
iii) Color changes
(a) Jaundice
(b) Pallor
(c) Cyanosis
iv) Rash
v) Pruritus
vi) Lesions
vii) Wounds: poor healing
viii) Inflammation
b) Eyes
i) Visual disturbances (e.g., blurring, diplopia)
ii) Blindness related to retinal hemorrhage
iii) Conjunctival pallor or inflammation
iv) Scleral hemorrhage
c) Ears
i) Vertigo
ii) Tinnitus
d) Nasopharynx and mouth
i) Epistaxis
ii) Dysphagia
iii) Gingival bleeding
iv) Painful lesions on mouth and lips
v) Sore or red, beefy tongue
vi) Sore throat
vii) Persistent hoarseness
viii) Cracks in corners of mouth (i.e., angular cheilitis)
e) Neck: nuchal rigidity
f) Lymph nodes
i) Swelling greater than 2 cm for longer than 2 weeks
ii) Tenderness
iii) Irregular and immovable
g) Cardiovascular
i) Chest pain
ii) Sternal tenderness
iii) Palpitations
iv) Known murmurs
h) Pulmonary
i) Exertional dyspnea
ii) Cough
iii) Sputum
iv) Orthopnea
v) Respiratory tract infections
vi) Hemoptysis
i) Gastrointestinal
i) Anorexia
ii) Abdominal pain and cramping

iii) Abdominal fullness
iv) Eructation
v) Bloody or black stools
vi) Vomiting of blood or coffee-ground material
vii) Ulcers: oral, esophageal, gastric
viii) Change in bowel habits
(a) Diarrhea
(b) Constipation
ix) Rectal pain or bleeding

j) Genitourinary
i) Hematuria
ii) Pyuria
iii) Abnormal menstrual flow: menorrhagia, amenorrhea
iv) Incontinence, dysuria, hesitancy, frequency
v) Urinary retention
vi) Pelvic or flank pain

k) Neurologic
i) Change in level of consciousness
ii) Confusion
iii) Irritability
iv) Memory loss
v) Headache
vi) Ataxia
vii) Sensory changes: paresthesia, anesthesia
viii) Syncope, vertigo

l) Back and extremities
i) Pain and/or tenderness in joints, back, shoulder, or bone
ii) Joint stiffness or swelling
iii) Muscle weakness

2. Past medical history
a. Surgical history
1) Splenectomy
2) Thymectomy
3) Tonsillectomy
4) Tumor removal
5) Total or partial gastrectomy
6) Surgical excision of duodenum
7) Organ or tissue transplant
8) Prosthetic heart valves
9) Response to dental extractions (e.g., excessive bleeding)

b. Medical problems
1) Anemia
2) Asthma
3) Autoimmune disease (e.g., lupus erythematosus)
4) Deep vein thrombosis or pulmonary embolus
5) Diabetes mellitus
6) HIV/AIDS
7) Liver disease
8) Malabsorption syndrome
9) Malignancy, especially leukemia, lymphoma, multiple myeloma
10) Mononucleosis
11) Problems with wound healing
12) Prolonged or excessive bleeding (e.g., after dental procedures, injury, or surgery)
13) Radiation therapy
14) Recent viral illness exposures or symptoms (e.g., exposure to children with Coxsackie virus, Epstein-Barr virus)
15) Recurrent infections
16) Renal failure
17) Sexually transmitted disease
18) Spleen disorders
19) Vitamin K deficiency

c. Allergies
1) Known allergies and type of reaction
a) Inhalants
b) Contactants
c) Injectables
d) Ingestibles
2) Transfusion with blood or blood products and reactions

d. Immunizations: types, dates, any adverse reactions

3. Family history
a. Congenital immune deficiency
b. Congenital bleeding disorder (e.g., hemophilia)
c. Congenital RBC dyscrasias (e.g., sickle cell disease)
d. Congenital anemia (e.g., thalassemia)
e. Asthma
f. Allergies
g. Anemia
h. Jaundice
i. Malignancies
j. Autoimmune disease (e.g., systemic lupus erythematosus [SLE], rheumatoid arthritis)

4. Social history
a. Relationship with spouse or significant other; family structure
b. Occupation
1) Occupational exposure to radiation
2) Occupational exposure to chemicals (e.g., lead, benzene, ethylene oxide, insecticides, vinyl chloride)
3) Military service; exposure to toxins
c. Educational level
d. Stress level and usual coping mechanisms; lifestyle changes
e. Recreational habits
f. Exercise habits
g. Dietary habits; dietary deficiency: iron, folic acid, vitamin B_{12}
h. Caffeine intake
i. Tobacco use: record as pack-years (number of packs per day times the number of years the patient has been smoking)
j. Alcohol use: record as alcoholic beverages consumed per month, week, or day
k. Recent foreign travel
l. Sexuality
1) Safe sex practices
2) Sexual preference: heterosexual; homosexual; bisexual

 3) Multiple sexual partners
 4) Sexual activity with prostitutes, homosexuals, or bisexuals
5. Medication history
 a. Agents used to treat existing hematologic conditions
 1) Drugs used for erythropoiesis: iron, vitamin B_{12}, pyridoxine, folic acid, recombinant human erythropoietin
 2) Drugs used for bleeding or clotting disorders: aspirin inhibitors, nonsteroidal antiinflammatory agents, aminocaproic acid (Amicar), cryoprecipitate, anticoagulants
 3) Antineoplastic agents for cancer or autoimmune disease
 4) Antiviral agents
 5) Antiretroviral medications
 6) Drugs to augment the immune system (e.g., interferon, interleukin-2, and colony-stimulating factors)
 7) Antibody preparations targeting autoimmune disorders (e.g., infliximab for Crohn's disease, rituximab for rheumatoid arthritis)
 b. Agents that may exert a negative effect on hematologic/immunologic system
 1) Allergy medication
 2) Analgesics
 a) Acetaminophen: may decrease platelets; may cause hemolytic anemia
 b) Antiinflammatory agents
 i) Antigout drugs (e.g., colchicine): may cause aplastic anemia
 ii) Aspirin: inhibits platelet aggregation; decreases macrophage activity
 iii) Corticosteroids (e.g., prednisone): suppresses the immune/ inflammatory process
 iv) Nonsteroidal (e.g., phenylbutazone [Butazolidin], ibuprofen [Motrin]): inhibits platelet aggregation; depresses bone marrow and may cause aplastic anemia; lyse T, B, and natural killer cells; inhibits interferon production; inhibits IL-1 and IL-2 production
 c) Opiates
 i) Heroin: may decrease platelets
 ii) Morphine sulfate: may decrease platelets
 3) Antibiotics
 a) Oral antibiotics: may kill vitamin K-producing bacteria in the GI tract
 b) All antibiotics may cause opportunistic infections by altering normal flora in GI tract, mouth, vagina, etc.; *Clostridium difficile* is an example frequently seen in critical care units that causes severe diarrhea.
 c) Tetracyclines: inhibit chemotaxis; inhibit activation of the lymphocytes
 d) Sulfonamides (including trimethoprim sulfamethoxazole [Bactrim]): inhibit chemotaxis; inhibit activation of the lymphocytes; may cause aplastic anemia; may decrease platelets
 e) Chloramphenicol: depresses WBC production; may cause aplastic anemia
 f) Penicillin: may decrease platelets
 g) Rifampicin: may decrease platelets
 4) Anticonvulsants
 a) Phenytoin (Dilantin): inhibits the effects of corticosteroids; may cause lymph node hyperplasia; may cause anemia or thrombocytopenia
 b) Phenobarbital: may cause aplastic anemia
 5) Antidysrhythmics
 a) Procainamide: may cause hemolytic anemia, thrombocytopenia; decreases production of WBCs
 b) Quinidine: may cause hemolytic anemia, thrombocytopenia
 c) Propranolol: inhibits platelet aggregation
 6) Antifungals
 a) Amphotericin B: may cause anemia or thrombocytopenia
 7) Antihypertensives
 a) Captopril (Capoten): may cause pancytopenia
 b) Methyldopa (Aldomet): may cause thrombocytopenia, anemia
 8) Antituberculins (e.g., para-aminosalicylic acid, isoniazid [INH])
 9) Diuretics
 a) Chlorothiazide (Diuril): may cause anemia or thrombocytopenia
 b) Furosemide (Lasix): may cause anemia or thrombocytopenia
 10) Heparin: may decrease platelets
 11) Histamine receptor antagonists (e.g., ranitidine): may decrease platelets
 12) Immunosuppressives
 13) Oral contraceptives and diethylstilbestrol: Estrogen products cause anemia.
 14) Oral hypoglycemic agents (e.g., chlorpropamide) may cause anemia or thrombocytopenia.
 15) Sympathomimetics (e.g., epinephrine): decrease chemotaxis; decrease WBC production and response to antigens; alter antibody production
 16) Anesthetic agents (e.g., halothane, nitrous oxide, cyclopropane): decrease phagocytosis and inhibit T cell function
 c. Nonprescribed drug use
 1) Over-the-counter drugs
 2) Vitamins, minerals, and herbs
 3) Substance abuse: injectable drug use, especially if needles are shared
 a) Intravenous drug use

b) Intramuscular steroid use
c) Intradermal "poppers"

Physical Examination

1. Vital signs
   a. Weight: weight loss
   b. Heart rate: tachycardia frequently seen with anemia, blood loss, or infection
   c. Blood pressure: hypotension seen with blood loss
   d. Temperature
      1) Hyperthermia frequently seen with infection but less likely to be seen in elderly patients
      2) Hypothermia frequently seen with anemia
2. Inspection
   a. Skin and appendages
      1) Color
         a) Pallor or flushing of mucous membranes and palmar creases
         b) Pallor of conjunctivae
         c) Cyanosis
         d) Jaundice
         e) Signs of inflammation
      2) Bleeding
         a) Petechiae
         b) Ecchymosis
         c) Purpura
         d) Mucous membrane bleeding
         e) Gingival bleeding
         f) Retinal hemorrhages
         g) Hemorrhage from orifices
         h) Blood in stool, urine, sputum
      3) Moisture
         a) Dry, rough skin (i.e., xeroderma)
         b) Moisture-related skin breakdown may occur at skin folds (e.g., axillae, groin, perineal areas); fungal infections are common in these areas.
      4) Lesions and wounds
         a) Rash
         b) Excoriated skin
         c) Leg ulcers
         d) IV catheter insertion site: erythema or inflammation
         e) Chest tube insertion site: erythema or inflammation
         f) Surgical or traumatic wounds: erythema, inflammation, or poor wound healing
         g) Orthopedic devices
         h) Drains
      5) Pitting edema of extremities
      6) Hair: alopecia
      7) Nail and nailbed
         a) Pallor of nailbeds
         b) Spoon nails
         c) Clubbing
         d) Slow capillary refill (greater than 3 seconds)
   b. Mouth
      1) Dryness of the mouth (i.e., xerostomia)
      2) Gingival and mucosal ulceration
      3) Swollen, reddened, bleeding gums
      4) Red, beefy tongue
      5) White coating on tongue (e.g., candidiasis, also called *thrush*)
      6) White, irregular lesions on lateral surfaces of tongue (oral hairy leukoplakia frequently seen in HIV-positive patients)
      7) Purplish lesions on tongue
   c. Gastrointestinal: nasogastric tube drainage
   d. Neuromuscular
      1) Decreased level of consciousness
      2) Pupil changes
      3) Decreased sensation
      4) Muscle weakness
3. Palpation
   a. Pulse amplitude
   b. Enlargement or tenderness of superficial lymph nodes
      1) Symptoms of benign or inflammatory lymph nodes include association with pain, movability, and regular borders.
      2) Malignant lymph nodes characterized by irregular shape, lack of movability, decreased discomfort
   c. Tenderness during sternal or rib palpation
   d. Tenderness during abdominal palpation
   e. Hepatomegaly
   f. Splenomegaly
4. Percussion
   a. Decreased deep tendon reflexes
   b. Diaphragmatic excursion
   c. Hepatomegaly
   d. Splenomegaly
5. Auscultation
   a. Cardiovascular
      1) Dysrhythmia
      2) S_3
      3) S_4
      4) Murmur
      5) Rub
      6) Bruits over carotids, aorta
   b. Pulmonary
      1) Crackles
      2) Pleural rub
   c. Abdomen
      1) Bowel sounds
      2) Peritoneal friction rub

Diagnostic Studies

1. Blood
   a. Hematology
      1) Red blood cells (RBC): normal $4.4\text{-}5.9 \times 10^6$/mL for males; $3.8\text{-}5.2 \times 10^6$/mL for females
         a) Quantity
            i) Elevated in dehydration, chronic hypoxemia, or high altitudes; may temporarily increase after a cold shower or with intense emotions
            ii) Decreased in bone marrow suppression, hemorrhage, anemias, leukemias, or hypothyroidism

b) Quality
   i) Size
      (a) Microcytic: RBCs too small
      (b) Macrocytic: RBCs too large
   ii) Color
      (a) Hypochromic: hemoglobin concentration too low
      (b) Hyperchromic: hemoglobin concentration too high
   iii) Types of anemia
      (a) Macrocytic, normochromic: pernicious anemia, folate deficiency
      (b) Microcytic, hypochromic: iron deficiency anemic
      (c) Normocytic, normochromic: aplastic anemia, posthemorrhagic anemia, hemolytic anemia, sickle cell anemia, and anemia of chronic illness; note that the RBCs are normal size and color but the numbers are insufficient

2) Reticulocyte count: normal 0.5-1.5% of RBC
   a) Young RBCs
   b) Assesses the responsiveness and potential of the bone marrow to respond to bleeding or hemolysis

3) Erythrocyte sedimentation rate (ESR or sed rate): normal 1-13 mm/hr for males, 1-20 mm/hr for females
   a) Nonspecific test; measures the amount of RBCs that settle in 1 hour
   b) Elevated in inflammatory processes (e.g., rheumatoid arthritis; malignancy; rheumatic fever; hemolytic anemia; thyroid disorders; autoimmune disorders; nephrotic syndrome)
   c) Decreased in polycythemia vera; hypofibrinogenemia; sickle cell anemia (not crisis); heart failure
   d) May be used to monitor trends in patients with chronic inflammatory diseases undergoing treatment

4) Hemoglobin: normal 13-18 g/dL for males; 12-16 g/dL for females
   a) Elevated in polycythemia which may occur in chronic hypoxia or high altitudes
   b) Decreased in anemia, hemorrhage

5) Hematocrit: normal 40-52% for males; 35-47% for females
   a) Elevated in dehydration or polycythemia
   b) Decreased with anemia, leukemia, or with normal hemoglobin and water overload

6) Red cell indices
   a) Mean corpuscular volume (MCV) (an average of size): normal 80-100 fL
      i) Decreased in iron deficiency, pernicious anemia
      ii) Increased in folic acid deficiency, high reticulocyte count
   b) Mean corpuscular hemoglobin (MCH) (an average of weight of hemoglobin in an RBC): normal 26.6-34 pg
      i) Decreased in iron deficiency, sickle cell anemia
      ii) Increased in polycythemia
   c) Mean corpuscular hemoglobin concentration (MCHC): normal 31.4-36.3 g/dL

7) Peripheral smear: evaluation of blood cell size, shape, and composition to provide insight but not confirmation of medical disorders
   a) Heinz bodies common with hemolytic anemia and portal hypertension
   b) Schistocytes present with disseminated intravascular coagulation
   c) Spherocytes occur after massive transfusion.
   d) Target cells present with iron deficiency, liver disease

8) White blood cells (WBC): 3500-11,000/mm^3
   a) Elevated in inflammation, infection, trauma, surgery, acute leukemia, stress
   b) Decreased in bone marrow depression (e.g., aplastic anemia, agranulocytosis, chronic leukemia, sepsis, chronic illness, autoimmune disorders)

9) Differential
   a) Neutrophils: normal 40-80%
      i) Elevated in infection; inflammatory processes; malignancy; trauma; hemorrhage; burns; tissue necrosis (e.g., myocardial infarction); ketoacidosis
      ii) Decreased in overwhelming infection; bone marrow depression; vitamin B_{12} or folic acid deficiency; hypersplenism
      iii) Presence of excessive bands rather than mature neutrophils signifies bacterial infection (termed a *left shift*).
      iv) Presence of grossly immature or malformed cells, called *blasts,* are indicative of leukemia.
   b) Eosinophils: normal 0-5%
      i) Elevated in:
         (a) Allergic conditions
            (i) Asthma
            (ii) Eczema
         (b) Eosinophilic leukemia
         (c) Autoimmune disorders
         (d) Parasitic infection, especially helminthic infections
         (e) Pulmonary disorders: pneumonia, inflammatory conditions
         (f) Skin rashes

ii) Decreased in:
(a) Adrenocortical stimulation
(b) Stress
(c) Cushing's syndrome
(d) Systemic lupus erythematosus

c) Basophils: 0-2%
i) Elevated in allergic conditions; inflammatory processes; graft rejection; acute leukemia; recent splenectomy
ii) Decreased in hyperthyroidism and long-term corticosteroid therapy

d) Monocytes: 3-8%
i) Elevated in chronic inflammatory conditions, viral infections, tuberculosis, ulcerative colitis, parasites
ii) Decreased in immunodeficiency disorders

e) Lymphocytes: 10-40%
i) Elevated in acute or chronic lymphocytic leukemia; chronic infections: bacterial and viral; multiple myeloma; mononucleosis; Cushing's syndrome
ii) Decreased in immunodeficiency disorders (e.g., AIDS; systemic lupus erythematosus; leukemia; antineoplastic drugs; steroids), prolonged critical illness or malnutrition, burns, sepsis
iii) Lymphocyte assays (Table 10-7)
(a) T cells
(b) B cells
(c) Natural killer cells

f) Changes in differential
i) Shift to the left: increased percentage of bands (i.e., immature neutrophils); seen in bacterial infection
ii) Shift to the right: increased percentage of segs (i.e., segmented neutrophils); seen in inflammation, pernicious anemia, viral illness, or hepatic disease
iii) Regenerative shift (shift to the left): elevated WBC with increased percentage of bands; indicative of stimulation of bone marrow

Table 10-7 Lymphocyte Assays

Lymphocyte Type	Percentage of Lymphocytes
Total T cells	70-80%
CD4 (helper T cells)	29-60%
CD8 (suppressor T cells)	18-42%
CD4/CD8 (helper/suppressor ratio)	0.8:2.9
Total B cells	10-20%

iv) Degenerative shift: decreased WBC with increased percentage of bands; indicative of bone marrow depression

10) Platelets: normal 150,000-400,000/mm^3; decreased in systemic lupus erythematosus, HIV infection, idiopathic thrombocytopenic purpura, sepsis, DIC
a) 50,000 to 100,000/mm^3: prolonged bleeding times, increased risk of bleeding after severe trauma or surgery
b) Below 50,000/mm^3: increased risk of bleeding after minor trauma
c) Below 20,000/mm^3: risk of spontaneous bleeding, including intracranial bleeding

11) Special hematology
a) Erythropoietin level: normal greater than 5-35 IU/L
i) Increased in anemia, chemotherapy, AIDS, renal cell carcinoma
ii) Decreased in polycythemia vera or chronic kidney disease
b) Ferritin level: normal 20-200 ng/mL
i) Iron precursor that demonstrates iron stores and ability to make new RBCs
ii) Decreased in iron-deficient anemia, nutritional deficiencies, and some bone marrow suppression
c) Iron level: normal 50-150 mcg/dL; reflects total iron, but not ability to create new iron, so this test is only used for iron evaluation in conjunction with ferritin level and iron-binding capacity or transferrin saturation
d) Total iron-binding capacity (TIBC): normal 250-410 mcg/dL
i) Reflects iron binding to hemoglobin
ii) Decreased with abnormal hemoglobin or anemia
e) Transferrin saturation: normal greater than 20%; provides an indication of available iron
f) Haptoglobin levels: normal 60-270 mg/dL in a fasting state; decreased in hemolytic anemias.
g) Hemoglobin variant/fetal hemoglobin: normal less than 1% of RBCs; used to detect or monitor the level of hemolysis in sickle cell disease

b. Clotting profile
1) Prothrombin time (PT): normal 12-15 seconds; assesses extrinsic coagulation pathway and the common pathway
a) International normalized ratio (INR): therapeutic INR is usually 2-3 but may be higher, depending on indications for anticoagulant therapy

            i) Mathematical calculation that accounts for the differences in sensitivity between reagents; standardizes PT values
    2) Activated partial thromboplastin time (aPTT): normal 25-38 seconds; assesses intrinsic coagulation pathway and the common pathway
    3) Activated clotting time (ACT): therapeutic ACT during procedures that require anticoagulation (e.g., PCI) is usually 300-350 seconds
        a) Bedside test used to monitor heparin-induced anticoagulation
        b) Sheath removal is generally delayed until ACT is less than 150 seconds.
    4) Thrombin time: normal 10-15 seconds; assesses time for thrombin to convert fibrinogen to a fibrin clot
        a) Used for monitoring fibrinolytic therapy (e.g., r-PA, rt-PA)
        b) Highly sensitive to minimal exposure to anticoagulants, and thus used for trending value rather than precise medication dose adjustment
    5) Bleeding time: normal 1-4 minutes; assesses platelet function
    6) Lee White clotting time: normal 6-12 minutes; rarely used nonspecific test for clotting abnormalities
    7) Fibrinogen level: normal 200-400 mg/dL
        a) Elevated in hypercoagulable states and inflammatory conditions; commonly increased in lymphoma, acute leukemia, autoimmune diseases
        b) Decreased in hypocoagulable states with propensity to bleed
        c) Chronic liver disease may cause increased or decreased levels
    8) Fibrin degradation products (FDPs) (also referred to as *fibrin split products (FSPs)*: normal 0-10 mcg/dL
        a) Elevated in excessive fibrinolysis (e.g., DIC)
    9) D-dimer: normal less than 250 ng/mL; elevated in DIC
        a) Differentiates DIC from abnormal fibrinogen produced by a failing liver
        b) Used to detect pulmonary embolism in some patients without factors that falsely increase D-dimer such as recent surgery, solid malignancies, autoimmune disease, and heart failure
    10) Specific factor assays: measure amounts of each factor in the blood
        a) Antithrombin III levels: normal greater than 50% of control; decreased in clotting disorders such as DIC
        b) Protein C levels: normal 60-130% of normal activity; decreased by heparin, DIC, liver disease
        c) Protein S levels: normal 70-150% of normal activity; decreased by heparin, DIC, liver disease
c. Serum proteins
    1) Total protein: normal 6-8 g/dL
    2) Albumin: normal 3.5-4.5 g/dL
    3) C-reactive protein: normal less than 0.8 mg/dL; nonspecific test for evaluating severity and course of inflammatory conditions
    4) Serum protein electrophoresis: immunoglobulin analysis (Table 10-8)
    5) Complement assay
        a) Components
            i) Total complement: normal 41-90 hemolytic units
            ii) C1 esterase inhibitor: normal 16-33 mg/dL
            iii) C3: normal 88-252 mg/dL in men; 88-206 mg/dL in females
            iv) C4: normal 12-72 mg/dL in men; 13-75 mg/dL in females
        b) Decreased total complement levels occurs in the following:
            i) Systemic lupus erythematosus (SLE)
            ii) Acute poststreptococcal glomerulonephritis
            iii) Acute serum sickness
            iv) Cirrhosis of the liver
            v) Multiple myeloma
            vi) Severe immunodeficiency
            vii) Rapidly rejecting allografts
        c) Elevated total complement levels occur in the following:
            i) Obstructive jaundice
            ii) Thyroiditis
            iii) Acute rheumatic fever
            iv) Rheumatoid arthritis
            v) Acute myocardial infarction
            vi) Ulcerative colitis
            vii) Diabetes mellitus
d. Chemistry
    1) Calcium: normal 8.5-10.5 mg/dL
    2) Bilirubin: normal total bilirubin 0.3-1.3 mg/dL
        a) Indirect (before being conjugated by liver): 0.1-1 mg/dL
        b) Direct (after being conjugated by liver): 0.1-0.3 mg/dL
e. Type and crossmatch
    1) Blood typing: determined by agglutination studies
    2) Rh factor determination
    3) Coombs' test: detects immune antibodies important in crossmatching
        a) Direct: normal negative; measures antibodies (IgG) attached to RBCs
        b) Indirect: normal negative; measures antibodies (IgG) in the serum
f. Human leukocyte antigens (HLA): evaluates tissue compatibility

Table 10-8 Immunoglobulin Analysis

Immunoglobulin	Increased	Decreased
IgG	• Infection • Hepatitis A • Glomerulonephritis • Rheumatoid arthritis • Systemic lupus erythematosus • AIDS • IgG myeloma	• Agammaglobulinemia • Chronic lymphocytic leukemia
IgM	• Hepatitis A and B • Chronic infections • SLE • Rheumatoid arthritis • Sjögren's syndrome • AIDS	• Hypogammaglobulinemia • Chronic lymphocytic leukemia • IgG myeloma • IgA myeloma • Agammaglobulinemia
IgA	• SLE • Rheumatoid arthritis • IgA myeloma	• IgA deficiency • Acute and chronic lymphocytic leukemia • Agammaglobulinemia • IgG myeloma • Chronic infections
IgE	• Allergic rhinitis • Allergic asthma • Parasitic infection	• IgA deficiency • Intrinsic asthma
IgD	• Eczema • Skin disorders	• Unknown

1) Tissue
   a) Complement-dependent cytotoxic assay
   b) Mixed lymphocyte culture
2) Crossmatching

g. Immune profile
   1) CD4 cell count: normal 800 cells/mm^3; varies with age
      a) Measured helper T cells
      b) Decreased in HIV infection and AIDS; assists in staging HIV infection
      c) Decreased with chronic corticosteroid therapy or immunosuppressive treatment
   2) T4/T8 (CD4/CD8) ratio
      a) Helper cells : suppressor/cytotoxic cells ratio: normal 1.8
      b) Normally more CD4 cells than CD8 cells
      c) Reverse ratio in HIV infection or AIDS

h. HIV antibody screening: normal negative
   1) Detects antibodies to HIV; present with exposure to HIV, but absence does not mean that the patient has not been exposed because time is required for development of antibodies
   2) Does not indicate immunity
   3) Types of tests
      a) Enzyme-linked immunosorbent assay (ELISA): screening test subject to error; up to 10% false-positive results
      b) Western blot: more specific than ELISA

i. HIV virus screening (e.g., polymerase chain reaction [PCR]: normal negative)

j. HIV viral load testing
   1) May range from imperceptible (less than 25-5000 copies of HIV/mL) to 1 million or more copies/mL; consider that the higher the viral load, the more rapid the damage from HIV
   2) Used to evaluate the effectiveness of antiretroviral therapy

2. Culture and sensitivity: various body secretions (e.g., blood, urine, wound secretions)
   a. Gram stain: identification of gram-positive or gram-negative bacteria
   b. Culture: identification of microorganism
   c. Sensitivity
      1) Minimum inhibitory concentration (MIC): the smallest concentration of antibiotic that effectively inhibits bacterial growth; reported as antibiotic concentration per mL of solution necessary for growth inhibition
      2) This is compared with the achievable blood level of the antibiotic.
         a) If this level is less than the MIC, the bacterium is considered resistant to that antibiotic.
         b) If this level is greater than the MIC, the bacterium is considered sensitive to that antibiotic.
         c) Certain antimicrobials are dosed to achieve a specific MIC level (e.g., vancomycin), while other blood levels are used to assess toxicity (e.g., aminoglycosides).
      3) Other factors, such as known adverse effects of the antibiotic, are also considered.

3. Urine
   a. RBCs: normal 0-2/low power field; RBCs in the urine may indicate trauma (e.g., renal calculi), severe thrombocytopenia, or bleeding disorder (e.g., DIC)
   b. WBCs: normal 0-4/low power field; WBCs in the catheterized urine specimen indicate urinary tract infection
   c. Bilirubin: normal none; urobilinogen indicates biliary obstruction or liver disease
4. Stool
   a. Blood: may be grossly bloody or guaiac positive in bleeding disorders
   b. Clostridial toxin assay: normal negative; positive indicates the presence of a toxin that is released by *Clostridium difficile*
5. Radiologic and radioisotope studies
   a. Chest x-ray: may show infiltrates indicative of infection or bleeding
   b. Flat plate of abdomen: may show gross bleeding or hematoma
   c. Lymphangiography: visualizes the lymph system after injection of a dye; assists in node assessment
   d. Isotopic lymphangiography: uses technetium 99m and is less invasive than radiographic lymphangiography
   e. Computed tomography (CT) scans: chest, liver, spleen; detection of enlarged lymph nodes
   f. Positron emission tomography (PET) scans: demonstrate metabolic activity and glucose uptake that can indicate the presence of malignancy, abnormal lymph nodes
6. Biopsy
   a. Bone marrow
      1) Aspirate reveals cell numbers and maturation to diagnose bone marrow suppression
      2) Biopsy of the bone and bone marrow is necessary for diagnosis of leukemia.
   b. Lymph node
      1) Open: direct visualization; performed in operating room
      2) Closed or needle: performed at bedside
   c. Synovial
   d. Biopsy of transplanted organs to look for indications of rejection
7. Anergy panel testing
   a. Administration of antigen for observation of a delayed inflammatory skin reaction
      1) Tuberculosis, mumps, *Candida*, and trichophytin are most frequently used.
      2) Mumps antigen is contraindicated for patients allergic to chicken or eggs.
   b. Normal response: a negative response to tuberculosis (unless the patient has been previously exposed to tuberculosis) and a positive reaction to several of the other antigens within 24-72 hours
   c. Abnormal responses
      1) Anergy: failure to respond to any of the injections
      2) Immunodeficiency: induration of less than 5 mm in diameter

Blood and Blood Component Administration

Actions

1. Replacement of circulating volume, blood, or blood component
2. Improvement of oxygen-carrying capacity (RBCs, whole blood)
3. Replenishment of clotting factors (fresh frozen plasma, cryoprecipitate) and platelets
4. Replenishment of granulocytes

Blood and Blood Products

See Table 10-9.

Collaborative Management

1. Administer blood safely.
   a. Insert or ensure patency of IV catheter; do not use a catheter (or lumen) smaller than 20 gauge.
   b. Ensure that the type and crossmatch has been done and blood or blood component is available.
   c. Assess vital signs; notify physician if temperature is 37.8° C (100° F) or higher.
   d. Request blood or blood component from blood bank when ready to administer it within 20-30 minutes; if you cannot begin the transfusion within 30 minutes after receiving it, return it to the blood bank.
   e. Check all of the following before administration of blood or blood component:
      1) Physician prescription for blood or blood product
      2) Consent form signed by the patient (according to hospital policy)
      3) Confirm the following with another registered nurse:
         a) Patient's name and hospital number on patient ID bracelet
         b) Type of blood component
         c) Patient's blood group and Rh type
         d) Donor's blood group and Rh type
         e) Unit number of blood or blood component
         f) Expiration date of the blood or blood component
   f. Sign the transfusion record, along with the RN who confirmed the above information.
   g. Prime the blood administration set with normal (0.9%) saline, allowing the normal saline to cover the filter; use only normal saline, do not use dextrose-containing solutions or lactated Ringer's solution.
   h. Warm the blood if indicated.

Table 10-9 Blood and Blood Products

Product	Contents	Compatibility Required	Uses	Volume/Unit	Comments
Whole blood	RBCs, WBCs, platelets, plasma, and clotting factors	ABO, Rh specific NOTE: In emergency situations, type-specific blood or O⁻ blood may be used	Restores blood volume and oxygen-carrying capacity	Approximately 500 mL	• Must be fresh (less than 4 hours old) to preserve platelet function • Administer over 2-4 hours • Best for hemorrhagic shock
Packed red blood cells	RBCs and 20% plasma	ABO, Rh specific preferred; ABO, Rh compatible required	Restores oxygen-carrying capacity	Approximately 250 mL	• Increases hemoglobin by 1 g/dL/unit and hematocrit by 2-3%/unit; this change takes at least 6-12 hours • Administer over 2-4 hours
Washed red blood cells	RBCs and 20% plasma with fewer WBCs and platelets than packed RBCs	ABO, Rh specific preferred; ABO, Rh compatible required	Restores oxygen-carrying capacity in patients previously sensitized by transfusions	Approximately 250 mL	• As for packed RBCs • Must be administered within 24 hours of washing
Leukocyte-poor RBCs	RBCs, plasma but no leukocytes	ABO, Rh specific preferred; ABO, Rh compatible required	Restores oxygen-carrying capacity in patients susceptible to febrile reactions	Approximately 250 mL	• As for packed RBCs
Platelets	Platelets, WBCs, plasma	ABO, Rh specific or compatible	Corrects low platelet levels to aid in clotting	Approximately 50 mL	• Administer 1 unit over 10 minutes • Will increase platelet count by 5000-10,000/mm³ • Agitate often as platelets tend to settle
Fresh frozen plasma (FFP)	Water, plasma proteins, clotting factors	Rh compatibility required; ABO compatibility preferred	Expands blood volume Restores clotting factor deficiencies Contains no platelets	Approximately 250 mL	• Takes 20 minutes to thaw • Must be given within 6 hours of thawing • Administer 1 unit over 1-2 hours or more rapidly if for hemorrhage
Granulocytes	WBCs, small amount of plasma	ABO, Rh compatible; HLA (human leukocyte antigen) compatible if possible	Restores granulocytes in life-threatening granulocytopenia	Approximately 300 mL	• Administer rapidly • Chills and fever may occur; steroids and antihistamines may be given; meperidine may be used for shivering • Administer over 2-6 hours
Cryoprecipitate	VIII, XIII, fibrinogen, fibronectin	ABO specific or compatible	Replaces clotting factors	Approximately 10 mL; usually 10 bags pooled	• Administer rapidly immediately after thawing • May administer 30 units at one time
Albumin	Albumin from plasma	No compatibility required	Provides volume expansion (no clotting factors)	5%: 200 or 500 mL 25%: 50 or 100 mL	• Administer 1 mL/min or more rapidly if patient is in shock • Chemically processed so no risk of hepatitis
Plasma protein fraction (PPF)	Albumin and globulin in saline solution	No compatibility required	Provides volume expansion (no clotting factors)	5%: 200-500 mL	• Administer 10 mL/min • Chemically processed so no risk of hepatitis

1) Blood may be warmed to avoid hypothermia in the patient receiving four or more units over 6 hours or in the patient who has tested positive for cold agglutinins.
2) Warm the blood to 32°-37° C, using a blood-warming device in these situations.

i. Clamp off the saline and start the blood or blood component.
j. Adjust rate to administer slowly 25-50 mL within the first 15 minutes.
k. Monitor for transfusion reaction (Table 10-10 and Box 10-1).
    1) Ask the patient to notify the nurse if he or she develops chills, low back pain, shortness of breath, nausea, sweating, itching, hives, or anxiety.
    2) Assess for clinical indications of transfusion reaction (Table 10-10).
    3) Take appropriate action for transfusion reactions (Table 10-10 and Box 10-2) if they occur.
l. Monitor vital signs every 15 minutes for the first hour and then every 30 minutes until transfusion is complete or according to hospital policy.
m. Adjust rate to infuse blood within 4 hours of initiating the infusion; FFP, platelets, and granulocytes are administered rapidly; if the blood slows, do the following:
    1) Ensure that the roller clamp is open.
    2) Increase the height of the blood bag.
    3) Gently squeeze the bag several times to agitate the blood cells.
    4) Gently squeeze the tubing and flashbulb.
    5) Remove dressing and check site.
    6) Close the blood and open the saline to allow 50-100 mL to irrigate the line, then restart the blood.
n. Flush administration set tubing with saline after transfusion is complete.
o. Disconnect the empty blood bag from the administration set and dispose of these according to hospital policy.

2. Monitor for adverse effects (Table 10-11) and complications.
    a. Complications
        1) Hepatitis
            a) Hepatitis B transmission has been reduced by mandatory testing of all donor blood for hepatitis B surface antigen.
            b) Non-A, non-B hepatitis (also referred to as type C hepatitis) accounts for 90% of transfusion-related hepatitis
        2) HIV
            a) HIV transmission through blood transfusion has been greatly reduced by screening for HIV antibody, which started in 1985, and by careful history taking of potential donors for risk factors for HIV.
        3) Cytomegalovirus (CMV)
            a) CMV usually is not a problem for immunocompetent patients but may be life-threatening in immunodeficient patients.
            b) Clinical indications of CMV infection include mild fever, mild splenomegaly, and atypical serum lymphocytes.
            c) CMV-negative blood products are indicated for immunodeficient patients.
        4) Transfusion-related acute lung injury or ARDS

Box 10-1 Clinical Indications of Blood Transfusion Reaction in an Unconscious or Sedated Patient

Tachycardia or bradycardia
Hypotension
Fever
Visible signs of hemoglobin in urine
Oliguria or anuria
Bleeding

Box 10-2 Nursing Actions for Suspected Transfusion Reaction

1. Stop transfusion
2. Maintain IV access with normal saline and new administration set
3. Reassure the patient; stay at the bedside
4. Notify physician and blood bank
5. Recheck blood numbers and type
6. Treat symptoms appropriately
7. Return unused portion of blood in blood bag and administration set to the blood bank
8. Collect and send blood and urine samples to the laboratory; send another urine specimen 24 hours after transfusion reaction
9. Document the transfusion reaction and treatment administered

Drugs Affecting Clotting

See Figure 10-5 on page 665.

Platelet Aggregation Inhibitors

1. Many drugs inhibit platelet aggregation as an adverse effect (e.g., nonsteroidal antiinflammatory agents, quinidine); others (Box 10-3) are prescribed for the specific purpose of impairing platelet aggregation to prevent the development of the platelet plug (i.e., white clot) and the intrinsic pathway.
2. Actions
    a. Inhibits platelet aggregation and platelet-mediated thrombosis
        1) Quality: inhibit platelet aggregation; though this effect has traditionally been thought to last as long as the platelet lives (i.e., 9-12

Table 10-10 Types of Transfusion Reactions

Type of Reaction	Cause	Clinical Indications	Timing	Treatment
Febrile (nonhemolytic) NOTE: most common type of transfusion reaction	Antigen-antibody reaction to WBCs, platelets, or plasma proteins in the blood product	• Fever (rise in temperature greater than 1° C) • Chills • Headache • Nausea, vomiting • Flushing • Anxiety • Muscle pain	Immediately or up to 6 hours after transfusion	• Stop transfusion • Keep vein open with saline • Notify physician and blood bank • Send blood specimens to blood bank • Antipyretics as indicated • Steroids may be prescribed • Washed or leukocyte-poor blood should be considered for future transfusions
Mild allergic (Type I hypersensitivity reaction)	Allergic reaction to plasma-soluble antigen in blood product	• Flushing • Itching • Urticaria • Hives	During transfusion or up to 1 hour after transfusion	• If febrile, stop transfusion • If afebrile, slow transfusion to keep-vein-open rate until advised by physician • Notify physician and blood bank • Monitor vital signs • Antihistamines as prescribed
Anaphylaxis (Type I hypersensitivity reaction)	Allergic reaction in patients with IgA deficiency sensitized to IgA through previous transfusion or pregnancy	• Anxiety • Urticaria • Facial edema • Dysphagia • Abdominal cramps, diarrhea • Urinary incontinence • Dyspnea • Stridor • Wheezing • Cyanosis • Chest pain or pulmonary edema may occur • Shock may occur • Cardiopulmonary arrest may occur	Immediately; after transfusion of only a few mL of blood	• Stop transfusion • Keep vein open with saline • Notify physician and blood bank • Oxygen • Antihistamines, steroids, and/or aqueous epinephrine as prescribed • Emergency airway and/or CPR may be necessary • Washed or leukocyte-poor blood or blood from IgA-deficient donor should be considered for future transfusions

Acute hemolytic (Type II hypersensitivity reaction)	ABO group incompatibility; antibodies in recipient's plasma attach to antigens in transfused RBCs, causing RBC destruction	• Burning sensation along vein
		• Lumbar pain
		• Chills
		• Fever
		• Flushing
		• Nausea, vomiting
		• Tachycardia, tachypnea
		• Hypotension (may be the only sign in unconscious patient)
		• May have:
		  • Dyspnea
		  • Chest pain
		  • Hemoglobinemia; hemoglobinuria
		  • Anuria
		  • Disseminated intravascular coagulation
		• Shock may occur
		• Cardiopulmonary arrest may occur
			Usually within 15 minutes after initiation of transfusion, but may occur anytime during transfusion; may be delayed if Rh incompatibility	• Stop transfusion
				• Keep vein open with saline
				• Notify physician and blood bank
				• Send blood unit and blood sample from the patient to the blood bank immediately
				• Monitor vital signs and urine output
				• Fluids for shock as prescribed
				• Diuretics (usually mannitol) may be prescribed especially if hemoglobinuria occurs
				• Monitor for acute renal failure and shock
				• Request new crossmatch

Table 10-10 Types of Transfusion Reactions—cont'd

Type of Reaction	Cause	Clinical Indications	Timing	Treatment
Delayed hemolytic	Alloimmune response causes slow hemolysis	• Fever • Mild jaundice • Purpura • Anemia	Days to weeks after completion of transfusion	• Monitor urine output and hemoglobin and hematocrit levels
Noncardiac pulmonary edema	Donor antibodies react with recipient HLA antigen	• Fever, chills • Dyspnea • Cough • Crackles • Hypoxemia • Shock	During transfusion or shortly after the transfusion	• Stop transfusion • Administer oxygen • Intubation and mechanical ventilation may be necessary • Steroids may be prescribed
Circulatory overload	Fluid administered faster that the cardiovascular system can accommodate	• Tachycardia • Hypertension • Headache • Jugular venous distention • Increased RAP, PAP, PAOP • Dyspnea • Cough • Crackles	During transfusion or shortly after the transfusion	• Administer RBCs no more rapidly than 4 mL/kg/hr unless severe hemorrhage occurring • Slow or stop transfusion • Continue IV saline slowly if transfusion discontinued • Position patient upright with legs over the side of bed • Oxygen as indicated • Diuretics or venous vasodilators as indicated
Sepsis	Transfusion of contaminated blood components (blood should be infused within 4 hours)	• Chills • Fever • Vomiting • Abdominal pain • Diarrhea (may be bloody) • Hypotension • Shock	During or after transfusion	• Stop the transfusion • Obtain cultures of patient's blood and send with remaining blood to blood bank • Antibiotics as prescribed • Fluids or steroids as prescribed • Vasopressors may be needed
Graft-versus-host disease	Occurs in immunodeficient patients who receive lymphocytes; involves donor's lymphocytes mounting an attack against the recipient's tissues	• Fever • Rash • Stomatitis • Hepatitis • Severe diarrhea • Bone marrow suppression • Infection • Lymphadenopathy • Hepatosplenomegaly	Days to weeks after transfusion	• Steroids as prescribed • Methotrexate or azathioprine (Imuran) may be prescribed

Box 10-3 Drugs Used to Decrease Platelet Aggregation

COX inhibitors (e.g., aspirin)
Phosphodiesterase inhibitors (e.g., dipyridamole [Persantine], cilostazol [Pletal])
ADP pathway inhibitors (e.g., ticlopidine [Ticlid], clopidogrel [Plavix], prasugrel [Effient])
GP IIb/IIIa platelet receptor blockers (e.g., abciximab [ReoPro], eptifibatide [Integrilin], tirofiban HCl [Aggrastat])
Combination agents (e.g., dipyridamole and aspirin [Aggrenox])
Dextran 40 (LMD)

days), evidence now suggests that the effect decreases after 24 hours

2) Quantity: may decrease the number of platelets, though this is an undesirable effect
   a) Referred to as *thrombotic thrombocytopenic purpura (TTP)*; treated by discontinuance of the offending drug and may require administration of platelets
   b) Monitor for and report petechiae, ecchymosis, or bleeding.

b. Cyclooxygenase (COX) inhibitors (e.g., aspirin) block synthesis of thromboxane A_2, inhibiting platelet aggregation.

Table 10-11 Potential Adverse Effects of Blood Transfusion

Complications	Clinical Indications	Prevention/Treatment

Citrate intoxication and hypocalcemia caused by binding of citrate with calcium	• Paresthesia of fingertips, circumoral area
	• Chvostek's sign
	• Trousseau's sign
	• Muscle cramps, tremors
	• Increased deep tendon reflexes (DTR), carpopedal spasm
	• Abdominal cramps, biliary colic
	• Confusion, psychosis
	• Memory loss
	• Laryngospasm, stridor
	• Tetany (characterized by cramps, twitching of the muscles, sharp flexion of the wrist and ankle joints, seizures)
	• ECG changes
	  • Prolonged QT interval
	  • Dysrhythmias
		• Monitor calcium in patients receiving multiple transfusion and/or patients with hepatic or renal disease
		• Administer 500 mg-1 g of calcium every 3-5 units of blood as prescribed

Hyperkalemia caused by hemolysis of stored blood and liberation of potassium
(NOTE: the older the blood, the higher the potassium in the blood)
	• Tachycardia progressing to bradycardia and cardiac arrest
	• Nausea, vomiting, intestinal colic, diarrhea
	• Muscle weakness progressing to flaccid paralysis
	• Numbness, tingling of extremities
	• Increased deep tendon reflexes
	• Fatigue
	• Lethargy, apathy, mental confusion
	• Respiratory muscle weakness may cause hypopnea, dyspnea
	• Respiratory distress
	• Oliguria
	• Decreased contractility, cardiac output
	• ECG changes
	  • Tall, peaked T waves
	  • Wide QRS complex
	  • Prolonged PR interval
	  • Flattened to absent P wave
	  • Bradycardia
	  • Dysrhythmias
		• Monitor potassium closely in patients receiving stored blood (especially patients with renal insufficiency)
		• Dextrose and insulin may be prescribed acutely for patients with cardiac effects of hyperkalemia

Loss of 2,3-DPG (2,3-DPG is a byproduct of glucose metabolism on the hemoglobin molecule; banked [refrigerated] blood is low in 2,3-DPG; 2,3-DPG encourages unloading between hemoglobin and oxygen)	• Clinical indications of hypoxia (e.g., tachycardia, dysrhythmias, cyanosis, restlessness, confusion)	• Especially a problem if massive amounts of banked blood are administered • Give fresh whole blood when possible for patients in need of multiple transfusions
Ammonia intoxication Occurs in older blood; especially a problem for patients with hepatic disease	• Decreased cardiac output: hypotension • Confusion • Altered level of consciousness • Elevated serum ammonia	• Avoid use of older blood, especially for massive transfusion • Monitor for ammonia intoxication in patients with hepatic disease
Dilutional coagulopathy	• Prolonged PT, aPTT • Bleeding from needle site, wound	• Administer 2 units FFP and/or platelets for every 10 units of packed RBCs as prescribed
Hypothermia	• Decrease in body temperature • Decrease in tissue delivery of oxygen caused by shift of the oxyhemoglobin dissociation curve to the left resulting in increased affinity between hemoglobin and oxygen	• Warm blood to 35-37° C if large quantities of blood are being administered

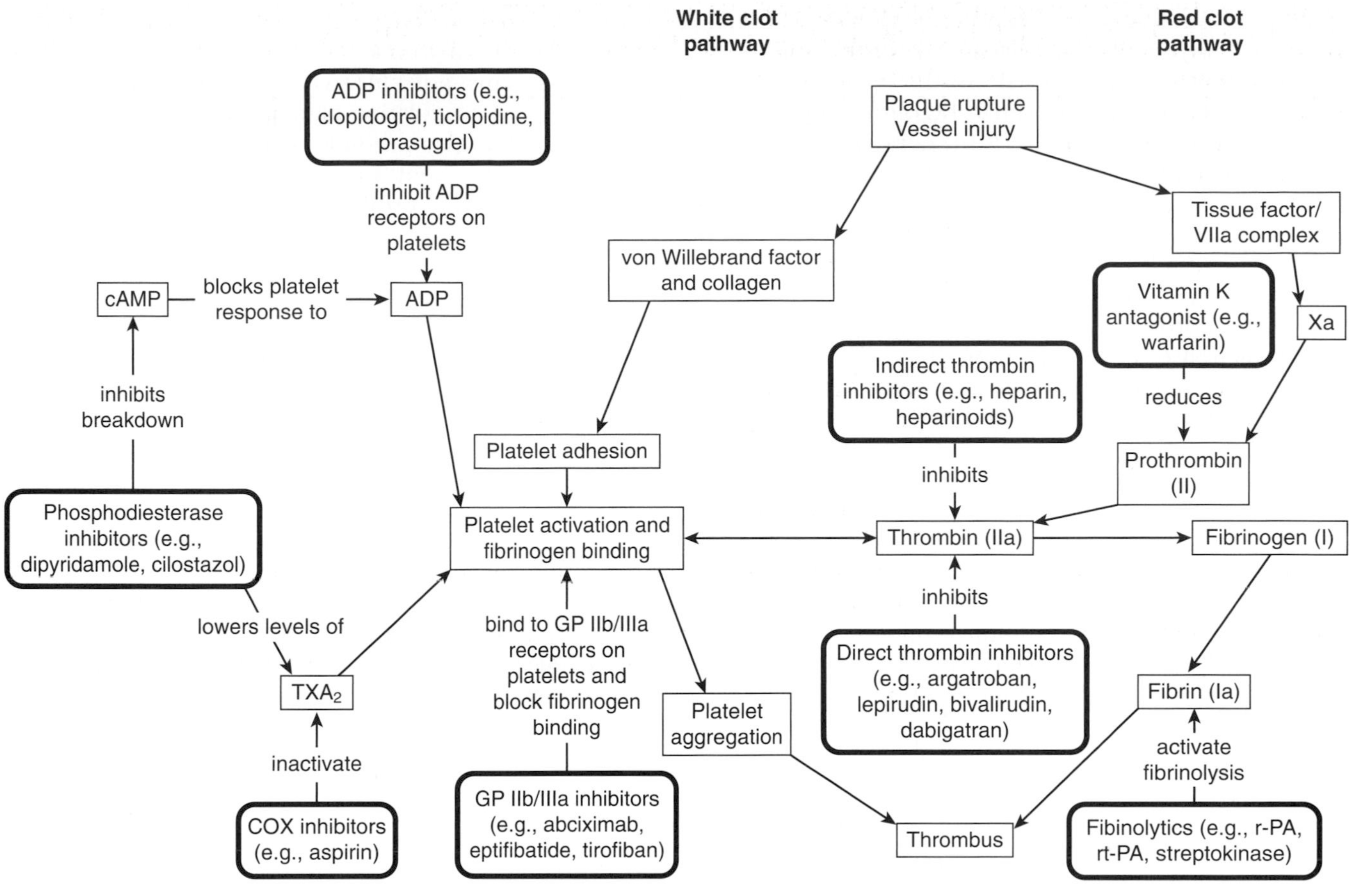

Figure 10-5 Drugs that affect clotting: Effects on pathways to thrombus formation. (Data from Bussard, M. E. [2002]. Reteplase: Nursing implications for catheter-directed thrombolytic therapy for peripheral vascular occlusions. *Crit Care Nurse, 22*[3], 57-63.)

c. ADP pathway inhibitors (e.g., ticlopidine [Ticlid], clopidogrel [Plavix], prasugrel [Effient]) block ADP from binding to its receptor, inhibiting platelet aggregation.

d. Phosphodiesterase inhibitors (e.g., dipyridamole [Persantine], cilostazol [Pletal]) increase cyclic adenosine monophosphate (cAMP) and lower levels of thromboxane A_2, inhibiting platelet aggregation.

e. Glycoprotein IIb/IIIa inhibitors (e.g., abciximab [ReoPro], eptifibatide [Integrilin], tirofiban HCl [Aggrastat]) block the glycoprotein IIb/IIIa platelet receptor; this interrupts the final common pathway for platelet aggregation by interfering with platelet aggregation via fibrinogen, von Willebrand factor, and fibronectin.

   1) Differences between these agents
      a) Half-life
         i) Abciximab: 10-30 minutes
         ii) Tirofiban: 120 minutes
         iii) Eptifibatide: 150 minutes
      b) Duration of platelet inhibition
         i) Abciximab causes the most significant and prolonged (i.e., usually 18-36 hours but may be up to a week) reduction in platelet aggregation.
         ii) Tirofiban and eptifibatide: 1-2 hours after cessation of infusion
      c) Effect of renal insufficiency on dosing
         i) Abciximab may be used with no adjustment.
         ii) Tirofiban requires dosage adjustment.
         iii) Eptifibatide is contraindicated if serum creatinine is 4 mg/dL or higher and requires dosage adjustment if serum creatinine is greater than 2 mg/dL.

3. Indications
   a. Oral agents
      1) Carotid artery disease for stroke prophylaxis (especially clopidogrel [Plavix], aspirin, or dipyridamole and ASA [Aggrenox])
      2) Peripheral arterial disease (especially cilostazol [Pletal])
      3) Postvascular surgery (especially dextran 40)
      4) Maintenance of coronary artery stent patency (especially clopidogrel [Plavix] or aspirin)

5) Acute coronary syndrome with or without myocardial infarction (especially aspirin)

b. Intravenous agents: GP IIb/IIIa platelet receptor blockers (e.g., abciximab [ReoPro], eptifibatide [Integrilin], tirofiban HCl [Aggrastat])
   1) Acute coronary syndrome (ACS) with or without percutaneous coronary intervention (PCI); note that abciximab is only used for ACS if PCI is planned within 24 hours
   2) PCI when risk for thrombosis is high (i.e., coronary artery stent placement)

4. Evaluation of effect: bleeding time
5. Reversal agent: no specific reversal agent; platelet transfusion may be indicated

Anticoagulants

1. Indirect thrombin inhibitors (e.g., unfractionated heparin [UFH] or low molecular weight heparin [LMWH]), heparinoid (e.g., danaparoid [Organ])
   a. Action: accelerates the formation of the antithrombin III-thrombin complex which deactivates thrombin and prevents the conversion of fibrinogen to fibrin
      1) Prevents extension of existing clots
      2) Decreases platelet aggregation
      3) Note that there is an unpredictable dose-response relationship with heparin, though prediction of response is improved with weight-dosing; there is a more predictable dose-response relationship with heparinoids.
   b. Indications
      1) Acute coronary syndrome (UFH or LMWH)
      2) Prevention or treatment of deep vein thrombosis (UFH, LMWH or danaparoid)
      3) Pulmonary embolism (UFH or LMWH)
      4) Peripheral arterial emboli (UFH)
      5) Transient ischemic attack or ischemic stroke (UFH)
      6) Disseminated intravascular coagulation with clinical evidence of thromboembolism (UFH)
      7) Maintenance of arterial patency after PCI or fibrinolytic therapy (UFH or heparinoid)
      8) Maintenance of arterial line patency (UFH)
      9) Patients with or at risk of HIT having PCI
   c. Differences between unfractionated and low-molecular-weight heparin
      1) LMWH is more potent at inactivating factor Xa than inactivating thrombin.
      2) LMWH has a longer half-life: 4-6 hours as compared to 1-2 hours for UFH.
      3) LMWH has 90% bioavailability, and UFH has only 30% bioavailability, which allows a more predictable anticoagulant response for LMWH.
      4) Less risk of heparin-induced thrombocytopenia (HIT) with LMWH than UFH
      5) Cost of LMWH is greater, but there is not a need for ongoing laboratory monitoring.
   d. Evaluation of effect
      1) Unfractionated heparin: aPTT, activated clotting time (ACT)
      2) Low-molecular-weight heparin: Monitoring of coagulation parameters is not required but may prolong PT and aPTT.
   e. Reversal agent: protamine
      1) 1 mg of protamine neutralizes approximately 100 units of heparin.
      2) Administer slowly to avoid hypotension.
2. Direct thrombin inhibitors (lepirudin [Refludan], argatroban [Acova], bivalirudin [Angiomax])
   a. Action: inhibit thrombin activity (note that there is a predictable dose-response relationship)
   b. Indications
      1) Heparin-induced thrombocytopenia and associated thromboembolic complications (specifically lepirudin and argatroban)
      2) Acute coronary syndrome undergoing PCI (specifically bivalirudin)
      3) Being evaluated for use in ischemic stroke, DIC, and MI
   c. Evaluation of effect: aPTT or activated clotting time (ACT)
   d. Reversal agent: none
3. Oral anticoagulants (e.g., warfarin [Coumadin])
   a. Actions: limits the availability of vitamin K, which is necessary for the formation of factors II (prothrombin), VII, IX, and X, along with the anticoagulant proteins C and S
      1) Prevents development of a clot
      2) Prevents extension of an existing clot and secondary thromboembolic complications
   b. Indications
      1) Deep vein thrombosis
      2) Valvular heart disease
      3) Arial dysrhythmias
      4) Postvalve replacement
   c. Evaluation of effect: PT, INR (Table 10-12)
   d. Reversal agent: vitamin K

Fibrinolytics

1. Action: activation of plasminogen to accelerate clot lysis
   a. Recombinant plasminogen activators (e.g., alteplase [Activase], reteplase [Retavase], tenecteplase [TNKase])

Table 10-12 Recommended INR for Selected Indications

Indication	INR
Prophylaxis for venous thrombosis	2-3
Treatment of venous thrombosis	2-3
Treatment of pulmonary embolism	2-3
Prevention of systemic embolism Tissue heart valves Acute MI Valvular heart disease Atrial fibrillation	2-3
Mechanical prosthetic valves	2.5-3.5

1) Activate plasminogen to plasmin, the active agent which breaks and degrades the fibrin clot (i.e., speeds up the normal process to allow early reperfusion)
2) Causes clot-specific lysis to reestablish flow; tenecteplase is the most fibrin specific, and reteplase is the least fibrin specific of these agents
3) Do not cause antigenicity because these are recombinant agents

b. Streptokinase (Streptase)
1) Activates plasminogen systemically and converts it to plasmin, which then degrades fibrin clots, fibrinogen, and other plasma proteins
2) Causes systemic lytic state

c. Comparison of half-life
1) Tenecteplase: ~20 minutes so dosed as a single bolus over 5 minutes
2) Reteplase: ~15 minutes so dosed as two boluses 30 minutes apart
3) Alteplase: ~5 minutes so dosed as a bolus followed by a 90-minute infusion
4) Streptokinase: ~20 minutes, but effects last 48-72 hours due to fibrinogen depletion; dosed as a 30-60-minute infusion

2. Indications
a. Myocardial infarction (within 6 hours or still having ischemic chest pain)
1) The goal is to have fibrinolytics initiated within 30 minutes of the patient's arrival to the emergency department because time is muscle.
a) Door
b) Data
c) Decision
d) Drug
2) Note that primary PCI is preferred if a cardiac catheterization laboratory and an interventional cardiologist is available; the goal is to have the catheter passing the stenosis within 60-90 minutes.

b. Ischemic stroke (within 3 hours): It is necessary to perform a CT to rule out hemorrhagic stroke and have that CT interpreted within the 3-hour window before administering the fibrinolytic; note that new evidence suggests that this time window may be extended to 4.5 hours for some subgroups.

c. Massive pulmonary embolism: as indicated by acute right ventricular failure, refractory hypoxemia, and/or hemodynamic instability

d. Acute arterial occlusion: typically administered intraarterially

Selected Drugs That Affect Clotting

See Table 10-13.

Coagulopathies

See Table 10-14.

Disseminated Intravascular Coagulation

Definition

1. A syndrome characterized by thrombus formation and hemorrhage secondary to overstimulation of the normal coagulation process leading to massive intravascular clotting with resultant depletion in clotting factors and platelets and risk for bleeding
2. DIC may be acute or chronic, but this discussion is limited to acute DIC.

Etiology

Always secondary

1. Vascular injury or inflammation
   a. Shock
   b. Vasculitis
   c. Giant hemangioma
   d. Dissecting aneurysm
   e. Toxemia of pregnancy
2. Infection and sepsis
   a. Bacterial
      1) Gram negative (e.g., *Escherichia coli*, meningococci)
      2) Gram positive (e.g., *Staphylococcus, Streptococcus*)
   b. Viral (e.g., influenza, herpes, cytomegalovirus, adenovirus)
   c. Rickettsial (e.g., Rocky Mountain spotted fever)
   d. Protozoal (e.g., malaria)
   e. Fungal (e.g., *Aspergillus, Candida, Histoplasma, Toxoplasma*)
3. Hematologic/immunologic
   a. Hemolytic blood transfusion reaction
   b. Massive blood transfusion
   c. Prolonged cardiopulmonary bypass
   d. Sickle cell crisis
   e. Thalassemia major
   f. Polycythemia vera
   g. Anaphylaxis
   h. Systemic lupus erythematosus
   i. Transplant rejection
4. Trauma
   a. Multiple traumas
   b. Burns
   c. Acute anoxia
   d. Heat stroke
   e. Crush injury
   f. Head injury
   g. Surgery
5. Neoplastic disorders
   a. Adenocarcinoma: produce the procoagulant mucin
      1) Pancreatic cancer
      2) Breast cancer
      3) Prostate cancer
      4) Ovarian cancer
      5) Lung cancer
      6) Colon cancer
      7) Stomach cancer
   b. Cancer of the urinary tract

Text continued on p. 675

Table 10-13 Selected Drugs that Affect Clotting

Drug	Administration	Adverse Effects	Nursing Implications
Glycoprotein IIb/IIIa Inhibitors			

Abciximab (ReoPro)	• IV injection: 0.25 mg/kg administered 10 minutes to 1 hour before the start of the percutaneous transluminal coronary angioplasty (PTCA) or atherectomy followed by infusion
	• IV infusion: 0.125 mcg/kg/min (10 mcg/min maximum) for 12 hours
		• Bleeding
		  • Intracranial hemorrhage
		  • Hematuria
		  • Hematemesis
		  • Bleeding at sheath site or other puncture point
		• Thrombocytopenia
		• Hypotension
		• Bradycardia
		• Nausea, vomiting, abdominal pain
		• Chest pain
		• Back pain
		• Headache
		• Pain at injection site
		• Allergic reaction, anaphylaxis (especially with repeat administration)
			• Monitor PT, aPTT or ACT, platelet count
			• Administer with aspirin and heparin therapy as prescribed
			• Note contraindications: patients with active internal bleeding, clinically significant bleeding in the GI or GU tract within the last 6 weeks, bleeding diathesis, history of CVA within the last 2 years or CVA with significant residual neurologic deficit, intracranial neoplasm, aneurysm, AV malformation, severe uncontrolled hypertension, oral anticoagulants within 7 days unless prothrombin time is less than 1.2 times control, thrombocytopenia, presumed or documented history of vasculitis, major surgery or trauma within the last 6 weeks, pericarditis, known hypersensitivity to abciximab or murine proteins
			• Use cautiously in patients who weigh less than 75 kg, patients older than 65 years of age, patients with a history of GI disease, patients receiving thrombolytics
			• Do not administer with dextran
			• Monitor oral secretions, sputum, vomitus, NG aspirate, stool, urine for blood
			• Limit venipuncture and urinary catheterization as much as possible; use IV catheter with saline lock for blood sampling; avoid noncompressible IV sites
			• Avoid nasotracheal and nasogastric tubes if possible
			• Avoid automatic BP cuffs
			• Administer platelets as prescribed for thrombocytopenia
			• Store refrigerated, do not shake (should be clear), administer through filter

Eptifibatide (Integrilin)	For acute coronary syndrome
	• IV injection: 180 mcg/kg over 1-2 minutes followed by:
	  • IV infusion: 2 mcg/kg/min for up to 72 hours; decreased to 0.5 mcg/kg/min during PCI and continued for 24 hours after PCI
	For percutaneous coronary intervention (PCI) without acute coronary syndrome
	• IV injection: 135 mcg/kg over 1-2 minutes before procedure followed by:
	• IV infusion: 0.5 mcg/kg/min for 24 hours
		• Bleeding
		  • Intracranial hemorrhage
		  • Hematuria
		  • Hematemesis
		  • Bleeding at sheath site
		• Hypotension
			• Monitor PT, aPTT or ACT, platelet count
			• Note contraindications: active internal bleeding, clinically significant bleeding in the GI or GU tract within the last 6 weeks, bleeding diathesis, history of CVA within the last 2 years or CVA with significant residual neurologic deficit, intracranial neoplasm, aneurysm, AV malformation, severe uncontrolled hypertension, oral anticoagulants within 7 days unless prothrombin time is less than 1.2 times control, thrombocytopenia, presumed or documented history of vasculitis, major surgery or trauma within the last 6 weeks, pericarditis, known hypersensitivity to eptifibatide, renal failure, thrombocytopenia
			• Administer with aspirin and heparin therapy as prescribed
			• Monitor oral secretions, sputum, vomitus, NG aspirate, stool, urine for blood
			• Limit venipuncture and urinary catheterization as much as possible; use IV catheter with saline lock for blood sampling; avoid noncompressible IV sites
			• Avoid nasotracheal and nasogastric tubes if possible
			• Avoid automatic BP cuffs
			• Administer platelets as prescribed for thrombocytopenia
			• Store refrigerated

Tirofiban HCl (Aggrastat)	• IV infusion: premixed as 25 mg in 500 mL; usual dose is 0.4 mcg/kg/min for 30 minutes and then continued at 0.1 mcg/kg/min (dosage is decreased in renal failure)	• Bleeding
		  • Intracranial hemorrhage
		  • Hematuria
		  • Hematemesis
		  • Bleeding at sheath site
		• Hypotension
		• Bradycardia
		• Pelvic pain
			• Monitor PT, aPTT or ACT, platelet count
			• Note contraindications: active internal bleeding, clinically significant bleeding in the GI or GU tract within the last 6 weeks, bleeding diathesis, history of CVA within the last 2 years or CVA with significant residual neurologic deficit, intracranial neoplasm, aneurysm, AV malformation, severe uncontrolled hypertension, oral anticoagulants within 7 days unless prothrombin time is less than 1.2 times control, thrombocytopenia, presumed or documented history of vasculitis, major surgery or trauma within the last month, pericarditis, known hypersensitivity to tirofiban
			• Use cautiously in patients who weigh less than 75 kg, patients older than 65 years of age, patients with a history of GI disease, patients receiving thrombolytics, patients with thrombocytopenia
			• Administer with aspirin and heparin therapy as prescribed
			• Limit venipuncture and urinary catheterization as much as possible; use IV catheter with saline lock for blood sampling; avoid noncompressible IV sites
			• Monitor oral secretions, sputum, vomitus, NG aspirate, stool, urine for blood

Indirect Thrombin Inhibitors			

Unfractionated heparin (UFH)	• Subcutaneous: usually prophylactic, dose is 5000 units every 12 hours (also called *miniheparin*)
	• IV injection: usually 80 units/kg (maximum 10,000 units) followed by infusion (only 60 units/kg recommended if patient is receiving fibrinolytics or GP IIb/IIIa inhibitors)
	• IV infusion: mix 25,000 units in 500 mL (50 units/mL) and infuse at 18 units/kg/hr (maximum 1000 units/hr) (only 12 units/kg recommended if patient is receiving fibrinolytics or GP IIb/IIIa inhibitors); dose is adjusted to achieve aPTT of 1.5-2.5 times the laboratory control
	• NOTE: The trend in IV weight-dosed heparin is to decrease the amount of heparin (60 units/kg for injection followed by 12 units/kg/hr for infusion) and desirable aPTT (45-60 seconds)
	• Maximum: 40,000 units/day
		• Hemorrhage with excessive aPTT
		• Hypertension or hypotension
		• Hypersensitivity reaction including bronchospasm
		• Fever
		• Hepatitis
		• Hyperkalemia especially in patients with renal failure
		• Thrombocytopenia (caused by immune response referred to as *heparin-induced thrombocytopenia [HIT]*)
			• Monitor aPTT and platelet count and for signs of hemorrhage
			  • Note petechiae and request platelet count if petechiae noted; heparin usually discontinued if platelet count is less than 100,000/mm^3
			    — Administer lepirudin (Refludan) or argatroban as prescribed for heparin-induced thrombocytopenia (HIT)
			• Note contraindications: known hypersensitivity, active bleeding, blood dyscrasias (except DIC), suspected intracranial hemorrhage, severe hypertension, peptic ulcer disease, open wounds, recent surgery, endocarditis, shock, threatened abortion
			• Use cautiously in alcoholism, liver disease, renal disease, older adults
			• Monitor oral secretions, sputum, vomitus, NG aspirate, stool, urine for blood
			• Ensure that protamine sulfate (antidote) is available
			• Avoid IM, arterial, or venous punctures if at all possible
			• Hold pressure for longer than usual if punctures are necessary
			• Do not discontinue suddenly: warfarin usually will have already been started and the PT within therapeutic range before heparin is discontinued
			• Do not aspirate before subcutaneous administration and do not massage after administration
			• Note that NTG interacts with heparin causing more heparin to be required to achieve therapeutic aPTT; monitor aPTT closely with significant NTG dosage changes or discontinuance

Continued

Table 10-13 Selected Drugs that Affect Clotting—cont'd

Drug	Administration	Adverse Effects	Nursing Implications
Low-molecular-weight heparin (LMWH)	Enoxaparin (Lovenox) • SC: 30 mg bid Dalteparin sodium (Fragmin) • SC: 2500 units daily starting 1-2 hours before surgery and repeated qd for 5-10 days postoperatively Ardeparin (Normiflo) • SC: 50 antifactor Xa units/kg every 12 hours beginning the evening before surgery and continued until the patient is ambulatory Tinzaparin sodium (Innohep) • SC: 175 antifactor Xa units/kg daily for approximately 6 days or until adequate anticoagulation with warfarin	• Bleeding • Epidural or spinal hematoma (especially when used with patients with epidural or spinal anesthesia) • Fever • Elevation of liver enzymes • Thrombocytopenia • Chest pain	• Note that LMW heparin does not require routine laboratory monitoring because it does not usually alter PT or aPTT • Note that contraindications and cautions are as for heparin • Obtain baseline platelet count; monitor for petechiae • Monitor oral secretions, sputum, vomitus, NG aspirate, stool, urine for blood • Ensure that protamine sulfate (antidote) is available • Avoid IM, arterial, or venous punctures if at all possible • Hold pressure for longer than usual if punctures are necessary • Administer deep subcutaneously but avoid IM injection
Direct Thrombin Inhibitors			

Lepirudin (Refludan)	• IV injection: 0.4 mg/kg (maximum 44 mg) administered over 15-20 seconds followed by IV infusion
	• IV infusion: 0.15 mg/kg/hr (maximum 16.5 mg/kg/hr) for 2-10 days
	• Reduce dosage in renal or hepatic disease
		• Bleeding
		• Anemia
		• Abnormal liver function studies
		• Skin reactions
			• Monitor PT, aPTT, CBC, and for signs of bleeding
			• Note that contraindications and cautions are as for heparin
			• Obtain baseline platelet count and aPTT; monitor aPTT every 4 hours
			  • Anticoagulant effects may increase as the duration of therapy increases
			  • Anticoagulant effects are increased in patients receiving platelet aggregation inhibitors, fibrinolytics, or other anticoagulants
			• Monitor oral secretions, sputum, vomitus, NG aspirate, stool, urine for blood
			• Avoid IM, arterial, or venous punctures if at all possible
			• Hold pressure for longer than usual if punctures are necessary
			• Gradually reduce the lepirudin dosage to reach an aPTT ratio just above 1.5 before initiating oral anticoagulant therapy

Argatroban (Acova)	• IV infusion: mix 250 mg in 250 mL of normal saline (1 mg/mL); administer initially at 2 mcg/kg/min; no loading dose is given • Maximum: 10 mcg/kg/min • Reduce dosage in hepatic disease; start at 0.5 mcg/kg/min	• Bleeding: gastrointestinal, genitourinary, intracranial • Allergic reaction • Dyspnea • Hypotension • Fever • Diarrhea • Sepsis • Cardiac arrest	• Monitor PT, aPTT, CBC, and for signs of bleeding • Note that contraindications and cautions are as for heparin • Obtain baseline platelet count and aPTT; monitor aPTT every 4 hours • Anticoagulant effects are increased in patients receiving platelet aggregation inhibitors, fibrinolytics, or other anticoagulants • Monitor oral secretions, sputum, vomitus, NG aspirate, stool, urine for blood • Avoid IM, arterial, or venous punctures if at all possible • Hold pressure for longer than usual if punctures are necessary • Protect infusion from direct sunlight
Bivalirudin (Angiomax)	• IV injection: 0.75-1 mg/kg followed by IV infusion • IV infusion: mix 250 mg in 250 mL of normal saline (1 mg/mL) and infuse at 1.75-2.5 mg/kg/hr for 4 hours then decrease infusion to 0.2 mg/kg/hr for an additional 14-20 hours if needed	• Bleeding • Back pain • Generalized pain • Headache • Nausea • Hypotension	• Monitor PT, aPTT, CBC, and for signs of bleeding • Note that contraindications and cautions are as for heparin • Obtain baseline platelet count and aPTT; ACT may also be used • Anticoagulant effects are increased in patients receiving platelet aggregation inhibitors, fibrinolytics, or other anticoagulants • Monitor oral secretions, sputum, vomitus, NG aspirate, stool, urine for blood • Avoid IM, arterial, or venous punctures if at all possible • Hold pressure for longer than usual if punctures are necessary • Protect infusion from direct sunlight

Vitamin K Antagonist			
Warfarin (Coumadin, Panwarfin)	• PO: 2-10 mg daily depending on PT and international normalized ratio (INR) • INR 2-3 — MI — DVT prophylaxis or treatment — Pulmonary embolus — Valvular heart disease — Atrial fibrillation — Tissue heart valve • INR 2.5-3.5 — Mechanical heart valve	• Hemorrhage with excessive PT • Agranulocytosis, leukopenia • Hepatitis • Diarrhea • Fever • Rash • Skin necrosis: occurs during the first several days of warfarin therapy; lesions occur on extremities, breasts, trunk, penis • Cholesterol microemboli causing purple toe syndrome	• Monitor PT and for signs of hemorrhage • Note contraindications: known hypersensitivity, bleeding disorders, leukemia, peptic ulcer disease, liver disease, severe hypertension, endocarditis, acute nephritis, blood dyscrasias, eclampsia, suspected intracranial hemorrhage, open wounds, recent surgery, threatened abortion • Use cautiously in alcoholism, pregnancy, lactation, during menses, during use of any drainage tube, in older adults, or in any patient in whom slight bleeding is dangerous • Ensure that vitamin K (AquaMephyton) is available • Avoid IM, arterial, or venous punctures if at all possible • Hold pressure for longer than usual if punctures are necessary • Monitor oral secretions, sputum, vomitus, NG aspirate, stool, urine for blood • Do not discontinue suddenly • Teach patient to avoid trauma and increase amounts of vitamin K (green leafy vegetables), and how to monitor for bleeding • Teach the patient to report fever or rash; usually necessitates discontinuance
Fibrinolytics			
Recombinant plasminogen activator (r-PA) reteplase (Retavase)	• IV injection of 10 units over 2 minutes initially followed by 10 units over 2 minutes after 30 minutes • Heparin administered concurrently	• Severe, spontaneous bleeding including potential cerebral, retroperitoneal, GU, GI bleeding, surface bleeding • Reperfusion dysrhythmias	• Monitor aPTT, PT, thrombin time, neurologic status, and for signs of hemorrhage • Note contraindications: active bleeding; history of cerebral hemorrhage, intracranial neoplasm, AV malformation or aneurysm; recent (within 2 months) intracranial or intraspinal surgery or trauma; known bleeding disorder; severe uncontrolled hypertension; prolonged CPR • Use cautiously in recent (within 10 days) major surgery, GI, GU bleeding, or trauma; hypertension with SBP greater than 180 mm Hg or DBP greater than 110 mm Hg; high likelihood of left heart thrombus; acute pericarditis; significant liver dysfunction; pregnancy; retinopathy; septic thrombophlebitis; advanced age (greater than 70-75 years); patients receiving oral anticoagulants; any condition in which bleeding constitutes a significant hazard or would be particularly difficult to manage because of its location • Identify indications of reperfusion in MI • Cessation of pain • ST segments descending back to baseline • Reperfusion dysrhythmias (ventricular ectopy including PVCs, VT or VF, accelerated idioventricular rhythm, junctional escape rhythms, bradycardia) • Early CK peak • Limit venipuncture and urinary catheterization as much as possible; use IV catheter with saline lock for blood sampling; avoid noncompressible IV sites • Avoid nasotracheal and nasogastric tubes if possible • Avoid automatic BP cuffs • Administer all drugs through existing IVs started before initiation of thrombolytic therapy or by mouth • Monitor oral secretions, sputum, vomitus, NG aspirate, stool, urine for blood • Bleeding precautions are maintained for 12-24 hours

Continued

Table 10-13 Selected Drugs that Affect Clotting—cont'd

Drug	Administration	Adverse Effects	Nursing Implications

Recombinant tissue plasminogen activator (rt-PA) alteplase (Activase)	For acute MI
	• IV injection: 15 mg followed by:
	• IV infusion: 0.75 mg/kg (not to exceed 50 mg) over next 30 minutes, followed by 0.5 mg/kg (not to exceed 35 mg) over the next 60 minutes
	• Heparin started within 1 hour of initial dose
	For ischemic stroke
	• Total dose: 0.9 mg/kg with maximum dose of 90 mg or less
	• IV injection: 10% of this total dose over 1 minute followed by:
	• IV infusion: remaining 90% of this total dose administered over 60 minutes
	• Anticoagulants and platelet aggregation inhibitors are not used for at least 24 hours
	For acute pulmonary embolism
	• IV infusion: 100 mg at 50 mg/hr for 2 hours
	For acute arterial occlusion
	• 0.05 to 0.1 mg/kg/hr by local intraarterial infusion
	• Reconstitution in sterile water only
		• Severe, spontaneous bleeding including potential cerebral, retroperitoneal, GU, GI bleeding, surface bleeding
		• Reperfusion dysrhythmias
			• Monitor aPTT, PT, thrombin time, fibrinogen, neurologic status, and for signs of hemorrhage
			• Note contraindications: active bleeding; history of cerebral hemorrhage, intracranial neoplasm, AV malformation or aneurysm; recent (within 2 months) intracranial or intraspinal surgery or trauma; known bleeding disorder; severe uncontrolled hypertension; prolonged CPR
			• Use cautiously in recent (within 10 days) major surgery, GI, GU bleeding, or trauma; hypertension with SBP greater than 180 mm Hg or DBP greater than 110 mm Hg; high likelihood of left heart thrombus; acute pericarditis; significant liver dysfunction; pregnancy; retinopathy; septic thrombophlebitis; advanced age (greater than 70-75 years); patients receiving oral anticoagulants; any condition in which bleeding constitutes a significant hazard or would be particularly difficult to manage because of its location
			• Monitor for indications of reperfusion in MI
			  • Cessation of pain
			  • ST segments descending back to baseline
			  • Reperfusion dysrhythmias (ventricular ectopy including PVCs, VT or VF, accelerated idioventricular rhythm, junctional escape rhythms, bradycardia)
			  • Early CK peak
			• Note that signs of reperfusion are much more subtle in PE and thrombotic stroke
			• Limit venipuncture and urinary catheterization as much as possible; use IV catheter with saline lock for blood sampling; avoid noncompressible IV sites
			• Administer all drugs through existing IVs started before initiation of thrombolytic therapy or by mouth
			• Avoid nasotracheal and nasogastric tubes if possible
			• Avoid automatic BP cuffs
			• Monitor oral secretions, sputum, vomitus, NG aspirate, stool, urine for blood
			• Bleeding precautions are maintained for 12-24 hours

Recombinant tissue plasminogen activator (rt-PA) tenecteplase (TNKase)	• IV injection over 5 seconds
	  • Less than 60 kg: 30 mg
	  • At least 60 but less than 70 kg: 35 mg
	  • At least 70 but less than 80 kg: 40 mg
	  • At least 80 but less than 90 kg: 45 mg
	  • At least 90 kg: 50 mg
	• Heparin administered concurrently
		• Severe, spontaneous bleeding including potential cerebral, retroperitoneal, GU, GI bleeding, surface bleeding
		• Reperfusion dysrhythmias
			• Monitor aPTT, PT, thrombin time, neurologic status, and for signs of hemorrhage
			• Note contraindications: active bleeding; history of cerebral hemorrhage, intracranial neoplasm, AV malformation or aneurysm; recent (within 2 months) intracranial or intraspinal surgery or trauma; known bleeding disorder; severe uncontrolled hypertension; prolonged CPR
			• Use cautiously in recent (within 10 days) major surgery, GI, GU bleeding, or trauma; hypertension with SBP greater than 180 mm Hg or DBP greater than 110 mm Hg; high likelihood of left heart thrombus; acute pericarditis; significant liver dysfunction; pregnancy; retinopathy; septic thrombophlebitis; advanced age (greater than 70-75 years); patients receiving oral anticoagulants; any condition in which bleeding constitutes a significant hazard or would be particularly difficult to manage because of its location
			• Identify indications of reperfusion in MI
			  • Cessation of pain
			  • ST segments descending back to baseline
			  • Reperfusion dysrhythmias (ventricular ectopy including PVCs, VT or VF, accelerated idioventricular rhythm, junctional escape rhythms, bradycardia)
			  • Early CK peak
			• Limit venipuncture and urinary catheterization as much as possible; use IV catheter with saline lock for blood sampling; avoid noncompressible IV sites
			• Avoid nasotracheal and nasogastric tubes if possible
			• Avoid automatic BP cuffs
			• Administer all drugs through existing IVs started before initiation of thrombolytic therapy or by mouth
			• Monitor oral secretions, sputum, vomitus, NG aspirate, stool, urine for blood
			• Bleeding precautions are maintained for 12-24 hours

Streptokinase (Streptase)	IV: mix 1.5 million units in 250 mL (6000 units/mL) • For acute MI, usual loading dose 750,000 units IV injection followed by 750,000 units IV infusion over next hour • For PE and arterial thromboembolism, usual loading dose 250,000 units over 30 minutes followed by 100,000 units/hr for up to 72 hours	• Allergic reaction (angioneurotic edema, pruritus, bronchospasm, dyspnea, hypotension, cyanosis, seizures, loss of consciousness) • Severe spontaneous bleeding • Cerebral, retroperitoneal, GU, GI, surface bleeding • Reperfusion dysrhythmias	• Monitor aPTT, PT, thrombin time, neurologic status, and for signs of hemorrhage • Note contraindications: patients who have had recent streptococcal infection or streptokinase within 6 months to 5 years • Note that indications in MI, contraindications, cautions, and signs of reperfusion after use for MI are as for r-PA or rt-PA • Administer diphenhydramine (Benadryl) and hydrocortisone sodium succinate (Solu-Cortef) if chance of allergic reaction • Limit venipuncture and urinary catheterization as much as possible; use IV catheter with saline lock for blood sampling; avoid noncompressible IV sites • Administer all drugs through existing IVs started before initiation of thrombolytic therapy or by mouth • Avoid nasotracheal and nasogastric tubes if possible • Avoid automatic BP cuffs • Monitor oral secretions, sputum, vomitus, NG aspirate, stool, urine for blood • Maintain bleeding precautions for 48-72 hours due to fibrinogen depletion seen with streptokinase

Table 10-14 Inherited and Acquired Coagulopathies

Cause of Coagulopathy	Pathophysiology	Treatment
Hereditary Coagulopathies		
Hemophilia A	• X-linked recessive disorder; though considered a hereditary disorder, may occur as a new mutation in factor VIII gene • Deficiency of factor VIII • Inadequate factor VIII-vWF complex • Inadequate platelet adhesion	• Either highly purified factor VIII concentrate or recombinant factor VIII administration • DDAVP stimulates the endothelial cells to release vWF and plasminogen activator
Hemophilia B (i.e., Christmas disease)	• X-linked recessive disorder • Deficiency of factor IX	• Highly purified factor IX
von Willebrand disease	• Types 1 and 2 are inherited as autosomal dominant traits, and type 3 is inherited as autosomal recessive deficiency of von Willebrand factor (vWF) • Decreased platelet adhesion	• Usually mild and does not require treatment though risk of bleeding is increased • Either highly purified factor VIII concentrate that contains vWF • DDAVP stimulates the endothelial cells to release vWF and plasminogen activator
Acquired Coagulopathies		
Vitamin K deficiency	• Inadequate synthesis and regulation of prothrombin, procoagulant factors (VII, IX, X), and anticoagulant regulators (proteins C and S)	• Parenteral administration of vitamin K • FFP in life-threatening hemorrhage or in preparation for emergency surgery
Liver disease	• Impaired clotting caused by diminished production of clotting factors, especially factor VII and less so factor IX • Impaired fibrinolysis caused by diminished production of plasminogen and alpha$_2$-antiplasmin • Decreased thrombopoietin results in decreased platelet production	• FFP • Platelets
Immune thrombocytopenic purpura (formerly known as *idiopathic thrombocytopenia purpura*)	Acute ITP • Secondary to infection, particularly viral, or other condition that results in large amounts of antigen in the blood, such as drug allergies or systemic lupus erythematosus • Antigen and antibodies form immune complexes that bind to receptors on platelets which causes platelet destruction in the spleen. Chronic ITP • Development of autoantibodies against platelet-specific antigens • Removal of the antibody-coated platelets removed by spleen	• Glucocorticoids • IV immunoglobulins • Splenectomy may be considered • Immunosuppressive agents may be used
Thrombotic thrombocytopenic purpura	• Platelets aggregate and cause occlusion of arterioles and capillaries within the microcirculation • Platelet consumption • Organ ischemia	• Plasma exchange with fresh frozen plasma • Glucocorticoids • Splenectomy may be considered • Immunosuppressive agents may be used
Disseminated Intravascular Coagulation (see pages 667, 675-678)		
Heparin-Induced Thrombocytopenia (see pages 678-680)		

   c. Sarcoma
   d. Leukemia
   e. Pheochromocytoma
6. Obstetric complications
   a. Abruptio placentae
   b. Retained dead fetus
   c. Retained placenta
   d. Septic abortion
   e. Hydatidiform mole
   f. Amniotic fluid embolism
   g. Acute fatty liver of pregnancy
   h. Toxemia
7. Embolism
   a. Pulmonary embolism
   b. Fat embolism
   c. Amniotic fluid embolism
8. Gastrointestinal and accessory organs
   a. Necrotizing enterocolitis
   b. Pancreatitis
   c. Obstructive jaundice
   d. Hepatitis
   e. Cirrhosis
   f. Acute hepatic failure
9. Pulmonary
   a. ARDS
   b. Pulmonary embolism
10. Toxins
   a. Snake bites
   b. Aspirin poisoning
   c. Impure IV drugs
11. Prosthetic devices
   a. LeVeen or Denver shunt
   b. Intraaortic balloon pump

Pathophysiology

See Figure 10-6.

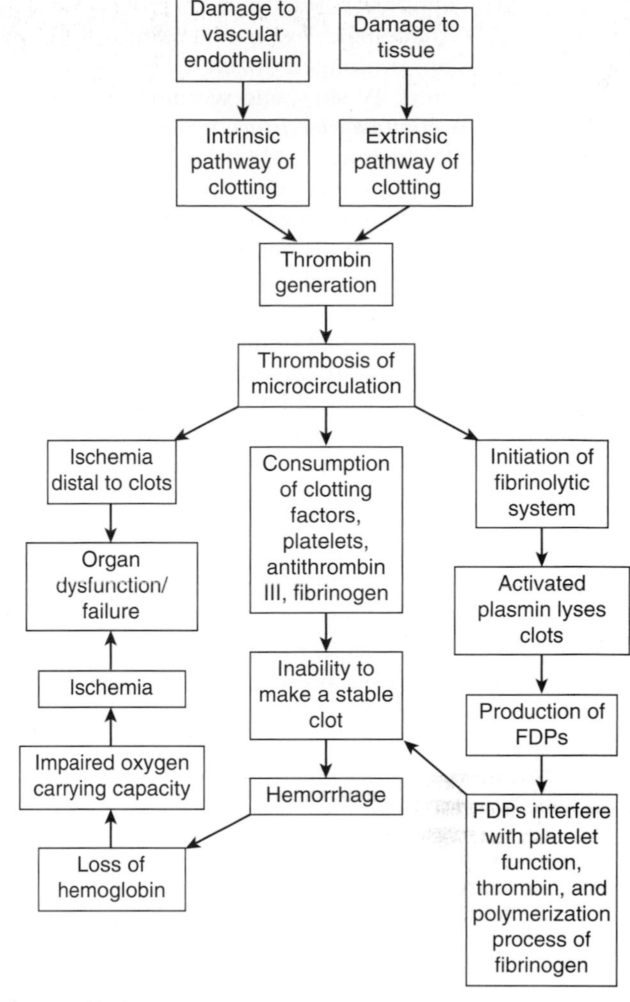

Figure 10-6 Pathophysiology of disseminated intravascular coagulation (DIC). *FDPs,* Fibrin degradation products.

Clinical Presentation

1. Subjective
   a. History of predisposing factor
   b. Symptoms related to ischemia
      1) Chest pain
      2) Dyspnea
      3) Abdominal pain
      4) Pain in digits
      5) Visual changes
      6) Headache
2. Objective
   a. Clinical indications of decreased perfusion (subjective included)
      1) Brain: change in level of consciousness, focal neurologic signs, seizures
      2) Heart: chest pain, ST segment elevation or depression, clinical indications of hypoperfusion
      3) Lung: dyspnea, chest pain, clinical indications of hypoxemia
      4) Kidney: decreased urine output, occult or gross hematuria, proteinuria, electrolyte imbalance
      5) GI tract: abdominal pain, diarrhea, occult or gross blood in stool
      6) Skin: acral cyanosis of toes, fingers, lips, nose, or ears; mottling, coldness, necrosis
   b. Clinical indications of platelet dysfunction
      1) Petechiae: frequently the first indication of DIC
      2) Ecchymoses
      3) Purpura
   c. Clinical indications of hemorrhage
      1) Tachycardia
         a) Initially postural only, then profound tachycardia
      2) Hypotension
         a) Initially narrowed pulse pressure
         b) Then postural hypotension
         c) Then profound hypotension
      3) Tachypnea
      4) Overt bleeding in a patient with no previous bleeding history
         a) Mucosal surfaces: gingival bleeding; epistaxis
         b) GU: Hematuria
         c) GI: Hematemesis, hematochezia, melena, guaiac-positive stool

d) Pulmonary: hemoptysis
e) Gynecologic: vaginal bleeding
f) Skin: prolonged oozing from puncture points, IV sites, and wounds (referred to as *surface bleeding*), bruising

5) Occult bleeding
   a) Swollen joints and joint pain may indicate bleeding into the joint.
   b) Abdominal distention and rebound tenderness may indicate intraperitoneal bleeding.
   c) Back pain, leg numbness, and hypotension may indicate retroperitoneal bleeding.
   d) Headache, change in level of consciousness, and pupillary changes may indicate intracerebral hemorrhage.
   e) Visual changes (e.g., blurred vision, loss of visual fields) may indicate retinal hemorrhage.
   f) Alterations in hemodynamic parameters: Right atrial pressure, pulmonary artery wedge pressure, and cardiac output/cardiac index may be decreased.

3. Diagnostic: All that bleeds is not DIC; diagnostic studies are definitive.
   a. Serum
      1) Platelet count: decreased (less than 150,000/mm^3); one of earliest findings
      2) Prothrombin time (PT): prolonged (usually greater than 40 seconds); less sensitive than other tests
      3) Activated partial prothrombin time (aPTT): prolonged (usually greater than 70 seconds); less sensitive than other tests
      4) Thrombin time: prolonged (greater than 15 seconds)
      5) Fibrinogen level: decreased by 50% or more or less than 200 mg/dL
         a) Used for patients who have contributing factors that do not permit monitoring platelet count
         b) Because fibrinogen is elevated in pregnancy, sepsis, and neoplastic conditions, a decrease of 50% is a more accurate indicator of DIC than an absolute value in these patients.
      6) Thrombin-antithrombin III (TAT) complex: decreased (usually less than 70% activity)
         a) Evaluates the activation of the coagulation system that occurs when thrombin is generated
         b) Decreased antithrombin III indicates accelerated coagulation.
      7) Fibrin degradation products (FDP): elevated (usually greater than 40 mcg/mL) but may be reported as positive at a number of dilutions; diagnostic for DIC is positive at greater than 100 dilutions (reported positive at 1 : 100)
         a) Measures the results of both fibrin and fibrinogen degradation
      8) D-dimer (end product of fibrin degradation): elevated (greater than 250 ng/mL) or positive at greater than 1 : 8 dilutions
         a) Specific to the results of fibrin degradation
         b) More specific for DIC than FDPs but less sensitive
            i) May be falsely positive postsurgical in certain malignancies, deep vein thrombosis, and pulmonary embolism
      9) Protamine sulfate test: strongly positive
         a) Protamine sulfate is added to plasma to see if fibrin strands are formed.
         b) A positive test reflects the formation of excessive amounts of thrombin.
      10) Clotting factor analysis: shows a decrease in factors I, V, VIII, and fibrinogen
      11) Peripheral smear: shows presence of schistocytes, helmet cells, and red cell fragments
      12) Hemoglobin and hematocrit: may be decreased if blood loss is significant
      13) Arterial blood gases: respiratory alkalosis initially progressing to metabolic acidosis due to lactic acidosis
      14) DIC scoring system using diagnostic tests (Table 10-15)
   b. Urine: may be positive for blood
   c. Stool: may be positive for blood
   d. Sputum: may be positive for blood

Collaborative Management

1. Identify and closely assess high-risk groups for clinical indications of DIC
   a. Monitor closely for thrombosis or bleeding.
      1) Note petechiae, ecchymosis, and acrocyanosis.
      2) Test nasogastric aspirate or vomitus, stools, and urine for blood.
      3) Monitor oral secretions, pulmonary secretions, and gums for bleeding.
      4) Monitor peripheral pulses and capillary refill.
   b. Monitor laboratory studies for diagnostic indications of DIC.
   c. Monitor closely for clinical indications of hypoperfusion or intracranial hemorrhage.
   d. Monitor hemodynamic parameters as indicated; insert indwelling urinary catheter to monitor hourly urine output.
2. Control underlying causative factors.
   a. Surgery
      1) Surgical débridement
      2) Abscess drainage
      3) Evacuation of the uterus
      4) Removal of tumor
   b. Antimicrobials for infection
   c. Antineoplastics for malignancy
3. Maintain airway, ventilation, and oxygenation.

Table 10-15 DIC Scoring System

Laboratory Test	0	1	2	3
Platelet count/nL	Greater than 100	Greater than 50	Less than 50	
D-dimer mcg/mL	Less than 1		1-5	Greater than 5
Fibrinogen g/L	Greater than 1	Less than 1		
Prothrombin index %	Greater than 70	40-70	Less than 40	

The DIC Scoring System requires the presence of a risk factor for DIC before the laboratory test results can be evaluated. If greater than or equal to 5, it is compatible with overt DIC. If less than 5, it is suggestive for nonovert DIC in a patient with an underlying disorder known to be associated with DIC.
Adapted from Taylor, F. B., Toh, C. H., Hoots, W. K., Wada, H., & Levi, M. (2001). Towards definition, clinical and laboratory criteria, and a scoring system for disseminated intravascular coagulation. *Thromb Haemost, 86:*1327-1330.

Table 10-16 Treatments for DIC

Treatment	Rationale	Controversy
Heparin	• Prevents further microclots and prevents platelet aggregation • Works with antithrombin III to neutralize circulating thrombin	• May perpetuate bleeding
Antithrombin III	• Works with heparin to neutralize circulating thrombin	• May perpetuate bleeding
Clotting factors • Fresh frozen plasma • Cryoprecipitate • Platelets	• Reestablishes normal hemostatic potential	• "Fuel to the fire" theory attests that until the clotting process is stopped, clotting factors just increase the thrombosis and microclotting
Epsilon-aminocaproic acid (Amicar)	• Blocks the fibrinolytic system so that stable clots are not degraded • Decreases amount of FDPs that act as anticoagulant	• Clearance of microclots from occluded vessels may be delayed • Indicated only in primary fibrinolysis

a. Administer oxygen to maintain PaO_2 of 80 mm Hg and SpO_2 of 95%.
b. Assist with intubation and mechanical ventilation as necessary.
c. Suction only as necessary and with low suction to avoid trauma to the tracheobronchial mucosa.

4. Correct hypovolemia, hypotension, hypoxia, and acidosis.
   a. Insert or ensure patency of peripheral intravenous catheter.
   b. Administer normal saline to replace volume until type and crossmatch are completed and blood is available.
   c. Administer volume replacement, inotropes, and/or vasopressors as prescribed to maintain MAP greater than 60 mm Hg.
5. Stop the microclotting to maintain perfusion and protect vital organ function.
   a. Administer intravenous heparin (usually 5-15 units/kg/hr) as prescribed; desirable aPTT is 1.5-2 times the control.
      1) Used primarily for patients with thrombosis who continue to bleed despite other rigorous treatment; often effective with underlying malignancy, acute promyelocytic leukemia, and purpura fulminans (may be seen in sepsis)
      2) Prevents further thrombosis in the microvasculature and prevents platelet aggregation; works with antithrombin III to neutralize circulating thrombin
      3) Continues to be controversial as it may potentiate or prolong bleeding, but it is thrombosis of small vessels, not hemorrhage, that has the greatest impact on morbidity and mortality in DIC
      4) Contraindicated in CNS or GI hemorrhage, DIC associated with hepatic failure, hemorrhagic obstetric causes (e.g., abruptio placentae), and recent surgical procedures
   b. Administer antithrombin III as prescribed: antithrombin III inhibits the action of thrombin; may be administered if antithrombin levels are low
   c. NOTE: Table 10-16 describes rationale and controversies regarding selected treatments.
6. Stop the bleeding by supporting coagulation.
   a. Administer blood products as prescribed to replace missing clotting factors.
      1) Platelets: Maintain platelet count above 50,000/mm^3; platelet replenishment is a priority to assist reinitiation of effective clotting.

a) Desmopressin acetate may be prescribed to improve platelet function when platelet dysfunction is due to dextran, nonsteroidal antiinflammatory agents, or aspirin; monitor for fluid overload, hyponatremia, and tachycardia.

2) Fresh frozen plasma (contains all clotting factors)
   a) Used for bleeding patients with markedly prolonged PT and aPTT
   b) Replenishes fibrinogen levels
3) Cryoprecipitate (contains factors VIII, XIII, and fibrinogen): maintains fibrinogen levels above 125 mg/dL
4) Packed red blood cells: may be needed if blood loss is significant
5) May potentiate or prolong the clotting (fuel-to-the-fire theory), so heparin may be given first

b. Administer hemostatic cofactors as prescribed.
   1) Vitamin K: needed for liver production of several clotting factors
   2) Folic acid: Deficiency may cause thrombocytopenia.
c. Administer an antifibrinolytic agent (epsilon aminocaproic acid [Amicar], tranexamic acid [Cyklokapron]) as prescribed for primary fibrinolysis.
   1) Should be avoided in all other situations because it may enhance deposition of fibrin in the microcirculation and macrocirculation and lead to fatal DIC
   2) Requires concurrent heparin therapy in DIC
d. Apply thrombin-soaked gauze, pressure dressings, and/or ice packs to control bleeding sites; the efficacy of topical hemostatics is unconfirmed.
e. Maintain normal body temperature because hypothermia contributes to coagulopathy and vasoconstriction, perpetuating tissue ischemia.
f. Maintain normal vascular volume because low circulating volume exacerbates effects of vascular clotting.

7. Treat ischemic pain.
   a. Administer analgesics as prescribed.
   b. Elevate ecchymotic limbs.
8. Maintain skin integrity and minimize tissue trauma.
   a. Provide meticulous skin care.
      1) Turn gently and frequently and assess skin during care
      2) Keep the skin moist with lubricating lotions.
      3) Utilize specialized beds as needed.
   b. Provide careful mouth care; use alcohol-free mouthwash and swabs.
   c. Provide careful perianal care; avoid rectal thermometers and suppositories.
   d. Alternate activity with rest; mobilize and ambulate patient progressively.
   e. Use an electric, rather than straight-edged, razor.
   f. Avoid tape if possible; use adhesive remover to remove tape.
   g. Apply local pressure to any break in skin integrity.
      1) Avoid intramuscular, subcutaneous infections.
      2) Use an existing vascular access for blood sampling whenever possible.
         a) If venous puncture is necessary, apply pressure for 3-5 minutes afterward.
         b) If arterial puncture is necessary, apply pressure for 10-15 minutes afterward.
   h. Reduce frequency of cuff BPs: An arterial line is ideal for pressure monitoring and obtaining blood specimens.
   i. Do not give ASA or NSAID due to the effect on platelet aggregation.
   j. Teach patient to avoid Valsalva maneuver; administer stool softeners to avoid constipation.
   k. Do not disturb any clot.
9. Provide psychological support and reassurance: Tell patient that treatment is being provided to stop the bleeding (hemorrhage causes extreme anxiety).
10. Monitor for complications.
   a. Intracerebral hemorrhage (a major cause of death)
   b. Hemorrhagic shock
   c. ARDS
   d. GI dysfunction
   e. Renal failure
   f. Infection or sepsis

Heparin-Induced Thrombocytopenia (HIT)

Definition

A prothrombotic disorder caused by a subset of antibodies against platelet factor 4 (PF4)/heparin complexes with strong platelet-activating properties

1. Differentiation between heparin-associated thrombocytopenia (HAT) and heparin-induced thrombocytopenia (HIT) (Table 10-17)

Etiology

Heparin administration or heparin-coated catheters

1. Risk is greater with unfractionated heparin (3-5%) than with low-molecular weight heparin (0.05%).
2. Risk is higher with bovine heparin than with porcine heparin.
3. Risk is higher in postoperative patients.
4. Risk is higher in patients with underlying vascular endothelial cell injury or venous stasis.

Pathophysiology

See Figure 10-7.

Clinical Presentation

1. Subjective: none
2. Objective
   a. Thrombotic events: reason for previous name of heparin-induced thrombosis and thrombocytopenia (HITT)
      1) Venous 4 times more likely than arterial

Table 10-17 Comparison of Nonimmune and Immune Heparin-Induced Thrombocytopenia

Characteristic	Nonimmune (previously referred to as *HIT-I*)	Immune (previously referred to as *HIT-II*)
Onset	Day 1-4 of heparin administration	Day 5-10 of heparin administration
Route and dose	Primarily with high dose of intravenous heparin	Any route or dose
Effect on platelets	90,000-150,000/mm^3 for 1-5 days	Greater than 50% drop from baseline on days 7-10
Course	Platelet count may normalize No thrombosis	Thrombosis May be associated with life-threatening complications
Mechanism	Direct toxic effect	Immune-mediated
Antibodies	No	Yes
Treatment	Observation	Cessation of heparin and nonheparin anticoagulants

Table 10-18 4Ts Scoring System for HIT

	2 Points	1 Point	0 Points
Thrombocytopenia	Platelet count fall greater than 50% from baseline AND platelet nadir greater than or equal to 20 × 10^9/L	Platelet count fall 30-50% from baseline AND platelet nadir 10-19 × 10^9/L	Platelet count fall less than 30% from baseline AND platelet nadir less than 10 × 10^9/L
Timing of fall in platelet count	Clear onset between days 5 and 10 OR less than or equal to 1 day if heparin exposure within previous 30 days	Fall in platelet count consistent with onset between days 5 and 10 but timing is not clear due to missing platelet counts OR onset after day 10 of heparin exposure OR fall in platelet count less than or equal to 1 day with prior heparin exposure 30-100 days ago	Fall in platelet count less than 4 days after recent heparin exposure
Thrombosis or related occurrence	New thrombosis, skin necrosis, or acute systemic reaction after UFH exposure	Progressive or recurrent thrombosis or unconfirmed but clinically suspected thrombosis	No thrombosis or thrombosis preceding heparin exposure
Thromobocytopenia: Possible other causes	None apparent	Possible other causes present	Probable other causes present

Score less than 4 = low probability of HIT; score of 4-5 = intermediate probability of HIT, score greater than 5 = high probability of HIT.
From Crowther, M. A., Cook, D. J., Albert, M., Williamson, D., Meade, M., Granton, J., et al. (2010). The 4Ts scoring system for heparin-induced thrombocytopenia in medical-surgical intensive care unit patients. *J Crit Care, 25*(2), 287-293.

a) Venous: deep vein thrombosis, pulmonary embolism, cerebral venous thrombosis, adrenal infarction
b) Arterial: myocardial infarction, thrombotic stroke, limb arterial occlusion, renal or mesenteric arterial thrombosis, aortic occlusion

b. Skin lesions, including petechiae
c. Acute systemic reactions
d. Bleeding is rare.

3. Diagnostic
   a. Platelet count less than 100,000/mm^3 or a 50% decrease from baseline platelet count
   b. Platelet activation (functional) assays: rely on the ability of the PF4/heparin antibody to activate platelets; less sensitive but more specific
      1) Serotonin release assay
      2) Platelet aggregation assay such as heparin-induced platelet aggregation
   c. Antigen assays: more sensitive but less specific
      1) Enzyme-linked immunoassay (ELISA) for PF4/heparin antibodies
   d. Platelet serotonin-release assay
4. Scoring system for HIT: 4Ts score (Table 10-18)

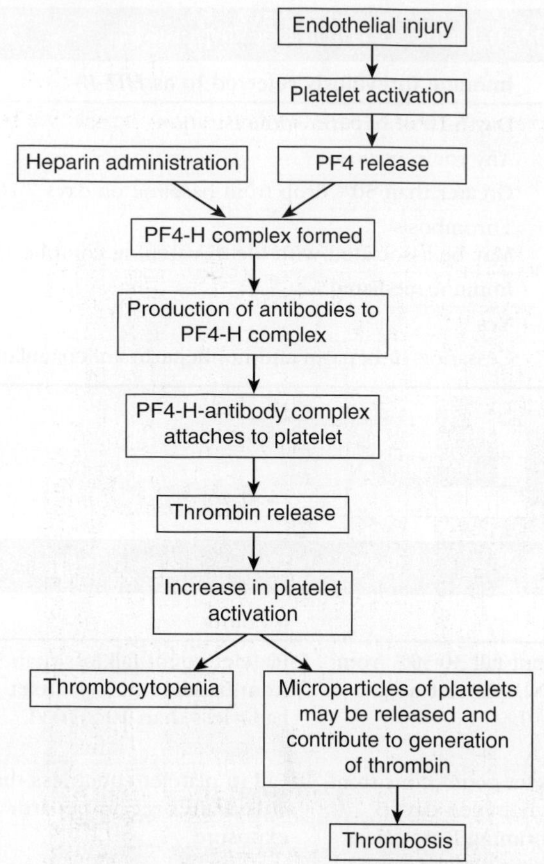

Figure 10-7 Pathophysiology of heparin-induced thrombocytopenia (HIT). *PF4-H,* Platelet factor 4/heparin.

Collaborative Management

1. Correct coagulopathy
   a. Discontinue offending agent (i.e., heparin).
   b. Administer an alternative anticoagulant (e.g., argatroban, lepirudin, danaparoid) as prescribed.
      1) Warfarin is contraindicated until platelet counts normalize because it decreases protein C activity and predisposes to microvascular thrombosis and limb gangrene.
   c. Plasmapheresis may be used to remove the pathogenic immunoglobulins.
2. Treat ischemic pain (as for DIC).
3. Maintain skin integrity and minimize tissue trauma (as for DIC).
4. Provide psychological support and reassurance (as for DIC).
5. Monitor for complications.
   a. Arterial or venous thrombosis
   b. Catheter-related thrombosis
   c. Pulmonary embolism
   d. Adrenal infarction and acute adrenal crisis
   e. Thrombotic stroke
   f. Myocardial infarction
   g. Mesenteric artery thrombosis

LEARNING ACTIVITIES

CHAPTER 10

1. Complete the following crossword puzzle.

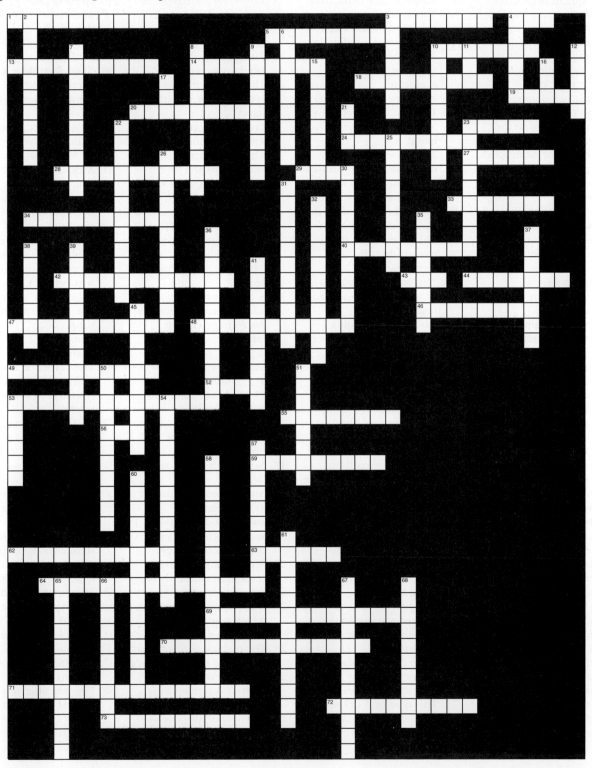

ACROSS

1. Complex physiologic process for termination of bleeding
3. The major physiologic effect of anemia
4. Characterized by widespread microclots, consumption of clotting factors and platelets, and impaired fibrinolysis (abbrev)
5. This mediator is released by the mast cell in allergic reactions
10. Activated plasminogen; the active agent in the fibrinolytic process
13. Movement of neutrophils and phagocytes through pores of small blood vessels
14. This type of anemia is associated with increased RBC destruction which causes jaundice
18. Factor X is sometimes referred to as ____ factor; deficient in hemophilia B
19. Increase in segmented neutrophils is referred to as a shift to the _____
20. This type of cell can engulf and digest microorganisms and cellular debris
23. The yellowish fluid that transports lymphocytes
24. The first sign of platelet dysfunction
27. The liquid portion of blood
28. Indirect thrombin inhibitor frequently used post-PCI (generic)
29. Increase in the number of immature neutrophils and other leukocytes in the blood is referred to as a shift to the ____
33. This type of immunity is mediated by B cells; involves the development of antigen-specific antibodies
34. A cascading system that can result in direct killing of invading organisms
40. The product of erythrocyte destruction
42. Leukocyte count that is higher than normal
43. The end result of fibrinolysis (abbrev)
44. These cells are fixed macrophages in the liver
46. This type of immunity is mediated by the T cell
47. This type of platelet analysis determines the ability of platelets to aggregate
48. A mature red blood cell
49. The percentage of RBCs in a given volume of blood
52. Anemia related to a deficiency of ____ causes nail changes and sores at the corners of the mouth
53. The main regulator of the platelet circulating mass
55. The granulocyte that releases heparin and histamine
56. The immunoglobulin most important in allergic reactions
59. Glycoprotein IIb/IIIa inhibitor frequently used before and after PCI (generic)
62. This mediator causes vasoconstriction, pulmonary vasoconstriction and platelet aggregation
63. Reduction in the total number of circulating erythrocytes or a decrease in the quality or quantity of hemoglobin
64. This blood product is administered to replace factor VIII in patients with hemophilia
69. A synonym for antibody; made by B cells
70. The process of erythrocyte production
71. A decrease in the number of platelets
72. A type of agranular leukocyte; B cells and T cells are examples
73. This type of T cell serves to modulate the immune response; increased in AIDS

DOWN

2. This type of granulocyte is most significant in allergic reactions
3. Parenteral anticoagulant that acts as an indirect thrombin inhibitor (generic)
4. The most specific laboratory test for DIC
6. The clotting pathway that is initiated by endothelial injury
7. Leukocyte count that is lower than normal
8. The movement of neutrophils and monocytes toward an antigen
9. These cells are decreased in ITP, DIC, and HIT
10. This electrolyte may increase with administration of banked blood
11. A drug frequently administered to decrease platelet aggregation (abbrev)
12. A platelet plug is sometimes referred to as a ____ clot
15. Chemical mediators of immunity and inflammation
16. The most abundant immunoglobulin
17. Normal adult hemoglobin (abbrev)
21. An autoimmune disorder in which an IgG autoantibody is formed and binds to and destroys the platelets (abbrev)
22. Sequential physiologic response that the body makes to injuries
23. Direct thrombin inhibitor which may be used for HIT (generic)
25. The clotting pathway that is initiated by tissue injury
26. This type of platelet analysis determines the number of platelets
30. A synonym for platelet
31. The adherence of phagocytes to the vessel wall
32. A leukocyte that releases granules when it ruptures
35. This sign may occur with hemolytic anemia
36. Heparin and _____ maintain the fluidity of the blood
37. Vitamin K antagonist; oral anticoagulant (generic)
38. This electrolyte may decrease with administration of banked blood
39. This coagulation study evaluates platelet function (2 words)
41. A cytokine synthesized by lymphocytes
45. This blood protein becomes fibrin when activated
50. Oral platelet aggregation inhibitor prescribed for several months after PCI with stents (generic)
51. This type of anemia is due to bone marrow suppression
53. The site of T cell distribution
54. This hormone is released from the kidney in response to low oxygen levels
57. This agranulocyte is the major phagocyte of the leukocytes
58. The first homeostatic mechanism
60. A common presenting symptom of leukemia and lymphoma
61. The process by which stem cells develop and differentiate into different types of blood cells
65. An immature erythrocyte
66. This type of anemia is caused by loss of intrinsic factor and malabsorption of vitamin B_{12}
67. The final stage of the clotting process
68. The reticulocyte count reflects activity of the ____ (2 words)

2. List the five major clinical indications of inflammation.
a. ______
b. ______
c. ______
d. ______
e. ______

3. Identify which type of hypersensitivity reaction the following situations demonstrate.

Example	Type
Skin testing for tuberculosis	
Poststreptococcal glomerulonephritis	
Anaphylaxis to penicillin	
Hemolytic blood transfusion reaction	

4. Complete the following table.

	Platelet Plug	Intrinsic Pathway	Extrinsic Pathway	Common Pathway	Fibrinolytic System
Activation					
Laboratory test					

5. Match the drug with the laboratory effect.

___ 1. Aspirin
___ 2. Heparin
___ 3. Warfarin
___ 4. rt-PA
___ 5. Streptokinase
___ 6. Clopidogrel

a. Prolonged bleeding time
b. Prolonged PT
c. Prolonged aPTT
d. Decreased fibrinogen levels
e. Increased fibrin degradation products
f. Increased INR

6. Identify the appropriate actions to take for suspected transfusion reaction.
a. ______
b. ______
c. ______
d. ______
e. ______
f. ______
g. ______
h. ______
i. ______

7. Identify the direction of change of the following laboratory values in DIC, ↑ or ↓.

Platelets	
PT	
aPTT	
Fibrin split products	
Factors V, VIII	
Fibrinogen	

8. Match the coagulopathy with the associated pathology.

___ 1. Hemophilia A
___ 2. Hemophilia B
___ 3. von Willebrand disease
___ 4. Heparin-induced thrombocytopenia
___ 5. Disseminated intravascular coagulation
___ 6. Liver disease
___ 7. Immune thrombocytopenic purpura
___ 8. Thrombotic thrombocytopenic purpura

a. Activation of thrombin and consumption of platelets and clotting factors
b. Binding of immune complexes to platelets which are then destroyed by the spleen
c. Deficiency of von Willebrand factor
d. Deficiency of factor VIII
e. Deficiency of factor IX
f. Development of heparin-platelet factor 4 complex which increases platelet activation and causes thrombocytopenia
g. Platelet aggregation and consumption
h. Inability to produce clotting factors

9. Discuss the controversy of the following therapies in the treatment of DIC.

a. Heparin	
b. Clotting factors	

Multisystem

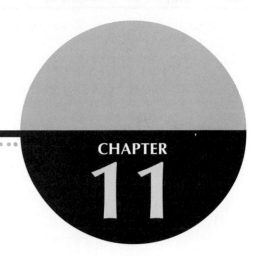

Shock

NOTE: The blueprint includes Cardiogenic Shock and Hypovolemic in Cardiovascular, Anaphylactic Shock in Hematology/Immunology, and Neurogenic Shock in Neurologic, but this text will discuss the similarities of all shock states together and then discuss their differences.

Definitions

1. Shock: the condition of insufficient perfusion of cells and vital organs, causing tissue hypoxia
   a. Perfusion is inadequate to sustain life, and this inadequate perfusion results in cellular, metabolic, and hemodynamic derangements.
   b. Note that shock is not a BP level, and the patient may not be significantly hypotensive, especially early in shock.
2. Systemic inflammatory response syndrome (SIRS): the systemic response to a variety of insults that begin as local inflammation; consider the vasodilation and increased capillary permeability of local inflammation as a normal healing process and the more global vasodilation and increased capillary permeability of SIRS as being life-threatening
3. Multiple organ dysfunction syndrome (MODS): a clinical syndrome in which progressive and potentially irreversible physiologic dysfunction of two or more organs or organ systems is induced by primary or secondary injury

Classification by Etiology

1. Hypovolemic: caused by inadequate intravascular volume
2. Cardiogenic: caused by impaired ability of the heart to pump blood effectively
   a. Note that some classification systems include a subgroup of cardiogenic shock referred to as *obstructive*, which is associated with poor filling of the heart.
3. Distributive: caused by massive vasodilation and a resultant relative hypovolemia
   a. Septic: resulting from massive vasodilation caused by release of mediators of the inflammatory process in response to overwhelming infection
   b. Anaphylactic: resulting from massive vasodilation caused by release of histamine in response to a severe allergic reaction
   c. Neurogenic: resulting from massive vasodilation caused by suppression of the sympathetic nervous system

Pathophysiology

1. Stages of shock
   a. Initial stage: subclinical hypoperfusion caused by inadequate delivery and/or inadequate extraction of oxygen
      1) Shock is initiated by decreased tissue oxygenation caused by any of the following:
         a) Decrease in circulating blood volume (hypovolemic)
         b) Decrease in ability of the heart to pump blood (cardiogenic)
         c) Decrease in vascular tone (distributive, may also be referred to as *vasogenic*)
      2) Cardiac output and index are decreased but there are no *clinical* indications of hypoperfusion; this decrease in cardiac output and index would be detected by invasive hemodynamic monitoring.
   b. Compensatory stage: attempts of the neuroendocrine systems to compensate and restore tissue perfusion to vital organs (Figure 11-1)
   c. Progressive stage: the inability of the compensatory mechanisms to maintain tissue perfusion (Figure 11-2)
   d. Refractory stage is irreversible and refractory to conventional therapy with manifestations of progressive organ dysfunction and/or failure (Figure 11-3).

Clinical Presentation (Table 11-1)

1. Initial stage: no clinical indications; expert nurse may detect that "something is different"
2. Compensatory stage: SNS stimulation

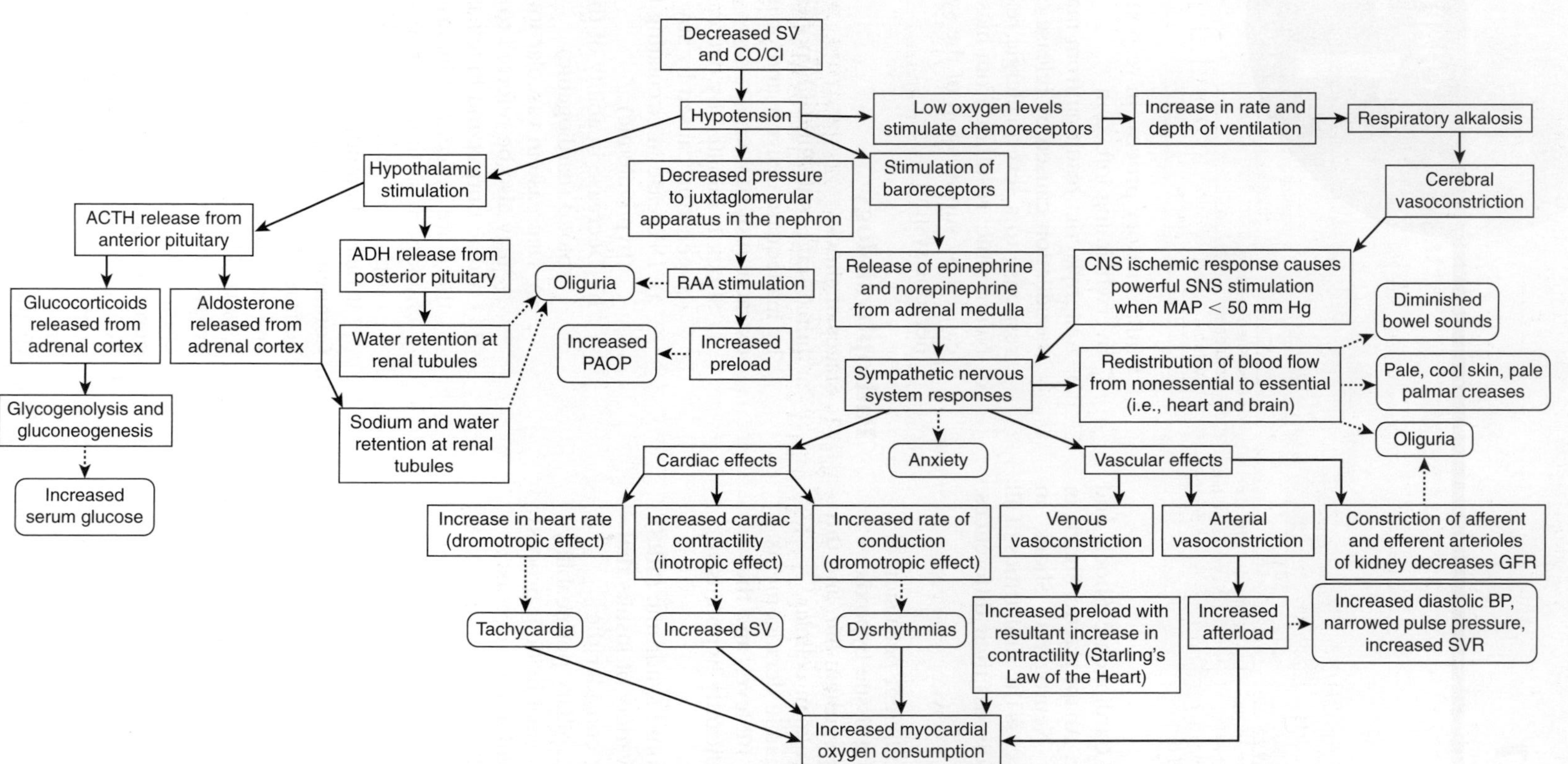

Figure 11-1 Pathophysiology of shock: Compensatory stage. Dotted lines connect pathology to clinical presentation. *ACTH,* Adrenocorticotropic hormone; *ADH,* antidiuretic hormone; *BP,* blood pressure; *CO/CI,* cardiac output/cardiac index; *CNS,* central nervous system; *GFR,* glomerular filtration rate; *PAOP,* pulmonary artery occlusive pressure; *RAA,* renin-angiotensin-aldosterone; *SV,* stroke volume; *SVR,* systemic vascular resistance.

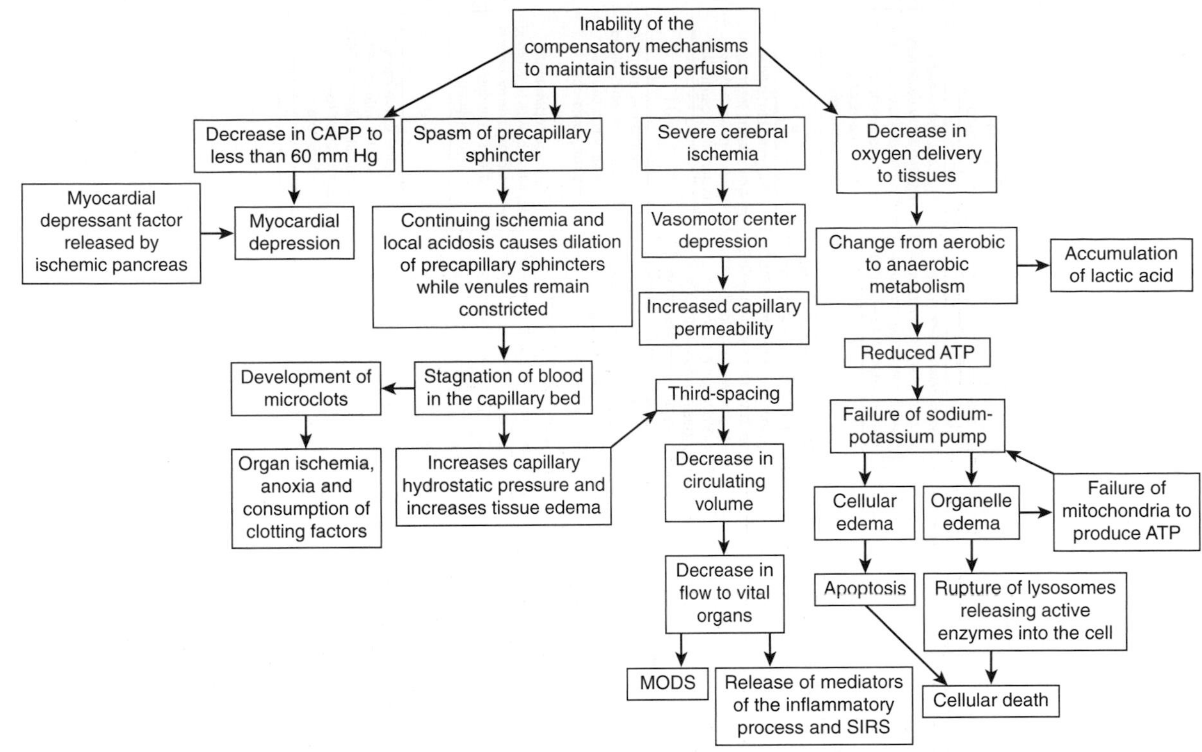

Figure 11-2 Pathophysiology of shock: Progressive stage. *ATP,* Adenosine triphosphate; *CAPP,* coronary artery perfusion pressure; *MODS,* multiple organ dysfunction syndrome.

Table 11-1 Clinical Presentation of the Stages of Shock

	Initial: Subclinical Hypoperfusion	**Compensatory: SNS Innervation**	**Progressive: Hypoperfusion**	**Refractory: Profound Hypoperfusion**
Cardiac index	2.2-2.5 L/min/m^2	2-2.2 L/min/m^2	Less than 2 L/min/m^2	Less than 1.8 L/min/m^2
Clinical indications	• No clinical indications of hypoperfusion but "something is different" • Detected by invasive hemodynamic monitoring	• Tachycardia • Narrowed pulse pressure • Tachypnea • Cool skin • Oliguria • Diminished bowel sounds • Restlessness → confusion	• Dysrhythmias • Hypotension • Tachypnea • Cold, clammy skin • Anuria • Absent bowel sounds • Lethargy → coma	• Life-threatening dysrhythmias • Hypotension despite potent vasopressors • ARDS • DIC • Hepatic dysfunction/failure • ATN • Mesenteric ischemia/infarction • Myocardial ischemia/infarction/ • Failure • Cerebral ischemia/infarction

a. Subjective
   1) Anxiety, fear, feeling of impending doom
   2) Thirst
b. Objective
   1) Tachycardia
   2) Blood pressure changes
      a) Systolic BP increases or stays the same while diastolic BP increases resulting in a decrease in pulse pressure
         i) Because diastolic BP is a reflection of arterial elasticity, the vasoconstriction caused by the SNS causes an elevation in diastolic BP and a narrowing of the pulse pressure earlier than a decrease in systolic BP or MAP.
      b) Orthostatic effects with the BP decreasing when the patient is repositioned from lying to sitting

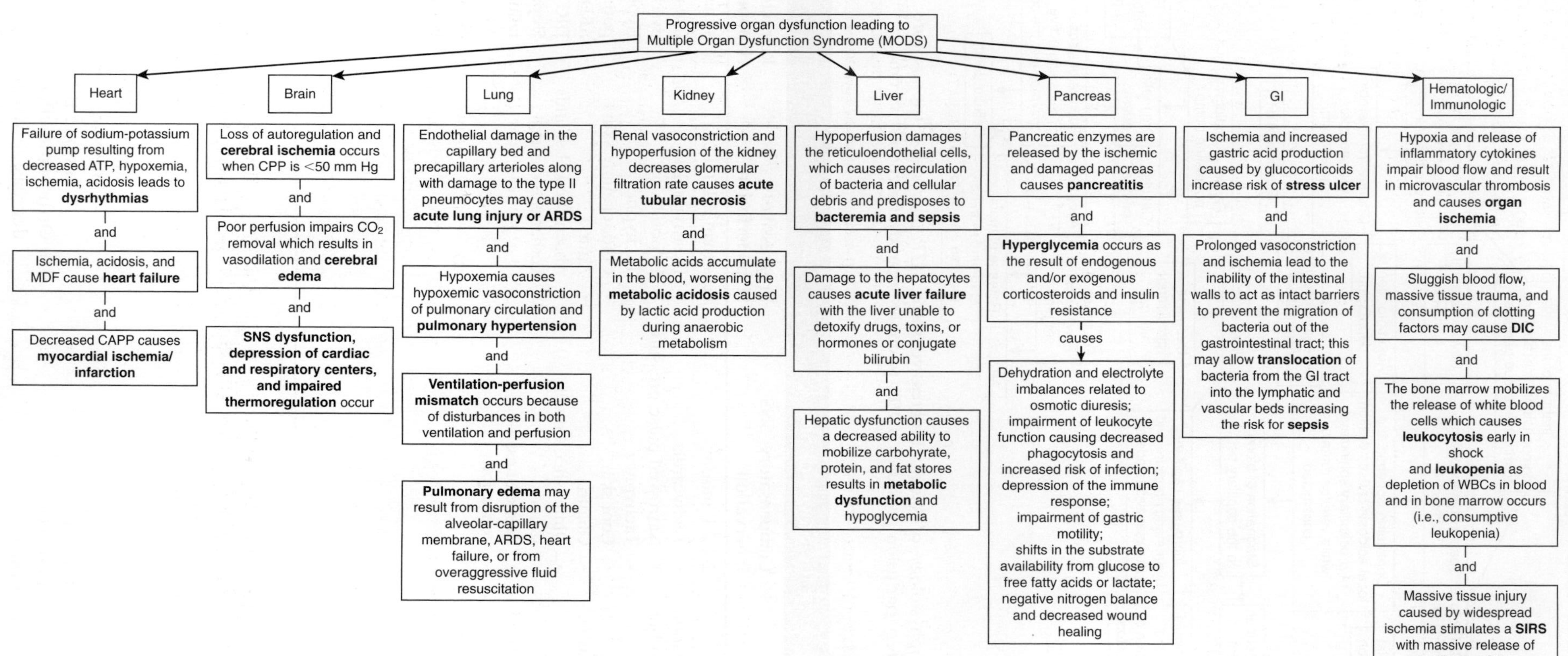

Figure 11-3 Pathophysiology of shock: Refractory stage. *ARDS,* Acute respiratory distress syndrome; *ATP,* adenosine triphosphate; *CAPP,* coronary artery perfusion pressure; *CPP,* cerebral perfusion pressure; *DIC,* disseminated intravascular coagulation; *GI,* gastrointestinal; *MDF,* myocardial depressant factor; *MODS,* multiple organ dysfunction syndrome; *SIRS,* systemic inflammatory response syndrome; *SNS,* sympathetic nervous system; *WBC,* white blood cell.

3) Tachypnea
4) Skin: cool, pale, clammy
5) GI: decreased bowel sounds
6) Renal: oliguria (i.e., less than 0.5 mL/kg/hr)
7) CNS: irritability, restlessness, confusion
   a) Even though the SNS shunts blood to the CNS, neurologic signs and symptoms occur early because the CNS is very sensitive to changes in oxygen and glucose.

3. Progressive stage: hypoperfusion
   a. Subjective
      1) Anorexia, nausea
      2) Chest pain and palpitations may occur.
      3) Dyspnea may occur.
   b. Objective
      1) Tachycardia, dysrhythmias
      2) Hypotension (MAP less than 70 mm Hg)
      3) Hypothermia (except in sepsis)
      4) Tachypnea
      5) Skin
         a) Bluish, mottled appearance
         b) Peripheral cyanosis
      6) GI: vomiting, absent bowel sounds
      7) Renal: anuria (i.e., negligible or less than 100 mL/24 hr)
      8) CNS: lethargy, coma
4. Refractory stage: profound hypoperfusion and evidence of MODS
   a. Heart
      1) Myocardial depression and hypotension
      2) Life-threatening dysrhythmias
      3) Myocardial ischemia/infarction: chest pain, ECG indicators of myocardial infarction, positive CK-MB and troponin
      4) Heart failure: S_3, crackles, dyspnea, JVD, hepatomegaly, edema, increased intracardiac pressures (i.e., PAP, PAOP)
      5) Cardiac arrest
   b. Brain
      1) Restlessness, confusion, altered level of consciousness
      2) Decrease in GCS of 1 or more
      3) Focal signs (e.g., hemiparesis or hemiplegia, aphasia) may be present.
   c. Lungs
      1) Hypoxemia with PaO_2/FiO_2 ratio of less than 250 mm Hg
      2) Decreased static compliance
         a) Increased work of breathing
         b) Increased peak and plateau pressure if patient on mechanical ventilation
      3) Diffuse pulmonary infiltrates on chest x-ray
      4) Necessity of mechanical ventilation with PEEP 7.5 cm H_2O or greater
   d. Kidney
      1) Urine output less than 0.5 mL/kg/hr
      2) Elevated BUN and creatinine
      3) Decreased urine creatinine clearance
   e. Gastrointestinal
      1) Diminished bowel sounds
      2) Poor tolerance of enteral feedings
      3) Occult or overt GI bleeding
   f. Liver
      1) Hypoglycemia
      2) Elevated bilirubin and jaundice
      3) Elevated AST, ALT, and LDH
      4) Decreased albumin
   g. Hematologic
      1) Decreased platelets
      2) Elevated aPTT/PT
      3) Decreased fibrinogen
      4) Positive D-dimer
      5) Bleeding in a patient without a prior history of bleeding; petechiae; blood in sputum, vomitus, nasogastric aspirate, urine, stool
   h. Metabolic
      1) Metabolic acidosis
      2) Serum lactate greater than 4
5. Hemodynamic parameters (Table 11-2)
   a. Decreased oxygen delivery to the tissues (DO_2): common to all forms of shock except early septic shock, in which DO_2 is increased, but extraction and utilization are impaired
      1) Oxygen delivery (DO_2) = CO × (Hgb × 1.34 × SaO_2) × 10
         a) Normal: approximately 1000 mL/min
      2) Oxygen delivery (DO_2I) = CI × (Hgb × 1.34 × SaO_2) × 10
         a) Normal: approximately 600 mL/min/m^2
   b. SvO_2 is valuable in assessment of shock states.
      1) Normal: 60-80%
      2) Decreased SvO_2 to less than 60% indicates a decrease in oxygen reserve caused by either a decrease in tissue oxygen delivery (DO_2)

Table 11-2 Hemodynamic Alterations in Shock

	Hypovolemic	Cardiogenic	Septic	Anaphylactic	Neurogenic
HR	High	High	High	High	Normal or low
BP	Normal → Low	Normal → Low	Low	Normal → Low	Normal → Low
CO/CI	Low	Low	High → Low	Normal → Low	Normal → Low
RAP/PAOP	Low	High	Low	Low	Low
SVR/SVRI	High	High	Low	Low	Low
SvO_2	Low	Low	High → Low	Low	Low

or an increase in tissue oxygen consumption (VO_2).
   a) Decrease in DO_2; decrease in SaO_2, CO, or hemoglobin
   b) Increase in VO_2: fever, agitation, seizures
c. Pulse pressure variation (dPP)
   1) Helpful in prediction of an increase in cardiac output induced by volume expansion prior to fluid administration
   2) May be measured via invasive arterial catheter
   3) dPP of 10-15% indicates fluid responsiveness
   4) Only reliable in mechanically ventilated patient; also predictive value lost when R-R intervals vary (e.g., atrial fibrillation) or if tidal volume varies breath to breath (Casserly, Read, & Levy, 2009)
d. Gastric tonometry or sublingual capnography may be used to assess tissue perfusion

6. Diagnostic
   a. Serum
      1) Sodium: increased early; increased or decreased late
      2) Potassium: decreased early; increased late
      3) Chloride: decreased early; increased late
      4) Bicarbonate: normal early; decreased late
      5) CO_2: normal early; decreased late
      6) Glucose: increased early; decreased late
      7) BUN: increased
      8) Creatinine: increased
      9) Total protein, albumin: decreased
      10) Bilirubin: increased late
      11) Amylase, lipase: increased late
      12) Ammonia: increased late
      13) CK: increased
      14) Liver enzymes (AST, ALT, LDH): increased
      15) Lactate: increased (should be done on arterial blood or central venous catheter [i.e., not from a vein with a tourniquet])
         a) Correlates with the degree of hypoperfusion
         b) Levels above 2 mmol/L are associated with increased mortality.
      16) Hemoglobin, hematocrit: decreased if due to hemorrhage
      17) Hematocrit: increased if due to cause other than hemorrhage
      18) WBC: increased early, decreased late
      19) PT, aPTT: may be prolonged
      20) Platelets: may be decreased
      21) Arterial blood gases: respiratory alkalosis progressing to metabolic acidosis; PaO_2 and SaO_2 may be decreased
      22) Blood cultures: may identify organism if septic shock
   b. Urine
      1) Urine creatinine clearance: decreased
      2) Urine specific gravity: increased early, decreased late
      3) Urine osmolality: increased early, decreased late
      4) Urine sodium: decreased
      5) Presence of heavy pigments
         a) Myoglobinuria occurs with muscle tissue destruction (e.g., crush injuries, muscle ischemia/necrosis, electrical burns, seizures).
         b) Hemoglobinuria occurs with mismatched blood transfusion reaction and fresh water near-drowning.
   c. Other diagnostic studies may be done to evaluate the reason for shock.

Collaborative Management

1. Maximize oxygen delivery to the tissues (Hgb, SaO_2, CO/CI).
   a. Maintain optimal hemoglobin and vascular volume; monitor and use CVP or PAOP when available.
      1) Two intravenous catheters should be inserted immediately, especially in cases of hemorrhage; these catheters should be short and large-gauge.
         a) Intraosseous route may be used to administer fluids and blood products when IV access cannot be obtained.
            i) Placement of rigid needle through the bone cortex into the medullary cavity
            ii) Preferred site is anterior aspect of the tibia 1-3 cm below the proximal tibial tuberosity
            iii) Requires immobilization of the limb
      2) Volume replacement for hypovolemic and vasogenic; may be necessary even in cardiogenic shock to achieve optimal PAOP
         a) Types of fluids used for fluid resuscitation (Box 11-1)
            i) Crystalloids: solutions with dextrose or electrolytes; safe, effective, inexpensive and usually the initial fluid type (Table 11-3)
            ii) Hypertonic crystalloids (e.g., 3% saline) has been advocated for trauma resuscitation, but there is no evidence of benefit of hypertonic crystalloid over isotonic crystalloid solutions (Patanwala, Amini, & Erstad, 2010)
            iii) Colloids: large molecule (protein or starch) solutions; considered when the patient's response to initial efforts are insufficient
               (a) Not only stay in the vascular space better than crystalloids but may contribute to intravascular colloidal oncotic pressure to pull more fluid into the vascular space
               (b) May be used in hypovolemic shock (except early burns) or

Box 11-1 Types of Fluids Used for Fluid Resuscitation

Crystalloids	Colloids	Blood and Blood Products
• Isotonic: NS; LR (D_5NS, D_5LR) • Hypotonic: ½NS (D_5½NS, D_5W) • Hypertonic: 3% saline; D_{10}W; TPN	• Albumin • Dextran 70/75 • Hetastarch (Hespan)	• Whole blood • Packed RBCs • Fresh frozen plasma

D_5LR, 5% dextrose in lactated Ringer's; *D_5NS,* 5% dextrose in normal saline; *D_5½NS,* 5% dextrose in 0.45% saline; *D_5W,* 5% dextrose in water; *D_{10}W,* 10% dextrose in water; *NS,* normal (0.9%) saline; *½NS,* 0.45% saline; *LR,* lactated Ringer's; *TPN,* total parenteral nutrition (usually 25% dextrose).

NOTE: Dextrose solutions are in parentheses because even though 5% dextrose adds to osmolality in the bottle or bag, this small amount of dextrose is metabolized so quickly when in the body that it should not be considered in the osmolality of the solution. So consider D_5NS as NS, D_5½NS as ½NS, and D_5W as water. This last example is why D_5W is avoided except in extreme hyperosmolar conditions. In significant volumes, D_5W will dilute electrolytes, particularly sodium, and potentially causes neurologic changes, including seizures.

Table 11-3 Crystalloids

	Isotonic	Hypotonic	Hypertonic
Osmolality	250-350 mOsm/L (which is similar to blood osmolality of 280-295 mOsm/L)	Less than 250 mOsm/L	Greater than 350 mOsm/L
Uses	• Tend to stay in the vascular space better than other crystalloids • Require replacement with 3 mL for every 1 mL lost because they equilibrate across fluid compartments	• Tend to leave the vascular space and replace the interstitial space better than the vascular space	• Pull fluid from the interstitial space into the intravascular space • Expand intravascular volume over isotonic crystalloid without the adverse effects of colloids • Monitor closely for clinical indications of fluid overload when these solutions are administered

Examples	0.9% saline
	• Composition
	  • 154 mEq of sodium
	  • 154 mEq of chloride
	  • Water
	• Osmolality is 289 mOsm/L
	• pH is 5.7
	• Large volumes may cause metabolic (hyperchloremic) acidosis
	Lactated Ringer's
	• Composition
	  • 130 mEq/L
	  • 109 mEq/L of chloride
	  • 4 mEq/L of potassium
	  • 3 mEq/L of calcium
	  • 28 mEq/L of lactate
	  • Water
	• Osmolality is 273 mOsm/L
	• pH 6.7
	• Lactate is added as a buffer to make the solution less acidic (than without the lactate)
	• Lactate is converted to bicarbonate by the liver, so large volumes may cause metabolic alkalosis; this solution should be avoided in patients who have liver disease
		Half normal (0.45%) saline
		• Composition
		  • 77 mEq of sodium
		  • 77 mEq of chloride
		  • Water
		D_5W
		• Composition
		  • 50 grams of dextrose
		  • Water
		• Note that though D_5W is isotonic in the bottle, the body quickly metabolizes the dextrose, and free water is left; avoid this solution except in extremely hyperosmolar patients (e.g., HHS, DI)
			Hypertonic (3% saline)
			• 513 mEq of sodium
			• 513 mEq of chloride
			D_{10}W (10% dextrose in water)
			• Composition
			  • 100 g of dextrose/L
			  • Water
			D_{50}W (50% dextrose in water)
			• Composition
			  • 25 grams of dextrose/50 mL ampule
			  • Water
			Total parenteral nutrition solution
			• Central
			  • 250 grams of dextrose/L
			  • Protein, electrolytes, vitamins vary
			  • Water
			• Peripheral
			  • 100 grams of dextrose/L
			  • Protein, electrolytes, vitamins vary
			  • Water

neurogenic shock; septic and anaphylactic shock are both associated with increased capillary permeability, so colloids should be avoided at least initially
(c) Examples
(i) Albumin: plasma protein component; most costly but least likely to cause complications
(ii) Dextran: contains polymers of high-molecular-weight polysaccharides; may cause coagulopathy by decreasing platelet aggregation; causes allergic reactions; may cause acute tubular necrosis and renal failure, but this is rare
(iii) Hetastarch: contains polymers of hydroxyethyl starch; may cause coagulopathy by decreasing platelet aggregation; may elevate serum amylase levels, but they return to normal 5-7 days after hetastarch

iv) Blood and blood products: used only to achieve a specific physiologic goal, such as to increase oxygen delivery or clotting capability
(a) Contain plasma proteins present to add to intravascular colloidal oncotic pressure; only solution that increases the CaO_2 (content of oxygen in arterial blood) because 97% of all oxygen is carried on the hemoglobin molecule
(b) Indicated when the patient has lost blood and there are clinical indications of hypoperfusion
(c) Blood should be used for patients with evidence of acute hemorrhage and hemodynamic instability or inadequate oxygen delivery (Napolitano et al., 2009).
(d) Transfusion should be considered if Hgb is less than 7 g/dL in critically ill patients requiring mechanical ventilation, in resuscitated critically ill trauma patients, and critically ill patients with stable cardiac disease (Napolitano et al., 2009)
(e) Major disadvantages of blood and blood products: cost and risk of blood transfusion reaction or blood-transmitted disease

b) Selection of solution for replacement
i) Colloids should not be used in situations with increased capillary permeability.
ii) In other situations, there is no difference in effectiveness (Perel & Roberts, 2011) and colloids are considerably more costly, so crystalloids are first choice in most situations
iii) Blood should be used only when specifically indicated because blood administration is associated with an increased risk of SIRS and mortality.

c) Volume
i) Typical fluid challenge is 250-500 mL of normal saline over 5 minutes.
ii) Monitor BP, CVP, and PAOP as available.
iii) Monitor for clinical indicators of fluid overload (e.g., dyspnea, jugular venous distention, S_3, systolic flow murmur, crackles).

3) Type and crossmatch immediately if patient is hemorrhaging; type-specific blood or O negative may be given in severe hemorrhage but may make future crossmatching more difficult.
4) Take care during fluid resuscitation to prevent hypothermia; fluids may need to be warmed if the patient's body temperature is low (35° C or less) at the initiation of fluid resuscitation or if multiple units of blood or multiple liters of IV fluids are needed.
5) Take care to avoid overresuscitation which is associated with increased incidence of bleeding, abdominal hypertension and abdominal compartment syndrome, MODS, and death.
a) In trauma patients, return of MAP to 70-80 mm Hg may cause clot disruption and increased bleeding; permissive hypotension with a MAP of 60 mm Hg is an approach that may be used until surgical intervention (Cottingham, 2006).
6) Administer venous vasodilators and/or diuretics as prescribed to decrease the preload (PAOP) in cardiogenic shock.

b. Maintain optimal cardiac contractility and cardiac output.
  1) Monitor ECG, MAP, RAP, PAP, PAOP, CO/CI, LVSWI, RVSWI, and neurologic status.
  2) Administer inotropes (e.g., dobutamine) as prescribed.
  3) Administer diuretics (e.g., furosemide) as prescribed.
  4) Administer vasoactive agents.
    a) Administer arterial vasodilators (e.g., nitroprusside [NTP]), to decrease afterload (SVR) and/or venous vasodilators (e.g., nitroglycerin [NTG]) to decrease preload (PAOP) as prescribed; these agents are typically needed in cardiogenic shock.
    b) Administer vasopressors as prescribed and in the lowest doses necessary to achieve desired effects (Table 11-4).
      i) Vasopressors are generally contraindicated in patients with cardiogenic shock because they increase afterload (SVR) and myocardial oxygen consumption; most useful in vasogenic forms of shock to maintain vascular tone
      ii) Vasopressors are sometimes used in an effort to maintain MAP above 60 mm Hg to maintain perfusion pressure, but by constricting the vessels they may actually decrease blood flow to organs, even though the MAP is higher.
  5) Correct metabolic acidosis because it affects cardiac contractility.
    a) Improve oxygenation and perfusion by improving Hgb, SaO_2, and Hgb.
    b) Administer sodium bicarbonate as prescribed; indicated only if pH is 7 or less
  6) Avoid overheating, which may cause vasodilation and decrease in preload.

c. Maintain optimal oxygen saturation.
  1) Monitor SpO_2, SvO_2, and arterial blood gases.
  2) Ensure adequate airway; endotracheal intubation is frequently necessary.
  3) Administer oxygen at 5-6 L/min initially.
    a) Higher concentrations may be necessary depending on SpO_2 and arterial blood gas values.
    b) CPAP or PEEP may be required for refractory hypoxemia.
  4) Initiate mechanical ventilation as prescribed for respiratory muscle fatigue, respiratory acidosis, and/or refractory hypoxemia.
  5) Monitor closely for changes in SpO_2, arterial blood gases, pulmonary vascular resistance, chest x-ray, and lung compliance indicative of ARDS.
  6) Assist with extracorporeal membrane oxygenation (ECMO) as required.

2. Minimize oxygen consumption of the tissues.
  a. Maintain patient comfort.
    1) Maintain bed rest and provide adequate rest periods.
    2) Administer analgesics and anxiolytics as required, but be cautious to avoid cumulative effect.
  b. Control body temperature.
    1) Treat hyperthermia with cooling blankets as necessary; set at 1° below patient's temperature to avoid drift and resultant shivering.
    2) Avoid overheating, which may increase myocardial oxygen consumption.
  c. Monitor work of breathing; initiate mechanical ventilation as prescribed for respiratory fatigue.
  d. Treat pain and anxiety.
    1) Administer analgesics and/or anxiolytics as prescribed and indicated.
    2) Provide patient and family support.
      a) Keep patient and family informed.
      b) Encourage the patient and family to discuss fear and concerns.
3. Prevent injury caused by decreased perfusion.
  a. Limit sedatives and other central nervous system (CNS) depressants.
  b. Administer drugs only IV because peripheral perfusion and drug absorption is impaired; central venous catheter with multiple-lumen catheter is preferred.
4. Maintain or improve nutritional status.
  a. Provide enteral feedings unless absolutely contraindicated (e.g., paralytic ileus or structural obstruction).
    1) Use of the GI tract is important to prevent bacterial translocation.
    2) Glutamine, arginine, and omega-3 fatty acids may be important in the prevention of sepsis, septic shock, SIRS, and MODS; arginine is contraindicated in sepsis.
  b. Provide parenteral feeding if enteral feedings are contraindicated or if parenteral supplementation of enteral feedings is needed to meet calorie and protein requirements.
  c. Closely monitor serum potassium, magnesium, and phosphate; replace or restrict as indicated.
  d. Add trace elements and vitamins as prescribed.
5. Maintain renal perfusion and glomerular filtration rate (GFR).
  a. Insert indwelling urinary catheter to monitor hourly urine output.
  b. Monitor BUN, creatinine, urine creatinine clearance, and urine sodium.
  c. Replace volume as indicated by CVP or PAOP.
  d. Monitor closely for change in color of urine which may indicate myoglobinuria or hemoglobinuria.
6. Maintain glycemic control.

Table 11-4 Selected Vasopressors

Drug	Administration	Adverse Effects	Nursing Implications
Norepinephrine bitartrate (Levophed)	• IV infusion: Mix 4 mg in 250 mL (16 mcg/mL) and infuse at 0.1-0.3 mcg/kg/min; titrate to BP response • Administer through central venous catheter if possible; if administered peripherally, use a large vein • Do not administer with alkaline solutions	• Bradycardia • Ventricular dysrhythmias • Hypertension • Anxiety • Headache • Tremor • Dizziness • Chest pain • Metabolic (lactic) acidosis • Severe vasoconstriction may cause renal or mesenteric necrosis • Local necrosis with high dosages or if infusion infiltrates	• Monitor HR, BP, ECG, urine output, neurologic status • Note contraindications: known hypersensitivity, ventricular fibrillation, tachydysrhythmias, pheochromocytoma, narrow-angle glaucoma • Use cautiously in peripheral vascular disease, hyperthyroidism, CAD, hypertension, psychoneurosis, diabetes, patients receiving MAO inhibitors or tricyclic antidepressants, and in older adults • Note that this drug may cause a fluid shift from intravascular to interstitial space, causing depletion of intravascular volume • Do not use discolored solution • Prevent extravasation because necrosis may occur; treat with phentolamine (Regitine)
Dopamine hydrochloride (Intropin)	• IV infusion: mix 400 mg in 250 mL (1600 mcg/mL) and infuse at 0.5-20 mcg/kg/min, depending on desired effect • Maximum: 20 mcg/kg/min • Administer through central venous catheter if possible; if administered peripherally, use a large vein • Do not administer with alkaline solutions	• Tachycardia • Ventricular ectopy • Hypertension or hypotension • Nausea, vomiting • Dyspnea • Headache • Palpitations • Chest pain in patients with CAD • Tissue necrosis with high dosages or extravasation	• Monitor HR, BP, ECG, PAP, PAOP, SVR, CI, urine output • Note contraindications: known hypersensitivity, uncorrected tachydysrhythmias, ventricular fibrillation, pheochromocytoma, hypertrophic cardiomyopathy, and in patients receiving MAO inhibitors • Use cautiously in peripheral vascular disease • Consider the cause of hypotension instead of automatically initiating dopamine to increase the blood pressure; improve perfusion by treating the cause of hypotension (e.g., volume replacement, inotropes, preload or afterload reduction) • Provide volume expansion during weaning; taper gradually to wean • Do not administer if discolored • Prevent extravasation because necrosis may occur; treat extravasation with phentolamine (Regitine)

Table 11-4 Selected Vasopressors—cont'd

Drug	Administration	Adverse Effects	Nursing Implications
Phenylephrine (Neo-Synephrine)	• IV infusion: mix 30 mg in 500 mL (60 mcg/mL); usual dose is 0.5-10 mcg/kg/min • Rapid onset and short duration • Preferred agent in patients with tachycardia	• Reflex bradycardia • Ventricular dysrhythmias • Hypertension • Nausea, vomiting • Paresthesia • Palpitations • Anxiety • Restlessness • Headache • Tremor • Chest pain	• Monitor BP, HR, ECG • Note contraindications: known hypersensitivity, ventricular fibrillation, tachydysrhythmias, pheochromocytoma, narrow-angle glaucoma • Use cautiously in older adults and those with hyperthyroidism, CAD, hypertension, psychoneurosis, diabetes mellitus, peripheral vascular disease • Prevent extravasation because necrosis may occur; treat with phentolamine (Regitine) • Treat reflex bradycardia with atropine • Discard if discolored or precipitate is present
Epinephrine hydrochloride (Adrenalin)	• IV infusion: mix 1 mg in 250 mL (4 mcg/mL) and infuse at 1-10 mcg/min (0.05-1 mcg/kg/min); titrate to desired effect • Administer through central venous catheter if possible; if administered peripherally, use a large vein • Do not administer with alkaline solutions	• Tachycardia • Dysrhythmias • Palpitations • Anxiety • Restlessness • Headache • Dizziness • Tremor • Cerebral hemorrhage • Chest pain • Hyperglycemia	• Monitor BP, HR, ECG • Note contraindications: glaucoma, organic brain damage, cardiomegaly • Use cautiously in older adults and those with hyperthyroidism, chest pain, hypertension, psychoneurosis, diabetes mellitus • Prevent extravasation because necrosis may occur; treat with phentolamine (Regitine) • Discard if discolored or precipitate is present
Vasopressin (Pitressin)	• IV infusion: 0.01- 0.04 units/min	• Bradycardia • Hypertension • Fever • Water intoxication (SIADH), hyponatremia • Nausea, abdominal cramps • Tremor • Headache • Seizures • Coma • Constriction of cardiac arteries, resulting in chest pain and myocardial ischemia	• Monitor HR, BP, daily weight, serum sodium • Note contraindications: known hypersensitivity, nephritis • Use cautiously in coronary artery disease

a. Recognize that hyperglycemia is related to stress and insulin resistance and occurs in patients without diagnosis of diabetes mellitus.

b. Maintain serum glucose at 140-180 mg/dL; note that though there has been considerable debate on the desirable serum glucose level over the last decade, the body of evidence related to this question indicates that there is no mortality benefit but increased hypoglycemia risk associated with glucose control maintained within the 80-110 [illegible]g/dL range (Sandrock & Albertson, 2010).

1) Measure serum [illegible]cose by point-of-care testing every h[illegible]il serum glucose is less than 180 [illegible]nd then every 4 hours.

a) Fingerstick [illegible]ents may be inaccurate i[illegible]tous, vasoconstric[illegible] poorly perfused patients; art[illegible]r venous catheter should be p[illegible] for sampling.

2) Administer insulin by infusion (usually 1 unit/mL) and adjust rate according to serum glucose level.
3) Administer $D_{10}W$ for hypoglycemia.
7. Monitor for complications.
   a. Dysrhythmias: close monitoring and appropriate antidysrhythmic agents depending on rhythm
   b. GI ulceration: stress ulcer prophylaxis with H_2 receptor antagonists or proton pump inhibitors
   c. Deep vein thrombosis: prophylaxis with low-molecular-weight heparin subcutaneously
   d. Mesenteric ischemia, infarction: monitoring for abdominal pain, bloody diarrhea; surgery required if intestinal perforation occurs
8. Monitor for indications of organ failure and multiple organ dysfunction syndrome (MODS).
   a. Acute lung injury progressing to respiratory distress syndrome (ARDS)
   b. Disseminated intravascular coagulation (DIC)
   c. Hepatic failure
   d. Acute tubular necrosis (ATN)
   e. Myocardial infarction
   f. Cerebral infarction
9. Provide emotional support to the patient and family.
   a. Inform the patient regarding what is going to occur and why.
   b. Provide the family with accurate information; maintain hope but do not give false reassurance.

Hypovolemic Shock

Definition

Shock caused by inadequate intravascular volume

Etiology

1. External losses
   a. Blood
      1) Gastrointestinal (e.g., esophageal varices, peptic ulcer, hemorrhoids)
      2) Genitourinary (e.g., antepartal or postpartum bleeding, hematuria)
      3) Amputations
      4) Major blood vessel disruption (may also be occult)
      5) Coagulopathy
         a) Congenital coagulopathy (e.g., hemophilia)
         b) Acquired coagulopathy (e.g., disseminated intravascular coagulation [DIC], excessive anticoagulation)
   b. Fluid
      1) Gastrointestinal (e.g., vomiting, diarrhea, nasogastric suction)
      2) Renal
         a) DKA
         b) HHS
         c) Diabetes insipidus
         d) Hypoaldosteronism (Addison's disease)
         e) Diuretics
         f) Osmotic dyes
      3) Cutaneous
         a) Burns
         b) Exudative wounds
         c) Excessive perspiration (e.g., heat exhaustion)
2. Internal sequestration
   a. Blood
      1) Hemoperitoneum or retroperitoneal (e.g., hemorrhagic pancreatitis, ruptured spleen, lacerated liver)
      2) Thoracic trauma with hemothorax, hemomediastinum
      3) Dissecting aortic aneurysm
      4) Pelvic or long bone fractures
   b. Fluid
      1) Ascites: peritonitis; pancreatitis; cirrhosis; intraabdominal malignancies (e.g., liver, ovarian)
      2) Pleural effusion
      3) Intestinal obstruction

Pathophysiology

See Figure 11-4.

Clinical Presentation

Same as for shock and including the following:
1. Subjective: history of precipitating factor
2. Objective
   a. Flat neck veins
   b. Abdominal girth
      1) Measure at same location on abdomen and mark with pen.
      2) One-inch increase in abdominal girth is equal to an increase in intraabdominal volume of 500-1000 mL.
   c. Daily weight
      1) Use same scale, same time of day, and same clothing and linens.
      2) One liter (1000 mL) is equal to 1 kg.
   d. Intake and output
      1) Consider insensible losses.
      2) Weigh dressings and convert to volume, using 1 kg equal to 1000 mL
      3) Include all drainage tubes.
   e. Parameters used for evaluation of severity of hemorrhagic shock (Table 11-5)
3. Hemodynamics: see Table 11-2
4. Diagnostic
   a. Hematocrit
      1) Elevated if due to dehydration
      2) Decreased if due to blood loss
   b. Diagnostic peritoneal lavage to detect intraabdominal bleeding
   c. Computerized tomography of chest or abdomen to detect source of bleeding

Collaborative Management

Same as for shock and including the following:
1. Identify high-risk patient, and monitor for clinical indications of hypoperfusion.
2. Treat the cause.

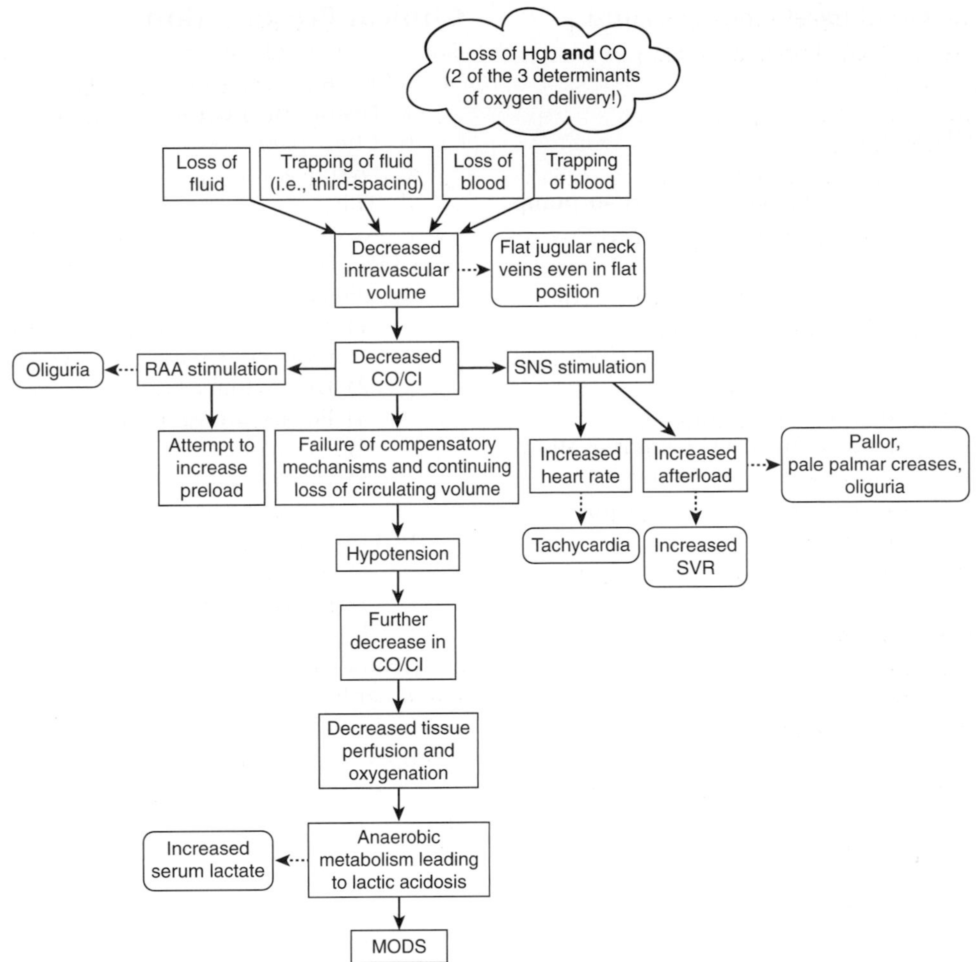

Figure 11-4 Pathophysiology of hypovolemic shock. Dotted lines connect pathology to clinical presentation. *CI,* Cardiac index; *CO,* cardiac output; *Hgb,* hemoglobin; *MODS,* multiple organ dysfunction syndrome; *RAA,* renin-angiotensin-aldosterone; *SNS,* sympathetic nervous system; *SVR,* systemic vascular resistance.

Table 11-5 Severity of Hemorrhagic Shock

Indicator	Class I	Class II	Class III	Class IV
Blood loss (% of blood volume)	Less than 15%	15-30%	30-40%	Greater than 40%
Blood loss (mL)	Less than 750 mL	750-1500 mL	1500-2000 mL	Greater than 2000 mL
Heart rate/min	Less than 100	Greater than 100	Greater than 120	140 or greater
Blood pressure	Normal	Normal	Decreased	Decreased
Pulse pressure	Widened or normal	Narrowed	Narrowed	Narrowed
Capillary refill	Normal	Delayed	Delayed	Delayed or absent
Ventilatory rate/min	14-20	20-30	30-40	Greater than 35
Urine output (mL/hr)	30 or greater	20-30	Less than 20	Negligible
Skin appearance	Cool, pink	Cool, pale	Cold, moist, pale	Cold, clammy, cyanotic
Neurologic status	Slightly anxious	Mildly anxious	Anxious, confused	Confused, lethargy

Adapted from American College of Surgeons (2008). *ATLS: Advanced trauma life support for doctors* (8th ed.). Chicago.

   a. Compress any compressible vessels.
   b. Surgery may be necessary to control bleeding.
   c. Antidiarrheals for diarrhea, insulin for hyperglycemia, etc.
3. Administer appropriate volume replacement.
   a. Two large-gauge intravenous catheters
   b. Normal saline at rapid rate initially; blood is indicated for class III and class IV when fluid loss is blood
   c. Monitor for fluid overload.
4. Utilize autotransfusion if appropriate; used primarily in chest trauma (or chest surgery)

to decrease the risk of transfusion-transmitted disease

Cardiogenic Shock

Definition

Shock caused by impaired ability of the heart to pump blood effectively

Etiology

1. Decreased contractility
   a. Coronary artery disease
      1) Acute MI
         a) Loss of 40% of left ventricular myocardium such as large anterior MI or acute MI in patient with history of previous MI or MIs and preexisting left ventricular dysfunction
      2) Myocardial ischemia with preexisting left ventricular dysfunction
   b. Myocardial contusion
   c. Cardiac surgery
   d. Dilated cardiomyopathy
   e. Myocarditis
   f. Severe HF
   g. Ventricular aneurysm
   h. Overdosage of myocardial depressant drugs (e.g., beta-blockers, calcium channel blockers, barbiturates)
   i. Stunned or hibernating myocardium: transient cardiogenic shock
      1) Cardiac surgery: related to hypothermia, cardioplegic arrest
      2) Reperfusion injury
      3) Post-CPR
      4) Hypoxemia
      5) Acidosis
      6) Hypoglycemia
      7) Electrolyte imbalance
   j. Acute rejection of cardiac transplant
2. Impaired filling
   a. Dysrhythmias
   b. Cardiac tamponade
   c. Noncompliant ventricle (e.g., left ventricular hypertrophy, right ventricular hypertrophy)
3. Impaired emptying (may be referred to as obstructive)
   a. Valvular dysfunction
      1) Chronic: stenosis or regurgitation
      2) Acute: papillary muscle rupture
   b. Ventricular septal rupture or rupture of ventricular free wall
   c. Intracardiac tumor
   d. Massive pulmonary embolism
   e. Tension pneumothorax
   f. Dissecting thoracic aortic aneurysm
   g. Coarctation of the aorta
   h. Restrictive or hypertrophic cardiomyopathy

Pathophysiology

See Figure 11-5.

Clinical Presentation

Same as for shock and including the following:

1. Subjective
   a. History of precipitating factor
   b. Chest pain
   c. Dyspnea
   d. Thirst
   e. Anxiety, fear, feeling of impending doom
2. Objectives
   a. Clinical indicators of LVF
      1) Tachycardia; note that this effect may be reduced if patient is receiving beta-blockers
      2) Dysrhythmias
      3) Pulsus alternans
      4) Tachypnea
      5) Heart sound changes: S_3
      6) Breath sound changes: crackles
   b. Clinical indicators of RVF
      1) Jugular venous distention
      2) Peripheral edema
      3) Hepatosplenomegaly
3. Hemodynamics: Table 11-2; defining characteristics of cardiogenic shock:
   a. CO/CI: less than 2 L/min/m^2
   b. RAP/PAP/PAOP increased; PAOP usually greater than 18 mm Hg
   c. SVR/SVRI increased; SVR usually greater than 2000 dynes/sec/cm^{-5}
4. Diagnostic
   a. Serum
      1) Enzymes and troponin: elevated if acute MI or myocardial contusion
      2) Electrolytes: note any abnormality
      3) Arterial blood gases: may reveal significant hypoxemia in pulmonary edema, respiratory acidosis as patient fatigues and acute respiratory failure occurs, and eventually metabolic acidosis with tissue hypoxia causing lactic acidosis
   b. ECG
      1) May reveal acute (i.e., ST segment elevation, pathologic Q waves) or old myocardial infarction (pathologic Q waves without ST segment elevation)
      2) May reveal ventricular aneurysm (i.e., persistent ST segment elevation in anterior leads)
      3) May reveal dysrhythmias
   c. Chest x-ray: may show pulmonary vascular congestion
   d. Cardiac catheterization
      1) May reveal cause of cardiogenic shock
      2) May reveal abnormal intracardiac pressures
   e. Echocardiography: may reveal cause of cardiogenic shock
      1) Ventricular wall motion abnormality
         a) Regional wall motional abnormality: myocardial in myocardial ischemia or infarction
         b) Global wall motion abnormality in cardiomyopathy or myocarditis

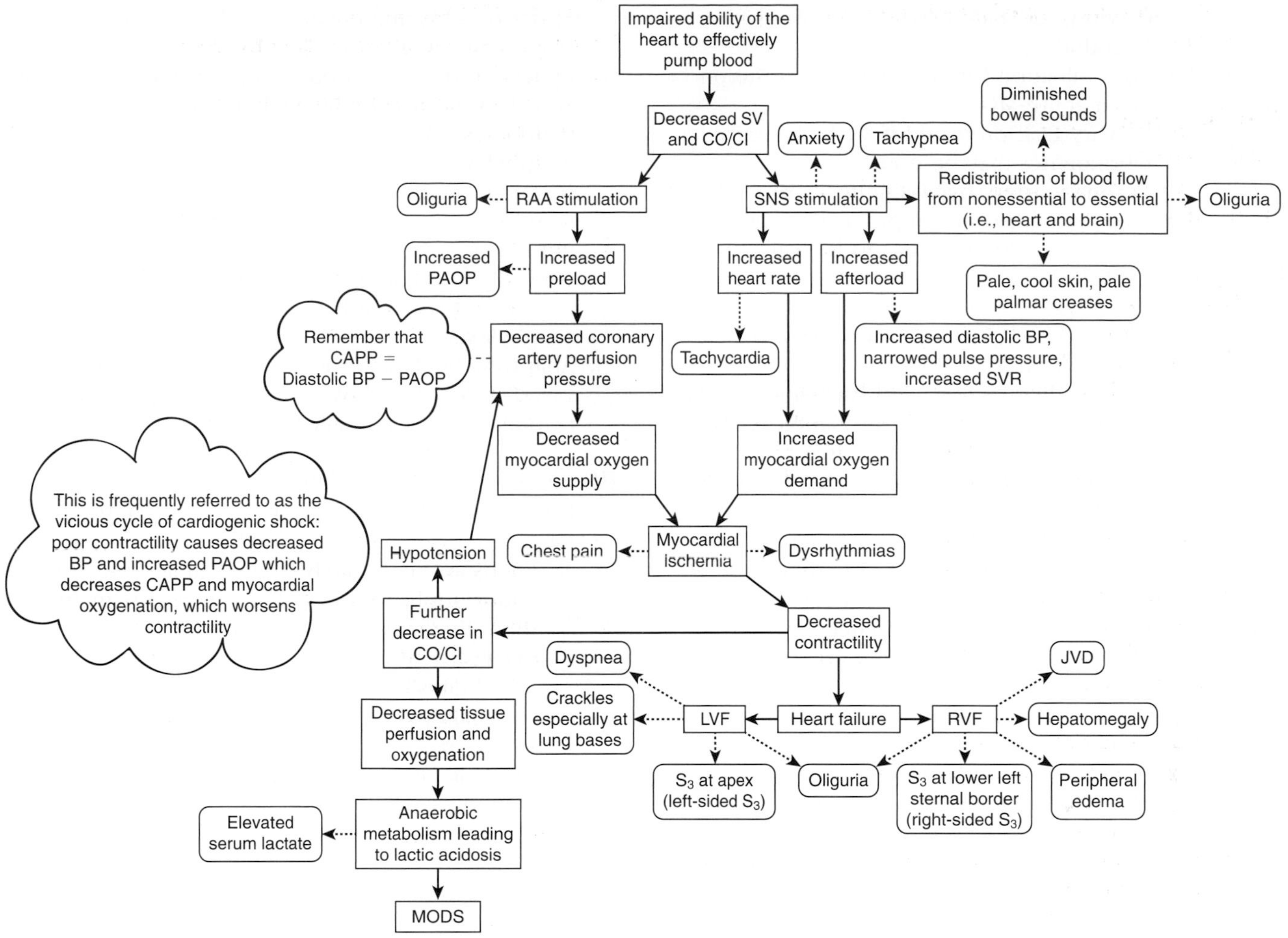

Figure 11-5 Pathophysiology of cardiogenic shock. Dotted lines connect pathology to clinical presentation. *BP,* Blood pressure; *CAPP,* coronary artery perfusion pressure; *CI,* cardiac index; *CO,* cardiac output; *LVF,* left ventricular failure; *MODS,* multiple organ dysfunction syndrome; *PAOP,* pulmonary artery occlusive pressure; *RAA,* renin-angiotensin-aldosterone; *RVF,* right ventricular failure; *SNS,* sympathetic nervous system; *SV,* stroke volume; *SVR,* systemic vascular resistance.

2) Valvular abnormality (e.g., ruptured ventricular septum, ruptured papillary muscle with acute mitral regurgitation)
3) Cardiac tamponade

Collaborative Management

Same as for shock and including the following:

1. Identify high-risk patient, and monitor for clinical indications of hypoperfusion; invasive hemodynamic monitoring if appropriate for early detection of changes in cardiac index
2. Prevent and treat the cause.
   a. Early reperfusion for acute MI
   b. Pericardiocentesis for cardiac tamponade
   c. Thrombolytics and anticoagulants for pulmonary embolus
   d. Surgery for removal of intracardiac tumors, valve replacement, septal repair, etc.
   e. Emergency decompression followed by chest tube for tension pneumothorax
3. Improve oxygenation.
   a. Oxygen by nasal cannula to achieve an SaO_2 of at least 95%; non-rebreathing face mask may be required to achieve this SaO_2 but is likely to increase dyspnea
   b. Mask CPAP may be helpful to improve oxygenation, especially for patients with significant pulmonary edema, but is likely to increase dyspnea.
   c. Intubation and mechanical ventilation may be required to decrease the work of breathing and improve ventilation and oxygenation.
4. Improve myocardial perfusion.
   a. Nitrates for ischemia while being careful not to decrease blood pressure and coronary artery perfusion pressure
      1) Remember that one nitroglycerin sublingually is 400 mcg, so titratable intravenous nitroglycerin is preferred.
      2) Ensure that patient has not taken an oral phosphodiesterase inhibitor such as sildenafil (Viagra), tadalafil (Cialis), vardenafil

(Levitra), udenafil (Zydena), or avanafil (Stendra).
   b. Prompt evaluation for emergency reperfusion options if acute MI
      1) Primary PCI: preferred if facilities available
      2) Fibrinolytics may be used.
      3) Coronary artery bypass graft (CABG)
5. Optimize cardiac output and improve tissue perfusion.
   a. Inotropes (e.g., dobutamine) to increase *contractility*
   b. Diuretics (e.g., furosemide) or venous vasodilators (e.g., nitroglycerin (NTG]) to decrease *preload* (PAOP)
   c. Arterial vasodilators (e.g., nitroprusside [NTP]) to decrease *afterload* if no contraindications
      1) Nitroprusside is contraindicated in acute myocardial ischemia due to the risk of coronary artery steal with shunting of blood from ischemic areas to nonischemic areas.
      2) Caution must be exercised with all arterial vasodilators in acute myocardial ischemia because they are likely to decrease aortic root pressure and coronary artery perfusion pressure.
      3) Careful titration of all vasodilators is required to maintain the MAP above the 60 mm Hg required to perfuse vital organs; afterload reduction may need to be achieved nonpharmacologically through the use of an IABP.
   d. Antidysrhythmics as required to control *heart rate*
      1) Anxiolytics (e.g., lorazepam [Ativan]) may be helpful to decrease heart rate by decreasing anxiety.
      2) Beta-blockers are contraindicated during cardiogenic shock states because they decrease contractility.
   e. Mechanical supports (e.g., intraaortic balloon pump [IABP]) (see Chapter 3, Figures 3-15 through 3-17 and Table 3-11) or ventricular assist devices (Table 3-23)
      1) IABP is especially helpful in patients who have very high afterload that is refractory to arterial vasodilators or who are too hypotensive to utilize arterial vasodilators to reduce afterload.
      2) IABP or ventricular assist devices may also serve as a bridge to transplant if the patient is a candidate for cardiac transplantation.
      3) Left ventricular assist device or biventricular assist device may be used; may be inserted percutaneously (i.e., Impella).
6. Register the patient for cardiac transplantation if appropriate.

Anaphylactic Shock

Definitions

1. Anaphylaxis: a systemic response to a specific antigen, usually occurring within 1 hour of exposure; this immunoglobulin E (IgE) mediated response is an example of a Type I hypersensitivity reaction, and prior exposure to the antigen is required which allows development of antibodies
2. Anaphylactoid reaction: an anaphylaxis-type reaction triggered by direct activation of the mast cell; this nonimmune response does not require previous exposure to the antigen; clinically indistinguishable from anaphylaxis, and acute treatment is the same as for anaphylaxis
3. Anaphylactic shock: shock resulting from massive vasodilation caused by release of histamine in response to a severe allergic reaction

Etiology

1. Examples of substances causing anaphylactic (IgE mediated) reactions
   a. Foods are more likely triggers in adolescents and young adults; most likely food triggers include the following:
      1) Fish
      2) Shellfish (e.g., shrimp, lobster, crab, scallops)
      3) Eggs
      4) Milk and milk products
      5) Soy
      6) Wheat
      7) Strawberries
      8) Legumes (e.g., peanuts, soybeans)
      9) Nuts (e.g., walnuts, pecans, cashews, almonds)
      10) Chocolate
      11) Food additives
         a) Artificial coloring
         b) Preservatives: sulfites and MSG
   b. Drugs
      1) ACE inhibitors (e.g., captopril, enalapril)
      2) Acetylcysteine (Mucomyst)
      3) Allergic extracts in hyposensitization therapy
      4) Allopurinol (Zyloprim)
      5) Anesthetics
         a) Local anesthetics: lidocaine, procaine, cocaine
         b) General anesthetics: thiopental, etomidate, ketamine
      6) Animal serums: antitoxins, antivenoms
      7) Antibiotics
         a) Beta-lactam antibiotics
            i) Penicillin
            ii) Cephalosporins
         b) Tetracycline
         c) Macrolides
      8) Barbiturates
      9) Blood and blood products: blood transfusion incompatibilities, albumin
      10) Enzymes
         a) Pancreatic
         b) Papaya enzyme

i) Chymopapain (used in chemical discectomy)
ii) Meat tenderizer
11) Insulin: pork or beef
12) Iodine-containing contrast media (e.g., Renografin)
13) Narcotics: morphine, meperidine, codeine
14) Neuromuscular blockers
15) Protamine sulfate
16) Thiazide diuretics (e.g., hydrochlorothiazide)
17) Vaccines
c. Venoms
1) Snakes
2) Hymenoptera (e.g., wasps, hornets, bees, yellow jackets, fire ants)
3) Spiders
4) Jellyfish
5) Stingrays
6) Deer flies
7) Scorpions
d. Other chemicals or biologicals
1) Materials (e.g., latex)
2) Hand lotions
3) Soap
4) Perfume
5) Iodine-containing solutions (e.g., Betadine)
6) Animal dander
2. Examples of substances causing anaphylactoid (non-IgE mediated) reactions
a. Drugs
1) Aspirin
2) Nonsteroidal antiinflammatory agents: aspirin, ibuprofen, indomethacin
3) Opiates
4) Thiamine
5) Dextran
6) Gamma globulin
b. Dyes
1) Radiopaque contrast media
2) Fluorescein

Pathophysiology

See Figure 11-6.

Clinical Presentation

Same as for shock and including the following:
1. Subjective
a. History of precipitating factor
b. Anxiety, vague uneasiness
c. Warmth
d. Nausea, abdominal cramping, abdominal pain
e. Chest tightness, palpitations
f. Dyspnea
g. Dizziness, vertigo
h. Pruritus
i. Feeling of a lump in throat
2. Objective
a. Cutaneous
1) An identifiable site of allergen exposure, bite, sting, or envenomation may be evident as localized redness, swelling, and pruritus.
2) May be generalized
a) Angioedema (edema of membranous tissues): swelling of eyes, lips, tongue, hands, feet, and genitalia
b) Flushing
c) Warm to hot skin
d) Urticaria
e) Conjunctival injection, tearing
f) Watery rhinorrhea, sneezing
g) Erythema more in upper extremities
b. Cardiovascular
1) Tachycardia
2) Hypotension
3) Dysrhythmias
4) ST and T wave changes consistent with ischemia
5) Shock
6) Cardiac arrest may occur.
c. Pulmonary
1) Hoarseness
2) Cough
3) Prolonged expiration
4) Breath sound changes: stridor, wheezing, crackles, rhonchi
5) Respiratory arrest may occur.
d. Neurologic
1) Restlessness
2) Headache
3) Paresthesia
4) Change in level of consciousness
5) Seizures
e. Genitourinary
1) Urinary incontinence
2) Urine output: may be decreased
3) Vaginal bleeding
f. GI
1) Dysphagia
2) Vomiting
3) Hyperactive bowel sounds
4) Diarrhea
3. Hemodynamics: Table 11-2
4. Diagnostic
a. Serum
1) IgE levels may be used to confirm allergic origin.
2) Eosinophils elevated
3) Arterial blood gases: initially respiratory alkalosis with hypoxemia, eventually respiratory and metabolic acidosis as hypoventilation and tissue hypoxia occur

Collaborative Management

Same as for shock and including the following:
1. Identify high-risk patient, and monitor for clinical indications of allergic reaction and hypoperfusion.
2. Provide CPR as required.
3. Maintain airway, oxygenation, and ventilation.
a. Airway

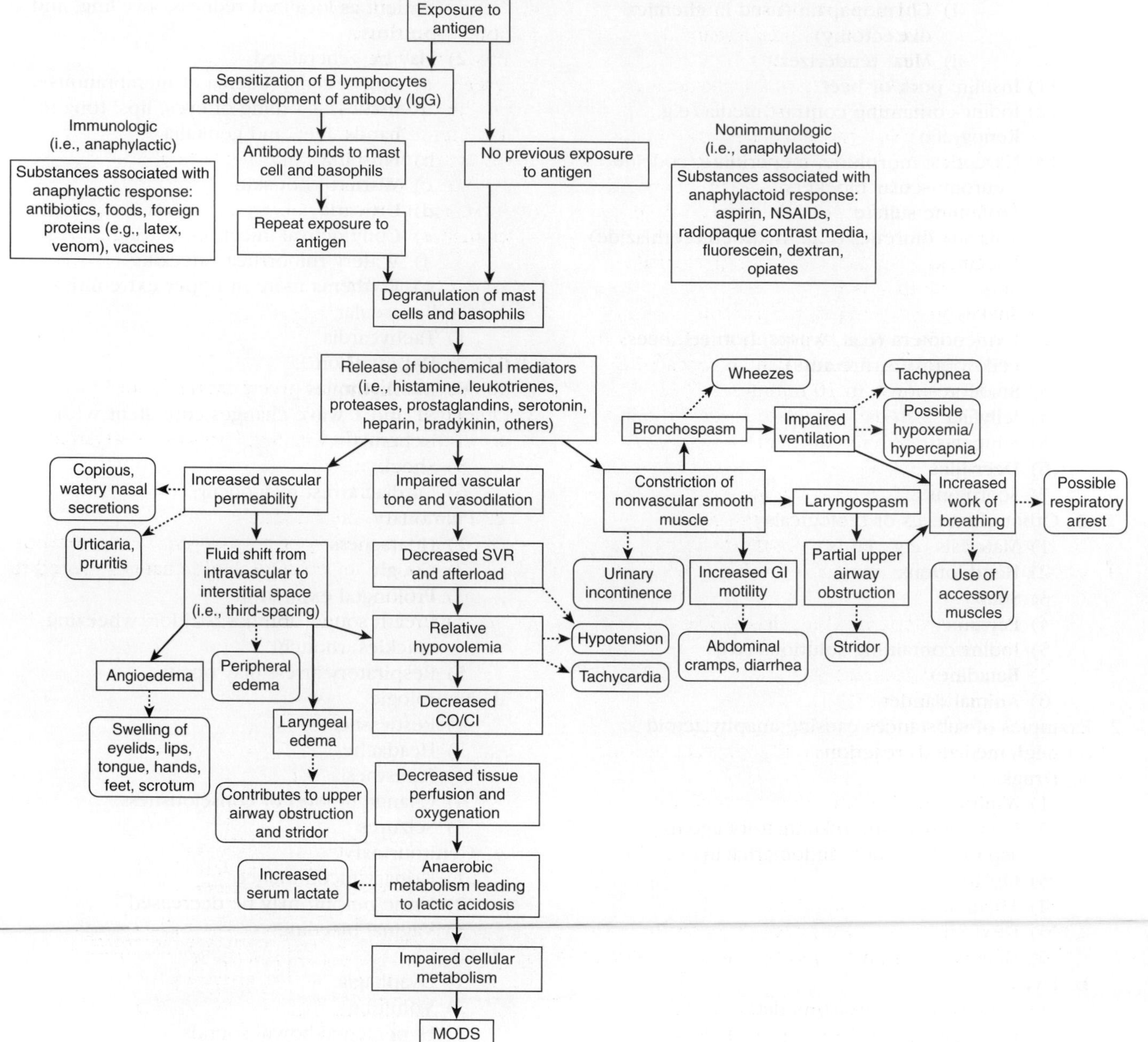

Figure 11-6 Pathophysiology of anaphylactic shock. Dotted lines connect pathology to clinical presentation. *CI,* Cardiac index; *CO,* cardiac output; *GI,* gastrointestinal; *NSAID,* nonsteroidal antiinflammatory drug; *SVR,* systemic vascular resistance.

1) Assess airway for clinical indications of angioedema (i.e., edema of uvula, respiratory distress, stridor, hypoxemia).
2) If angioedema is present, assist with endotracheal tube insertion early to prevent complete airway obstruction; cricothyrotomy may be necessary because of laryngeal edema.

b. Oxygen at 5-6 L initially; adjust to maintain SpO_2 at 95% unless contraindicated; 100% nonrebreathing mask may be required, but the mask may increase the sensation of dyspnea

c. Mechanical ventilation as prescribed

4. Remove the offending agent or slow absorption of antigen.

a. Removal of stinger if anaphylaxis is due to a sting and if the stinger can be removed easily without squeezing

b. Ice if due to sting or bite

c. Discontinuance of infusion of dye, drug, or blood

d. Dermal decontamination with soap and water if skin exposure to allergen

e. Gastric lavage not recommended to remove an ingested antigen

5. Modify or block the effects of biochemical mediators.

a. Sympathomimetic agents

1) Epinephrine

a) Intravenous

i) IV injection: 0.1 mg (100 mcg) over 5-10 minutes initially if clinical indications of cardiovascular compromise are present; stop injection if dysrhythmias or chest pain occur
ii) IV infusion: 1-4 mcg/min if inadequate response to IV injection
b) Intramuscular: 0.3-0.5 mg every 5-10 minutes for patients with less severe symptoms; thigh injection preferred over upper arm
2) Glucagon 3.5-5 mg IV for patients taking beta-blockers with hypotension refractory to epinephrine and fluids; can be repeated if no BP response in 10 minutes
a) Glucagon can stimulate an increase in heart rate and contractility even with beta-blockade.
b) Monitor for nausea, vomiting, hypokalemia, and hyperglycemia.
b. Crystalloids: 1-2 L of normal saline
c. Antihistamines as prescribed to block histamine receptors
1) Diphenhydramine (Benadryl) 25-50 mg IV, IM, or PO
2) Ranitidine (Zantac) 50 mg IV or famotidine (Pepcid) 20 mg IV
d. Steroids as prescribed to stabilize mast cells, decrease capillary permeability, prevent delayed reaction
1) Methylprednisolone sodium succinate (Solu-Medrol) 100 mg IV or hydrocortisone sodium succinate (Solu-Cortef) 100 to 200 to 500 mg IV
2) Prednisone 40-60 mg PO daily
e. Bronchodilators as prescribed to reverse the bronchoconstriction caused by histamine, SRS-A, and bradykinin
1) Albuterol, intermittent or continuous nebulizer for wheezing refractory to epinephrine
2) Ipratropium bromide (Atrovent) or magnesium may also be used.
6. Maintain MAP and tissue perfusion: fluids, inotropes, and/or vasopressors may be necessary.

Neurogenic Shock

Definition

Shock resulting from massive vasodilation caused by suppression of the sympathetic nervous system

Etiology

1. Cervical spinal cord injury (most common cause); note that this is not the same as spinal shock which is loss of neurologic function below the level of the injury but not necessarily associated with inadequate tissue perfusion
2. Head injury
3. Insulin shock
4. General anesthesia
5. Spinal anesthesia
6. Epidural block
7. Drugs
   a. Barbiturates
   b. Phenothiazines
   c. Sympathetic blocking agents (e.g., antihypertensives)
8. Exposure to unpleasant circumstances (e.g., fright or pain)

Pathophysiology

See Figure 11-7.

Clinical Presentation

1. Subjective: history of precipitating factor
2. Objective
   a. Bradydysrhythmias; may progress to asystole
   b. Hypotension
   c. Hypothermia
   d. Skin warm, dry, flushed
   e. Neurologic deficit (e.g., paralysis below level of spinal cord injury, neurologic changes related to head injury)
3. Hemodynamics: see Table 11-2

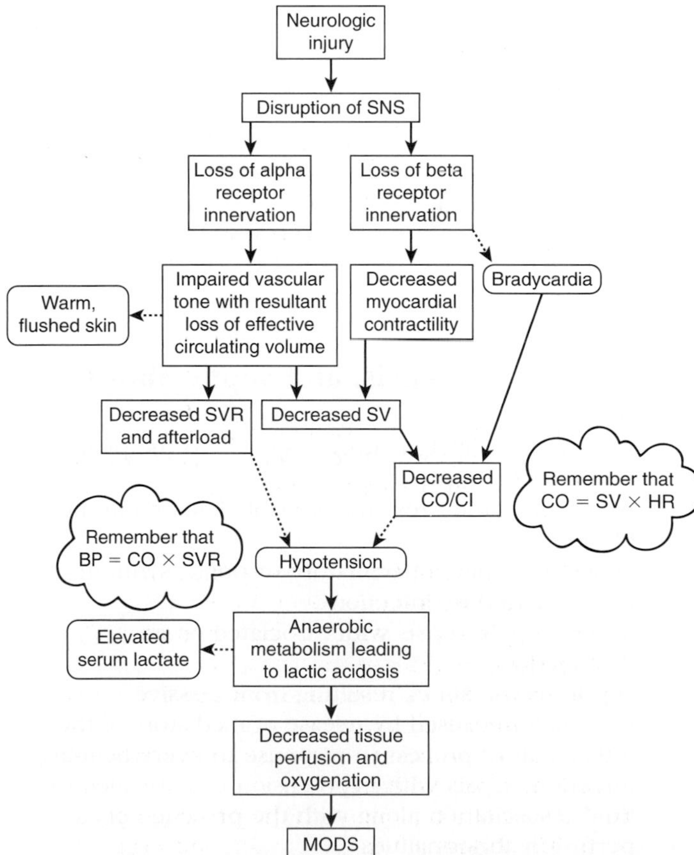

Figure 11-7 Pathophysiology of neurogenic shock. Dotted lines connect pathology to clinical presentation. *BP,* Blood pressure; *CI,* cardiac index; *CO,* cardiac output; *HR,* heart rate; *MODS,* multiple organ dysfunction syndrome; *SNS,* sympathetic nervous system; *SV,* stroke volume; *SVR,* systemic vascular resistance.

Collaborative Management

Same as for shock and including the following:

1. Identify high-risk patient, and monitor for clinical indications of hypoperfusion.
2. Prevent and treat the cause.
   a. Suspected spinal cord injury
      1) Early immobilization of the spine with suspected spinal injury
      2) Elevate the head of the bed to 30 degrees to decrease spinal cord edema.
   b. Anesthesia: reverse anesthesia, rewarm
   c. Insulin shock
      1) Monitor for clinical indications of hypoglycemia and measure serum glucose as required.
      2) Administer 10-15 grams of carbohydrate if the patient is conscious or 50 mL of $D_{50}W$ if unconscious.
3. Maintain MAP and tissue perfusion.
   a. Maintain MAP greater than 70 mm Hg.
      1) Fluids
         a) Crystalloids: Hypertonic saline may be used.
         b) Colloids: Albumin traditionally has been advocated, but recent studies and a meta-analysis show no benefit to the use of colloids, including in patients with neurologic problems.
         c) Monitor closely for pulmonary or cerebral edema.
      2) Inotropes and/or vasopressors may be necessary.
   b. Maintain heart rate 60-100/min: atropine and/or a pacemaker may be necessary.
4. Treat hypothermia if necessary.
5. Prevent venous stasis and deep vein thrombosis: anticoagulants (e.g., low dose heparin) as prescribed

Sepsis, Severe Sepsis, and Septic Shock

Definitions

1. Infection: an inflammatory response to the presence of microorganisms
2. Bacteremia: the presence of viable bacteria in the blood
3. Sepsis: systemic inflammatory response syndrome (SIRS) caused by infection
4. Severe sepsis: sepsis with associated organ dysfunction
5. Septic shock: shock resulting from massive vasodilation caused by release of mediators of the inflammatory process in response to overwhelming infection; sepsis with hypotension despite adequate fluid resuscitation along with the presence of perfusion abnormalities

Etiology

1. Factors that cause immunosuppression
   a. Extremes of age
   b. Malnutrition
   c. Alcoholism or drug abuse
   d. Debilitation
   e. Malignancy
   f. AIDS
   g. History of splenectomy
   h. Chronic health problems (diabetes mellitus, liver disease, heart disease [e.g., coronary artery disease or heart failure], renal failure)
   i. Bone marrow suppression
   j. Immunosuppressive therapies (e.g., immunosuppressive drugs, antineoplastic drugs, antibiotic therapy, corticosteroids)
2. Factors that cause bacteremia and septicemia
   a. Invasive procedures and devices
   b. Pulmonary procedures
   c. Diagnostic procedures
   d. Surgical procedures or wounds
   e. Traumatic wounds or burns
   f. Genitourinary infection
   g. Untreated GI disease (cholelithiasis, intestinal obstruction, appendicitis, diverticulitis)
   h. Peritonitis
   i. Food poisoning
   j. Prolonged hospitalization
   k. Translocation of GI bacteria: NPO status, decreased peristalsis, and GI ischemia contribute to proliferation of gastrointestinal bacteria and translocation of these bacteria into blood or lymph
3. Microorganisms
   a. Gram-negative bacteria (*most likely)
      1) *Escherichia coli**
      2) *Klebsiella*
      3) *Enterobacter**
      4) *Pseudomonas aeruginosa**
      5) *Proteus mirabilis*
      6) *Enterococcus*
      7) *Serratia marcescens*
      8) *Bacteroides* organisms
      9) *Haemophilus influenzae*
   b. Gram-positive organisms
      1) *Staphylococcus aureus*
      2) *Staphylococcus epidermidis*
      3) *Streptococcus pneumoniae*
      4) *Clostridium* organisms
      5) *Pneumococcus*
   c. Less likely
      1) Viruses
      2) Fungi
      3) *Rickettsia*
      4) *Spirochaeta*
      5) Protozoa
      6) Parasites

Pathophysiology

See Figure 11-8.

Clinical Presentation

1. Documented or suspected infection
2. Altered mental status
3. Hyperglycemia

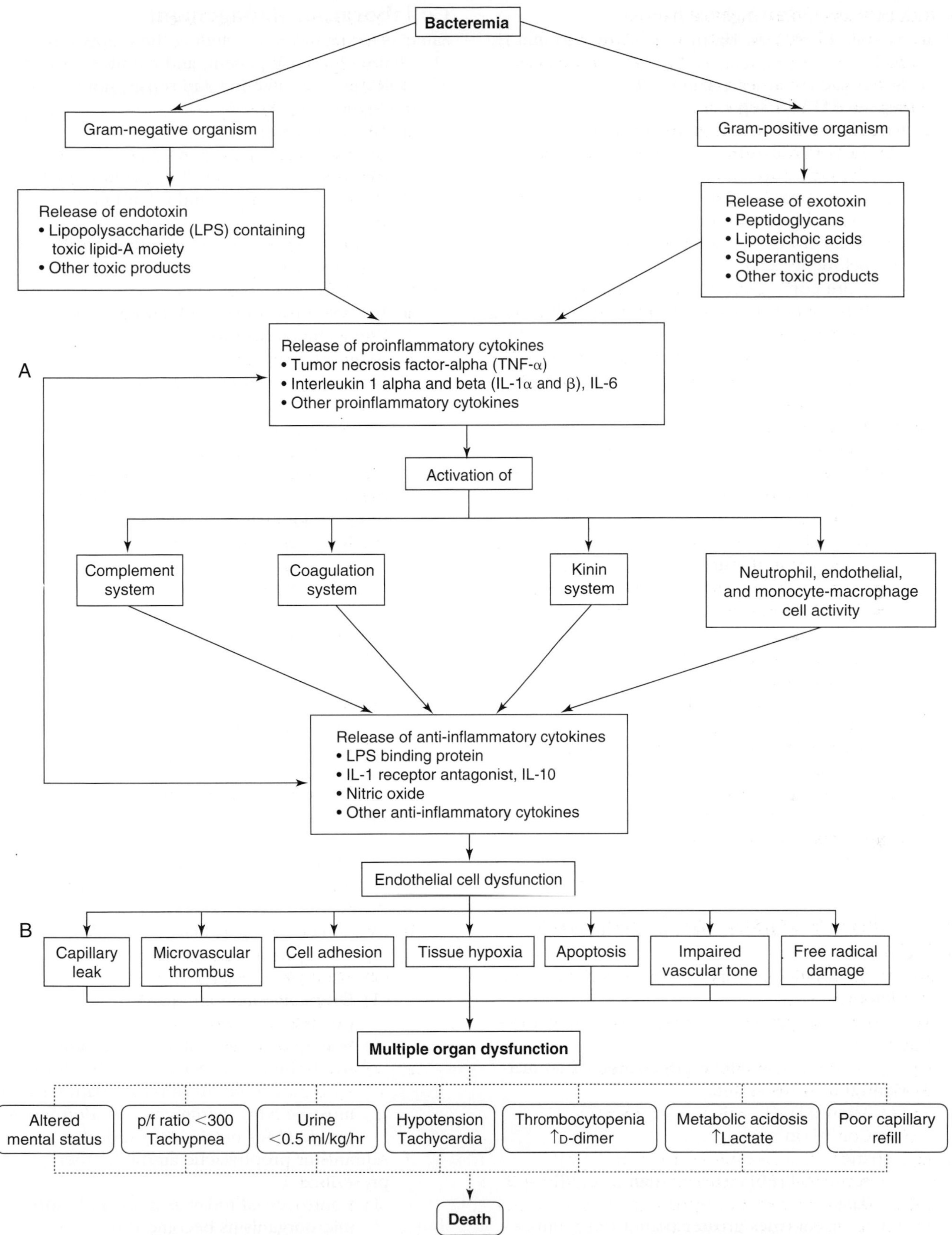

Figure 11-8 Pathophysiology of sepsis/septic shock. Dotted lines connect pathophysiology to clinical presentation. p/f, PaO_2/ FiO_2. (**A,** From Lazaron, V., & Barke, R.A. [1999]. Gram-negative bacterial sepsis and the sepsis syndrome. *Urol Clin North Am, 26*(4), 687-699. **B,** Copyright © 2003, Eli Lilly and Company. All rights reserved. Reprinted with permission from Eli Lilly and Company.)

4. Clinical indications of global hypoxia
   a. Systolic BP 90 mm Hg or less or MAP 65 mm Hg or less
   b. Serum lactate at least 4 mmol/L
5. Evidence of SIRS if sepsis
   a. Criteria for SIRS (2 or more of the following):
      1) Tachycardia (greater than 90 beats/min)
      2) Hyperpnea (respiratory rate above 20 breaths/min or $PaCO_2$ below 32 mm Hg)
      3) Hyperthermia (temperature above 38° C or 100.4° F) or hypothermia (temperature below 36° C or 96.8° F) (hypothermia is more common in elderly patients)
      4) WBC above 12,000 cells/mm^3 or below 4000 cells/mm^3 or more than 10% immature neutrophils (i.e., bands)
6. Evidence of infection, sepsis, and acute organ dysfunction if severe sepsis
   a. Cardiovascular
      1) Systolic BP 90 mm Hg or less or MAP 70 mm Hg or less for 1 hour despite fluid resuscitation
   b. Respiratory
      1) PaO_2/FiO_2 less than 250
      2) Bilateral infiltrates on chest x-ray
      3) Need for mechanical ventilation and PEEP greater than 7.5 cm H_2O
   c. Renal
      1) Doubling of baseline creatinine or 2 times upper limit of normal
      2) Urine output less than 0.5 mL/kg/hr for 1 hour despite adequate fluid resuscitation
   d. Hematologic
      1) Platelet reduction
         a) Thrombocytopenia less than 100,000 platelets/mm^3
         b) Decrease of platelets by 50% from highest value in last 3 days
      2) INR greater than 1.2
      3) PTT/aPTT greater than upper limit of normal
      4) Increased D-dimer
   e. Metabolic
      1) pH less than 7.3 (or base deficit greater than 5)
      2) Serum lactate above upper limit of normal
   f. Central nervous system
      1) Altered LOC
      2) Confusion
   g. Hepatic
      1) Serum bilirubin greater than 2 mg/dL for 2 days
      2) Liver enzymes greater than 2 times upper limit of normal
7. Evidence of infection, sepsis, and hypotension if septic shock
   a. Sepsis with hypotension despite adequate fluid resuscitation along with the presence of perfusion abnormalities
8. Hemodynamics: Table 11-2

Collaborative Management

Same as for shock and including the following:

1. Identify high-risk patient, and monitor for clinical indications of infection and sepsis; note any of the following:
   a. Hyperthermia
   b. Increase in respiratory rate
   c. Elevated glucose caused by insulin resistance
   d. Poor gastric motility and retention of enteral feedings
   e. Elevated serum lactate despite clinical picture of increased cardiac output
2. Prevent infection and sepsis.
   a. Use good handwashing techniques and prevent cross-contamination.
   b. Avoid intrusive procedures if possible.
   c. Participate in early identification of focus of infection.
      1) Monitor color, characteristics of sputum, urine, stools, wounds, etc.
      2) Culture secretions and wounds as indicated.
   d. Prepare patient for surgery as indicated for any of the following:
      1) Removal of all necrotic tissue
      2) Drainage of abscess
      3) Early débridement of burn eschar
      4) Prompt stabilization of fractures to minimize soft tissue damage, inflammation, infection
   e. Perform meticulous oral and airway care; silent aspiration of oral, nasopharyngeal, and sinus secretions around the endotracheal tube cuff occurs and is a cause of nosocomial pneumonia.
   f. Perform meticulous intravenous, intraarterial, pulmonary arterial, and urinary catheter care according to Centers for Disease Control (CDC) guidelines or hospital policy.
   g. Perform meticulous wound care as indicated by type and appearance of wound.
   h. Avoid NPO status to prevent translocation of enteric bacteria into the lymphatics and vascular bed.
      1) Enteral feedings should be given if at all possible.
      2) Selective gut decontamination (gut sterilization) has been advocated for use with parenteral nutrition for patients that must be NPO; parenteral nutrition would be provided for nutritional support.
   i. Administer prophylactic antibiotic therapy as prescribed.
      1) Controversial today as more and more microorganisms become resistant to available antibiotic therapy
      2) Many physicians prefer to have clinical indications of infection before prescribing antibiotic therapy.
   j. Prevent ventilator-associated pneumonia.
3. Restore tissue perfusion and normalize cellular metabolism.

a. Provide early goal-directed therapy during first 6 hours after severe sepsis or septic shock are recognized (Figure 11-9).
   1) Indications
      a) Suspected or confirmed infection
      b) Two or more indications of SIRS
      c) MAP less than 65 mm Hg after 20 mL/kg fluid bolus OR serum lactate of at least 4 mmol/L
   2) Goals include the following:
      a) CVP of 8-12 mm Hg
      b) MAP of 65 mm Hg or greater
      c) $ScvO_2$ or SvO_2 of 70% or greater
      d) Urine output greater than 0.5 mL/kg/hr
   3) Resuscitation and management (Marik, 2011; Nguyen et al., 2007; Dellinger et al., 2004; Rivers et al., 2001)
      a) Intubation and mechanical ventilation when required for respiratory distress; utilize the following settings to avoid ventilator-induced lung injury (VILI)
         i) Tidal volume at 6 mL/kg
         ii) Peak inspiratory plateau pressure of no more than 30 cm H_2O
      b) Antimicrobial agents following blood cultures
         i) Cultures
            (a) One blood draw should be percutaneous.

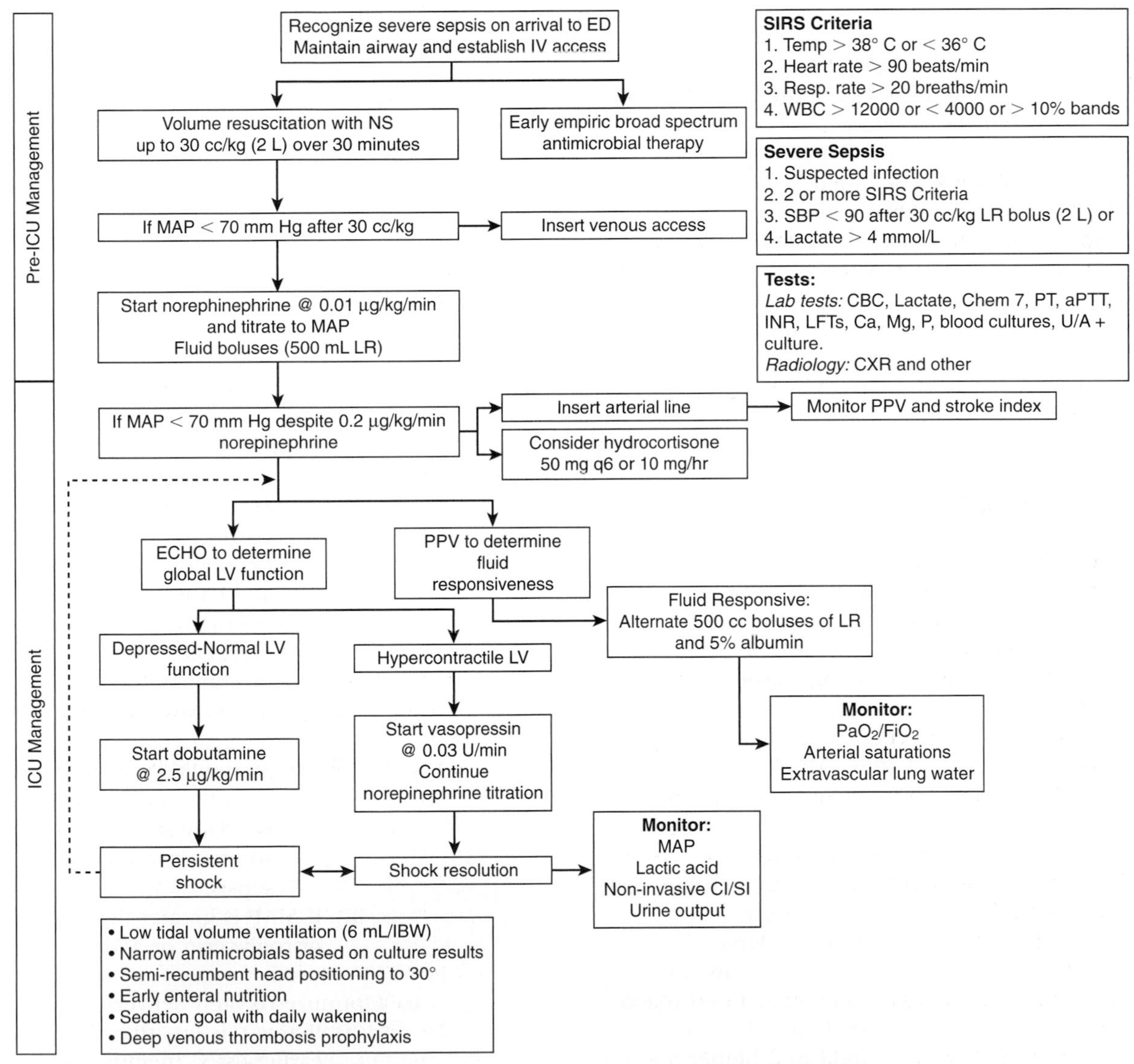

Figure 11-9 Suggested initial approach to the management of patients with severe sepsis and septic shock. *Ca,* Calcium; *CI,* cardiac index; *ED,* emergency department; *IBW,* ideal body weight; *ICU,* intensive care unit; *INR,* international normalized ratio; *LFT,* liver function test; *LR,* lactated Ringer's; *LV,* left ventricular; *MAP,* mean arterial pressure; *Mg,* magnesium; *NS,* normal saline; *P,* phosphate; *PPV,* pulse pressure variation; *PT,* prothrombin time; *aPTT,* activated partial prothrombin time; *SBP,* systolic blood pressure; *SI,* stroke index; *SIRS,* systemic inflammatory response syndrome; *U/A,* urinalysis; *WBC,* white blood cell. (Adapted from Marik, P. E. [2011]. Surviving sepsis: Going beyond the guidelines. *Ann Intensive Care, 1*[1], 17.)

(b) One blood draw should be through each vascular access that has been in place more than 48 hours.
(c) Other cultures from other sites (e.g., CSF, pulmonary secretions, urine, wound) may be indicated as possible sources of infection.

ii) Antimicrobials
(a) Initiated within 1 hour of recognition of severe sepsis; it is not necessary to wait for cultures
(b) Broad-spectrum antimicrobials guided by clinical presentation, likely microorganism, and local and institutional susceptibility guidelines (Levins, 2010)
(c) Reassessed after 48-72 hours

c) Preload correction
i) If CVP less than 8 mm Hg: crystalloid fluid boluses until CVP 8-12 mm Hg
(a) Colloids are not indicated and may be harmful.
(b) Hypertonic crystalloids are also not recommended at this time.

ii) If CVP more than 15 mm Hg and MAP greater than 110 mm Hg: nitroglycerin until CVP less than 12 or MAP less than 90 mm Hg

d) Afterload correction
i) If MAP is less than 65 mm Hg after 2 L of crystalloids, vasopressors should be used as necessary to maintain a MAP of at least 65 mm Hg; if diastolic BP is less than 40 mm Hg, vasopressors should be started immediately and concurrently with fluid resuscitation (Marik, 2011)
(a) Norepinephrine (2-20 mcg/min) is frequently advocated as the initial agent.
(b) Dopamine (5-20 mcg/kg/min) may also be used.
(i) A recent large, prospective multicenter randomized controlled trial (SOAP trial) indicated higher mortality with use of dopamine versus norepinephrine; this same study also found a higher mortality in patients with shock receiving steroids and dopamine (DeBacker et al., 2010).
(ii) Low-dose dopamine (less than 5 mcg/kg/min) was previously thought to provide renal protection and is currently not advocated.
(c) Phenylephrine is preferred if heart rate is greater than 120 beats/min.
(d) Vasopressin at 0.03 units/min should be added if the patient remains hypotensive despite a reasonable dose of norepinephrine.
(i) Very low doses (0.01-0.04 units/min) of vasopressin have been shown to improve MAP in septic shock.
(ii) Terlipressin, a longer-acting synthetic analog of vasopressin, has a longer half-life and similar hemodynamic effects to vasopressin.
(e) Arterial catheter for continuous monitoring of blood pressure is indicated.

ii) Corticosteroids should be considered if patient is vasopressor dependent.
(a) Cosyntropin stimulation test is recommended: baseline cortisol level, ACTH 250 mcg IV, remeasurement of cortisol at 30 and 60 minutes; change in cortisol of less than 9 mcg/dL suggests adrenal insufficiency
(b) If cosyntropin stimulation test is negative, hydrocortisone 50 mg IV every 6 hours along with fludrocortisone 50 mcg PO daily is recommended for adrenal insufficiency in severe sepsis.

iii) If MAP is greater than 110 mm Hg, nitroglycerin or hydralazine may be used.

e) Optimize oxygen delivery.
i) If $ScvO_2$ is less than 70% after earlier-listed therapies and hemoglobin is less than 10 g/dL, red blood cells may be indicated.
(a) Platelets are indicated if platelet counts are less than 5000/mm^3 or when less than 30,000/mm^3 if there is significant risk for bleeding.

ii) If $ScvO_2$ is less than 70% after earlier-listed therapies and hemoglobin is greater than 10 g/dL, dobutamine or dopamine is indicated.
iii) If heart rate is more than 120 beats/min, digoxin may be considered.

b. Decrease inflammation and antithrombotic aspects of sepsis.
   1) Corticosteroids as prescribed
   2) Control of serum glucose as described in the general discussion of shock

4. Treat infection and neutralize toxins.
   a. Administer antimicrobials as prescribed.
   b. Prepare the patient for surgery as requested.
      1) Drainage of abscess
      2) Débridement of wound
      3) Reduction of fractures
   c. Use experimental therapies as prescribed; may only be available for compassionate use
      1) Monoclonal antibodies to endotoxin may neutralize endotoxins and prevent mediator release.
      2) Plasmapheresis may be used to remove endotoxin and/or bacterial byproducts.
      3) Extracorporal membrane oxygenation (ECMO)
5. Control hyperthermia.
   a. Monitor core body temperature.
   b. Administer antipyretics as indicated with recognition that fever is an important defense mechanism (Cunha, 2012).
      1) Indications for treatment of fever
         a) Severe cardiopulmonary disease with body temperatures greater than 38.8° C (102° F)
         b) Brain injury
         c) Extreme hyperpyrexia (i.e., body temperature greater than 41.1° C [106° F])
      2) Treatment guidelines
         a) Reduce temperatures slowly to 38.8° C (102° F) to prevent chills and rebound increase in body temperature.
         b) Use antipyretics (e.g., acetaminophen) and environmental cooling methods such as fans.
   c. Utilize cooling blankets and tepid soaks.
6. Monitor for complications of shock and clinical indications of organ failure.

Systemic Inflammatory Response Syndrome (SIRS) and Multiple Organ Dysfunction Syndrome

Definitions

1. Systemic inflammatory response syndrome: "Widespread inflammation (or clinical response to that inflammation) that can occur in patients with such diverse disorders as infection, pancreatitis, ischemia, multiple trauma, shock, or immunologically-mediated organ injury" (Bone, Sprung, & Sibbald, 1992)
2. Multiple organ dysfunction syndrome: "Presence of altered organ function in an acutely ill patient such that homeostasis cannot be maintained without intervention" (Bone, Sprung, & Sibbald, 1992); progressive impairment of two or more organ systems
   a. "Primary multiple organ dysfunction syndrome occurs when there is a direct injury to the organ that becomes dysfunctional" (Bone, Sprung, & Sibbald, 1992)
   b. "Secondary multiple organ dysfunction syndrome occurs as a consequence of trauma or infection in one part of the system that results in the systemic inflammatory response and dysfunction of organs elsewhere" (Bone, Sprung, & Sibbald, 1992)

Etiology

1. SIRS
   a. Mechanical tissue damage: trauma, burns, crush injuries, surgical procedures
   b. Abscesses: intraabdominal and intracranial
   c. Ischemic/necrotic tissue: prolonged shock, MI, pancreatitis, DIC
   d. Microbial invasion: immunosuppressed states, surgery/trauma, community exposure, nosocomial exposure
   e. Endotoxin release: gram-negative sepsis, translocation of bacteria from gut (sepsis is the most common single etiologic factor, but 40-50% of MODS patients do not have positive blood cultures)
   f. Global perfusion deficits: shock and cardiopulmonary arrest
   g. Regional perfusion deficits: vascular injury, vascular repair procedures, thromboembolic events
2. MODS
   a. Primary due to acute direct injury to an organ or organs
   b. Secondary due to SIRS

Pathophysiology

See Figure 11-10.

Clinical Presentation

1. SIRS
   a. Criteria (2 or more of the following) (Bone, 1991):
      1) Tachycardia (greater than 90 beats/min)
      2) Hyperpnea (respiratory rate above 20 breaths/min or $PaCO_2$ below 32 mm Hg)
      3) Hyperthermia (temperature above 38° C or 100.4° F) or hypothermia (temperature below 36° C or 96.8° F) (NOTE: hypothermia is more common in elderly patients)

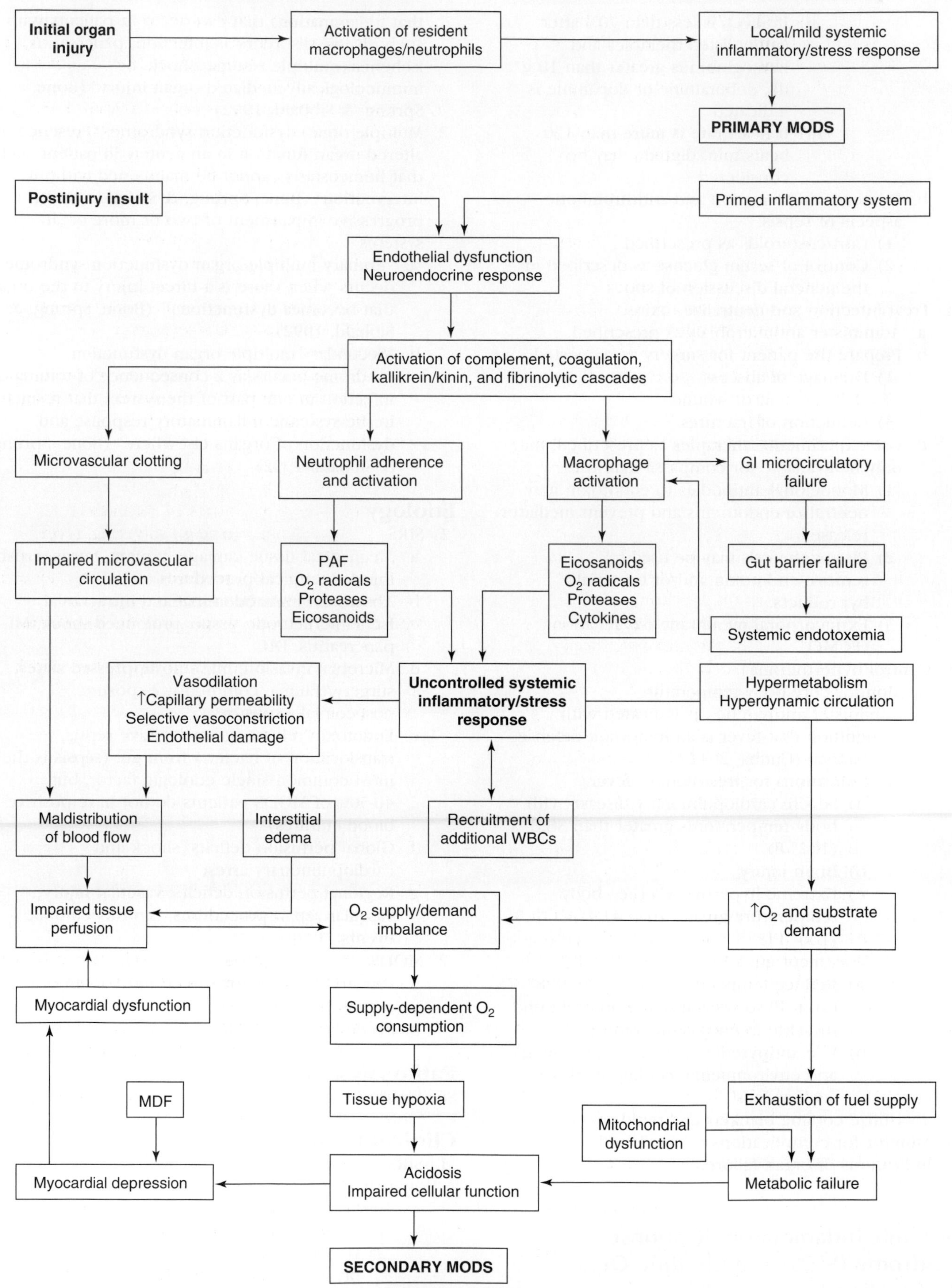

Figure 11-10 Pathophysiology of multiple organ dysfunction syndrome (MODS). *GI,* Gastrointestinal; *MDF,* myocardial depressant factor; *PAF,* platelet-activating factor; *WBC,* white blood cell. (From McCance, K. L., & Huether, S. E. [2010]. *Pathophysiology. The biologic basis for disease in adults and children* [6th ed.]. St. Louis: Mosby.)

4) WBC above 12,000 cells/mm^3 or below 4000 cells/mm^3 or more than 10% bands
b. Systems assessment (Table 11-6)
2. MODS: dysfunction of more than one of the following organs:
a. Pulmonary (ARDS): absence of pulmonary embolism or bilateral pneumonia with the following:
1) Predisposing factor such as sepsis
2) Unexplained hypoxemia
3) Bilateral pulmonary infiltrates consistent with pulmonary edema
4) PaO_2/FiO_2 ratio less than 300
5) PAOP less than 18 mm Hg (to rule out cardiac pulmonary edema)
b. Hematologic (DIC): absence of liver failure, major hematoma, or anticoagulation therapy with the following:
1) Fibrin degradation products (FDPs) greater than 1:40 or D-dimer greater than 2 mg/L
2) Thrombocytopenia or a 25% drop from a previous value
3) aPTT prolonged
4) INR greater than 1.2
5) May have clinical evidence of bleeding
c. Renal: absence of diuretic within 2 hours of urine analysis with the following:
1) Urine output less than 0.5 mL/kg/min
2) Serum creatinine abnormal and urinary sodium greater than 40 mmol/L
3) If previous renal insufficiency, an increase in creatinine by 2 mg/dL not due to myoglobinuria
d. Hepatobiliary: absence of preexisting liver disease with the following:
1) Serum bilirubin greater than 2 mg/dL for 2 days
2) Alkaline phosphatase, ALT, AST, gamma-glutamyl transferase (GGT) over twice laboratory normal
e. Central nervous system: absence of sedation or paralyzing agents that would alter the patient's ability to respond with decrease in Glasgow coma score by one point
f. Metabolic: serum lactate level increased
g. Degrees of organ dysfunction are described in Table 11-7.

Collaborative Management

1. Prevent and treat infection (see Septic Shock section).
2. Maximize oxygen delivery to the tissues (see Shock section).
a. Maintain cardiac index within normal limits. (NOTE: Current research has not shown increasing the CI to 4.5 L/min/m^2 or greater to be effective in reducing mortality.)
1) Administer fluids: Crystalloids are used because capillary permeability is increased.
2) Administer inotropes (e.g., dobutamine) as prescribed.
3) Administer vasopressors (e.g., dopamine, norepinephrine) as prescribed when SVR is very low and adequate filling volume has been established.
b. Maintain hematocrit at approximately 30-32%.
1) Administer blood and blood products as prescribed.
2) Correct coagulopathies; administer fresh frozen plasma, platelets, and vitamin K as prescribed.
c. Maintain SaO_2 greater than 95%.
1) Ensure adequate airway.
2) Administer oxygen as needed.
3) Initiate mechanical ventilation as needed; PEEP may also be necessary.
d. Monitor SvO_2.
1) Decreased SvO_2 to less than 60% indicates that oxygen delivery is impaired or oxygen consumption is increased.
a) Assess SaO_2.
b) Assess cardiac output/index.
c) Assess hemoglobin.
d) Assess for causes of increased consumption (e.g., shivering, fever, seizures).
2) Increased SvO_2 to greater than 80% indicates that oxygen extraction is impaired.
3. Minimize oxygen consumption of the tissues (see Shock section).
4. Maintain or improve nutritional status (see Shock section).
5. Monitor for complications.
a. Shock (if not caused by shock)
b. Organ failure
c. Death

Multisystem Trauma

Definitions

1. Trauma: injury to the body caused by acute exposure to mechanical, thermal, electrical, or chemical energy
a. Unintentional causes include vehicular collision, falls, burns, or firearm, recreational, or occupational mishap
b. Intentional: deliberate acts of violence such as shootings, stabbings, assaults, and child or elder abuse
2. Mechanism of injury: circumstances and energy forces that produced the trauma
a. Blunt trauma
1) Caused by the following forces:
a) Acceleration or deceleration: occurs with increased velocity or speed of a moving object followed by a sudden decrease
b) Shearing: occurs when two oppositely directed parallel forces are applied to tissue
c) Compression: occurs when a squeezing inward pressure is applied to tissues

Table 11-6 Systems Assessment with Potential Inflammatory/Immune Impact and Complications

System	Risk Factors	Impact on IIR	Assessment	Potential Complications
CNS	• Invasive drains • ICP monitoring • Surgical incision • Cranial nerve involvement • Spinal cord injury	• Increased microbial access • IIR activation • Impaired natural defenses	• LOC, GCS • CCP • Inflammation at wound • Respiratory depression • Skin breakdown	• CNS infection • Aspiration • Corneal abrasions • Skin breakdown
Pulmonary	• Artificial airway • Mechanical ventilation • Barotrauma • High FiO_2 levels	• Bypass of natural airway defenses • Increased microbial access • Activation of alveolar macrophages with toxic mediator release • Altered surfactant production	• Dyspnea • Use of accessory muscles • Thick, discolored sputum • Wheezes, crackles, rhonchi • Decreased compliance • Increased V/Q mismatching • Increased intrapulmonary shunt infiltrates on chest x-ray • Respiratory acidosis (↓pH, ↑ $PaCO_2$) • Hypoxemia (↓PaO_2, ↓ SaO_2, SpO_2) • Hypoxia (↓SvO_2, ↑ lactate)	• Aspiration • Atelectasis • Pneumonia • ARDS • Oxygen toxicity
CV	• Invasive monitoring • Poor perfusion	• Increased microbial access • Tissue ischemia → IIR activation with third-spacing and edema • Cellular activation and mediator release	• Changes in HR, BP, CO/CI, PAP, PAOP, CVP/RAP, SVR • Cold, pale skin • Inflammation at access sites • Diminished pulses • Narrowed pulse pressure • Urine output • Dysrhythmias • Myocardial ischemia or infarction • Positive cardiac isoenzymes, troponin • ↑ Lactate	• Reperfusion injury • Cellulitis • Bacteremia/sepsis • Endothelial damage and clotting abnormalities
GI	• Nasogastric tube • Antacid therapy • H_2-blocker therapy • Stress ulceration • Antibiotics • Ileus	• Gastric pH → bacterial colonization • IIR activation • Inhibition of normal flora's protective function • Inability to clear bacterial load	• Bowel sounds • Upper or lower GI bleeding • Abdominal distention • Diarrhea • Constipation, impaction • Ileus • Stress ulceration/erosion • Guaiac + stool • Enteric organisms on blood culture • Jaundice • Ascites • Drug clearance • Abnormal bleeding • Liver enzymes • Hypoglycemia • Ammonia • Plasma proteins • Clotting factors • Hepatomegaly/splenomegaly	• Colonization of esophagus and tracheobronchial tree • Pneumonia • Overgrowth of pathogenic organisms in the GI tract (e.g., *Clostridium difficile*) • Translocation of bacteria to the lymph and blood

Table 11-6 Systems Assessment with Potential Inflammatory/Immune Impact and Complications—cont'd

System	Risk Factors	Impact on IIR	Assessment	Potential Complications
GU	• Bladder catheter • Antibiotics • Hyperglycemia	• Increased microbial access • Altered normal flora in vagina • Promotion of yeast growth	• Changes in urine output • Malodorous urine or vaginal discharge • Peripheral edema • CVP/RAP, PAP, PAOP • BUN and creatinine • Metabolic acidosis (↓ pH, ↓ HCO_3)	• Urinary tract infection • Septicemia • *Candida* infections

Adapted from Huddleston Secor, V. (1996). *Multiple organ dysfunction & failure: Pathophysiology and clinical implications* (2nd ed.). St Louis: Mosby.

ARDS, Acute respiratory distress syndrome; *BP,* blood pressure; *BUN,* blood urea nitrogen; *CCP,* cerebral perfusion pressure; *CNS,* central nervous system; *CO/CI,* cardiac output/cardiac index; *CV,* cardiovascular; *CVP/RAP,* central venous pressure/right atrial pressure; *FiO_2,* fraction of inspired oxygen; *GCS,* Glasgow Coma Score; *GI,* gastrointestinal; *GU,* genitourinary; *H_2,* histamine type 2 receptor; *HCO_3,* bicarbonate; *HR,* heart rate; *ICP,* intracranial pressure; *IIR,* inflammatory/immune response; *LOC,* level of consciousness; *$PaCO_2$,* partial pressure of carbon dioxide in arterial blood; *PaO_2,* partial pressure of oxygen in arterial blood; *PAOP,* pulmonary artery occlusive pressure; *PAP,* pulmonary artery pressure; *SaO_2,* oxygen saturation of hemoglobin in arterial blood; *SpO_2,* oxygen saturation of hemoglobin by pulse oximetry; *SvO_2,* oxygen saturation of hemoglobin in venous blood; *SVR,* systemic vascular resistance.

Table 11-7 Definitions of Degrees of Organ Dysfunction

			Organ Dysfunction			
Organ System	**Parameter**	**Normal**	**Mild**	**Moderate**	**Severe**	**Extreme**
CV	Systolic BP (mm Hg)	Greater than 90	Less than 90 but fluid responsive	Less than 90, not fluid responsive	Less than 90, not fluid responsive	Less than 90, not fluid responsive
	Arterial pH	At least 7.3	At least 7.3	At least 7.3	Less than 7.3	Less than 7.2
Pulmonary	PaO_2/FiO_2 (mm Hg)	Greater than 400	301-400	201-300	101-200	Less than 100
CNS	GCS	15	13-14	10-12	7-9	At least 6
Coagulation	Platelet count (1000/mL)	Greater than 120	81-102	51-80	21-50	Less than or equal to 20
Renal	Creatinine (mg/dL)	Less than 1.5	1.5-1.9	2-3.4	3.5-4.9	Less than or equal to 5
Hepatic	Bilirubin (mg/dL)	Less than 1.2	1.2-3.5	3.6-7	7.1-14	Greater than 14

From Bone, R. C. (1997). Managing sepsis: What treatments can we use today? *J Crit Illn, 12*(1):15.

2) Results in more injuries and more types of injury such as contusions, lacerations, fractures, or ruptures of solid tissue masses
3) Tends to be more difficult to manage because more structures are injured, frequently occult presentation so diagnosis may be delayed, and results in more significant complications

b. Penetrating trauma
1) Caused by direct contact with an instrument that cuts the skin, such as stabbing with a sharp object, bullet wound, high-pressure injections, or foreign object impalement
2) Results in injury to fewer body structures

3. Kinematics: the physics of trauma; the relationship between energy and trauma
a. Newton's first law of motion: a body at rest will remain at rest unless acted upon by an outside force (i.e., principle of inertia) and a body in motion will remain in motion traveling in a straight line unless acted upon by an outside force (i.e., principle of momentum)
b. Energy can be changed from one form to another, but it can neither be created nor destroyed.
1) Consider that the transformation of the kinetic energy of a moving object (e.g., motor vehicle) that suddenly stops causes damage to the motor vehicle and occupants.
a) Four collisions occur in vehicle collisions.
i) A: auto collision
ii) B: body collision
iii) C: cavity contents collision
iv) D: debris collision

c. Kinetic energy: the energy of motion

1) Formula:

$$(Mass \times Velocity^2)/2$$

2) Consider that doubling the size of an object results in doubling the kinetic energy, and doubling the velocity quadruples the kinetic energy; this explains why a bullet (small mass with significant velocity) can cause such tissue damage.
3) Force applied slowly over a large surface area results in less tissue destruction than that same force applied to a small surface area

Predisposing Factors

1. Blunt trauma
   a. Vehicular collision motor vehicle, motorcycle, bicycle, watercraft, pedestrian struck by motor vehicle
   b. Falls
   c. Assault
   d. Industrial mishaps
   e. Blast force
   f. Sports-related injuries
2. Penetrating trauma
   a. Gunshot wounds
   b. Stab wounds
   c. Impalement
   d. Projectiles
3. Alcohol is a major factor in both intentional and unintentional trauma; in 40% of all traffic-related fatalities, the driver has an elevated blood-alcohol concentration (Schulman, 2009)
4. Another risk to vehicular safety is talking on cellular phones or texting while driving.

Mechanism of Injury

1. Motor vehicle collision
   a. Useful information
      1) Speed of vehicle(s)
      2) Size of vehicle(s)
      3) Location of impact
         a) Head-on
         b) Rear impact
         c) Lateral
         d) Ejection
         e) Rollover
      4) Position of patient in vehicle before and after the impact
         a) If thrown from the vehicle, distance from the vehicle
      5) Use of safety devices
         a) Lap belt
         b) Shoulder belt
         c) Child car seat
         d) Air bags
            i) Did they deploy?
            ii) Location: front or side
      6) Damage to vehicle
         a) Indications of impact
            i) Bent steering wheel
            ii) Broken windshield
            iii) Broken rearview mirror
            iv) Broken gearshift
      7) Smoke or fumes on scene
      8) Condition of other occupants
   b. Anticipated injury
      1) By type of collision (Table 11-8)
      2) By position in vehicle
         a) Driver may strike steering column, instrument panel, gearshift, rearview mirror, windshield, pillar between windshield and door, and door

Table 11-8 Anticipated Injuries in Motor Vehicle Collisions

Type of Collision	Anticipated Injuries
Head-on: up-and-over pathway	• Cervical spine compression injury • Skull fractures, traumatic brain injury • Rib, sternal fractures, flail chest • Pulmonary contusion, pneumothorax, hemothorax • Myocardial contusion • Liver, spleen, duodenum, diaphragmatic lacerations • Great vessel tear
Head-on: down-and-under pathway	• Cervical spine flexion injury • Laryngeal trauma • Carotid shearing • Rib, sternal fractures, flail chest • Pulmonary contusion, pneumothorax, hemothorax • Myocardial contusion • Aortic tears • Pelvic or acetabular fractures • Femur, tibia, fibula fractures
Rear-end	• Whiplash • Rib, sternal fractures, flail chest • Pulmonary contusion, pneumothorax, hemothorax
Lateral	• Cervical ligamentous injuries • Lateral rib fractures, flail chest • Pulmonary contusion, pneumothorax, hemothorax • Spleen or liver lacerations • Pelvic, hip, acetabular fractures • Humerus and clavicle fractures
Ejections	• Skull fractures, traumatic brain injury • Cervical and thoracic spine compression fractures • Rib fracture, pneumothorax, hemothorax • Liver, spleen, pancreas lacerations • Aortic tears • Pelvic fractures, straddle fractures

Adapted from Schulman, C. S. (2009). Trauma. In K. K. Carlson (Ed.), *Advanced critical care nursing*. St. Louis: Saunders.

i) Facial laceration, facial bone fractures
ii) Scalp lacerations, skull fracture, traumatic brain injury
iii) Spinal injuries
iv) Chest wall lacerations, pulmonary contusion, rib, clavicle or sternal fractures, pneumohemothorax
v) Thoracic aorta tear
vi) Abdominal wall lacerations, rupture or avulsion of liver, spleen, kidney, pancreas, bowel, and bladder
vii) Fractured humerus, radius, ulna, wrist, hand
viii) Fractured pelvis, hip dislocation, fractured femur, tibia, fibula, ankle, foot, ligamentous injury to knee

b) Front seat passenger: higher incidence of head and abdominal injuries and upper torso fractures but fewer thoracic injuries and lower torso fractures
c) Rear seat passenger: similar to front seat passenger if not restrained

c. Injury caused by protective devices (Shulman, 2009)
1) Lap belt only worn
a) Fractured ribs, sternum, clavicle
b) Myocardial contusion
c) Aortic tear
d) Mesenteric tear, bowel perforation
e) Bladder rupture
f) Lower thoracic or lumbar vertebral fracture
2) Shoulder harness only
a) Cervical spine injuries
b) Abrasions to neck, chest, abdomen
c) Carotid artery injuries
d) Laryngeal injuries
3) Air bag deployment
a) Cervical spine injuries
b) Bag slap injuries to face and neck
c) Temporary hearing deficit
d) Corneal abrasion, corneal burns, retinal detachment
e) Respiratory distress or anaphylaxis from inhaled particles from within the bag and propellant
f) Upper extremity contusion
g) Fracture or dislocation of thumb or wrist

2. Motorcycle collision
a. Useful information
1) Deformity of the motorcycle
2) Stationary objects impacted
3) Helmet: Cracks in helmet are likely to result in significant brain injury.
b. Anticipated injury
1) Traumatic brain injury is the leading cause of death, especially if rider is not wearing a helmet.
2) Tibial and radial injuries are most common injury.
3) Facial fractures
4) Spinal injuries, especially thoracic
5) Pulmonary injuries (i.e., pulmonary contusion, pneumothorax, hemothorax)
6) Pelvic fractures result from straddling position; may have coexisting bladder or urethral injury
7) Traumatic amputation
8) Specific to type of impact
a) Head-on: Bike flips forward so rider strikes or travels over the handlebars.
i) Injury to abdomen and chest as rider strikes handlebars
ii) Bilateral femur fractures
iii) Head and neck injuries
b) Angular: Cycle hit at an angle and collapses on the rider.
i) Tibia and fibula fractures; may be open
ii) Crushed legs
iii) Ankle dislocation
c) Ejection: Rider is thrown off motorcycle.
i) Serious injury likely, especially head injury
d) Laying the bike down
i) Fractures, abrasions, crush injuries, road burns to lower leg

3. Bicycle collision
a. Useful information: forward, sideward, or backward unseating
b. Anticipated injury
1) If over the handlebars, facial injuries and/or fractures, head injury
2) Blunt trauma caused by handlebars
a) Serious abdominal injury may not be apparent until later in children.
3) Fractures of the feet from spokes of wheel
4) Straddle injuries such as vaginal tears, scrotal injuries, perineal contusions, anal or rectal injuries
5) Injury to rider from rearview mirror extending from truck or van can cause serious, even fatal, injury to the head, neck, or face.

4. Watercraft collision
a. Useful information
1) Description of event: collision with another boat or obstruction with an object in the water or on shore
b. Anticipated injury
1) Drowning
2) Hypothermia
3) Other injuries as for ejection from a vehicle

5. Pedestrian struck by motor vehicle
a. Useful information: type of vehicle
b. Anticipated injury: three points of impact
1) Bumper
a) Adult: impact to lower leg
i) Tibia and fibula fractures

b) Child: leg
i) Femur, tibia, and fibula fractures
2) Hood
a) Adult: as the person bends, impact to lower abdomen, pelvis, or upper femur
i) Thoracic injuries
ii) Abdominal injuries
iii) Spinal fractures
iv) Hip, pelvis, or femur fractures
b) Child: head, chest, or abdominal injury; very small children are knocked down and under the vehicle and then run over
3) Ground: head, cervical spine, chest, or abdominal injuries
c. Waddell's triad: the combination of injuries that often occurs when a child is struck by a car
1) Chest
2) Head
3) Femurs

6. Falls
a. Useful information
1) Distance of fall: a fall from more than three times the person's height results in significant injury (McSwain, 2000)
2) Surface of impact
3) Area of body that made initial impact
4) If objects were struck during the fall
5) Patient's activity before and after fall
b. Anticipated injury
1) Compression fractures: os calcis (i.e., heel), femur, tibia, fibula, pelvis, lumbar spine; may be referred to as "Don Juan syndrome"
2) Bilateral wrist (Colles) fractures if arms are forward for protection in forward propulsion
3) Vascular injuries: pelvis and thorax
4) Renal injury

7. Sports-related injuries
a. Useful information
1) Impact to patient
2) Damaged equipment
3) Previous training (or lack of training) of patient
4) Use of protective equipment
b. Anticipated injury: dependent upon sport (Table 11-9)

8. Penetrating injury
a. Useful information
1) Wounding agent (e.g., knife, bullet, arrow, ice pick)
2) Number and location of wounds
3) Size and length of the agent
4) If gunshot, caliber and distance of the weapon from the patient
a) Low-velocity bullets travel at less than 1000 feet per second (fps).
b) Medium-velocity bullets travel at 1000-2000 fps.
c) High-velocity bullets travel at greater than 2000 fps.

Table 11-9 Potential Anticipated Injuries in Selected Sports

Sport	Anticipated Injuries
Baseball	• Skull fracture, traumatic brain injury • Ocular injuries • Extremity fractures • Lacerations • Sprains • Strains
Basketball	• Lower extremity sprains, strains, fractures • Lacerations • Contusions
Boxing	• Skull fracture, traumatic brain injury (cumulative) • Ocular injuries • Nasal fractures • Hand fractures • Lacerations
Bungee jumping	• Impact-related injuries (may be major) • Intraocular hemorrhages • Spinal fractures, spinal cord injury • Peroneal nerve injury • Soft tissue injury
Football	• Spinal fractures, spinal cord injuries • Skull fracture, traumatic brain injury • Knee strains, ligament tears • Fractures • Lacerations
Gymnastics	• Spinal fractures, spinal cord injuries • Extremity fractures • Sprains • Strains
Horseback riding	• Skull fracture, traumatic brain injury • Crush wounds
Ice hockey	• Facial fractures • Soft tissue injuries • Lacerations
Inline skating	• Skull fracture, traumatic brain injury • Wrist fractures • Lower extremity fractures
Running	• Lower extremity injuries • Sprains • Strains
Skiing	• Skull fracture, traumatic brain injury • Lower extremity fractures • Hypothermia, frostbite

Adapted from Revere, C. (2002). Mechanisms of injury. In L. Newberry (Ed.), *Sheehy's emergency nursing: Principles and practice* (5th ed.). St. Louis: Mosby.

5) Trajectory
6) Contaminants
b. Anticipated injury: dependent upon previously indicated factors

9. Injury related to machinery
a. Useful information
1) Location of injury
2) Length of time since injury or extrication

3) Function of the machine
4) Potential contaminants

b. Anticipated injury: depends on previous information

Pathophysiology

1. Hemorrhage: may be overt or occult
   a. Caused initially by injury but secondarily by coagulopathy
   b. Results in decreased oxygen delivery to tissues (DO_2)
      1) Decrease in cardiac output due to loss of circulating blood volume
      2) Loss of hemoglobin to carry oxygen
2. Hypoperfusion
   a. Caused by decrease in hemoglobin and cardiac output which results in a decrease in DO_2
   b. Results in the following:
      1) Organ ischemia and possible organ failure
      2) Rhabdomyolysis with muscle ischemia, necrosis, or crush injury
      3) Bowel ischemia with resultant translocation of intestinal bacteria into lymphatics or vascular bed, potentially causing sepsis
      4) Acidosis
3. Hypothermia: Most trauma patients arrive in the ED with hypothermia.
   a. Caused by the following:
      1) Exposure: lack of clothing
      2) Open body cavities, especially if long surgery required
      3) Administration of refrigerated blood
      4) Administration of room-temperature intravenous fluids
      5) Alcohol
   b. Results in the following:
      1) Shift in oxyhemoglobin dissociation curve that impairs tissue oxygen delivery
      2) Shivering which increases oxygen consumption
      3) Impairs platelet function and causes coagulopathy that perpetuates hemorrhage
      4) Increased blood viscosity
      5) Myocardial depression
      6) Acidosis
4. Hypertension (compartment)
   a. Potential intracranial hypertension and brain herniation
   b. Abdominal hypertension and abdominal compartment syndrome
   c. Compartment syndrome

Clinical Presentation

This is specific to the injury.

Collaborative Management

1. Initiate primary survey to identify and treat life-threatening conditions
   a. A: airway
   b. B: breathing
   c. C: circulation
   d. D: disability
   e. E: exposure
2. Provide resuscitation measures (Talbert, 2005)
   a. A: airway and B: breathing
      1) Maintain airway, oxygenation, and ventilation.
         a) Jaw thrust until cervical spine has been cleared either clinically or radiologically; then may use head tilt–chin lift
            i) Note that any patient with blunt or penetrating trauma above the nipple line must have the cervical spine immobilized with assessment of the airway (Fultz & Sturt, 2005).
         b) Oropharyngeal (if no gag reflex) or nasopharyngeal (if basal skull fracture is not suspected) to hold the tongue away from the hypopharynx in patients with altered LOC
         c) Intubation may be required; RSI methods should be utilized
         d) Oxygen by whatever delivery method necessary to maintain SpO_2 of 95%: may be nasal cannula, 100% non-rebreathing mask, or intubation with mechanical ventilation with PEEP
   b. C: circulation
      1) Control of bleeding
         a) Pressure on site or artery above site
         b) Reinforcement and stabilization of impaled object before surgical procedure for removal
         c) Emergent surgery may be required.
      2) Maintain adequate circulation and perfusion.
         a) IV access with two large-bore catheters for fluid and medication administration
      3) Fluid replacement
         a) Crystalloids: usually 0.9% saline or lactated Ringer's solution
         b) Red packed cells or other blood products as prescribed
         c) Should be given early if significant blood loss is suspected to prevent tissue hypoxia; replacement of platelets, clotting factors, and calcium should be considered especially if multiple transfusions are given
         d) Colloids generally are not recommended in trauma.
   c. D: disability
      1) Neurologic assessment, including Glasgow Coma Score, and protection of the cervical spine
   d. E: environment
      1) Expose: Remove all clothing but do not leave patient uncovered; care must be taken to prevent or treat hypothermia.
      2) Evacuate if necessary: Prompt transfer should be achieved if the patient's needs are

beyond the resources available at the facility.

3. Conduct secondary survey to identify serious threats that may require emergency surgery or emergency procedures.
   a. F
      1) Full set of vital signs
      2) Focused adjuncts
         a) Cardiac monitoring
         b) Pulse oximetry to measure SpO_2
         c) Nasogastric or orogastric tube to low suction if indicated and not contraindicated
         d) Indwelling urinary catheter if indicated and not contraindicated
         e) Diagnostic studies
            i) Serum
               (a) CBC with differential, hemoglobin, hematocrit
               (b) Chemistry profile including glucose, BUN, creatinine
               (c) Coagulation profile
               (d) Serum lactate
               (e) Toxicology including alcohol
               (f) Type and crossmatch
            ii) Urine
               (a) Pregnancy test if female of childbearing age
               (b) Toxicology
            iii) Diagnostic imaging
               (a) Spine
               (b) Chest
               (c) Pelvis
               (d) Focused assessment sonography for trauma (FAST)
            iv) CT scan
               (a) Head
               (b) Chest
               (c) Abdomen
            v) Diagnostic peritoneal lavage (DPL) or diagnostic peritoneal aspiration (DPA)
      3) Facilitate family presence.
         a) Facilitate and support family's involvement.
         b) Provide explanations about procedures.
         c) Support family's emotional and spiritual needs.
   b. G: Give comfort measures
      1) Positioning for comfort
      2) Anxiolytics
      3) Analgesics: NSAID, narcotics, anesthetics
      4) Ice if appropriate
      5) Splinting and stabilization of fractures
      6) Cutaneous stimulation (e.g., massage)
      7) Distraction (e.g., music)
   c. H
      1) History
         a) Prehospital: MIVT
            i) Mechanism of injury
            ii) Injuries sustained
            iii) Vital signs
            iv) Treatment initiated and response
         b) Past medical history
      2) Head-to-toe assessment
   d. I: Inspect posterior surfaces while maintaining cervical spine protection
4. Continue assessment during admission; frequency dependent upon patient acuity
   a. ABCs
   b. Vital signs: blood pressure, pulse, respiratory rate, and temperature
   c. Oxygen saturation
   d. Respiratory effort and excursion
   e. Cardiac rate and rhythm
   f. Pain and discomfort level
   g. Accurate intake and output
   h. Serum electrolytes
   i. Level of consciousness
   j. Close monitoring for progression of symptoms
5. Reverse hypothermia
   a. Passive warming
      1) Removal of wet linens and clothing
      2) Application of warm blankets
   b. Active external warming: convection blankets (e.g., Bair Hugger)
   c. Active internal warming
      1) Warm IV fluid
      2) Warm humidified oxygen
      3) Lavage of stomach, chest, colon, and/or bladder with warm isotonic fluids
      4) Peritoneal lavage with warm isotonic fluids
      5) Extracorporeal systems such as hemodialysis, cardiopulmonary bypass, or continuous arteriovenous or venovenous warming
   d. Monitoring for afterdrop (i.e., decrease in core body temperature that occurs as warming causes more blood to move through cold tissues)
   e. Monitoring for hypotension caused by vasodilation with rewarming
6. Reverse acidosis
   a. Measures to treat underlying cause of decrease in tissue delivery (DO_2)
      1) Hemoglobin
         a) Stop the bleeding: apply pressure, prepare patient for surgery, etc.
         b) Administer blood and blood products as prescribed.
      2) Cardiac output
         a) Administer isotonic fluids and blood and blood products.
         b) Administer vasopressors (e.g., phenylephrine [Neo-Synephrine], norepinephrine [Levophed], dopamine [Intropin]) as prescribed.
            i) Vasopressors should be used only when hypotension persists despite adequate fluid resuscitation.

ii) Phenylephrine causes the least tachycardia of these vasopressors; norepinephrine causes less tachycardia than does dopamine.
c) Administer inotropic agents (e.g., dobutamine) to improve contractility as prescribed.
3) SaO_2
a) Ensure airway, ventilation, and oxygenation to maintain SaO_2 at least 95%.
b. Treatment of hypothermia that can impair oxygen delivery to the tissues
c. Avoidance of the use of sodium bicarbonate unless the pH is less than 7; adverse effects of sodium bicarbonate include the following:
1) Shifts the oxyhemoglobin dissociation curve to the left, impairing the dissociation of oxygen from the hemoglobin at the tissue level, which may worsen metabolic acidosis
2) Increased CO_2 production that may cause or worsen respiratory acidosis
3) Hypokalemia by shifting potassium from serum to intracellular space
4) Hypocalcemia by increasing the amount of calcium bound to albumin, thereby reducing ionized calcium

7. Correct coagulopathy
a. Treat hypothermia that can adversely affect platelet function
b. Replace clotting factors as prescribed.
8. Assist with measurement and treatment of compartment hypertension (e.g., intracranial hypertension, abdominal hypertension, compartment syndrome).
9. Treat infection (if present) and prevent sepsis.
a. Antimicrobials as prescribed
b. Tetanus prophylaxis if indicated
c. Dressing of wounds
d. Stabilization of fractures
10. Identify, prevent, and treat rhabdomyolysis.
a. Identification of high-risk patient (e.g., crush injuries, muscle ischemia/necrosis, electrical burns, sustained generalized seizures)
b. Detection of change in color of urine (e.g., brownish, tea-colored); laboratory confirmation of myoglobinuria
c. Isotonic fluids, diuretics (e.g., mannitol [Osmitrol]), and alkalinization of the urine, using intravenous sodium bicarbonate as prescribed
d. Hemodialysis or continuous renal replacement therapy (e.g., continuous venovenous hemodialysis) may be required
11. Monitor for complications
a. Shock
b. Multiple organ dysfunction syndrome
1) ARDS
2) DIC
3) Renal failure
4) Hepatic failure
5) Myocardial failure
6) Cerebral failure
c. Infection/sepsis/septic shock
d. Deep vein thrombosis and pulmonary embolism
e. Other complications specific to organ injury

Drug Intoxication and Poisoning

Definition

Drug ingestion in amounts greater than recommended or the ingestion or absorption of a substance toxic to the human body

Etiology

1. Accidental or intentional overdosage of prescribed medication
a. Intentional overdosage often involves more than one agent; frequently includes alcohol and/or illegal drugs
b. Intentional overdosage may be a suicide attempt or an attention-seeking behavior (i.e., suicide gesture).
c. Accidental overdosage may be due to knowledge deficit regarding drug dosing or confusion.
2. Accidental overdosage of illegal drugs
a. Overdosage frequently caused by changes in drug purity or potency.
b. Patient may be mentally ill and have tendency to be violent.
3. Ingestion/absorption of poison or toxin

Pathophysiology

Dependent upon the following:
1. Drug ingested
a. Fatal drug intoxications are most likely to be caused by analgesics, antidepressants, carbon monoxide, and cardiovascular drugs.
2. Amount of drug(s) or toxin ingested or absorbed
3. Time from ingestion to treatment
4. Preexisting condition of patient: cardiovascular, hepatic, or renal disease may increase drug effect by impairing biotransformation and excretion

Clinical Presentation (Table 11-10)

1. Subjective: for drug-specific symptoms, see Table 11-10
a. History of drug ingestion or exposure to toxin
1) Ask the patient why the overdosage occurred; listen carefully.
2) Patients are frequently inaccurate related to drug ingestion and may minimize or exaggerate the amount of the drug; verify information with family, friends, police officers, and paramedics.
3) Identify the following:
a) Drug or toxin
b) Route
c) Dose
d) Length of time elapsed since drug or toxin

Text continued on p. 729

Table 11-10 Drugs and Toxins

Drug or Toxin	Clinical Presentation of Intoxication	Specific Collaborative Management

Acetaminophen	Stage 1: first 24 hours
	• May be asymptomatic
	• Anorexia, nausea, vomiting
	• Diaphoresis
	• Malaise
	• Pallor
	Stage 2: 24-72 hours
	• Nausea, fatigue, malaise
	• Signs of hepatotoxicity may occur: liver enzymes elevated, bilirubin may be elevated, right upper quadrant pain
	• Gradual return to normal may occur
	Stage 3: 72-96 hours
	• Anorexia, nausea, vomiting
	• Hepatic failure
	  • More likely if ethanol consumption, malnutrition, short-term fasting
	  • Jaundice, elevated bilirubin
	  • Hepatosplenomegaly
	  • Prolonged PT, GI bleeding
	  • Hypoglycemia
	  • Metabolic acidosis
	  • Hepatic encephalopathy: confusion → coma
	• Acute tubular necrosis and renal failure may develop
	• Dysrhythmias and shock may occur
	• Death may result from severe metabolic disturbances, cerebral edema, coagulopathy
	Stage 4: 4 days-2 weeks
	• Gradual return of liver function in patients who recover
		• Gastric lavage only if within 1 hour of ingestion
		• Activated charcoal (single dose) if patient arrives within 4-6 hours after ingestion (though activated charcoal does adsorb N-acetylcysteine and reduces its peak serum levels, the loading dose of N-acetylcysteine does not need to be increased)
		• N-acetylcysteine (Mucomyst) 140 mg/kg initially, then 70 mg/kg every 4 hours × 17 doses to total of 1330 mg/kg
		  • If given PO, dilute in juice or carbonated beverage; if given via nasogastric or duodenal tube, dilute 3 to 1 with juice or carbonated beverage
		    — May cause anorexia, nausea, vomiting, diarrhea; repeat dose if vomiting occurs within 1 hour
		  • IV preparation (Acetadote) has recently been approved; 20-hour protocol
		• Treat vomiting with metoclopramide (Reglan); ondansetron (Zofran) or droperidol (Inapsine) for refractory vomiting
		• Monitor for bleeding; vitamin K may be prescribed especially if hepatic failure occurs
		• Dextrose (e.g., $D_{50}W$) may be needed for hypoglycemia
		• Antidysrhythmics may be needed
		• Registration for hepatic transplantation if indicated

Barbiturates • Pentobarbital (Nembutal) • Phenobarbital (Luminal) • Secobarbital (Seconal)	• Bradycardia, cardiac dysrhythmias • Hypotension • Hypothermia • Respiratory depression → respiratory arrest • Headache • Nystagmus, dysconjugate eye movements • Dysarthria • Ataxia • Depressed deep tendon reflexes • Confusion, stupor, coma • Hemorrhagic blisters • Gastric irritation (chloral hydrate) • Pulmonary edema (meprobamate) • Hypertonicity, hyperreflexia, myoclonus, seizures (methaqualone)	• Gastric lavage only if within 1 hour of ingestion • Multiple doses of activated charcoal, with cathartic added to first dose • Phenobarbital: sodium bicarbonate to alkalinize the urine and increase rate of barbiturate excretion; maintain urine pH greater than 7.5 • Monitor potassium, calcium, and magnesium levels • Anticonvulsants (e.g., diazepam, phenytoin, phenobarbital) for seizures • Hemodialysis or hemoperfusion may be required

Table 11-10 Drugs and Toxins—cont'd

Drug or Toxin	Clinical Presentation of Intoxication	Specific Collaborative Management

Benzodiazepines
• Diazepam (Valium)
• Flurazepam (Dalmane)
• Lorazepam (Ativan)
• Midazolam (Versed)
• Oxazepam (Serax)
	• Hypotension
	• Respiratory depression
	• Diminished or absent bowel sounds
	• Decreased deep tendon reflexes (DTRs)
	• Confusion, drowsiness, stupor, coma
		• Gastric lavage only if within 1 hour of ingestion
		• Activated charcoal (single dose)
		• Flumazenil (Romazicon), a benzodiazepine receptor antagonist, may be prescribed
		  • Contraindicated if patient has coingested tricyclic antidepressants; use cautiously if patient has history of long-term use of benzodiazepines
		  • Monitor for seizures, agitation, flushing, nausea, and vomiting as side effects of flumazenil
		• Intubation and mechanical ventilation may be necessary

Beta-blockers	• Sinus bradycardia, arrest, block • Junctional escape rhythm • AV nodal block • Bundle branch block (usually right) • Hypotension • Heart failure • Cardiogenic shock • Cardiac arrest • Decreased LOC • Seizures • Respiratory depression, apnea • Bronchospasm • Hyperglycemia or hypoglycemia	• Gastric lavage only if within 1 hour of ingestion • Multiple doses of activated charcoal, with cathartic added to first dose • Bowel irrigation if sustained-release preparations ingested • Atropine, epinephrine, dopamine, or isoproterenol for bradycardia and hypotension; temporary pacing may be required • Glucagon 3-5 mg IV, IM, or subcutaneously, followed by infusion of 1-5 mg/hr • $D_{50}W$ for hypoglycemia • Anticonvulsants (e.g., diazepam, phenobarbital) for seizures; phenytoin is contraindicated
Calcium channel blockers	• Sinus bradycardia, arrest, block • SA blocks (diltiazem) • AV blocks (verapamil) • Hypotension • Heart failure • Confusion, agitation, dizziness, lethargy, slurred speech • Seizures • Nausea, vomiting • Paralytic ileus • Hyperglycemia	• Gastric lavage only if within 1 hour of ingestion • Activated charcoal; multiple doses, with cathartic added to first dose, if massive ingestion or ingestion of sustained-release preparations • Bowel irrigation if sustained-release preparations ingested • Calcium chloride 5 (500 mg)-10 (1 g) mL of 10% solution • Atropine, epinephrine, dopamine, or isoproterenol for bradycardia and hypotension; temporary pacing may be required • Glucagon 3-5 mg IV, IM, or subcutaneously, followed by infusion of 1-5 mg/hr • Anticonvulsants (e.g., diazepam, phenytoin, phenobarbital) for seizures
Cannabinoids • Hashish • Marijuana	• Euphoria • Slowed thinking and reaction time • Confusion • Impaired balance and coordination	• Supportive care

Continued

Table 11-10 Drugs and Toxins—cont'd

Drug or Toxin	Clinical Presentation of Intoxication	Specific Collaborative Management

Carbon monoxide
• Note: The affinity between carbon monoxide and hemoglobin is approximately 200 times the affinity between oxygen and hemoglobin
	• Dysrhythmias
	• Impaired hearing or vision
	• Pallor; cherry-red skin coloring may be seen
	• Elevated HbCO levels; normal 0-3% for nonsmoker and 3-8% for smoker
	  • 10-20%: mild headache, flushing, dyspnea or angina on vigorous exertion, nausea, dizziness
	  • 20-30%: throbbing headache, nausea, vomiting, weakness, dyspnea on moderate exertion, ST segment depression
	  • 30-40%: severe headache, visual disturbances, syncope, vomiting
	  • 40-50%: tachypnea, tachycardia, chest pain, worsening syncope
	  • 50-60%: chest pain, respiratory failure, shock, seizures, coma
	  • 60-70%: respiratory failure, shock, coma, death
		• Removal from contaminated area
		• Oxygenation
		  • 100% oxygen via mask initially; CPAP by mask may be utilized
		  • Intubation and mechanical ventilation until HbCO level is less than 5%; PEEP may be utilized
		  • Hyperbaric oxygen (at 3 atmospheres) as soon as available if:
		    — HbCO greater than 25%
		    — HbCO greater than 15% and if history of cardiovascular disease, acute ECG changes, or CNS symptoms
		• Fluids, diuretics, urine alkalinization to treat myoglobinuria if present
		• Anticonvulsants (e.g., diazepam, phenytoin, phenobarbital) for seizures

Caustic poisoning • Acids (e.g., battery acid, drain cleaners, hydrochloric acid) • Alkalis (e.g., drain cleaners, refrigerants, fertilizers, photographic developers)	• Burning sensation in the oral cavity, pharynx, esophageal area • Dysphagia • Respiratory distress: dyspnea, stridor, tachypnea, hoarseness • Soapy-white mucous membrane Acid • Oral ulcerations and/or blisters • May have signs of gastric perforation (e.g., abdominal pain, distention, absent bowel sounds, rebound tenderness) • May have signs of shock Alkali • May have signs of esophageal perforation (e.g., chest pain, subcutaneous emphysema)	• Diluent: flush mouth with copious volumes of water; drink water or milk (approximately 250 mL) • Do not induce vomiting or perform gastric lavage • Esophagogastroscopy to assess damage • Corticosteroids may be prescribed for alkali poisoning
Cocaine, including "crack" cocaine	• Tachycardia, dysrhythmias, conduction defects • Hypertension or hypotension • Tachypnea or hyperpnea • Cocaine-induced MI • Pallor or cyanosis • Euphoria, hyperexcitability, anxiety • Headache • Hyperthermia, diaphoresis • Nausea, vomiting, abdominal pain • Dilated but reactive pupils • Confusion, delirium, hallucinations • Seizures • Coma • Respiratory arrest	• Swabbing of inside of nose to remove any residual drug if cocaine was snorted • Bowel irrigation for "body packers" • Anxiolytics (e.g., lorazepam, diazepam • Anticonvulsants (e.g., benzodiazepine, phenytoin, phenobarbital) for seizures • Antidysrhythmics, usually lidocaine; calcium channel blockers may also be used (they may also help with coronary artery spasm) • Antihypertensives: vasodilators (e.g., nitroprusside [Nipride]) • Vasopressors (e.g., norepinephrine) for hypotension • Hypothermia blanket, ice packs, ice-water sponge baths for hyperthermia • Dantrolene (Dantrium) may be prescribed for malignant hyperthermia • Fluids, diuretics, urine alkalinization to treat myoglobinuria if present

Table 11-10 Drugs and Toxins—cont'd

Drug or Toxin	Clinical Presentation of Intoxication	Specific Collaborative Management

Cyanide	• Anxiety, restlessness, hyperventilation initially
	• Bradycardia followed by tachycardia
	• Hypertension followed by hypotension
	• Dysrhythmias
	• Bitter almond odor to breath
	• Cherry red mucous membranes
	• Nausea
	• Dyspnea
	• Headache
	• Dizziness
	• Pupil dilation
	• Confusion
	• Stupor, seizures, coma, death
	• Elevated cyanide level
	  • 0.5 mcg/mL or less: asymptomatic
	  • 0.5-1 mcg/mL: tachycardia, flushing
	  • 1-2.5 mcg/mL: agitation or decreased LOC
	  • 2.5-3 mcg/mL: coma
	  • More than 3 mcg/mL: potentially fatal
		• 100% oxygen initially by mask
		  • Hyperbaric oxygen may be needed
		  • Intubation and mechanical ventilation is frequently necessary
		• Supportive care if only anxiety, restlessness, hyperventilation
		• Discontinuance of causative agent (e.g., nitroprusside)
		• Antidotes for more serious symptoms
		  • Amyl nitrite by inhalation
		  • Sodium nitrite IV
		  • Sodium thiosulfate IV
		• Gastric lavage only if within 1 hour of ingestion
		• Activated charcoal if cyanide was ingested
		• Flushing of eyes and/or skin with water if dermal contamination; removal and isolation of clothing
		• Fluids, vasopressors for BP support
		• Anticonvulsants (e.g., diazepam, phenytoin, phenobarbital) for seizures
		• Antidysrhythmics (e.g., lidocaine) for ventricular dysrhythmia, atropine for bradydysrhythmias
		• Sodium bicarbonate for severe metabolic acidosis
		• Vitamin B_{12} may be prescribed

Digitalis preparations	• Anorexia
	• Nausea
	• Vomiting
	• Headache
	• Restlessness
	• Visual changes
	• Sinus bradycardia, block, or arrest
	• PAT with AV block
	• Junctional tachycardia
	• AV blocks: 1st, 2nd Type I, 3rd
	• PVCs: bigeminy, trigeminy, quadrigeminy
	• Ventricular tachycardia: especially bidirectional
	• Ventricular fibrillation
		• Gastric lavage only if within 1 hour of ingestion
		• Multiple-dose activated charcoal, with cathartic added to first dose
		• Cholestyramine
		• Bowel irrigation for large ingestions
		• Correction of hypoxia, electrolyte imbalance (especially potassium)
		• Treatment of dysrhythmias
		  • For symptomatic bradydysrhythmias and blocks
		    — Atropine
		    — External pacemaker
		  • For symptomatic tachydysrhythmias
		    — Lidocaine
		    — Phenytoin
		    — Magnesium if hypomagnesemia or hyperkalemia present
		    — Cardioversion at lowest effective voltage and only if life-threatening dysrhythmias exist
		    — Defibrillation for ventricular fibrillation
		    — Verapamil if SVT
		• Digoxin immune Fab (Digibind) if greater than 10 mg ingested (adult), serum digoxin greater than 10 ng/mL, or serum potassium greater than 5 mEq/L
		• Monitor closely for exacerbation of condition for which digitalis was being used (i.e., increase in heart rate, heart failure)

Continued

Table 11-10 Drugs and Toxins—cont'd

Drug or Toxin	Clinical Presentation of Intoxication	Specific Collaborative Management
Dissociative anesthetics • Ketamine • Phencyclidine (PCP)	• Tachycardia • Hypertensive crisis initially; may cause hypotension later • Hyperthermia • Agitation, hyperactivity • Nystagmus • Blank stare • Hypoglycemia • Violent, psychotic behavior • Ataxia • Seizures • Myoglobinuria, renal failure • Lethargy, coma • Cardiac arrest	• Quiet environment • Gastric lavage only if within 1 hour of ingestion • Activated charcoal • Gastric suction • Benzodiazepines (e.g., diazepam) for anxiety and agitation • Antidysrhythmics if required • Antihypertensives: vasodilators (e.g., nitroprusside [Nipride]) • Hypothermia blanket, ice packs, ice-water sponge baths for hyperthermia • Dantrolene (Dantrium) may be prescribed for malignant hyperthermia • Anticonvulsants (e.g., diazepam, phenytoin, phenobarbital) for seizures • Haloperidol (Haldol) for acute psychotic reactions • Fluids and diuretics for myoglobinuria; sodium bicarbonate is contraindicated because urinary alkalinization interferes with urinary elimination of PCP
Ethanol (i.e., grain) alcohol	Increased ethanol concentration (mg/dL) • Less than 25: sense of warmth and well-being, talkativeness, self-confidence, mild incoordination • 25-50: euphoria, decreased judgment and control • 50-100: decreased sensorium, worsened coordination, ataxia, decreased reflexes and reaction time • 100-250: nausea, vomiting, ataxia, diplopia, slurred speech, visual impairment, nystagmus, emotional lability, confusion, stupor • 250-400: stupor or coma, incontinence, respiratory depression • Greater than 400: respiratory paralysis, loss of protective reflexes, hypothermia, death Note: There is a wide variability between these signs/symptoms and blood ethanol levels; these signs/symptoms are for a non–alcohol-dependent person Also: • Alcohol odor to breath • Hypoglycemia • Seizures • Metabolic acidosis	• Gastric lavage if within 1 hour of ingestion • Fluid and electrolyte replacement (potassium, magnesium, calcium may be needed) • Anticonvulsants (e.g., diazepam, phenytoin, phenobarbital) for seizures • Monitor blood glucose and administer glucose for hypoglycemia and multivitamins, including thiamine and folic acid • Note: Thiamine is necessary for the brain to utilize glucose; thiamine deficiency in alcoholic patients may cause Wernicke's encephalopathy • Hemodialysis may be necessary

Table 11-10 Drugs and Toxins—cont'd

Drug or Toxin	Clinical Presentation of Intoxication	Specific Collaborative Management
Ethylene glycol (i.e., antifreeze)	First 12 hours after ingestion • Appears "drunk" without the odor of ethanol on breath • Nausea, vomiting, hematemesis • Focal seizures, coma • Nystagmus, depressed reflexes, tetany • Metabolic acidosis with increased anion gap 12-24 hours after ingestion • Tachycardia • Mild hypertension • Pulmonary edema • Heart failure • 24-72 hours after ingestion • Flank pain, costovertebral tenderness • Acute renal failure	• Gastric lavage only if within 1 hour of ingestion • 10% ethanol in D_5W IV to maintain serum ethanol level at 100-200 mg/dL • Fomepizole (Antizol) intravenously may be used instead of ethanol • Fluid and electrolyte replacement (particularly calcium, but potassium and magnesium may also be needed) • Sodium bicarbonate for severe metabolic acidosis • Glucose for hypoglycemia and multivitamins, including thiamine, folic acid, and pyridoxine • Note: Thiamine is necessary for the brain to utilize glucose; thiamine deficiency in alcoholic patients may cause Wernicke's encephalopathy • Anticonvulsants (e.g., diazepam, phenytoin, phenobarbital) for seizures • Hemodialysis may be needed
Hallucinogens (e.g., D-lysergic acid diethylamide [LSD])	• Tachycardia, hypertension • Hyperthermia • Anorexia, nausea • Headaches • Dizziness • Agitation, anxiety • Impaired judgment • Distortion and intensification of sensory perception • Toxic psychosis • Dilated pupils • Rambling speech • Polyuria	• Reassurance • Quiet environment with soft lighting • If ingested orally: activated charcoal may be used • Benzodiazepines (e.g., diazepam, lorazepam) for anxiety and agitation • Anticonvulsants (e.g., phenytoin, phenobarbital) for seizures • Restraints only if necessary to protect patient
Inhalants • Gases such as butane, propane, aerosol propellants, nitrous oxide • Nitrites such as amyl nitrate, butyl nitrate, cyclohexyl nitrate • Solvents such as paint thinner, gasoline, glue	• Mental status changes • Depression • Muscle weakness • Memory impairment • CNS damage • Sudden death	• Oxygen • Supportive care
Isopropyl (i.e., rubbing) alcohol	• Gastrointestinal distress (e.g., nausea, vomiting, abdominal pain) • Headache • CNS depression, areflexia, ataxia • Respiratory depression • Hypothermia; hypotension	• Gastric lavage only if within 1 hour of ingestion • Gastric suction • Hemodialysis may be needed • Fluids and vasopressors for hypoperfusion

Continued

Table 11-10 Drugs and Toxins—cont'd

Drug or Toxin	Clinical Presentation of Intoxication	Specific Collaborative Management
Lithium	Mild • Vomiting, diarrhea • Lethargy, weakness • Polyuria, polydipsia • Nystagmus • Fine tremors Severe • Hypotension • Severe thirst • Tinnitus • Hyperreflexia • Coarse tremors • Ataxia • Seizures • Confusion • Coma • Dilute urine, renal failure • Heart failure	• Gastric lavage only if within 1 hour of ingestion • Hydration with normal saline • Anticonvulsants (e.g., phenytoin, phenobarbital) for seizures • Bowel irrigation • Hemodialysis may be necessary • Treatment of nephrogenic diabetes insipidus with amiloride (Midamor)
Methanol (i.e., wood) alcohol	• Nausea and vomiting • Hyperpnea, dyspnea • Visual disturbances ranging from blurring to blindness • Speech difficulty • Headache • CNS depression • Motor dysfunction with rigidity, spasticity, and hypokinesis • Metabolic acidosis with anion gap	• Gastric lavage only if within 1 hour of ingestion • 10% ethanol in D_5W IV to maintain serum ethanol level at 100-200 mg/dL • Sodium bicarbonate for severe metabolic acidosis • Hemodialysis if visual impairment, base deficit greater than 15, renal insufficiency, or blood methanol concentration greater than 30 mmol/L

Methemoglobinemia (caused by nitrites, nitrates, sulfa drugs, local anesthetics such as benzocaine, and others)	• Tachycardia
	• Fatigue
	• Nausea
	• Dizziness
	• Cyanosis in the presence of a normal PaO_2; failure of cyanosis to resolve with oxygen therapy
	• Dark red or brown blood
	• Elevated methemoglobin levels
	  • 15-30%: nausea, headache, dizziness, fatigue, headache, cyanosis
	  • 30-50%: tachycardia, tachypnea, dyspnea, weakness, marked cyanosis
	  • 50-70%: dysrhythmias, respiratory depression, seizures, coma
	  • Greater than 70%: potentially fatal
		• Oxygen
		• Removal of cause
		  • Stop nitroglycerin, nitroprusside, sulfa drugs, anesthetic agents, or other causative agents
		  • Gastric lavage only if within 1 hour of ingestion
		  • Multiple-dose activated charcoal, with cathartic added to first dose if agent ingested
		• Methylene blue
		  • If stupor, coma, angina, or respiratory depression or if level greater than 30%
		  • Administered at 1-2 mg/kg over 5 minutes; repeated at 1 mg/kg if patient still symptomatic after 30-60 minutes; total dose should not exceed 7 mg/kg
		• Ascorbic acid may be administered in large doses

Table 11-10 Drugs and Toxins—cont'd

Drug or Toxin	Clinical Presentation of Intoxication	Specific Collaborative Management
Opioids and opiates • Cocaine • Fentanyl • Heroin • Methadone • Morphine • Opium	• Bradycardia • Hypotension • Decreased level of consciousness • Respiratory depression → respiratory arrest • Hypothermia • Miosis • Diminished bowel sounds • Needle tracks, abscesses • Seizures • Pulmonary edema (especially with heroin)	• Gastric lavage only if within 1 hour of ingestion • Activated charcoal • Bowel irrigation for "body packers" • Naloxone (Narcan) 0.4-2 mg IV, IM, or transtracheally or nalmefene (Revex) 0.5 mg IV • Duration of action of naloxone is 1-2 hours; nalmefene has a duration of action of 4-8 hours (heroin and morphine 4-6 hours, meperidine 2-4 hours) • Anticonvulsants (e.g., diazepam, phenytoin, phenobarbital) for seizures • Intubation and mechanical ventilation may be required; PEEP may be needed for pulmonary edema
Organophosphate and carbamate (cholinesterase inhibitors)	• Bradycardia • Nausea, vomiting, diarrhea • Abdominal pain and cramping • Increased oral secretions • Dyspnea • Slurred speech • Constricted pupils • Visual changes • Unsteady gait • Urinary incontinence • Poor motor control • Twitching • Change in level of consciousness • Seizures	• Gastric lavage only if within 1 hour of ingestion • Activated charcoal if ingested • Washing of skin with soap and water and then ethyl alcohol if dermal contamination; removal and isolation of clothing • Atropine 1-2 mg IV or IM; repeated as required • Pralidoxime chloride (Protopam) 1-2 g IV over 15-30 minutes followed by infusion of 10-20 mg/kg may be used for organophosphates • Anticonvulsants (e.g., diazepam, phenytoin, phenobarbital) for seizures
Petroleum distillates	• Flushed skin • Hyperthermia • Vomiting • Diarrhea • Abdominal pain • Tachypnea • Dyspnea • Cyanosis • Coughing • Breath sound changes: crackles, rhonchi, diminished breath sounds • Staggering gait • Confusion • CNS depression or excitation	• Washing of skin with soap and water if dermal contamination; removal and isolation of clothing • Oxygen • Positioning on left side • Bronchodilators may be required • Antiemetics

Continued

Table 11-10 Drugs and Toxins—cont'd

Drug or Toxin	Clinical Presentation of Intoxication	Specific Collaborative Management

Salicylates	Initial
	• Hyperthermia
	• Burning sensation in mouth or throat
	• Change in level of consciousness
	• Petechiae
	Later
	• Hyperventilation (respiratory alkalosis)
	• Nausea, vomiting, epigastric pain, GI bleeding
	• Thirst
	• Tinnitus
	• Diaphoresis
	Late
	• Hearing loss
	• Motor weakness
	• Vasodilation and hypotension
	• Oliguria, renal failure
	• Pulmonary edema, respiratory depression → respiratory arrest
	• Metabolic acidosis
	• Prolonged PT, bleeding time
	• Hypokalemia, hypocalcemia
		• Gastric lavage only if within 1 hour of ingestion
		• Multiple-dose activated charcoal, with cathartic added to first dose
		• Bowel irrigation if enteric-coated salicylates ingested
		• Fluids with dextrose (e.g., D_5½NS) to maintain urine output at 2 mL/kg/hr
		• Hypothermia blanket, ice packs, ice-water sponge baths for hyperthermia
		  • Dantrolene (Dantrium) may be prescribed for malignant hyperthermia
		• Sodium bicarbonate to alkalinize the urine and increase rate of salicylate excretion; maintain urine pH greater than 7.5
		  • Monitor potassium, calcium, and magnesium levels
		• Hemodialysis may be necessary
		• Monitoring for bleeding; vitamin K may be needed
		• Monitoring and correction of potassium, calcium levels
		• Anticonvulsants (e.g., diazepam, phenytoin, phenobarbital) for seizures
		• H_2 receptor blocker or proton pump inhibitor for gastric ulcer prophylaxis

Stimulants
• Amphetamines (e.g., biphetamine, Dexedrine)
• Methylenedioxymeth-amphetamine (MDMA) (i.e., Ecstasy) (NOTE: 3, 4-Methylenedioxyamphetamine (MDA) is also sometimes called Ecstasy)
• Methamphetamine (i.e., meth)
• Methylphenidate (Ritalin)
• Gamma-hydroxybutyrate (GHB) (i.e., liquid ecstasy, liquid X)
	• Tachycardia
	• Hypertension or hypotension
	• Tachypnea
	• Dysrhythmias
	• Hyperthermia, diaphoresis
	• Dilated but reactive pupils
	• Dry mouth
	• Urinary retention
	• Headache
	• Paranoid-type psychotic behavior
	• Hallucinations
	• Hyperactivity, anxiety
	• Hyperactive deep tendon reflexes, tremor, seizures
	• Confusion, stupor, coma
		• Calm, quiet environment
		  • Avoid overstimulation of patient
		  • Do not speak loudly or move quickly
		  • Do not approach from behind
		  • Avoid touching the patient unless you are sure it is safe
		• Gastric lavage only if within 1 hour of ingestion
		• Activated charcoal (single dose)
		• Diazepam (Valium) or lorazepam (Ativan) for agitation
		• Phentolamine (Regitine) for hypertension
		• Anticonvulsants (e.g., diazepam, phenytoin, phenobarbital) for seizures
		• Antidysrhythmics (e.g., lidocaine) for ventricular dysrhythmias
		• Haloperidol (Haldol) for acute psychotic reactions
		• Hypothermia blanket, ice packs, ice-water sponge baths for hyperthermia
		  • Dantrolene (Dantrium) may be prescribed for malignant hyperthermia

Table 11-10 Drugs and Toxins—cont'd

Drug or Toxin	Clinical Presentation of Intoxication	Specific Collaborative Management
Tricyclic antidepressants (TCAs) • Amitriptyline (Elavil) • Desipramine (Norpramin) • Doxepin (Sinequan) • Imipramine (Tofranil) • Nortriptyline (Aventyl) • Trimipramine (Surmontil)	Anticholinergic • Tachycardia, palpitations • Dysrhythmias • Hyperthermia • Headache • Restlessness • Mydriasis • Dry mouth • Nausea, vomiting • Dysphagia • Decreased bowel sounds • Urinary retention • Decreased deep tendon reflexes • Restlessness, euphoria • Hallucinations • Seizures • Coma Anti-alpha adrenergic • Hypotension • QT prolongation and quinidine-like dysrhythmias (including torsades de pointes) • AV and bundle branch blocks • Clinical indications of heart failure	• Gastric lavage only if within 1 hour of ingestion • Activated charcoal if agent ingested • Sodium bicarbonate to alkalinize the urine and increase rate of TCA excretion; maintain urine pH greater than 7.5 • Monitor potassium, calcium, magnesium levels • Hyperventilation may be used to produce alkalosis • Physostigmine (Antilirium) may be prescribed • Cardioversion, defibrillation, pacemaker as needed for dysrhythmias; avoid quinidine, lidocaine, digitalis; phenytoin or beta-blockers may be used to shorten QRS duration; overdrive pacing for torsades de pointes • Anticonvulsants (e.g., diazepam, phenytoin, phenobarbital) for seizures • Fluids and vasopressors for hypotension • Bethanechol (Urecholine) for urinary retention

e) Reason for exposure (e.g., dose confusion, suicide attempt, inadvertent exposure to toxin)
f) Previous exposure to drug or toxin
g) Source
i) Prescription
ii) Over the counter
iii) Street

b. May have history of depression or psychiatric illness
c. May have history of previous drug overdosage/toxin ingestion
d. May have history of chemical dependency
e. May have history of complicated drug regimen with or without confusion
f. Note any history of cardiovascular, renal, or hepatic disease.

2. Objective: Focus assessment on the following (for drug-specific signs, see Table 11-10)
a. Vital signs
b. Mental status
c. Seizures
d. Pupils
e. Ventilation
f. Skin and mucous membranes
g. Peristalsis
h. Odors
i. Urine color
j. Also note:
1) Needle marks
2) Evidence of self-injury (e.g., cutting on forearms)
k. Physiologic grading of the severity of poisoning (Table 11-11)

3. Diagnostic
a. Toxicology
1) Rapid drug screens (qualitative)
a) Serum
i) Acetaminophen
ii) Ethanol
iii) Salicylates
iv) Tricyclic antidepressants
b) Urine
i) Amphetamines
ii) Barbiturates
iii) Benzodiazepines
iv) Cannabinoids
v) Cocaine
vi) Methadol
vii) Opiates
viii) Phencyclidine
ix) Propoxyphene
2) Quantitative drug levels may be required to determine appropriate treatment
a) Carbamazepine
b) Carbon monoxide
c) Digoxin
d) Ethylene glycol
e) Lithium
f) Methanol

Table 11-11 Physiologic Grading of the Severity of Poisoning

Severity	Signs and Symptoms: Stimulant Poisoning	Signs and Symptoms: Depressant Poisoning
Grade 1	Agitation, anxiety, diaphoresis, hyperreflexia, mydriasis, tremors	Ataxia, confusion, lethargy, weakness, verbal, able to follow commands
Grade 2	Confusion, fever, hyperactivity, hypertension, tachycardia, tachypnea	Mild coma (nonverbal but responsive to pain), brainstem and deep tendon reflexes intact
Grade 3	Delirium, hallucinations, hyperpyrexia, tachydysrhythmias	Moderate coma (respiratory depression, unresponsive to pain), some but not all reflexes absent
Grade 4	Coma, cardiovascular collapse, seizures	Deep coma (apnea, cardiovascular depression), all reflexes absent

Data from Irwin, R. S., & Rippe, J. M. (2003). *Irwin and Rippe's intensive care medicine* (Vol. 5). Philadelphia: Lippincott Williams & Wilkins.

g) Methemoglobin
h) Phenytoin
i) Theophylline

b. Arterial blood gases
   1) Respiratory acidosis caused by hypoventilation when drugs or toxin depress ventilation
   2) Metabolic acidosis
      a) With increased anion gap
         i) Paraldehyde, ethylene glycol, methanol, toluene, salicylates
         ii) Agents which cause hypoxia and resultant increase in serum lactate
      b) With decreased anion gap: lithium, bromide, iodide
c. ECG: dysrhythmias frequently seen, depending on the drug or toxin
d. Flat plate of abdomen (i.e., KUB): to assess for presence of radiopaque agents
e. CT scan: may be done to rule out pathology
f. Lumbar puncture: may be done to rule out pathology

Collaborative Management

1. Maintain airway, oxygenation, and ventilation.
   a. Administer oxygen, dextrose, thiamine, and naloxone (Narcan) (sometimes referred to as a *coma cocktail*) for altered mental status with no known cause.
      1) Administer oxygen to reverse hypoxemia as a cause of loss of consciousness.
         a) Goal is to achieve a SaO_2 of 95% unless contraindicated; if history of COPD, goal is to achieve a SaO_2 of 90%.
         b) Contraindicated if the herbicide paraquat is ingested because it is likely to increase alveolar injury caused by oxygen free radicals
      2) Administer dextrose to reverse possible hypoglycemia as the cause of loss of consciousness.
         a) Usual dose is 50-100 mL of 50% dextrose IV.
      3) Administer thiamine to prevent Wernicke's encephalopathy, especially if there is a history of alcoholism or chronic drug abuse.
         a) Usual dose is 50-100 mg IV or IM.
         b) Also helpful in ethylene glycol intoxication because thiamine may prevent formation of toxic metabolites
      4) Administer naloxone (Narcan) to reverse possible opiate intoxication as a cause of loss of consciousness
         a) Dose is usually 1 to 2 mg IV, IM, or transtracheally.
            i) Dose of up to 10 mg may be required.
            ii) Consider half-life of naloxone and the half-life of the opiate given; may require redose
         b) Goal is to reverse the CNS and respiratory depression, not full consciousness.
         c) Sudden narcotic withdrawal occurs in patients with opiate intoxication so caution must be exercised to prevent the patients from injuring themselves or health care providers.
   b. Maintain head tilt–chin lift position to maintain open airway; use jaw thrust technique if cervical spine injury may exist.
   c. Use an oropharyngeal or a nasopharyngeal airway to keep the tongue away from the hypopharynx.
      1) Choose appropriate airway: oropharyngeal airways should not be used in conscious patients due to their propensity to cause vomiting by stimulating the gag reflex.
      2) Place patient in a left side-lying position.
      3) Have suction equipment available.
   d. Assist with endotracheal intubation if gag and cough reflexes are depressed or if gastric lavage is initiated in lethargic patient.
   e. Monitor breath sounds and chest x-ray for aspiration and pulmonary edema.
   f. Administer oxygen therapy; adjust flow rate or oxygen concentration to keep SpO_2 approximately 95% unless contraindicated; in patients with chronic hypercapnia, adjust flow rate or oxygen concentration to keep SpO_2 approximately 90%.

g. Assist with initiation of mechanical ventilation for acute respiratory failure or respiratory failure and respiratory acidosis.

2. Maintain cardiovascular function.
   a. Monitor ECG rhythm for conduction changes or dysrhythmias, especially if tricyclic antidepressant (TCA) overdosage.
   b. Administer antidysrhythmic agents as prescribed.
   c. Assist with treatment of hypotension if required.
      1) Insertion of intravenous catheter
      2) Treatment of hypovolemia with infusion of isotonic crystalloids
      3) Administration of vasopressors for vasodilation
         a) Alpha stimulants for tricyclic antidepressants
         b) Alpha and beta stimulants for beta-blocker or calcium channel blocker intoxication
         c) Calcium may be administered for calcium channel blocker intoxication.
   d. Assist with treatment of hypertension if required.
      1) Sedation with benzodiazepine as prescribed
      2) Alpha-beta blocker (e.g., labetalol [Normodyne]) as prescribed for hypertension with tachycardia
      3) Peripheral vasodilator if hypertension with normal heart rate or bradycardia
   e. Apply blankets or forced air rewarming (e.g., Bair Hugger) if needed for hypothermia.
3. Assist with treatment of seizures if required.
   a. Airway maintenance including intubation if necessary, oxygen to maintain SaO_2 of at least 95%, ventilation with manual resuscitation bag if necessary
   b. Provision of protection from injury
   c. Serum glucose and administration of dextrose if indicated
   d. Anticonvulsants as prescribed; benzodiazepines (e.g., diazepam, lorazepam, or midazolam) are used initially
4. Assist with treatment of hyperthermia if required.
   a. Removal of clothing and fans; moistening of skin with fanning may be helpful
   b. Neuromuscular paralysis may be necessary because heat is frequently associated with excessive muscle rigidity.
   c. Reversal of drug with antidote if available
   d. Dantrolene (Dantrium) may be prescribed in some situations
5. Prevent further absorption of drug or toxin depending on the route of absorption.
   a. Eye: immediate irrigation of the eyes with large quantities of isotonic saline
   b. Skin
      1) Protect yourself with gloves, gown, and goggles.
      2) Remove and discard clothing.
      3) Rinse with water until skin pH is normal if toxin is a strong acid or alkaline.
      4) Wash body with soap and water.
   c. Ingestion
      1) Induced emesis using ipecacuanha (Ipecac): not recommended
      2) Gastric lavage: usually only performed when the patient arrives within 60 minutes of ingestion of drug or toxin
         a) Assist with endotracheal intubation prior to gastric lavage in patients who have a decreased level of consciousness and a diminished gag reflex.
         b) Consider contraindications.
            i) Ingestion of hydrocarbons or corrosives
               (a) Use dilution: Give water or milk (usually approximately 250 mL).
            ii) Airway cannot be protected.
            iii) Seizures
         c) Use large-bore (32-40 French) orogastric tube (Ewald)
            i) Viscous lidocaine on tube may decrease gag reflex.
            ii) Confirm placement by aspirating gastric contents.
         d) Place patient in a left side-lying, head-down position; have suction equipment available.
         e) Use approximately 5-10 L of warm tap water; inject 150-200 mL at a time and aspirate completely before injecting any more lavage fluid.
         f) Monitor for potential complications (e.g., esophageal or gastric perforation, aspiration pneumonitis, laryngospasm, epistaxis, hypothermia, hyponatremia).
         g) Do not remove tube until after activated charcoal has been given.
      3) Adsorbent therapy
         a) Administer activated charcoal as prescribed: usually 0.5-1 g/kg.
            i) Indicated if patient has ingested a potentially toxic amount of drug or toxin that binds to charcoal
            ii) Contraindications
               (a) More than an hour after ingestion of the drug or toxin; may be used if more than 1 hour since ingestion of a significant overdosage of a drug that slows gastric emptying as long as the airway is protected
               (b) Substance not bound to charcoal, including the following:

(i) Metal salts: iron, lithium, potassium
(ii) Alcohols: ethanol, ethylene glycol, glycol, methanol
(iii) Hydrocarbons, solvents, corrosives, acids, alkalis
(iv) Pesticides
(v) Cyanide
(c) Airway cannot be protected.
(d) Oral antidote is given.

iii) Multiple doses as prescribed
(a) Usually administered as 0.5 g/kg of body weight every 2-6 hours until serum drug level is normal
(b) Indicated for life-threatening overdosage of the following agents:
(i) Carbamazepine (Tegretol)
(ii) Dapsone
(iii) Theophylline
(iv) Phenobarbital
(v) Quinine

iv) Cathartics: necessity and safety now questioned so likely to be prescribed only with multiple doses of activated charcoal
(a) Administer sorbitol with first dose of activated charcoal as prescribed.
(b) Repeated doses may cause intractable diarrhea.

4) Bowel irrigation
a) Administer nonabsorbable, osmotically active solution (e.g., polyethylene glycol lavage electrolyte solution [GoLYTELY, Colyte]) as prescribed orally or by nasogastric tube; usually at a rate of 1-2 L/hr for 4-6 hours or until the patient has clear stools
b) Indications
i) Large ingestions of drugs or toxins not adsorbed to activated charcoal
ii) Large ingestions of sustained-release or enteric-coated drugs
iii) "Body packers" and "body stuffers"; surgical intervention may also be required in these situations
(a) "Body packers" swallow condoms or balloons filled with a drug to smuggle it.
(b) "Body stuffers" swallow drugs to prevent detection by police; these drugs are not specially prepared to prevent absorption in the GI tract so they present great risk of overdosage.
iv) Formed concretions of drugs in the GI tract
c) Contraindicated if the patient has significant gastrointestinal pathology or dysfunction
d) Monitor for vomiting.

5) Assist with gastroscopy if indicated: may be necessary to remove coalesced mass of pills

6. Facilitate removal of drug.
a. Forced diuresis: Intravenous fluids and osmotic or loop diuretics were used to cause a forced osmotic diuresis in ethanol, methanol, ethylene glycol intoxication in the past, but this is no longer recommended.
b. Urine alkalinization
1) Intravenous sodium bicarbonate is used.
2) Indicated for salicylates, tricyclic antidepressants, phenobarbital, chlorpropamide
3) Goal is urine pH of 7.5-8.5
4) Monitoring of potassium is required.
c. Acidification of the urine was previously used for PCP and amphetamines but is currently avoided due to incidence of rhabdomyolysis and resultant myoglobinuria that may cause acute renal failure.
d. Hemodialysis or hemoperfusion as prescribed
1) Indications for hemodialysis include the following:
a) Heavy metals
b) Salicylate intoxication with severe acid-base imbalance or seizures unresponsive to treatment
c) Severe poisoning of a dialyzable drug (Box 11-2)
d) Ingestion of an agent known to produce delayed toxicity
e) Drug-induced renal or hepatic toxicity
2) Hemoperfusion is more effective for drugs that are bound to plasma proteins, but it is not effective in correcting acid-base imbalances.
a) May be used for the following:
i) *Amanita* (mushroom) poisoning
ii) Carbamazepine
iii) Colchicine

Box 11-2 Selected Dialyzable Drugs/Toxins

Acetaminophen
Alcohols: ethanol, ethylene glycol, methanol
Amphetamines
Antibiotics (most)
Barbiturates
Electrolytes: potassium, calcium, magnesium
Lithium
Phenobarbital
Salicylates
Theophylline

iv) Phenobarbital
v) Theophylline
3) Hemodialysis and hemoperfusion both require double-venous vascular catheter.
e. Appropriate antidote if available and prescribed (listed where applicable in Table 11-10)
7. Maintain renal function.
   a. Administer intravenous fluids to maintain urine output at 0.5 to 1 mL/kg/hr.
   b. Monitor for myoglobinuria; administer fluids and diuretics as prescribed.
8. Monitor hepatic function, liver function studies, and coagulation studies.
9. Monitor for complications.
   a. Acute respiratory failure due to respiratory depression
   b. Aspiration pneumonitis
   c. Dysrhythmias
   d. Hypotension
   e. Heart failure
   f. Nephrotoxicity, acute renal failure
   g. Hepatotoxicity, acute hepatic failure
   h. Gastrointestinal ileus, bleeding, or perforation
   i. Seizures
   j. Coma, neurologic injury
   k. Hyperthermia or hypothermia
   l. Fluid and electrolyte imbalance
   m. Acid-base imbalance
   n. Repeat overdosage
10. Ensure appropriate psychological counseling.
   a. Allow patient to express feelings; maintain a noncondemning approach.
   b. Monitor environment for safety hazards; maintain suicide precautions if indicated.
   c. Refer the patient to a substance abuse program if appropriate.
   d. Request psychiatric consultation for destructive behavior if appropriate.

Asphyxia

Definition

1. A condition in which there is inadequate delivery, uptake, and/or utilization of oxygen by the body's tissues and cells; may be accompanied by an increase of carbon dioxide (Graham, 2011)

Etiology

1. Choking (i.e., nose, mouth, and/or upper pharynx occluded by an object or body part such as a hand) (e.g., pillow, hand, plastic bag)
2. Upper airway obstruction (e.g., foreign body, angioedema)
3. Trauma to airways (e.g., fracture of larynx)
4. Aspiration including drowning
5. Strangulation (e.g., manual, ligature, choke hold)
6. Hanging (i.e., force applied to neck primarily as the result of the victim's body weight)
7. Compression (i.e., external force on the chest and/or abdomen)
8. Positional (i.e., position of the body causes airway restriction, vascular compromise, or breathing fatigue) (e.g., upside-down suspension, crucifixion)
9. Inhalation of smoke and poisonous gases (e.g., cyanide, carbon monoxide, hydrogen sulfide)
10. Chemical asphyxia (i.e., ingestion or injection of drugs or toxins that interfere with oxygenation to tissues and cells)
   a. Cyanide including thiocyanate associated with nitroprusside administration
   b. Methemoglobinemia associated with nitrates and nitrites (e.g., nitroglycerine, nitroprusside, nitric oxide) and local anesthetics (e.g., Cetacaine, Lidocaine)

Pathophysiology

1. Interruption in the normal exchange of oxygen and carbon dioxide between the lungs and the outside air
2. Hypoxia and hypercapnia
3. Restriction of blood flow or altered hemodynamics
4. Cellular derangement
5. Cellular death
6. Cardiac arrest and death

Clinical Presentation

1. Subjective: history of potential cause of asphyxia
2. Objective
   a. Irregular and disturbed respirations or a complete absence of breathing
   b. Congestion of the face and cyanosis
   c. Facial edema
   d. Petechiae on eyelids, conjunctivae, sclerae, face, and gums
   e. Ligature mark or bruising around neck may be evident.
3. Diagnostic: Radiographic examination of the neck may reveal fracture of hyoid bone or larynx.

Collaborative Management

1. Treat the cause.
   a. Removal of airway obstruction
   b. Positioning for adequate chest excursion
   c. Removal from toxic environment
   d. Appropriate antidote for toxins
2. Establish airway and ensure adequate oxygenation and ventilation.
   a. Airway management that is likely to include endotracheal intubation or cricothyrotomy
   b. Oxygen at 100% initially and then adjusted to ensure SaO_2 of at least 95%
   c. Mechanical ventilation may be necessary.
3. Assess for cardiovascular impairment, and treat dysrhythmias and/or impaired cardiac output.

LEARNING ACTIVITIES

CHAPTER 11

1. Complete the following crossword puzzle related to shock, SIRS, and MODS.

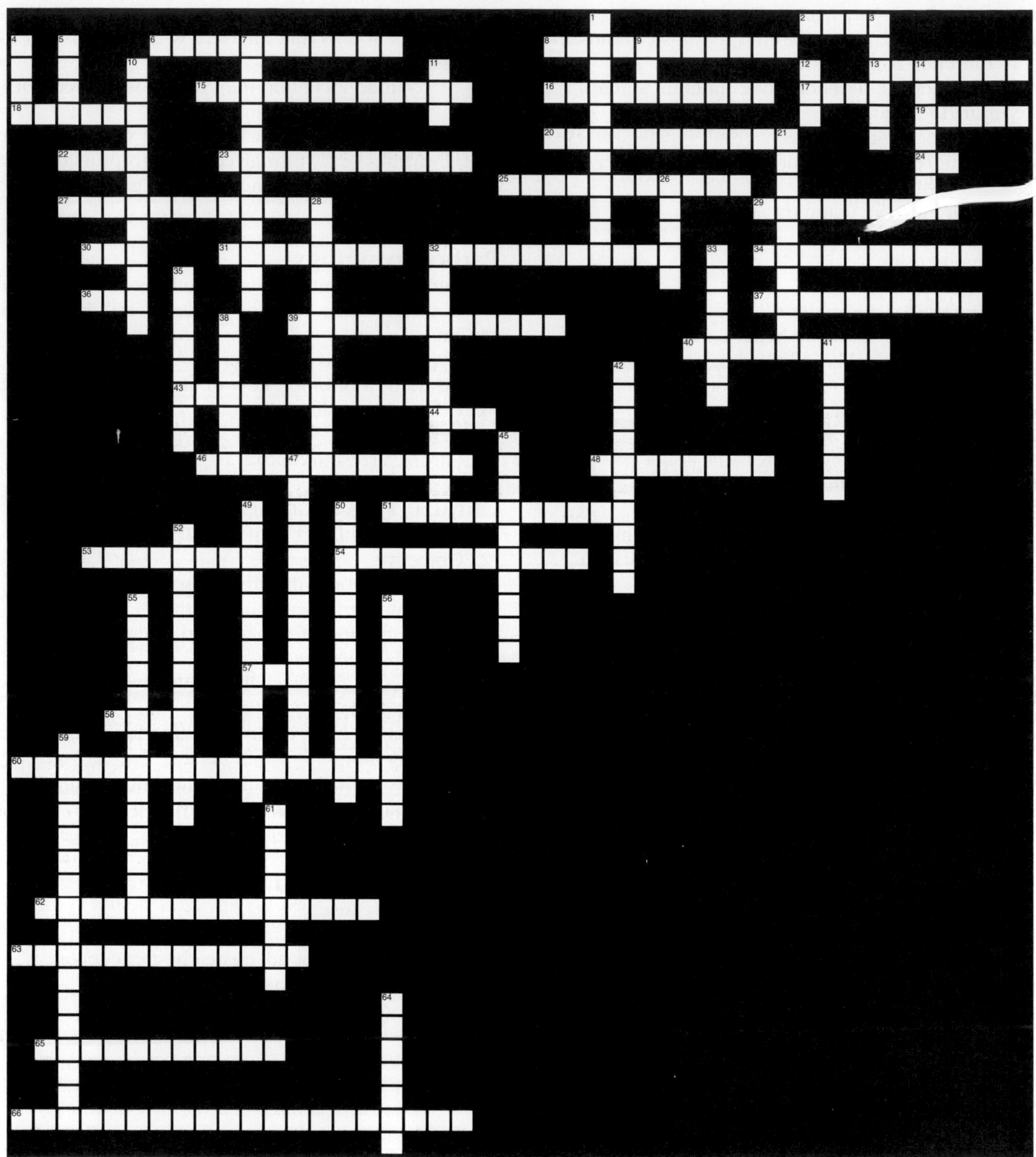

ACROSS

2. The frequently fatal result of SIRS; previously referred to as multisystem organ failure (abbrev)
6. Type of shock caused by loss of intravascular volume
8. This stage of septic shock is also referred to as late or cold septic shock
13. These legumes are a common cause of anaphylactic shock
15. This category of shock includes the three forms of shock that result in massive vasodilation and resultant relative hypovolemia
16. The drug most commonly associated with anaphylactic shock (generic)
17. Crystalloids are generally preferred over colloids for fluid resuscitation due to the lower ____ of crystalloids
18. Infection with SIRS
19. This type of intravenous infusion is required for hemorrhage to the point of hypoperfusion
20. A complication of administering large volumes of IV fluid and blood, which may cause shifting of the oxyhemoglobin dissociation curve to the left
22. This hemodynamic parameter differentiates between hypovolemic and cardiogenic shock and between cardiac and noncardiac pulmonary edema (abbrev)
23. An alkaline buffer used for severe metabolic acidosis
24. The most common cause of cardiogenic shock (abbrev)
25. The stage of shock when compensatory mechanisms are no longer effective in maintaining tissue perfusion
27. This stage of shock is associated with fever, increased CO/CI, and decreased SVR
29. The mediator seen in anaphylactic shock that causes vasodilation and increased capillary permeability
30. The branch of the autonomic nervous system responsible for the early compensatory response to hypoperfusion in shock (abbrev)
31. Vasopressor that increases risk of tachycardia and dysrhythmia (generic)
32. The type of shock caused by the inability of the heart to pump effectively
34. The stage of shock associated with irreversible organ damage
36. The hemodynamic parameter that is increased in hypovolemic and cardiogenic shock (abbrev)
37. A colloid solution that contains large starch molecules; may transiently elevate serum amylase levels
39. Alternative route for fluid administration when IV access cannot be obtained
40. Conditionally essential amino acid advocated in critically ill patients; may be added to enteral feedings or given in an immune boosting formula
43. Third-spacing is the shift of fluid from the intravascular space to the _____ space, pleural space, pericardial space, and peritoneal space
44. S_3, crackles, and dyspnea are manifestations of ____ seen in cardiogenic shock (abbrev)
46. This type of shock is caused by IgE and the release of histamine and other mediators
48. DO_2 is oxygen _____
51. Tension pneumothorax and cardiac tamponade are examples of this subtype of cardiogenic shock
53. Urine output of less than 0.5 mL/kg/hr
54. The decrease in BP when the patient is repositioned from lying to standing is referred to as ____ changes or being tilt positive
57. The type of acute kidney injury seen in MODS (abbrev)
58. A systemic response of the immune system to microorganism, tissue trauma, toxins, and burns (abbrev)
60. This type of mismanagement may contribute to ARDS
62. H_1 receptor antagonist (generic)
63. The movement of GI bacteria through the bowel wall and into the lymphatics
65. VO_2 is oxygen _____
66. This complication of shock is manifested by bloody diarrhea (2 words)

DOWN

1. The first-line drug for anaphylactic shock (generic)
3. This type of shock is associated with mediator release in response to overwhelming infection
4. The type of acute respiratory failure seen in MODS (abbrev)
5. A mechanical therapy used in cardiogenic shock to increase coronary artery perfusion pressure and decrease afterload (abbrev)
7. This type of drug may be used to decrease preload or afterload in cardiogenic shock (plural)
9. The type of coagulopathy seen in MODS (abbrev)
10. This type of drug may be used in vasogenic shock to restore normal vascular tone (plural)
11. JVD, peripheral edema, and hepatomegaly are manifestations of ____ seen in cardiogenic shock (abbrev)
12. Preferred method of reperfusion for acute MI (abbrev)
14. The plasma protein with the greatest effect on plasma oncotic pressure
21. Swelling beneath the surface of the skin or mucous membranes associated with anaphylaxis; most often on the face, hands, feet, genitals, and airways
26. The condition of insufficient perfusion of cells and vital organs
28. The stage of shock dominated by neuroendocrine responses to hypoperfusion
32. This type of IV fluid contains solutes and may be categorized as hypotonic, isotonic, or hypertonic
33. Skin appearance in progressive and refractory stages of shock
35. Type of intravenous fluids that are used to increase intravascular colloidal oncotic pressure
38. A colloid solution that contains large starch molecules; affects platelet aggregation
41. This stage of shock is associated with a decrease in tissue oxygenation but no clinical indications of hypoperfusion
42. The presence of viable bacteria in the blood
45. The inotropic agent used most often in cardiogenic shock (generic)
47. A consequence of hemolytic blood transfusion reaction; may cause renal failure
49. An anaphylactic-like reaction that does not require previous exposure; not mediated by IgE, probably triggered by the complement system
50. The consequence of muscle destruction; may cause renal failure
52. The increased or normal systolic BP, along with the increased diastolic BP, causes the decrease in ____ seen in compensatory stage of shock (2 words)
55. First choice of vasopressor in septic shock (generic)
56. The type of shock caused by suppression of the sympathetic nervous system
59. Predominant acid-base disorder in shock (2 words)
61. This drug may be used for anaphylaxis in patients who have been receiving beta-blockers (generic)
64. Elevated serum ____ is an indication of lactic acidosis

2. Identify which type of shock the following pathologic conditions or procedures may cause.

Condition	Hypovolemic	Cardiogenic	Septic	Anaphylactic	Neurogenic
Myocardial infarction					
Bee sting					
Head injury					
Diarrhea					
Pulmonary embolism					
Ruptured gallbladder					
Esophageal varices					
Ruptured papillary muscle					
Insulin shock					
Ascites					
IVP dye					
Spinal cord injury					
Invasive procedures					
Burns					
Blood transfusion reaction					
Spinal anesthesia					
Trauma					
Malnutrition					
Chemotherapy					

3. Match the pathophysiology with the type of shock.

___ 1. Anaphylactic
___ 2. Cardiogenic
___ 3. Hypovolemic
___ 4. Neurogenic
___ 5. Septic

a. Massive vasodilation caused by the release of inflammatory mediators in response to overwhelming infection
b. Inability of the heart to effectively pump
c. Inadequate intravascular volume
d. Vasodilation caused by the release of histamine from mast cells
e. Vasodilation resulting from suppression or loss of the sympathetic nervous system

4. Identify the following signs/symptoms of shock as occurring during the compensatory, progressive, and/or refractory stages of shock.

Sign/Symptom	Compensatory	Progressive	Refractory
Tachycardia			
Dysrhythmias			
Cool, pale skin			
Disseminated intravascular coagulation			
Mottling of extremities			
Neurologic changes: lethargy, coma			
Oliguria			
Anuria			
Acute respiratory distress syndrome			
Narrow pulse pressure			
Profound hypotension despite vasopressors			
Dysrhythmias			
Hypotension			
Decreased bowel sounds			
Thirst			
Neurologic changes: irritability, confusion			
Nausea			
Neurologic changes: coma; focal signs			

5. Complete this table by putting ↑, ↓, or normal in the empty cells.

Type of Shock	CO/CI	RAP/PAP/PAOP	SVR	SvO_2
Hypovolemic				
Cardiogenic				
Septic				
Anaphylactic				
Neurologic				

CI, Cardiac index; *CO,* cardiac output; *PAOP,* pulmonary artery occlusive pressure; *PAP,* pulmonary artery pressure; *RAP,* right atrial pressure; SvO_2, oxygen saturation of venous blood; *SVR,* systemic vascular resistance.

6. List two fluids in each category.

Crystalloids		
Isotonic		
Hypotonic		
Hypertonic		
Colloids		
Blood or blood products		

7. Match these general treatments of shock with the factor of oxygen delivery or consumption that they are intended to affect.

___ 1. Isotonic crystalloids
___ 2. Red blood cells
___ 3. Oxygen
___ 4. Mechanical ventilation
___ 5. Inotropic agents
___ 6. Sedation
___ 7. PEEP
___ 8. Surgical intervention to stop bleeding
___ 9. Treatment of metabolic acidosis
___ 10. Hypothermia

a. Improved DO_2 by improving SaO_2
b. Improved DO_2 by improving hemoglobin
c. Improved DO_2 by improving cardiac output
d. Diminished VO_2

8. Match the following specific therapies with the type of shock for which they may be used. You may list more than one therapy for each form of shock, and the therapies may be used more than once.

___ 1. Anaphylactic
___ 2. Cardiogenic
___ 3. Hypovolemic
___ 4. Neurogenic
___ 5. Septic

a. Intravenous fluids
b. Corticosteroids
c. Blood
d. Vasopressors
e. Inotropes
f. Intraaortic balloon pump (IABP)
g. Pacemaker
h. Epinephrine
i. Antihistamines
j. Antimicrobials
k. Treatment of cause
l. Oxygen
m. Vasodilators

9. Match the sign/symptom of dysfunction with the organ that is dysfunctional.

___ 1. Brain
___ 2. Heart
___ 3. Blood
___ 4. Kidneys
___ 5. Liver
___ 6. Lungs

a. Decreased Pao_2/FiO_2 ratio
b. Oliguria
c. Hypoglycemia
d. Decrease in Glasgow Coma Scale score
e. Prolonged PT, aPTT, decreased platelets
f. Increased PAOP

10. Complete the following table that describes the four physiologic alterations that are likely to be seen in systemic inflammatory response syndrome. The criteria for systemic inflammatory response syndrome are two of these four parameters.

Heart rate	Greater than ____			
Respiratory rate	Greater than ____	OR	$PaCO_2$	Less than ____
Temperature	Greater than ____	OR	Less than ____	
WBC	Greater than ____	OR	Less than ____	

11. Identify the three actions which may be used in toxicities/overdosages to decrease absorption of the toxin or drug.

a. ______________________________

b. ______________________________

c. ______________________________

12. Match the following antidotes to the appropriate drug or toxin.

___ 1. Methemoglobinemia
___ 2. Cyanide
___ 3. Methanol
___ 4. Organophosphates
___ 5. Carbon monoxide
___ 6. Acetaminophen
___ 7. Benzodiazepines (e.g., diazepam)
___ 8. Opiates (e.g., morphine sulfate)
___ 9. Ethylene glycol
___ 10. Beta-blocker
___ 11. Digoxin
___ 12. Calcium channel blockers

a. Glucagon
b. 100% oxygen, hyperbaric oxygenation if possible
c. Digibind
d. Fomepizole (Antizol)
e. Ethanol
f. Methylene blue
g. Calcium
h. Amyl nitrate
i. Atropine
j. Acetylcysteine (Mucomyst)
k. Flumazenil (Romazicon)
l. Naloxone (Narcan)

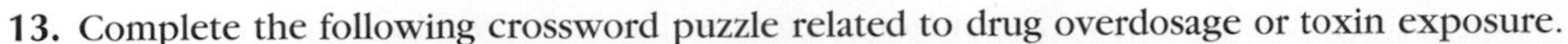

13. Complete the following crossword puzzle related to drug overdosage or toxin exposure.

ACROSS

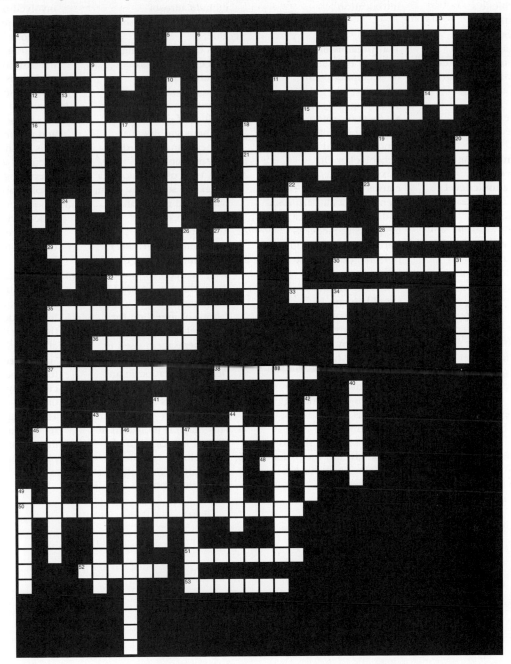

2. Bowel irrigation with this solution is used for OD of sustained-release drugs (trade)
5. High pressure; this type of oxygen therapy is used in carbon monoxide poisoning
7. Dilution is used if this type of chemical is ingested
8. This calcium channel blocker is most frequently used for cocaine-induced coronary artery spasm (generic)
11. This device may be required for the bradycardia seen in beta-blocker or calcium channel blocker OD
13. This dissociative agent is associated with violent behavior (abbrev)
14. This radiologic procedure may be used to identify the presence of radiopaque agents (abbrev)
15. Antidotes for opiates (generic)
16. This complication of drug overdose is the result of excessive muscle rigidity
21. This type of blood screen is done to determine what drugs have been ingested
23. Type of antidepressant which may cause torsades de pointes, especially at toxic levels
25. Increased in stage 2 or 3 of acetaminophen overdose
27. This drug is used for malignant hyperthermia that occurs in some drug overdosages (generic)
28. Osmotic laxative added to first dose of activated charcoal if multiple doses are going to be used
29. This electrolyte is given for calcium channel blocker OD
30. Accidental exposure to a toxic substance
32. This type of syndrome may cause generalized seizures
33. This B vitamin must be given with dextrose to

malnourished patients to prevent Wernicke's encephalopathy
35. The affinity between hemoglobin and this substance is much greater than the affinity between hemoglobin and oxygen (2 words)
36. New antidote used for ethylene glycol toxicity (trade)
37. Usually intentional but may be inadvertent exposure to a toxic level of a substance
38. Known as the "hug drug"
45. This condition causes hypoxia and may be caused by nitrates, sulfa drugs, and local anesthetics
48. This antidote is given if digoxin level is greater than 10 ng/mL (trade)
50. This procedure is used to assess injury after ingestion of caustic agents
51. Drug used for the treatment of bradycardia (generic)
52. Pinpoint pupils
53. May be used intravenously in methanol or ethylene glycol intoxication

DOWN

1. This organ is most likely to be injured by acetaminophen overdose
2. This drug can stimulate the beta-receptors even in the presence of beta-blockade; used for beta-blocker OD
3. Toxicity of this drug causes nystagmus, tremors, ataxia, seizures, and nephrogenic diabetes insipidus (generic)
4. Carbon monoxide poisoning causes the skin to be very _____
6. This type of consult should always be requested for patients with drug overdosage
7. This therapy may be used to detoxify heavy metal poisoning
9. The greatest risk with ingestion of petroleum distillates
10. This antidote for benzodiazepines should not be given if the patient has coingested tricyclic antidepressants
12. Category of toxins that include aerosol propellants, paint thinner, glue
17. This blood cleansing procedure is more effective than hemodialysis for plasma protein bound drugs
18. Antidote for methemoglobinemia (generic and 2 words)
19. Dilated pupils
20. This type of behavior is a danger to staff; may occur with rapid reversion of sedating drugs
22. Antidote for acetaminophen (trade)
24. Procedure to flush the drug or toxin from the stomach; may be used if the patient arrives within 1 hour of ingestion for most substances
26. Adsorbent agent used in drug overdose
31. Drug intoxication in an attempt to get attention is referred to as a suicide _____
34. This "gap" is increased in alcohol intoxication
35. Hemoglobin saturated with carbon monoxide rather than oxygen
39. The drug most often involved in intentional and unintentional drug overdose in U.S.
40. This drug may cause necrosis and perforation of the nasal septum and may cause MI (generic)
41. This type of overdose causes metabolic acidosis and respiratory alkalosis
42. This toxin causes chemical asphyxia by interfering with cellular respiration
43. Blood cleansing procedure that may be used to remove some drugs or toxins from the blood
44. A coma cocktail consists of oxygen, _____, thiamine, and naloxone
46. Insecticides are frequently this type that causes cholinergic effect
47. Sedative-hypnotic toxidromes are usually caused by this type of drug
49. This complication requires airway maintenance and protection from injury

Behavioral/Psychosocial

CHAPTER 12

Physical Assessment and Examination

Chief Complaint
Identify chief complaint.

History of Present Illness
Identify current symptoms.

Current Medications
Include dose, type, how long the medication has been ordered, time last taken, and any changes related to medication use. Identify current use/abuse of substances including prescribed, over-the-counter, alcohol, and other drugs.

Past Medical History
1. Previous illnesses or injuries
2. Previous hospitalizations
3. Review of body systems
4. Allergies

Social History
1. Family structure: Identify who makes or influences health care decisions.
2. Substance abuse history
3. Support system: These are the individuals who are in regular contact with the patient, and may include immediate or extended family or friends.
4. Educational level
5. Responsibilities: This may include job, financial, spouse, parents, children, and pets.
6. Major family traumas

Mental Status Exam
1. Presentation
    a. Dress (e.g., is it clean, age appropriate, fit, and appropriate for the season)
    b. Eye contact (consistent, intermittent, poor)
    c. General appearance (e.g., hygiene and grooming)
    d. Motor activity (purposeful, restless, tremulous, cooperative)
2. Affect: the emotion that the patient demonstrates
    a. Anxious, worried
    b. Flat: demonstrates no emotion
    c. Inappropriate: Emotions demonstrated are not consistent with the situation or maturity.
    d. Labile: Emotions demonstrated fluctuate high to low rapidly and inconsistently without respect to the situation.
    e. Guarded: appears wary or overly cautious in conversation
    f. Normal: emotions consistent with the situation and conversation
3. Mood: the emotion that the patient reports
    a. Hostile
    b. Depressed
    c. Elated
    d. Anxious
    e. Agitated
4. Speech
    a. Pressured: rapid, forced speech
    b. Slurred
    c. Loud
    d. Soft
    e. Patterns
    f. Idiosyncrasies
5. Thought processes
    a. Blocking: cessation in the flow of thought or speech
    b. Flight of ideas: leap from one idea to another, distracted from thoughts and speech by things in the environment
    c. Looseness of association: no logical connection between sentences
    d. Circumstantial: thoughts or speech that contains excessive details about the topic but finally reaches the intended point
    e. Tangential: thoughts that are logical and directed that may be related to the topic but take off in a different direction and do not address the question or specific topic
6. Thought content
    a. Suspicious
    b. Hopeless
    c. Guilty

d. Delusion: persistent belief or perception held by a person despite evidence to the contrary; examples include the following:
    1) Being controlled
    2) Grandeur
    3) Persecution
    4) Nihilistic
    5) Somatic
e. Ideation (thought): Assess for any distortion of thought in addition to thoughts or plan of suicide or homicide; bringing up this topic will not cause the patient to have these thoughts.

7. Perceptual disturbances
    a. Hallucinations: sensory perceptions that do not result from an external stimulus and occur in an awake state
        1) Normal hallucinations
            a) Hypnagogic: associated with the semiconsciousness immediately preceding sleep
            b) Hypnopompic: associated with the semiconsciousness preceding waking
        2) Abnormal hallucinations (Table 12-1)
    b. Illusion: a false interpretation of an external sensory stimulus (e.g., a coat hanging over a chair is perceived as a person sitting there)
8. Cognition
    a. Orientation: person, place, time, and situation
    b. Memory
        1) Immediate: minutes
        2) Short term: hours to days
        3) Long term: weeks to years
    c. Intelligence: cognitive ability
    d. Concentration: the ability to focus and pay attention
    e. Judgment: the ability to make sound decisions
    f. Insight: the understanding one has of the current situation
9. Diagnostic studies to rule out medical conditions and/or substance abuse
    a. CBC
    b. Hemoglobin
    c. Hematocrit
    d. Thyroid panel
    e. Liver and renal function
    f. Drug toxicology
    g. Pregnancy exam for women 10-50 years old
    h. Urinalysis

Table 12-1 Types of Abnormal Hallucinations

Type	Perception of:
Auditory	Voices or other sounds
Visual	Images
Gustatory	Taste
Tactile	Touch
Olfactory	Odors
Kinesthetic	Bodily movement
Somatic	Something occurring within one's own body

Psychosocial Characteristics (Erikson, 1968)

Young Adulthood (18-40 Years of Age)

1. Intimacy versus self-isolation or self-absorption
2. Developmental tasks
    a. Accepts self
    b. Establishes independence
    c. Establishes a vocation to make worthwhile contributions
    d. Learns to appraise and express love responsibly
    e. Establishes intimate bond with another
    f. Establishes and manages residence
    g. Finds congenial social group
    h. Decides on option of a family
    i. Formulates philosophy of life
    j. Establishes role in community

Middle Adulthood (40-60 Years of Age)

1. Generativity versus self-absorption and stagnation
2. Developmental tasks
    a. Develops new satisfaction as a mate
    b. Supportive to mate
    c. Develops sense of unity with mate
    d. Assists offspring to become happy, responsible adults
    e. Takes pride in accomplishments of self and mate
    f. Balances work with other roles; assists aging parents
    g. Achieves social and civic responsibility
    h. Maintains active organizational membership
    i. Accepts physical changes of middle age
    j. Makes an art of friendship
    k. Balances leisure with service pursuits
    l. Develops more depth of personal philosophy by reevaluating values and examining assets

Older Adulthood (60 Years of Age to Death)

1. Integrity versus despair
2. Developmental tasks
    a. Continued self-development
    b. Adapts to family responsibilities
    c. Maintains self-worth, pride, and usefulness
    d. Deals with loss of spouse, friends, upcoming end to life

Basic Human Needs

Basic needs may be the same, but the manner in which they are fulfilled depends on personal abilities, environment, and life experience.

Maslow's Hierarchy of Needs

Progressive; primary needs must be met before dealing with higher-level needs (Table 12-2).

Human Needs of the Critically Ill Patient

See Figure 12-1.

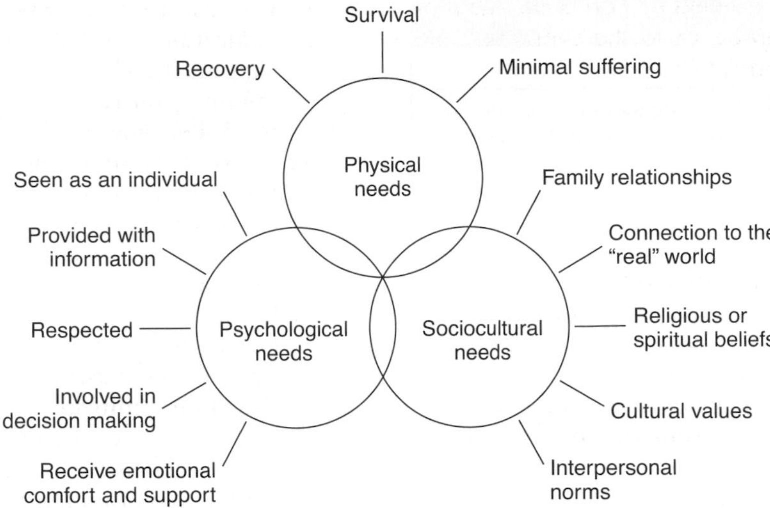

Figure 12-1 Human needs of the critically ill patient. (From Kinney, M. et al. [1998]. *AACN's clinical reference for critical care nursing* [4th ed.]. St. Louis: Mosby.)

Table 12-2 Maslow's Hierarchy of Needs

Physiologic	Oxygen, food, water, and sleep
Safety and security	Protection and freedom from anxiety
Love and belonging	Freedom from loneliness and alienation
Esteem and recognition	Freedom from a sense of worthlessness, inferiority, and helplessness
Self-actualization	Aesthetic needs, self-fulfillment, creativity, and spirituality

From Maslow, A. (1968). *Toward a psychology of being* (2nd ed.). Princeton, MA: Van Nostrand.

Box 12-1 Potential Stressors in the Critical Care Setting

Threat of death
Threat of disability
Threat of body image alteration
Pain or discomfort
Separation from family and loved ones
Loss of usual role in family, community, workplace
Loss of autonomy
Loss of privacy and/or dignity
Powerlessness and loss of control over environment
Sleep disturbances
Sensory overload
Sensory deprivation
Inability to communicate (if aphasic or intubated)

Adapted from Urden, L., Stacy, K., & Lough, M. (2010). *Critical care nursing: Diagnosis and management* (6th ed.). St. Louis: Mosby.

Responses to Illness and Environment

Stress

1. Definition: mental, emotional, or physical tension or strain
2. Stressors in the critical care setting (Box 12-1)
   a. Distress: stress as a result of noxious stimuli
   b. Eustress: stress as a result of nonthreatening stimuli
3. Admission to a critical care unit is frightening and anxiety producing.
4. Sensory deprivation and sensory overload are stress factors within a critical care unit.
5. Interventions to decrease or eliminate stress
   a. Maintain a calm, restful environment.
   b. Provide for as much independence of the patient as possible.
   c. Provide contact with reality and outside world.
   d. Encourage use of coping mechanisms (Table 12-3 and Table 12-4).

Table 12-3 Coping Mechanisms for Stress

Type	Example
Action	Taking walks, cleaning house, gardening, singing
Cognitive	Problem solving, reading about issue
Spiritual	Prayer
Interpersonal	Talking with support person
Emotional	Use of psychological defense mechanisms (Table 12-4)

Anxiety

See Anxiety Section.

Loneliness

1. Definition: discomfort caused by separation from significant relationships, places, events, and objects
2. Manifestations may include crying and withdrawal.

Table 12-4 Psychological Defense Mechanisms

Defense Mechanism	Description
Suppression	Conscious, deliberate forgetting of unacceptable or painful thoughts, impulses, feelings, or acts
Repression	Unconscious, involuntary forgetting of unacceptable or painful thoughts, impulses, feelings, or acts
Denial	Treating obvious reality factors as though they do not exist because they are consciously intolerable
Rationalization	Attempting to justify feelings, behavior, and motives that would otherwise be intolerable, by offering a socially acceptable, intellectual, and apparently logical explanation for an act or decision
Compensation	Making extra effort to achieve in one area to offset real or imagined deficiencies in another area
Sublimation	Directing energy from unacceptable drives into socially acceptable behavior
Projection	Unconsciously attributing one's own unacceptable qualities and emotions to others
Regression	Going back to an earlier level of emotional development and organization
Withdrawal	Separating oneself from interpersonal relationships in order to avoid emotional expression or responsiveness

3. Interventions to decrease loneliness
   a. Encourage participation in decision making and self-care.
   b. Encourage discussion of fears and asking of questions.
   c. Encourage the patient to talk about his or her life, family, work, or pet.
   d. Ask the family to bring in familiar and loved objects.

Powerlessness
1. Definition: a perceived lack of control over the outcome of a specific situation or problem and the patient's perception that any action he or she takes will not affect the outcome
2. May be manifested by apathy, withdrawal, resignation, fatalism, lack of decision making, aggression, or anger
3. Interventions to decrease feelings of powerlessness
   a. Recognize the potential for feelings of powerlessness; particularly at risk are individuals who usually are in a position of power or control in their daily life.
   b. Support the patient's sense of control by offering alternatives related to activity times, treatment times, diet, routine hygiene, diversionary activities, and visitation.
   c. Assist the patient in identifying activities that he or she can perform independently.
   d. Keep the patient informed about his or her treatment.
   e. Encourage the patient's involvement in decision making related to treatment.
   f. Increase the patient's control as his or her condition improves.

Sensory Overload
1. Definition: increased frequency and intensity of stimulation of the senses with nonmeaningful stimuli
2. Contributing factors: constant noise and lights, alarms, chatter of unfamiliar voices
3. Intervention: Eliminate or limit nonmeaningful sensory stimulation.

Sensory Deprivation
1. Definition: decreased frequency, intensity, or variety of stimulation of the senses with meaningful stimuli
2. Contributing factors: absence of windows, clocks, and calendars; constant noise, lights, technical language, and lack of familiar faces; deprivation of familiar touches, sounds, smells, and tastes of their usual environment
3. Interventions
   a. Encourage family visitation.
   b. Encourage the family to bring familiar objects to the hospital.
   c. Place calendar and clock where the patient can see them.

Anger
1. Definition: feeling of great displeasure, hostility, and exasperation
2. May be manifested by clenching of teeth or muscles, avoidance of eye contact, sarcasm, insulting comments, screaming, argumentativeness, and demanding behavior
3. Interventions to decrease feelings of anger
   a. Assist in identifying the cause of anger.
   b. Give the patient permission to be angry.
   c. Assist the patient in identifying appropriate ways to express the anger.

Depression
1. Definition: feeling of sadness and hopelessness
2. May be manifested by loss of interest in people, dissatisfaction, difficulty making decisions, and crying; patient may say that he or she is a failure, being punished, or is considering hurting himself or herself
3. Interventions to decrease feelings of depression

a. Provide information necessary to identify the patient's needs and to realistically visualize the future.
b. Inspire hope and facilitate coping.

Denial

1. Definition: refusal to acknowledge the truth; allows the patient to come to grips with reality a little at a time
2. Denial may be manifested by shrugging off symptoms, refusing to discuss the illness, appearing cheerful, and verbalizing the illness while ignoring restrictions.
3. Interventions
   a. Allow the patient to express his or her feelings.
   b. Do not confront the patient with the truth.

Near-Death Experience (NDE)

1. Definition: a vivid series of events reported by some individuals after periods of clinical death
2. Manifestations may include the following events:
   a. Time interval without feeling
   b. Separation of mind and body
   c. Propulsion through space or a long, dark tunnel
   d. Interaction with a bright light
   e. Meeting an escort (often a decreased family member or friend) who accompanies the patient to a warm, peaceful, bright area
   f. Experiencing a life review
   g. The choice of whether to go back or being told to go back
   h. Return to the body
3. Interventions
   a. Be alert for indications that the patient has had a NDE, especially if the patient has experienced cardiac arrest, electrophysiologic studies, or any life-threatening crisis; the patient may do any of the following:
   b. Say, "I had the strangest dream," or something similar.
   c. Be angry, withdrawn, or unusually calm.
   d. Provide the patient with an opportunity to discuss the experience, such as, "Did anything happen when you were very sick yesterday that you want to talk about?"
   e. Explore your own feelings about NDE.
   f. Listen to the patient and avoid judgment.
   g. Reassure the patient who has a NDE that he or she is not "crazy" and that many persons have had this experience.
   h. Refer the patient to books to read or a support group if available.

General Principles of Care

1. Focus on initial signs and symptoms, methods of assessment for specific disorders, principles of safe care and pharmacologic agents appropriate to the presentation
2. Emergency personnel are frequently confronted by individuals or families who appear out of control, in a state of extreme distress, confused, or numb.
3. It is the job of the clinician to assess the reason behind the distress, diagnose any accompanying disorders, treat effectively, and release, refer, or hospitalize the person for additional care.

Therapeutic Milieu

1. An environment where the focus is designed to heal
   a. Healthy social interactions
   b. Respect for all persons
   c. Recognition of patient's rights
   d. Freedom of speech
   e. Sense of support
   f. Honesty in interactions
2. Staff responsibilities
   a. Adhere to schedules.
   b. Maintain safety at all times.
   c. Focus interactions and activities on growth and understanding.
   d. Encourage responsibility; allow the patient to do for self as much as possible.
   e. Inform patient of all changes.
   f. Incorporate patients in the government of environment.
3. Ethical care
   a. Fundamental concept used in making decisions for patient care
      1) Each patient must be treated equal and fair with respect to patient dignity.
      2) Provide no harm (i.e., nonmalfeasance) and do what is in the patient's best interest (i.e., beneficence).
      3) Be honest with the patient and build a trusting relationship.
      4) Impartial treatment of all patients (i.e., justice)
      5) Patients have the independence and freedom to select their treatment (i.e., autonomy).
   b. Patients with a psychiatric emergency have the same rights as other patients to make decisions; it is the health care provider's responsibility to intervene in the freedom of decision making if the patient's safety is at risk (Hamilton, 2007). Short-acting medications can be administered against the patient's will only if the patient is posing an imminent risk to self or others.
   c. Care should be provided in accordance with the provider's standards of care as defined on a state-by-state basis.
4. Confidentiality
   a. Health care agencies and providers must provide confidentiality and privacy of an individual's health care information that is collected and maintained; only those needing the information to provide further care are permitted access.
   b. Health Insurance Portability and Accountability Act (HIPAA) of 1996
      1) Protects the privacy of an individual's identifiable health information and identifiable information

   2) Requirements must be followed by each institution.
5. Civil rights
   a. Civil rights protect an individual from unfair treatment or discrimination because of race, color, national origin, disability, age, gender, or religion.
   b. Civil rights laws ensure that everyone has equal access to and opportunity to participate in certain health care and human services programs without facing unlawful discrimination.
   c. Patients with mental illness have the same patient rights as any other patient.
   d. Hospitalization of the Mentally Ill Act of 1964: All patients in public or private hospitals have a right to treatment (Hamilton, 2007).

Crisis

1. Definition: a state that occurs when one's usual ways of coping are inadequate to deal with the stress (Caplan, 1970)
   a. Involves an attempt to regain equilibrium
   b. Self-limited and allows for growth
2. Types of crises
   a. Situational crises
      1) Occurs suddenly
      2) Can be devastating
      3) Is not part of normal development
         a) Motor vehicle collisions
         b) Acts of nature such as a tornado or flood
         c) Sexual assault
         d) Robbery
         e) Legal difficulties
         f) Separation or divorce
         g) Unemployment
         h) Terminal illness diagnosis
   b. Maturational crises
      1) Occurs over time
      2) Recognized as common and occurs as part of normal development such as:
         a) Pregnancy
         b) Childbirth
         c) Adolescence
         d) Leaving home
         e) Marriage
         f) Midlife events
         g) Aging
         h) Death
3. Stages
   a. Shock and disbelief
   b. Disorganization: may be demanding, irrational, angry
   c. Reorganization: difficulty making decisions, forced to confront critical questions
   d. Resolution
4. Clinical indications of crisis
   a. Crying, screaming
   b. Angry, pacing, hitting out at others
   c. Silent, unresponsive to questions, appears in shock
5. Crisis intervention
   a. Alleviate crisis state.
      1) Many will abate over time without interventions.
      2) Problem-solving techniques for others
      3) End result is to return person to precrisis functioning.
   b. Utilize interventions that have been shown to be helpful.
      1) Listen to the patient's story.
      2) Offer empathy.
      3) Ask about attempts to cope.
         a) Identify coping behaviors that have been successful in the past.
         b) Identify current attempts to cope, such as friends, family, prayer, crying, substance use or abuse.
         c) Suicidal thoughts or plans
      4) Aid the patient in organization of the next few hours or days.
      5) Ensure that basic needs, such as safety, nutrition and sleep, are being met.
      6) Connect the patient to support services or family support.

Anxiety Disorders

Definition/Description

1. Anxiety: a state of uneasiness, apprehension, and worry
   a. Subjective experience that differs from one individual to another
   b. Both physiologic and psychological components
   c. Person often does not know cause
   d. Unpleasant emotional state with increased feelings of tension and helplessness
2. Types of anxiety disorders include the following:
   a. Panic disorder: sudden-onset anxiety in the form of fear and panic (i.e., panic attack)
   b. Phobia: irrational or illogical fear of an object, situation, or event
   c. Obsessive-compulsive disorder (OCD): recurrent, persistent, intrusive thoughts and feelings (obsessions), coupled with behaviors that are ritualistic and repetitive (compulsions)
   d. Posttrauma stress disorder (PTSD): persistent or repeated reexperiencing of a traumatic event that has occurred in the past through thoughts and memories that induce an anxiety response
   e. Substance-induced anxiety disorder: anxiety symptoms that develop with substance withdrawal or within a month of substance-abuse cessation

Predisposing Factors

1. Genetic predisposition
2. Preexisting diseases
   a. Physical: hyperthyroidism, hyperparathyroidism, pheochromocytoma, vestibular disorders,

seizure disorders, arrhythmias, and other cardiac disorders
   b. Psychological: major depressive disorder
3. Developmental causes
   a. Children: separation from parents, perceived loss of love
   b. Adolescents: peer pressure related to appearance, substance abuse, pressure to achieve, puberty
   c. Adults: life changes such as marriage, divorce, childbirth, menopause, career pressures, loss of parents
   d. Older adult: loss of spouse, significant other, or friends; diminished independence and health
   e. Exposure to high levels of stress over time
   f. Sleep deprivation
   g. Acute changes in health status
   h. Related to substance use: This may include CNS stimulants (i.e., cocaine, amphetamine, and caffeine) and withdrawal from CNS depressants (i.e., alcohol and barbiturates).
   i. Trauma

Pathophysiology (Yates, 2009)

1. Not well understood
2. Thought to be caused by a disruption of modulator within the central nervous system (CNS)
3. Several neurotransmitter systems are thought to be involved.
   a. Serotonin
   b. Norepinephrine
   c. Gamma-aminobutyric acid (GABA)
   d. Peptides
   e. Corticotropin
4. Autonomic nervous system mediates the majority of the symptoms.

Clinical Presentation

1. Subjective
   a. May have history of:
      1) Excessive anxiety or worry for more than 6 months
      2) Inability to control feelings
      3) Three or more of the following symptoms:
         a) Restlessness, keyed up
         b) Fatigue
         c) Difficulty concentrating
         d) Irritability
         e) Muscle tension
         f) Sleep disturbances: difficulty falling or staying asleep, not rested
         g) Sexual problems
      4) Apprehensive, fearfulness, helplessness
      5) Tightness in chest, shortness of breath
      6) Dizziness
      7) Choking feeling
2. Objective
   a. Tachycardia, tachypnea, may have elevated BP
   b. Pallor
   c. Tremors
   d. Dilated pupils, nystagmus
3. Diagnostic
   a. Serum blood and urine drug screen as indicated
   b. ECG: may show dysrhythmias, particularly sinus tachycardia, PACs, PVCs
   c. Other diagnostic studies to rule out medical conditions

Collaborative Management

1. Maintain airway, breathing, and ventilation.
   a. Oxygen by nasal cannula at 2-6 L/min if indicated to maintain SpO_2 of 95% unless contraindicated; in patients with COPD, use pulse oximetry to guide oxygen administration to SpO_2 of ~90%
   b. IV access for fluid and medication administration if indicated
2. Provide a safe, quiet environment.
   a. Decrease stimulation by providing a quiet, darkened room.
   b. Assess psychiatric status, especially suicidal ideation and agitation level.
   c. Ensure continuous observation.
3. Establish a trusting relationship.
   a. Maintain a calm manner when approaching the patient.
   b. Acknowledge patient's feelings and fears.
   c. Use a calm tone, speak clearly and distinctly.
   d. Maintain eye contact when speaking with the patient.
   e. Communicate honestly.
   f. Assist in problem solving.
4. Reduce anxiety.
   a. Anxiolytics as directed (e.g., diazepam [Valium], lorazepam [Ativan], chlordiazepoxide [Librium])
   b. Benzodiazepines are synergistic with alcohol, so assess for recent alcohol usage.
   c. Beta-blockers may also be prescribed.
   d. Antidepressants as prescribed
5. Monitor for complications.
   a. Dysrhythmias
   b. Suicide
   c. Paradoxical reaction to medications, particularly benzodiazepines.

Trauma/Violence/Abuse

Definition

1. Injury caused by violence, accidental injuries, or criminal activity
2. Abuse: mistreatment of another (can be physical, mental, or emotional)
3. Neglect: lack of care for physical, mental, or emotional well-being.
4. Sexual assault

Predisposing Factors

1. Substance abuse
2. Stress reactions
3. Inability to cope
4. Direct intent to injure (i.e., assault)
5. History of trauma, violence or abuse

Clinical Presentation
1. Subjective: Utilize collaborative information provided by family, friends, and significant others.
   a. Pain related to injury
   b. Extreme emotional distress
      1) May be unable to report symptoms
      2) Injury and history of incident may not seem to match.
      3) Inconsistency with the report of what happened prior to coming into the ED or changes in the story
2. Objective
   a. Sudden unexpected physical or emotional injury
      1) Injury can be obvious or not obvious.
   b. Clinical presentation related to location and severity of injury
   c. Bruises in various stages may indicate physical abuse.
   d. Injury with identifiable pattern (e.g., cigarette burn)
3. Diagnostic
   a. Serum: tests to rule out medical concerns
   b. Forensic testing as indicated (e.g., DNA)
   c. Evidence collection following chain of evidence if associated with a crime; photos as indicated
   d. Radiographic films of injured areas; radiographic films that show old fractures may indicate abuse
   e. CT scans as indicated; noncontrast head CT if hemorrhage suspected
   f. Other diagnostic studies to rule out other causes

Age-Related Considerations
1. Adult (likely causes): gunshot wounds, lacerations, fractures, rape, penetrating injuries, domestic violence, single car collision.
2. Elder (likely causes): fractures, nutritional deficits, domestic violence, self-injuries, neglect

Collaborative Management
1. Maintain airway, breathing, and ventilation.
   a. Oxygen by nasal cannula at 2-6 L/min if indicated to maintain SpO_2 of 95% unless contraindicated; in patients with COPD, use pulse oximetry to guide oxygen administration to SpO_2 of ~90%
   b. Artificial airway and mechanical ventilation may be necessary, depending on severity of injury.
   c. IV access for fluid and medication administration if indicated
2. Ensure patient safety.
   a. Assessment of psychiatric status, especially suicidal ideation
   b. Clothing and other personal articles must be secured as a protection of chain of evidence if there are potential legal ramifications.
      1) Be aware of duty-to-protect regulations for health care providers.
   c. Notification of authorities if abuse/neglect suspected
   d. Maintenance of safe environment for patient
   e. Protection against unwanted visitors or potential abusers who may attempt to control care
   f. Documentation of what patient reports using exact quotes
3. Relieve pain and discomfort.
   a. Position of comfort
   b. Analgesics
   c. Complementary therapies such as heat and cold
4. Prepare patient and assist with procedures as indicated by type, location, and severity of injury.
   a. Determination of what the patient wishes if able to comprehend situation
5. Monitor for complications: dependent upon type, location, and severity of injury
   a. Homicide
   b. Suicide

Antisocial Personality
Definition/Description
1. An adult (18 years of age and older) with a childhood history of conduct disorder
2. Pervasive disregard for and violation of the rights of others
3. Exhibits three or more of the following:
   a. Unlawful behavior resulting in potential for or history of arrests
   b. Deceitfulness/lying
   c. Impulsive/restless
   d. Irritable/aggressive
   e. Irresponsibility/blame
   f. Lack of remorse
   g. Callous/arrogant/disregard for others
4. Not due to schizophrenia or mania (DSM-IV-TR) (APA, 2000)

Predisposing Factors
1. Gender: Both, although predominately female
2. Familial: Biological relatives of females with the disorder
3. Somatization disorders
4. Substance-related disorders
5. Risks
   a. More likely than the general population to die prematurely by violence (suicide/homicide/accidents) (APA, 2000)
   b. Harm to self or others
   c. Unit/staff/milieu disruption: These individuals may pit staff members against each other and/or create chaos on the unit.

Collaborative Management
1. Ensure therapeutic milieu.
   a. Use a calm, nonjudgmental approach.
   b. Maintain therapeutic relational boundaries.
   c. Clearly explain and consistently enforce rules and behavioral expectations.
   d. Clearly communicate plan of care with patient.
   e. Establish communication within the health care team so that patient issues, concerns, and

progress are clearly communicated with each other and that a consistent approach is used.
2. Maintain a safe environment for patient, other patients, staff, and visitors.
   a. Assessment of psychiatric status, especially suicidal ideation
   b. Removal of any object that can be used for harm

Dementia

Definition

1. A chronic global deterioration of cognitive functioning. (Table 12-5)
2. Results from a disorder of the brain or an organic disease
3. May be accompanied by personality, behavioral, emotional, and functional change
4. Chronic or progressive in nature

Predisposing Factors

1. Aging
2. Cerebrovascular disease
3. Brain tumors
4. Alzheimer's disease
5. Hypothyroidism
6. Hypercalcemia
7. Neurosyphilis
8. HIV infection
9. Substance abuse
10. Normal-pressure hydrocephalus
11. Subdural hematoma
12. Deficiency in any of the following:
    a. Folic acid
    b. Vitamin B_{12}
    c. Niacin

Table 12-5 Delirium versus Dementia

	Delirium	Dementia
Onset	Rapid: hours to days	Gradual: months to years
Orientation	Impaired	Impaired
Memory	Impaired: short-term and remote	Predominantly short-term memory impaired; remote memory stays intact
Level of consciousness	Disturbed, often fluctuates over 24-hour period	Alert, steady
Sleep/wake cycle	Erratic, disturbed over the course of the day, no patterns	No acute change; however, day/night reversal is common over time
Etiology	Evidence of general medical condition, trauma, substance use/withdrawal, or toxin	No evidence of medical illness, trauma, substance use/withdrawal, or toxin to account for changes
EEG	Diffuse slowing	Slowing may occur
Duration	Brief (if effectively treated)	Chronic
Symptoms	Fluctuate over 24 hours	Consistent pattern
Sensory/perception	Hallucinations common	Misidentification, delusions

Pathophysiology

1. Dependent upon etiology
2. A chronic global deterioration of cognition
3. Cognitive malfunctioning preceded by deterioration in the following:
   a. Emotional control
   b. Social behavior
   c. Motivation
4. Cognitive malfunctioning in the following:
   a. Memory
   b. Intellect
   c. Learning
   d. Orientation
   e. Comprehension
   f. Calculation
   g. Language
   h. Judgment

Clinical Presentation

1. Subjective
   a. Memory loss
   b. Confusion
   c. Decline in cognitive functioning and judgment
2. Objective
   a. Lack of orientation to situation, time, place, and person
   b. Aphasia
   c. Apraxia
   d. Agnosia
   e. Behavioral disturbances
   f. Shallow to flat affect
   g. Focal neurologic signs
      1) Exaggeration of deep tendon reflexes
      2) Extensor plantar response
      3) Pseudobulbar palsy
      4) Gait abnormalities
      5) Weakness of an extremity
3. Diagnostic
   a. Mini mental status exam (Folstein, Folstein, & McHugh, 1975)
   b. Other diagnostic studies to rule out other causes

Collaborative Management

1. Maintain airway, breathing, and ventilation.
   a. Oxygen by nasal cannula at 2-6 L/min if indicated to maintain SpO_2 of 95% unless contraindicated; in patients with COPD, use pulse oximetry to guide oxygen administration to SpO_2 of ~90%
   b. IV access for fluid and medication administration if indicated

2. Provide safe environment.
   a. Assessment of psychiatric status, especially suicidal ideation and sensory status, such as hearing and visual deficits
   b. Quiet room with minimal stimulation, which allows continuous observation
   c. Use of patient's name during conversation
   d. Conversations should be kept simple and short
   e. Frequent reorientation to person and place
   f. Determination of additional information to ensure safety
      1) Interview family for additional information.
      2) Evaluate risk for making unsafe decisions.
      3) Evaluate potential for wandering and falling.
   g. Restraints should be avoided if possible but may be required to ensure patient safety.
3. Monitor for complications.
   a. Violence
   b. Falls
   c. Decreased awareness of environment
   d. Decreased self-care

Delirium

Definition/Description

1. An acute change (hours to days) in consciousness and cognition not due to dementia (see Table 12-5)
2. May result from or be related to: a general medical condition (trauma, infection); use/abuse of or withdrawal from a prescribed, illegal, or over-the-counter substance; exposure to a toxin; or a combination of these.
3. May be accompanied by personality, behavioral, emotional, and functional change
4. Acute and fluctuating in nature

Predisposing/Risk Factors

1. Age: Children and the elderly are more susceptible to delirium.
2. Gender: males at higher risk.
3. History of delirium
4. Existing dementia

Pathophysiology

1. Dependent upon etiology
2. An acute (hours to days) deterioration of cognition with fluctuating level of awareness
3. Prodromal symptoms:
   a. Emotional: anxiety, irritability
   b. Behavioral: restlessness
   c. Cognition: disorientation
   d. Sleep/wake cycle disturbance
4. Cognitive malfunctioning in the following:
   a. Memory
   b. Intellect
   c. Learning
   d. Orientation
   e. Comprehension
   f. Calculation
   g. Language
   h. Judgment

Clinical Presentation

1. Subjective
   a. Memory loss
   b. Confusion
   c. Decline in cognitive functioning, judgment
2. Objective
   a. Lack of orientation to situation, time, place, and person
   b. Behavioral disturbances
   c. Functional decline
   d. Progression if underlying etiology not effectively treated: stupor, coma, seizures, death
3. Diagnostic
   a. Mini mental status exam (Folstein, Folstein, & McHugh, 1975)
   b. Diagnostic studies to determine cause of delirium

Collaborative Management

1. Maintain airway, breathing, and ventilation.
   a. Oxygen by nasal cannula at 2-6 L/min if indicated to maintain SpO_2 of 95% unless contraindicated; in patients with COPD, use pulse oximetry to guide oxygen administration to SpO_2 of ~90%
   b. IV access for fluid and medication administration if indicated
2. Provide safe environment.
   a. Quiet room with minimal stimulation, which allows continuous observation
   b. Use of patient's name during conversation
   c. Conversations should be kept simple and short.
   d. Frequent reorientation to person, place, time and situation.
   e. Determination of additional information to ensure safety
      1) Interview family for additional information.
      2) Presence of familiar persons may be calming and helpful.
      3) Evaluate risk for making unsafe decisions.
      4) Evaluate potential for falling.
   f. Restraints should be avoided if possible but may be required to ensure patient safety.
3. Monitor for complications.
   a. Violence
   b. Falls
   c. Decreased awareness of environment
   d. Decreased self-care (e.g., feeding, toileting, hygiene)

ICU Delirium

Definition

1. Confusion or psychosis associated with the critical care environment
2. Also called ICU psychosis, postcardiotomy delirium, postoperative psychosis, intensive care delirium, acute confusion, and impaired psychological response
3. Usually occurs after 48 hours in the critical care unit; usually clears within 48 hours after transfer from the critical care unit

Contributing Factors

1. Sleep deprivation
2. Sensory deprivation
3. Sensory overload
4. Age
5. Severe illness
6. History of mental illness or psychological problems
7. Noise
8. Isolation
9. Immobilization
10. Cardiopulmonary bypass
11. Prolonged surgery
12. Electrolyte imbalance
13. Hypothermia
14. Endocrine disorders
15. Medications especially corticosteroids

Clinical Presentation

1. Altered consciousness
2. Decreased attention span
3. Disorientation, confusion
4. Memory loss
5. Labile emotions
6. Perceptual distortions such as hallucinations, paranoia
7. Combativeness

Collaborative Management

1. Eliminate possible causes.
    a. Plan uninterrupted sleep time; do not awaken the patient unless truly necessary.
        1) In a study by Tamburri, DiBrienza, Zozula, and Redeker (2004), the mean number of care interactions per night was 42.6, and patient had 2-3 hours of uninterrupted sleep on only 6% of the nights observed.
    b. Provide continuity of nursing staff to lessen the number of adjustments required by the patient.
    c. Reorient the patient frequently.
    d. Decrease noise level on alarms, and decrease extraneous conversation and other noise; earplugs may also be used.
        1) The Environmental Protection Agency (EPA) (1974) recommends that daytime noise levels in a hospital not exceed 45 dB and that nighttime levels not exceed 35 dB.
    e. Adjust lighting to simulate night and day, and maintain sleep-wake cycles while allowing for short naps throughout the day.
2. Provide frequent reorientation.
    a. Place a clock and calendar in the room.
    b. Encourage the family to visit and reorient the patient.
    c. Encourage placement of personal belongings at bedside.

Failure to Thrive (FTT)

Definition

1. A syndrome manifested by physiologic, psychological, and functional decline that can be seen in individuals of all ages, although more commonly seen in children and elderly populations; if untreated, it can lead to death; the discussion below is limited to the adult
2. Diagnosis by exclusion: rule out infection, malignancy, abscess, endocrine imbalance, malnutrition, dehydration, renal failure, electrolyte imbalance, and complications of polypharmacy

Predisposing Factors

1. Infection
2. Diminished cell-mediated immunity
3. Hip fractures (and other large bone fractures)
4. Decubitus ulcers
5. Abuse/neglect
6. Chronic progressive health problems
7. Medications associated with FTT
    a. Anticholinergic
    b. Antiepileptic
    c. Benzodiazepine
    d. Beta-blockers
    e. Central alpha antagonists
    f. Chronic steroid use
    g. Diuretics
    h. Glucocorticoids
    i. Neuroleptics
    j. Opioids
    k. Selective serotonin reuptake inhibitors (SSRIs)
    l. Tricyclic antidepressants
    m. More than four prescription medications
8. Medical conditions associated with FTT
    a. Cancer
    b. Chronic lung diseases
    c. Chronic mental illness
    d. Chronic progressive neurodegenerative diseases
    e. Chronic renal insufficiency
    f. Cirrhosis/hepatitis
    g. Heart failure
    h. Depression
    i. Dementia
    j. Diabetes
    k. Dysphagia
    l. Gastrointestinal surgery
    m. Hip fracture
    n. Inflammatory bowel disease
    o. Myocardial infarction
    p. Psychosis
    q. Recurrent infections (i.e., UTI, pneumonia)
    r. Rheumatologic disease
    s. Sepsis
    t. Stroke
    u. Tuberculosis

Pathophysiology

Dependent on the underlying physical condition

Clinical Presentation

1. Subjective
    a. History of impaired functional status
        1) Progressive functional decline
        2) Selective inactivity

3) Chronic bed rest
4) Social withdrawal/isolation
b. Depression
c. Socioeconomic factors: social network, relationships, family support, living situation, financial resources, abuse, neglect, recent loss
2. Objective
a. Malnutrition
1) Weight loss greater than 5% of baseline
2) Decreased appetite
b. Cognitive loss
c. Muscle weakness
3. Diagnostic
a. Serum
1) CBC
2) Electrolytes
3) BUN and creatinine
4) Glucose
5) Albumin
6) Lipid profile
7) Immune profile
8) C-reactive protein levels
9) Blood culture may be indicated
10) Thyroid-stimulating hormone level
b. Chest x-ray
c. MRI

Collaborative Management
1. Improve functional ability.
a. Utilize team approach: nurse, physician, dietitian, speech therapist, social worker, mental health specialist, and physical therapist.
b. Provide nutritional supplementation and support to meet energy and nutritional needs.
c. Facilitate high-intensity resistance exercise training.
d. Teach/provide appropriate adaptive techniques and devices.
e. Encourage the patient to participate in decision making and exercise control.
2. Treat identifiable illness and, wherever possible, choose interventions with the least risks or negative side effects.
3. Provide support and education for family and significant others.

Developmental Delays
Definition
A condition in which one's developmental age lags significantly behind one's chronological age; developmental delays are often seen in individuals with developmental disorders, including mental retardation, learning disorders, and pervasive developmental disorders

Predisposing Factors
1. Genetic
2. Chromosomal abnormality
3. Pregnancy and perinatal problems
4. Environmental: exposure to toxins, deprivation, abuse, neglect
5. Medical conditions or trauma in infancy/childhood
6. Unknown or undetermined cause or factors

Pathophysiology
Varies depending on the cause

Clinical Presentation
1. Mental retardation: diagnosis and onset of symptoms occur before age 18
a. Sub average general intellect (IQ) less than 70
1) Mild: IQ level 50-55 to 70
2) Moderate: IQ level 35-40 to 50-55
3) Severe: IQ level 20-25 to 35-40
4) Profound: IQ level less than 20-25
b. Functional limitation in two of the following: communication, self-care, home living, social/interpersonal skills, use of community resources, self-direction, functional academic skills, work, leisure, health and safety
2. Learning disorders: Academic achievement is significantly lower than expected for age, schooling, and level of intelligence.
3. Pervasive developmental disorders
a. These include autistic disorder, Asperger's disorder, childhood disintegrative disorder, and Rett's disorder.
b. Impairment in at least one of the following areas relative to the individual's developmental level or mental age: reciprocal social interaction skills, communication skills, or stereotyped behavior, interests and activities (APA, 2000)

Collaborative Management
1. Establish effective communication.
a. Ensure that conversations with the patient are consistent with the developmental functioning level of the patient.
b. Include the patient in conversations; avoid talking around, over, or above the patient's developmental functioning level.
c. Use appropriate pain assessment tools; the Wong-Baker FACES™ Pain Rating Scale or the Eland Color Scale may be used (Baldridge & Andrasik, 2010).
2. Involve patient, family, and other care providers in decision making.
a. Clearly explain all treatments and procedures prior to doing them; it may also be helpful to talk the patient through the procedure/treatment as you proceed.
b. Engage the family, friends, and care providers with whom the patient has a relationship in planning and providing care as appropriate. They often know the patient best, and are a great resource for approaches, communication strategies and techniques, and activities that are most successful with the patient.
3. Reduce anxiety and provide comfort.
a. Have familiar objects for comfort in acute settings; may include specific pictures, books, toys, or items of personal value

b. Provide simple structured tasks for the individual that create an opportunity for successful completion.
c. Monitor the level of stimulation and its impact on the patient; adjust accordingly.

Depression

Definition

Disturbance of mood associated with anhedonia (loss of interest/pleasure in usual activities) or an increase in sadness or negative thinking not associated with medication withdrawal, bereavement, or another medical condition.

Predisposing Factors

1. Genetic predisposition
2. Severe psychosocial stressors
3. Hormonal imbalance
4. Sudden increase or decrease in substance use
5. Medical conditions such as diabetes, myocardial infarction, carcinomas, or stroke
6. Medication side effects

Pathophysiology (Bhalla, Moraille-Bhalla, & Aronson, 2009)

1. Not well defined but thought to be a disturbance in CNS serotonin activity
2. Dysregulation of neurotransmitter system
3. Serotonin deficiency
4. Norepinephrine and dopamine are also thought to be involved.

Clinical Presentation

1. Subjective: symptoms last longer than 2 months
   a. Presence of depressed mood (irritability in a child or adolescent) or anhedonia (loss of interest or pleasure)
   b. Expressions of the following:
      1) Guilt, worthlessness, hopelessness
      2) Feelings of suicide
      3) Recurrent thoughts of death
   c. History of attempted suicide, thoughts or plans of suicide, or recurrent thoughts of death.
   d. Sleep disturbance: insomnia, hypersomnia, feeling unrested
   e. Low energy/fatigue
   f. Inability to concentrate
   g. Changes in appetite
   h. Weight loss/gain
   i. Decreased libido
   j. Amenorrhea
   k. Constipation
   l. Psychomotor symptoms
      1) Psychomotor agitation: restless, need to keep moving
      2) Psychomotor retardation: generalized slowing down of movements, physical reactions, and speech.
2. Objective
   a. Appearance indicative of poor hygiene, lack of concern regarding appearance
   b. Flat affect
   c. Tearful
   d. Quiet speech
   e. Little eye contact
   f. Psychomotor retardation
   g. Evidence of psychotic symptoms (i.e., hallucinations, delusions)
3. Diagnostic
   a. Serum blood and urine drug screen
   b. Serum alcohol
   c. Thyroid function test to rule out hypothyroidism
   d. CBC with differential to rule out anemia
   e. CT scan and possible MRI of the head to rule out medical cause

Collaborative Management

1. Maintain airway, breathing, and ventilation.
   a. Oxygen by nasal cannula at 2-6 L/min if indicated to maintain SpO_2 of 95% unless contraindicated; in patients with COPD, use pulse oximetry to guide oxygen administration to SpO_2 of ~90%
   b. IV access for fluid and medication administration if indicated
2. Provide safe environment.
   a. Assessment of psychiatric status especially suicidal ideation
   b. Quiet room with minimal stimulation, which allows continuous observation
   c. Nonjudgmental approach
   d. Frequent contacts to assure patient of staff concern
   e. If suicide is a concern, someone to stay with patient at all times
3. Assist with treatment of depression.
   a. Antidepressant therapy
   b. Counseling
   c. Electroconvulsant therapy
   d. Light therapy
   e. Transcranial magnetic stimulation
4. Monitor for complications.
   a. Violent behavior
   b. Suicide

Mania

Definitions

1. Mania: elevated, irritable, or expansive mood
   a. Episode of irritable or elevated mood lasting at least 1 week
   b. Marked impairment in functioning
   c. Symptoms are not due to substance or general medical condition
2. Bipolar: a combination of mood swings from mania to depression

Predisposing Factors

1. Genetic predisposition
2. Severe psychosocial stressors

3. Hormonal imbalance
4. Sudden decrease in substance use

Pathophysiology

Thought to involve the dysregulation of neurotransmitters

Clinical Presentation

1. Subjective
   a. History of manic or hypomanic episodes
   b. Racing thoughts
   c. Little need for sleep
   d. Increase in use of prescribed or illegal drugs to calm down
   e. Risky behaviors
   f. Abuse of credit cards and reckless spending
   g. Multiple sex partners
   h. Arrests
   i. Interference with job performance
   j. Unrealistic future plans
   k. Previous suicide attempts: past and current plans
2. Objective
   a. Fidgeting, pacing
   b. Difficulty staying on topic; flight of ideas
   c. Elation or euphoria; laughing
   d. Grandiosity
   e. May have injuries
3. Diagnostic
   a. Serum blood and urine drug screen
   b. Serum alcohol
   c. ECG: tachycardia, atrial dysrhythmias, PACs, PVCs
   d. Other diagnostic studies to rule out other causes

Collaborative Management

1. Maintain airway, breathing, and ventilation.
   a. Oxygen by nasal cannula at 2-6 L/min if indicated to maintain SpO_2 of 95% unless contraindicated; in patients with COPD, use pulse oximetry to guide oxygen administration to SpO_2 of ~90%
   b. IV access for fluid and medication administration if indicated
2. Provide safe environment.
   a. Assessment of psychiatric status especially suicidal ideation
   b. Quiet room with minimal stimulation, which allows continuous observation
   c. Nonjudgmental approach
   d. Restraints should be avoided if possible but may be required to ensure patient safety.
3. Control mania.
   a. Antipsychotics for psychosis, if present, until mood stabilizers take effect.
   b. Anticonvulsants for regulation of mood (helps stabilize mania and depression in bipolar)
   c. Antidepressants for depression
   d. Beta-blockers to block effects of catecholamines
   e. Counseling to deal with cycling of moods, behavior, and interpersonal relationships
4. Monitor for complications: self-injury or suicide.

Psychosis

Definition

1. A severe psychiatric disorder characterized by personality disorganization, loss of contact with reality, and deterioration of normal social functioning
2. Acute or chronic: lasting from a few days to several months
3. May be functional or organic

Predisposing Factors

1. Functional type: severe depression, mania, schizophrenic disorder, or brief psychotic episode
2. Organic type
   a. Ingestion of toxic substance
   b. Shock or trauma
   c. Dementia: slow onset
   d. Delirium: rapid onset

Pathophysiology

Poorly understood

Clinical Presentation

1. Subjective: may report any of the following:
   a. Previous history of psychotic episodes
   b. Confusion or amnesia
   c. Paranoid ideation
   d. Fears about safety
   e. Loss of energy
   f. Self-medication
2. Objective
   a. Positive symptoms
      1) Delusions
      2) Hallucinations: usually auditory
   b. Negative symptoms
      1) Avolition: inability to initiate activities (including self-care)
      2) Alogia: absence of speech
      3) Anhedonia: lack of pleasure
      4) Flat affect: absence of emotional responses
   c. Disorganized speech or incoherence
   d. Conversation shows confusion, loss of touch with reality, loss of orientation to time, place, and person
   e. Increased agitation or bizarre behavior
   f. Grossly exaggerated behaviors
   g. Psychomotor retardation (i.e., visible generalized slowing down of movements, physical reactions, and speech)
3. Diagnostic
   a. Urinalysis especially if person is elderly female
   b. Urine and serum drug screens
   c. CT scan if changes have been rapid
   d. Other diagnostic studies to rule out other causes

Collaborative Management

1. Maintain airway, breathing, and ventilation
   a. Oxygen by nasal cannula at 2-6 L/min if indicated to maintain SpO_2 of 95% unless contraindicated; in patients with COPD, use pulse oximetry to guide oxygen administration to SpO_2 of ~90%
   b. IV access for fluid and medication administration if indicated
2. Provide safe environment.
   a. Assessment of psychiatric status especially suicidal ideation
   b. Quiet room with minimal stimulation, which allows continuous observation.
   c. Nonjudgmental approach
   d. Conversations should be kept simple, short, reality based, and concrete.
   e. Acknowledgement of patient's delusion and/or hallucinations while maintaining reality (e.g., "I believe that you are hearing voices, but I do not hear them").
   f. Avoidance of arguing with patient about his or her experience; provide support for the feelings that may be generated (e.g., "It must be frightening to hear those voices.")
   g. Frequent reorientation to person, place, time and situation
   h. Restraints should be avoided if possible but may be required to ensure patient safety.
3. Assist with management of psychosis.
   a. Antipsychotic medications to reduce psychosis
   b. Anxiolytic medications may be used adjunctively with antipsychotic medications to reduce anxiety and/or induce sleep.
   c. Consult with the patient's current psychiatrist or refer to a psychiatrist if patient has not been previously treated for psychosis.
4. Monitor for complications.
   a. Extrapyramidal symptoms (EPS)
   b. Neuroleptic malignant syndrome
   c. Incontinence
   d. Coma

Substance Use Disorders

Definitions/Descriptions

1. Substance dependence: maladaptive pattern of substance use, leading to clinically significant impairment or distress as manifested by three or more of the following, occurring at any time in the same 12-month period (DSM TR diagnostic criteria)
   a. Tolerance
   b. Substance is taken in larger amounts or over a longer period than was intended.
   c. Persistent desire or unsuccessful efforts to cut down or control
   d. Much time spent in activities necessary to obtain the substance.
   e. Important social, occupational, or recreational activities are given up or reduced because of usage.
   f. Use is continued despite knowledge of physical or psychological problems caused by usage.
2. Substance abuse: pattern of continued substance use causing clinically significant impairment in one or more of the following areas, once or more in a 12-month period (APA, 2000).
   a. Failure to fulfill role obligations at work, home, or school
   b. Substance use in physically hazardous situations
   c. Substance-related legal problems
   d. Social or interpersonal problems related to the substance use

Predisposing Factors

1. Subjective
   a. Family history of substance abuse or dependence
   b. Inability to cope effectively
   c. Group modeling especially in adolescence
   d. Genetic predisposition
   e. Related history of usage
   f. History of request for help with addictions
   g. Report of emotional distress
2. Objective
   a. May be weeping
   b. Drug seeking behavior: a pattern of seeking a particular medication (e.g., narcotic pain medication or tranquilizers) without an organic basis; may demonstrate abusive or threatening behavior when denied drugs

Clinical Presentation

1. Subjective
   a. Self-report of use
   b. Family/friends report use.
   c. Request for help with addictions
   d. Emotionally distressed, weeping
2. Objective
   a. Person exhibits intoxication or erratic behavior including impaired judgment, aggression, mood lability.
   b. Speech can be slurred or rambling.
   c. Unsteady gait
   d. Nystagmus
   e. Impaired memory or attention
   f. Stupor or coma
3. Diagnostic: serum and urine drug screens

Collaborative Management

1. Maintain airway, breathing, and ventilation.
   a. Oxygen by nasal cannula at 2-6 L/min if indicated to maintain SpO_2 of 95% unless contraindicated; in patients with COPD, use pulse oximetry to guide oxygen administration to SpO_2 of ~90%
   b. IV access for fluid and medication administration if indicated
2. Provide safe environment.
   a. Assessment of psychiatric status especially suicidal ideation

b. Close monitoring for progression of symptoms; the Clinical Institute Withdrawal Assessment of Alcohol Scale (CIWA-Ar) is a widely accepted tool to facilitate assessing and treating alcohol withdrawal (Sullivan et al., 1989).
c. Quiet room with minimal stimulation, which allows continuous observation
d. Determination of suicidal ideation and/or plan for suicide
e. Restraints should be avoided if possible but may be required to ensure patient safety.
f. Prevent seizures: benzodiazepines as prescribed.

3. Monitor for complications.
   a. Cardiac dysrhythmias
   b. Hypertension or hypotension
   c. Respiratory depression
   d. Seizures
   e. Coma

Substance Abuse Withdrawal

Definition

1. A substance-specific syndrome due to the cessation of (or reduction in) substance use that has been heavy and prolonged (APA, 2000)
2. Causes clinically significant distress or impairment
3. Unrelated to a general medical condition or another mental disorder

Predisposing Factors

Cessation of use of a substance that has been heavy and prolonged

Clinical Presentation

Two or more of the following develop within hours to a few days following cessation:

1. Autonomic hyperactivity
2. Hand tremors
3. Insomnia
4. Nausea or vomiting
5. Visual, tactile, or auditory hallucinations
6. Psychomotor agitation
7. Anxiety
8. Seizures

Collaborative Management

1. Maintain airway, breathing, ventilation, and circulation.
   a. Assessment of vital signs: blood pressure, pulse, respiratory rate, and temperature; vital signs every 15-30 minutes until stable
   b. Assessment of cardiac rate and rhythm
   c. Oxygen by nasal cannula at 2-6 L/min if indicated to maintain SpO_2 of 95% unless contraindicated; in patients with COPD, use pulse oximetry to guide oxygen administration to SpO_2 of ~90%
   d. IV access for fluid and medication administration if indicated
2. Provide safe environment.
   a. Assessment of psychiatric status especially suicidal ideation
   b. Quiet room with minimal stimulation, which allows continuous observation
   c. Nonjudgmental attitude
   d. Conversations should be kept simple and short.
   e. Frequent reorientation to person and place
   f. Restraints should be avoided if possible but may be required to ensure patient safety.
   g. Benzodiazepines as prescribed to prevent seizures
3. Monitor for complications.
   a. Delirium tremors (DTs)
   b. Death

Suicide and Homicide

Definitions

1. Suicide: willful taking of one's own life
2. Homicide: taking of another's life
3. Either may be premeditated or impulsive

Predisposing Factors

1. Family history
2. Prior attempts at suicide
3. Substance abuse
4. Depression
5. Physical illnesses
6. Violent environmental factors
7. Anniversary of suicide/death of a loved one.

Clinical Presentation

1. Subjective
   a. Suicidal or homicidal thoughts (may be unconscious)
   b. May have a plan
   c. If the method is substance overdose, need to determine time and type of substance
2. Objective: dependent upon mechanism of injury
3. Diagnostic: serum toxicology to determine serum levels if overdose

Collaborative Management

1. Maintain airway, breathing, and ventilation.
   a. Oxygen by nasal cannula at 2-6 L/min if indicated to maintain SpO_2 of 95% unless contraindicated; in patients with COPD, use pulse oximetry to guide oxygen administration to SpO_2 of 90%
   b. Artificial airway and mechanical ventilation may be necessary depending on severity of injury.
   c. IV access for fluid and medication administration if indicated
2. Provide safe environment.
   a. Assessment of psychiatric status especially suicidal ideation
   b. Quiet room with minimal stimulation, which allows continuous observation

1) Patient should not be left alone.
2) Environment to be cleared of any potential items that could be used for self-harm or harm to others.

c. Nonjudgmental approach
d. Restraints should be avoided if possible but may be required to ensure patient safety.
e. Immediate medical crisis needs to be resolved before dealing with mental health issues.
f. Support to family members

3. Prepare for surgery or other treatment if indicated.
4. Monitor for complications.
   a. Injury
   b. Death

LEARNING ACTIVITIES

CHAPTER 12

1. Complete the following crossword puzzle related to psychosocial conditions.

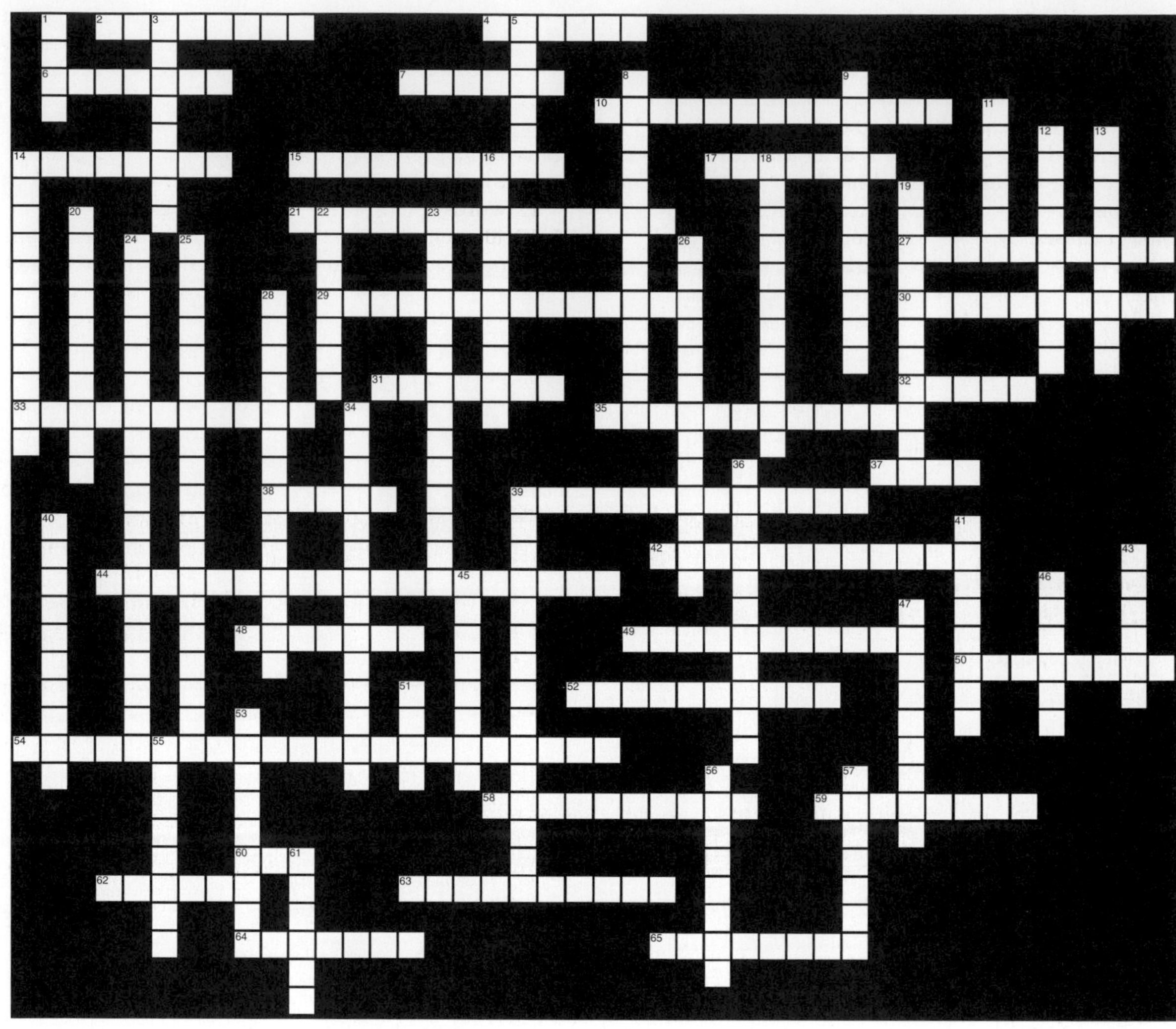

ACROSS

2. Sensory ____ is an increased frequency and intensity of stimulation of the senses with nonmeaningful stimuli
4. Emotions are said to be ____ when they fluctuate high to low rapidly and inconsistently without respect to the situation
6. The inability to recognize or identify objects despite intact sensory function
7. This hierarchy of needs contends that physiologic needs for oxygen and nutrients take priority over love and belonging
10. A perceived lack of control over the outcome of a specific situation or problem
14. Stress in response to noxious stimuli
15. Brief test of specific aspects of cognitive function
17. A language disturbance seen in dementia
21. Sensory perceptions when there is no sensory stimuli
27. Unconscious, involuntary forgetting of unacceptable or painful thoughts, impulses, feelings, or acts
29. This class of drugs is also used for mood stabilization
30. This type of personality is associated with a pervasive disregard for and violation of the rights of others (abbrev)
31. According to Erikson, older adulthood is focused on integrity versus ____
32. Elevated or irritable mood of at least 1 week duration
33. To person, place, time, and situation
35. Cognitive ability
37. Persistent or repeated reexperiencing of a traumatic event that has occurred in the past which induces an anxiety response (abbrev)
38. Physical, mental, or emotional mistreatment of another
39. Non-goal-directed speech that leaps from one idea to another (3 words)
42. Stressors expected as part of normal growth and development

44. Condition in which one's developmental age lags significantly behind one's chronological age (2 words)
48. This disorder is characterized by feelings of helplessness and tension
49. Directing energy from unacceptable drives into socially acceptable drives
50. According to Erikson, young adulthood is focused on ____ versus self-isolation
52. Discomfort caused by separation from significant relationships, places, events, and objects
54. Thought process in which there is no logical connection between sentences (3 words)
58. Unconsciously attributing one's own unacceptable qualities and emotions to others
59. An acute change (hours to days) in consciousness and cognition not due to dementia
60. Recurrent, persistent, intrusive thoughts and feelings coupled with ritualistic and repetitive behaviors (abbrev)
62. State that occurs when one's usual ways of coping are inadequate to deal with the stress
63. Going back to an earlier level of emotional development
64. Willful taking of one's own life
65. Ability to make sound decisions

DOWN

1. Affect is said to be ____ if it demonstrates no emotion
3. Stress in response to nonthreatening stimuli
5. Absence of speech
8. Ability to focus and pay attention
9. Medications that decrease anxiety
11. A spiritual form of coping mechanism
12. These are fixed false beliefs
13. Inability to initiate activities, which is seen in psychosis
14. Sensory ____ is a decreased frequency, intensity, or variety of stimulation of the senses with meaningful stimuli
16. Logical, directed thought that may "circle the topic" but does not make a point or answer the intended question
18. Hallucination that occurs upon awakening
19. A state of sorrow over the loss of a loved one
20. Alteration in mood characterized by sadness and negative self-concept
22. The inability to perform motor activities despite intact motor function
23. Thoughts or speech that contain excessive details about a topic but finally reach the intended point
24. Tolerance to a substance and inability to stop use (2 words)
25. Vivid events reported by some individuals after clinical death; may report bright light, dark tunnel, and presence of deceased loved ones (3 words)
26. Talking with a support person would be this type of coping mechanism
28. This type of drug is administered to decrease the risk of seizures during substance withdrawal
34. Recurrent substance use resulting in a failure to fulfill major role obligations at work, home, or school (2 words)
36. This type of crisis occurs suddenly in response to an unexpected stressful event
39. Syndrome manifested by physiologic, psychological, and functional decline that can be seen in individuals of all ages (3 words)
40. Hallucinations are this type of disturbance
41. Involuntary cessation in the flow of thought or speech
43. Demonstrated emotion
45. A chronic global deterioration of cognition
46. Patients with mania have this type of thoughts
47. Lack of pleasure
51. The emotion that the patient reports
53. Characterized by hallucinations and delusions
55. There is an increase in this type of thinking in depression
56. Willful taking of another person's life
57. Not attending to the emotional, physical, or mental care needs of another who cannot care for himself or herself
61. Treating obvious reality factors as though they do not exist because they are consciously intolerable

2. **Match the following hallucinations with the correct definition.**

____ 1. Auditory	a. Feeling sensations when not being touched
____ 2. Visual	b. Seeing images that are not present
____ 3. Gustatory	c. Smelling odors that are not present
____ 4. Hypnopompic	d. Perceiving a taste without an identifiable cause
____ 5. Tactile	e. Hearing voices or sounds that are not there
____ 6. Olfactory	f. Vivid dreamlike hallucination upon awakening
____ 7. Kinesthetic	g. Perceiving movement of the body without cause
____ 8. Somatic	h. Feeling that something is occurring within one's own body

3. **List 5 age-related considerations for older adults with psychological emergencies.**

a. ____
b. ____
c. ____
d. ____
e. ____

4. **Match the level of Maslow's Hierarchy of Needs to the example.**

____ 1. Physiologic	a. Art and music
____ 2. Safety and security	b. Water
____ 3. Love and belonging	c. Promotion at work
____ 4. Esteem and recognition	d. Marriage
____ 5. Self-actualization	e. Home security

5. Identify the assessment findings in each of the following conditions that would help you distinguish it from the others.

Condition	Subjective Assessment	Objective Assessment
Anxiety disorder		
Depression		
Mania		
Hallucinations		
Psychosis		
Dementia		
Delirium		

6. Mr. D is a 67-year-old widower of 2 years who retired 3 months ago from his position as a mechanical engineer. He lives alone in his home of 30 years. His son has accompanied him to the ED. He presents to the ED unshaven and disheveled with poor eye contact. He mumbles in response to questions in soft, low tones and is difficult to understand. He keeps stating that he is in awful shape, he has no memory, is of no good use to himself or anyone else, and they should just let him die. When pressed to do so, he reluctantly identifies the correct year, date, and day. He is aware he has been brought to a hospital. His sleep is erratic, his appetite is poor, he has generalized weakness, and his gait is unsteady. His son reports that his father typically is meticulous about his appearance and is very articulate. He states that he last saw his father 2 weeks ago when they had gone out to dinner and had done some grocery shopping. At that time, Mr. D was well groomed, walking steadily and independently, and actively involved in their conversation, his son said. He is concerned that his father has had a stroke or is getting dementia.
   a. What additional information might you need about Mr. D?
   b. What lab tests might be helpful?
   c. What would be a preliminary diagnosis for Mr. D and what are the data that support that diagnosis?
   d. What would be priority care issues for Mr. D?

7. Ms. B is a 21-year-old college student who is brought to the ED by the local police for running naked though her neighborhood. She is cooperative, although she insists that she does not need to be in the hospital. She reports that she feels great, hasn't slept in 2 days, and is not sleepy. She states, "I need to be free, like the birds and the bees." When asked for identification, she responds, "I am a daughter of the world." You notice that she has several bruises and many superficial cuts and scrapes on her body and feet.
   a. What additional information might you need about Ms. B?
   b. What lab tests might be helpful?
   c. What are potential diagnoses for Ms. B and what data support that diagnosis?
   d. What would be priority care concerns for Ms. B?

8. Mr. P is a 65-year-old businessman who was admitted in acute respiratory failure. He is intubated and has been on a mechanical ventilator for 2 days. Tonight he is restless and confused. He appears frightened and is pulling at catheters and tubes.

a. What is the most likely cause of Mr. P's symptoms?

____

____

b. What are the most likely contributing factors?

____

____

c. What are the priorities of care for Mr. P?

____

____

Professional Caring and Ethical Practice

CHAPTER 13

Critical Care Nursing: General Concepts

Nursing

1. Definition: "Nursing is the protection, promotion, and optimization of health and abilities, prevention of illness and injury, alleviation of suffering through the diagnosis and treatment of human response, and advocacy in the care of individuals, families, communities, and populations." (ANA, 2012a)
2. The nursing process (ANA, 2012b)
   a. Assessment: collecting and analyzing physical, psychological, and sociocultural data about a patient
   b. Diagnosis: making a clinical judgment about the client's response to actual or potential health conditions or needs
   c. Planning: setting short-term and long-term goals with the patient and developing a plan of care to achieve those goals
   d. Implementation: supervising or carrying out the actual care plan
   e. Evaluation: continuous assessment of the effectiveness of the care plan and the patient's status; the care plan is modified as needed

Critical Care Nursing

1. Critical care nursing is "that specialty within nursing that deals specifically with human responses to life-threatening problems" (AACN, 2012a).
   a. Standards for Acute and Critical Care Nursing Practice are available at *www.aacn.org*
2. A critical care nurse is "a licensed professional nurse who is responsible for ensuring that acutely and critically ill patients and their families receive optimal care" (AACN, 2012a).
3. Critical care patients are "those patients who are at high risk for actual or potential life-threatening health problems. The more critically ill the patient, the more likely he/she is to be highly vulnerable, unstable and complex, thereby requiring intense and vigilant nursing care" (AACN, 2012a).
4. While critical care nursing is generally practiced in a critical care specialty unit such as an intensive care unit, AACN asserts that "critical care nurses work wherever critically ill patients are found" (AACN, 2012a).

The Future of Nursing

1. The Institute of Medicine (2010) recently published a report regarding the future of nursing.
   a. Four key messages are:
      1) Nurses should practice to the full extent of their education and training.
      2) Nurses should achieve higher levels of education and training through an improved education system that promotes seamless academic progression.
      3) Nurses should be full partners with physicians and other health care professionals in redesigning health care in the United States.
      4) Effective workforce planning and policy making require better data collection and information infrastructure.
   b. Eight recommendations are:
      1) Remove scope-of-practice barriers.
      2) Expand opportunities for nurses to lead and diffuse collaborative improvement efforts.
      3) Implement nurse residency programs.
      4) Increase the proportion of nurses with a baccalaureate degree to 80% by 2020.
      5) Double the number of nurses with a doctorate by 2020.
      6) Ensure that nurses engage in lifelong learning.
      7) Prepare and enable nurses to lead change to advance health.
      8) Build an infrastructure for the collection and analysis of interprofessional health care workforce data.

2. This report with recommendations has been supported by ANA (ANA, 2012d).

Clinical Judgment

Description

"Clinical reasoning, which includes clinical decision making, critical thinking and a global grasp of the situation, coupled with nursing skills acquired through a process of integrating education, experiential knowledge and evidence-based guidelines." (AACN, 2012b)

Decision Making

1. Involves a number of steps by which information is assimilated, integrated, weighed, and valued to arrive at the selection of a course of action from among a number of possible alternatives
2. Steps in the decision-making process
   a. Information collection and problem identification
   b. Identification of possible solutions or actions
   c. Analysis of the possible consequences of each solution or action
   d. Selection of the best possible solution or action for implementation
   e. Implementation of the solution or action
   f. Evaluation of the results

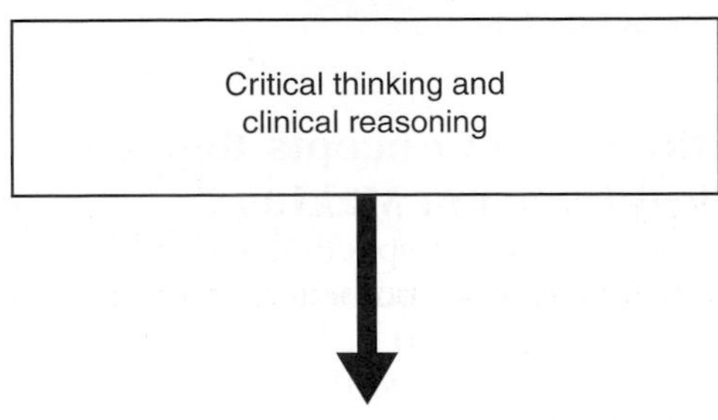

Figure 13-1 Relationship between clinical judgment, clinical reasoning, and critical thinking. (From Alfaro-Lefevre, R. [2013]. *Critical thinking, clinical reasoning, and clinical judgment: A practical approach* [5th ed.]. St. Louis: Saunders.)

Critical Thinking, Clinical Judgment, and Clinical Reasoning

1. Definitions
   a. Critical thinking: "a disciplined process that requires validation of data, including any assumptions that may influence your thoughts, and then careful reflection on the entire process while evaluating the effectiveness of what you have determined is the necessary action to take" (Jackson et al., 2006)
   b. Clinical judgment: "the development of opinions in the clinical practice setting, based on experience and knowledge, to guide the decisions you will make regarding the care of the patient" (Jackson et al., 2006)
   c. Clinical reasoning: use of "clinically specific data regarding specific populations or disease processes and making evaluations regarding their meaning" (Jackson et al., 2006)
2. Relationship between clinical judgment, clinical reasoning, and critical thinking (Figure 13-1)
3. Nine key questions of clinical judgment (Alfaro-LeFevre, 1995)
   a. What outcomes are expected in this person, family, or group when the plan of care is terminated?
   b. What problems or issues must be addressed to achieve these outcomes?
   c. What are the circumstances?
   d. What knowledge is required?
   e. How much room is there for error?
   f. How much time do I have?
   g. What resources can help me?
   h. Whose perspectives must be considered?
   i. What is influencing my thinking?
4. Strategies enhancing critical thinking (Alfaro-LeFevre, 1995); consider these strategies in the improvement of your own critical thinking as well as when working with your preceptees
   a. Anticipate the questions others might ask.
   b. Ask, "Why?"
   c. Ask, "What else?"
   d. Ask, "What if?"
   e. Paraphrase in your own words.
   f. Compare and contrast.
   g. Organize and reorganize information.
   h. Look for flaws in your thinking.
   i. Ask someone else to look for flaws in your thinking.
   j. Develop good inquiry skills.
   k. Revisit information periodically.
   l. Replace the phases "I don't know" or "I'm not sure" with "I need to find out."
   m. Turn errors into learning opportunities.
   n. Share your errors; they are valuable to help others learn.

Clinical Knowledge and Skills by System

Refer to Chapters 2-12.

Advocacy/Moral Agency

Description

"Working on another's behalf and representing the concerns of the patient/family and nursing staff; serving as a moral agent in identifying and helping to resolve ethical and clinical concerns within and outside the clinical setting." (AACN, 2012b)

Definitions and Concepts Related to Ethical Decision Making

1. Advocacy refers to respecting and supporting the basic values, rights, and beliefs of the critically ill patient (AACN, 2012a).
   a. The nurse should do the following (AACN, 2012a):
      1) Respect and support the right of the patient or the patient's designated surrogate to autonomous informed decision making.
      2) Intervene when the best interest of the patient is in question.
      3) Help the patient obtain necessary care.
      4) Respect the values, beliefs, and rights of the patient.
      5) Provide education and support to help the patient or the patient's designated surrogate make decisions.
      6) Represent the patient in accordance with the patient's choices.
      7) Support the decisions of the patient or the patient's designated surrogate or transfer care to an equally qualified critical care nurse.
      8) Intercede for patients who cannot speak for themselves in situations that require immediate action.
      9) Monitor and safeguard the quality of care the patient receives.
      10) Act as liaison between the patient, the patient's family, and health care professionals.
2. Moral agency: ability to serve as a moral agent in identifying and resolving ethical and clinical concerns (Curley, 1998)
3. Ethics: systems of valued behaviors and beliefs that govern proper conduct to ensure the protection of an individual's rights; involves judgments that help to differentiate right from wrong or indicate how things ought to be
4. Values: personal beliefs about the truth and the worth of thoughts, objects, and behavior
5. Accountability: answerability or responsibility
   a. Personal accountability: to oneself and the patient
   b. Public accountability: to employer, community, and society
6. Ethical principles
   a. Autonomy: an individual's obligation to respect a person's right of self-determination, independence, and freedom
      1) The nurse must be willing to respect the patient's right to make decisions about his or her own care, even if the nurse does not agree with those decisions.
      2) Limitations to autonomy include the following:
         a) When the rights of one person interfere with another individual's rights, health, or well-being
         b) When there is a high probability that a person may self-injure or injure others
   b. Beneficence: an individual's obligation to do good
      1) Conflicts that may occur include the following decisions:
         a) What is best for another person
         b) Who should make the decision
         c) Long-term or short-term benefit (a temporary harm may eventually produce a greater good)
   c. Nonmaleficence: an individual's obligation to do no harm, intentionally or unintentionally
      1) It includes protecting mentally incompetent persons, nonresponsive persons, children, and any other person who cannot protect himself or herself.
      2) This principle is not absolute; an example of a conflict related to nonmaleficence is when surgical trauma causes an ultimate cure or improvement in the patient's condition.
   d. Veracity: an individual's obligation to tell the truth and to not intentionally deceive or mislead the patient
      1) This principle is not absolute; an example of a conflict related to veracity is when telling the patient the truth may cause harm.
   e. Justice: an individual's obligation to be fair to all people
      1) Individuals have the right to be treated fairly and equally regardless of race, sex, marital status, medical diagnosis, social standing, economic level, or religious belief; also includes equal access to health care for all
   f. Paternalism: an individual's obligation to assist another person in making a decision when that person does not have sufficient data or expertise
      1) Undesirable when the entire decision is taken away from the patient
   g. Fidelity: an individual's obligation to be faithful or loyal to agreements and responsibilities that the individual has accepted
      1) It is one of the key elements of accountability.
      2) A conflict may occur between fidelity to patients and fidelity to employer, government, and society.
   h. Confidentiality: an individual's responsibility to respect privileged information
      1) Access to patient data is limited to those individuals with a "need to know."
      2) Others wishing access to patient data must have the patient's permission.
      3) Information about the patient (status and/or presence in the health care institution) is limited to those persons whom the patient has identified.

4) The patient has the right to access his or her medical record; if this occurs while the patient is still hospitalized, a nurse should be available to explain entries about which the patient has questions.
5) Computerized patient records introduce new challenges to ensuring the confidentiality of patient data.
   a) Never give out your password.
   b) Never leave unattended a computer terminal where you have signed in; log off when leaving the terminal,
   c) Do not allow anyone to view the screen while you are viewing patient data.
   d) Do not view things that you don't "need to know."

Ethical Approaches: The Basis for Ethical Decisions

1. Deontology: Actions are right or wrong based on a set of morals or rules.
   a. Emphasizes duty or obligation to another person
   b. Only acceptable ethical theory for decision making in health care
2. Teleology: Actions are right or wrong based on the action's consequences and usefulness; it looks at outcome; the end justifies the means.
3. Utilitarianism: The morally right thing to do is whatever produces the greatest good for the greatest number; it is derived from teleology.
4. Egoism: Actions are right or wrong based on self-interest and self-preservation.
5. Paternalism: Beneficence should take precedence over autonomy.
6. Social contract theory: People give up some rights to a government in exchange for social order.
7. Natural law: Actions are morally or ethically right when they are in accord with human nature.

Moral Distress

When one knows the right thing to do but cannot pursue the right action; obstacles may be internal or external

1. Contributes to nurses feeling dissatisfied with their work and even leaving nursing (AACN, 2012c)
2. Four A's to rise above moral distress (Wavra, 2006)
   a. Ask: Determine whether the nurse is experiencing moral distress.
      1) Expressions of anger, resentment, and frustration
      2) Statements such as "Why are we doing this?"
      3) Physical symptoms such as change in weight, sleep patterns, and depression
   b. Affirm.
      1) Acknowledge the distress.
      2) Affirm professional obligations to act as described in the ANA Code of Ethics for Nurses.
   c. Assess.
      1) Identify sources and severity of moral distress.
      2) Assess readiness to act by analyzing risks and benefits.
   d. Act.
      1) Prepare personally and professionally to act.
      2) Take action based on self-exploration regarding obligations, responsibilities, and risks.
      3) Anticipate setbacks and manage accordingly.

Ethical Dilemmas

Situation that requires a choice between two or more equally undesirable alternatives

1. Characteristics of an ethical dilemma (Curtin, 1982)
   a. The problem cannot be solved using only empirical data.
   b. The problem is so perplexing that it is difficult to decide what facts and data should be used to make the decision.
   c. There are far-reaching effects to the decision.
2. Conflicts related to rights of the individual: autonomy versus paternalism
   a. Informed consent
   b. Technology versus quality of life
   c. Resuscitate versus do not resuscitate (DNR)
   d. Behavior control
      1) May be misused to suppress personal freedom (e.g., use of restraints or sedating drugs)
      2) Individual's right to freedom may conflict with society's obligation to maintain social order.
3. Conflicts related to resource allocations: justice versus utilitarianism
   a. Triage decisions
   b. Quality-of-life decisions
   c. Inability to pay and/or lack of health insurance
   d. Organ transplantation decisions
      1) Living donors: rights of donor, recipient, families, and society
      2) Choice of one recipient over another: potential for elitism
      3) Utilization of health care resources: tremendous cost of organ transplantation
      4) Designation of death: when can an organ or organs be removed
4. Conflicts related to the role of the nurse: veracity versus fidelity
   a. Withholding therapy
   b. Right to die
      1) Positive euthanasia (also referred to as active euthanasia or mercy killing): life support systems are withdrawn or a medication, treatment, or procedure is used to cause death (e.g., assisted suicide)
      2) Negative euthanasia (also referred to as passive euthanasia): no extraordinary or heroic life-support measures are used to

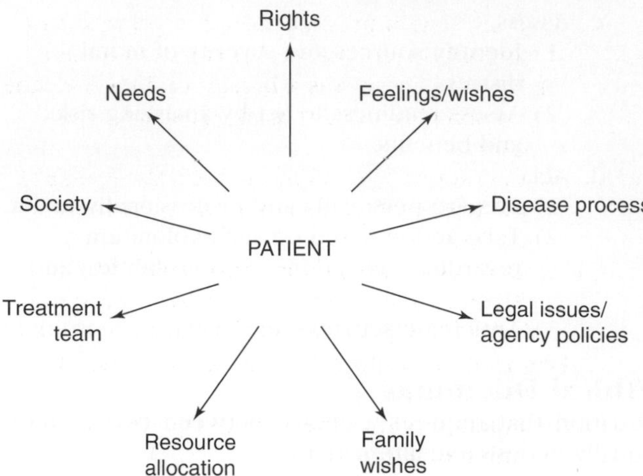

Figure 13-2 Factors affecting ethical issues and ethical decision making in nursing. (From Kinney, M. et al. [1998]. *AACN's clinical reference for critical care nursing* [4th ed.]. St Louis: Mosby.)

save a person's life (e.g., do-not-resuscitate [DNR] orders)

5. Conflicts related to personal values: professional integrity versus personal ethical and moral beliefs
   a. Nurse participation in treatments or therapies against the nurse's ethical or moral beliefs (e.g., abortion)
   b. Nurse providing care for patients whose practices are against the nurse's ethical or moral beliefs (e.g., domestic violence)

Factors Affecting Ethical Issues and Decision Making

See Figure 13-2.

Ethical Codes

Guidelines which outline the nurse's responsibility to the patient, to the employer, and to society

1. American Nurses Association (ANA) Ethical Code for Nurses (Box 13-1)

Rights

1. Ethical rights (moral rights)
   a. Based on moral or ethical principle
   b. Backed by general opinion of society or culture
   c. Often privileges allotted to certain individuals or groups of individuals
2. Legal rights: life, liberty, property, individual freedoms, and due process
   a. Based on a legal entitlement to some good or benefit
   b. Guaranteed by laws and, if violated, can be upheld in the legal system
3. Entitlements: statutory rights for a defined group (e.g., Medicare)
4. The American Hospital Association (AHA) Patient's Bill of Rights has been replaced by a patient information brochure titled "The Patient Care Partnership" which identifies the following expectations during a hospital stay (AHA, 2003).
   a. High-quality hospital care
   b. A clean and safe environment
   c. Involvement in your care
   d. Protection of your privacy
   e. Help with your bill and filing insurance claims

Box 13-1 American Nurses Association Code of Ethics for Nurses (ANA, 2001)

1. The nurse, in all professional relationships, practices with compassion and respect for the inherent dignity, worth, and uniqueness of every individual, unrestricted by considerations of social or economic status, personal attributes, or the nature of health problems.
2. The nurse's primary commitment is to the patient, whether an individual, family, group, or community.
3. The nurse promotes, advocates for, and strives to protect the health, safety, and rights of the patient.
4. The nurse is responsible and accountable for individual nursing practice and determines the appropriate delegation of tasks consistent with the nurse's obligation to provide optimum patient care.
5. The nurse owes the same duties to self as to others, including the responsibility to preserve integrity and safety, to maintain competence, and to continue personal and professional growth.
6. The nurse participates in establishing, maintaining, and improving health care environments and conditions of employment conducive to the provision of quality health care and consistent with the values of the profession through individual and collective action.
7. The nurse participates in the advancement of the profession through contributions to practice, education, administration, and knowledge development.
8. The nurse collaborates with other health professionals and the public in promoting community, national, and international efforts to meet health needs.
9. The profession of nursing, as represented by associations and their members, is responsible for articulating nursing values, for maintaining the integrity of the profession and its practice, and for shaping social policy.

From American Nurses Association (2001). *Code of ethics for nurses with interpretative statements*. Washington, DC: American Nurses Publishing.

Legal Issues

1. Sources of law
   a. A constitution establishes the basis of a governing system.
   b. Statutes are laws that govern.
      1) Made, voted on, and passed by legislative bodies
      2) Nurse practice acts are statutes.
         a) Define and limit the practice of nursing
         b) May vary state to state but all must be consistent with federal provisions and statutes

   c. Administrative agencies (e.g., state boards of nursing) create rules and regulations that enforce statutory laws.
   d. Court decisions are made when the courts interpret legal issues that are in dispute.
   e. Common law consists of statements made by courts, sometimes decades in the past, when no statute exists governing the particular matter.
2. Types of court cases
   a. Criminal: charges filed by the state or federal attorney general for crimes committed against an individual or society
      1) Burden of proof is on the filing agency; the defendant is presumed innocent and must be proven guilty beyond reasonable doubt.
      2) Consequences if found guilty include imprisonment or even death.
      3) An example would be a nurse who intentionally administered drugs that caused a patient's death,
   b. Civil: One individual sues another.
      1) Burden of proof to be found liable is a preponderance of the evidence.
      2) Consequences are monetary.
      3) An example would be a nurse sued for wrongful death because he or she failed to do something that would have prevented the death.
      4) Intentional torts
         a) Definition: A tort is a legal wrong committed against a person or property, independent of a contract, that renders the person who commits it liable for damages in a civil action; an intentional tort is a direct invasion of someone's legal rights.
         b) Examples include assault, battery, false imprisonment, invasion of privacy, defamation, and slander.
   c. Administrative: charges filed by a state or federal governmental agency (e.g., state board of nursing)
      1) Burden of proof to be found guilty is a preponderance of the evidence.
      2) Consequences may be monetary, disciplinary, or loss of privileges (e.g., professional license).
      3) An example would be failure to obtain a new license at the predetermined time.
3. Malpractice (i.e., professional negligence)
   a. Definition: failure to do something that a reasonable and prudent professional would do, or doing something that a reasonable and prudent professional would not do; an unintentional tort
      1) Reasonable and prudent: average judgment, foresight, intelligence, and skill that would be expected of a person with similar training and experience
   b. Elements that must be present for a professional to be held liable for malpractice
      1) Duty: The nurse had a duty to provide care and follow an acceptable standard of care.
      2) Breach: There was a breach of duty (i.e., the nurse failed to adhere to the standard of care).
      3) Causation: The failure to meet the standard of care must have caused injury to the patient.
      4) Damages: The patient must have suffered injuries as a result of the nurse's breach of duty.
   c. Avoidance of malpractice claims (Marquis and Huston, 2011)
      1) Practice within the scope of your state's nurse practice act.
      2) Follow your institution's policies and procedures.
      3) Model your practice after established practice standards and scientific evidence.
      4) Make patients' rights and welfare the priority.
      5) Make rational decisions based on the biological, psychological, and social sciences and be aware of laws and legal doctrines
      6) Practice within your area of competence.
      7) Continue to update and upgrade your technical skills and seek specialty certification.
      8) Purchase professional liability insurance and know the limits of your policy.
      9) Document thoroughly in the patient's record.
         a) Document
            i) Patient status with factual observations along with time, date, and signature (may be electronic signature)
            ii) Any deviations from standard practice and reasons for such deviations
            iii) Notification of physician for changes in status and the physician's response
         b) Common problems made in documentation
            i) Omissions without explanation
            ii) Vague and ambiguous language
            iii) Unapproved abbreviations
            iv) Error correction
            v) Spelling and grammar errors
            vi) Illegibility
            vii) Time inconsistencies (especially with electronic documentation systems)
4. Consent
   a. Blanket consent: The person gives permission for routine and customary care; this type of consent is required prior to admission.
   b. Informed consent: The person gives consent for a specific procedure.

1) The physician or advanced practice registered nurse (APRN) informs the patient and ensures that he or she understands the following:
   a) Explanation of the treatment/procedure
   b) Expected results/benefits
   c) Risks involved
   d) Alternatives, including absence of treatment
   e) Name of person performing the treatment/procedure
   f) That the patient may withdraw consent at any time
2) It is the responsibility of the person who will perform the procedure to obtain informed consent, but the nurse may witness the patient's signature on the consent form; the nurse has an ethical responsibility to notify the person who will perform the procedure if the nurse believes that the patient does not understand the procedure.

c. Implied consent: The patient is unable to sign, but treatment is needed immediately and the treatment is in the patient's best interest.

5. Incident reports
   a. These are internal documents completed for any unusual occurrence, including errors.
   b. These reports should include facts about the incident and the care given to the patient, such as diagnostic studies, medications, and consults.
   c. Avoid statements of guilt or blame in the incident report and do not allude to the incident report in the patient's medical record.
      1) Note that there is a national trend to fully disclose all errors to the patient and some studies have found fewer lawsuits when the patient was informed of the error.
6. Terms related to end-of-life care
   a. Advance directive: a legal document that expresses the patient's preferences related to end-of-life issues
      1) Must be developed by a competent adult (i.e., 18 years of age or older)
      2) Must be witnessed by two people
      3) May be revoked verbally, in writing, or by destruction of the document at any time
      4) Becomes effective when the person is certified to be terminally ill or have an irreversible condition with loss of decision-making capability
      5) Does not contraindicate the use of treatments for pain or suffering
   b. Living will: a directive that expresses what the patient wants done if he or she becomes terminally ill and is not able to make health care decisions
   c. Durable power of attorney for health care: a directive that designates someone to make health care decisions for the patient if the patient is unable to make the decisions

Caring Practices

Nursing activities that are responsive to the uniqueness of the patient and family and that create a compassionate and therapeutic environment with the aim of promoting comfort and preventing suffering. (AACN, 2012b)

Death and Dying

1. Definition: Dying is a psychophysiologic process that ultimately terminates in death for the individual and grieving for significant others
2. Stages of death and dying (Kübler-Ross, 1969) (Table 13-1)
3. Interventions to assist the patient to cope with death and dying
   a. Develop a personal philosophy of death in order to deal effectively with dying patients and living families.
   b. Do not eliminate hope.
      1) Hope is the expectation that a desire will be fulfilled.
      2) Hope aids in the tolerance of pain and suffering throughout the dying process.
   c. Encourage the patient and family to discuss their fears and concerns; listen attentively.
   d. Provide your presence and your compassion.
   e. Provide comfort measures and analgesia.
4. Interventions to assist the family
   a. Allow the family to be with the patient.
   b. Encourage the family to participate in the care of the patient.
   c. Reassure the family of the patient's analgesia and comfort.
   d. Provide information about the patient's status frequently, especially when death is imminent.
   e. Encourage ventilation of anxiety, fears, and concerns.
   f. Ensure a private, comfortable area for the family.
   g. Refer the family to other sources of support, such as the chaplain, social worker, and support group.

Pain Management

1. Definition of pain: anything the patient says it is; it occurs whenever the patient says it does (McCaffery, 1968)

Table 13-1 Stages of Death and Dying

Stage	The Patient May Say:
Shock and disbelief	"I can't be dying; you're wrong" "No, not me"
Denial	"Most people with this disease die but not me"
Anger	"Me? What have I done to deserve this"
Bargaining	"If I do this. . .; let me live until. . ."
Depression	"What's the use"
Acceptance	"I'm ready to die"

Kübler-Ross, E. (1969). *On death and dying*. New York: Macmillan.

a. Acute pain: pain that follows injury and ends when healing occurs; an example is surgical pain
b. Chronic pain: pain that lasts longer than the normal healing period; an example is low back pain
c. Neuropathic pain: chronic pain caused by nerve damage; an example is diabetic neuropathy
2. Assessment
   a. Self-report
      1) Pain scales
         a) Numerical (0-10) pain scale
         b) Wong-Baker FACES™ scale
         c) Verbal graphic rating scale
         d) Behavioral Pain Scale (Table 13-2)
      2) Guidelines for teaching your patient to use a pain rating scale (McCaffery, 2002)
         a) Explain the purpose of the scale.
         b) Explain the increments of the scale.
         c) Explain what is meant by "pain."
         d) Ask the patient to give an example of pain to practice using the scale.
         e) Ask the patient to practice using the scale to rate the pain.
         f) Assist the patient to set a goal for an acceptable level of pain.
   b. Verbal cues: moaning, crying
   c. Nonverbal cues: rubbing, splinting, guarding
   d. Facial expressions: grimacing, frowning
   e. Physiologic signs: tachycardia, elevated blood pressure, tachypnea (NOTE: These do not always occur, especially when pain is chronic.)
3. Pharmacologic management
   a. Pharmacologic agents:
      1) Opioids (e.g., morphine, fentanyl, hydromorphone)

Table 13-2 Behavioral Pain Scale

Item	Description	Score
Facial expression	Relaxed	1
	Partially tightened (e.g., brow lowering)	2
	Fully tightened (e.g., eyelid closing)	3
	Grimacing	4
Upper limbs	No movement	1
	Partially bent	2
	Fully bent with finger flexion	3
	Permanently retracted	4
Compliance with ventilation	Tolerating movement	1
	Coughing but tolerating	2
	Fighting ventilator	3
	Unable to control ventilation	4
Total score		**3-12**

From Payen, J.-F., Bru, O., Bosson, J. L., Lagrasta, A., Novel, E., Deschaux, I., et al. (2001). Assessing pain in critically ill sedated patients using a behavioral pain scale. *Crit Care Med, 29*(12), 2258-2263.

      2) Nonsteroidal antiinflammatory agents (e.g., ibuprofen, ketorolac)
      3) Local anesthetics (e.g., lidocaine, bupivacaine)
   b. Drug delivery methods used in critical care areas
      1) Analgesia
         a) Oral agents, especially sustained-release agents
         b) Intravenous
            i) Continuous infusion
            ii) Intermittent injection
            iii) Patient-controlled: usually consists of a continuous infusion with patient-controlled injection for breakthrough pain
         c) Epidural
            i) Continuous infusion
            ii) Patient-controlled: usually consists of a continuous infusion with patient-controlled injection for breakthrough pain
      2) Regional anesthesia
         a) Transdermal
         b) Peripheral nerve catheter: delivers local anesthetic directly to the nerve sheath
         c) Intrapleural: delivers local anesthetic directly to the parietal pleura
4. Nonpharmacologic
   a. Application of heat or cold
   b. Relaxation techniques
   c. Distraction (e.g., music, television, reading, needlepoint, coloring, drawing, writing, visitors)
   d. Other complementary therapies as described later

Complementary Therapies

Therapies used in conjunction with conventional therapies; most are intended to cause relaxation, decrease anxiety, and augment pain management

1. Progressive muscle relaxation (PMR)
   a. Involves progressive tensing and relaxing of successive muscle groups, frequently accompanied by diaphragmatic breathing
   b. Helps the patient eventually sense muscle tension without having to progress through the tensing and relaxing of successive muscle groups
   c. Decreases stress and anxiety
   d. Frequently accompanied by diaphragmatic breathing
2. Breathing
   a. Involves instruction, practice, and encouragement in the use of breathing techniques, such as diaphragmatic breathing or pursed-lip breathing
   b. Decreases stress and anxiety; may improve effectiveness of ventilation, especially in dyspneic patients
3. Meditation
   a. Involves intentional concentration and repetition of a word, phrase, or muscular activity

b. Encourages use of a word or phrase that holds a special meaning for the patient
c. Decreases stress and anxiety

4. Co-meditation
   a. Involves concentrating on certain sounds, images, or words
      1) An assistant utters the words, which frequently are in a script written by the patient
      2) Efforts are made to synchronize the words with the rhythm of the patient's exhalations
   b. Decreases stress and anxiety
5. Guided imagery
   a. Involves focusing and directing the imagination through the use of specific words and suggestions
   b. Identify the patient's concept of a relaxing location or situation and verbally guide the patient's thoughts there.
   c. Decreases stress, fear, and anxiety; enhances the immune system
6. Massage
   a. Involves a technique of controlled touch to manipulate soft tissue
   b. Effects are dependent on the type and speed of movements, the pressure exerted by the hands, fingers, or thumbs, and the area of the body being massaged.
   c. Decreases stress and anxiety, reduces muscle tension and spasm, reduces edema, causes release of endorphins to augment pain relief
   d. Aromatherapy and music may enhance the effectiveness.
7. Hypnosis
   a. Involves suggestion to enable a person to experience the imaginary as real, allowing deep relaxation
   b. Decreases stress and anxiety
8. Biofeedback
   a. Involves use of conscious mental effort to control involuntary body functions, such as BP, heart rate, and respiratory rate
      1) A biofeedback instrument is used initially to alert the patient to the cues that signal a developing symptom (e.g. tension in neck and shoulders); audible tones are given.
      2) Relaxation techniques are taught to decrease muscle tension.
   b. Decreases stress and anxiety and causes muscle relaxation
9. Therapeutic (or healing) touch
   a. Involves the transfer of energy from the practitioner's hands to the patient, without actually touching, to potentiate the healing process of one who is ill or injured
   b. Consists of the following steps: centering, assessment, unruffling, modulating, and evaluation
   c. Used to help restore the balance of the energy field and to provide additional energy to be used for healing
10. Purposeful touch
    a. Involves hand holding, stroking, or patting a patient's arm, hand, or face, placing one's hand on the patient's shoulder, placing one's arm around the patient's shoulder, or hugging
    b. May also be referred to as *affective touch, comforting touch,* or *empathetic touch*
    c. Reduces stress and communicates encouragement, support, or affection
11. Music therapy
    a. Involves use of music to soothe and relax
    b. Identify the patient's music preferences; any simple, repetitive, low-pitched music is appropriate for relaxation.
    c. The most soothing music has a ¾ beat; chants, folk songs, and lullabies are very relaxing.
    d. Causes endorphin release, distraction from pain or anxiety, and relaxation; improves quantity and quality of sleep
12. Aromatherapy
    a. Involves the use of essential oils extracted from flowers, leaves, stalks, fruits, and roots for therapeutic purposes
    b. May be used in massage, baths, compresses, or inhalation
    c. Effects vary depending on the essential oil used; may alter mood, reduce anxiety, cause relaxation, cause decongestion, reduce inflammation, increase circulation, or relieve pain
13. Pet therapy
    a. Involves visits by the patient's own pet or by pet-visitation animals (usually dogs)
    b. Decreases stress and anxiety, may decrease heart rate and blood pressure
    c. Adhere to specific guidelines to ensure the safety and security of the patient, families, and staff.
14. Humor
    a. Involves using word and images to elicit laughter
    b. Decreases stress and anxiety, enhances the patient's ability to cope and feelings of well-being, decreases tension in a difficult situation, causes endorphin release, augments the immune system, causes muscle relaxation
    c. Involves judgment for appropriateness
       1) Start by determining the patient's receptiveness to humor and asking about what type of humor he or she appreciates
       2) Consider timing of humor; inappropriate during a crisis or when laughing will cause pain
       3) Some forms of humor are inappropriate, such as humor that demeans (e.g., racial or ethnic jokes) or sexually oriented humor (e.g., "dirty" jokes).
15. Acupuncture
    a. Involves the insertion of needles into specific points in the body for therapeutic purposes; may also involve use of heat (moxibustion),

pressure (acupressure), or electromagnetic energy to stimulate acupuncture points
   b. Causes endorphin release and decrease in pain

Rest Requirement

1. Sleep quality is poor and sleep deprivation is a common problem for patients in critical care units.
   a. Causes (Holley, 2010; Matthews, 2011)
      1) Long periods in bed
      2) Supine position with little or no activity
      3) Little or no light variation
      4) Patient-ventilator asynchrony
      5) Pain with inadequate analgesia
      6) Dyspnea
      7) Pharmacologic agents which cause agitation or wakefulness
      8) Note that while sedatives, hypnotics, and analgesics cause the appearance of sleep, it is unclear as to whether this "sleep" has the same restorative qualities as normal physiologic sleep.
   b. In a study by Tamburri, DiBrienza, Zozula, and Redeker (2004), the mean number of care interactions per night was 42.6, and patients had 2-3 hours of uninterrupted sleep on only 6% of the nights observed.
   c. Recommendations to improve sleep quality in the critical care unit (Holley, 2010)
      1) Promote wakefulness during the day.
      2) Use sedatives judiciously, especially during the day.
      3) Decrease light and noise during the night.
      4) Minimize disruptions and awakenings during the night.
2. Noise control
   a. Noise can produce serious physical and psychological stress and may impair the healing process; the Environmental Protection Agency (1974) recommends that daytime noise levels in a hospital not exceed 45 dB and that nighttime levels not exceed 35 dB.
      1) In 2005, the average daytime sound level in 2005 was 72 dB and average nighttime sound level was 60 dB (Choiniere, 2010). Decrease volume on alarms and decrease extraneous conversation and other noise; earplugs also may be used.
   b. Recommendations to reduce noise in the critical care unit (Choiniere, 2010)
      1) Half of hospital sound peaks are directly related to human behavior with staff conversations being the most disturbing noise to patients; staff should be educated and encouraged to reduce volume of conversation and close doors during reports.
      2) Reduce volume of alarms, phones, beepers, televisions, and music.
      3) Eliminate overhead pages.
      4) Limit the number of visitors to two at a time.
      5) Note and correct noisy carts.
      6) Design units with improved sound acoustics, decentralized nurses' stations, and single-patient rooms.

The Family of the Critically Ill Adult

1. Definition: individuals who are relatives or significant others with whom the patient shares an established relationship
2. Assessment
   a. Availability of family
   b. Structure and communication patterns within the family
      1) Role of patient within the family
      2) Primary decision maker
      3) Family spokesperson
      4) Conflicts within the family
   c. Perceptions and understanding
      1) Knowledge of patient's condition
      2) Past experience with critical care
      3) Past experience with similar health situations (e.g., MI, cancer)
      4) Need for information about the patient
      5) Expectations of patient's outcome
   d. Coping patterns
      1) Previous responses to crises
      2) Usual coping mechanism
   e. Family resources and needs related to resources
      1) Transportation
      2) Lodging
      3) Finances
      4) Spirituality
   f. Family health maintenance needs
      1) Dietary
      2) Hygiene
      3) Rest/sleep
      4) Medications
3. Stressors
   a. Observation of a loved one in a life-threatening situation
   b. Overwhelming technology in the critical care environment
   c. Separation from the family member
   d. Financial impact
4. Most important needs of families (Leske, 1991)
   a. To have questions answered honestly
   b. To be assured the best care possible is being given to the patient
   c. To know the prognosis
   d. To feel there is hope
   e. To know specific facts about the patient's progress
   f. To be called at home about changes in the patient's condition
   g. To know how the patient is being treated medically
   h. To feel that hospital personnel care about the patient
   i. To receive information about the patient daily
   j. To have understandable explanations
   k. To know exactly what is being done for the patient

l. To know why things were done for the patient
m. To see the patient frequently
n. To talk to the doctor every day
o. To be told about transfer plans

5. Responses
   a. Fear of death, pain, and discomfort of their loved one
   b. Anxiety
   c. Financial concerns
   d. Fear of temporary or permanent changes in the roles of the patient and other family members
   e. Severe dysfunction: argumentativeness, aggression, intoxication, guilt, blame, verbal or physical abuse toward health care workers
6. Interventions
   a. Provide information about the status of the patient; on request, at designated times, including during visiting hours, at the time of any significant change in condition
   b. Be available during family visitation to answer questions and provide explanations.
   c. Encourage family members to make notes regarding information that the physicians or nurses have given or questions that they would like to ask during the next interaction with the nurse or physician.
   d. Encourage the designation of one family member to phone or be phoned who then will communicate to the other family members.
   e. Provide a brochure describing the unit, usual activities, visitation policies, and other useful information.
   f. Introduce yourself and ask names and relationships of family members.
   g. Identify family members by name if possible.
   h. Use touch therapeutically as indicated and allowed by the family members.
   i. Individualize visiting times based on the needs and response of the patient and the family.
      1) In a recent AACN practice alert, it is stated that "evidence shows that the unrestricted presence and participation of a support person can enhance patient and family satisfaction, because it improves the safety of care." (AACN, 2011)
      2) Previous cited concerns about unrestricted visiting hours that have not been supported through research (AACN, 2011)
         a) Physiologic stress for the patient
         b) Barriers to the provision of care
         c) Exhaustion of family and friends
         d) Increased risk of infection
      3) Benefits of flexible visitation for the patient include the following (AACN, 2011):
         a) Decreased anxiety
         b) Decreased confusion and agitation
         c) Reduced cardiovascular complications
         d) Decreased length of stay in the critical care unit
         e) Improved feelings of security
         f) Increased satisfaction
         g) Increased quality and safety
      4) Benefits of flexible visitation for the family include the following (AACN, 2011):
         a) Increased satisfaction
         b) Decreased anxiety
         c) Improved communication
         d) Improved understanding of the patient
         e) More opportunities for participation in care
   j. Explain to the family if visitation is interrupted or postponed by a procedure or crisis.
   k. Warn the family and explain the reason for a patient's unusual behavior (e.g., confusion).
   l. Encourage family members to talk to and touch the patient, hold the patient's hand, and express their feelings.
   m. Involve the family in decision making.
   n. Encourage family participation in care if they desire.
   o. Respect the cultural beliefs and rituals of the family; accommodate these beliefs and rituals if at all possible.
   p. Encourage family members to take care of their own basic needs (eating, sleeping, and attending to hygiene).
   q. Provide a comfortable area for visitors, close to the unit, with bathroom facilities and a telephone; have private area available for family meetings and family-physician discussion.
   r. Encourage participation in a support group if available.
   s. Be empathetic; empathy is a "special emotion that comes as the result of a close identification and connection with another person" (Dracup & Bryan-Brown, 1999).
7. Family presence for invasive procedures and resuscitation interventions
   a. Family members should be given the option of presence at the bedside (AACN, 2010).
   b. Benefits
      1) Less anxiety about what is happening to the patient
      2) More likely to believe that everything possible was being done
      3) Greater ability to provide emotional support to the patient
      4) Studies have shown that almost all family members would be present again if a similar event were to occur and patients reported feeling comfort and support because the family member(s) were present.
   c. Commonly stated concerns that have *not* been demonstrated in research studies on the subjects
      1) Disruption in the delivery of emergency care
      2) Adverse psychological effects to the family
   d. Role of family facilitator is recommended (Mangurten et al., 2005).

1) Prepares the family and explains that patient care is the priority
2) Provides the family with personal protective equipment if appropriate
3) Escorts family members (maximum of 2) to the bedside and remains with the family to provide comfort measures, facilitate seeing, touching, and talking to the patient, and provide opportunities for asking questions
4) Escorts family members from the room if they become ill, disruptive, or overwhelmed
5) Provides debriefing, comfort, and answers to questions after medical procedures or resuscitation

8. Guidelines for giving bad news
   a. Present information clearly; ask if there are any questions.
   b. Avoid euphemisms such as "passed" because they may be misunderstood; also avoid platitudes such as "he's better off now."
   c. Be silent if you don't know what to say; offer your presence.
   d. Offer to call the family's pastor, priest, rabbi, or other religious leader; honor the family's cultural and religious beliefs.
   e. Monitor the family for any physical complaints because stress may cause exacerbation of any preexisting condition.
   f. Provide privacy for saying goodbye and assist as the family packs the deceased's belongings; explain what to expect so they will not be surprised.
   g. If the patient is a candidate to be an organ donor, work with the organ donation coordinator to discuss donation and organ procurement with the family.
9. Guidelines for giving bad news by phone
   a. Ask for the closest family member by name.
   b. Introduce yourself: name, title, and hospital.
   c. Inform the closest family member of the incident that caused the patient to be brought to the hospital or of a change in status if the patient has been in the hospital.
   d. Ask if the family member can come to the hospital; suggest that he or she come to the hospital with another relative or friend if possible.
   e. Avoid telling the family by phone that the patient has died, but tell the truth if they ask; if the family lives a long distance from the hospital, they need to be informed of the death by phone, preferably by the physician but it may be the responsibility of the nurse in some situations.
   f. If the patient is a candidate to be an organ donor, work with the organ donation coordinator to discuss donation and organ procurement with the family.

Collaboration

Description

Working with others in a way that promotes and encourages each person's contributions toward achieving optimal and realistic patient/family goals; collaboration involves intradisciplinary and interdisciplinary work with colleagues and community (AACN, 2012b)

Definitions

1. Collaboration: working together
   a. Attributes of an effective team (Yoder-Wise, 2011)
      1) Working environment: informal, comfortable, and relaxed
      2) Discussion: focused and shared by almost everyone
      3) Objectives: well understood and accepted
      4) Listening: respectful, facilitation of participation
      5) Ability to handle conflict: comfortable with disagreement, open discussion of conflicts
      6) Decision making: usually reached by consensus, general agreement necessary for action, dissenters free to voice opinions
      7) Criticism: frequent, frank, and constructive
      8) Leadership: shared; changes from time to time
      9) Assignments: clearly stated, accepted by all despite disagreements
      10) Feelings: freely expressed and open for discussion
      11) Self-regulation: frequent and ongoing, focused on solutions
   b. Basic rules to create synergy (Yoder-Wise, 2011)
      1) Establish a clear purpose.
      2) Listen actively.
      3) Be compassionate.
      4) Tell the truth.
      5) Be flexible.
      6) Commit to resolution.
2. Collaborative practice: when members of the medical and nursing professions, together with members of other related health care disciplines, work together to assure quality patient and family care; includes the following critical aspects
   a. Sharing in planning, decision making, problem solving, goal setting, and responsibility
   b. Communicating openly and respectfully
   c. Coordinating
   d. Cooperating
   e. Recognizing and accepting of separate and interrelated spheres of practice
3. Consultation: process of seeking, giving, and receiving help; may be formal (written) or informal (verbal)

Essential Elements of Collaboration

1. Communication
2. Trust

3. Respect
4. Understanding and acceptance of team members' roles
5. Competence
6. Shared responsibility and accountability
7. Shared goal setting
8. Flexibility
9. Administrative support

Components of Collaborative Practice

1. Unit co-directors: a physician and a nurse
2. Collaborative practice committee
3. Primary nurse and primary physician
4. Autonomy for clinical decision making
5. Integrated patient records
6. Multidisciplinary review of care

Blocks to Collaboration

1. Nurses and physicians
   a. Authoritative (sometimes aggressive) physicians
   b. Nonassertive (sometimes submissive) nurses
   c. Team members satisfied with traditional hierarchy
2. Misunderstanding or lack of understanding regarding the role and practice of professional nursing
   a. Nurses have their own license; they do not practice under the license of the physician.
   b. Physicians cannot discipline or fire nurses employed by the hospital.
   c. Nursing is not medicine; these are two separate and interrelated professions; if an umbrella term is needed, let it be *health care*, not *medicine*.
   d. Nurses have independent functions as well as dependent functions; they can perform these independent functions without a physician's order (*prescription* is a much better word than *order*).
   e. Nursing research has established a unique body of scientific knowledge.
   f. Nursing practice is controlled by nurses through state nurse practice acts, not by physicians.
3. Ineffective or lack of communication between the professions
4. Lack of administrative support
5. Systems issues

Strategies for Improving Collaboration

1. Evaluate current interdisciplinary relationships in your institution and on your unit.
   a. Are team members sought out for communication about the patient?
   b. Is communication peer to peer?
   c. Is there recognition of each team member's role in enhancing patient outcomes?
   d. Are team members willing to accept responsibility and accountability for patient outcomes?
   e. What are the steps taken when conflicts arise between team members?
2. Establish a multidisciplinary critical care committee co-chaired by a nurse and a physician.
   a. Disciplines have equal representation and decision making.
   b. The committee should handle issues related to practice, communication, and improving effectiveness or efficiency of clinical care.
3. Establish multidisciplinary professional activities such as the following:
   a. Rounds
   b. Patient records
   c. Orientation
   d. Education programs
   e. Quality and safety programs
   f. Task forces for problem resolution
   g. Research
4. Establish a professional nursing environment
   a. Assurance of competency
   b. Knowledge of and ability to articulate the unique role of nursing
   c. Encouragement of professional development of nursing staff

Communication

1. Types of communication
   a. Spoken
   b. Nonverbal
   c. Symbolic gestures
   d. Written words
   e. Visual images
   f. Multimedia
2. Rules for good communication
   a. Be clear in your mind as to what you want to communicate.
   b. Deliver the message as succinctly as possible.
   c. Ensure that the message has been clearly and correctly understood; ask for feedback.
3. Pitfalls (Yoder-Wise, 2011)
   a. Advice giving
   b. Making others wrong
   c. Defensiveness
   d. Judging the other person
   e. Patronizing
   f. Giving false reassurance
   g. Asking "why" questions
   h. Blaming others

Conflict Resolution

1. Types of conflict (Yoder-Wise, 2011)
   a. Intrapersonal: within a person
   b. Intergroup: between two or more groups
   c. Interpersonal: between two or more people
2. The conflict process
   a. Frustration
   b. Conceptualization
   c. Action
   d. Outcomes
3. Common strategies
   a. Avoiding: Parties involved in the conflict do not acknowledge it or try to resolve it.

   b. Cooperating: One party sacrifices and allows the other party to win.
   c. Smoothing: Another person calms the parties involved in the conflict.
   d. Competing/Coercing: One party pursues what it wants at the expense of the other party.
   e. Negotiating/Compromising: Each party gives up something it wants.
   f. Collaborating: All parties set aside their original goals and work together to establish a common goal.
4. Guidelines for dealing with interpersonal conflict
   a. Communicate with the angry person.
   b. Identify common goals (e.g., quality patient care).
   c. Discuss only one issue at a time; don't bring up old issues and anger.
   d. Discuss facts, not opinions, judgments, or what others are saying; don't make personal attacks.
   e. Communicate with the person involved; do not engage others in the conflict or jump to a higher organizational level.

Delegation

1. Definition: "achieving performance of care outcomes for which you are accountable and responsible by sharing activities with other individuals who have the appropriate authority to accomplish the work" (Yoder-Wise, 2011)
   a. Direct delegation: The delegation is the result of the RN actively deciding what to delegate.
   b. Indirect delegation: The decision to delegate is the result of organizational protocols that designate specific tasks as appropriate for another to perform.
2. Process (ANA & NCSBN, n.d.)
   a. Assess and plan the delegation, based on the patient needs and available resources.
   b. Communicate directions to the delegate, including any unique patient requirements and characteristics as well as clear expectations regarding what to do, what to report, and when to ask for assistance.
   c. Surveillance and supervision of the delegation, including the level of supervision needed, implementation, and follow-up to problems or a changing situation
   d. Evaluation and feedback to consider the effectiveness of the delegation, including any need to adjust the plan of care
3. The five rights of delegation (ANA & NCSBN, n.d.)
   a. The right task
   b. Under the right circumstances
   c. To the right person
   d. With the right directions and communication
   e. Under the right supervision and evaluation
4. Delegation to unlicensed assistive personnel (UAP) (ANA & NCSBN, n.d.)
   a. Recognize what may not be delegated.
      1) Initial and subsequent nursing assessments requiring the professional judgment of a registered nurse
      2) Determination of nursing diagnoses, care goals, care plans, and progress
      3) Interventions that require the knowledge and skill of a registered nurse
   b. Be aware of the job description, skills, and knowledge of the individual.
   c. Never delegate any task that requires the skill or knowledge of a registered nurse.

Systems Thinking

Description

The body of knowledge and tools that allow the nurse to appreciate the care environment from a perspective that recognizes the holistic interrelationship that exists within and across health care systems

System

1. Definition: "A collection of interdependent elements that interact to achieve a common purpose" (Nolan, 1998)
2. Nursing is one aspect to patient care; nurses must work together with other members of the health care team and understand the organizational structure of the institution.
3. AACN (2005) is committed to fostering work and care environments that are "safe, healing, humane and respectful of the rights, responsibilities, needs, and contributions of all people—including patients, their families and nurses"; the standards for establishing and sustaining health work environments are as follows:
   a. Nurses must be as proficient in communication skills as they are in clinical skills.
   b. Nurses must be relentless in pursuing and fostering true collaboration.
   c. Nurses must be valued and committed partners in making policy, directing and evaluating clinical care, and leading organizational operations.
   d. Staffing must ensure the effective match between patient needs and nurse competencies.
   e. Nurses must be recognized and must recognize others for the value each brings to the work of the organization.
   f. Nurse leaders must fully embrace the imperative of a healthy work environment, authentically live it, and engage others in its achievement.

Types of Organizational Structure

1. Bureaucracy: formal, centralized, hierarchical
   a. Rules, policies, and procedures ensure consistency and promote efficiency and productivity.
   b. Communication and decisions flow from top to bottom with limited employee autonomy.
2. Flat: less formal and hierarchical than bureaucratic organizations

a. Fewer rules and policies than bureaucratic organizations
b. Provides authority to make decisions at the point of interaction with the client

3. Matrix: focus on product and function
   a. Hybrid of bureaucratic and flat structures
   b. Sometimes referred to as product line management
4. Self-governance: organizational structure that allows the staff to govern themselves
   a. Sometimes referred to as *professional practice models*
   b. Authority, responsibility, and accountability belong to the nurse delivering care.
5. Shared-governance: organizational structure with governance shared by staff and management

Patient Care Delivery Systems: Methods Nurses Use

See Table 13-3.

Delivery-of-Care Models

1. Patient-centered care
   a. Goal: provide patients a "seamless" health care experience and decrease fragmentation of care; focus is meeting the needs of the patient
   b. Key components
      1) Care for each patient coordinated by an RN or case manager
      2) Cross training of staff to provide up to 90% of patient services
      3) Assignment of ancillary personnel to patient care units
      4) Team approach between licensed and unlicensed members
      5) Location of services closer to the patient
   c. Benefits
      1) To hospital
         a) Reduction in management layers
         b) Emphasis on shared governance and self-directed work teams.
      2) To patient
         a) Interaction with fewer health care providers
         b) Improved coordination of care to enhance quality of care and increase patient satisfaction
      3) To society: reduction of health care costs
2. Family-centered care
   a. Definition: an approach to care that recognizes the role and the needs of patients' family members
   b. Goal: allow the patient and family members to maintain their normal roles as much as possible, including communication between the interdisciplinary team and patient and family members
   c. Considers the nurse, patient, and family as partners in the care of the patient and the impact of the patient's illness on the family unit
   d. Several studies cited in Davidson (2009) showed reduced anxiety, depression, and posttraumatic stress disorder and increased satisfaction.
3. Cooperative care
   a. Similar to that of home health care: the patient and the family are in charge
   b. Goal: early self-management by providing patients with a wellness-oriented hospital environment
   c. Hospital environment viewed as an extension of the home rather than as an interruption.
   d. An integrated, multidisciplinary health care team focusing on therapeutic care and education

Table 13-3 Patient Care Delivery Systems

	Functional Nursing	Team Nursing	Primary Nursing	Total Patient Care
Description	Task oriented; nurses perform tasks (e.g., charge, medicine, treatments) as assigned	Group oriented; team leader (RN) with team members deliver care to a group of patients	Patient oriented; nurse is responsible for all aspects of care for assigned patients; accountable for care delivered during entire hospitalization	As for Primary Nursing except that the nurse is accountable for care delivered during the entire shift
Advantages	• Cost effective • Each person becomes efficient at specific tasks	• Cost effective • Increased staff satisfaction	• Increased staff satisfaction, though nurses may be dissatisfied with the number of nonnursing tasks that do not require their degree of skill and knowledge • Improved quality of care • Improved continuity of care in primary nursing	
Disadvantages	• Fragmented nursing care • Diminished continuity of care • Diminished staff satisfaction	• Diminished continuity of care • Team leader must have leadership skills, especially effective delegation skills	• Efficacy questionable because an RN is very expensive and is performing tasks that do not require the skill and knowledge of an RN; use of unlicensed assistive personnel to perform nonnursing tasks increases efficacy • Restricted opportunity for evening and night shift nurses to be assigned as "primary nurse"	

allows response to patient's need in a timely manner.
   e. Patients have the right and responsibility to participate in their own health care as full partners to maximize their ability for self-management on discharge.
   f. Inclusion of the patient's family and support system as care partners during the hospital stay leads to more humanistic hospital care and enhances the potential for improved treatment compliance and self-management after discharge.
4. Holistic care
   a. Designed for the chronically ill patient with complex medical conditions that require frequent acute care admissions; addresses the physical, mental, emotional, and spiritual health of the patient and family—mind, body, and spirit
   b. Goal: maximize wellness, minimize complications, and provide an inner peace
   c. Includes common holistic therapies such as relaxation therapy, humor, massage, music, art, recreation, imagery, and pet therapy to reduce physiologic and psychological stress
   d. Characteristics of the holistic team include:
      1) Excellent psychosocial and physical assessment skills
      2) Informed, flexible practitioners
      3) Ability to manage without the security of routines
      4) Mature and refined interpersonal skills and self-awareness
      5) Knowledge of family theory and the impact of illness on family functioning
5. Transitional care (also known as *subacute care*)
   a. Developed to provide the need for a more cost-effective approach to the treatment of patients with complex medical conditions and rehabilitation needs
   b. Goal: to achieve desired outcomes in a low-cost humane setting
   c. Severity of the patient's condition requires:
      1) Frequent on-site visits from the physician
      2) Professional nursing care
      3) Significant ancillary services
      4) Outcomes-focused, interdisciplinary approach using a professional team
      5) Complex medical and/or rehabilitation care
6. Case management
   a. Definition: a strategy to coordinate care, maintain quality, and contain cost with emphasis on coordination and prioritization of all needed services; though a designated case manager may provide comprehensive care for patients with complex health problems, all nurses have case management responsibilities
   b. Tools
      1) Critical paths: a grid that outlines critical events expected to happen each day of the patient's hospitalization based on the Diagnosis-Related Group (DRG) classification
      2) Care Multidisciplinary Action Plan (MAP): a combination of a nursing care plan and critical path

Change Process

1. Change is one constant in health care organizations.
2. Types of change
   a. Unplanned: reactive process to change that was not planned
   b. Planned: active process with predetermined goals; intentional, thought-out, mutual goal setting, equal power distribution; there are many models of planned change (Table 13-4)
3. The change agent: the person who works to bring about the change
   a. Key qualities of effective change agents
      1) Excellent communication skills
      2) Observational skills to monitor change
      3) Knowledge of group dynamics
      4) Perceptive nature about political issues
      5) Supportive attitude toward change participants
      6) Ability to establish trusting relationships
   b. Tips for leading change (Kotter, 1995)
      1) Involve all stakeholders in the process of planning for the change.
      2) Share the vision and create goals.
      3) Select a change model; different models will work better for different change processes.
      4) Identify champions among each of the major groups of stakeholders.
      5) Identify facilitators and barriers and adjust your plan accordingly.
      6) Create a detailed plan but be flexible.

Response to Diversity

Description

The sensitivity to recognize, appreciate, and incorporate differences into the provision of care

Cultural Diversity

1. Definitions
   a. Diversity: those differences that make each person unique; includes national origin, religion, age, gender, sexual orientation, race, ethnicity, education, socioeconomic status, and abilities/disabilities
   b. Culture: the learned, shared, and transmitted values, beliefs, and practices of a particular group that guide thinking, actions, behaviors, interactions with others, emotional reactions to daily living, and one's world view; subculture: a recognizable segment of a larger cultural group that shares some characteristics of the larger group but with unique features of its own
   c. Cultural sensitivity: a learned skill in which a person has an awareness of and appreciation for

Table 13-4 Selected Models for Planned Change

Author	Steps in the Planned Change Process
Lewin (1951) Model of Change	• Status quo (diagnose the problem) • Unfreezing (develop the solutions) • Disequilibrium (overcome resistance) • Moving (implement change) • Refreezing (reestablish balance) • Equilibrium
Lippitt, Watson, & Westley (1958) Seven Phases of Planned Change	• Aware of the need for change • Development of a relationship between client system and change agent • Definition of the change problem • Establishment of change goals and exploration of options for achievement • Implementation of the plan for change • Acceptance and stabilization of the change • Redefinition of the relationships of the change entities
Havelock (1973) Six Phases of Planned Change	• Building a relationship • Diagnosing the problem • Acquiring relevant resources • Choosing the solution • Gaining acceptance • Stabilizing the innovation and generating self-renewal
Rogers (1995) Diffusion of Innovation Model	• Knowledge • Persuasion • Decision • Implementation • Confirmation
Prochaska (2000) and Prochaska et al (2001) Transtheoretical Model	• Precontemplation: the individual is not thinking of change • Contemplation: the individual is thinking of but not committed to change in the near future • Preparation: the individual intends to change in the near future • Action: the individual actively attempts to change • Maintenance: the individual sustains the change over time
Kotter (1995) Process for Leading Change	• Establish a sense of urgency • Form a powerful guiding coalition • Create a vision • Communicate the vision • Empower others to act on the vision • Plan for and create short-term wins • Consolidate improvements and produce still more change • Institutionalize new approaches
Berwick (2003) From Description to Prescription	• Find sound innovations • Find and support innovators • Invest in early adopters • Make early adopter activity observable • Trust and enable reinvention • Create slack for change • Lead by change

another's cultural uniqueness; also referred to as *ethnosensitivity*

d. Cultural competence: "a set of congruent behaviors, attitudes, and policies that come together in a system, agency, or among professionals that enables effective work in cross-cultural situations" (HRSA, 2001)

e. Culturally congruent nursing care: use of cognitively based nursing techniques that incorporate an individual's cultural values, beliefs, and lifeway; these techniques facilitate, assist, support, and/or enable an individual toward health and well-being or to face illness or death in culturally meaningful ways

f. Race: a group of people related by common descent of heredity who have similar physical characteristics such as skin color, facial form, and eye shape

g. Ethnic group: subset of culture; a smaller group that identifies itself as distinct because of shared characteristics, such as culture, language, traditions, appearance, and social heritage

h. Nationality: a people from a place with specified political and geographic boundaries

i. Customs: patterns and practices within a cultural group that encompass collective learned behaviors (includes diet and health behaviors)
j. Rituals: culturally prescribed codes of behavior (may guide practices and decisions including health and wellness)
k. Values: personal standards of what is good or useful in relationship to oneself and to others
l. Norms: commonly shared customs and standards of behavior that are acceptable within a given group of people
m. Cultural paradigms: abstract explanation used by a cultural group to account for major life events
n. Enculturation: the process by which culture is transmitted from one generation to the next by means of social learning
o. Acculturation: the process by which an individual or group takes on the behaviors and practices of the dominant culture; factors that influence the degree and pace of an individual's acculturation include length of time in the new culture, age, economic/educational status, and discriminatory practices of the dominant culture
p. Ethnocentrism: the belief that one's own ethnic group, way of life, beliefs, and values are superior to others
q. Cultural imposition: the practice of imposing one's cultural beliefs upon others with the belief that they are best or superior
r. Cultural relativism: the attitude that the differences in ways of doing things hold equal validity
s. Cultural pain: the discomfort and suffering experienced by an individual or group resulting from the insensitivity of others who have different beliefs and/or cultural norms

2. Significance
   a. Of the developed countries in the world, the United States has the greatest increase in population and diversity of inhabitants; immigration accounts for at least one third of the increase.
      1) The percentage of whites of European origin (the dominant culture in the United States) will continue to decline, creating a more multicultural power base.
      2) U.S. Census Bureau population projections indicate that non-Hispanic whites will no longer compose the majority of the population in 2042 (U.S. Census Bureau, 2011)
   b. Nurses must be aware that issues of culture, race, gender, and socioeconomics strongly influence health status and utilization of the health care system.
      1) Culturally inappropriate care and inattention to cultural differences in care may negatively affect health outcomes.
      2) Individuals from different cultures and illegal immigrants often delay seeking medical attention because of language, cost, and cultural barriers; these delays often result in more serious conditions.
   c. Health care reform is resulting in cultural competence guidelines and enforcement by state agencies.
3. Aspects of cultural sensitivity
   a. Acknowledgment that cultural diversity exists
   b. Avoidance of stereotypes with appreciation of the uniqueness of each patient, with culture as one aspect that enhances uniqueness
   c. Respect of the unfamiliar
   d. Appreciation that cultural values are ingrained and difficult to change
   e. Modification of care to include consistency with the patient's culture
   f. Examination of personal cultural beliefs and values
   g. Realization that the patient's health practices may be very different from yours but that each cultural group has health practices that attempt to improve health and temper illness
   h. Recognition that all people within a cultural group do not respond to illness the same; there is diversity within cultures
4. Cultural assessment
   a. Assess degree of acculturation (e.g., how well language of the dominant culture is spoken, language spoken in the home, length of time in country, food preferences).
   b. Encourage the patient to discuss cultural beliefs and practices; definitions of health/illness and origin of illnesses may differ within cultures.
   c. Make efforts to respect and understand different communication styles.
   d. Honor time and value orientation.
   e. Provide privacy according to individual needs; be aware that in many cultures, it is extremely important for family members to be present during assessments.
   f. Identify the decision maker within families; it may be someone other than the patient.
   g. Recognize that patients' reactions to pain are sometimes culturally driven.
   h. Be aware of biological variations among cultures, such as body structure, skin/hair color, population-specific diseases, and psychological coping characteristics.
   i. Recognize that dietary/religious practices and cultural taboos have important implications related to nursing care.
   j. Identify hobbies.
   k. Note cultural practices and modify care as necessary.
5. Cultural phenomena impacting nursing care (Figure 13-3 and Table 13-5)
6. Cultural aspects of pain
   a. Pain is not purely a neurophysiologic response; cultural, social, and psychological denominators influence pain.

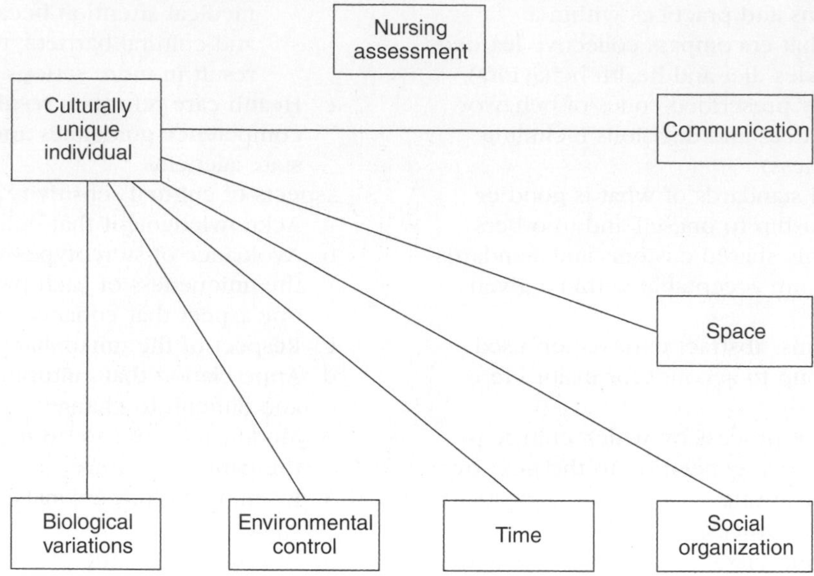

Figure 13-3 Application of cultural phenomena to nursing care and nursing practice. (From Giger, J. [2013]. *Transcultural nursing: Assessment and intervention* [6th ed.]. St. Louis: Mosby.)

b. Pain intensity, expression, tolerance, and expected responses from caretakers are influenced by culture.
c. A patient's attitude and beliefs about pain are determined by culture.
d. Each culture has its own language of distress.
   1) Facial expressions
   2) Sounds
   3) Changes in activity
   4) Words to describe feelings
e. Nurses must always remember that regardless of the patient's cultural background, pain is what the patient says it is and it occurs when he or she says it does.
   1) All pain should be considered "real" and treated compassionately.
   2) Be aware that patients who do not verbally express the presence of pain may not be pain free.

7. Drug polymorphism
   a. Age, drug, gender, body size, and body composition affect individual responses to drugs.
   b. Factors that influence drug polymorphism vary among ethnic groups and can be categorized as environmental, genetic, and cultural; these do not include all the aspects that affect a patient's response to drugs but raise awareness regarding possible differences in response.
   c. Drug metabolism is genetically determined.
   d. Race may affect response; also called *genetic polymorphism*
   e. Environmental factors include diet, alcohol, smoking, malnutrition, vitamin deficiencies, stress, fever, and physiologic rhythms; each of these can affect drug absorption.
   f. Cultural factors include values, beliefs, compliance, family influence, and prior drug experience; patients may be taking herbal or homeopathic remedies that can alter response to drug absorption.
   g. Nurses must become familiar with drugs that affect patients of different ethnicity.
8. Cultural behaviors relevant to nursing care (Table 13-6)
   a. Respect and embrace diversity among the patient and health care team members.
   b. Have a cultural reference available on your unit.
   c. Have a list of employees who speak another language and are willing to assist with translation and how to contact them.
9. Problems in providing culturally congruent health care; all of the following issues can lead to poor health outcomes:
   a. Stereotyping, prejudice, ignoring blind spots, and labeling
   b. Personal biases and bigotry
   c. Cultural differences, patients being labeled by nurses as "the difficult patient and/or family"
   d. Lack of interpreters and educational materials in patient's language
   e. Lack of diversity among nursing staff
   f. Lack of time (with culturally congruent care, listening to stories is important)
   g. Lack of flexibility with teaching methods

Religious Diversity

1. Definitions
   a. Spirituality: a basic human phenomenon that helps create meaning in the world
      1) Encompasses a person's ideology, view of the world, and meaning of life

Table 13-5 Cultural Phenomena Affecting Nursing Care

Nations of Origin	Communication	Space	Time Orientation	Social Organization	Environmental Control	Biological Variation
Asian • China • Hawaii • Philippines • Korea • Japan • Southeast Asia (Laos, Cambodia, Vietnam)	• National language preference • Dialects, written characters • Use of silence • Nonverbal and contextual cuing	• Noncontact people	• Present	• Family: hierarchical structure, loyalty • Devotion to tradition • Many religions, including Taoism, Buddhism, Islam, and Christianity • Community social organizations	• Traditional health and illness beliefs • Use of traditional medicines • Traditional practitioners: Chinese doctors and herbalists	• Liver cancer • Stomach cancer • Coccidioidomycosis • Hypertension • Lactose intolerance
African • West Coast (as slaves) • Many African countries • West Indian Islands • Dominican Republic • Haiti • Jamaica	• National languages • Dialect: pidgin, Creole, Spanish, and French	• Close personal space	• Present over future	• Family: many female, single parent • Large, extended family networks • Strong church affiliation within community • Community social organizations	• Traditional health and illness beliefs • Folk medicine tradition • Traditional healer: root-worker	• Sickle cell anemia • Hypertension • Cancer of the esophagus • Stomach cancer • Coccidioidomycosis • Lactose intolerance
Europe • Germany • England • Italy • Ireland • Other European countries	• National languages • Many learn English immediately	• Noncontact people • Aloof • Distant • Southern countries: closer contact and touch	• Future over present	• Nuclear families • Extended families • Judeo-Christian religions • Community social organizations	• Primary reliance on modern health care system • Traditional health and illness beliefs • Some remaining folk medicine traditions	• Breast cancer • Heart disease • Diabetes mellitus • Thalassemia
Native American • 500 Native American tribes • Aleuts • Eskimos	• Tribal languages • Use of silence and body language	• Space very important and has no boundaries	• Present • Community social organizations	• Extremely family oriented • Biological and extended families • Children taught to respect traditions	• Traditional health and illness beliefs • Folk medicine tradition • Traditional healer: medicine man	• Accidents • Heart disease • Cirrhosis of the liver • Diabetes mellitus
Hispanic countries • Spain • Cuba • Mexico • Central and South America	• Spanish or Portuguese primary language	• Tactile relationships • Touch • Handshakes • Embracing • Value physical presence	• Present	• Nuclear family • Extended families • Compadrazgo godparents • Community social organizations	• Traditional health and illness beliefs • Folk medicine tradition • Traditional healers: curandero, espiritisco, portera, señoro	• Diabetes mellitus • Parasites • Coccidioidomycosis • Lactose intolerance

Compiled by Rachel Spector, RN, PhD, from Davidhizer, R., & Giger, J. (1999). *Transcultural nursing: Assessment and intervention* (3rd ed.). St. Louis: Mosby.

Table 13-6 Cultural Behaviors Relevant to Nursing Care

Cultural Group	Cultural Variations (Common Belief/ Practice)	Nursing Implications
African Americans	• Dialect and slang terms require careful communication to prevent error (e.g., "bad" may mean "good")	• Question the client's meaning or intent
Mexican Americans	• Eye behavior is important. An individual who looks at and admires a child without touching the child has given the child the "evil eye"	• Always touch the child you are examining or admiring
American Indian	• Eye contact is considered a sign of disrespect and is thus avoided	• Recognize that the client may be attentive and interested even though eye contact is avoided
Appalachians	• Eye contact is considered impolite or a sign of hostility • Verbal patter may be confusing	• Clarify statements
American Eskimos	• Body language is important • The individual seldom disagrees publicly with others • Client may nod yes to be polite, even if not in agreement	• Monitor own body language closely, as well as client's, to detect meaning
Jewish Americans	• Orthodox Jews consider excess touching, particularly from members of the opposite sex, offensive	• Establish whether client is an Orthodox Jew and, if so, avoid excessive touch
Chinese Americans	• Individual may nod head to indicate yes or shake head to indicate no • Excessive eye contact indicates rudeness • Excessive touch is offensive	• Ask questions carefully and clarify responses • Avoid excessive eye contact and touch
Filipino Americans	• Offending people is to be avoided at all cost • Nonverbal behavior is important	• Monitor nonverbal behaviors of self and client, being sensitive to physical and emotional discomfort or concerns of the client
Haitian Americans	• Touch is used in conversation • Direct eye contact is used to gain attention and respect during communication	• Use direct eye contact when communicating
East Indian Hindu Americans	• Be aware that men may view eye contact by women as offensive • Avoid eye contact	• Women avoid eye contact as a sign of respect
Vietnamese Americans	• Avoidance of eye contact is a sign of respect • The head is considered sacred; it is not polite to pat the head • An upturned palm is offensive in communication	• Limit eye contact • Touch the head only when mandated and explain clearly before proceeding to do so • Avoid hand gesturing

From Giger, J. (2013). *Transcultural nursing: Assessment and intervention* (6th ed.). St. Louis: Mosby.

2) It gives an individual a sense of inner peace and harmony

b. Spiritual distress: disruption in the life principle that pervades a person's entire being and integrates and transcends one's biological and psychosocial nature

c. Religion: a specific unified system of an expression of the belief in and reverence for a supernatural power accepted as the creator and governor of the universe

d. Religious symbols: symbols used in the expression of faith (e.g., rosary, prayer cloth, prayer rug, medicine bundles, red ribbon, charms, "the garment")

e. Meditation: a devotional exercise of contemplation

f. Prayer: an intimate conversation between an individual and God or other Higher Being

g. Hope: to wish for something with expectation of its fulfillment

h. Faith: confident belief in the truth of a person, idea, or thing (e.g., God); belief not based on logical proof or material evidence

2. Significance
   a. Exclusion of the important role of spirituality for patients and families can impact on recovery and health.
   b. Care of the whole person enhances healing and health.
   c. Spiritual beliefs of providers may be an important consideration for many patients when selecting a health care provider.
3. Causes of spiritual distress
   a. Separation from religious and cultural ties
   b. Challenged belief and value systems
   c. Sense of meaninglessness or purposelessness
   d. Remoteness from God
   e. Disrupted spiritual trust
   f. Moral or ethical nature of therapy
   g. Sense of guilt and shame
   h. Intense suffering
   i. Unresolved feelings about death
   j. Anger toward God
4. Aspects of spiritual sensitivity include the following:
   a. Perform exploration of your own values and beliefs.
   b. Acknowledge that you may not agree with every aspect of the patient's spiritual beliefs and practices; be nonjudgmental and respect the patient's right to worship the Supreme Being of his or her choice.
   c. Develop good listening skills; encourage patient to discuss spiritual concerns.
   d. Know your limits; if you are uncomfortable discussing spiritual needs with the patient or praying with the patient, contact the patient's personal spiritual advisor or consult the hospital chaplain service as requested by the patient and/or family.
   e. Schedule physical care to allow religious rituals and practices.
   f. Respect the patient's rights and privacy.
   g. Increase your knowledge regarding different faiths (Table 13-7 identifies selected faiths and nursing implications).
5. Perform spiritual needs assessment.
   a. Assess the patient's spiritual or religious beliefs, values, and practices.
   b. Listen for verbal cues regarding spirituality (e.g., referring to God/spiritualist, talking about church, prayer, or synagogue)
   c. Note the presence of religious symbols (e.g., crucifix, Star of David, Bible, Torah, Qur'an, or other spiritual books, prayer cloth) in room during interview.
   d. Listen for expressions of spiritual distress (expressed hopelessness or guilt, crying, sleep disturbances, disrupted spiritual trust, loss of meaning and purpose in life).
   e. Be alert to comments related to spiritual concerns or conflicts (e.g., "Why me God?" or "I'm being punished for my sins").
   f. Determine if there are religious or spiritual practices (such as communion) that the patient wishes to participate in during hospitalization,
   g. Identify specific religious concerns such as dietary needs or refusal of blood.

Table 13-7 Religious Beliefs of Selected Religions and Appropriate Nursing Interventions

Religion	Belief	Interventions
Catholicism	• God does not cause suffering, but allows it for furthering human growth • Baptism is necessary for salvation	• Inform patient that Holy Communion is available • Have Catholic priest/deacon available to perform Anointing of the Sick • If patient is close to death and a Catholic religious representative is not available, any Christian may perform the baptism and then notify the priest immediately • Make all efforts to leave religious symbols (e.g., rosary) in place
Christian Scientist	• Sin, sickness, and death can be overcome by a full understanding of the divine principle of Jesus' teaching and healing • Disease and illness is a delusion of the nonspiritual mind and can be overcome by prayer	• Be aware that medical care may be refused • May utilize the services of physicians for the purpose of setting bones, treatment of malignancies, and delivering babies • Pain medications may be accepted for severe pain only • There is no clergy or priesthood
Hinduism	• Illness may result from misuse of the body or sins from a previous lifetime • Meditation and prayer must be done at specific times throughout the day • Females cannot be left in the presence of an unfamiliar male	• Plan care around religious practices • Provide same-sex caregivers • Provide vegetarians meals as requested • May refuse medication by capsule since many capsules are made from beef • Allow the family to wash the family member's body following death if desired; do not remove any sacred threads that are placed on the body

Continued

Table 13-7 Religious Beliefs of Selected Religions and Appropriate Nursing Interventions—cont'd

Religion	Belief	Interventions
Islam (Muslim)	• Submit to Allah's will in matters of health • Prayer and washing required five times a day • The left hand is considered unclean; food will not be handled with the left hand	• Provide privacy and plan care to accommodate prayer times • Educate regarding pain-reducing techniques • Provide diet with dietary restrictions as requested • Pork and some other foods prohibited • May refuse to take capsules since many are made from pork • Follow patient and family wishes regarding therapies; prolonging life by life-support machinery is often seen as unacceptable • Allow family to stay with relative during process of dying • Allow to wash body after death • Turn deceased person's face toward the right
Jehovah's Witnesses	• Opposed to transfusions of blood obtained from a blood bank and some blood products (the source of the soul is believed to be in the blood) • Opposed to eating foods to which blood has been added • Do not celebrate national holidays (including Christmas), birthdays, or salute flags; it is believed that violators will spend an eternity in nothingness	• Assess the patient's religious beliefs and practices before administering blood or blood products • Most Witnesses carry cards indicating types of acceptable transfusions • "Mature minors," according to Jehovah's Witness standards, may refuse blood transfusions • Be aware that the patient may refuse surgical or medical interventions that will require blood transfusion • Consider the use of volume expanders such as saline, lactated Ringer's solution, hetastarch (Hespan) • Implement blood-conservation strategies, especially in children • Consult hematologist and/or medical centers familiar with bloodless medicine and surgery management, if needed • Respect patient and family decisions to refuse blood products • Avoid foods to which blood has been added (e.g., certain sausages, lunch meats) • Avoid attempts to involve the patient in preparations for celebrations of national holidays

Judaism	• Sabbath begins at sundown on Friday and ends at sundown on Saturday
	• There is hope for recovery until death is imminent
	• May not eat non-kosher foods
	• Orthodox Jews: work of any kind is prohibited on the Sabbath, including driving or using the telephone
	• Orthodox Jews: prayer is required three times a day
	• A person must stay with a critically ill or dying family member until death so that the soul will not feel alone
		• Provide kosher diet as requested
		• Provide privacy and plan care considering prayer times
		• Allow a relative to stay with the dying patient
		  • Notify rabbi/rebbe according to family's wishes
		  • Caregivers should leave the body untouched for approximately one-half hour after death to allow the soul to depart
		  • After death, by Judaic law, the body cannot be left alone
		  • Autopsies generally are not allowed unless required by law
		• Assist and respect practices of the Sabbath
		• Do not shave body hair of Hasidic Jews
		• Hasidic/Orthodox: provide same-sex caregivers

Seventh-Day Adventist	• Sabbath is recognized as dusk on Friday to dusk on Saturday. • The body is a temple of God and should be kept healthy	• Provide diet with dietary restrictions as requested • The church encourages a vegetarian diet • Be aware that the patient may avoid seafood, meat, caffeine, alcohol, drugs, and tobacco • Protein and iodine deficiency may occur • Be aware that the patient may refuse procedures (medical or surgical) that occur on the Sabbath

6. Provide care that is sensitive to the patient's spiritual/religious needs.
   a. Convey a caring, nonjudgmental attitude.
   b. Inform the patient and family of the availability of spiritual/religious services (e.g., pastoral care, chapel, religious services, religious books, communion, baptism, last rites).
   c. Inform the patient and family of policies related to clergy visitation.
   d. Provide privacy and opportunities for religious practices, such as prayer and meditation.
   e. Prepare the patient for desired religious rituals.
   f. Join in prayer for reading of scripture if comfortable.
      1) If you are comfortable praying with the patient and family, the following suggestions may be helpful:
         a) Trust God or other Higher Power to enable you to know what to do and what to say.
         b) Really listen to the patient so that you know the patient's and family's greatest concerns.
         c) Explore the spiritual needs of the patient; ask the patient what he or she would like for God or other Higher Power to do.
         d) Keep prayers realistic (e.g., comfort versus miraculous healing).
         e) Be sensitive and respectful.
         f) Hold the patient's hand or stroke his or her arm, if culturally appropriate.
      2) If you are not comfortable praying with or providing other spiritual support for the patient and family, call the patient's spiritual advisor or a representative of pastoral care to pray with or comfort the patient and family.
   g. Notify the chaplain or patient's spiritual advisor of the patient's spiritual distress (with the patient's permission).
   h. Provide honest information to aid in informed decision making when spiritual beliefs and therapeutic regimens are in conflict.
7. Problems in providing spirituality-sensitive health care
   a. Avoiding or minimizing the role of spirituality in patient healing
   b. Treating religious beliefs as mental illness
   c. Failing to involve patient and family in decision making
   d. Giving information that can lead to false hope
   e. Failing to allow the patient an opportunity to work through grief

Generational Diversity

1. Each generation has a peer personality that lends itself to a collective mind-set (Johnson & Romanello, 2005) (Table 13-8).
2. Avoid overgeneralizing; not everyone in each age group fits the description (or every aspect of the description) of the age group.

Clinical Inquiry or Innovator/Evaluator

Description

The ongoing process of questioning and evaluating practice, providing informed practice, and innovating through research and experiential learning

Evidence-Based Practice (EBP)

1. Definition: the integration of the following:
   a. Best evidence
   b. Clinician expertise
   c. Patient values
   d. Circumstances
2. Five-step process for ensuring that clinical decisions are based on best evidence (Straus, Glasziou, Richardson, & Haynes, 2011)
   a. Converting information into clear questions
      1) PICOT format frequently is used (Melnyk & Fineout-Overholt, 2011)
         a) P: problem or population
         b) I: intervention
         c) C: comparison intervention
         d) O: outcome
         e) T: timing
      2) Remember: the best questions come from clinicians
   b. Seeking evidence to answer those questions
      1) Published research reports
         a) Use search engines such as CINAHL, Pub Med/MEDLINE, and Google scholar.
         b) Scour the bibliographies of the studies that you found helpful.
      2) Unpublished research reports
         a) Consult known researchers regarding the issue.
         b) Important because research studies with statistically insignificant results are frequently not published; either the researcher chooses not to publish or the report is rejected for publication (i.e., publication bias)
   c. Evaluating (critically appraising) the evidence for its validity (truthfulness) and usefulness; grading the evidence considers the following:
      1) Quality: the aggregate of quality ratings for individual studies, predicated on the extent to which bias was minimized (i.e., level of evidence)
         a) Study designs
            i) Traditional hierarchy of evidence based on study designs
               (a) Randomized controlled trials (double-blinded)
               (b) Nonblinded randomized clinical trials
               (c) Nonrandomized clinical trials
               (d) Prospective cohort studies

Table 13-8 Characteristics of Today's Generations

Generation	Born Between	Characteristics
Silent Generation (sometimes called the Veteran Generation): ~10% of today's workforce	1925 and 1942	• Tend to be hard working, thrifty, disciplined • Value traditional • Appreciate conformity, consistency, and uniformity at work and value the system over the individual • Tend to work at large corporations that offer security and reward longevity • Prefer direct orders • Prefer assignments that are structured and task oriented
Baby Boomers: ~45% of today's workforce	1943 and 1960	• Tend to be rebellious and questioning of the status quo • Equate work with self-worth • Are driven and dedicated; willing to work overtime • May be resistant to technology • Prefer facilitation • Prefer assignments that require flexibility, independent thinking, and creativity
Generation X: ~30% of today's workforce	1961 and 1981	• Tend to be ironic, cynical, resourceful • Balance work and leisure time; less likely to work overtime • Are more independent; do not belong to any group • Are comfortable with technology • Embrace diversity • Adapt well to change • Attempt to attain several goals at once • Prefer coaching with feedback and credit for accomplishments • Prefer assignments that allow self-direction
Millennials (sometimes called Nexters or Generation Y): 15% of today's workforce	1982 and 2002	• Tend to be optimistic, assertive, self-confident, friendly • Accept authority and prefer to be led • Are cooperative team players; prefer to work in groups and teams • Have difficulty focusing on one task; prefer to multitask • Are very technology savvy • Prefer collegiality and mentoring • Prefer assignments that challenge and stretch their capabilities

(e) Case-control studies
(f) Case reports
(g) Expert opinion (including consensus groups)

ii) Randomized controlled trials are considered the "gold standard," but many nursing questions are not answered using quantitative techniques.

b) Sample size
c) Control of extraneous variables

2) Quantity: the magnitude of effect, numbers of studies, and sample size or power (i.e., strength of evidence)
3) Consistency: the extent to which similar findings are reported using similar and different study designs
4) Relevance: the study question's similarity to the clinical question and the extent to which the findings from the study can be applied in other clinical settings to different patients
5) There are many grading scales used to grade sources of evidence; the AACN system has recently been modified (Table 13-9).

Table 13-9 AACN Levels of Evidence

Level	Description
A	Meta-analysis of multiple controlled studies or meta-analysis of qualitative studies with results that consistently support a specific action, intervention, or treatment
B	Well-designed controlled studies, both randomized and nonrandomized, with results that consistently support a specific action, intervention, or treatment
C	Qualitative studies, descriptive or correlational studies, integrative reviews, systematic reviews, or randomized controlled trials with inconsistent results
D	Peer-reviewed professional organizational standards with clinical studies to support recommendations
E	Theory-based evidence from expert opinion or multiple case reports
M	Manufacturers' recommendations only

From Armola, R. et al. (2009). AACN Levels of Evidence: What's New? *Crit Care Nurse,* 29(4), 70-73.

d. Integrating findings with clinical expertise, patient values, and circumstances and, if appropriate, applying these findings
e. Evaluating performance and the outcomes of the clinical practice

The Cycle of Knowledge Transformation Using the ACE Star Model (Stevens, 2004)

See Figure 13-4.

1. Discovery
   a. Primary goal of nursing research: develop a specialized, scientifically based body of nursing knowledge to facilitate improvement in patient care
   b. Definitions
      1) Scientific method: systematic approach to solving problems that controls variables and biases
      2) Basic research: research with purpose to advance knowledge; helps in understanding relationships among phenomena
      3) Applied research: research with purpose to solve a particular problem; helps in making decisions or evaluating techniques
      4) Variable: a measurable concept that varies among the subjects in a research study
         a) Independent variable: the concept that is being observed, introduced, or manipulated in a research study; may be referred to as the *treatment variable*
         b) Dependent variable: the concept that is being observed for a change after the intervention
         c) Extraneous variable: concept that is not being studied but may or may not be relevant to the results of the study; this variable can affect the dependent variable and interfere with research results
      5) Hypothesis: statement that predicts a relationship among two or more variables; may be simple, complex, directional, nondirectional, or null
   c. Research types
      1) Quantitative research: deductive process that tests hypotheses and examines cause-and-effect relationships to examine specific phenomena; emphasizes facts and data to validate or extend existing knowledge
         a) Experimental: uses randomization and a control group to test the effects of an intervention
         b) Quasi-experimental: involves manipulation of variables but lacks a comparison group or randomization
         c) Nonexperimental
            i) Descriptive: describes situations, experiences, and phenomena as they exist
            ii) Ex post facto (correlational): describes relationships between variables
      2) Qualitative: inductive process used to understand phenomena in a defined context; emphasizes development of new insights, theory, and knowledge
         a) Relies less on numbers and measurements and more on nursing strategies, interpersonal communication techniques, intuition, and collaboration between nurse and patient to discover underlying relationships
         b) Includes case studies, open-ended questions, field studies, and participant observation
   d. Steps in the research process
      1) Formulate the research problem.
      2) Review related literature.
      3) Formulate the hypothesis.
      4) Select the research design.
      5) Identify the population to be studied.
      6) Specify methods of data collection.
      7) Design the study.
      8) Conduct the study.
      9) Analyze the data.
      10) Interpret the results.
      11) Communicate the findings.
      12) Utilize the findings to improve patient care.
   e. Ethical responsibilities related to nursing research studies
      1) Protect the rights of research subjects.
      2) Ensure that the potential benefits of the study outweigh any potential risk to the subjects.
      3) Submit the proposed study for review by the investigational review committee.
      4) Obtain informed consent from each subject.
   f. Nursing responsibilities related to research
      1) Identify problem areas and research questions for investigation.
      2) Assist in collection of data as requested.
      3) Read and interpret reports of nursing research.
      4) Assess the quality of nursing research studies and applicability to practice.

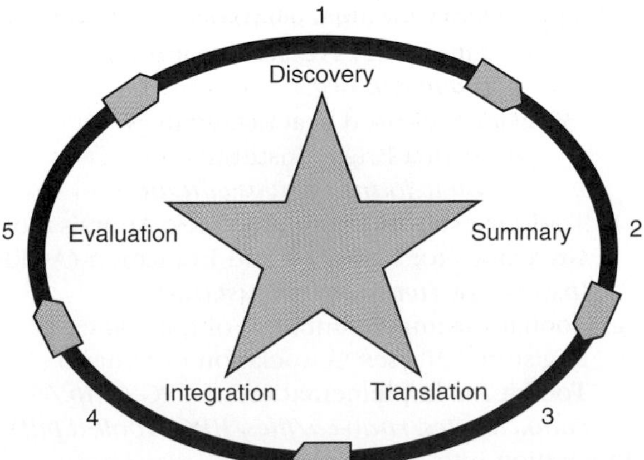

Figure 13-4 ACE Star Model of Knowledge Transformation. (From Stevens, K. R. [2004]. *ACE Star Model of EBP: Knowledge transformation.* Retrieved August 12, 2012, from http://www.acestar.uthscsa.edu/acestar-model.asp

5) Apply research findings to change clinical practice and improve patient care.
6) Share research findings with peers.
7) Design and conduct nursing research.

2. Evidence summary: systematic reviews
   a. Definition: a summary of all evidence related to a specific research question using a rigorous method
      1) Quantitative systematic reviews are conducted using meta-analysis statistical techniques
      2) Qualitative systematic reviews are a descriptive summary of the review of existing studies
   b. Advantage to using systematic reviews (Stevens, 2001)
      1) Provides a usable form because the studies included in the systematic review already have been critically appraised so that high-quality studies are included; more usable for the following:
         a) For clinicians making clinical decisions
         b) For policy makers making policy decisions
         c) For administrations making economic decisions
         d) For researchers making decisions about future research designs
      2) Shortens time between research and clinical implementation
      3) Provides a distillation of large quantities of information into a manageable form with a recommendation for clinical practice
   c. Finding systematic reviews
      1) Agency for Healthcare Research and Quality: *www.ahrq.gov*
      2) The Cochrane Collaboration *www.cochrane.org*
      3) The Campbell Collaboration: *www.campbellcollaboration.org*
      4) The Joanna Briggs Institute: *www.joannabriggs.edu.au/*
3. Translation into practice recommendations: clinical practice guidelines (CPGs)
   a. Definition: a statement based on the best scientific evidence designed to assist clinical decision making about appropriate health care for specific clinical circumstances; Stevens (2004) states that CPGs explicitly articulate the link between the clinical recommendation and the strength of supporting evidence
   b. Advantage of CPG: "can help to overcome the barriers to research use because they eliminate the need to search for journal articles, overcome nurses' limited skills in critical analysis, and minimize the impact of research jargon and unfamiliar terminology because most guidelines are published as clinical application documents." (Ciliska, Pinelli, DiCenso, & Cullum, 2001)
      1) CPG may be incorporated into standards of care, care MAPs, policies and procedures, and protocols
   c. Topics of CPG
      1) A condition (e.g., MI)
      2) A symptom (e.g., chest pain)
      3) A clinical procedure (e.g., PCI)
   d. Purposes of CPG
      1) Encourage treatment that offers individual patients maximum likelihood of benefit and minimum harm and is acceptable in terms of cost
      2) Reduce inappropriate variations in practice
         a) Common reasons for variations
            i) Variations in clinical decision making
            ii) Differing approaches to problem solving
            iii) Varied routines and standards
            iv) Availability of resources
            v) Lack of consensus related to appropriate treatment for given conditions
      3) Promote the delivery of evidence-based health care
      4) Provide ready evaluation criteria by which health care professionals can be made accountable for clinical performance
      5) Reduce the cost of health care
   e. Finding CPG
      1) Governmental agencies
         a) National Guideline Clearinghouse: *www.guidelines.gov*
         b) Scottish Intercollegiate Guideline Network (SIGN): *www.sign.ac.uk/guidelines/index.html*
      2) Select professional associations with EBP resources
         a) Sigma Theta Tau International (STTI): *www.nursingknowledge.org*
         b) American Association of Critical-Care Nurses: *www.aacn.org*
         c) Registered Nurses' Association of Ontario: *www.rnao.org/bestpractices*
         d) Emergency Nurses Association: *www.ena.org*
      3) Evidence-based practice centers
         a) Joanna Briggs Institute: *www.joannabriggs.edu.au*
   f. Tool for evaluation of guidelines: Appraisal of Guidelines for Research and Evaluation (AGREE) Instrument *(www.agreetrust.org)*
   g. Toolkit for implementation of guidelines: Registered Nurses' Association of Ontario Toolkit for Implementation of CPG (*http://rnao.ca/sites/rnao-ca/files/BPG_Toolkit.pdf*)
4. Integration into practice
   a. Select an EBP change model (e.g., Iowa Model of EBP to Promote Quality Care, Stetler Model of Research Utilization, Rosswurm-Larrabee Model of EBP, Johns Hopkins EBP Conceptual Model).

b. Consider organizational barriers to EBP.
c. Utilize organizational strategies to facilitate EBP.
   1) Foster an environment that values inquiry and critical thinking.
      a) Encouragement of formal education
      b) Provision of time to read research and evaluate applicability to setting
      c) Provision of access to the Internet, e-journals, library, and photocopying
      d) Provision of opportunities to attend conferences, continuing education, and in-service education, including education regarding critical appraisal of research
      e) Addition of scholarship to the nurse's role so that dissemination through local, regional, and national presentations and publication is encouraged and expected
      f) Establishment of nursing leadership to spearhead EBP activities, such as a nurse researcher, clinical nurse specialist, or nurse practitioner
      g) Encouragement of the questioning of the status quo and nursing rituals
      h) Development of collaborative teams across disciplines; "EBP is a multidisciplinary practice" (Gray, 1997)
   2) Communicate the expectation of EBP
      a) Incorporation of EBP activities in job descriptions, performance appraisals, merit raises, and career ladders promotions.
      b) Leaders asking, "Why are you doing that?" "Why are you doing that in that way?" "What is the evidence?"
      c) Requirement of evidence for practice changes and revision of policies, procedures, and protocols
   3) Increase nurse autonomy over practice.
      a) Decentralization of administration
      b) Establishment of shared governance with appropriate nursing department council and committee structures
      c) Establishment of unit-level EBP committees
   4) Eliminate the gap between research and practice (NOTE: The gap between research and practice is estimated to be approximately 10 years).
      a) Establishment of more joint appointments between academic and practice settings
      b) Appointment of a nurse researcher on staff
      c) Utilization of expert consultants as necessary
      d) Provision of support for EBP committees and research activities
      e) Development of research presentations (e.g., Nursing Research Grand Rounds)
      f) Establishment of journal clubs
      g) Publication of a monthly research newsletter
   5) Utilize resources appropriately
      a) Commitment of expertise, money, and time to EBP activities, including having adequate staffing
      b) Use of systematic reviews and implementation of clinical practice guidelines

5. Evaluation of the impact of EBP
   a. Formative evaluation: assessment during the change process to ensure that the change has actually occurred and preliminary effects
   b. Summative evaluation: assessment at the completion of the change process to evaluate the impact of the change; possible evaluation criteria may include the following:
      1) Patient health outcomes such as length of stay or quality of life
      2) Patient satisfaction
      3) Staff satisfaction
      4) Cost-benefit impact

Quality Management (QM) and Improvement (QI)

1. Goals
   a. Quality management emphasizes achievement of optimal patient outcomes along with the involvement of employees in the process of monitoring quality, identifying problems, and devising solutions
   b. Quality improvement emphasizes progressive improvement through innovation
2. Areas of focus (Yoder-Wise, 2011)
   a. Customer rather than provider
   b. Prevention rather than detection
   c. System rather than individual
3. Principles (Yoder-Wise, 2011)
   a. QM is most effective within a flat, democratic organizational structure.
   b. Managers and workers must be committed to QI.
   c. Emphasis is on improving systems and processes rather than assigning blame.
   d. Customers ultimately define quality; others involved in definition of quality include governmental agencies, accreditation agencies, and third-party payers.
   e. QI focuses on outcomes.
   f. Decisions must be based on data.
4. QI process
   a. Identify the needs.
   b. Assemble a multidisciplinary team.
   c. Collect data to measure current status.
      1) Structure evaluation: examines the components of services, such as the setting and environment, that affect quality of care
      2) Process evaluation: examines activities and behaviors of the health care provider (e.g., nurse)

3) Outcome evaluation: measures changes in patients
   a) The "five Ds" (Elinson, 1987)
      i) Death
      ii) Disease
      iii) Disability
      iv) Discomfort
      v) Dissatisfaction
   b) Other indicators that are more positive and broader in scope (e.g., functional status, quality of life)
   c) Clinical indicators should reflect desired outcomes and represent high-quality care delivery.

d. Establish outcomes.
   1) Comparison of observed practice with expectations
      a) Retrospective review: examination of completed health care delivery by reviewing charts, conducting conferences or interviews, and reviewing questionnaires
      b) Concurrent review: evaluation of a patient's health status (outcome audit) or management (process) while ongoing by chart reviews, interviews, and observation of the patient
   2) Benchmarks
      a) Reference points or standards against which performance or achievements can be compared
   3) Sources of standards
      a) Internal policies and procedures
      b) State nurse practice acts
      c) Accrediting bodies (e.g., The Joint Commission [TJC])
      d) Professional associations (e.g., American Nurses Association [ANA])
      e) Governmental agencies (Agency for Healthcare Research and Quality [AHRQ])
      f) Award criteria (Magnet, Beacon, & Baldwin)
      g) Other hospitals
   4) Nursing Minimum Data Set: collection of essential nursing information for comparisons across patient populations
      a) Nursing care
         i) Nursing diagnosis
         ii) Nursing intervention
         iii) Nursing outcome
         iv) Intensity of nursing care
      b) Demographics
         i) Personal identification
         ii) Date of birth
         iii) Sex
         iv) Race and ethnicity
         v) Residency
      c) Service
         i) Unique facility or service agency number
         ii) Unique health record number of the patient
         iii) Unique number of a principal registered nurse provider
         iv) Episode, admission, or encounter date
         v) Discharge or termination
         vi) Disposition of patient or client
         vii) Expected payer for most of the bill
   5) National Database of Nursing Quality Indicators (NDNQI)
      a) Developed by the American Nurses Association to promote and facilitate the standardization of information submitted by hospitals across the United States on nursing quality and patient outcomes
      b) Provides comparison data from similar hospitals and units (e.g., teaching status, number of beds, type of patient care unit)
      c) Nursing-Sensitive Indicators: those indicators that capture care or its outcomes most affected by nursing care (ANA, 2012d)
         i) Mix of RNs, LPNs, and unlicensed staff caring for patients in acute care settings
         ii) Total nursing care hours provided per patient day
         iii) Pressure ulcer rate
         iv) Patient falls
         v) Restraints
         vi) Patient satisfaction with pain management
         vii) Patient satisfaction with educational information
         viii) Patient satisfaction with overall care
         ix) Patient satisfaction with nursing care
         x) Nosocomial infection rate
         xi) Nurse staff satisfaction
         xii) Nursing turnover

e. Select and implement a plan to reconcile discrepancies between observations and expectations.

f. Evaluate the implementation of the plan and the achievement of outcomes.

5. Rapid cycle change for improvement
   a. The Model for Improvement (Figure 13-5) is advocated by the Institute for Healthcare Improvement for accelerating improvement.
   b. The model has two parts: (IHI, 2011)
      1) Three fundamental questions that can be addressed in any order:
         a) What are we trying to accomplish?
         b) How will we know that the change is an improvement?
         c) What changes can we make that will result in improvement?

What are we trying to accomplish?

Setting aims
Improvement requires setting aims. The aim should be time-specific and measurable; it should also define the specific population of patients that will be affected.

How will we know that a change is an improvement?

Establishing measures
Teams use quantitative measures to determine if a specific change actually leads to an improvement.

What changes can we make that will result in improvement?

Selecting changes
All improvement requires making changes, but not all changes result in improvement. Organizations therefore must identify the changes that are most likely to result in improvement.

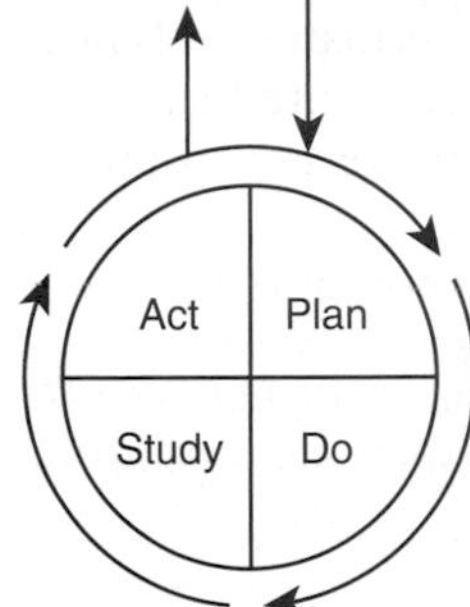

Testing changes
The Plan-Do-Study-Act (PDSA) cycle is shorthand for testing a change in the real work setting—by planning it, trying it, observing the results, and acting on what is learned. This is the scientific method used for action-oriented learning.

Implementing changes
After testing a change on a small scale, learning from each test, and refining the change through several PDSA cycles, the team can implement the change on a broader scale—for example, for an entire pilot population or on an entire unit.

Spreading changes
After successful implementation of a change or package of changes for a pilot population or an entire unit, the team can spread the changes to other parts of the organization or in other organizations.

Figure 13-5 Model for Improvement. (From Langley, G. L., Nolan, K. M., Nolan, T. W., Norman, C. L., & Provost, L. P. [1996]. *The improvement guide: A practical approach to enhancing organizational performance*. San Francisco: Jossey-Bass Publishers.)

2) The Plan-Do-Study-Act (PDSA) cycle to test and implement changes in real work settings

c. Members of the improvement team should be multidisciplinary and are critical to a successful improvement effort.

Patient Safety

1. Recent focus on the impact of medical error on patient outcomes through several publications of the Institute of Medicine (Page, 2004; Kohn, Corrigan, & Donaldson, 2000)
2. The Joint Commission has recently been establishing annual National Patient Safety Goals.
3. The Quality and Safety Education for Nurses (QSEN) project has established competencies for nursing and has proposed targets for knowledge, skills, and attitudes (QSEN, 2012).
   a. Categories
      1) Patient-centered care
      2) Teamwork and collaboration
      3) Evidence-based practice
      4) Quality improvement
      5) Safety
      6) Informatics
   b. Prelicensure and graduate program competencies are intended to be incorporated into curricula.
4. Medication errors
   a. Nurses are most likely to be involved in medication errors than any other form of medical errors.
   b. Prevention of medication errors (Dennison, 2005)
      1) Individual responsibility
         a) Ten rights
            i) Right patient: Use two patient identifiers (i.e., not patient's room and bed number)
            ii) Right drug
            iii) Right dose
            iv) Right time
            v) Right route
            vi) Right reason
            vii) Patient's right to education
            viii) Patient's right to refuse
            ix) Patient evaluation: Clarify titration parameters.
            x) Right documentation
         b) Reporting of errors and near-hits so that system analysis can occur and prevent future errors
      2) Systems thinking
         a) Nonpunitive culture
         b) Adherence to policies, procedures, and protocols
            i) Avoidance of unapproved abbreviations, trailing zeros
            ii) Avoidance of verbal orders; if necessary, a verbal repeat should be used for confirmation
            iii) Label with drug being administered
               (a) Bag
               (b) Pump chamber (using channel labels on infusion pump if available)
               (c) Tubing
         c) Use of information
            i) Patient information (e.g., laboratory values, vital signs); electronic patient record is preferred because the record is available to more than one health care professional simultaneously
            ii) Drug information: Use up-to-date medication references such as Micromedex, Epocrates, and drug books that are updated annually.
         d) Use of technology
            i) Automated dispensing devices
            ii) Bar-code point of care (BPOC)

iii) Computerized provider order entry (CPOE)
iv) "Smart" pumps with guardrails to alert the nurse of too high or too low dose

e) Standardization
   i) Restriction of formulary (i.e., do you really need to have three GP IIb/IIIa inhibitors or will one or two suffice?)
   ii) Standardization of infusion concentrations (i.e., avoid double, triple, quadruple concentration)
   iii) Standardization of equipment (e.g., infusion pumps)

f) Pharmacist
   i) Review of all prescriptions
   ii) Presence on unit and on rounds

g) Medication reconciliation

h) Environment control
   i) Adequate lighting
   ii) Noise reduction
   iii) Distraction avoidance
   iv) Clean, clutter-free, organized space for preparation of medications

i) Teamwork
   i) Clarification of any unclear prescription
   ii) Utilization of independent double-checks of drug, dose, calculation, patient identity, infusion rate, and appropriate line for all high-alert medications (Box 13-2)
      (a) "Check this *with* me" is unacceptable because it causes confirmation error (i.e., you see what you expect to see).
      (b) Also applies to dose changes of high-alert drugs
   iii) Use of time-out if there is a question about the safety of the drug for this patient, at this time, at this dose, by this route; never administer a drug that is unsafe
   iv) Documentation and communication of changes in patient response or adverse drug events

Box 13-2 High-Alert Medication Infusions Frequently Administered in Critical Care Areas

Classes/Categories of Medications

Adrenergic agonists (e.g., epinephrine, norepinephrine, dopamine, dobutamine)
Adrenergic antagonists (e.g., esmolol)
Anesthetic agents (e.g., propofol)
Anticoagulants (e.g., heparin, bivalirudin, argatroban, lepirudin)
Antidysrhythmics (e.g., amiodarone, lidocaine)
Antineoplastic agents
Dextrose, hypertonic, 20% or greater
Electrolyte solutions (e.g., potassium chloride, potassium phosphate, magnesium sulfate, hypertonic sodium chloride)
Fibrinolytics (e.g., streptokinase, anistreplase, alteplase, tenecteplase)
Glycoprotein IIb/IIIa inhibitors (e.g., eptifibatide)
Inotropic agents (e.g., milrinone)
Liposomal forms of drugs (e.g., liposomal amphotericin B)
Moderate sedation agents (e.g., midazolam, lorazepam, diazepam)
Narcotics/opiates
Neuromuscular blocking agents (e.g., atracurium, vecuronium, cisatracurium, pancuronium)
Total parenteral nutrition solutions
Vasodilators (e.g., nitroglycerin, nitroprusside, nesiritide)

Adapted from Institute for Safe Medication Practices. *ISMP's List of high-alert medications.* Available at: http://www.ismp.org/Tools/highalertmedications.pdf.

Peer Review

1. Component of professional autonomy and development
2. Purpose is to ensure quality and safety through maintaining standards of care.
3. Process is defined by a representative goal of nurses; it does not replace annual performance reviews by nursing leadership.
4. Six principles (Haag-Heitman & George, 2011)
   a. A peer is someone of the same rank.
   b. Peer review is practice-focused.
   c. Feedback is timely, routine, and a continuous expectation.
   d. Peer review fosters a continuous learning culture of patient safety and best practice.
   e. Feedback is not anonymous.
   f. Feedback incorporates the nurse's developmental stage.

Facilitator of Learning of Patient/Family Educator

Description

The ability to facilitate patient and family learning

Definitions

1. Teaching; the process of facilitating learning; an interaction designed to help a person learn to do something that he or she is currently unable to do; a two-way interaction
2. Learning; the process by which a person becomes capable of doing something he or she could not do before, including a wide range of behavior from motor skills to intellectual skills; an emotional experience which can be negative or positive, traumatic, or pleasant

3. Patient education: the process of teaching patients and their families about an illness, treatment, and other health-related matters, including how to adhere to the regimen and helping them change their behavior.

Reasons for Patient Education

1. Because the patient has a need and a right to know those things that are relevant to his or her condition, disease, or situation
2. To produce changes in knowledge, skills, attitudes, appreciation, and understanding
3. To promote and improve health
4. To encourage the patient to assume responsibility for disease management
5. To prevent illness and complications
6. To aid in coping with illness and adaptation to change
7. To promote compliance with the therapeutic regimen
8. To reduce anxiety (including family stress and anxiety)
9. To reduce the number of visits to the physician's office and/or emergency department and the number and length of hospitalizations
10. To comply with regulatory requirements

Principles of Adult Education

1. Qualities of the adult learner: a self-directed independent person who becomes ready to learn when the need to know or to perform is experienced; characteristics of the adult learner are likely to include the following:
   a. Goal-oriented
   b. Less flexible
   c. Requires longer time in the performance of learning tasks
   d. Impatient in the pursuit of objectives
   e. Finds little use for isolated facts
   f. Strives for recognition and success
   g. Has multiple responsibilities, all of which draw upon his or her time
   h. Experienced in the "school of life"
   i. Requires a more constant and ideal learning environment
   j. Usually comes to the teaching program on a voluntary basis
   k. Wishes to be involved in mutual planning of learning experiences
   l. Likes to participate in diagnosing needs for learning, formulating learning objectives, and evaluating learning
   m. Expects a climate of mutual respect, trust, and collaboration that supports learning
2. Educational concepts useful with adults
   a. Pacing
      1) Allow adults to set their own pace, if possible.
      2) Tasks or methods involving significant time pressure are likely to be difficult for adults.
   b. Arousal anxiety
      1) Some degree of arousal is necessary for learning; however, older adults may become anxious in a learning situation.
      2) Allow individuals an opportunity to become familiar with a situation.
      3) Minimize the role of competition and evaluation.
   c. Fatigue
      1) Some tasks may produce considerable mental or physical fatigue, a problem likely to particularly affect older adults.
      2) Shorten the instruction sessions or provide frequent rest breaks.
   d. Difficulty: Arrange materials from the simple to the complex in order to build the individual's confidence and skills.
   e. Errors: Structure the tasks so errors are avoided and do not have to be unlearned.
   f. Practice: Provide an opportunity for practice on similar but different tasks; such practice helps to develop generalizable skills.
   g. Feedback: Provide information on the adequacy of previous responses.
   h. Cues
      1) Materials should be presented to compensate for the potential sensory problems of older adults.
      2) Direct attention toward the relevant aspects of the task.
      3) Reduce the level of irrelevant information to a minimum.
   i. Organization
      1) Learning and remembering often require that information be grouped or related in some way.
      2) Instruct individuals in the use of various mnemonic techniques (e.g., mental images, verbal associations) which may be used to elaborate or organize the material.
   j. Relevance/experience
      1) People learn and remember what is important to them.
      2) Attempt to make the task relevant to the individual's concerns.
      3) Performance is likely to be facilitated to the extent that the individuals are able to integrate the new information with known information.

Barriers to Teaching/Learning

1. Nurse factors: lack of time, lack of knowledge, or consideration of teaching as a lower priority than physical care
2. Physician interference (i.e., not wanting the nurse to teach the patient)
3. Patient factors
   a. Physiologic factors
      1) Instability
      2) Sedation
      3) Pain

b. Lack of availability (e.g., procedures, physical therapy)
c. Psychological factors (e.g., anxiety, pain)
d. Poor language or reading skills
e. Sensory deficits: vision, hearing
f. Poor manual dexterity for psychomotor skills
g. Attitudes and beliefs that conflict with teaching

Teaching/Learning Process

1. Assessment
   a. Readiness to learn
      1) Desire to know (e.g., asking questions)
      2) Absence of acute distress (e.g., pain, dyspnea)
      3) Adequate energy
   b. Sensory deficits (e.g., use of eyeglasses, hearing aid)
   c. Educational level and reading ability
   d. Learning style
      1) Environment
         a) Formal or informal
         b) Tolerance to distraction
      2) Alone or in a group
      3) Preferred learning mode
         a) Reading: print materials
         b) Seeing: pictorial materials
         c) Listening: auditory
         d) Manipulating: tactile, kinesthetic
2. Plan
   a. Identify objectives; parts of the objective should include the following:
      1) What should the learner be able to do? (behavior)
         a) Cognitive
         b) Affective
         c) Psychomotor
      2) How well should the learner be able to do it? (the criteria)
      3) Under what conditions should the learner be able to do it? (the condition)
   b. Identify content to teach.
      1) Language and terminology
      2) Health care system: personnel; organization and structure; routines and procedures; norms and expectations; immediate environment
      3) Basic anatomy and physiology of affected body system
      4) Diagnosis, disease process
      5) Therapy: treatments, medications, diet, activity, personal health habits
      6) Prevention of complications
      7) Skills (e.g., insulin administration, pulse-taking)
      8) Community resources
   c. Determine methods.
      1) Individual or group
         a) Use individual method when you are assessing patient's knowledge, when family members or friends try to dominate teaching sessions, and when the information you'll teach provokes anxiety or is considered a topic not generally discussed in public.
         b) Individual methods include programmed instruction, reading materials, AV aids, and one-to-one instruction.
         c) Group sessions lessen feelings of alienation and being "different"; learners learn from other learners.
         d) Patient-operated groups and self-help groups offer the benefit of encouraging patients to share coping techniques and useful hints.
         e) Group teaching saves time and money.
         f) Family members gain support from health professionals and other patients and their families.
         g) Combinations may be helpful to meet the patient's individual needs.
      2) Teaching methods: The teacher of adults is a facilitator more than a teacher and uses various methods.
         a) Lecture
            i) May be in group session, on videotape, or on closed-circuit TV
            ii) Is usually no longer than 20 minutes
            iii) Includes the introduction to establish the need to know, the body to deliver content that needs to be known, and the summary to review what was covered
         b) Discussion
            i) Helps the patient to ask any questions about information that is in doubt
            ii) Guides the nurse to assess what the patient needs to know
         c) Audiovisuals
            i) Includes visual and auditory stimulation to teach content
         d) Printed materials
            i) May be used in place of other techniques but should include a discussion with the nurses after reading for clarification of content
            ii) May be used as a supplement to other methods
            iii) Useful as an aid to review at a later date
            iv) Should be written at no higher than sixth grade level and lower if possible (Institute for Healthcare Advancement, 2012)
            v) Need to be in patient's language
         e) Explanations
            i) Give only as much information as requested
            ii) Ask for feedback
         f) Exploration: Encourage patient to answer own questions.

g) Demonstration and return demonstration
   i) Used when the patient must learn a new skill
   ii) Describe what you are going to do, then do it while the patient observes; then talk to patient through the process while the patient does it; finally have the patient perform the skill while the patient tells you what he or she is doing.
h) Role-playing
   i) Provides practice in a safe setting
   ii) Useful to see how others might respond

3. Implement
   a. Assign one person to teach the patient to minimize confusion, contradiction, and incompleteness.
   b. Schedule teaching sessions according to the patient's receptiveness; let the patient set the pace and choose topics of most interest first.
   c. Provide ideal setting: Control the environment.
   d. Know your subject area: Be competent and confident.
   e. Speak the patient's language: Minimize use of medical terminology.
   f. Consider your presentation style.
      1) Keep the presentations of material short.
      2) Place key points up front.
      3) Use verbal headings.
      4) Summarize at the end.
      5) Obtain feedback and request questions.
   g. Include "why" where appropriate.
   h. Use visual aids.
   i. Remember that successful learning takes time and reinforcement.
   j. Provide a means for the patient to learn more, such as written information for reading and review, resource groups, and an outpatient program.
   k. Coordinate education through written teaching plans, patient care conferences, and documentation.
      1) Written teaching plans should include the following:
         a) Objectives
         b) Content
         c) Teaching methods
         d) Methods of evaluation
      2) Documentation should include the following:
         a) Objectives
         b) Content outline
         c) Method used
         d) Evaluation of learning
            i) Objective met
            ii) Objective partially met: needs reinforcement
            iii) Objective not met: needs repeat
         e) Comments
         f) Signature
4. Evaluate learning using any of the following methods:
   a. Written tests
   b. Oral evaluation
   c. Return demonstration
   d. Analysis of physical findings (e.g., serum glucose, weight)
   e. Follow-up questionnaire

Education for Low-Literacy Individuals

1. Definition: adults with poorly developed skills in reading, writing, listening, and speaking
2. Assessing literacy level
   a. Individuals reading at a fifth-grade or higher level are considered literate; hand printing instructions and asking the patient to read them back to you is a nonthreatening way to assess reading ability.
   b. Incongruent behavior may signal a literacy problem; be alert for behavior that does not match the reported level of understanding.
   c. Low-literacy materials are preferred for low-literacy individuals.
3. Teaching strategies for low-literacy patients
   a. Identify and eliminate or minimize stress, anxiety, or other distractions before teaching.
   b. Correct misconceptions that affect learning.
   c. Personalize the health message and explain the need for the information.
   d. Relate information to patient's past experiences and actively involve the patient and family in discussions.
   e. Consider qualities of poor readers and utilize teaching strategies that are helpful (Table 13-10).

Table 13-10 Qualities of Poor Readers and Appropriate Teaching Strategies

Qualities of Poor Readers	Teaching Strategies
Take words literally	Explain the meaning of all words
Read slowly; miss meaning	Use common words and examples
Skip over uncommon words	Use examples, review content frequently
Miss content	Describe content first, use verbal heading and visuals
Tire quickly	Use short segments

LEARNING ACTIVITIES

CHAPTER 13

1. Complete the following crossword puzzle.

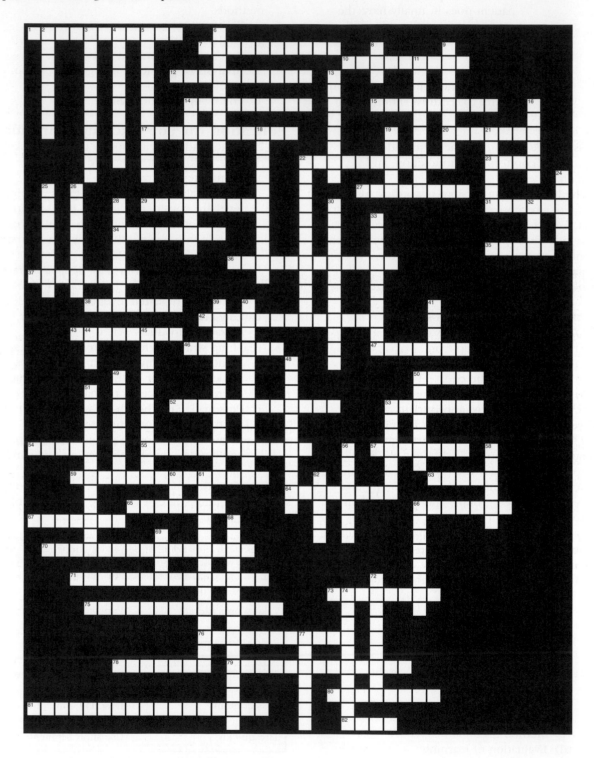

ACROSS

1. Involves use of conscious mental effort to control involuntary body function, such as BP, heart rate, respiratory rate
7. A nurse who was born in 1950 would be in this generational group
10. The type of variable that is the response or outcome the researcher would like to explain or predict
12. This method is a systematic approach to solving problems that controls variables and biases
14. A reference point against which performance can be compared
15. Ethical approach that asserts that actions are right or wrong based on consequences
17. The third point on the ACE Star model
20. An ethical ____ is a situation that requires a choice between two undesirable alternatives
22. Failing to do something that a reasonable and prudent professional would do or doing something that a reasonable and prudent professional would not do
23. To wish for something with the expectation of its fulfillment
27. The right to self-determination
29. Includes behavior, criteria, and condition
31. A collection of interdependent elements that interact to achieve a common purpose
34. This type of thinking is controlled, purposeful, and goal-directed reasoning
35. Belief not based on logical proof or material evidence
36. The process of seeking, giving, and receiving help
37. This type of consent is voluntarily given after the patient has been given required information
38. Culturally prescribed codes of behavior
42. When one knows the right thing to do but cannot pursue the right action (2 words)
43. The process of facilitating learning
46. Learned, shared, and transmitted values, beliefs, and practices of a particular group that guides thinking
47. The second point on the ACE Star model is the ____ of evidence
50. One of the recommendations of the IOM publication *The Future of Nursing* is to remove the barriers on the ____ of nursing practice
52. A basic human phenomenon that helps create meaning in the world
53. Focusing and directing the imagination through the use of specific words and suggestions
54. One way to eliminate the gap between research and practice is to establish _____ appointments between academic and clinical facilities
55. Type of research that uses randomization and a control group to test the effects of an intervention
57. Patterns and practices within a cultural group that encompass collective learned behaviors
59. The ethical approach that asserts that actions are right or wrong based on the greatest good for the greatest number
63. Type of charges that could be filed if a nurse unintentionally causes a patient's death
64. The obligation to tell the truth
65. The obligation to be fair to all people
66. Type of research to solve a particular problem
67. This type of consent applies when the patient cannot give consent but treatment is needed immediately
70. Critical care nurses deal with human responses to ____ problems
71. The fourth point on the ACE Star model
73. The kind of evidence that is "best" if it is available
75. The obligation to do no harm
76. Assault, battery, and defamation are all examples of this type of tort
78. Nursing care delivery system where one nurse has accountability for the patient's care during the entire hospitalization
79. The process by which an individual or group takes on the behaviors and practices of the dominant culture
80. The obligation to be faithful to agreements and responsibilities accepted
81. Quantitative research design that does not utilize a control group or randomization
82. A collection of essential nursing information for comparison across patient populations (abbrev)

DOWN

2. Type of consent that must be obtained prior to inclusion as a subject in a study
3. A statutory right of a defined group
4. Ethical approach that asserts that actions are right or wrong based on a set of morals or rules
5. Insertion of needles into specific points in the body for therapeutic purposes
6. To assist an individual to make a decision when he or she does not have the data or expertise
8. A statement designed to assist the clinician in making decisions about the appropriate health care for specific clinical situations (abbrev)
9. The first point on the ACE Star model is discovery of _____
11. Achieving performance of care outcomes for which you are accountable and responsible by sharing activities with other individuals who have the appropriate authority to accomplish the work
13. A concept examined in a research study
14. The obligation to do good
16. An intimate conversation between an individual and God or other Higher Being
18. Type of variable that is the presumed cause of the change in the dependent variable
19. Format for posing clinical questions (abbrev)
21. Systems of valued behaviors and beliefs that govern proper conduct
22. Statistical technique for conducting quantitative systematic reviews; yields a summary statistic
24. Using words and images to elicit laughter
25. The process by which a person becomes capable of doing something he or she could not previously do
26. Specific unified system of an expression of the belief in and reverence for a supernatural power accepted as the creator and governor of the universe
28. This type of report is completed for errors or other unusual occurrences
30. Use of scents for therapeutic purposes
32. A legal wrong committed against a person or property
33. Statement that predicts a relationship among two or more variables
39. Working together
40. M level on the AACN Level of Evidence scale includes recommendations from ____
41. Process for rapid cycle change (abbrev)
44. The integration of best evidence, clinician expertise, patient values, and circumstances (abbrev)
45. Quality _____ emphasizes innovation
48. Type of research that takes place in the individual's natural setting with emphasis on

understanding human experience; results in words or phrases

49. Type of charges that would be filed if a nurse intentionally caused a patient's death
50. A nurse practice act is an example of a ____
51. Type of research that controls study variables as much as possible and has objective and measurable data collection; results in numbers
53. A goal for fostering EBP is to create a spirit of ____
56. The nursing ____ is assess, diagnose, plan, implement, and evaluate
58. Personal beliefs about the truth and the worth of thoughts, objects, and behaviors
60. The "gold standard" of evidence (abbrev)
61. Answerability or responsibility
62. Quality, quantity, and consistency are used to ____ the evidence
66. Working on another's behalf
68. The obligation to respect privileged information
69. A group of people related by common descent of heredity who have similar physical characteristics
72. Nursing____ indicators are those indicators that capture care or the outcomes most affected by nursing care
74. The fifth point on the ACE Star model
77. Type of evaluation or review that might look at a physiologic parameter

2. List the six steps of the decision-making process.

a. ____________________

b. ____________________

c. ____________________

d. ____________________

e. ____________________

f. ____________________

3. Match the situation with the ethical concept demonstrated.

___ 1. Veracity
___ 2. Confidentiality
___ 3. Autonomy
___ 4. Nonmaleficence
___ 5. Fidelity
___ 6. Justice
___ 7. Advocacy

a. The new surgical resident has made three attempts to place a central venous catheter in an elderly patient. The nurse insists that no more attempts be made until the attending physician is present.
b. The nurse makes a medical error but the patient suffers no harm. She reports the error and completes an incident report.
c. The patient has decided that he does not want to be intubated again. You ensure that his wishes are recorded and honored.
d. The nurse explains to the patient that care will still be provided despite the fact that he has no health insurance.
e. The nurse's next-door neighbor is in the hospital. She visits him, but she does not read his chart.
f. The nurse begins on time, takes only the allotted time for lunch, and leaves after completion of work and report.
g. The confused patient keeps reaching for his endotracheal tube. The nurse applies soft restraints to prevent self-extubation.

4. Match the ethical approach to the statement that best describes a "right" decision using the approach.

___ 1. Utilitarianism
___ 2. Egoism
___ 3. Deontology
___ 4. Paternalism
___ 5. Social contract
___ 6. Natural law
___ 7. Teleology

a. When it results in the most good for the most people
b. When it results in a positive outcome
c. When it is the best thing in the opinion of the decision maker
d. When it provides significant benefit to the decision maker
e. When it is in accordance with human nature
f. When it is inherently right morally
g. When some rights must be lost for the greater good of society

5. List eight complementary therapies that are helpful with patients with stress, anxiety, or pain.

a. ______

b. ______

c. ______

d. ______

e. ______

f. ______

g. ______

h. ______

6. List five of the most important needs of families as identified by the classic work of Leske.

a. ______

b. ______

c. ______

d. ______

e. ______

7. List five of the essential elements of collaboration.

a. ______

b. ______

c. ______

d. ______

e. ______

8. Describe a change model and how you might use it to make a change that you feel is needed on your unit.

______

9. Note whether the following statements are True or False.

a. The nurse's own values and beliefs will not affect his or her sensitivities with patients	
b. Pain is influenced by culture	
c. Race is not a factor in drug absorption and action	
d. It is never appropriate for a nurse to pray with a patient; the chaplain should be called	
e. Physical care should always take precedence over psychosocial and spiritual care	

10. Match the religion with the implication.

___ 1. Islam (Muslim)
___ 2. Catholicism
___ 3. Judaism
___ 4. Hinduism
___ 5. Christian Scientist
___ 6. Seventh-Day Adventist
___ 7. Jehovah's Witnesses

a. Provide kosher diet as requested
b. Opposed to blood transfusions
c. Provide same-sex caregivers
d. Medical care may be refused; prayer is used as the primary treatment of illness
e. The patient must be baptized before death
f. Procedures may be refused between dusk on Friday and dusk on Saturday
g. The patient's head is turned to the right after death

11. Match the following activities with the appropriate point on the ACE Star Model for Knowledge Transformation. Points may be used more than once.

___ 1. Developing a clinical practice guideline for a common clinical condition or procedure
___ 2. Designing and conducting a research study when the available evidence base is inadequate
___ 3. Conducting a systematic review of available evidence related to a clinical issue
___ 4. Initiation of an evidence-based clinical change
___ 5. Appraisal of the impact of an evidence-based clinical change
___ 6. Conducting a literature search for available evidence related to a clinical question

a. Discovery
b. Summary
c. Translation
d. Implementation
e. Evaluation

12. List five ways to share research findings with colleagues.

a. ______________________________
b. ______________________________
c. ______________________________
d. ______________________________
e. ______________________________

13. List five qualities of an adult learner.

a. ______________________________
b. ______________________________
c. ______________________________
d. ______________________________
e. ______________________________

LEARNING ACTIVITIES ANSWERS

CHAPTER 2

1.

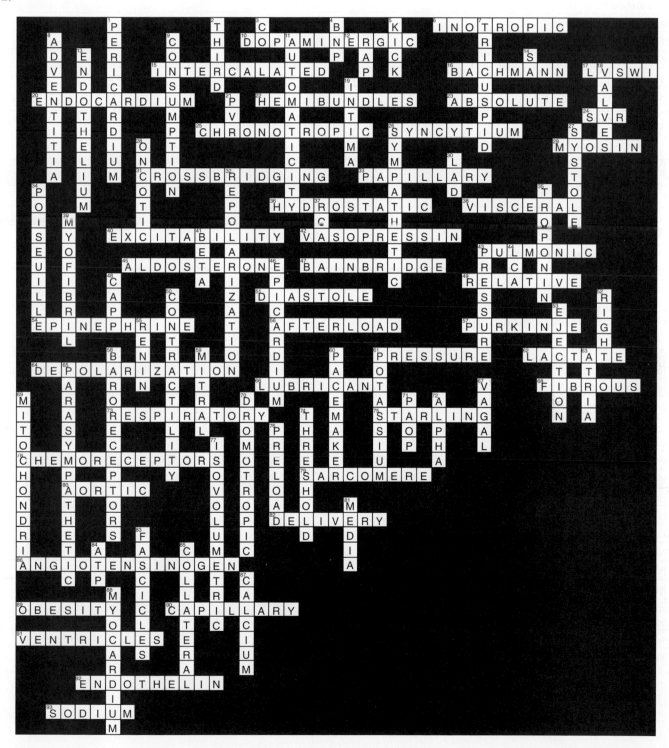

2.

Structure	Coronary Artery
Anterior left ventricle	LAD
AV node	Most commonly RCA; less commonly LCA
Bundle branches	LAD
Inferior left ventricle	RCA
Lateral left ventricle	LCA
Left atrium	LCA
Posterior left ventricle	Most commonly RCA; less commonly LCA
Right atrium	RCA
Right ventricle	RCA
SA node	Most commonly RCA; less commonly LCA
Septum	LAD

3.

Myocardial Oxygen Supply	Myocardial Oxygen Demand
Coronary artery patency	Heart rate
Diastolic pressure	Preload
Diastolic time	Afterload
Oxygen extraction: hemoglobin; SaO_2	Contractility

4. Remember that you were asked to identify primary effects. If you gave answers other than these, perhaps you were thinking of the secondary effects, especially those mediated by the SNS or the resultant effect of a decrease in preload on contractility.

Conditions				
Aortic stenosis	___Heart Rate	___Preload	↑ LV Afterload	___Contractility
Bradydysrhythmias	↓ Heart Rate	↑ Preload	___Afterload	___Contractility
Cardiac tamponade	___Heart Rate	↓ Preload	___Afterload	___Contractility
Cardiogenic shock	___Heart Rate	↑ Preload	↑ Afterload	↓ Contractility
Cardiomyopathy	___Heart Rate	___Preload	___Afterload	↓ Contractility
Heart failure	___Heart Rate	↑ Preload	↑ Afterload	↓ Contractility
Hypertension	___Heart Rate	___Preload	↑ LV Afterload	___Contractility
Hypovolemia	___Heart Rate	↓ Preload	___Afterload	___Contractility
Left ventricular myocardial infarction	___Heart Rate	___Preload	___Afterload	↓ Contractility
Neurogenic shock	↓ Heart Rate	↓ Preload	↓ Afterload	___Contractility
Pulmonary hypertension	___Heart Rate	___Preload	↑RV Afterload	___Contractility
Right ventricular myocardial infarction	___Heart Rate	↑RV Preload ↓LV Preload	___Afterload	↓ Contractility
Septic shock - early	___Heart Rate	↓ Preload	↓ Afterload	↑ Contractility
Septic shock - late	___Heart Rate	↓ Preload	↓ Afterload	↓ Contractility
Tachydysrhythmias	↑ Heart Rate	↓ Preload	___Afterload	___Contractility

Treatments				
Aminophylline	___Heart Rate	___Preload	↓RV Afterload	___Contractility
Digoxin (Lanoxin)	↓ Heart Rate	___Preload	___Afterload	↑ Contractility
Dobutamine (Dobutrex)	___Heart Rate	↓ Preload	↓ Afterload	↑ Contractility
Dopamine (3-5 mcg/kg/min)	↑ Heart Rate	___Preload	___Afterload	↑ Contractility
Dopamine (5-10 mcg/kg/min)	↑ Heart Rate	___Preload	↑ Afterload	↑ Contractility
Dopamine (>10 mcg/kg/min)	↑ Heart Rate	___Preload	↑ Afterload	___Contractility
Fluid challenge	___Heart Rate	↑ Preload	___Afterload	___Contractility
Furosemide (Lasix)	___Heart Rate	↓ Preload	↓RV Afterload	___Contractility
Intraaortic balloon pump	___Heart Rate	___Preload	↓ Afterload	___Contractility
Isoproterenol (Isuprel)	↑ Heart Rate	↓ Preload	↓ Afterload	↑ Contractility
Milrinone (Primacor)	___Heart Rate	↓ Preload	↓ Afterload	↑ Contractility
Nesiritide (Natrecor)	___Heart Rate	↓ Preload	↓ Afterload	___Contractility
Nitroglycerin	___Heart Rate	↓ Preload	* Afterload	___Contractility
Nitroprusside (Nipride)	___Heart Rate	↓ Preload	↓ Afterload	___Contractility
Phenylephrine (Neo-Synephrine)	___Heart Rate	___Preload	↑ Afterload	___Contractility
Propranolol (Inderal)	↓ Heart Rate	___Preload	___Afterload	↓ Contractility
Vasopressin (Pitressin)	___Heart Rate	___Preload	↑ Afterload	___Contractility

*Nitroglycerin will decrease afterload if dosage is greater than 1 mcg/kg/min or approximately 70 mcg/min in a 70-kg patient.

5.

b 1. Increase in heart rate, contractility, conductivity
d 2. Dilation of the renal and mesenteric arteries
a 3. Vasoconstriction
c 4. Vasodilation and bronchodilation

6.

c 1. $Alpha_1$
d 2. $Beta_1$
a 3. $Beta_2$
b 4. Dopaminergic

7.

Parameter	Formula
a. Cardiac output (CO)	heart rate (HR) × stroke volume (SV)
b. Stroke index (SI)	cardiac index (CI) ÷ heart rate (HR)
c. Blood pressure (BP)	cardiac output (CO) × systemic vascular resistance (SVR)
d. Coronary artery perfusion pressure (CAPP)	diastolic BP – pulmonary artery occlusive pressure (PAOP)
e. Mean arterial pressure (MAP)	[BP systolic + (BP diastolic × 2)] ÷ 3
f. Systemic vascular resistance (SVR)	[(MAP – RAP) × 80] ÷ CO
g. Delivery of oxygen to the tissues (DO_2)	Hgb × SaO_2 × CO × 13.4

8.

k 1. S_1
i 2. S_2
a 3. Physiologic split of S_2
f 4. Paradoxical split of S_2
b 5. Fixed, wide split of S_2
h 6. S_3
m 7. S_4
c 8. Pericardial friction rub
j 9. Midsystolic click
g 10. Holosystolic murmur
d 11. Systolic ejection murmur
l 12. Early diastolic murmur
e 13. Mid- to late-diastolic murmur

9.

Condition	Timing	Location	Pitch
Mitral regurgitation	Systolic	Mitral (apex)	High
Mitral stenosis	Diastolic	Mitral (apex)	Low
Aortic regurgitation	Diastolic	Aortic (base)	High
Aortic stenosis	Systolic	Aortic (base)	High
Mitral valve prolapse	Systolic	Mitral (apex)	High
Papillary muscle dysfunction or rupture	Systolic	Mitral (apex)	High
Ventricular septal defect or rupture	Systolic	LLSB	High

NOTES:
1) To figure out timing, consider when the valve would have been open or closed. For example, in mitral regurgitation, the mitral valve would not be closed when it should be closed which is during systole so this is a systolic murmur. Another example would be that the aortic valve would not be open when it should be open in aortic stenosis so this is also a systolic murmur.
2) To figure out location, consider the auscultatory areas; a mitral valve problem would cause a murmur in the mitral auscultatory area which is at the apex.
3) To figure out pitch, remember that all murmurs are high-pitched except murmurs of AV valve stenosis (i.e., mitral or tricuspid stenosis).

10.

k 1. Normal sinus rhythm
e 2. Sinus bradycardia
j 3. Sinus tachycardia
b 4. Premature atrial contraction
f 5. Atrial fibrillation
c 6. Atrial flutter
p 7. Supraventricular tachycardia
g 8. Premature junctional contraction
h 9. Junctional escape rhythm
m 10. Accelerated junctional rhythm
o 11. Junctional tachycardia
d 12. Premature ventricular complex
n 13. Accelerated idioventricular rhythm
t 14. Ventricular tachycardia
s 15. Ventricular fibrillation
i 16. Asystole
a 17. First-degree AV block
l 18. Second-degree AV block, type I
q 19. Second-degree AV block, type II
r 20. Third-degree AV block

11.

a. Ventricular fibrillation
b. Sinus bradycardia with wide QRS (BBB should be assessed for on 12-lead ECG)
c. Supraventricular tachycardia; this is a regular narrow QRS tachycardia with no discernible P waves; the P waves could be hidden in the QRS or T wave so there is no way to identify where above the ventricle the rhythm originates but the rate of 180/min suggests an atrial origin.
d. Idioventricular (escape) rhythm
e. Underlying sinus rhythm (atrial rate is 90/min); there is a third-degree AV block with a ventricular escape rhythm (ventricular rate is 35/min)
f. Underlying rhythm is sinus rhythm (atrial rate is 80/min); there is a second-degree type I (Wenckebach) AV block present; conduction ratio is 3:2 and ventricular rate is 40-50/min
g. Ventricular tachycardia (monomorphic)
h. Underlying rhythm is sinus tachycardia (atrial rate is 145/min); there is a second-degree type II block present; conduction ratio is variable but the PR interval of the conducted P wave is consistent
i. Sinus rhythm with two unifocal PVCs

12.

g 1. Acute myocardial infarction
k 2. Hypercalcemia
n 3. Hyperkalemia
b 4. Hypocalcemia
l 5. Hypokalemia
e 6. Left atrial enlargement
f 7. Left bundle branch block
h 8. Left ventricular hypertrophy
d 9. Pericarditis
m 10. Variant angina
j 11. Right atrial enlargement
i 12. Right bundle branch block
c 13. Right ventricular hypertrophy
a 14. Wellens syndrome

13.

g 1. II, III, aVF
e 2. V_{4R}
b 3. I, aVL
f 4. V_1, V_2
a 5. V_3, V_4
c 6. V_5, V_6
d 7. V_8, V_9

14.

a. LBBB: Note indicative changes of BBB in V_6 (LV lead) and the wide QRS is totally below the isoelectric line in V_1.
b. RBBB: Note indicative changes of BBB in V_1 (RV lead) and the wide QRS is totally above the isoelectric line in V_1.

15.

a. Right axis deviation: Note negative QRS in I and positive QRS in aVF. Right atrial enlargement: Note tall, peaked P wave in lead II and dominant initial component of the P wave in V_1. Right ventricular hypertrophy: Note dominant R in V_1 along with RAD, RAE, and strain pattern (i.e., asymmetric T wave inversion in V_1 and V_2).
b. Normal axis: Note positive QRS in I and isoelectric QRS in aVF. Left atrial enlargement: Note wide, notched P wave in lead II. Left ventricular hypertrophy: Note deep S wave (must be doubled since voltage was halved when the ECG was recorded) in V_1 and tall R wave in V_5. To check for voltage criteria, add the S in V_1 or V_2 and the R in V_5 or V_6. Since the sum is greater than 35 mm (40 in this case), voltage criteria for LVH is met.

16.

a. Normal axis: Note positive QRS in I and positive QRS in aVL. ST segment elevation is noted from V_1 - V_6. Pathologic Q waves are noted in V_2 and V_3. There is a small R wave in V_1 so the negative wave in that lead is an S wave. This ECG shows evidence of hyperacute anterior MI with injury extending to the septal and lateral walls.

b. Left axis deviation: Note positive QRS in I and negative QRS in aVF. ST segment elevation and pathologic Q waves are noted in II, III, and aVF indicative of acute inferior MI. Reciprocal changes in the V leads (ST segment depression from V_1-V_5) suggests posterior wall involvement also. Posterior wall leads are indicated.

17.

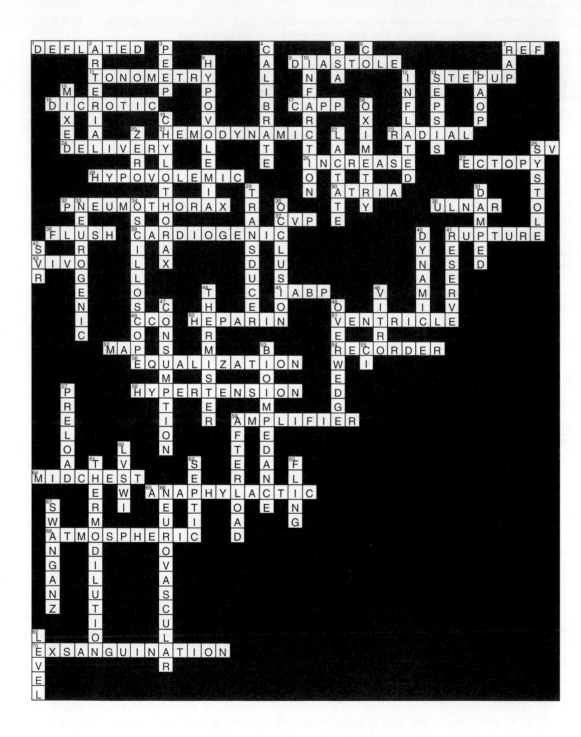

18.

i 1. Cardiac tamponade
h 2. Noncardiac pulmonary edema
g 3. Cardiac pulmonary edema
b 4. Rupture of interventricular septum
d 5. Pulmonary hypertension
c 6. Papillary muscle rupture
a 7. Right ventricular MI
f 8. Cardiogenic shock
e 9. Hypovolemic shock

19.

a.

Parameter	↑, ↓, or Normal	Parameter	↑, ↓, or Normal
BP: 88/70 mm Hg	↓	SV: 23 ml/beat	↓
MAP: 76 mm Hg	Normal	SI: 14 ml/m²/beat	↓
HR: 128 beats/min	↑	SVR: 1813 dynes/sec/cm⁻⁵	↑
RAP: 8 mm Hg	↑	SVRI: 3022 dyncs/sec/cm⁻⁵	↑
PAP: 42/26 mm Hg	↑	PVR: 240 dynes/sec/cm⁻⁵	Normal
PAm: 31 mm Hg	↑	PVRI: 400 dynes/sec/cm⁻⁵	Normal
PAOP: 22 mm Hg	↑	LVSWI: 10.3 g • m/m²	↓
CO: 3.0 L/min	↓	RVSWI: 2.7 g • m/m²	↓
CI: 1.8 L/min/m²	↓	SvO_2: 51%	↓
SaO_2: 88%	↓	DO_2I: 318 ml/min/m²	↓

Implications and treatment goals: Patient A is in cardiogenic shock as evidenced by the low cardiac index, increased PAOP and RAP, along with the increase in SVR and SVRI. Myocardial oxygen demand is being increased by the increased heart rate, increased preload (note PAOP and RAP), and increased afterload (note SVR). Treatment priorities at this time are to increase contractility (dobutamine), decrease preload (dobutamine will affect preload to some degree but careful IV titration of nitroglycerin or the administration of furosemide may be required), and decrease afterload (IABP may be used since even careful titration of an arterial vasodilator such as nitroprusside may drop the MAP to below 60 mm Hg which is required to perfuse vital organs).

b.

Parameter	↑, ↓, or Normal	Parameter	↑, ↓, or Normal
BP: 92/70 mm Hg	↓	SV: 24 ml/beat	↓
MAP: 77 mm Hg	Normal	SI: 13 ml/m²/beat	↓
HR 122 beats/min	↑	SVR: 2097 dynes/sec/cm⁻⁵	↑
RAP: 1 mm Hg	↓	SVRI: 4053 dynes/sec/cm⁻⁵	↑
PAP: 20/6 mm Hg	↓	PVR: 221 dynes/sec/cm⁻⁵	Normal
PAm: 11 mm Hg	↓	PVRI: 427 dynes/sec/cm⁻⁵	Normal
PAOP: 3 mm Hg	↓	LVSWI: 13.1 g • m/m²	↓
CO: 2.9 L/min	↓	RVSWI: 1.8 g • m/m²	↓
CI: 1.5 L/min/m²	↓	SvO_2: 50%	↓
SaO_2: 95% on 5 L/min via nasal cannula	Normal with supplemental O_2	DO_2I: 134 ml/min/m²	↓
Hgb: 7 g/dL	↓		

Implications and treatment goals: Patient B is in hypovolemic shock evidenced by the low cardiac index with low PAOP and RAP. Heart rate and SVR and SVRI are elevated due to sympathetic nervous system stimulation. The current treatment priority is to replace blood volume because surgery has been accomplished to stop the blood loss. Considering that the primary fluid loss was blood, blood replacement in the form of either whole blood or packed cells is required along with the normal saline as a primary crystalloid. Hemoglobin is critical for oxygen delivery to the tissues and his history of coronary artery disease accentuates this need. Notice how profound the DO_2 is reduced since the hemoglobin and the cardiac output are insufficient to adequately deliver oxygen to the tissues.

CHAPTER 3

1.

f 1. Ventricular fibrillation
g 2. Stable monomorphic ventricular tachycardia
a 3. Asystole
h 4. Symptomatic bradycardia
i 5. Pulseless electrical activity
d 6. Stable SVT
c 7. Acute-onset atrial fibrillation
f 8. Pulseless ventricular tachycardia
j 9. Junctional tachycardia
h 10. Complete heart block with ventricular escape rhythm
b 11. Sinus tachycardia
e 12. Torsades de pointes

2.

Adenosine (Adenocard)	Unclassified
Amiodarone (Cordarone)	III
Atropine	Unclassified
Digoxin	Unclassified
Diltiazem (Cardizem)	IV
Dofetilide (Tikosyn)	III
Esmolol (Brevibloc)	II
Flecainide (Tambocor)	IC
Ibutilide (Corvert)	III
Lidocaine (Xylocaine)	IB
Metoprolol (Lopressor)	II
Procainamide (Pronestyl)	IA
Propranolol (Inderal)	II
Quinidine	IA
Sotalol (Betapace)	II & III
Verapamil (Calan)	IV

3.

a. 24 mL/hr
b. 2 mcg/kg/min
c. 5 mcg/kg/min
d. 10 mL/hr
e. 30 mL/hr
f. 45 mL/hr

4.

AOO	VVI		a. DVI
VVI	VAT		b. VDD
AAI	VAT	VVI	c. DDD

5.

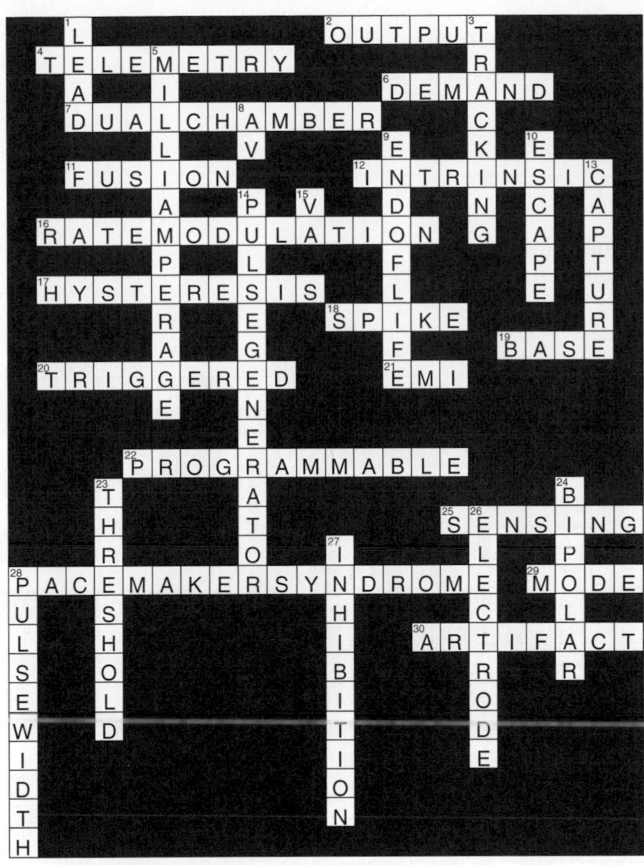

6.

a. Interpretation: VVI with normal function; complex #4 is a PVC and it is sensed appropriately
b. Interpretation: DVI function with failure to sense; complex #5 shows atrial pacing with an intrinsic ventricular complex that is not sensed
c. Interpretation: VVI with intermittent failure to capture; after the third paced complex, there is a nonconducted pacing spike; after the fourth paced complex, there is a nonconducted pacing spike

7.

Nonmodifiable	Modifiable
Heredity	Hypertension
Advancing age	Diabetes mellitus or glucose intolerance
Male gender	Hyperlipidemia
	Hyperhomocysteinemia
	Sedentary lifestyle
	Stress
	Obesity
	Cigarette smoking
	Oral contraceptives (especially in smokers)

8.

a 1. Fibrinolytics
a 2. Percutaneous interventional procedures (PCI)
g 3. ACE inhibitors
d, c 4. Nitroglycerin
c 5. Calcium channel blockers
b, h 6. Beta-blockers
e, h 7. ASA
e, f 8. Heparin
e 9. Glycoprotein IIb/IIIa inhibitors
i, j 10. Intraaortic balloon pump (IABP)

9.

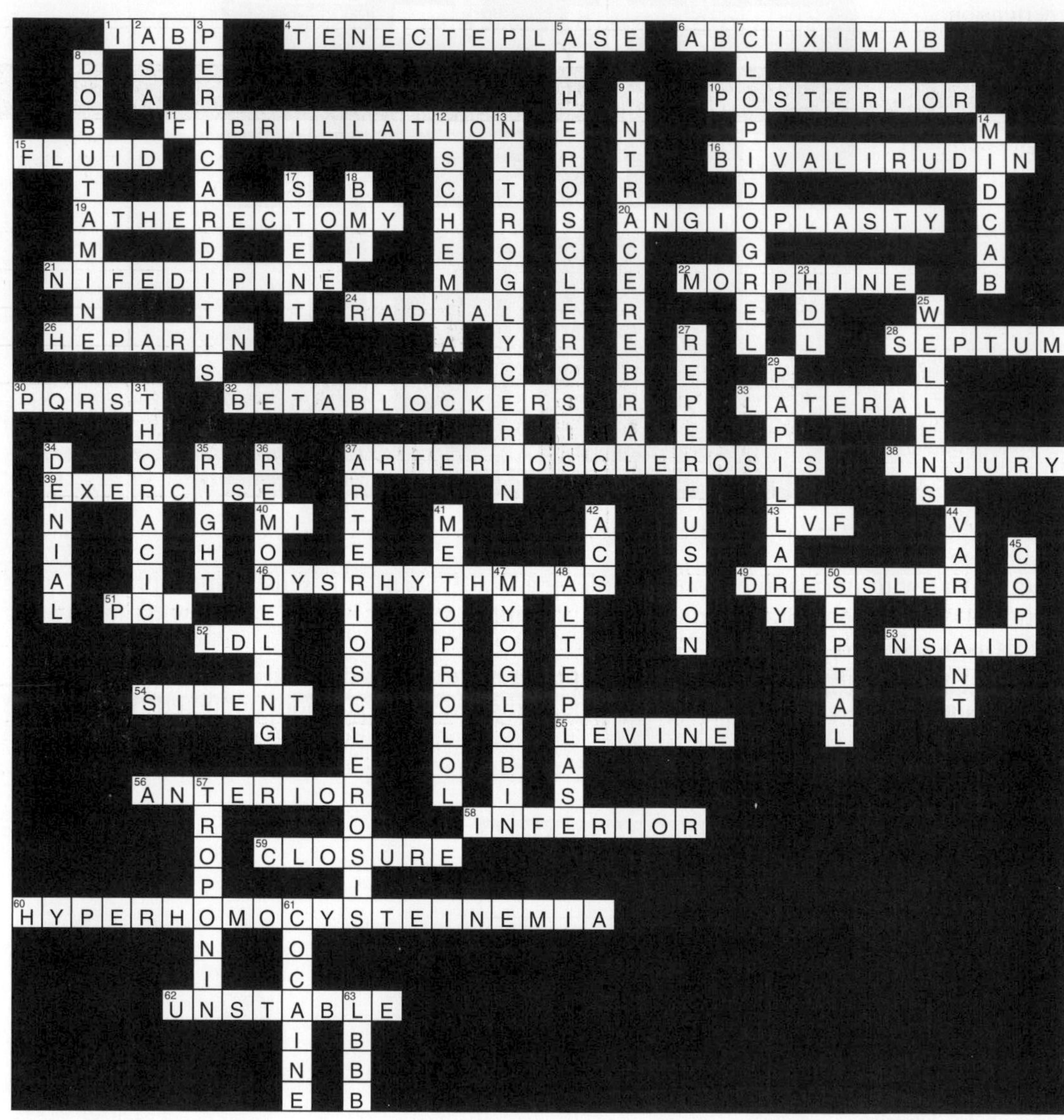

10.

a, b, d, g, j, m 1. Right ventricular failure
b, c, g, l 2. Left ventricular failure
e 3. Left ventricular MI
a, f 4. Right ventricular MI
a, e, h, n 5. Cardiac tamponade
g 6. Valvular dysfunction
i, k 7. Chronic arterial insufficiency

11.

Causes	Left	Right
Aortic stenosis	✓	
Cardiac tamponade	✓	✓
Cardiomyopathy	✓	✓
Mitral stenosis	✓ (Forward failure)	✓ (Backward failure)
Myocardial infarction (left)	✓	
Myocardial infarction (right)		✓
Pulmonary embolism	✓ (Forward failure)	✓ (Backward failure)
Pulmonary hypertension		✓
Systemic hypertension	✓	
Sign/Symptom	**Left**	**Right**
Abnormal liver function studies		✓
Ascites		✓
Atrial dysrhythmias	✓	✓
Crackles audible over lungs	✓	
Dyspnea	✓	
Elevated PAOP	✓	
Elevated RAP		✓
Hepatomegaly		✓
Jugular venous distention		✓
Mental confusion	✓	
Murmur of mitral regurgitation	✓	
Murmur of tricuspid regurgitation		✓
Orthopnea	✓	
Peripheral edema		✓
S_3, S_4 at apex	✓	
S_3, S_4 at sternum		✓
Weight gain	✓	✓

12.

a. 1) Increases coronary artery perfusion pressure
   2) Decreases afterload
b. 1) Aortic regurgitation
   2) Aortic aneurysm
c. Diastole
d. Systole
e. 1) Ischemia of left arm
   2) Renal ischemia

13.

A. Assisted aortic end-diastolic pressure
B. Unassisted aortic end-diastolic pressure
C. Assisted systole
D. Unassisted systole
E. Diastolic augmentation

14.

a. Yes. EF less than 40%
b. Systolic. This is pump failure as evidenced by S_3.
c. Because she has acute decompensated heart failure, IV diuretics would be warranted. Aldactone, an aldosterone antagonist, would likely be helpful. She is already receiving an ACE inhibitor. Inotropic agents may be used.

d. Continuous renal replacement therapy, such as continuous venous-venous hemofiltration, might be used. Cardiac resynchronization therapy with a biventricular pacemaker may be indicated. Also, a frank discussion of end-of-life care with the patient and family is indicated.
e. D

15.

Drug	Arterial Dilator	Venous Dilator
Clevidipine (Cleviprex)	✓	
Dobutamine (Dobutrex)	✓	✓
Fenoldopam (Corlopam)	✓	
Hydralazine (Apresoline)	✓	
Milrinone (Primacor)	✓	✓
Minoxidil (Loniten)	✓	
Morphine sulfate		✓
Nifedipine (Procardia)	✓	✓
Nitroglycerin (less than 1 mcg/kg/min)		✓
Nitroglycerin (greater than 1 mcg/kg/min)	✓	✓
Nitroprusside (Nipride)	✓	✓
Phentolamine (Regitine)	✓	✓
Prazosin (Minipress)	✓	✓

16.

a.
- BP 220/140 mm Hg
- Left ventricular failure (dyspnea, tachypnea, S_3, crackles, hypoxemia, pulmonary edema on chest x-ray)
  - (NOTE: You would expect tachycardia, but remember that the beta-blocker has prevented this sympathetic nervous system compensatory mechanism.)
- Left ventricular hypertrophy (displaced PMI, cardiomegaly on chest x-ray, ventricular strain and large R waves in left ventricular leads)
- Renal insufficiency (decreased urine output, elevated BUN and creatinine maintaining the normal 10:1 ratio)
- Occipital headache

b. Indomethacin (Indocin) and other nonsteroidal antiinflammatory agents inhibit the synthesis of prostaglandins (which are vasodilators) so they increase BP and cause sodium and fluid retention
c. Heart, brain, kidney, retina
d. Yes. Hypertensive emergency warrants an admission to a critical care unit.
e. Reduction of MAP by 25%
f.

Vasodilator	Nitroprusside, nitroglycerin, hydralazine, nicardipine
ACE inhibitor	Enalapril
Alpha-blocker	Phentolamine
Beta-blocker	Esmolol
Alpha- and beta-blocker	Labetalol

g. 24 mL/min; since this would result in a significant fluid gain, a more concentrated infusion would be recommended
h.
- Nausea, vomiting, abdominal pain: patient report
- Headache, tinnitus: patient report
- Coronary artery steal: evidence of myocardial ischemia such as chest pain, ST segment elevation
- Nitroprusside-induced intrapulmonary shunt: decrease in SpO_2, decrease in SaO_2 and PaO_2 on ABGs
- Methemoglobinemia: decrease in SpO_2, decrease in SaO_2 on ABGs, increase in methemoglobin levels
- Thiocyanate toxicity: metabolic acidosis, confusion, hyperreflexia, seizures, elevated thiocyanate levels

i. No. Nifedipine has never been FDA-approved for sublingual (or bite and swallow) use and is no longer recommended because of the precipitous drops in BP that may occur.
j. Labetalol would have been preferable because nitroprusside's effect of causing direct vasodilation may increase intracranial pressure.

k.

- Murmur of aortic regurgitation (high-pitched diastolic murmur) heard best in aortic (second right intercostal space at the right sternal border) area
- BP differences from left arm to right arm or left leg to right leg
- "Ripping" or "tearing" chest pain
- Chest pain that radiates to the back
- Hypotension or shock
- Widening of mediastinum on chest x-ray

17.

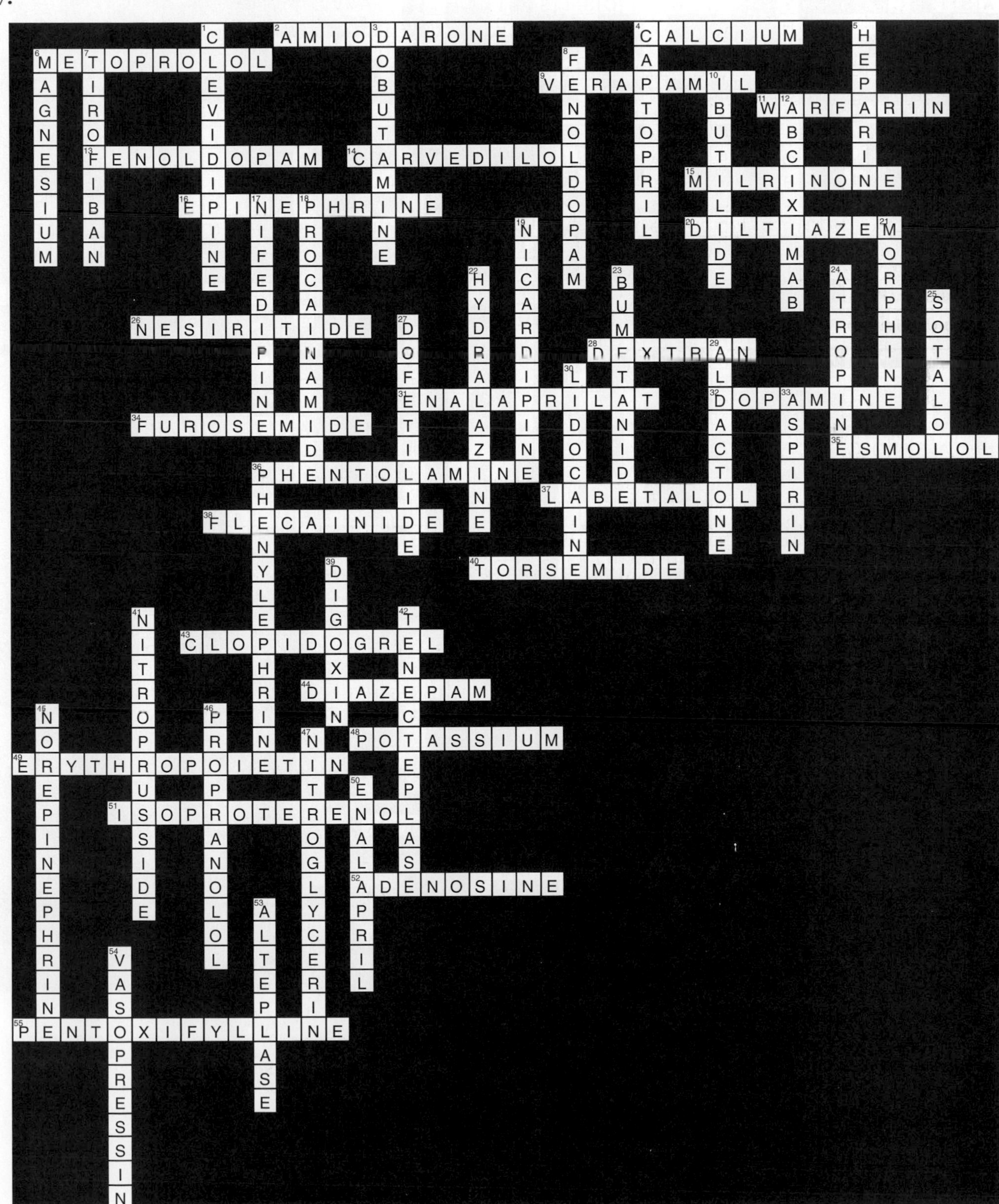

CHAPTER 4

1.

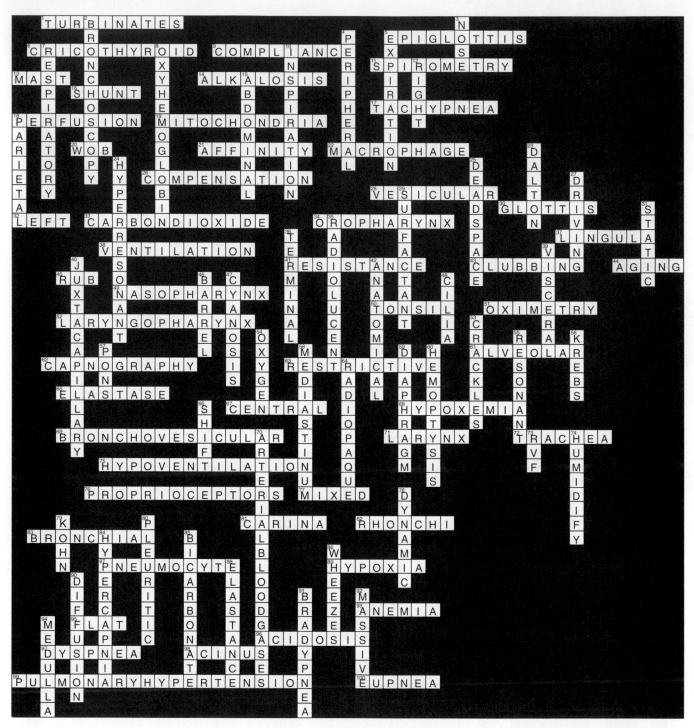

2.

	Primary	Accessory
Inspiration	Diaphragm External intercostals	Scalene Sternocleidomastoid
Expiration	None; expiration is normally passive	Internal oblique External oblique Rectus abdominis Internal intercostals Transverse abdominis

3.

	Left	Right
Increased 2,3-DPG		x
Hypothermia	x	
Hypercapnia		x
Hyperthermia		x
Acidosis		x
Decreased 2,3-DPG	x	
Hypocapnia	x	
Alkalosis	x	
Hypophosphatemia	x	
Massive blood transfusion	x	

4.

Driving pressure of oxygen = $FiO_2 \times$ barometric pressure so FiO_2 of $1.0 \times$ barometric pressure at sea level of 760 mm Hg so driving pressure of oxygen = 760 mm Hg
$PAO_2 = FiO_2\ (Pb - 47) - (PaCO_2/\ 0.8)$ so $1.0\ (760 - 47) - 37/0.8$ so $PAO_2 = 1.0 \times (760{-}47) - 50/0.8$ so $713 - 50$ so $PAO_2 = 663$ mm Hg
A:a gradient = $PAO_2 - PaO_2$ so $663 - 60$ so A:a gradient = 603 mm Hg
Estimated shunt = A:a gradient $\times$ 0.05 so estimated shunt $\cong$ 30% (remember that normal is $\approx$ 5%)
P/F ratio = PaO_2/FiO_2 so 60/1.0 so P/F ratio = 60 mm Hg (remember that P/F ratio of less than 200 is characteristic of ARDS)

5.

	Restrictive	Obstructive
Obesity hypoventilation syndrome	x	
Asthma		x
Pneumothorax	x	
Atelectasis	x	
Pneumonia	x	
Kyphoscoliosis	x	
Pulmonary edema	x	
Mucus plugs		x
Lung cancer (bronchial)		x
Lung cancer (parenchymal)	x	
Chronic bronchitis		x
Artificial airway		x
Bronchospasm		x

6.

Condition	Breath Sound Change or Changes
Emphysema	Diminished breath sounds
Atelectasis	Diminished breath sounds Bronchial or bronchovesicular breath sounds Crackles
Pneumonia	Diminished breath sounds Bronchial or bronchovesicular breath sounds Rhonchi may be present
Chronic bronchitis	Rhonchi Wheezes may also be present
Pneumothorax	Diminished or absent breath sounds
Pulmonary fibrosis	Diminished breath sounds Crackles
Asthma	Wheezes Rhonchi
Pulmonary edema	Crackles Wheezes (referred to as *cardiac asthma*) may be present
Pleurisy	Pleural friction rub
Hemothorax	Diminished or absent breath sounds
Pleural effusion	Diminished breath sounds
Pulmonary embolism	Crackles Pleural friction rub if pulmonary infarction develops

7.

b 1. Nailbed clubbing
c 2. Stridor
h 3. Crackles on auscultation
a, i 4. Hyperresonance to percussion
e 5. Dullness to percussion
i 6. Absent breath sounds
e 7. Increased tactile fremitus on palpation
g 8. Rhonchi on auscultation
d 9. Pleural friction rub on auscultation
e 10. Bronchovesicular breath sounds auscultated over peripheral lung
f 11. Wheezes on auscultation

8.

b 1. V_T
d 2. TLC
e 3. FVC
f 4. RV
a 5. FEV_1
c 6. VC
h 7. FRC
g 8. RSBI

9.

Tidal volume	~7 mL/kg
Vital capacity	Greater than 15 mL/kg
Maximal inspiratory pressure	Less than (more negative than) −60 cm H_2O
PaO_2	80-100 mm Hg
SaO_2	Greater than 95%
SvO_2	60%-80%

10.

a.	Respiratory acidosis
b.	Metabolic alkalosis
c.	Respiratory acidosis (but with elevated bicarbonate; chronic compensated respiratory acidosis with decompensation)
d.	Metabolic alkalosis
e.	Respiratory alkalosis
f.	Metabolic acidosis

11.

	pH	$PaCO_2$	HCO_3^-	PaO_2	Answer
1.	7.30	54	26	64	Respiratory acidosis with hypoxemia
2.	7.48	30	24	96	Respiratory alkalosis
3.	7.30	40	18	85	Metabolic acidosis
4.	7.50	40	33	92	Metabolic alkalosis
5.	7.35	54	30	55	Compensated respiratory acidosis with significant hypoxemia
6.	7.21	60	20	48	Mixed disorder: respiratory and metabolic acidosis with significant hypoxemia
7.	7.54	25	30	95	Mixed disorder: respiratory alkalosis and metabolic alkalosis
8.	7.40	58	33	72	Mixed disorder: respiratory acidosis and metabolic alkalosis*
9.	7.40	30	18	89	Mixed disorder: respiratory alkalosis and metabolic acidosis*
10.	7.40	40	24	98	Normal
11.	7.33	40	21	62	Metabolic acidosis with hypoxemia
12.	7.34	60	34	70	Respiratory acidosis with partial compensation and hypoxemia
13.	7.29	32	15	98	Metabolic acidosis with partial compensation
14.	7.52	28	22	95	Respiratory alkalosis with partial compensation
15.	7.49	48	38	72	Metabolic alkalosis with partial compensation and hypoxemia

*Without history and previous gases, what looks like a mixed disorder could be compensation and vice-versa. Remember that midline pH makes a mixed disorder with both an acidosis and an alkalosis more likely, while a leaning pH makes compensation more likely.

12.

a. The term hypoxemia indicates that there is decreased oxygen in the blood while hypoxia indicates that there is decreased oxygen in the tissue.

b. Because hypoxemia indicates a decrease in blood oxygen, blood parameters are used, such as PaO_2 (less than 80 mm Hg) or SaO_2 or SpO_2 (less than 95%).

c. Clinical indications of oxygen deficit are not evident until the tissues are deficient. The brain is a very sensitive indicator of low oxygen so restlessness and confusion are indications that brain oxygen levels are low. The adrenal glands are also sensitive to low oxygen levels and they release catecholamines to cause tachycardia and tachypnea. Central cyanosis may also occur. Serum arterial lactate levels would increase due to the shift to anaerobic from aerobic metabolism.

d. Absolutely. Since hypoxemia is present when PaO_2 is less than 80 mm Hg and SaO_2 is less than 95%, the tissues are still able to maintain normal oxygen levels by increasing the amount of oxygen that they extract. This would be reflected by a decrease in SvO_2. Generally, consider a PaO_2 of less than 60 mm Hg and SaO_2 of less than 90% as consistent with both hypoxemia AND hypoxia. You can also relate this to the oxyhemoglobin dissociation curve because PaO_2 of 60 mm Hg and SaO_2 of 90% is when the curve changes from horizontal to vertical so any decrease in PaO_2 results in a more significant decrease in SaO_2.

e. Absolutely. Even with a normal PaO_2 and SaO_2, if the hemoglobin or cardiac output/index is reduced, oxygen delivery to the tissues is deficient and hypoxia occurs. Some other factors to be considered are shift of the oxyhemoglobin dissociation curve to the left, decreased extraction by the tissues such as occurs in sepsis, and then local perfusion issues such as peripheral vascular disease.

13.

Problem	Preferred Artificial Airway
Tongue against hypopharynx	Oropharyngeal or nasopharyngeal
Need for frequent nasotracheal suctioning	Nasopharyngeal
Inability to open mouth (e.g., seizure)	Nasopharyngeal
Facial or jaw fracture	Nasopharyngeal or nasotracheal tube
Complete upper airway obstruction when endotracheal intubation is impossible (e.g., laryngeal edema or spasm, tracheal fracture)	Cricothyrotomy or tracheostomy
Need for sealed airway (e.g., mechanical ventilation or potential for aspiration)	Endotracheal tube or tracheostomy LMA but less protection from aspiration
Need for long-term lower airway access and sealed airway	Tracheostomy

NOTE: Nasal cannulation should be short-term only because of the risk of sinus infection.

14.

d 1. Non-rebreathing mask
e 2. Venturi mask
a 3. Nasal cannula
b 4. Tracheostomy collar
c 5. Partial rebreathing mask

15.

i 1. Control
q 2. Assist-control
e 3. Synchronized intermittent mandatory ventilation
a 4. Pressure support ventilation
j 5. Pressure-controlled ventilation
d 6. Independent lung ventilation
h 7. High-frequency ventilation
f 8. Pressure-regulated volume-controlled
c 9. Bi-PAP
g 10. Airway pressure release ventilation
m 11. Tidal volume
o 12. Positive end-expiratory pressure
k 13. Sigh
p 14. Peak inspiratory pressure
n 15. FiO_2
b 16. Plateau pressure
l 17. Continuous positive airway pressure

16.

a. Increase the driving pressure of oxygen
b. Decrease surface tension
c. Decrease intrapulmonary shunt (alveolar recruitment)
d. Aid in prevention of ventilator-induced lung injury

17.

	High Pressure	Low Exhaled Volume
Cuff leak		x
Bronchospasm	x	
Need for suctioning	x	
Disconnect		x
Water condensation in tubing	x	
Pneumothorax	x	
ARDS	x	

18.

a. Spontaneous tidal volume: <u>at least 5 mL/kg</u>
b. Spontaneous vital capacity: <u>at least 10 mL/kg</u>
c. Maximal inspiratory pressure: <u>greater than (more negative than) −25 cm H_2O</u>
d. PaO_2 of at least <u>60 mm Hg</u> on a FiO_2 of no greater than <u>0.5</u> with no more than <u>5</u> cm H_2O PEEP.
e. Rapid shallow breathing index: <u>less than or equal to 105 breaths/min/L</u>

19.

	Patient A	Patient B
Age	38	64
Gender	F	M
Diagnosis	asthma	ARDS
IBW	60 kg	75 kg
ABGs	FiO_2 of 0.28 pH 7.42 $PaCO_2$ 39 mm Hg HCO_3 25 mEq/L PaO_2 88 mm Hg SaO_2 98%	FiO_2 of 0.6 with 10 cm H_2O PEEP pH 7.32 $PaCO_2$ 50 mm Hg HCO_3 23 mEq/L PaO_2 55 mm Hg SaO_2 88%
Spontaneous V_T	350 mL	300 mL
Spontaneous Vital Capacity	650 mL	600 ml
Spontaneous Minute Ventilation	7 L	10.8 L
NIF	−40 cm H_2O	−20 cm H_2O
Spontaneous Respiratory Rate (f)	20/min	36/min
Rapid Shallow Breathing Index (RSBI)	57 breaths/min/L	120 breaths/min/L
Ready for weaning?	Yes	No

Calculations: To calculate the minute ventilation, you would multiply the tidal volume by the respiratory rate. To calculate the RSBI, you would divide the respiratory rate (frequency) by the spontaneous tidal volume (V_T) in liters so in patient A, f of 20 is divided by 0.35.

Decision-making: Patient A is ready for weaning and extubation. Patient B is not ready for weaning and extubation. Note that Patient B's V_T is less than 5 mL/kg of IBW, his vital capacity is less than 10 mL/kg, and his minute ventilation is more than 10 L. His RSBI is greater than 105 breaths/min/L (should be less than 105). His ABGs show mild respiratory acidosis which is likely to worsen should mechanical ventilation not be continued. His oxygenation status is still impaired despite FiO_2 of 0.6 and 10 cm H_2O of PEEP. Also, his VC and NIF both indicate that his coughing ability is impaired and he will likely not be able to clear his airways if extubated.

CHAPTER 5

1.

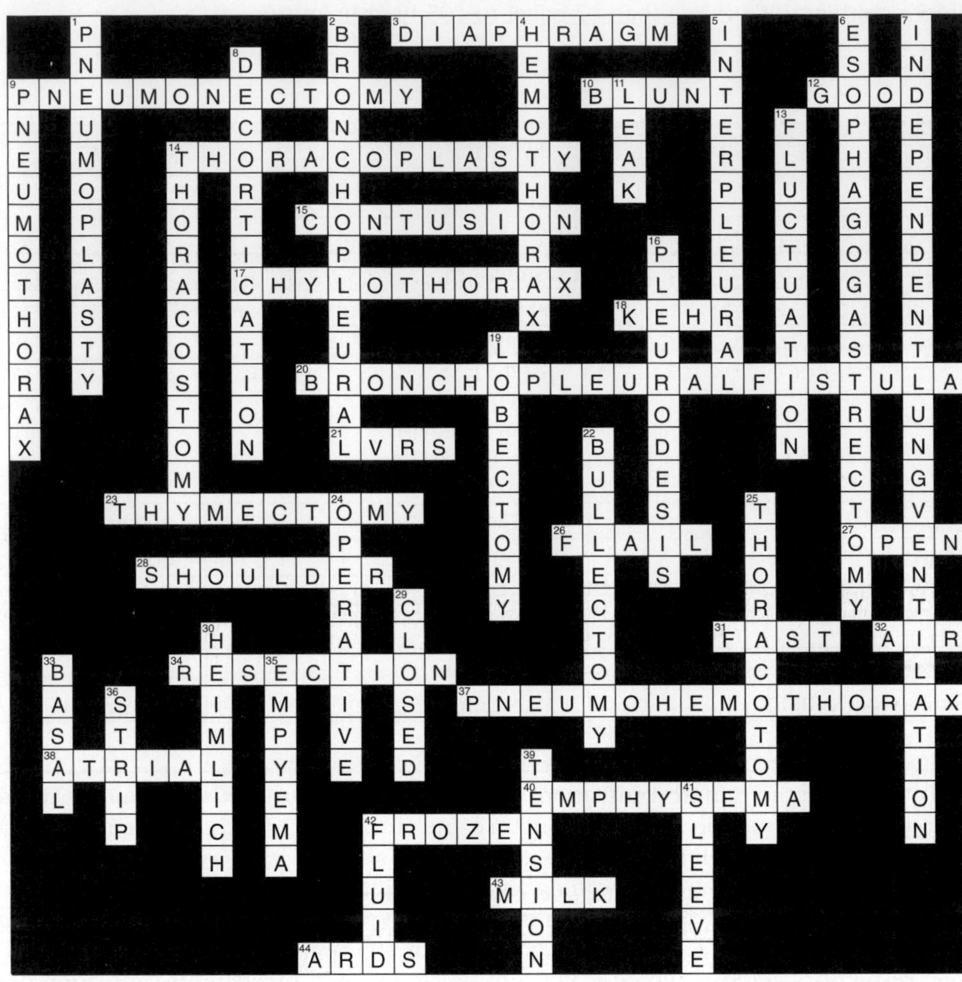

2. Any 10 of the following:

Acute respiratory distress syndrome (early)
Aminoglycosides
Amyotrophic lateral sclerosis
Anesthesia
Aspiration pneumonitis
Asthma
Atelectasis
Chest trauma
CNS depressant drugs
COPD with acute exacerbation
Cystic fibrosis
Epiglottis
Fat embolism
Guillain-Barré syndrome
Head trauma
Kyphoscoliosis
Morbid obesity
Multiple sclerosis
Muscle paralytics
Muscular dystrophy
Myasthenia gravis
Near-drowning
Neuromuscular blocking drugs
Organophosphate poisoning
Pleural effusion
Pneumonia
Pneumothorax
Poliomyelitis
Pulmonary edema
Pulmonary embolism
Pulmonary fibrosis
Sleep apnea
Smoke inhalation
Spinal cord injury
Status asthmaticus
Surgery: especially thoracic, abdominal, flank incision
Tracheal obstruction

3.

d 1. Upper airway obstruction
f 2. Airway secretions
i 3. Overdosage of narcotics
h 4. Bronchospasm
b, c 5. Pneumothorax
a, b 6. Pneumonia
j 7. Postoperative pain
g 8. ARDS
e 9. Myasthenic crisis
b 10. Atelectasis

4.

a. No, because CO_2 is more diffusible than O_2. A great clinical example is early pulmonary embolism which causes hypoxemia due to a perfusion and therefore diffusion defect. In early PE, the PaO_2 and SaO_2 are decreased but the patient is hyperventilating so the $PaCO_2$ is actually decreased. $PaCO_2$ is a reflection of ventilation, and the PaO_2 is a reflection of oxygenation.

b. Yes, because of the effect of Dalton's law. Since the formula for PAO_2 (partial pressure of oxygen in the alveolus) is:

$$[FiO_2 \text{ (barometric pressure} - \text{the pressure of water vapor)}] - (PaCO_2 \div 0.8)$$

any increase in $PaCO_2$ would decrease the PAO_2 and therefore the PaO_2. A great clinical example is COPD or any other cause of hypoventilation. When the $PaCO_2$ increases, the PaO_2 decreases unless the patient is receiving supplemental oxygen which would increase the driving pressure of oxygen and normalize the PaO_2 even if the $PaCO_2$ is increased. This is why the two types of acute respiratory failure are hypoxemic normocapnic (as explained in **a.** above) and hypoxemic hypercapnic (as explained in **b.** above).

5. Any five in each column.

Pulmonary	Nonpulmonary
Chest trauma: pulmonary contusion	Sepsis (No. 1 cause)
Near-drowning	Shock or prolonged hypotension
Hypervolemia, pulmonary edema	Septic shock
Inhalation of toxic gases and vapors	Hypovolemic shock
Smoke	Anaphylactic shock
Chemicals	Cardiogenic shock
Oxygen toxicity	Neurogenic shock
Pneumonia	Multisystem trauma
Aspiration pneumonitis	Burns
Radiation pneumonitis	Cardiopulmonary bypass
Pulmonary embolism	Disseminated intravascular coagulation (DIC)
Radiation	Toxemia of pregnancy
Drugs: bleomycin	Acute pancreatitis
	Diabetic coma
	Head injury
	Drug overdosage
	Multiple blood transfusions

6.

b, d 1. Pulmonary hypertension
a 2. Intrapulmonary shunt
b, e 3. Ventilation/perfusion mismatch
a, d 4. Diffusion defect
a, c 5. Pulmonary edema

7.

Staphylococcus aureus	CAP, HCAP
Serratia marcescens	HCAP
Escherichia coli	HCAP
Legionella pneumophila	CAP, HCAP
Proteus mirabilis	HCAP
Bacteroides fragilis	CAP
Hantavirus	CAP

8.

1. Elevate the head of the bed 45 degrees.
2. Ensure appropriate positioning of feeding tube.
3. Keep cuff of endotracheal tube inflated to 20-30 cm H_2O pressure.

9.

Stage	PaO_2	$PaCO_2$	pH	Acid-Base Imbalance
I	↔	↓	↑	Respiratory alkalosis
II	↓	↓	↑	Respiratory alkalosis and mild to moderate hypoxemia
III	↓	↔	↔	Moderate hypoxemia
IV	↓	↑	↓	Respiratory acidosis and critical hypoxemia

10.

Classification	Example
1. $Beta_2$ adrenergic agonists	Salmeterol (Serevent) Metaproterenol (Alupent, Metaprel) Albuterol (Proventil, Ventolin) Pirbuterol (Maxair) Bitolterol (Tornalate) Terbutaline (Brethine, Brethaire)
2. Anticholinergic agents	Ipratropium bromide (Atrovent)
3. Methylxanthines	Aminophylline Theophylline (Theobid, Quibron) Oxtriphylline (Choledyl SA)
4. Electrolyte	Magnesium

11. Any three in each column.

Hypercoagulability	Alteration in Blood Vessel	Venous Stasis
Malignancy	Trauma	Prolonged bed rest or immobilization
Oral contraceptives high in estrogen: especially in smokers	IV drug use	Obesity
Dehydration and hemoconcentration	Aging	Advanced age
Fever	Vasculitis	Burns
Sickle-cell anemia	Varicose veins	Pregnancy
Pregnancy	Diabetes mellitus	Postpartum period
Polycythemia vera	Atherosclerosis	Congestive heart failure
Thrombocytopenia	Inflammatory process	Myocardial infarction

Hypercoagulability	Alteration in Blood Vessel	Venous Stasis
Abrupt discontinuance of anticoagulants		Bacterial endocarditis
Sepsis		Recent surgery especially legs, pelvis, or abdomen
		Thrombus formation in heart (AF)
		Cardioversion

12.

e 1. Forward failure of left ventricle
a, d 2. Pulmonary hypertension
a, d 3. Occlusion of pulmonary blood supply
b 4. Backward failure of right ventricle
c 5. Low levels of antithrombin III
f 6. V/Q mismatch

13.

Parameter	↑, ↓, or Normal	Parameter	↑, ↓, or Normal
BP: 112/84 mm Hg	Normal	SV: 40 mL/beat	↓
MAP: 93 mm Hg	Normal	SI: 25 mL/m^2/beat	↓
HR 110 beats/min	↑	SVR: 1364 dynes/sec/cm^{-5}	Normal
RAP: 18 mm Hg	↑	SVRI: 2182 dynes/sec/cm^{-5}	Normal
PAP: 55/32 mm Hg	↑	PVR: 618 dynes/sec/cm^{-5}	↑
PAm: 40 mm Hg	↑	PVRI: 989 dynes/sec/cm^{-5}	↑
PAOP: 6 mm Hg	Normal	LVSWI: 30 gm • m/m^2	↓
CO: 4.4 L/min	Normal	RVSWI: 7 gm • m/m^2	Normal
CI: 2.75 $L/min/m^2$	Normal	SvO_2: 58%	↓
SaO_2: 85% on 5 L/min by nasal cannula	↓	DO_2I: 470 $mL/min/m^2$	↓

Implications and treatment goals: The hemodynamic parameters confirm pulmonary hypertension. Note the increase in PAd with a normal PAOP. Remember that if the PAd is more than 5 mm Hg above the PAOP, pulmonary hypertension exists. The increased PVR is further evidence of pulmonary hypertension. Sympathetic nervous system stimulation has caused the tachycardia and the high SVR. Considering her history, you would suspect pulmonary embolism as the cause. V/Q scan or spiral CT would be indicated to aid in the diagnosis of a pulmonary embolism. Arterial blood gases should be analyzed for degree of hypoxemia. Treatment goals for this patient include improving oxygenation (100% by non-rebreathing mask would probably be required and the patient may need to be intubated if fatigue and $PaCO_2$ increases), reestablishing pulmonary perfusion (fibrinolytics are indicated in this patient because she does have acute right ventricular failure and refractory hypoxemia), and prevent extension of the clot and reocclusion (heparin). Note that it has been 2 weeks since her surgery, which is long enough for the surgical clot to have been lysed by the natural fibrinolytic process so fibrinolytics are not contraindicated on that basis. If fibrinolytics are contraindicated for other reasons, pulmonary artery catheter aspiration or fragmentation of the clot may be attempted. Surgical pulmonary embolectomy is associated with a relatively high mortality and should be avoided if possible.

14.

c 1. Pulmonary contusion
f 2. Flail chest
b 3. Simple pneumothorax
e 4. Hemothorax
a 5. Tension pneumothorax
d 6. Diaphragmatic rupture

15.

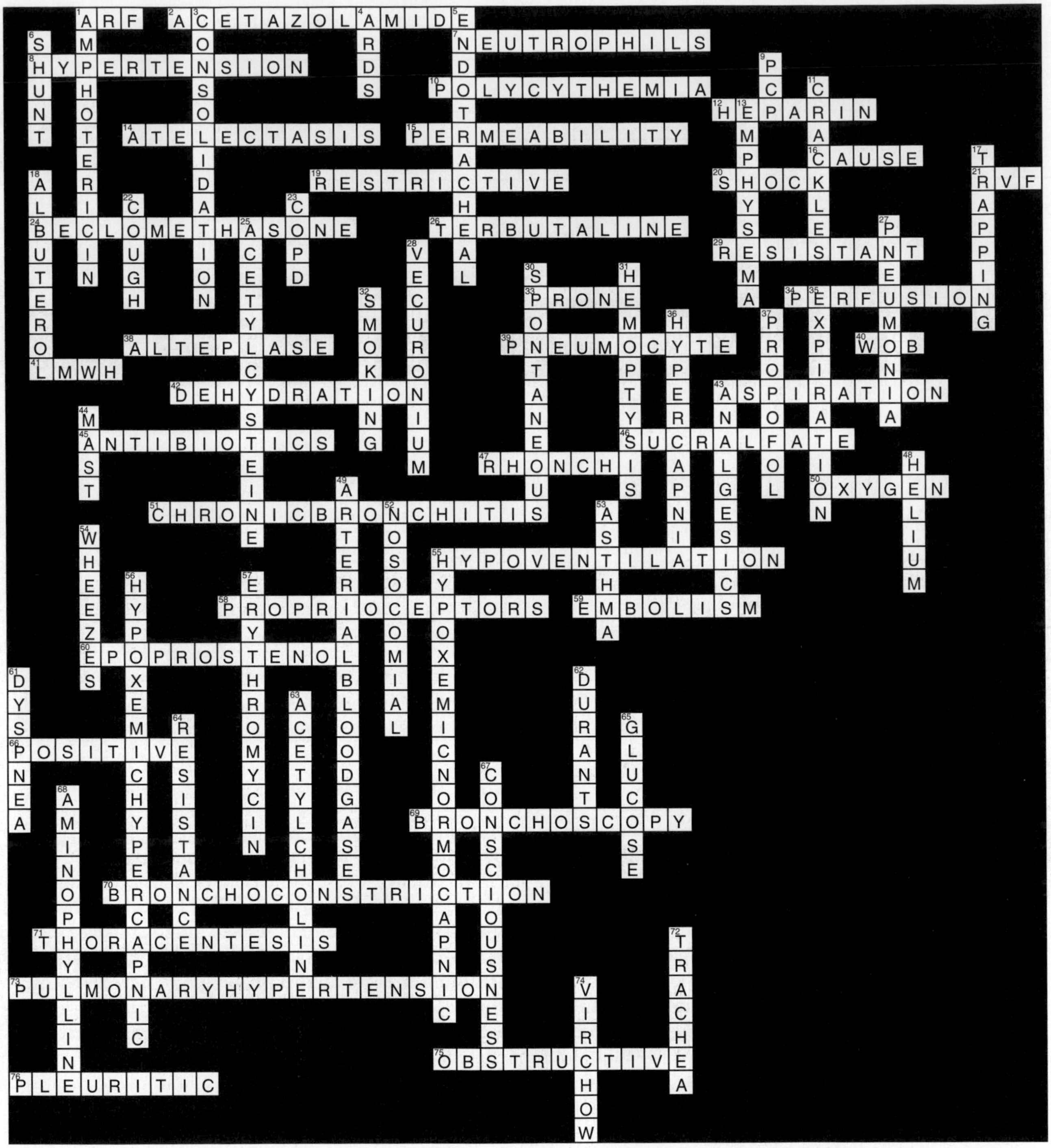
1 ARF
2 ACETAZOLAMIDE
7 NEUTROPHILS
8 HYPERTENSION
10 POLYCYTHEMIA
12 HEPARIN
14 ATELECTASIS
15 PERMEABILITY
16 CAUSE
19 RESTRICTIVE
20 SHOCK
21 RVF
24 BECLOMETHASONE
26 TERBUTALINE
29 RESISTANT
33 PRONE
34 PERFUSION
38 ALTEPLASE
39 PNEUMOCYTE
40 WOB
41 LMWH
42 DEHYDRATION
43 ASPIRATION
45 ANTIBIOTICS
46 SUCRALFATE
47 RHONCHI
50 OXYGEN
51 CHRONICBRONCHITIS
55 HYPOVENTILATION
58 PROPRIOCEPTORS
59 EMBOLISM
60 EPOPROSTENOL
66 POSITIVE
69 BRONCHOSCOPY
70 BRONCHOCONSTRICTION
71 THORACENTESIS
73 PULMONARYHYPERTENSION
75 OBSTRUCTIVE
76 PLEURITIC
1 AMPHOTERICIN
3 CONSOLIDATION
4 ARDS
5 ENDOTRACHEAL
6 SHUNT
9 PCO
11 CRACKLES
13 EMPHYSEMA
17 TRAPPING
18 ALBUTEROL
22 COUGH
23 COPD
25 ACETYLCYSTEINE
27 PNEUMONIA
28 VECURONIUM
30 SPONTANEOUS
31 HEMOPTYSIS
32 SMOKING
35 EXPIRATION
36 HYPERCAPNIA
37 PROPOFOL
43 ANALGESIC
44 MAST
48 HELIUM
49 ARTERIALBLOODGASE
52 NOSOCOMIAL
53 ASTHMA
54 WHEEZES
55 HYPOXEMICNORMOCAPNIC
56 HYPOXEMICHYPERCAPNIC
57 ERYTHROMYCIN
61 DYSPNEA
62 DURANT
63 ACETYLCHOLINE
64 RESISTANCE
65 GLUCOSE
67 CONSCIOUSNESS
68 AMINOPHYLLIN
72 TRACHEA
74 VIRCHOW

CHAPTER 6

1.

2.

k 1. Anterior frontal lobe
j 2. Posterior frontal lobe
g 3. Parietal lobe
c 4. Occipital lobe
f 5. Temporal lobe
d 6. Cerebellum
b 7. Medulla
e 8. Hypothalamus
i 9. Wernicke's area
l 10. Thalamus
h 11. Limbic system
a 12. Broca's area

3.

To calculate mean arterial pressure:

$[SBP + (DBP \times 2)] \div 3: 80 + (2 \times 50) = 180,$
then divide by $3 = 60$

To calculate cerebral perfusion pressure:

$MAP - ICP: 60 - 20 = 40$ mm Hg

Should you be concerned? YES! CPP less than 50 is associated with loss of autoregulation, hypoperfusion of the brain, and anoxic encephalopathy.

4.

	Sympathetic	Parasympathetic
Bronchodilation	x	
Coronary artery dilation	x	
Hypersalivation		x
Increased blood glucose	x	
Increased perspiration	x	
Increased intestinal motility		x
Pupil constriction		x
Tachycardia	x	

5.

Pattern	Site of Lesion
CNS hyperventilation	Lower midbrain or upper pons
Cheyne-Stokes	Cerebral hemispheres, basal ganglia, cerebellar lesion, or upper brainstem
Cluster (or Biot's)	Lower pons or upper medulla
Ataxic	Medulla
Apneustic	Mid to lower pons

6.

Cranial Nerve	Name	Method of Assessment
I	Olfactory	• Evaluate the patient's ability to identify familiar odors
II	Optic	• Evaluate visual acuity using Snellen chart or newsprint • Evaluate the optic disk during funduscopic examination
III	Oculomotor	• Evaluate the ability to open eyes widely • Check size, shape, position, and reactivity of the pupils • Have patient follow your finger with his or her eyes through the six cardinal positions of gaze • Look for abnormal eye movement (i.e., nystagmus)
IV	Trochlear	• Have patient follow your finger with his or her eyes through the six cardinal positions of gaze
V	Trigeminal	• Evaluate ability of the patient to detect light touch, superficial pain, and temperature on forehead, cheeks, and jaw • Touch the cornea with a wisp of cotton and check for bilateral blink • Palpate the strength of the masseter muscles with the patient clinching his or her teeth and the strength of the temporal muscles with the patient squeezing his or her eyes shut
VI	Abducens	• Have patient follow your finger with his or her eyes through the six cardinal positions of gaze
VII	Facial	• Ask the patient to smile and assess symmetry • Test the patient's ability to taste salt and sugar on the anterior tongue
VIII	Acoustic	• Evaluate ability of the patient to hear when speaking at normal voice tones • Note any vertigo, nystagmus, nausea, vomiting, pallor, sweating, hypotension
IX	Glossopharyngeal	• Evaluate patient's ability to speak; note any hoarseness • Look for bilateral elevation of the palate with phonation • Test the patient's ability to taste sour and bitter on the posterior tongue • Evaluate the patient's ability to swallow • Test the gag reflex by stroking the palate with a tongue blade and looking for reflex gag • Evaluate cough reflex by touching the hypopharynx with a suction catheter
X	Vagus	• Tested with glossopharyngeal
XI	Spinal accessory	• Ask the patient to shrug his or her shoulders as you push down on them with your hands • Palpate the sternocleidomastoid and trapezius muscles for size and symmetry
XII	Hypoglossal	• Look for midline alignment when the patient protrudes his or her tongue • Look for fasciculations of the tongue

7.

1. Neck twisting or flexion
2. Valsalva maneuver
3. Airway obstruction
4. Pain or noxious stimuli
5. Disturbing conversation
6. Noise
7. Bright lights
8. Tight tracheostomy ties or cervical collar
9. Seizure activity
10. Hyperthermia

8.

Intervention	What Is Decreased?
1. Hyperventilation to cause respiratory alkalosis	Blood
2. Maintenance of euvolemia	Brain edema
3. Mannitol	Brain edema
4. Furosemide	Brain edema, CSF
5. Ventriculostomy and CSF drainage	CSF
6. Barbiturate coma	Blood

9.

k 1. Brainstem lesion
h 2. Chronic subdural hematoma
i 3. Subarachnoid hemorrhage
j 4. Status epilepticus
g 5. Dural tear
e 6. Postcraniotomy
l 7. Upper motor neuron lesion
a 8. Meningeal irritation
d 9. Intracranial hypertension
m 10. Basal skull fracture
c 11. Guillain-Barré syndrome
b 12. Myasthenia gravis
f 13. Hydrocephalus

10.

GCS: 4
Hunt and Hess aneurysm grade: V

11.

	Vasospasm	Rebleed
Occurs either immediately after the bleed or between 7-10 days after the bleed		x
Caused by calcium influx into the vessel	x	
Occurs any time after 3 days	x	
Treated by hypervolemic hemodilution and calcium channel blockers	x	
Caused by lysis of the protective clot		x
Prevented by early clipping if the patient is stable enough		x

12.

1. Dose: 0.9 mg/kg with maximum dose of less than or equal to 90 mg with the initial bolus being 10% of this total dose over 1 minute and the remaining 90% of this total dose infused over 60 minutes
2. Time frame: within 4.5 hours of the initial symptoms
3. Adjuvant therapy: no anticoagulants or platelet aggregation agents for the first 24 hours
4. Additional contraindications: awakening with symptoms (eliminates ability to determine time of onset of symptoms) and seizure at onset of symptoms (increases risk that the stroke is hemorrhagic rather than ischemic)
5. Additional contraindications including seizure at symptom onset and awakening with symptoms

13.

Bacterial meningitis	• Elevated pressure • Increased WBC • Normal or elevated protein • Decreased glucose • Cloudy appearance
Viral meningitis	• Elevated pressure • Normal or increased WBC • Normal or elevated protein • Clear appearance
Subarachnoid hemorrhage	• Elevated protein • Bloody appearance if acute • Dark amber (xanthochromic) if more than 5 days old

14.

Observations to Make

Any five of the following:

Preceding events: Was there an aura?

Onset:

- Body movements
- Deviation of head and eyes
- Chewing and salivation
- Posture of body
- Sensory changes

Tonic and clonic phases:

- Progression of movements of the body
- Skin color and airway
- Pupillary changes
- Incontinence
- Duration of each phase

Level of consciousness during seizure

- Postictal phase:
- Duration
- General behavior
- Memory of events
- Orientation
- Pupillary changes
- Headache
- Aphasia
- Injuries

Duration of entire seizure

Medications given and response

Interventions

Any five of the following:

- Do not leave patient; provide privacy
- Loosen clothing
- Open airway but do not try to pry mouth open; nasopharyngeal or nasotracheal airways may be used if necessary
- Turn patient to side
- Administer oxygen
- Do not restrain; gentle guiding of extremities is acceptable
- Pad side rails with blankets or pillows
- Administer anticonvulsants (e.g., diazepam, phenytoin)
- Reorient patient after seizure
- Clean patient if incontinence has occurred
- Allow patient to sleep

15.

e 1. Amyotrophic lateral sclerosis
b 2. Guillain-Barré
a 3. Muscular dystrophy
c 4. Multiple sclerosis
d 5. Myasthenia gravis

16.

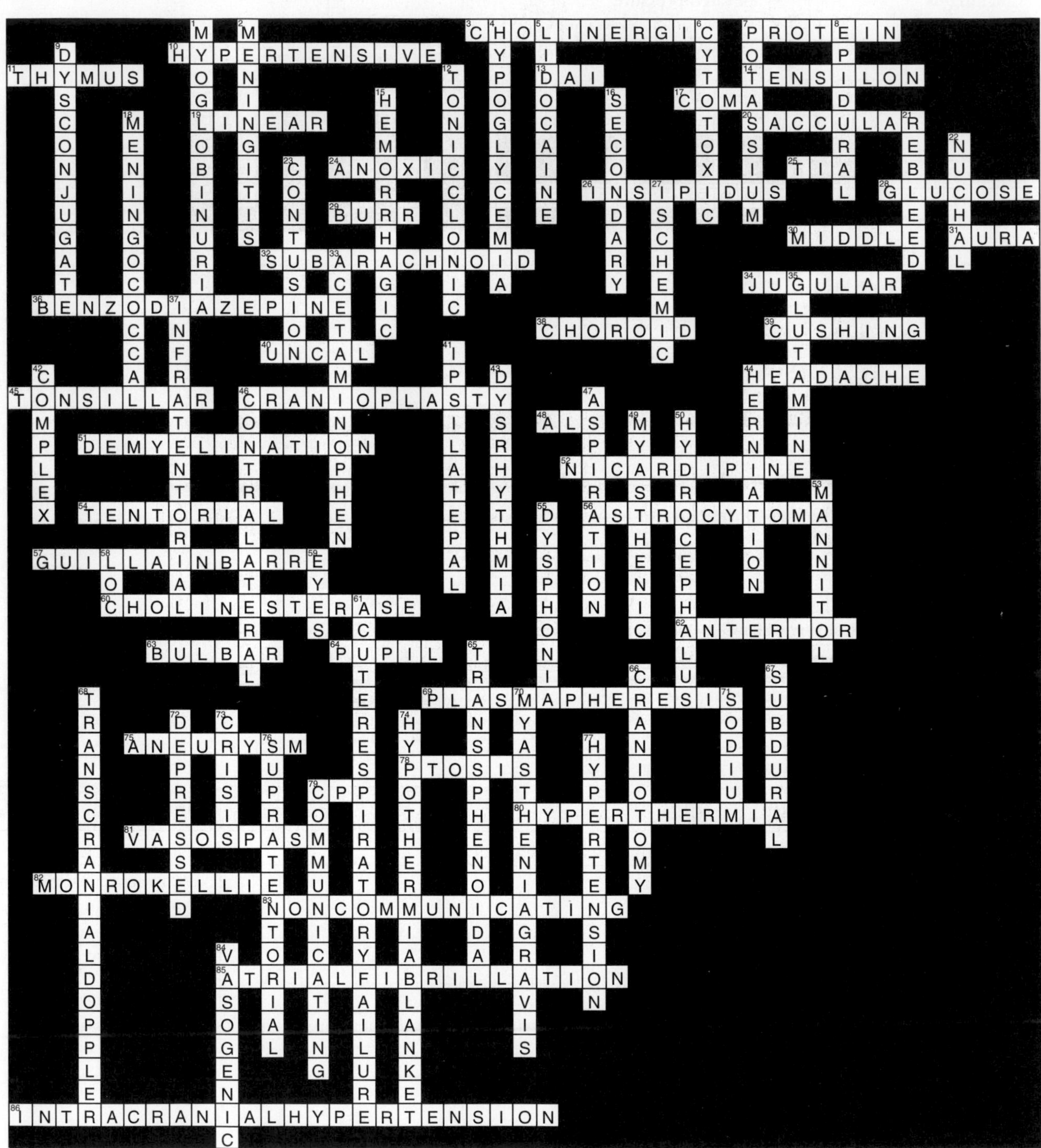

CHAPTER 7

1.

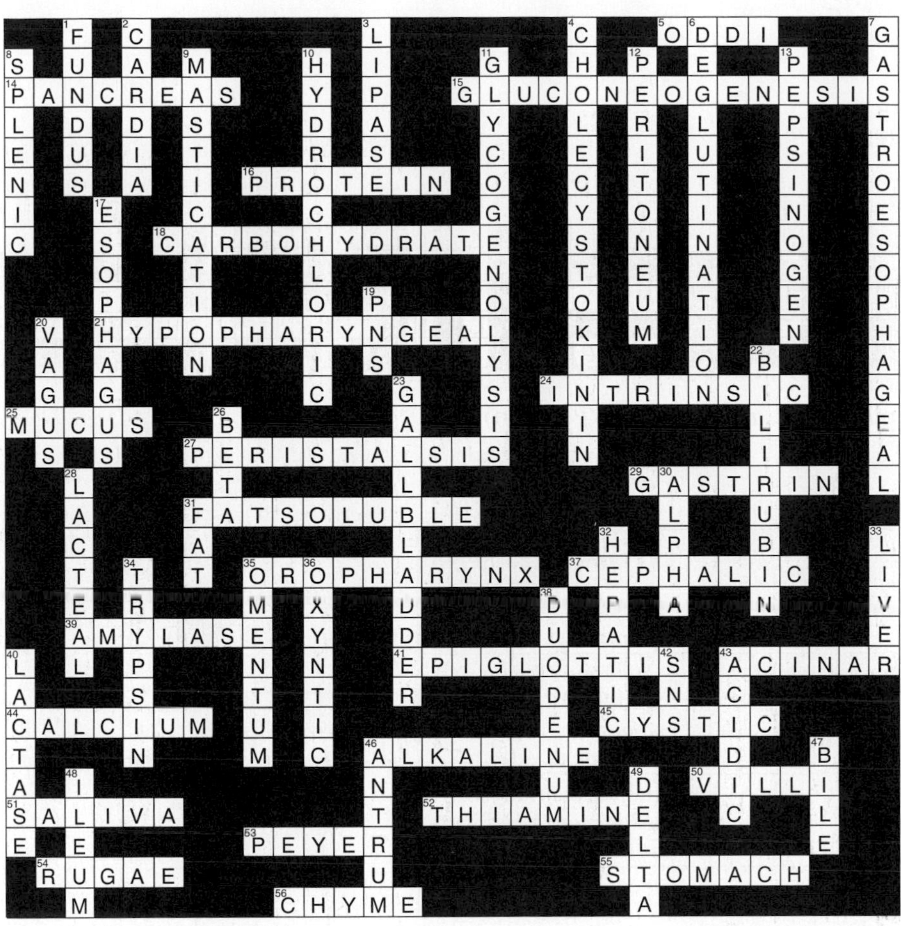

2.

Sign	Description	Indicates
Ballance's	Dullness over right flank with patient on left side	Ruptured spleen
Grey Turner's	Ecchymosis to flank	Retroperitoneal bleeding
Cullen's	Ecchymosis around umbilicus	Intraperitoneal bleeding
Coopernail's	Ecchymosis of scrotum or labia	Pelvic fracture
Kehr's	Left shoulder pain	Splenic rupture
Chvostek's	Spasm of the facial muscles elicited by tapping on the facial nerve	Hypocalcemia
Trousseau's	Carpal spasm induced by inflating a BP cuff on the upper arm to a pressure exceeding systolic blood pressure	Hypocalcemia

3.

a. Liver disease (e.g., cirrhosis, hepatitis)
b. Biliary obstruction (e.g., cholelithiasis)
c. Excessive hemolysis (e.g., hemolytic blood transfusion reaction)

4. The half-life of serum prealbumin is 2-3 days versus albumin with a half-life of 10-20 days. Therefore, serum transferrin will show improvement or decline more quickly.

5. 2428 calories

6.

a. Administer oxygen (maintain SaO_2 of at least 95%)
b. Insert at least two large-gauge (16 or 18) intravenous catheters
c. Obtain blood samples for H&H and type and crossmatch
d. Initiate normal saline infusion initially and then blood when prescribed and available

7.

a. Peptic ulcer
b. Esophageal varices
c. Mallory-Weiss tear
d. Gastritis
e. Vascular tumor

8.

a. Sclerotherapy of varices
b. Ligation of varices
c. Intrahepatic (e.g., TIPS) or portosystemic shunt
d. Balloon tamponade
e. Octreotide (Sandostatin) or vasopressin (Pitressin)

9.

Type	Example
Antacids	Maalox Mylanta
Histamine (H_2) receptor antagonists	Cimetidine (Tagamet) Ranitidine (Zantac) Famotidine (Pepcid) Nizatidine (Axid)
Proton pump inhibitors	Omeprazole (Prilosec) Lansoprazole (Prevacid) Esomeprazole (Nexium)
Mucosal barrier	Sucralfate (Carafate)

10.

a, f 1. Splenic engorgement
Remember that splenic engorgement causes thrombocytopenia and therefore clotting abnormalities.
g 2. Stretching of the liver capsule
d 3. Decrease in the metabolism of testosterone
c 4. Decrease in metabolism of aldosterone
a, c 5. Decrease in production of plasma proteins
Remember that many plasma proteins are actually clotting factors.
e 6. Decrease in metabolism of estrogen
a 7. Decreased production of clotting factors
b 8. Decrease in conjugation and excretion of bilirubin

11.

Indicated	Contraindicated
Aldosterone antagonist (potassium-sparing)	Thiazide

12. Any five of the following:
- Abdominal surgery
- Acute cholecystitis
- Hypokalemia
- Intestinal distention
- Intestinal ischemia
- Narcotics (e.g., morphine)
- Pancreatitis
- Pelvic abscess
- Peritonitis
- Pleuritis
- Pneumonia
- Sepsis
- Severe trauma
- Spinal cord injury
- Subphrenic abscess
- Ureteral distention

13. Any five of the following:
- Abdominal pain
- Rebound tenderness
- Abdominal distention
- Rigid "boardlike" abdomen
- Diminished bowel sounds
- Fever
- Leukocytosis
- Nausca, vomiting

14.

Sign/Symptom	Condition
Elevated lipase, amylase	Acute pancreatitis
Sudden, painless hematemesis	Esophageal varices
Decreased protein	Acute pancreatitis, liver disease, malnutrition
Rebound tenderness	Peritonitis
Jaundice	Liver disease, biliary obstruction, hemolysis
Hypocalcemia	Acute pancreatitis
Bleeding tendencies	Liver disease
Elevated ammonia	Hepatic failure, hepatic encephalopathy
Bloody diarrhea	Intestinal infarction
Hyperbilirubinemia	Liver disease, biliary obstruction, hemolysis
Fetor hepaticus	Hepatic failure
High-pitched rushing bowel sounds	Small bowel obstruction
Succussion splash	Pyloric obstruction
Management	**Condition**
Irrigate NG tube until clear	Upper GI bleed
Neomycin and lactulose	Hepatic failure; hepatic encephalopathy
Sclerosis during endoscopy	Esophageal varices
Aldosterone antagonist diuretics	Hepatic failure; hepatic encephalopathy
NPO status	Pancreatitis
Sengstaken-Blakemore tube	Esophageal varices
Volume and blood replacement	GI bleed
Billroth I or II	Gastric ulcer

15.

CHAPTER 8

1.

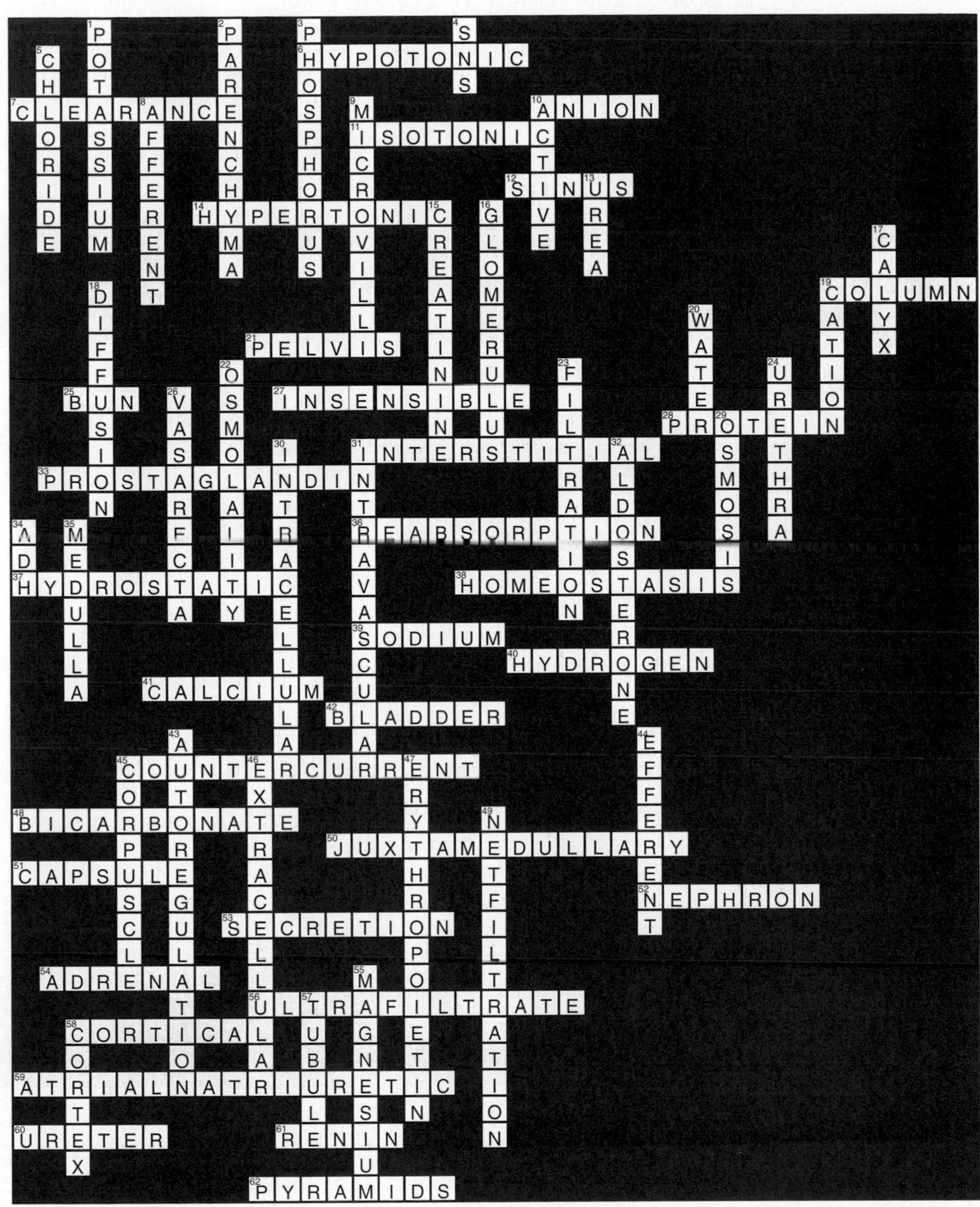

2.

7 Ureters
1 Glomerulus
4 Loop of Henle
3 Proximal convoluted tubule
8 Bladder
2 Bowman's capsule
6 Collecting ducts
5 Distal convoluted tubule
9 Urethra

3.

Water moves by the process of osmosis.
Electrolytes move by the process of diffusion.
The sodium-potassium pump is an example of active transport.
The use of a pushing pressure, such as hydrostatic pressure, is called filtration.

4.

Serum osmolality is 433 mOsm/kg which indicates severe dehydration. This is an example of a hyperglycemic hyperosmolar state caused by glucose intolerance associated with recent initiation of high-glucose enteral feedings.

5.

a. Potassium
b. Potassium, calcium, magnesium
c. Calcium
d. Calcium, phosphorus
e. Magnesium, phosphorus
f. Potassium, chloride

6.

Condition	Normal Anion Gap	Increased Anion Gap
Shock		×
Renal failure		×
Diarrhea	×	
Diabetic ketoacidosis		×
Salicylate overdose		×
Renal tubular acidosis	×	
Rhabdomyolysis		×
Carbonic anhydrase inhibitors	×	
Ethylene glycol poisoning		×

7.

a. Volume depletion (i.e., prerenal)
b. Catabolism
c. GI hemorrhage

8.

Sign/Symptom	Excess (Hyper)	Deficit (Hypo)
Sodium		
Weight gain	×	
Abdominal cramps		×
Flushed, dry skin	×	
Postural hypotension		×
Headache		×
Hypertension	×	
Potassium		
Flat T waves, prominent U waves		×
Decreased GI motility, paralytic ileus		×
Intestinal colic, diarrhea	×	
Muscle cramps → flaccid paralysis		×
Decreased cardiac contractility	×	
Tall, peaked T waves, widened QRS complex	×	

Sign/Symptom	Excess (Hyper)	Deficit (Hypo)
Calcium		
Tetany		×
Decreased deep tendon reflexes	×	
Neuromuscular weakness, flaccidity	×	
Seizures		×
Bone or flank pain	×	
Laryngospasm		×
Phosphorus		
Tetany	×	
Fatigue		×
Chest pain		×
Dyspnea		×
Increased deep tendon reflexes	×	
Abdominal cramps	×	
Magnesium		
Decreased deep tendon reflexes	×	
Anorexia, nausea, vomiting		×
Cardiopulmonary arrest	×	
Lethargy	×	
Dysrhythmias, especially torsades de pointe		×
Facial flushing	×	

9.

a. Hypercalcemia
b. Hypokalcmia
c. Hypomagnesemia

10.

a. A patient receiving regular doses of furosemide.
   1. Hypovolemia
   2. Hyponatremia
   3. Hypokalemia
   4. Hypocalcemia
   5. Hypomagnesemia
   6. Metabolic alkalosis (due to hypochloremia and hypokalemia)

b. A patient with persistent vomiting.
   1. Hypovolemia
   2. Hyponatremia
   3. Hypokalemia
   4. Metabolic alkalosis (due to hypochloremia and hypokalemia)

c. A patient with acute kidney injury (oliguric phase).
   1. Hypervolemia
   2. Hyponatremia
   3. Hyperkalemia
   4. Hypocalcemia
   5. Hyperphosphatemia
   6. Hypermagnesemia
   7. Metabolic acidosis

d. A patient with diabetic ketoacidosis (before treatment).
   1. Hyperkalemia
   2. Hypophosphatemia
   3. Hypermagnesemia
   4. Metabolic acidosis

e. A patient receiving multiple units of banked blood.
   1. Hyperkalemia
   2. Hypocalcemia
   3. Hypomagnesemia

11. Any three of the following:
BUN greater than 100 mg/dL
Volume overload especially with pulmonary edema
Uncontrollable hyperkalemia
Uncontrollable hyperphosphatemia
Uncontrollable acidosis
Pericarditis
Seizures or coma
Symptomatic uremia

12.

Condition	Prerenal	Intrarenal	Postrenal
Acute pyelonephritis		×	
Benign prostatic hypertrophy			×
Contrast dyes		×	
Diuretics	×	×	
Aminoglycosides		×	
Glomerulonephritis		×	
Goodpasture's syndrome		×	
Hemorrhage	×		
Hepatorenal syndrome	×		
Hypersensitivity reactions	×	×	
Intraabdominal tumor			×
Malignant hypertension		×	
Neurogenic bladder			×
Prolonged hypotension		×	
Renal calculi			×
Rhabdomyolysis with myoglobinuria		×	
Septic shock	×		

13.

Characteristic	Oliguric Phase	Diuretic Phase	Both
Elevated BUN			×
Hyperkalemia			×
Metabolic acidosis			×
Volume deficit		×	
Volume excess	×		

14.

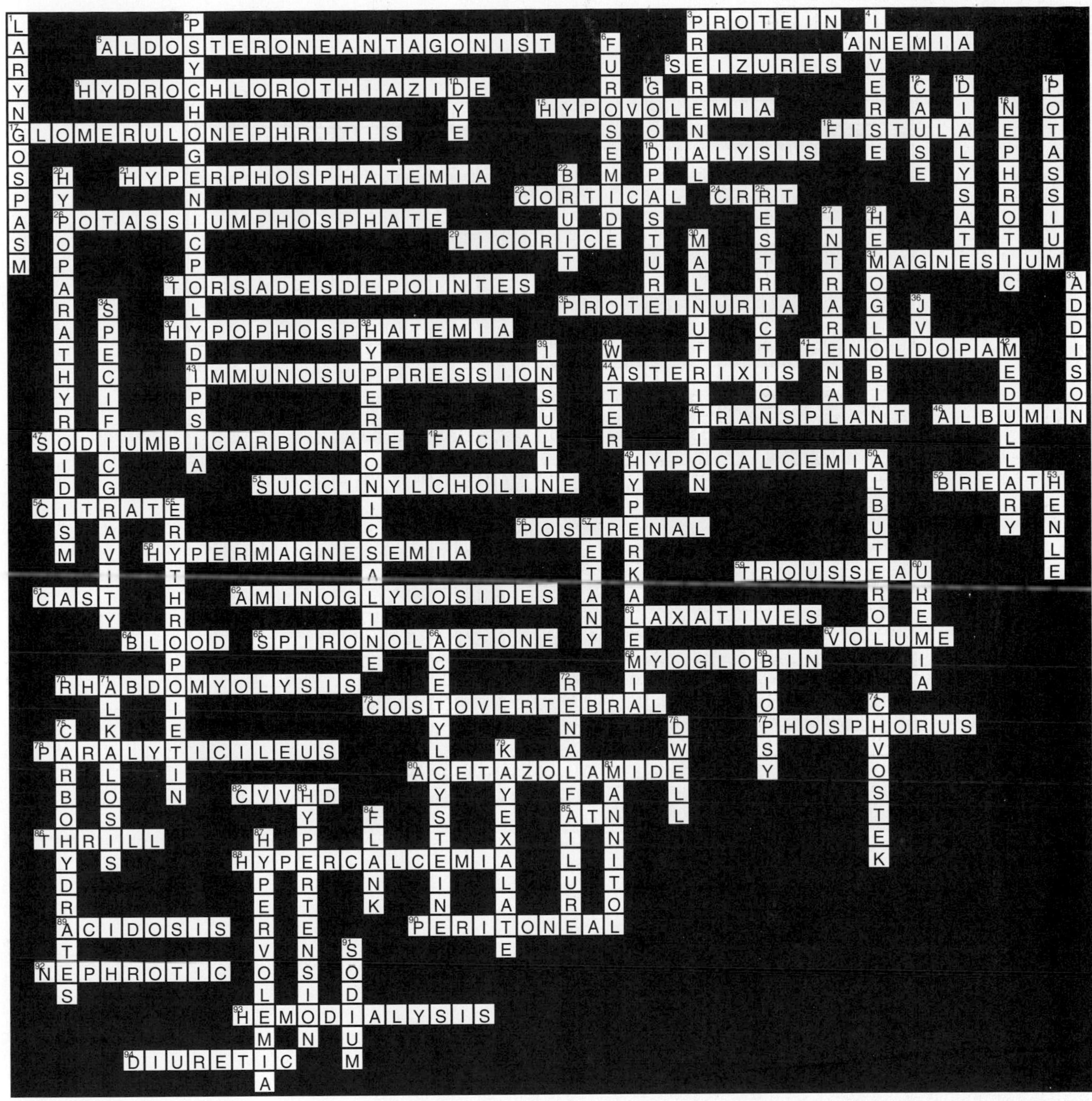

CHAPTER 9

1.

2.

Lithium	Decrease
Alcohol	Decrease
Chlorpropamide (Diabinese)	Increase
Positive pressure ventilation	Increase
Chlorpromazine (Thorazine)	Decrease
Phenytoin (Dilantin)	Decrease
Hydrochlorothiazide (HydroDIURIL)	Increase
Anesthetic agents	Increase
Demeclocycline (Declomycin)	Decrease
Beta stimulants	Increase
Morphine sulfate	Increase

3.

	DI	SIADH
Serum ADH	Decreased (if neurogenic DI)	Increased (if neurogenic SIADH)
Urine output	Greater than 200 mL/hr	Less than 0.5 mL/kg/hr
Urine specific gravity	Less than 1.005	Greater than 1.03
Urine osmolality	Low	High
Serum osmolality	Greater than 295 mOsm/L	Less than 280 mOsm/L
Serum sodium	Greater than 145 mEq/L	Less than 135 mEq/L
Right atrial/pulmonary artery occlusive pressures	RAP less than 2 mm Hg; PAOP less than 4 mm Hg	RAP greater than 6 mm Hg; PAOP greater than 12 mm Hg

4.

To calculate the serum osmolality: (serum sodium [158]) × 2 + (BUN [32] ÷ 2.6]) + (serum glucose [110] ÷18) = serum osmolality of 334.4 mOsm/kg. The most likely cause of the increase in urine output and the laboratory findings is diabetes insipidus.

5.

	DKA	HHS
Type of diabetes mellitus	1	2 or nondiabetic with intolerance to glucose load (e.g., enteral feeding)
Onset	Gradual or sudden	Gradual
Typical serum glucose range	600 mg/dL	1100 mg/dL
Presence of ketosis	Positive	Negative or minimal
pH	Acidosis	Normal or minimally acidotic
Anion gap	Increased	Normal
Respiratory pattern	Kussmaul's (rapid and deep)	Normal or tachypneic (rapid and shallow)
Breath odor	Acetone (fruity)	Normal
Serum osmolality	295-330 mOsm/kg	330-450 mOsm/kg
Serum sodium	Decreased, normal, or increased	Normal or increased
Serum potassium	Increased initially; drops with rehydration and correction of acidosis	Decreased
BUN	Mildly increased	Severely increased
Average fluid deficit	4-8 L	8-15 L

6.

Serum glucose greater than 300 mg/dL	Both
Kussmaul's respirations	DKA
pH less than 7.3	DKA
Positive serum and urine ketones	DKA
Abdominal pain	DKA
Dehydration	Both
Lethargy → coma	Both
Serum glucose greater than 600 mg/dL	HHS

7.

Headache	Hypoglycemia
Serum glucose greater than 300 mg/dL	DKA
Abdominal pain	DKA
Cold, clammy skin	Hypoglycemia
Nervousness, tremors	Hypoglycemia
Polyuria	DKA
Lethargy → coma	DKA
Seizures → coma	Hypoglycemia
Glycosuria	DKA
Tachycardia	Both
Agitation, difficulty with concentration	Hypoglycemia
Weakness, fatigue	DKA
Fruity breath	DKA
Serum glucose less than 50 mg/dL	Hypoglycemia

8.

c, f 1. Neurogenic DI
b, e 2. Nephrogenic DI
c, d, h 3. DKA
c, d, h 4. HHS
a 5. Hypoglycemia
i, g 6. SIADH

CHAPTER 10

1.

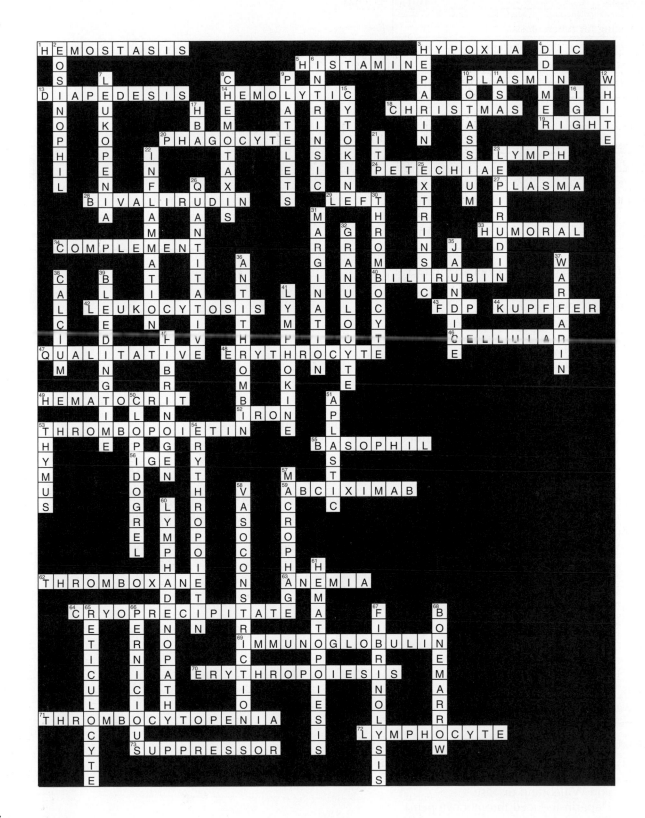

2.

a. Warmth
b. Redness
c. Swelling
d. Pain
e. Loss of function

3.

Example	Type
Skin testing for tuberculosis	IV
Poststreptococcal glomerulonephritis	III
Anaphylaxis to penicillin	I
Hemolytic blood transfusion reaction	II

4.

	Platelet Plug	Intrinsic Pathway	Extrinsic Pathway	Common Pathway	Fibrinolytic System
Activation	Intimal defect	Hageman factor (XII)	Tissue thromboplastin (III)	Stuart-Prower factor (X)	Tissue plasminogen activator
Laboratory Test	Bleeding time	aPTT	PT	aPTT, TT	Fibrin split products

5. Match the drug with the laboratory effect.

a 1. Aspirin
c 2. Heparin
b, f 3. Warfarin
e 4. rt-PA
d, e 5. Streptokinase
a 6. Clopidogrel

6.

a. Stop transfusion
b. Maintain IV access with normal saline and new administration set
c. Reassure the patient; stay at the bedside
d. Notify physician and blood bank
e. Recheck blood numbers and type
f. Treat symptoms appropriately
g. Return unused portion of blood in blood bag and administration set to the blood bank
h. Collect and send blood and urine samples to the laboratory; send another urine specimen 24 hours after transfusion reaction
i. Document the transfusion reaction and treatment administered

7.

Platelets	↓
PT	↑
aPTT	↑
Fibrin split products	↑
Factors V, VIII	↓
Fibrinogen	↓

8. Match the coagulopathy with the associated pathology.

d 1. Hemophilia A
e 2. Hemophilia B
c 3. von Willebrand disease
f 4. Heparin-induced thrombocytopenia
a 5. Disseminated intravascular coagulation
h 6. Liver disease
b 7. Immune thrombocytopenic purpura
g 8. Thrombotic thrombocytopenic purpura

9.

a. Heparin	May perpetuate bleeding
b. Clotting factors	May perpetuate clotting

CHAPTER 11

1.

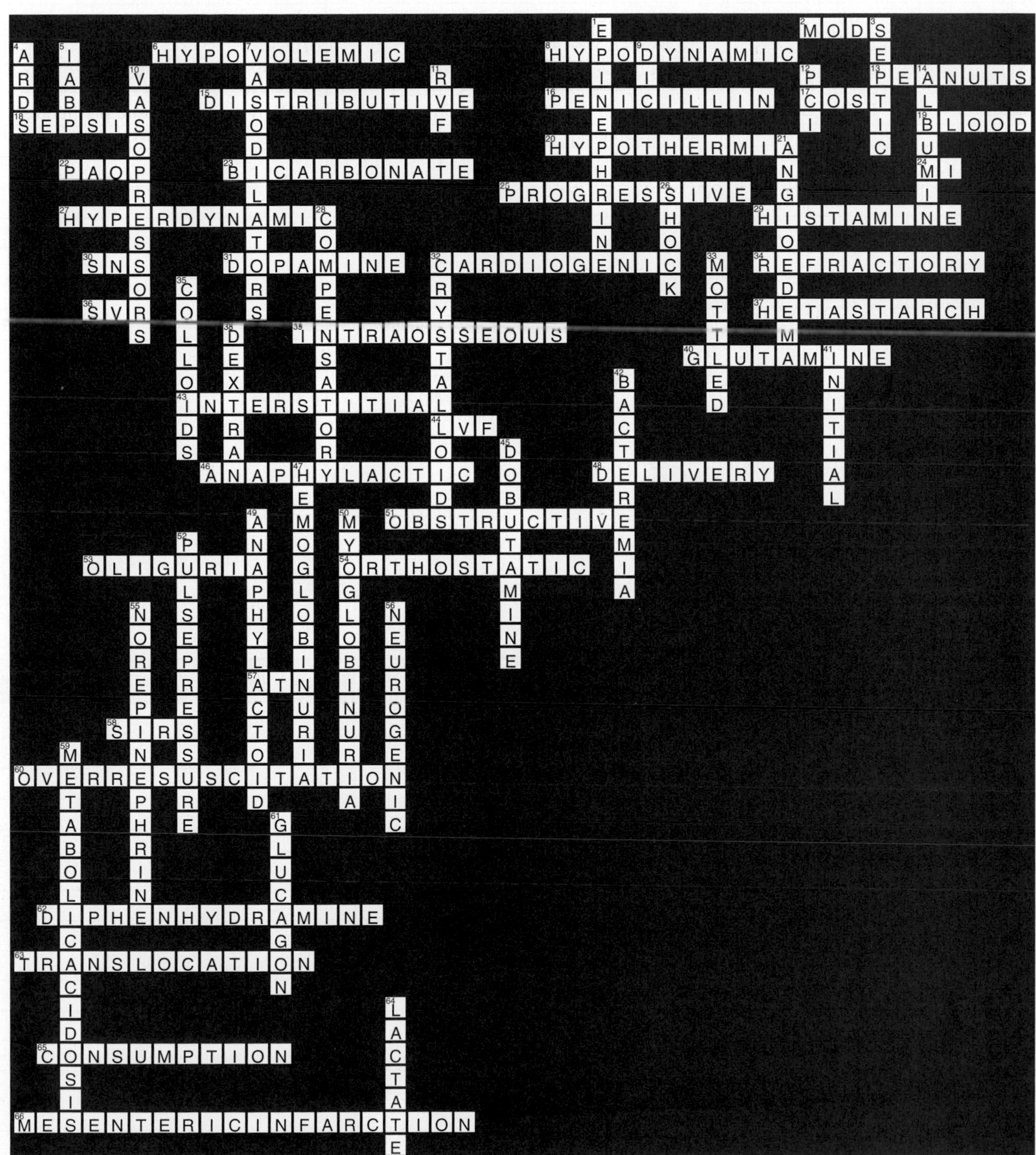

2.

Condition	Hypovolemic	Cardiogenic	Septic	Anaphylactic	Neurogenic
Myocardial infarction		✓			
Bee sting				✓	
Head injury					✓
Diarrhea	✓				
Pulmonary embolism		✓			
Ruptured gallbladder			✓		
Esophageal varices	✓				
Ruptured papillary muscle		✓			
Insulin shock					✓
Ascites	✓				
IVP dye				✓	
Spinal cord injury					✓
Invasive procedures	✓		✓		
Burns	✓		✓		
Blood transfusion reaction				✓	
Spinal anesthesia					✓
Trauma	✓		✓		
Malnutrition			✓		
Chemotherapy			✓		

3.

d 1. Anaphylactic
b 2. Cardiogenic
c 3. Hypovolemic
e 4. Neurogenic
a. 5. Septic

4.

Sign/Symptom	Compensatory	Progressive	Refractory
Tachycardia	✓	✓	
Dysrhythmias		✓	✓
Cool, pale skin	✓		
Disseminated intravascular coagulation			✓
Mottling of extremities		✓	✓
Neurologic changes: lethargy, coma		✓	✓
Oliguria	✓		
Anuria		✓	✓
Acute respiratory distress syndrome			✓
Narrow pulse pressure	✓		
Profound hypotension despite vasopressors			✓
Hypotension		✓	✓
Decreased bowel sounds	✓	✓	
Thirst	✓	✓	
Neurologic changes: irritability, confusion	✓		
Nausea		✓	

5.

Type of Shock	CO/CI	RAP/PAP/PAOP	SVR	SvO_2
Hypovolemic	↓	↓	↑	↓
Cardiogenic	↓	↑	↑	↓
Septic	↑	↓	↓	↑
Anaphylactic	↓	↓	↓	↓
Neurologic	↓	↓	↓	↓

CI, cardiac index; *CO*, cardiac output; *PAOP*, pulmonary artery occlusive pressure; *PAP*, pulmonary artery pressure; *RAP*, right atrial pressure; *SVR*, systemic vascular resistance; SvO_2, oxygen saturation of venous blood.

6.

Crystalloids		
Isotonic	Normal (0.9%) saline	Lactated Ringer's
Hypotonic	Half-normal (0.45%) saline	5% dextrose in water
Hypertonic	3% saline	10% dextrose in water
Colloids	Albumin	Dextran 70
Blood or blood products	Whole blood	Red blood cells

7.

c 1. Isotonic crystalloids
b, c 2. Red blood cells
a 3. Oxygen
a 4. Mechanical ventilation
c 5. Inotropic agents
d 6. Sedation
a 7. PEEP
b 8. Surgical intervention to stop bleeding
c 9. Treatment of metabolic acidosis
d 10. Hypothermia

8.

a, b, d, h, i, k, l	1. Anaphylactic
e, f, k, l, m, and possibly g	2. Cardiogenic
a, k, l, and possibly c	3. Hypovolemic
a, d, k, l and possibly g	4. Neurogenic
a, d, j, k, l, and possibly b and e	5. Septic

9.

d 1. Brain
f 2. Heart
e 3. Blood
b 4. Kidneys
c 5. Liver
a 6. Lungs

10.

Heart rate	Greater than 90 beats/min			
Respiratory rate	Greater than 20 beats/min	OR	$PaCO_2$	Less than 32 mm Hg
Temperature	Greater than 38°C (100.4°F)	OR	Less than 36°C (96.8°F)	
WBC	Greater than 12,000 cells/mm^3	OR	Less than 4000 cells/mm^3	

11.

a. Gastric lavage
b. Activated charcoal
c. Cathartic

12.

f 1. Methemoglobinemia
h 2. Cyanide
e 3. Methanol
i 4. Organophosphates
b 5. Carbon monoxide
j 6. Acetaminophen
k 7. Benzodiazepines (e.g., diazepam)
l 8. Opiates (e.g., morphine sulfate)
d 9. Ethylene glycol
a 10. Beta-blocker
c 11. Digoxin
g 12. Calcium channel blockers

13.

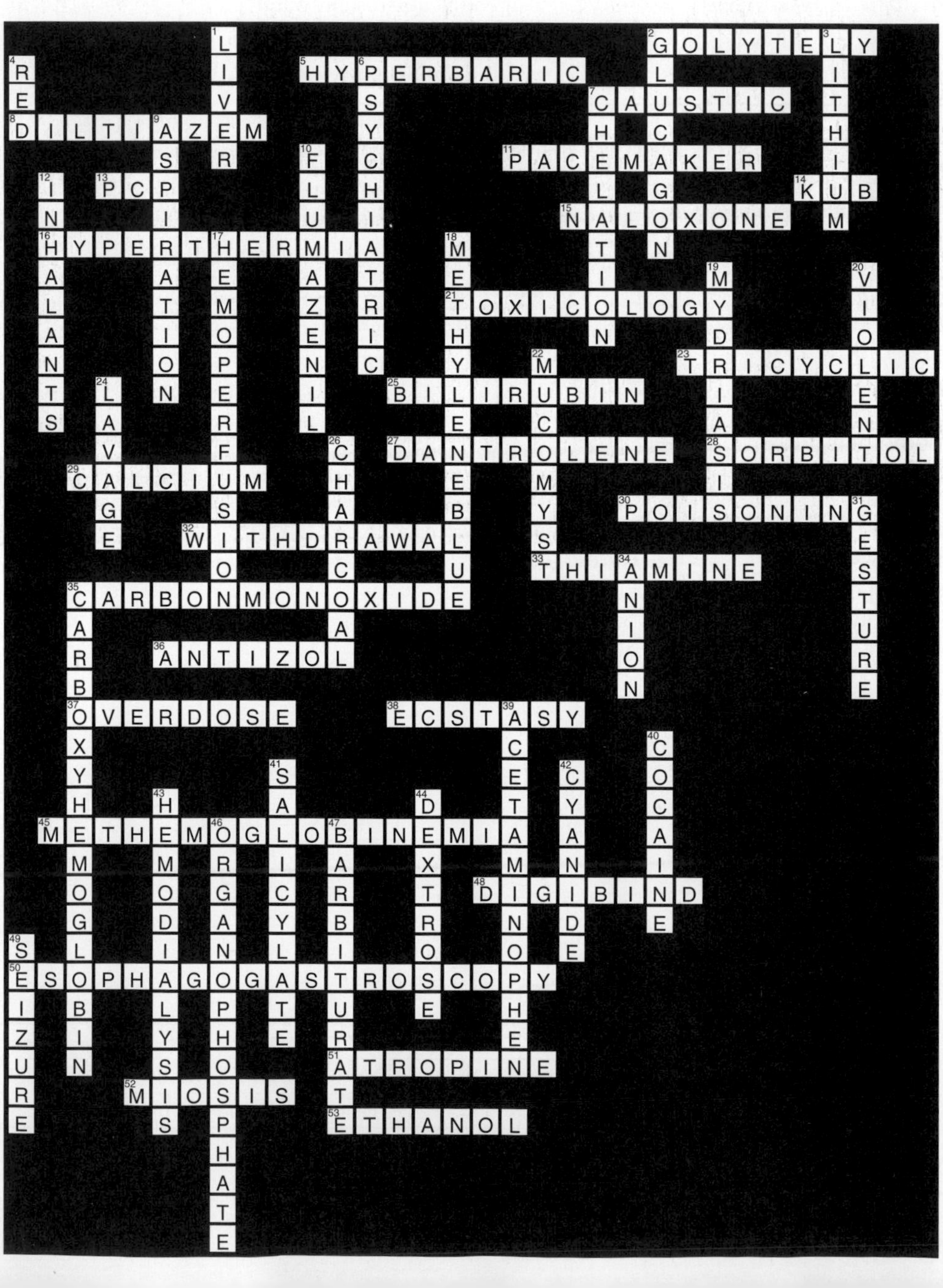

CHAPTER 12

1.

2.

e 1. Auditory
b 2. Visual
d 3. Gustatory
f 4. Hypnopompic
a 5. Tactile
c 6. Olfactory
g 7. Kinesthetic
h 8. Somatic

3.

a. Possibility of neglect or abuse
b. Accidental substance abuse related to poor eyesight or decreasing cognitive function
c. Medications take longer to clear due to aging renal function and may cause elderly patients to appear depressed or have flat affect.
d. Intentional substance abuse related to loneliness
e. Depression common in elderly patients with personal loss or faced with losing independence

4.

b 1. Physiologic
e 2. Safety and security
d 3. Love and belonging
c 4. Esteem and recognition
a 5. Self-actualization

5.

Condition	Subjective Assessment	Objective Assessment
Anxiety disorder	• Apprehension, nervousness • Tremors • Tightness in chest • Dizziness	• Tachycardia, elevated BP, tachypnea • Dilated pupils
Depression	• Hopeless feeling • Inability to concentrate • Low energy, fatigue, loss of appetite • Depressed mood • Decreased libido • Recurrent thought of death	• Appearance sloppy • Flat affect • Tearful • Little eye contact • Slowness of movement • Quiet
Mania	• Racing thoughts • Risky or reckless behaviors • Little need for sleep	• Increased activity • Flight of ideas • Distractibility • Elation • Grandiosity
Hallucinations	• Patient reports having visions or hearing voices	• Patient is talking or responding to voices or other perceptual disturbances
Psychosis	• Paranoid ideas • Confusion or amnesia • Fears about safety	• Delusions, hallucinations • Agitation or bizarre behavior • Appears out of touch with reality • Inability to initiate activities • Lack of pleasure
Dementia	• Memory loss • Speech impairment • Decline in cognitive function	• Decrease in orientation and judgment • Aphasia • Apraxia • Agnosia • Shallow affect • Gradual onset • Chronic
Delirium	• Disorientation • Hallucinations • Acute onset	• Etiology identified; may include medical condition, trauma, substance use/withdrawal, toxins • Fluctuating level of consciousness

6.

a. Does he have a history of medical or emotional issues?
Is he currently taking any medication?
Completion of neurologic exam

b. CBC/electrolyte panel
Toxicology screen
Urinalysis

c. Delirium as evidenced by acute mental status change
Rule out depression: No reported medical cause for the change. He is oriented to person, place, and time.
Rule out sepsis, stroke, and substance use: There is no evidence for this, but, given the rapid change, these and other causes of delirium should be ruled out.
Most likely not dementia due to acute onset

d. Safety
Physical stabilization: Assess vital signs and labs, and intervene as indicated. If no abnormality is identified, consider a mental health issue such as depression.
Emotional stabilization: Consider initiating treatment for depression if no physical problems are identified.

7.

a. How long has she been exhibiting these behaviors?
Has she had episodes of this nature previously?
Is she eating on a regular basis?
Is she sleeping on a regular basis?
Has she been harmed by someone else?
Has she had thoughts of hurting herself or anyone else?
Is she having any hallucinations?
Has she had any prescribed medication?
Has she used any over-the-counter substance?
Has she used any alcohol or other drugs?
Has she been physically ill?

b. CBC/electrolyte panel
Thyroid level
Drug screen for alcohol, marijuana, and other hallucinogens

c. Delirium: need to rule out medical cause of change of behavior
Mood disorder, such as mania, based on current symptoms and no physical cause identified

d. Safety
Physical stabilization: Treat any medical issues identified; normalize sleep/eat schedule.
Emotional stabilization

8.

a. ICU delirium

b. Most likely cause is sleep deprivation, but other causes should be investigated, including looking at what drugs the patient is receiving or withdrawing from that may be factors.

c. Safety: prevention of self-extubation and self-harm
Elimination of causes: uninterrupted sleep to allow REM sleep, extubation and transfer as soon as possible, reduction of noise, maintenance of normal light-dark cycles.

CHAPTER 13

1.

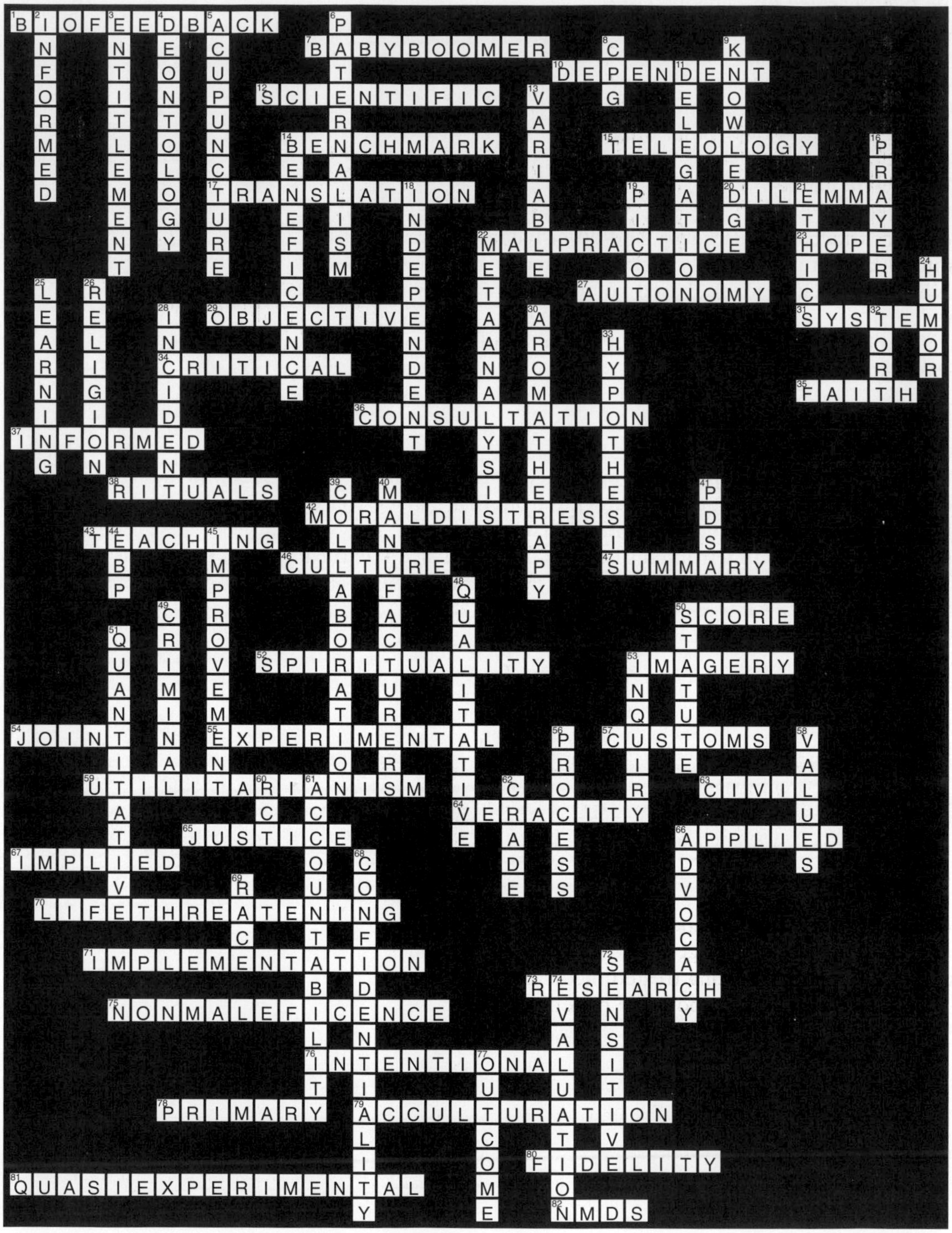

2.

a. Information collection and problem identification
b. Identification of possible solutions or actions
c. Analysis of the possible consequences of each solution or action
d. Selection of the best possible solution or action for implementation
e. Implementation of the solution or action
f. Evaluation of the results

3.

b 1. Veracity
e 2. Confidentiality
c 3. Autonomy
g 4. Nonmaleficence
f 5. Fidelity
d 6. Justice
a 7. Advocacy

4.

a 1. Utilitarianism
d 2. Egoism
f 3. Deontology
c 4. Paternalism
g 5. Social contract
e 6. Natural law
b 7. Teleology

5. Any eight of the following:
Progressive muscle relaxation (PMR)
Breathing
Meditation
Co-meditation
Guided imagery
Massage
Hypnosis
Biofeedback
Therapeutic (or healing) touch
Purposeful touch
Music therapy
Aromatherapy
Pet therapy
Humor
Acupuncture

6. Any five of the following:
To have questions answered honestly
To be assured the best care possible is being given to the patient
To know the prognosis
To feel there is hope
To know specific facts about the patient's progress
To be called at home about changes in the patient's condition
To know how the patient is being treated medically
To feel hospital personnel care about the patient
To receive information about the patient daily
To have understandable explanations
To know exactly what is being done for the patient
To know why things were done for the patient
To see the patient frequently
To talk to the doctor every day
To be told about transfer plans

7. Any five of the following:
Communication
Trust
Respect
Understanding and acceptance of team members' roles
Competence
Shared responsibility and accountability
Shared goal-setting
Flexibility
Administrative support

8.

You could have chosen any of the change models in Table 13-4 and described how you would implement each aspect of the model to change practice.

9.

a. False
b. True
c. False
d. False
e. False

10.

g 1. Islam (Muslim)
e 2. Catholicism
a 3. Judaism
c 4. Hinduism
d 5. Christian Scientist
f 6. Seventh-Day Adventist
b 7. Jehovah's Witnesses

11.

c 1. Developing a clinical practice guideline for a common clinical condition or procedure
a 2. Designing and conducting a research study when the available evidence base is inadequate
b 3. Conducting a systematic review of available evidence related to a clinical issue
d 4. Initiation of an evidence-based clinical change
e 5. Appraisal of the impact of an evidence-based clinical change
a 6. Conducting a literature search for available evidence related to a clinical question

12.

a. Bulletin boards for current articles
b. Journal clubs
c. Patient care conferences
d. Protocol and procedure development
e. Care paths

13. Any five of the following:
Goal-oriented
Less flexible
Requires longer time in the performance of learning tasks
Impatient in the pursuit of objectives
Finds little use for isolated facts
Strives for recognition and success
Has multiple responsibilities, all of which draw upon his or her time
Experienced in the "school of life"
Requires a more constant and ideal learning environment
Usually comes to the teaching program on a voluntary basis
Wishes to be involved in mutual planning of learning experiences
Likes to participate in diagnosing needs for learning, formulating learning objectives, and evaluating learning
Expects a climate of mutual respect, trust, and collaboration that supports learning

References and Recommended Reading

Abay, M. C., Reyes, J. D., Everts, K., & Wisser, J. (2007). Current literature questions the routine use of low-dose dopamine. *AANA J, 75*(1), 57–63.

Abrahamian, F. M., Deblieux, P. M., Emerman, C. L., Kollef, M. H., Kupersmith, E., Leeper, K. V., Jr., et al. (2008). Health care-associated pneumonia: Identification and initial management in the ED. *Am J Emerg Med, 26*(6 Suppl), 1–11.

Ackerman, M. H., & Mick, D. J. (2006). Technologic approaches to determining proper placement of enteral feeding tubes. *AACN Adv Crit Care, 17*(3), 246–249.

Adams, H. P., del Zoppo, G., Alberts, M. J., et al. (2007). American Heart Association guidelines for the early management of adults with ischemic stroke. *Stroke, 38*, 1655–1711.

Adhikari, N. K., Burns, K. E., Friedrich, J. O., Granton, J. T., Cook, D. J., & Meade, M. O. (2007). Effect of nitric oxide on oxygenation and mortality in acute lung injury: Systematic review and meta-analysis. *BMJ, 334*(7597), 779.

Adoni, A., & McNett, M. (2007). The pupillary response in traumatic brain injury: A guide for trauma nurses. *J Trauma Nurs, 14*(4), 191–196; quiz 197-198.

Aehlert, B. (2002). *ECGs made easy* (2nd ed.). St. Louis: Mosby.

Afshari, A., Brok, J., Moller, A. M., & Wetterslev, J. (2010a). Aerosolized prostacyclin for acute lung injury (ALI) and acute respiratory distress syndrome (ARDS). *Cochrane Database Syst Rev*, (8), CD007733.

Afshari, A., Brok, J., Moller, A. M., & Wetterslev, J. (2010b). Inhaled nitric oxide for acute respiratory distress syndrome (ARDS) and acute lung injury in children and adults. *Cochrane Database Syst Rev*, 2010(7), CD002787.

Ahrens, T. (2010). Stroke volume optimization versus central venous pressure in fluid management. *Crit Care Nurse, 30*(2), 71–73.

Albert, N. M., & Lewis, C. (2008). Recognizing and managing asymptomatic left ventricular dysfunction after myocardial infarction. *Crit Care Nurse, 28*(2), 20–37; quiz 38.

Alderson, P., Schierhout, G., Roberts, I., & Bunn, F. (2004). Colloids versus crystalloids for fluid resuscitation in critically ill patients. Retrieved May 31, 2005, from *www.medscape.com/viewarticle/485370_print*.

Alfaro-LeFevre, R. (2003). *Critical thinking in nursing: A practical approach* (3rd ed.). Philadelphia: Saunders.

Alspach, J. (2006). *Core curriculum for critical care nursing* (6th ed.). Philadelphia: Saunders.

Altman, M. (2011). Let's get certified: Best practices for nurse leaders to create a culture of certification. *AACN Adv Crit Care, 22*(1), 68–75.

American Association of Critical-Care Nurses and AACN Certification Corporation. (2003). Safeguarding the patient and the profession: The value of critical care nurse certification. *Am J Crit Care, 12*(2), 154–164.

American Association of Critical-Care Nurses. (2004). Practice alert: Pulmonary artery pressure measurement. Retrieved December 21, 2006, from *http://www.aacn.org//AACN/practiceAlert.nsf/Files/PAPMonitoring4-7-04/$file/PAPMonitoring.pdf*.

American Association of Critical-Care Nurses. (2005). AACN standards for establishing and sustaining healthy work environments. Retrieved August 13, 2012, from *http://www.aacn.org/aacn/pubpolcy.nsf/Files/HWEStandards/$file/HWEStandards.pdf*.

American Association of Critical-Care Nurses. (2008). Ventilator associated pneumonia. Retrieved June 24, 2011, from *http://www.aacn.org/WD/Practice/Docs/PracticeAlerts/Ventilator%20Associated%20Pneumonia%201-2008.pdf*.

American Association of Critical-Care Nurses. (2010). AACN Practice Alert. Family presence during resuscitation and invasive procedures. Retrieved August 13, 2012, from *http://www.aacn.org/WD/Practice/Docs/PracticeAlerts/Family%20Presence%2004-2010%20final.pdf*.

American Association of Critical-Care Nurses. (2010). Certification exam handbook. Retrieved July 11, 2010, from *http://www.aacn.org/WD/Certifications/Docs/certexamhandbook.pdf*

American Association of Critical-Care Nurses. (2011). AACN Practice Alert. Family presence: visitation in the adult ICU Retrieved. August 13, 2012, from *http://www.aacn.org/WD/practice/docs/practicealerts/family-visitation-adult-icu-practicealert.pdf*.

American Association of Critical-Care Nurses. (2012a). About critical care nursing. Retrieved August 10, 2012, from *http://www.aacn.org/wd/pressroom/content/aboutcriticalcarenursing.pcms?menu=*.

American Association of Critical-Care Nurses. (2012b). Certification Exam Handbook Retrieved August 10, 2012, from *http://www.aacn.org/WD/Certifications/Docs/certexamhandbook.pdf*.

American Association of Critical-Care Nurses. (2012c). Moral distress. Retrieved August 13, 2012, from *http://www.aacn.org/wd/practice/content/ethic-moral.content*.

American Heart Association. (2006). *Advanced cardiac life support manual*. American Heart Association: Author.

American Hospital Association. (2003). *The patient care partnership. Understanding expectations, rights and responsibilities*. Chicago: Author.

American Nurses Association & National Council of State Boards of Nursing. (n.d.). Joint statement on delegation. Retrieved August 13, 2012, from *https://www.ncsbn.org/Joint_statement.pdf*.

American Nurses Association. (1999). Nursing-sensitive quality indicators for acute care settings and ANA's safety & quality initiative. Retrieved August 2, 2006, from *http://www.nursingworld.org/readroom/fssafe99.htm*.

American Nurses Association. (2001). *Code of ethics for nurses with interpretative statements*. Washington, DC: American Nurses Publishing.

American Nurses Association. (2012a). What is nursing? Retrieved August 10, 2012, from *http://www.nursingworld.org/EspeciallyForYou/What-is-Nursing*.

American Nurses Association. (2012b). The nursing process. Retrieved August 10, 2012, from *http://www.nursingworld.org/EspeciallyForYou/What-is-Nursing/Tools-You-Need/Thenursingprocess.html*.

American Nurses Association. (2012c). ANA applauds IOM's release of 'Future of Nursing' report. Retrieved August 12, 2012, from *http://www.capitolupdate.org/index.php/2010/10/ana-applauds-ioms-release-of-future-of-nursing-report*.

American Nurses Association. (2012d). Nursing-sensitive indicators. Retrieved August 12, 2012, from *http://www.nursingworld.org/MainMenuCategories/ThePracticeofProfessionalNursing/PatientSafetyQuality/Research-Measurement/The-National-Database/Nursing-Sensitive-Indicators_1*.

American Psychiatric Association. (2000). *Diagnostic and statistical manual of mental disorders* (4th ed.). Washington, D.C.: American Psychiatric Association.

Amerine, E. (2007). Get optimum outcomes for acute pancreatitis patients. *Nurse Pract, 32*(6), 44–48.

Anderson, E. M., Spencer, D. D., & Walroth, T. A. (2008). Community-acquired pneumonia. A review of current practice guidelines. *Adv Emerg Nurs J, 30*(3), 209–217.

Andrews, P., & Habashi, N. M. (2010). Weaning patients from the mechanical ventilator: The nurse's role. *American Nurse Today, 5*(3), 11–14.

Andris, A. (2010). Pancreatitis: Understanding the disease and implications for care. *AACN Adv Crit Care, 21*(2), 195–204.

Angelo, T. A., & Cross, K. P. (1993). *Classroom assessment techniques: A handbook for college teachers*. Hoboken, NJ: Jossey-Bass.

Anthony, K., Wiencek, C., Bauer, C., Daly, B., & Anthony, M. K. (2010). No interruptions please: Impact of a No Interruption Zone on medication safety in intensive care units. *Crit Care Nurse, 30*(3), 21–29.

Armola, R. R., Bourgault, A. M., Halm, M. A., Board, R. M., Bucher, L., Harrington, L., & Medina, J. (2009). Upgrading the American Association of Critical-Care Nurses' evidence-leveling hierarchy. *Am J Crit Care, 18*(5), 405–409.

Armola, R. R., Bourgault, A. M., Halm, M. A., Board, R. M., Bucher, L., Harrington, L., & Medina, J. (2009). AACN levels of evidence: What's new? *Crit Care Nurse, 29*(4), 70–73.

Arnold, J. J., & Williams, P. M. (2011). Anaphylaxis: Recognition and management. *Am Fam Physician, 84*(10), 1111–1118.

Arrich, J. (2007). Clinical application of mild therapeutic hypothermia after cardiac arrest. *Crit Care Med, 35*(4), 1041–1047.

Ashworth, A., & Klein, A. A. (2010). Cell salvage as part of a blood conservation strategy in anaesthesia. *Br J Anaesth, 105*(4), 401–416.

Augustyn, B. (2007). Ventilator-associated pneumonia: Risk factors and prevention. *Crit Care Nurse, 27*(4), 32–36, 38-39; quiz 40.

Bagshaw, S. M., Uchino, S., Bellomo, R., Morimatsu, H., Morgera, S., Schetz, M., et al. (2009). Timing of renal replacement therapy and clinical outcomes in critically ill patients with severe acute kidney injury. *J Crit Care, 24*(1), 129–140.

Baguley, I. J., Heriseanu, R. E., Cameron, I. D., et al. (2008). A critical review of the pathophysiology of dysautonomia following traumatic brain injury. *Neurocrit Care, 8*, 293–300.

Baird, M. S., & Bethel, S. (2010). *Manual of critical care nursing. Nursing interventions and collaborative management* (6th ed.). St. Louis: Mosby.

Baldridge, K. H., & Andrasik, F. (2010). Pain assessment in people with intellectual or developmental disabilities. *Am J Nurs, 110*(12), 28–35; quiz 36-27.

Barbera, J. A., & Blanco, I. (2009). Pulmonary hypertension in patients with chronic obstructive pulmonary disease: Advances in pathophysiology and management. *Drugs, 69*(9), 1153–1171.

Barill, T. P. (2003). An ECG primer. Retrieved April 4, 2010, from *http://www.nursecom.com/ECGprimer.pdf*.

Barker, E. (2008). *Neuroscience nursing. A spectrum of care* (3rd ed.). St. Louis: Mosby.

Barr, F. (2010). Nursing peer review: Raising the bar on quality. *American Nurse Today, 5*(9), 46–48.

Barrantes, F., Tian, J., Vazquez, R., Amoateng-Adjepong, Y., & Manthous, C. A. (2008). Acute kidney injury criteria predict outcomes of critically ill patients. *Crit Care Med, 36*(5), 1397–1403.

Barst, R. J., Gibbs, J. S., Ghofrani, H. A., Hoeper, M. M., McLaughlin, V. V., Rubin, L. J., et al. (2009). Updated evidence-based treatment algorithm in pulmonary arterial hypertension. *J Am Coll Cardiol, 54*(1 Suppl), S78–S84.

Bass, N. M., Mullen, K. D., Sanyal, A., Poordad, F., Neff, G., Leevy, C. B., et al. (2010). Rifaximin treatment in hepatic encephalopathy. *N Engl J Med, 362*(12), 1071–1081.

Bauman, M. (2009). Noninvasive ventilation makes a comeback. *American Nurse Today, 4*(4), 20–25.

Baumhover, N., & Hughes, L. (2009). Spirituality and support for family presence during invasive procedures and resuscitations in adults. *Am J Crit Care, 18*(4), 357–366; quiz 367.

Becattini, C., Lignani, A., & Agnelli, G. (2010). New anticoagulants for the prevention of venous thromboembolism. *Drug Des Devel Ther, 4*, 49–60.

Bederson, J. B., Connolly, E. S., Batjer, H. H., et al. (2009). Guidelines for the management of subarachnoid hemorrhage: A statement for healthcare professionals from a special writing group of the Stroke Council, American Heart Association. *Stroke, 40*, 1–32.

Bel, E. H., Sousa, A., Fleming, L., Bush, A., Chung, K. F., Versnel, J., et al. (2011). Diagnosis and definition of severe refractory asthma: An international consensus statement from the Innovative Medicine Initiative (IMI). *Thorax, 66*(10), 910–917.

Bell, R. L., Ovadia, P., Abdullah, F., Spector, S., & Rabinovici, R. (2001). Chest tube removal: End-inspiration or end-expiration? *J Trauma, 50*(4), 674–677.

Benner, P. (2003). Beware of technologic imperatives and commercial interests that prevent best practices! *Am J Crit Care, 12*(5), 469–471.

Bentley, M. L., Corwin, H. L., & Dasta, J. (2010). Drug-induced acute kidney injury in the critically ill adult: Recognition and prevention strategies. *Crit Care Med, 38*(6 Suppl), S169–S174.

Bergman, K., & Bay, E. (2010). Mild traumatic brain injury/concussion: A review for ED nurses. *J Emerg Nurs, 36*(3), 221–230.

Bergman, K., Maltz, S., & Fletcher, J. (2010). Evaluation of moderate traumatic brain injury. *J Trauma Nurs, 17*(2), 102–108.

Bernstein, A. D., Daubert, J. C., Fletcher, R. D., Hayes, D. L., Luderitz, B., Reynolds, D. W., et al. (2002). The revised NASPE/BPEG generic code for antibradycardia, adaptive-rate, and multisite pacing. North American Society of Pacing and Electrophysiology/British Pacing and Electrophysiology Group. *Clin Electrophysiol, 25*(2), 260–264.

Berwick, D. M. (2003). Disseminating innovations in health care. *JAMA, 289*(15), 1969–1975.

Bhalla, R. N., Moraille-Bhalla, P., & Aronson, S. C. (2009). Depression. *Emedicine*, Retrieved on November 14, 2009, from *http://emedicine.medscape.com/article/286759-overview*.

Bielefeldt, S. (2009). The rules of transfusion: Best practices for blood product administration. *American Nurse Today, 4*(2), 27–30.

Bockenstedt, T. L., Baker, S. N., Weant, K. A., & Mason, M. A. (2012). Review of vasopressor therapy in the setting of vasodilatory shock. *Adv Emerg Nurs J, 34*(1), 16–23.

Bone, R. C. (1991). Let's agree on terminology: Definitions of sepsis. *Crit Care Med, 19*(7), 973–976.

Bone, R., Sprung, C., & Sibbald, W. (1992). Definitions for sepsis and organ failure. *Crit Care Med, 20*(6), 724.

Boucher, B. A., & Hannon, T. J. (2007). Blood management: A primer for clinicians. *Pharmacotherapy, 27*(10), 1394–1411.

Bourgault, A. (2008). AACN practice alert. Dysrhythmia monitoring. Retrieved March 30, 2011, from *http://www.aacn.org/WD/Practice/Docs/PracticeAlerts/Dysrhythmia_Monitoring_04-2008.pdf*.

Bourgault, A. M., & Halm, M. A. (2009). Feeding tube placement in adults: Safe verification method for blindly inserted tubes. *Am J Crit Care, 18*(1), 73–76.

Bourgault, A. M., Ipe, L., Weaver, J., Swartz, S., & O'Dea P. J. (2007). Development of evidence-based guidelines and critical care nurses' knowledge of enteral feeding. *Crit Care Nurse, 27*(4), 17–22, 25-19; quiz 30.

Boutou, A. K., Abatzidou, F., Tryfon, S., Nakou, C., Pitsiou, G., Argyropoulou, P., et al. (2011). Diagnostic accuracy of the rapid shallow breathing index to predict a successful spontaneous breathing trial outcome in mechanically ventilated patients with chronic obstructive pulmonary disease. *Heart Lung, 40*(2), 105–110.

Bowman, A., Greiner, J. E., Doerschug, K. C., Little, S. B., Bombei, C. L., & Comried, L. M. (2005). Implementation of an evidence-based feeding protocol and aspiration risk reduction algorithm. *Crit Care Nurs Q, 28*(4), 324–333; quiz 334-325.

Boyd, J. H., Forbes, J., Nakada, T. A., Walley, K. R., & Russell, J. A. (2011). Fluid resuscitation in septic shock: A positive fluid balance and elevated central venous pressure are associated with increased mortality. *Crit Care Med, 39*(2), 259–265.

Boyle, M., & Baldwin, I. (2010). Understanding the continuous renal replacement therapy circuit for acute renal failure support: A quality issue in the intensive care unit. *AACN Adv Crit Care, 21*(4), 367–375.

Bratcher, J. R. (2010). How do critical care nurses define a "good death" in the intensive care unit? *Crit Care Nurs Q, 33*(1), 87–99.

Bream-Rouwenhorst, H. R., Beltz, E. A., Ross, M. B., & Moores, K. G. (2008). Recent developments in the management of acute respiratory distress syndrome in adults. *Am J Health Syst Pharm, 65*(1), 29–36.

Bridges, E. (2006). Pulmonary artery pressure monitoring. When, how, and what else to use. *AACN Adv Crit Care, 17*(3), 286–305.

Bridges, E. (2009). AACN practice alert. Pulmonary artery/central venous pressure measurement. Retrieved April 7, 2010, from *http://www.aacn.org/WD/Practice/Docs/PracticeAlerts/PAP_Measurement_05-2004.pdf.*

Broden, C. C. (2009). Acute renal failure and mechanical ventilation: Reality or myth? *Crit Care Nurse, 29*(2), 62–75; quiz 76.

Brodkey, M. B., Ben-Zacharia, A. B., & Reardon, J. D. (2011). Living well with multiple sclerosis. [Review]. *Am J Nurs, 111*(7), 40–48; quiz 49-50.

Brower, R. G., Lanken, P. N., MacIntyre, N., Matthay, M. A., Morris, A., Ancukiewicz, M., et al. (2004). Higher versus lower positive end-expiratory pressures in patients with the acute respiratory distress syndrome. *N Engl J Med, 351*(4), 327–336.

Brunetti, J. (2008). A brief overview of some of the changes of the American Heart Association's guidelines for cardiopulmonary resuscitation and emergency cardiovascular care. *Crit Care Nurs Clin North Am, 20,* 245–250.

Brush, K. A. (2007). Abdominal compartment syndrome: The pressure is on. *Nursing, 37*(7), 36–41; quiz 40-31.

Brush, K. A. (2007). Measuring intra-abdominal pressure. *Nursing, 37*(7), 42–44.

Bulger, E. M., May, S., Brasel, K. J., Schreiber, M., Kerby, J. D., Tisherman, S. A., et al. (2010). Out-of-hospital hypertonic resuscitation following severe traumatic brain injury: A randomized controlled trial. *JAMA, 304*(13), 1455–1464.

Burns, S. M. (2005). Mechanical ventilation of patients with acute respiratory distress syndrome and patients requiring weaning: The evidence guiding practice. *Crit Care Nurse, 25*(4), 14–23; quiz 24.

Burns, S. M. (2008). Pressure modes of mechanical ventilation: The good, the bad, and the ugly. *AACN Adv Crit Care, 19*(4), 399–411.

Calder, S. (2008). Clinical pearls and pitfalls of electrocardiogram interpretation in acute myocardial infarction. *J Emerg Nurs, 34(4),* 324–329.

Calendrillo, T. (2009). Team building for a healthy work environment. *Nurs Manage, 40*(12), 9–12.

Cannon-Diehl, M. R. (2010). Emerging issues for the postbariatric surgical patient. *Crit Care Nurs Q, 33*(4), 361–370.

Cannon-Diehl, M. R. (2010). Transfusion in the critically ill: Does it affect outcome? *Crit Care Nurs Q, 33*(4), 324–338.

Caplan, G. (1970). *Theory and practice of mental health consultation*. New York: Basic Books.

Carlson, K. K. (Ed.). (2009). *Advanced critical care nursing*. St. Louis: Saunders.

Cary, A. H. (2001). Certified registered nurses: Results of the study of the certified workforce. *Am J Nurs, 101*(1), 44–52.

Cason, C. L., Tyner, T., Saunders, S., & Broome, L. (2007). Nurses' implementation of guidelines for ventilator-associated pneumonia from the Centers for Disease Control and Prevention. *Am J Crit Care, 16*(1), 28–36; discussion 37; quiz 38.

Casserly, B., Read, R., & Levy, M. M. (2009). Hemodynamic monitoring in sepsis. *Crit Care Clin, 25*(4), 803–823, ix.

Casserly, B., Read, R., & Levy, M. M. (2011). Hemodynamic monitoring in sepsis. *Crit Care Nurs Clin North Am, 23,* 149–169.

Cecil, S., Chen, P. M., Callaway, S. E., Rowland, S. M., Adler, D. E., & Chen, J. W. (2011). Traumatic brain injury: Advanced multimodal neuromonitoring from theory to clinical practice. *Crit Care Nurse, 31*(2), 25–36.

Cerda, J., Lameire, N., Eggers, P., Pannu, N., Uchino, S., Wang, H., et al. (2008). Epidemiology of acute kidney injury. *Clin J Am Soc Nephrol, 3*(3), 881–886.

Chen, L. (2010). A literature review of intensive insulin therapy and mortality in critically ill patients. *Clin Nurse Spec, 24*(2), 80–86.

Chng, Y., & Kosowsky, J. (2004). A triage algorithm for the rapid clinical assessment and management of emergency department patients presenting with chest pain. *Crit Pathw Cardiol, 3*(3), 154–157.

Chobanian, A. V., Bakris, G. L., Black, H. R., Cushman, W. C., Green, L. A., Izzo, J. L., Jr., et al. (2003). The seventh report of the Joint National Committee on Prevention, Detection, Evaluation, and Treatment of High Blood Pressure: The JNC 7 report. *JAMA, 289*(19), 2560–2572.

Choiniere, D. B. (2010). The effects of hospital noise. *Nurs Adm Q, 34*(4), 327–333.

Choudhary, P., & Amiel, S. A. (2011). Hypoglycaemia: Current management and controversies. *Postgrad Med J, 87*(1026), 298.

Chrysochoou, G., Marcus, R. J., Sureshkumar, K. K., McGill, R. L., & Carlin, B. W. (2008). Renal replacement therapy in the critical care unit. *Crit Care Nurs Q, 31*(4), 282–290.

Ciliska, D. K., Pinelli, J., DiCenso, A., & Cullum, N. (2001). Resources to enhance evidence-based nursing practice. *AACN Clinical Issues, 12*(4), 520–528.

Ciliska, D. K., Pinelli, J., DiCenso, A., & Cullum, N. (2001). Resources to enhance evidence-based nursing practice. *AACN Clinical Issues, 12*(4), 520–528.

Clark, J. D. (2010). Isopropyl alcohol intoxication. *J Emerg Nurs, 36*(1), 81–82.

Collins, T. A. (2011). Packed red blood cell transfusions in critically ill patients. *Crit Care Nurse, 31*(1), 25–33; quiz 34.

Connolly, E. S., Jr., Rabinstein, A. A., Carhuapoma, J. R., Derdeyn, C. P., Dion, J., Higashida, R. T., Vespa, P. (2012). Guidelines for the management of aneurysmal subarachnoid hemorrhage: A guideline for healthcare professionals from the American Heart Association/American Stroke Association. *Stroke, 43*(6), 1711–1737.

Connor, K. A. (2010). New intravenous antibiotics: A focused pharmacotherapy update. *AACN Adv Crit Care, 21*(3), 237–240; quiz 242.

Connors, A. F., Speroff, T., Dawson, N. V., Thomas, C., Harrell, F. E., Wagner, D., et al. (1996). The effectiveness of right heart catheterization in the initial care of critically ill patients. *JAMA, 276*(11), 889–897.

Cook, A. M., & Weant, K. A. (2007). Pharmacologic strategies for the treatment of elevated intracranial pressure. Focus on metabolic suppression. *Adv Emerg Nurs J, 29*(4), 309–318.

Cook, A., Laughlin, D., Moore, M., North, D., Wilkins, K., Wong, G., et al. (2009). Differences in glucose values obtained from point-of-care glucose meters and laboratory analysis in critically ill patients. *Am J Crit Care, 18*(1), 65–71; quiz 72.

Cook, L. K., & Clements, S. L. (2011). Emergency: Stroke recognition and management. *Am J Nurs, 111*(5), 64–69.

Cooper, B. E. (2008). Review and update on inotropes and vasopressors. *AACN Adv Crit Care, 19*(1), 5–13; quiz 14-15.

Corbridge, S., & Corbridge, T. C. (2010). Asthma in adolescents and adults. *Am J Nurs, 110*(5), 28–38; quiz 39-40.

Cotter, G., Cotter, O. M., & Kaluski, E. (2008). Hemodynamic monitoring in acute heart failure. *Crit Care Med, 36*(1), S40–S43.

Cottingham, C. A. (2006). Resuscitation of traumatic shock: A hemodynamic review. *AACN Adv Crit Care, 17*(3), 317–326.

Coughlin, R. M. (2008). Recognizing aortic dissection: A race against time. *American Nurse Today, 3*(4), 31–36.

Cranwell-Bruce, L. A. (2008). Antihypertensives. *MEDSURG Nurs, 17*(5), 337–342.

Craven, D. E. (2006). Preventing ventilator-associated pneumonia in adults: Sowing seeds of change. *Chest, 130*(1), 251–260.

Craven, D. E. (2006). What is healthcare-associated pneumonia, and how should it be treated? *Curr Opin Infect Dis, 19*(2), 153–160.

Crowther, M. A., Cook, D. J., Albert, M., Williamson, D., Meade, M., Granton, J., et al. (2010). The 4Ts scoring system for heparin-induced thrombocytopenia in medical-surgical intensive care unit patients. *J Crit Care, 25*(2), 287–293.

Cunha, B. A. (2008). Sepsis and septic shock: Selection of empiric antimicrobial therapy. *Crit Care Clin, 24*, 313–334.

Cunha, B. A. (2012). Fever myths and misconceptions: The beneficial effects of fever as a critical component of host defenses against infection. *Heart Lung, 41*(1), 99–101; author reply 199.

Curley, M. A. Q. (2007). *Synergy: The unique relationship between nurses and patients*. Indianapolis, IN: Sigma Theta Tau International.

Curley, M. A. Q. (1998). Patient-nurse synergy: Optimizing patients' outcomes. *Am J Crit Care, 7*(1), 64–72.

Curtis, J. R., Cook, D. J., Sinuff, T., White, D. B., Hill, N., Keenan, S. P., et al. (2007). Noninvasive positive pressure ventilation in critical and palliative care settings: Understanding the goals of therapy. *Crit Care Med, 35*(3), 932–939.

Dager, W. E., Sanoski, C. A., Wiggins, B. S., & Tisdale, J. E. (2006). Pharmacotherapy considerations in advanced cardiac life support. *Pharmacotherapy, 26*(12), 1703–1729.

Daly, M. L. (2009). Stopping a COPD flare-up. *American Nurse Today, 4*(8), 40–41.

Darovic, G. (2002). *Hemodynamic monitoring: Invasive and noninvasive clinical application* (3rd ed.). Philadelphia: Saunders.

Daschner, F., Kappstein, I., Engles, I., Reuschenbach, K., Pfesterer, J., & Kreig, N. (1988). Stress ulcer prophylaxis and ventilation pneumonia: Prevention by antibacterial cytoprotective agents. *Infect Control Hosp Epidemiol, 9*, 59–65.

Davenport, A., Bouman, C., Kirpalani, A., Skippen, P., Tolwani, A., Mehta, R. L., et al. (2008). Delivery of renal replacement therapy in acute kidney injury: What are the key issues? *Clin J Am Soc Nephrol, 3*(3), 869–875.

Davidson, J. E. (2009). Family-centered care: Meeting the needs of patients' families and helping families adapt to critical illness. *Crit Care Nurse, 29*(3), 28–34; quiz 35.

Davis, D. P., Idris, A. H., Sise, M. J., Kennedy, F., Eastman, A. B., Velky, T., et al. (2006). Early ventilation and outcome in patients with moderate to severe traumatic brain injury. *Crit Care Med, 34*(4), 1202–1208.

Davison, D. L., Chawla, L. S., Selassie, L., Jones, E. M., McHone, K. C., Vota, A. R., et al. (2010). Femoral-based central venous oxygen saturation is not a reliable substitute for subclavian/internal jugular-based central venous oxygen saturation in patients who are critically ill. *Chest, 138*(1), 76–83.

Day, L. (2009). Questions on organ donation and hastening death. *Am J Crit Care, 18*(4), 377–380.

De Backer, D., Biston, P., Devriendt, J., Madl, C., Chochrad, D., Aldecoa, C., et al. (2010). Comparison of dopamine and norepinephrine in the treatment of shock. *N Engl J Med, 362*(9), 779–789.

de Smet, A. M., Kluytmans, J. A., Cooper, B. S., Mascini, E. M., Benus, R. F., van der Werf, T. S., et al. (2009). Decontamination of the digestive tract and oropharynx in ICU patients. *N Engl J Med, 360*(1), 20–31.

De Waele, J. J., De Laet, I., Kirkpatrick, A. W., & Hoste, E. (2011). Intra-abdominal hypertension and abdominal compartment syndrome. *Am J Kidney Dis, 57*(1), 159–169.

DeKeyser Ganz, F., Fink, N. F., Raanan, O., Asher, M., Bruttin, M., Nun, M. B., et al. (2009). ICU nurses' oral-care practices and the current best evidence. *J Nurs Scholarsh, 41*(2), 132–138.

Del Zoppo, G. J., Saver, J. L., Jauch, E. C., et al. (2009). Expansion of the time window for treatment of acute ischemic stroke with intravenous tissue plasminogen activator: A science advisory from the American Heart Association/American Stroke Association. *Stroke, 40*, 2945–2948.

Dellinger, R. P., Carlet, J. M., Masur, H., Gerlach, H., Calandra, T., Cohen, J., et al. (2004). Surviving sepsis campaign guidelines for management of severe sepsis and septic shock. *Crit Care Med, 32*(3), 858–873.

Dennison, R. D. (2005). Creating an organizational culture for medication safety. *Nurs Clin North Am, 40*(1), 1–23.

Dennis-Rouse, M. D., & Davidson, J. E. (2008). An evidence-based evaluation of tracheostomy care practices. *Crit Care Nurs Q, 31*(2), 150–160.

Depew, C. L., & McCarthy, M. S. (2007). Subglottic secretion drainage: A literature review. *AACN Adv Crit Care, 18*(4), 366–379.

Dernaika, T. A., Keddissi, J. I., & Kinasewitz, G. T. (2009). Update on ARDS: Beyond the low tidal volume. *Am J Med Sci, 337*(5), 360–367.

Derrick, D. (2009). The "broken heart syndrome": Understanding Takotsubo cardiomyopathy. *Crit Care Nurse, 29*(1), 49–57, quiz 58.

Deshmukh, M., & Yafai, S. (2008). Interpreting noncontrast head CT. *Adv Emerg Nurs J, 30*(4), 297–302.

De-Souza, D. A., & Greene, L. J. (2005). Intestinal permeability and systemic infections in critically ill patients: Effect of glutamine. *Crit Care Med, 33*(5), 1125–1135.

Despins, L. A. (2009). Patient safety and collaboration of the intensive care unit team. *Crit Care Nurse, 29*(2), 85–91.

Deutschman, C. S., & Neligan, P. J. (2010). *Evidence-based practice of critical care*. Philadelphia: Saunders.

Devlin, J. W., Boleski, G., Mlynarek, M., Nerenz, D. R., Peterson, E., Jankowski, M., et al. (1999). Motor activity assessment scale: A valid and reliable sedation scale for use with mechanically ventilated patients in an adult surgical intensive care unit. *Crit Care Med, 27*(7), 1271–1275.

Dirkes, S. (2011). Acute kidney injury: Not just acute renal failure anymore? *Crit Care Nurse, 31*(1), 37–49; quiz 50.

Dirkes, S., & Hodge, K. (2007). Continuous renal replacement therapy in the adult intensive care unit: History and current trends. *Crit Care Nurse, 27*(2), 61–66, 68-72, 74-80; quiz 81.

Dracup, K., & Bryan-Brown, C. W. (1999). Empathy: A challenge for critical care. *American Journal of Critical Care, 8*(4), 204–205.

Drew, B. (2007). Pulling it all together. Case studies on ECG monitoring. *AACN Adv Crit Care, 18*(3), 305–317.

Drew, D. J., & St Marie, B. J. (2011). Pain in critically ill patients with substance use disorder or long-term opioid use for chronic pain. *AACN Adv Crit Care, 22*(3), 238–254; quiz 255-236.

Druding, M. C. (2000). Integrating hemodynamic monitoring and physical assessment. *Dimens Crit Care Nurs, 19*(4), 25–30.

Dumont, C. P., & Tiep, B. L. (2002). Using a reservoir nasal cannula in acute care. *Crit Care Nurse, 22*, 41–46.

Dumont, C., & Hardware, J. (2009). Teaching patients to tame their hypertension. *American Nurse Today, 4*(7), 20–25.

Dunn, H., Anderson, M. A., & Hill, P. D. (2010). Nighttime lighting in intensive care units. *Crit Care Nurse, 30*(3), 31–37.

Dykes, P. C., Rothschild, J. M., & Hurley, A. C. (2010). Medical errors recovered by critical care nurses. *J Nurs Adm, 40*(5), 241–246.

Eastes, L. E. (2010). Alcohol withdrawal syndrome in trauma patients: A review. *J Emerg Nurs, 36*(5), 507–509.

El Khoury, M. Y., Panos, R. J., Ying, J., & Almoosa, K. F. (2010). Value of the PaO:FiO ratio and Rapid Shallow Breathing Index in predicting successful extubation in hypoxemic respiratory failure. *Heart Lung, 39*(6), 529–536.

Elinson, J. (1987). Advances in health assessment discussion panel. *J Chronic Dis, 40*(Suppl 1), 83S–91S.

El-Khatib, M. F., Zeineldine, S., Ayoub, C., Husari, A., & Bou-Khalil, P. K. (2010). Critical care clinicians' knowledge of evidence-based guidelines for preventing ventilator-associated pneumonia. *Am J Crit Care, 19*(3), 272–276.

Ellis, K. C. (2008). Keeping asthma at bay. *American Nurse Today, 3*(2), 20–26.

Elpern, E. H., Killeen, K., Ketchem, A., Wiley, A., Patel, G., & Lateef, O. (2009). Reducing use of indwelling urinary catheters and associated urinary tract infections. *Am J Crit Care, 18*(6), 535–541; quiz 542.

Emergency Nurses Association. (2007). *Emergency nursing core curriculum* (6th ed.). Philadelphia: Saunders.

Environmental Protection Agency. (1974). Information on levels of environmental noise requisite to protect public health and welfare with an adequate margin of safety. Retrieved August 13, 2012, from *http://www.nonoise.org/library/levels74/levels74.htm*.

Epstein, E. G. (2012). Preventive ethics in the intensive care unit. *AACN Adv Crit Care, 23*(2), 217–224.

Erdemoglu, M., Kuyumcuoglu, U., Kale, A., & Akdeniz, N. (2010). Factors affecting maternal and perinatal outcomes in HELLP syndrome: Evaluation of 126 cases. *Clin Exp Obstet Gynecol, 37*(3), 213–216.

Erikson, E. (1968). *Identity, youth and crisis*. New York: W. W. Norton.

Evenson, L., & Farnsworth, M. (2010). Skilled cardiac monitoring at the bedside: An algorithm for success. *Crit Care Nurse, 30*(5), 14–22.

Faith, K., & Chidwick, P. (2009). Role of clinical ethicists in making decisions about levels of care in the intensive care unit. *Crit Care Nurse, 29*(2), 77–84.

Falise, J. P. (2007). True collaboration: interdisciplinary rounds in nonteaching hospitals–it can be done! *AACN Adv Crit Care, 18*(4), 346–351.

Fan, J. Y., Kirkness, C., Vicini, P., Burr, R., & Mitchell, P. (2008). Intracranial pressure waveform morphology and intracranial adaptive capacity. *Am J Crit Care, 17*(6), 545–554.

Farwell, A. L. (2010). Saving muscle: Evidence-based strategies for reducing door-to-balloon times for ST-segment elevation myocardial infarction patients. *J Emerg Nurs, 36*(3), 231–237.

Favaloro, E. J. (2010). Laboratory testing in disseminated intravascular coagulation. *Semin Thromb Hemost, 36*(4), 458–467.

Fawcett, J. (2008). Bipolar disorder: Manic-depressive illness. *Merck Manuals Online*, Retrieved on November 15, 2009, from *http://www.merck.com/mmhe/sec07/ch101/ch101c.html*.

Feider, L. L., Mitchell, P., & Bridges, E. (2010). Oral care practices for orally intubated critically ill adults. *Am J Crit Care, 19*(2), 175–183.

Feldstein, C. (2007). Management of hypertensive crises. *Am J Crit Care, 14*(2), 135–139.

Field, J. M., Hazinski, M. F., Sayre, M. R., Chameides, L., Schexnayder, S. M., Hemphill, R., et al. (2010). Part 1: executive summary: 2010 American Heart Association guidelines for cardiopulmonary resuscitation and emergency cardiovascular care. *Circulation, 122*(18 Suppl 3), S640–S656.

Fisher, E. M., & Brown, D. K. (2010). Hepatorenal syndrome: Beyond liver failure. *AACN Adv Crit Care, 21*(2), 165–186.

Fitzpatrick, J. C., Campo, T. M., Graham, G., & Lavandero, R. (2010). Certification, empowerment, and intent to leave current position and the profession among critical care nurses. *Am J Crit Care, 19*(3), 218–229.

Fletcher, B., & Thalinger, K. K. (2010). Prasugrel as antiplatelet therapy in patients with acute coronary syndromes or undergoing percutaneous coronary intervention. *Crit Care Nurse, 30*(5), 45–54.

Folan, L., & Funk, M. (2008). Measurement of thoracic fluid content in heart failure. *AACN Adv Crit Care, 19*(1), 47–55.

Folstein, M. F., Folstein, S. E., & McHugh, P. R. (1975). "Mini-mental state": A practical method for grading the cognitive state of patients for the clinician. *J Psychiatr Res, 12*, 189–198.

Fournier, M. (2009). Perfecting your acid-base balancing act. *American Nurse Today, 4*(1), 17–22.

Fox, L., Kirkendall, C., & Craney, M. (2010). Continuous ST-segment monitoring in the intensive care unit. *Crit Care Nurse, 30*(5), 33–44.

Frazier, S. (2008). Hemodynamic monitoring. In D. K. Moser & B. Riegel (Eds.), *Cardiac nursing* (pp. 705–736). Philadelphia: Saunders.

Friedlander, R. M. (2007). Arteriovenous malformations of the brain. *N Engl J Med, 356*, 2704–2712.

Friend, L. (2012). Ethical decision making in the emergency department: the Golden Rule. *J Emerg Nurs, 38*(3), 251–253.

Fultz, J., & Sturt, P. A. (2005). *Mosby's emergency nursing reference* (3rd ed.). St. Louis: Mosby.

Funk, M., Wood, K., Valderrama, A. L., & Dunbar, S. B. (2007). Supraventricular dysrhythmias: Nursing research to improve health outcomes. *J Cardiovasc Nurs, 22*(3), 196–217.

Galie, N., Hoeper, M. M., Humbert, M., Torbicki, A., Vachiery, J. L., Barbera, J. A., et al. (2009). Guidelines for the diagnosis and treatment of pulmonary hypertension. *Eur Respir J, 34*(6), 1219–1263.

Gallagher, J. J. (2010). Intra-abdominal hypertension: Detecting and managing a lethal complication of critical illness. *AACN Adv Crit Care, 21*(2), 205–219.

Gando, S., Iba, T., Eguchi, Y., Ohtomo, Y., Okamoto, K., Koseki, K., et al. (2006). A multicenter, prospective validation of disseminated intravascular coagulation diagnostic criteria for critically ill patients: Comparing current criteria. *Crit Care Med, 34*(3), 625–631.

Garcia, R., Jendresky, L., Colbert, L., Bailey, A., Zaman, M., & Majumder, M. (2009). Reducing ventilator-associated pneumonia through advanced oral-dental care: A 48-month study. *Am J Crit Care, 18*(6), 523–532.

Gardetto, N., & Carroll, K. (2007). Management strategies to meet the core heart failure measures for acute decompensated heart failure: A nursing perspective. *Crit Care Nurs Q, 30*(4):307–320.

George, J. N. (2010). Management of immune thrombocytopenia: Something old, something new. *N Engl J Med, 363*(20), 1959–1961.

George, K. J. (2008). A systematic approach to care: Adult respiratory distress syndrome. *J Trauma Nurs, 15*(1), 19–24.

Gheorghiade, M., Zannad, F., Sopko, G., Klein, L., Pina, I. L., Konstam, M. A., et al. (2005). Acute heart failure syndromes: Current state and framework for future research. *Circulation, 112*(25), 3958–3968.

Gin-Sing, W. (2010). Pulmonary arterial hypertension: A multidisciplinary approach to care. *Nurs Stand, 24*(38), 40–47.

Goldhill, D. R., Imhoff, M., McLean, B., & Waldmann, C. (2007). Rotational bed therapy to prevent and treat respiratory complications: A review and meta-analysis. *Am J Crit Care, 16*(1), 50–61; quiz 62.

Goldstein, L. B., Bushnell, C. D., Adams, R. J., Appel, L. J., Braun, L. T., Chaturvedi, S., et al. (2011). Guidelines for the primary prevention of stroke: A guideline for healthcare professionals from the American Heart Association/American Stroke Association. *Stroke, 42*(2), 517–584.

Gonzalez, C. E., Carroll, D. L., Elliott, J. S., Fitzgerald, P. A., & Vallent, H. J. (2004). Visiting preferences of patients in the intensive care unit and in a complex care medical unit. *American Journal of Critical Care, 13*(3), 194–198.

Graham, M. (2011). Pathology of asphyxial death. Retrieved June 24, 2012, from *http://emedicine.medscape.com/article/1988699-overview?src=emailthis#showall*.

Grannito, M. H., Norton, C. K., Sher, R., & Baldia, C. (2010). Takotsubo cardiomyopathy. Implications for nursing practice. *Adv Emerg Nurs J, 32*(1), 83–91.

Grap, M. J. (2009). Not-so-trivial pursuit: Mechanical ventilation risk reduction. *Am J Crit Care, 18*(3), 198.

Gray, J. A. M. (1997). *Evidence-based healthcare: How to make health policy and management decisions*. London: Churchill Livingstone.

Greinacher, A., & Selleng, K. (2010). Thrombocytopenia in the intensive care unit patient. *Hematology Am Soc Hematol Educ Program, 2010*, 135–143.

Griffin, S., & Logue, B. (2009). Takotsubo cardiomyopathy: A nurse's guide. *Crit Care Nurse, 29*(5), 32–43.

Guimond, M. E., Sole, M. L., & Salas, E. (2009). TeamSTEPPS. *Am J Nurs, 109*(11), 66–68.

Gusa, D., Miers, A., & Pfimmer, D. (2007). Using the FOUR score scale to assess comatose patients. *American Nurse Today, 2*(6), 18–19.

Guthrie, D. W., Guthrie, R. A., Hinnen, D., & Childs, B. P. (2011). It's time to abandon the sliding scale. *J Fam Pract, 60*(5), 266–270.

Gyamlani, G., & Geraci, S. A. (2007). Secondary hypertension due to drugs and toxins. *South Med J, 100*(7), 692–699; quiz 700, 708.

Haag-Heitman, B. & George, V. (2011). Nursing peer review: Principles and practice. *American Nurse Today*, 6(9), 48–52.

Hacke, W., Kaste, M., Bluhmki, E., et al. (2008). Thrombolysis with alteplase 3 to 4.5 hours after acute ischemic stroke. *Neurocrit Care, 359*(13), 1317–1329.

Halm, M. A. (2007). To strip or not to strip? Physiological effects of chest tube manipulation. *Am J Crit Care, 16*(6), 609–612.

Halm, M. A. (2008). The healing power of the human-animal connection. *Am J Crit Care, 17*(4), 373–376.

Halm, M. A. (2009). Relaxation: A self-care healing modality reduces harmful effects of anxiety. *Am J Crit Care, 18*(2), 169–172.

Halm, M. A., & Armola, R. (2009). Effect of oral care on bacterial colonization and ventilator-associated pneumonia. *Am J Crit Care, 18*(3), 275–278.

Halm, M. A., & Krisko-Hagel, K. (2008). Instilling normal saline with suctioning: Beneficial technique or potentially harmful sacred cow? *Am J Crit Care, 17*(5), 469–472.

Hamel, J. (2011). A review of acute cyanide poisoning with a treatment update. *Crit Care Nurse, 31*(1), 72–81; quiz 82.

Hamilton, P. M. (2007). Psychiatric emergencies: Caring for people in crisis. *Nursing CEU.com*, Retrieved on August 29, 2012, from *http://www.nursingceu.com/courses/358/index_nceu.html.*

Hammond, B. B. (2010). Four steps to reducing door-to-balloon time. *J Emerg Nurs, 36*(3), 217–220.

Hansen, L., Goodell, T. T., Dehaven, J., & Smith, M. (2009). Nurses' perceptions of end-of-life care after multiple interventions for improvement. *Am J Crit Care, 18*(3), 263–271; quiz 272.

Hanzik, J. (2008). Treatment of symptomatic severe hypertension in the emergency department. An acute finding of a chronic condition. *Adv Emerg Nurs J, 30*(3), 242–251.

Happ, M. B., Garrett, K., Thomas, D. D., Tate, J., George, E., Houze, M., Sereika, S. (2011). Nurse-patient communication interactions in the intensive care unit. *Am J Crit Care, 20*(2), e28–40.

Harding, A. (2010). Stroke scales you can use. *J Emerg Nurs, 36*(1), 40–52.

Harding, A. D. (2010). Poison control in the emergency department. *J Emerg Nurs, 36*(3), 242–245.

Hart, A. M., Patti, A., Noggle, B., Haller-Stevenson, E., & Hines, L. B. (2008). Acute respiratory infections and antimicrobial resistance. *Am J Nurs, 108*(6), 56–65.

Hartog, C. S., Bauer, M., & Reinhart, K. (2011). The efficacy and safety of colloid resuscitation in the critically ill. *Anesth Analg, 112*(1), 156–164.

Harvey, M. A., & Davidson, J. (2011). Long-term consequences of critical illness: a new opportunity for high-impact critical care nurses. *Crit Care Nurse, 31*(5), 12–15.

Havelock, R. (1973). *The change agent's guide to innovation in education*. Englewood Cliffs, NJ: Educational Technology Publications.

Haymore, J. (2004). A neuron in a haystack. Advanced neurologic assessment. *AACN Clin Issues, 15*(4), 568–581.

Hays, A. J., & Wilkerson, T. D. (2010). Management of hypertensive emergencies: A drug therapy perspective for nurses. *AACN Adv Crit Care, 21*(1), 5–14.

Hazinski, M. F., Nolan, J. P., Billi, J. E., Bottiger, B. W., Bossaert, L., de Caen, A. R., et al. (2010). Part 1: Executive summary: 2010 International consensus on cardiopulmonary resuscitation and emergency cardiovascular care science with treatment recommendations. *Circulation, 122*(16 Suppl 2), S250–S275.

Health Resources and Services Administration. (2001). Cultural competence works. Using cultural competence to improve the quality of health care for diverse populations and add value to managed care arrangements. Retrieved from *http://www.hrsa.gov/financeMC/ftp/cultural-competence.pdf.*

Hearrell, C. L. (2011). Advocacy: nurses making a difference. *J Emerg Nurs, 37*(1), 73–74.

Henneman, E. A., & Cardin, S. (2002). Family-centered critical care: A practical approach to making it happen. *Critical Care Nurse, 22*(6), 12–19.

Henzler, D., Cooper, D. J., Tremayne, A. B., Rossaint, R., & Higgins, A. (2007). Early modifiable factors associated with fatal outcome in patients with severe traumatic brain injury: A case control study. *Crit Care Med, 35*(4), 1027–1031.

Herlihy, B. (2007). *The human body in health and illness* (3rd ed.). Philadelphia: Saunders.

Hermanides, J., Vriesendorp, T. M., Bosman, R. J., Zandstra, D. F., Hoekstra, J. B., & Devries, J. H. (2010). Glucose variability is associated with intensive care unit mortality. *Crit Care Med, 38*(3), 838–842.

Herzig, S. J., Howell, M. D., Ngo, L. H., & Marcantonio, E. R. (2009). Acid-suppressive medication use and the risk for hospital-acquired pneumonia. *JAMA, 301*(20), 2120–2128.

Higgins, P. A., Daly, B. J., Lipson, A. R., & Guo, S. E. (2006). Assessing nutritional status in chronically critically ill adult patients. *Am J Crit Care, 15*(2), 166–176; quiz 177.

Hill, K. M. (2009). Mitral valve repair: A new choice. *American Nurse Today*, 4(5), 8–10.

Himmelfarb, J., Joannidis, M., Molitoris, B., Schietz, M., Okusa, M. D., Warnock, D., et al. (2008). Evaluation and initial management of acute kidney injury. *Clin J Am Soc Nephrol, 3*(4), 962–967.

Hoeper, M. M., Barbera, J. A., Channick, R. N., Hassoun, P. M., Lang, I. M., Manes, A., et al. (2009). Diagnosis, assessment, and treatment of non-pulmonary arterial hypertension pulmonary hypertension. *J Am Coll Cardiol, 54*(1 Suppl), S85–S96.

Hoesch, R. E., Koenig, M. A., & Geocadin, R. G. (2008). Coma after global ischemic brain injury: Pathophysiology and emerging therapies. *Crit Care Clin, 24*(1), 25–44, vii-viii.

Holcomb, S. S. (2007). Stopping the destruction of acute pancreatitis. *Nursing, 37*(6), 42–47; quiz 47-48.

Holley, A. B. (2010). Sleep in the ICU. Retrieved August 13, 2012, from *http://www.medscape.com/viewarticle/723907.*

Holzinger, U., Feldbacher, M., Bachlechner, A., Kitzberger, R., Fuhrmann, V., & Madl, C. (2008). Improvement of glucose control in the intensive care unit: An interdisciplinary collaboration study. *Am J Crit Care, 17*(2), 150–156.

Horne, E. M., & Gordon, P. M. (2009). Taking aim at hypertensive crises. *Nursing, 39*(3), 48–53.

House, D. T., & Ramirez, E. G. (2008). Emergency management of asthma exacerbations. *Adv Emerg Nurs J, 30*(2), 122–138.

Hung, O. L., Shih, R. D. (2011). Antiepileptic drugs: The old and the new. *Emerg Med Clin N Am, 29*, 141–150.

Hunt, C. W. (2010). Immune thrombocytopenia purpura. *MEDSURG Nurs, 19*(4), 237–239.

Hunt, S. A., Baker, D. W., Chin, M. H., Cinquegrani, M. P., Feldman, A. M., Francis, G. S., et al. (2001). ACC/AHA guidelines for the evaluation and management of chronic heart failure in the adult: Executive summary, a report of the American College of Cardiology/American Heart Association Task Force on Practice Guidelines (Committee to Revise the 1995 Guidelines for the Evaluation and Management of Heart Failure): Developed in collaboration with the International Society for Heart and Lung Transplantation; endorsed by the Heart Failure Society of America. *Circulation, 104*(24), 2996–3007.

Hunt, W. E., & Hess, R. M. (1968). Surgical risks as related to time of intervention in the repair of intracranial aneurysms. *Journal of Neurosurgery, 28*:14.

Hutchison, R., & Rodriguez, L. (2008). Capnography and respiratory depression. *Am J Nurs, 108*(2), 35–39.

Imazio, M., Trinchero, R., & Shabetai, R. (2007). Pathogenesis, management, and prevention of recurrent pericarditis. *J Cardiovasc Med (Hagerstown), 8*(6):404–410.

Institute for Healthcare Advancement. (2012). What is health literacy? Retrieved August 13, 2012, from *www.iha4health.org.*

Institute for Healthcare Improvement. (2011). Science of improvement: How to improve. Retrieved October 1, 2012, from *http://www.ihi.org/knowledge/Pages/HowtoImprove/ScienceofImprovementHowtoImprove.aspx*.

Institute for Healthcare Improvement. (2005). Implement the ventilator bundle. Retrieved June 13, 2011, from *http://www.ihi.org/IHI/Topics/CriticalCare/IntensiveCare/Changes/ImplementtheVentilatorBundle.htm*.

Institute for Healthcare Improvement. (2006). What is a bundle? Retrieved June 13, 2011, from *http://www.ihi.org/IHI/Topics/CriticalCare/IntensiveCare/ImprovementStories/WhatIsaBundle.htm*.

Institute of Medicine. (2010). The future of nursing: Leading change, advancing health. Retrieved March 30, 2012, from *http://www.iom.edu/Reports/2010/The-Future-of-Nursing-Leading-Change-Advancing-Health.aspx*.

Iwai, K., Uchino, S., Endo, A., Saito, K., Kase, Y., & Takinami, M. (2010). Prospective external validation of the new scoring system for disseminated intravascular coagulation by Japanese Association for Acute Medicine (JAAM). *Thromb Res, 126*(3), 217–221.

Jackson, M., Ignatavicius, D. D., & Case, B. (2006). *Conversations in critical thinking and clinical judgment*. Boston: Jones and Bartlett.

Jacobson, C. (2006). Tools for teaching arrhythmias: Wide QRS beats and rhythms. *AACN Adv Crit Care, 17*(3), 353–358.

Jacobson, C. (2007). Narrow QRS complex tachycardias. *AACN Adv Crit Care, 18*(3), 264–274.

Jacobson, C. (2007). Tools for teaching arrhythmias: Wide QRS beats and rhythms. Part I: P waves, fusion, and capture beats. *AACN Adv Crit Care, 17*(4), 462–465.

Jacobson, C. (2007). Tools for teaching arrhythmias: Wide QRS beats and rhythms. Part II: QRS morphology clues. *AACN Adv Crit Care, 18*(1), 91–96.

Jacobson, C. (2008). ECG diagnosis of acute coronary syndrome. *AACN Adv Crit Care, 19*(1), 101–108.

Jacobson, C. (2008). Myocardial infarction mimics ST segments. *AACN Adv Crit Care, 19*(2), 245–248.

Jacobson, C. (2009). Understanding atrioventricular blocks. Part I: First-degree and second-degree atrioventricular blocks. *AACN Adv Crit Care, 19*(4), 479–484.

Jacobson, C. (2009). Understanding atrioventricular blocks. Part II: High-grade and third-degree atrioventricular blocks. *AACN Adv Crit Care, 20*(1), 112–116.

Jauch, E. C., Cucchiara, B., Adeoye, O., Meurer, W., Brice, J., Chan, Y. Y., et al. (2010). Part 11: Adult stroke: 2010 American Heart Association guidelines for cardiopulmonary resuscitation and emergency cardiovascular care. *Circulation, 122*(18 Suppl 3), S818–S828.

Jeffrey, S. (2010). New AHA/ASA guidelines on management of intracerebral hemorrhage. Retrieved July 12, 2011, from *http://www.medscape.com/viewarticle/726066*.

Jenko, M., Gonzalez, L., & Alley, P. (2010). Life review in critical care: possibilities at the end of life. *Crit Care Nurse, 30*(1), 17–27; quiz 28.

Jessup, M., Abraham, W. T., Casey, D. E., Feldman, A. M., Francis, G. S., Ganiats, T. G., et al. (2009). 2009 Focused update: ACCF/AHA guidelines for the diagnosis and management of heart failure in adults: A report of the American College of Cardiology Foundation/American Heart Association Task Force on Practice Guidelines: Developed in collaboration with the International Society for Heart and Lung Transplantation. *Circulation, 119*(14), 1977–2016.

Johnson, C. (2009). Peril on the periphery. *American Nurse Today, 4*(6), 28–30.

Johnson, K. (2009). AACN practice alert. ST segment monitoring. Retrieved March 30, 2011, from *http://www.aacn.org/WD/Practice/Docs/PracticeAlerts/ST_Segment_Monitoring_05-2009.pdf*.

Johnson, S. A., & Romanello, M. L. (2005). Generational diversity. Teaching and learning approaches. *Nurse Educator, 30*(5), 212–216.

Jones, B., Higginson, R., & Santos, A. (2010). Critical care: Assessing blood pressure, circulation and intravascular volume. *Br J Nurs, 19*(3), 153, 155–159.

Kabes, A. M., Graves, J. K., & Norris, J. (2009). Further validation of the nonverbal pain scale in intensive care patients. *Crit Care Nurse, 29*(1), 59–66.

Kacmarek, R. M., Wiedemann, H. P., Lavin, P. T., Wedel, M. K., Tutuncu, A. S., & Slutsky, A. S. (2006). Partial liquid ventilation in adult patients with acute respiratory distress syndrome. *Am J Respir Crit Care Med, 173*(8), 882–889.

Kallenbach, J., Gutch, C. F., Stoner, M. H., & Corea, A. L. (2011). *Review of hemodialysis for nurses and dialysis personnel* (8th ed.). St. Louis: Mosby.

Kaplow, R. (2011). Creating a culture to promote nursing specialty certification. *AACN Adv Crit Care, 22*(1), 23–24.

Kaplow, R., & Reed, K. D. (2008). The AACN synergy model for patient care: A nursing model as a force of magnetism. *Nurs Econ, 26*(1), 17–25.

Kendall-Gallagher, D., & Blegen, M. A. (2009). Competency and certification of registered nurses and safety of patients in intensive care units. *Am J Crit Care, 18*(2), 106–116.

Kenny, D. J., & Goodman, P. (2010). Care of the patient with enteral tube feeding: An evidence-based practice protocol. *Nurs Res, 59*(1 Suppl), S22–S31.

Keough, V. & Pudelek, B. (2001). Blunt chest trauma: Review of selected pulmonary injuries focusing on pulmonary contusion. *AACN Clinical Issues: Advanced Practice in Acute & Critical Care, 12*(2):270–281.

Kesecioglu, J. (2010). Farewell to exogenous surfactant therapy in acute lung injury/acute respiratory distress syndrome! Or, must we start all over again? *Crit Care Med, 38*(7), 1606–1607.

Keske, L. A., & Letizia, M. (2010). *Clostridium difficile* infection: Essential information for nurses. *MEDSURG Nurs, 19*(6), 329–332; quiz 333.

Keyrouz, S. G., & Diringer, M. N. (2007). Clinical review: Prevention and therapy for vasospasm in subarachnoid hemorrhage. *Crit Care, 11*(4), 220–229.

Keys, V. A. (2011). Alcohol withdrawal during hospitalization. *Am J Nurs, 111*(1), 40–44; quiz 45-46.

Khalid, I., Doshi, P., & DiGiovine, B. (2010). Early enteral nutrition and outcomes of critically ill patients treated with vasopressors and mechanical ventilation. *Am J Crit Care, 19*(3), 261–268.

Kiekkas, P. (2011). Peak fever: Helpful or harmful? *Heart Lung, 40*(3), 272–273.

Kimball, E. J., Baraghoshi, G. K., Mone, M. C., Hansen, H. J., Adams, D. M., Alder, S. C., et al. (2009). A comparison of infusion volumes in the measurement of intra-abdominal pressure. *J Intensive Care Med, 24*(4), 261–268.

Kinney, M., Dunbar, S., Brooks-Brunn, J. A., Molter, N., & Vitello-Cicciu, J. (1998). *AACN clinical reference for critical care nursing* (4th ed.). St. Louis: Mosby.

Kirchhoff, K. T., & Faas, A. I. (2007). Family support at end of life. *AACN Adv Crit Care, 18*(4), 426–435.

Kirkness, C. J. (2005). Cerebral blood flow monitoring in clinical practice. *AACN Clin Issues, 16*(4), 476–487.

Kirkness, C. J., & Thompson, H. J. (2009). Brain tissue oxygen monitoring in traumatic brain injury: Cornerstone of care or another brick in the wall? *Crit Care Med, 37*(1), 371–372.

Kirkness, C. J., Burr, R. L., & Mitchell, P. H. (2009). Intracranial and blood pressure variability and long-term outcome after aneurysmal subarachnoid hemorrhage. *Am J Crit Care, 18*(3), 241–251.

Kirkness, C. J., Burr, R. L., Cain, K. C., Newell, D. W., & Mitchell, P. H. (2006). Effect of continuous display of cerebral perfusion pressure on outcomes in patients with traumatic brain injury. *Am J Crit Care, 15*(6), 600–609; quiz 610.

Kitchens, C. S. (2009). Thrombocytopenia and thrombosis in disseminated intravascular coagulation (DIC). *Hematology Am Soc Hematol Educ Program*, 240–246.

Kjonegaard, R., Fields, W., & King, M. L. (2010). Current practice in airway management: A descriptive evaluation. *Am J Crit Care, 19*(2), 168–173; quiz 174.

Kohn, L. T., Corrigan, J. M., & Donaldson, M. S. (Eds.). (2000). *To err is human. Building a safer health system*. Washington, DC: National Academy Press.

Kohtz, C., & Thompson, M. (2007). Preventing contrast medium-induced nephropathy. *Am J Nurs, 107*(9), 40–49; quiz 49-50.

Kollef, M. H. (2004). Prevention of hospital-associated pneumonia and ventilator-associated pneumonia. *Crit Care Med, 32*(6), 1396–1405.

Kollef, M. H., Afessa, B., Anzueto, A., Veremakis, C., Kerr, K. M., Margolis, B. D., et al. (2008). Silver-coated endotracheal tubes and incidence of ventilator-associated pneumonia: The NASCENT randomized trial. *JAMA, 300*(7), 805–813.

Kollef, M. H., Morrow, L. E., Baughman, R. P., Craven, D. E., McGowan, J. E., Jr., Micek, S. T., et al. (2008). Health care-associated pneumonia (HCAP): A critical appraisal to improve identification, management, and outcomes—proceedings of the HCAP Summit. *Clin Infect Dis, 46*(Suppl 4), S296–S334; quiz 335-298.

Kollef, M. H., Zilberberg, M. D., Shorr, A. F., Vo, L., Schein, J., Micek, S. T., et al. (2011). Epidemiology, microbiology and outcomes of healthcare-associated and community-acquired bacteremia: A multicenter cohort study. *J Infect, 62*(2), 130–135.

Kotter, J. P. (1995). Leading change: Why transformation efforts fail. *Harvard Business Review, 73*(1), 59–68.

Kraut, J. A., & Xing, S. X. (2011). Approach to the evaluation of a patient with an increased serum osmolal gap and high-anion-gap metabolic acidosis. *Am J Kidney Dis, 58*(3), 480–484.

Kübler-Ross, E. (1969). *On death and dying*. New York: Macmillan.

Kushner, F. G., Hand, M., Smith, S. C., Jr., King, S. B., 3rd, Anderson, J. L., Antman, E. M., et al. (2009). 2009 Focused updates: ACC/AHA guidelines for the management of patients with ST-elevation myocardial infarction (updating the 2004 guidelines and 2007 focused update) and ACC/AHA/SCAI guidelines on percutaneous coronary intervention (updating the 2005 guidelines and 2007 focused update): A report of the American College of Cardiology Foundation/American Heart Association Task Force on Practice Guidelines. *Circulation, 120*(22), 2271–2306.

Lahm, T., McCaslin, C. A., Wozniak, T. C., Ghumman, W., Fadl, Y. Y., Obeidat, O. S., et al. (2010). Medical and surgical treatment of acute right ventricular failure. *J Am Coll Cardiol, 56*(18), 1435–1446.

Laird, P., & Ruppert, S. D. (2011). Acute respiratory distress syndrome—a case study. *Crit Care Nurs Q, 34*(2), 165–174.

Langley, G. L., Nolan, K. M., Nolan, T. W., Norman, C. L., & Provost, L. P. (1996). *The improvement guide: A practical approach to enhancing organizational performance*. San Francisco: Jossey-Bass Publishers.

Lantz, M. (2008). Failure to thrive. *Clinical Geriatrics*, Retrieved on August 29, 2012 from *http://50.28.4.237/articles/Failure-Thrive?page=0,0.*

Larson, A. M. (2010). Diagnosis and management of acute liver failure. *Curr Opin Gastroenterol, 26*(3), 214–221.

Lauck, S., Mackay, M., Galte, C., & Wilson, M. (2008). A new option for the treatment of aortic stenosis: Percutaneous aortic valve replacement. *Crit Care Nurse, 28*(3), 40–51.

Ledesma, C. R. (2011). Relationship-based care: a new approach to caring. *Nurs Manage, 42*(4), 40–43.

Lehne, R. (2009). *Pharmacology for nursing care* (7th ed.). St. Louis: Saunders.

Lemke, D. M. (2007). Sympathetic storming after severe traumatic brain injury. *Crit Care Nurse, 27*(1), 30–37; quiz 38.

Leske, J. (1991). Overview of family needs after critical illness: from assessment to intervention. *AACN Clinical Issues in Critical Care Nursing, 2*(2), 220–229.

Levi, M. (2010). Disseminated intravascular coagulation: A disease-specific approach. *Semin Thromb Haemost, 36*(4), 363–365.

Levins, T. T. (2010). Shock: Early recognition and management. *J Emerg Nurs, 36*(4), 300–301.

Lewin, K. (1951). *Field theory in social sciences*. New York: Harper.

Lim, W. S., van der Eerden, M. M., Laing, R., Boersma, W. G., Karalus, N., Town, G. I., et al. (2003). Defining community acquired pneumonia severity on presentation to hospital: An international derivation and validation study. *Thorax, 58*(5), 377–382.

Link, M. S., Atkins, D. L., Passman, R. S., Halperin, H. R., Samson, R. A., White, R. D., et al. (2010). Part 6: Electrical therapies: Automated external defibrillators, defibrillation, cardioversion, and pacing: 2010 American Heart Association guidelines for cardiopulmonary resuscitation and emergency cardiovascular care. *Circulation, 122*(18 Suppl 3), S706–S719.

Lippi, G., & Cervellin, G. (2010). Disseminated intravascular coagulation in trauma injuries. *Semin Thromb Haemost, 36*(4), 378–387.

Lippitt, R., Watson, J., & Westley, B. (1958). *The dynamics of planned change*. New York: Harcourt, Brace and Company.

Lo, G. K., Juhl, D., Warkentin, T. E., Sigouin, C. S., Eichler, P., & Greinacher, A. (2006). Evaluation of pretest clinical score (4 T's) for the diagnosis of heparin-induced thrombocytopenia in two clinical settings. *J Thromb Haemost, 4*(4), 759–765.

Lowenstein, D.H., Alldredge, B.K. (1998). Status epilepticus. *N Engl J Med, 338*(14), 970–976.

Lucidarme, O., Seguin, A., Daubin, C., Ramakers, M., Terzi, N., Beck, P., et al. (2010). Nicotine withdrawal and agitation in ventilated critically ill patients. *Crit Care, 14*(2), R58.

Lyerla, F., LeRouge, C., Cooke, D. A., Turpin, D., & Wilson, L. (2010). A nursing clinical decision support system and potential predictors of head-of-bed position for patients receiving mechanical ventilation. *Am J Crit Care, 19*(1), 39–47.

Magder, S. (2007). Invasive intravascular hemodynamic monitoring: Technical issues. *Crit Care Clin, 23*, 401–414.

Makic, M. B., VonRueden, K. T., Rauen, C. A., & Chadwick, J. (2011). Evidence-based practice habits: Putting more sacred cows out to pasture. *Crit Care Nurse, 31*(2), 38–61; quiz 62.

Maloney-Wilensky, E., Gracias, V., Itkin, A., et al. (2009). Brain tissue oxygen and outcome after severe traumatic brain injury: A systematic review. *Crit Care Med, 37*(6), 1–7.

Mangurten, J. A., Scott, S. H., Guzzetta, C. E., Sperry, J. S., Vinson, L. A., Hicks, B. A., Scott, S. M. (2005). Family presence: Making room. *Am J Nurs, 105*(5), 40–49.

Manuel, A., & Maynard, N. D. (2009). Nutritional support. Retrieved November 1, 2011, from *http://www.medscape.com/viewarticle/703713.*

March, K. (2005). Intracranial pressure monitoring: Why monitor? *AACN Clin Issues, 16*(4), 456–475.

Marik, P. E. (2011). Surviving sepsis: Going beyond the guidelines. *Ann Intensive Care, 1*(1), 17.

Marik, P.E., Baram, M., Vahid, B. (2008). Does central venous pressure predict fluid responsiveness? A systematic review of the literature and a tale of seven mares. *Chest, 134*, 172–178.

Marini, J., & Wheeler, A. (2010). *Critical care medicine: The essentials* (4th ed.). Philadelphia: Lippincott Williams & Wilkins.

Marks, P. W. (2009). Coagulation disorders in the ICU. *Clin Chest Med, 30*(1), 123–129, ix.

Marquis, B. L., & Huston, C. J. (2011). *Leadership roles and management functions in nursing. Theory and application* (7th ed.). Philadelphia: Lippincott Williams & Wilkins.

Martin, B. (2010). Family presence during resuscitation and invasive procedures. Retrieved April 19, 2011, from *http://www.aacn.org/WD/Practice/Docs/PracticeAlerts/Family%20Presence%2004-2010%20final.pdf.*

Martin, B., Armola, R., & McQuillan, K. (2010). AACN practice alert. Severe sepsis: Initial recognition and resuscitation. Retrieved June 5, 2012, from *http://www.aacn.org/WD/Practice/Docs/PracticeAlerts/Severe%20Sepsis.pdf.*

Martin, G. S. (2006). Pulmonary artery catheterization. Retrieved April 7, 2010, from *http://www.medscape.org/viewarticle/521197*.

Martin, R. K. (2010). Acute kidney injury: Advances in definition, pathophysiology, and diagnosis. *AACN Adv Crit Care, 21*(4), 350–356.

Maselli, D. J., & Restrepo, M. I. (2011). Strategies in the prevention of ventilator-associated pneumonia. *Ther Adv Respir Dis, 5*(2), 131–141.

Maslow, A. (1968). *Toward a psychology of being* (2nd ed.). Princeton, MA: Van Nostrand.

Matthews, E. E. (2011). Sleep disturbances and fatigue in critically ill patients. *AACN Adv Crit Care, 22*(3), 204–224.

McAdam, J. L., & Puntillo, K. (2009). Symptoms experienced by family members of patients in intensive care units. *Am J Crit Care, 18*(3), 200–209; quiz 210.

McAdams-Jones, D. (2008). Reversing SIADH. *American Nurse Today, 3*(9), 40.

McAtee, M. E. (2011). Cardiogenic shock. *Crit Care Nurs Clin North Am, 23*(4), 607–615.

McCaffery, M. (1968). *Nursing practice theories related to cognition, bodily pain and main environment interactions*. Los Angeles: University of California, Los Angeles.

McCaffery, M. (2002). Teaching your patient to use a pain rating scale. *Nursing2002, 32*(8), 17.

McCance, K. L., & Huether, S. E. (2009). *Pathophysiology. The biologic basis for disease in adults and children* (6th ed.). St. Louis: Elsevier Mosby.

McClintick, C. (2008). Open pneumothorax resulting from blunt thoracic trauma: A case report. *J Trauma Nurs, 15*(2), 72–76.

McCowan, C. (2007). Hypertensive emergencies. *EMedicine*, Retrieved November 4, 2008, from *http://www.emedicine.com/emerg/TOPIC267*.

McCoy, C., & Johnson, K. (2011). Behavioral emergencies: A closer look. *J Emerg Nurs, 37*(1), 104–108.

McCulloch, B. (2009). Takotsubo cardiomyopathy. *AACN Adv Crit Care, 20*(2), 194–200.

McGowan, C. M. (2011). Legal aspects of end-of-life care. *Crit Care Nurse, 31*(5), 64–69.

McKean, S. (2009). Induced moderate hypothermia after cardiac arrest. *AACN Adv Crit Care, 20*(4), 343–355.

McKinley, M. G. (2009). Recognizing and responding to acute liver failure. *Nursing, 39*(3), 38–44; quiz 44-35.

McNett, M. (2007). A review of the predictive ability of Glasgow Coma Scale scores in head-injured patients. *J Neurosci Nurs, 39*(2), 68–75.

McNett, M. M., & Gianakis, A. (2010). Nursing interventions for critically ill traumatic brain injury patients. *J Neurosci Nurs, 42*(2), 71–77; quiz 78-79.

McNett, M., Doheny, M., Sedlak, C. A., & Ludwick, R. (2010). Judgments of critical care nurses about risk for secondary brain injury. *Am J Crit Care, 19*(3), 250–260.

McRae, M. E., Rodger, M., & Bailey, B. A. (2009). Transcatheter and transapical aortic valve replacement. *Crit Care Nurse, 29*(1), 22–37; quiz 38.

McSwain, N. E. (2000). Kinematics of trauma. In K. L. Mattox, D. V. Feliciano, & E. E. Moore (Eds.), *Trauma* (pp. 127–152). New York: McGraw-Hill.

Medina, D. L., Sumter, D., George, J., Rushenberg, J., & Leonard, C. (2007). Reducing door-to-balloon times in acute myocardial infarction. *J Emerg Nurs, 33(4)*, 336–341.

Mehta, R. L., Pascual, M. T., Soroko, S., & Chertow, G. M. (2002). Diuretics, mortality, and nonrecovery of renal function in acute renal failure. *JAMA, 288*(20), 2547–2553.

Mellott, K. G., Grap, M. J., Munro, C. L., Sessler, C. N., & Wetzel, P. A. (2009). Patient-ventilator dyssynchrony: Clinical significance and implications for practice. *Crit Care Nurse, 29*(6), 41–55.

Melnyk, B. M., & Fineout-Overholt, E. (2011). *Evidence-based practice in nursing and healthcare. A guide to best practice*. Philadelphia: Lippincott Williams & Wilkins.

Merhaut, S., & Trupp, R. J. (2010). Cardiorenal dysfunction. *AACN Adv Crit Care, 21*(4), 357–364; quiz 365-356.

Metheny, N. (2009). Verification of feeding tube placement (blindly inserted). Retrieved July 3, 2011, from *http://www.aacn.org/WD/Practice/Docs/PracticeAlerts/Verification_of_Feeding_Tube_Placement_05-2005.pdf*.

Metheny, N. A. (2006). Preventing respiratory complications of tube feedings: Evidence-based practice. *Am J Crit Care, 15*(4), 360–369.

Metheny, N. A. (2008). Residual volume measurement should be retained in enteral feeding protocols. *Am J Crit Care, 17*(1), 62–64.

Metheny, N. A., Clouse, R. E., Chang, Y. H., Stewart, B. J., Oliver, D. A., & Kollef, M. H. (2006). Tracheobronchial aspiration of gastric contents in critically ill tube-fed patients: Frequency, outcomes, and risk factors. *Crit Care Med, 34*(4), 1007–1015.

Metheny, N. A., Schallom, L., Oliver, D. A., & Clouse, R. E. (2008). Gastric residual volume and aspiration in critically ill patients receiving gastric feedings. *Am J Crit Care, 17*(6), 512–519; quiz 520.

Miller, J., & Mink, J. (2009). Acute ischemic stroke: Not a moment to lose. *Nursing, 39*(5), 37–42; quiz 42-33.

Mirski, M. A., & Varelas, P. N. (2008). Seizures and status epilepticus in the critically ill. *Crit Care Clin, 24*(1), 115–147, ix.

Mitchell, M., Chaboyer, W., Burmeister, E., & Foster, M. (2009). Positive effects of a nursing intervention on family-centered care in adult critical care. *Am J Crit Care, 18*(6), 543–552; quiz 553.

Moore, K. M. (2011). The four horsemen of the apocalypse of trauma. *J Emerg Nurs, 37*(3), 294–295.

Moorman, L. P. (2010). Implantable cardioverter-defibrillator: Not just another device. *American Nurse Today, 5*(1), 12–14.

Morelli, A., Teboul, J. L., Maggiore, S. M., Vieillard-Baron, A., Rocco, M., Conti, G., et al. (2006). Effects of levosimendan on right ventricular afterload in patients with acute respiratory distress syndrome: A pilot study. *Crit Care Med, 34*(9), 2287–2293.

Mortimer, D. S., & Jancik, J. (2006). Administering hypertonic saline to patients with severe traumatic brain injury. *J Neurosci Nurs, 38*(3), 142–146.

Morton, P. G., & Fontaine, D. K. (2009). *Critical care nursing. A holistic approach* (9th ed.). Philadelphia: Lippincott Williams & Wilkins.

Moseley, M. J., Allen, D., & Martell, M. (2010). Electrocardiogram lead selection using critical thinking. *Dimens Crit Care Nurs, 29*(6), 253–258.

Munro, C. L., Grap, M. J., Jones, D. J., McClish, D. K., & Sessler, C. N. (2009). Chlorhexidine, toothbrushing, and preventing ventilator-associated pneumonia in critically ill adults. *Am J Crit Care, 18*(5), 428–437; quiz 438.

Mutchner, L. (2007). The ABCs of CPR again. *Am J Nurs, 107*(1), 60–70.

Napolitano, L. M., Kurek, S., Luchette, F. A., Corwin, H. L., Barie, P. S., Tisherman, S. A., et al. (2009). Clinical practice guideline: Red blood cell transfusion in adult trauma and critical care. *Crit Care Med, 37*(12), 3124–3157.

Narayan, M. C. (2010). Culture's effects on pain assessment and management. *Am J Nurs, 110*(4), 38–47; quiz 48-39.

National Council of State Boards of Nursing. (1996). Assuring competence. Retrieved May 20, 2002, from *www.ncsbn.org/public/resources/ncsbn_competence_two.htm*.

National Institutes of Health. (2008). ARDSnet mechanical ventilation protocol summary. Retrieved June 29, 2011, from *http://www.ardsnet.org/system/files/6mlcardsmall_2008update_final_JULY2008.pdf*.

National Kidney Foundation. (2002). KDOQI clinical practice guidelines for chronic kidney disease: Evaluation, classification, and stratification. Retrieved January 2, 2012, from *http://www.kidney.org/professionals/KDOQI/guidelines_ckd/p4_class_g1.htm*.

Ndefo, U. A., Erowele, G. I., Ebiasah, R., & Green, W. (2010). Clevidipine: A new intravenous option for the management of acute hypertension. *Am J Health Syst Pharm, 67*(5), 351–360.

Neal, A., Twibell, R., Osborne, K., & Harris, D. (2010). Providing family-friendly care - even when stress is high and time is short. *American Nurse Today, 5*(11), 9–12.

Neithercott, T. (2011). 6 ways to prevent and treat low blood glucose. *Diabetes Forecast, 64*(4), 46–47.

Nelson, D. P., & Plost, G. (2009). Registered nurses as family care specialists in the intensive care unit. *Crit Care Nurse, 29*(3), 46–52; quiz 53.

Nelson, J. M. (2010). Recognizing, preventing, and managing delirium in hospital patients. *American Nurse Today, 5*(11), 43–45.

NeSmith, E., Weinrich, S., Andrews, J., Medeiros, R., Hawkins, M., Weinrich, M., et al. (2011). Substance use and the systemic inflammatory response syndrome (SIRS) following trauma. *J Trauma Nurs, 18*(2), 79–86.

Neumar, R. W., Otto, C. W., Link, M. S., Kronick, S. L., Shuster, M., Callaway, C. W., et al. (2010). Part 8: Adult advanced cardiovascular life support: 2010 American Heart Association guidelines for cardiopulmonary resuscitation and emergency cardiovascular care. *Circulation, 122*(18 Suppl 3), S729–S767.

Nguyen, H. B., Corbett, S. W., Steele, R., Banta, J., Clark, R. T., Hayes, S. R., et al. (2007). Implementation of a bundle of quality indicators for the early management of severe sepsis and septic shock is associated with decreased mortality. *Crit Care Med, 35*(4), 1105–1112.

Nolan, T. W. (1998). Understanding medical systems. *Annals of Internal Medicine, 128*(4), 293–298.

Norton, C. K., & Linenfelser, P. (2009). Patient with intracranial subarachnoid hemorrhage requiring an endovascular coiling procedure. *Adv Emerg Nurs J, 31*(1), 12–18.

Norton, C. K., Hobson, G., & Kulm, E. (2011). Palliative and end-of-life care in the emergency department: guidelines for nurses. *J Emerg Nurs, 37*(3), 240–245.

Nyquist, P., Stevens, R. D., & Mirski, M. A. (2008). Neurologic injury and mechanical ventilation. *Neurocrit Care, 9*(3), 400–408.

O'Connor, R. E., Brady, W., Brooks, S. C., Diercks, D., Egan, J., Ghaemmaghami, C., et al. (2010). Part 10: Acute coronary syndromes: 2010 American Heart Association guidelines for cardiopulmonary resuscitation and emergency cardiovascular care. *Circulation, 122*(18 Suppl 3), S787–S817.

Ojiako, K., Shingala, H., Schorr, C., & Gerber, D. R. (2008). Famotidine versus pantoprazole for preventing bleeding in the upper gastrointestinal tract of critically ill patients receiving mechanical ventilation. *Am J Crit Care, 17*(2), 142–147.

Olson, D. M., Thoyre, S. M., Peterson, E. D., & Graffagnino, C. (2009). A randomized evaluation of bispectral index-augmented sedation assessment in neurological patients. *Neurocrit Care, 11*(1), 20–27.

O'Malley, P. (2010). Vasopressors in septic shock: A possible deadly intervention. *Clin Nurse Spec, 24*(5), 235–237.

Oman, K. S., & Duran, C. R. (2010). Health care providers' evaluations of family presence during resuscitation. *J Emerg Nurs, 36*(6), 524–533.

Osman, D., Ridel, C., Ray, P., et al. (2007). Cardiac filling pressures are not appropriate to predict hemodynamic response to volume challenge. *Crit Care Med, 35*(1), 64–68.

Owens, A. P., 3rd, & Mackman, N. (2010). Tissue factor and thrombosis: The clot starts here. *Thromb Haemost, 104*(3), 432–439.

Pagana, K. D., & Pagana, T. J. (2010). *Mosby's manual of diagnostic and laboratory tests* (4th ed.). St. Louis: Mosby Elsevier.

Page, A. (Ed.). (2004). *Keeping patients safe. Transforming the work environment for nurses.* Washington, DC: The National Academies Press.

Palevsky, P. M. (2008). Indications and timing of renal replacement therapy in acute kidney injury. *Crit Care Med, 36*(4 Suppl), S224–S228.

Palmer, B. (2011). Systematic cardiac rhythm strip analysis. *MEDSURG Nurs, 20*(2), 96–97.

Palmer, J. L., & Metheny, N. A. (2008). Preventing aspiration in older adults with dysphagia. *Am J Nurs, 108*(2), 40–48; quiz 49.

Palmieri, R. L. (2007). Responding to primary brain tumor. *Nursing, 37*(1), 36–42; quiz 43.

Palmieri, R. L. (2009). Unlocking the secrets of locked-in syndrome. *Nursing, 39*(7), 22–29; quiz 29-30.

Palmieri, R. L. (2009). Wrapping your head around cranial nerves. *Nursing, 39*(9), 24–30; quiz 30-21.

Pannu, N., & Nadim, M. K. (2008). An overview of drug-induced acute kidney injury. *Crit Care Med, 36*(4 Suppl), S216–S223.

Pannu, N., Klarenbach, S., Wiebe, N., Manns, B., & Tonelli, M. (2008). Renal replacement therapy in patients with acute renal failure: A systematic review. *JAMA, 299*(7), 793–805.

Park, G., Coursin, D., Ely, E. W., England, M., Fraser, G. L., Mantz, J., et al. (2001). Balancing sedation and analgesia in the critically ill. *Crit Care Clin, 17*, 1015–1027.

Patanwala, A. E., Amini, A., & Erstad, B. L. (2010). Use of hypertonic saline injection in trauma. *Am J Health Syst Pharm, 67*(22), 1920–1928.

Pavlish, C., Brown-Saltzman, K., Hersh, M., Shirk, M., & Nudelman, O. (2011). Early indicators and risk factors for ethical issues in clinical practice. *J Nurs Scholarsh, 43*(1), 13–21.

Pavlish, C., Brown-Saltzman, K., Hersh, M., Shirk, M., & Rounkle, A. M. (2011). Nursing priorities, actions, and regrets for ethical situations in clinical practice. *J Nurs Scholarsh, 43*(4), 385–395.

Payen, J.-F., Bru, O., Bosson, J. L., Lagrasta, A., Novel, E., Deschaux, I., et al. (2001). Assessing pain in critically ill sedated patients using a behavioral pain scale. *Critical Care Medicine, 29*(12), 2258–2263.

Pearlman, M. K., Tanabe, M. B., Mycyk, D. N., & Stone, D. B. (2008). Evaluating disparities in door-to-EKG time for patients with noncardiac chest pain. *J Emerg Nurs, 34(5).* 414–418.

Peberdy, M. A., Callaway, C. W., Neumar, R. W., Geocadin, R. G., Zimmerman, J. L., Donnino, M., et al. (2010). Part 9: Post-cardiac arrest care: 2010 American Heart Association guidelines for cardiopulmonary resuscitation and emergency cardiovascular care. *Circulation, 122*(18 Suppl 3), S768–S786.

Peiffer, K. M. (2007). Brain death and organ procurement. *Am J Nurs, 107*(3), 58–67; quiz 68.

Perel, P., & Roberts, I. (2011). Colloids versus crystalloids for fluid resuscitation in critically ill patients. *Cochrane Database Syst Rev, 2011*(3), 1–62. CD000567.

Perkins, G. D., Gao, F., & Thickett, D. R. (2008). In vivo and in vitro effects of salbutamol on alveolar epithelial repair in acute lung injury. *Thorax, 63*(3), 215–220.

Pickham, D., & Drew, B. (2008). QT/QTc interval monitoring in the emergency department. *J Emerg Nurs, 34*(5), 428–434.

Pierrakos, C., & Vincent, J. L. (2010). Sepsis biomarkers: A review. *Crit Care, 14*(1), R15.

Pluta, A., Gutkowski, K., & Hartleb, M. (2010). Coagulopathy in liver diseases. *Adv Med Sci, 55*(1), 16–21.

Polanco, P. M., & Pinsky, M. R. (2006). Practical issues of hemodynamic monitoring at the bedside. *Surg Clin North Am, 86*, 1434–1466.

Polderman, K. H. (2009). Mechanisms of action, physiological effects, and complications of hypothermia. *Crit Care Med, 37*(7 Suppl), S186–S202.

Polly, D. M., Paciullo, C. A., & Hatfield, C. J. (2011). Management of hypertensive emergency and urgency. *Adv Emerg Nurs J, 33*(2), 127–136.

Povlishock, J.T., Bullock, M.R., Hillered, L.T., et al. (2007). Guidelines for the management of severe traumatic brain injury (3rd ed.). *J Neurotrauma, 24(*1), 1–106.

Powers, C. M. (2011). Use of alteplase beyond 3 hours of ischemic stroke onset. *Adv Emerg Nurs J, 33*(1), 65–70.

Priziola, J. L., Smythe, M. A., & Dager, W. E. (2010). Drug-induced thrombocytopenia in critically ill patients. *Crit Care Med, 38*(6 Suppl), S145–S154.

Prochaska, J. M. (2000). A transtheoretical model for assessing organizational change: A study of family service agencies' movement to time-limited therapy. *Family in Society: The Journal of Contemporary Human Services, 81*(1), 76–85.

Prochaska, J. M., Prochaska, J. O., & Levesque, D. A. (2001). A transtheoretical approach to changing organizations. *Administration and Policy in Mental Health, 28*(4), 247–261.

Protacio, J. (2010). Patient-directed music therapy as an adjunct during burn wound care. *Crit Care Nurse, 30*(2), 74–76.

Pustavoitau, A., & Stevens, R. D. (2008). Mechanisms of neurologic failure in critical illness. *Crit Care Clin, 24*(1), 1–24, vii.

Pyle, K., & Wavra, T. (2007). Quality indicators for critical care. *AACN Adv Crit Care, 18*(3), 229–243.

Pyle, K., Pierson, G., Lepman, D., & Hewett, M. (2007). Keeping cardiac arrest patients alive with therapeutic hypothermia. *American Nurse Today, 2*(7), 32–37.

Pyne, C. C. (2004). Classification of acute coronary syndromes using the 12-lead electrocardiogram as a guide. *AACN Clin Issues, 15*(4), 558–567.

Quality and Safety Education for Nurses. (2012). Quality and safety competencies. Retrieved August 13, 2012, from *http://www.qsen.org/competencies.php*.

Rachel, M. M. (2012). Accountability: A concept worth revisiting. *American Nurse Today, 7*(3), 36–39.

Radovich, P. (2008). Buying time for patients with acute liver failure. *American Nurse Today, 3*(11), 10–11.

Ramsay, M., Savege, T., Simpson, B., & Goodwin, R. (1974). Controlled sedation with alphaxalone-alphadolone. *Bri Med J, 2*, 656.

Rattray, J. E., & Hull, A. M. (2008). Emotional outcome after intensive care: Literature review. *J Adv Nurs, 64*(1), 2–13.

Rauen, C. A., & Wolfe, A. C. (2009). Cardiac contusion and the 12-lead ECG. *AACN Adv Crit Care, 20*(3), 301–304.

Realsen, J. M., & Chase, H. P. (2011). Recent advances in the prevention of hypoglycemia in type 1 diabetes. *Diabetes Technol Ther, 13*(12), 1177–1186.

Reina, M. L., Reina, D. S., & Rushton, C. H. (2007). Trust: The foundation for team collaboration and healthy work environments. *AACN Adv Crit Care, 18*(2), 103–108.

Reinhardt, M. R. (2010). Subarachnoid hemorrhage. *J Emerg Nurs, 36*(4), 327–329.

Reising, D. (2012). Make your nursing care malpractice-proof. *American Nurse Today, 7*(1), 24–30.

Reising, D. L., & Neal, R. S. (2005). Enteral tube flushing. *Am J Nurs, 105*(3), 58–63; quiz 63-54.

Reuter, D. A., Kirchner, A., Felbinger, T. W., et al. (2003). Usefulness of left ventricular stroke volume variation to assess fluid responsiveness in patients with reduced cardiac function. *Crit Care Med, 31*(5), 1399–1404.

Revere, C. (2002). Mechanisms of injury. In L. Newberry (Ed.), *Sheehy's emergency nursing: Principles and practice* (5th ed.). St. Louis: Mosby.

Rhoney, D., & Peacock, W. F. (2009). Intravenous therapy for hypertensive emergencies, part 1. *Am J Health Syst Pharm*, 66(15), 1343–1352.

Rhoney, D., & Peacock, W. F. (2009). Intravenous therapy for hypertensive emergencies, part 2. *Am J Health Syst Pharm*, 66(16), 1448–1457.

Riba, A. (2008). Evidence-based performance and quality improvement in the acute cardiac care setting. *Critical Care Clinics, 24*, 201–229.

Ricci, Z., & Ronco, C. (2008). Dose and efficiency of renal replacement therapy: Continuous renal replacement therapy versus intermittent hemodialysis versus slow extended daily dialysis. *Crit Care Med, 36*(4 Suppl), S229–S237.

Rice, T. W., & Wheeler, A. P. (2009). Coagulopathy in critically ill patients. Part 1: Platelet disorders. *Chest, 136*(6), 1622–1630.

Richards, N. M., & Stahl, M. A. (2007). Ventricular assist devices in the adult. *Crit Care Nurs Q, 30*(2), 104–118; quiz 119-120.

Richmond, T. S., & Ulrich, C. (2007). Ethical issues of recruitment and enrollment of critically ill and injured patients for research. *AACN Adv Crit Care, 18*(4), 352–355.

Riddle, E., Bush, J., Tittle, M., & Dilkhush, D. (2010). Alcohol withdrawal: Development of a standing order set. *Crit Care Nurse, 30*(3), 38–47; quiz 48.

Riker, R., Picard, J., & Fraser, G. (1999). Prospective evaluation of the Sedation-Agitation Scale for adult critically ill patients. *Crit Care Med, 27*, 1325.

Rivers, E., Nguyen, B., Havstad, S., Ressler, J., Muzzin, A., Knoblich, B., et al. (2001). Early goal-directed therapy in the treatment of severe sepsis and septic shock. *N Engl J Med, 345*(19), 1368–1377.

Roberts, M. (2010). Clinical utility and adverse effects of amiodarone therapy. *AACN Adv Crit Care, 21*(4), 333–338.

Robertson, R.G. & Montagnini, M. (2004). Geriatric failure to thrive. *Am Fam Physician, 70*, 343–350.

Robichaux, C. (2012). Developing ethical skills: From sensitivity to action. *Crit Care Nurse, 32*(2), 65–72.

Rodrigo, G. J. (2009). Predicting response to therapy in acute asthma. *Curr Opin Pulm Med, 15*(1), 35–38.

Roe, E. (2012). Practical strategies for death notification in the emergency department. *J Emerg Nurs, 38*(2), 130–134; quiz 200.

Rogers, E. M. (1995). *Diffusion of innovations* (4th ed.). New York: Free Press.

Roitberg, B. Z., Hardman, J., Urbaniak, K., Merchant, A., Mangubat, E. Z., Alaraj, A., et al, (2008). Prospective randomized comparison of safety and efficacy of nicardipine and nitroprusside drip for control of hypertension in the neurosurgical intensive care unit. *Neurosurgery, 63*(1), 115–120; discussion 120-111.

Rondina, M. T., Walker, A., & Pendleton, R. C. (2010). Drug-induced thrombocytopenia for the hospitalist physician with a focus on heparin-induced thrombocytopenia. *Hosp Pract (Minneap), 38*(2), 19–28.

Rosen, M. J., & Senicola, W. (2007). PA catheter controversy. *American Nurse Today, 2*(6), 25–27.

Rosenthal, G., Hemphill, J. C., Sorani, M., et al. (2008). Brain tissue oxygen tension is more indicative of oxygen diffusion than oxygen delivery and metabolism in patients with traumatic brain injury. *Crit Care Med, 36*(6), 1917–1924.

Rost, N. S., Smith, E. E., Chang, Y., et al. (2008). Prediction of functional outcome in patients with primary intracerebral hemorrhage: The FUNC score. *Stroke, 39*, 2304–2309.

Rushton, C. H. (2007). Respect in critical care: A foundational ethical principle. *AACN Adv Crit Care, 18*(2), 149–156.

Rushton, C. H., & Penticuff, J. H. (2007). A framework for analysis of ethical dilemmas in critical care nursing. *AACN Adv Crit Care, 18*(3), 323–329.

Rylah, B., & Vercueil, A. (2010). Intensive therapy of the patient with liver disease. *Br J Hosp Med (Lond), 71*(7), 377–381.

Sabol, V. K. (2004). Nutrition assessment of the critically ill adult. *AACN Clin Issues, 15*(4), 595–606.

Sanborn, C. (2009). Controlling blood glucose in hospital patients. *American Nurse Today, 4*(6), 10–12.

Sandau, K. E., Sendelbach, S., Frederickson, J., & Doran, K. (2010). National survey of cardiologists' standard of practice for continuous ST-segment monitoring. *Am J Crit Care, 19*(2), 112–123.

Sandrock, C. E., & Albertson, T. E. (2010). Controversies in the treatment of sepsis. *Semin Respir Crit Care Med, 31*(1), 66–78.

Savage, M., & Hilton, L. (2010). Managing diabetic ketoacidosis in adults: New national guidance from the JBDS. *J Diabetes Nurs, 14*(6), 220–225.

Scheibly, K. (2010). Indications for implantation of cardiac pacemakers. *AACN Adv Crit Care, 21*(2), 227–232.

Scheibly, K. (2010). Pacemaker timing and electrocardiogram interpretation. *AACN Adv Crit Care, 21*(4), 386–396.

Scheibly, K. (2010). Systematic assessment of basic pacemaker function. *AACN Adv Crit Care, 21*(3), 322–328.

Schmalenberg, C., & Kramer, M. (2009). Nurse-physician relationships in hospitals: 20,000 nurses tell their story. *Crit Care Nurse, 29*(1), 74–83.

Schulenburg, M. (2007). Management of hypertensive emergencies: Implications for the critical care nurse. *Crit Care Nurs Q, 30*(2), 86–93.

Schulman, C. S. (2009). Trauma. In K. K. Carlson (Ed.), *Advanced critical care nursing* (pp. 1134–1188). St. Louis: Saunders.

Selleng, K., Warkentin, T. E., & Greinacher, A. (2007). Heparin-induced thrombocytopenia in intensive care patients. *Crit Care Med, 35*(4), 1165–1176.

Shackell, E., & Gillespie, M. (2009). The oxygen supply and demand framework: A tool to support integrative learning. *Dynamics, 20*(4), 15–19.

Shannon, D., Hallinan, W., Massey, H. T., & Ackerman, M. H. (2006). Mechanical circulatory support devices. *AACN Adv Crit Care, 17*(4), 368–372.

Shaughnessy, K. (2007). Massive pulmonary embolism. *Crit Care Nurse, 27*(1), 39–50; quiz 51.

Shearer, A., Boehmer, M., Closs, M., Dela Rosa, R., Hamilton, J., Horton, K., et al. (2009). Comparison of glucose point-of-care values with laboratory values in critically ill patients. *Am J Crit Care, 18*(3), 224–230.

Shigemitsu, H., & Afshar, K. (2007). Aspiration pneumonias: Under-diagnosed and under-treated. *Curr Opin Pulm Med, 13*(3), 192–198.

Shindler, D. M. (2007). Practical cardiac auscultation. *Crit Care Nurs Q, 30*(2), 166–180.

Shorr, A. F., Chan, C. M., & Zilberberg, M. D. (2011). Diagnostics and epidemiology in ventilator-associated pneumonia. *Ther Adv Respir Dis, 5*(2), 121–130.

Shorr, A. F., Zilberberg, M. D., Micek, S. T., & Kollef, M. H. (2008). Prediction of infection due to antibiotic-resistant bacteria by select risk factors for health care-associated pneumonia. *Arch Intern Med, 168*(20), 2205–2210.

Short, J. (2010). Use of dexmedetomidine for primary sedation in a general intensive care unit. *Crit Care Nurse, 30*(1), 29–38; quiz 39.

Siela, D. (2008). Chest radiograph evaluation and interpretation. *AACN Adv Crit Care, 19*(4), 444–473; quiz 474-445.

Sihler, K. C., & Napolitano, L. M. (2010). Complications of massive transfusion. *Chest, 137*(1), 209–220.

Simonneau, G., Robbins, I. M., Beghetti, M., Channick, R. N., Delcroix, M., Denton, C. P., et al. (2009). Updated clinical classification of pulmonary hypertension. *J Am Coll Cardiol, 54* (1 Suppl), S43–S54.

Simpson, S. Q., Peterson, D. A., & O'Brien-Ladner, A. R. (2007). Development and implementation of an ICU quality improvement checklist. *AACN Adv Crit Care, 18*(2), 183–189.

Siow, E. (2008). Enteral versus parenteral nutrition for acute pancreatitis. *Crit Care Nurse, 28*(4), 19–25, 27-31; quiz 32.

Smith, M. M. (2010). Emergency: Variceal hemorrhage from esophageal varices associated with alcoholic liver disease. *Am J Nurs, 110*(2), 32–39; quiz 40-31.

Smithburger, P. L., Kane-Gill, S. L., Nestor, B. L., & Seybert, A. l. (2010). Recent advances in the treatment of hypertensive emergencies. *Crit Care Nurse, 30*(5), 24–31.

Soat, M. (2009). Aortic aneurysm: Causes, clues, and treatment options. *American Nurse Today, 4*(7), 7–9.

Sole, M. L., Aragon, D., Bennett, M., & Johnson, R. L. (2008). Continuous measurement of endotracheal tube cuff pressure: How difficult can it be? *AACN Adv Crit Care, 19*(2), 235–243.

Sole, M. L., Klein, D. G., & Moseley, M. J. (2009). *Introduction to critical care nursing* (5th ed.). Philadelphia: Saunders.

Sole, M. L., Penoyer, D. A., Su, X., Jimenez, E., Kalita, S. J., Poalillo, E., et al. (2009). Assessment of endotracheal cuff pressure by continuous monitoring: A pilot study. *Am J Crit Care, 18*(2), 133–143.

Solseng, T., Vinson, H., Gibbs, P., & Greenwald, B. (2008). In vitro formation of biofilms on Lopez enteral feeding valves: Implications for critical care patients and nurses. *Crit Care Nurse, 28*(1), 37–41.

Spangler, S. (2008). Pericarditis, acute. *EMedicine*, Retrieved November 3, 2008, from *http://www.emedicine.com/med/TOPIC1781.HTM*.

Spaniol, J. R., Knight, A. R., Zebley, J. L., Anderson, D., & Pierce, J. D. (2007). Fluid resuscitation therapy for hemorrhagic shock. *J Trauma Nurs, 14*(3), 152–160; quiz 161-152.

Speroni, K. G., Lucas, J., Dugan, L., O'Meara-Lett, M., Putman, M., Daniel, M., et al. (2011). Comparative effectiveness of standard endotracheal tubes vs. endotracheal tubes with continuous subglottic suctioning on ventilator-associated pneumonia rates. *Nurs Econ, 29*(1), 15–20, 37.

Sprung, C. L., Brezis, M., Goodman, S., & Weiss, Y. G. (2011). Corticosteroid therapy for patients in septic shock: Some progress in a difficult decision. *Crit Care Med, 39*(3), 571–574.

Stahl, M. A., & Richards, N. M. (2009). Update on ventricular assist device technology. *AACN Adv Crit Care, 20*(1), 26–34.

Staudinger, T., Bojic, A., Holzinger, U., Meyer, B., Rohwer, M., Mallner, F., et al. (2010). Continuous lateral rotation therapy to prevent ventilator-associated pneumonia. *Crit Care Med, 38*(2), 486–490.

Stephens, E. (2007). Peripheral vascular disease. *EMedicine*, Retrieved November 3, 2008, from *http://www.emedicine.com/emerg/TOPIC862*.

Stern, S. (2002). Angina pectoris without chest pain: Clinical implications of silent ischemia. *Circulation, 106*(15), 1906–1908.

Stevens, K. R. (2004). ACE Star Model of EBP: Knowledge transformation. Retrieved August 12, 2012, from *http://www.acestar.uthscsa.edu/acestar-model.asp*.

Stevens, K. R. (2001). Systematic reviews: The heart of evidence-based practice. *AACN Clinical Issues, 12*(4), 529–538.

Stevenson, L. W., & Perloff, J. K. (1989). The limited reliability of physical signs for estimating hemodynamics in chronic heart failure. *JAMA, 261*(6), 884–888.

Stich, J. C., & Cassella, D. M. (2009). Getting inspired about oxygen delivery devices. *Nursing, 39*(9), 51–54.

Stockley, R. A., O'Brien, C., Pye, A., & Hill, S. L. (2009). Relationship of sputum color to nature and outpatient management of acute exacerbations of COPD. *Chest, 136*(5 Suppl), e30.

Stonecypher, K. (2010). Ventilator-associated pneumonia: The importance of oral care in intubated adults. *Crit Care Nurs Q, 33*(4), 339–347.

Storm, L. A., Koh S., & Frey L. (2010). New antiepileptic drugs: Lacosamide, rufinamide, and vigabatrin. *Curr Treat Options Neurol, 12*, 287–299.

Straus, S. E., Glasziou, P., Richardson, W. S., & Haynes, R. B. (2011). *Evidence-based medicine: How to practice and teach it* (4th ed.). Edinburgh: Churchill Livingstone.

Stringham, R., & Shah, N. R. (2010). Pulmonary arterial hypertension: An update on diagnosis and treatment. *Am Fam Physician, 82*(4), 370–377.

Stromborg, M., Niebuhr, B., Prevost, S., Fabrey, L., Muenzen, P., Spence, C., et al. (2005). Specialty certification: More than a title. *Nurs Manage, 36*(5), 36.

Stunkard, M. E., Pikul, V. T., & Foley, K. (2011). Hyperosmolar hyperglycemic syndrome with rhabdomyolysis. *Clin Lab Sci, 24*(1), 8–13.

Suarez, J. I., Tarr, R.W., & Selman, W.R. (2006). Aneurysmal subarachnoid hemorrhage. *N Engl J Med, 354*, 387–396.

Sullivan, J. T., Sykora, K., Schneiderman, J., Naranjo, C. A., & Sellers, E. M. (1989). Assessment of alcohol withdrawal: The revised Clinical Institute Withdrawal Assessment for Alcohol scale (CIWA-AR). *Br J Addict, 84*, 1353–1357.

Sutton, L., & Chapman-Novakofski, K. (2011). Hypoglycemia education needs. *Qual Health Res, 21*(9), 1220–1228.

Sweat, M. T. (2011). How can I give spiritual care to patients in ICU? *J Christ Nurs, 28*(1), 50.

Tachjian, A., Maria, V., & Jahangir, A. (2010). Use of herbal products and potential interactions in patients with cardiovascular disease. *J Am Coll Cardiol, 55*(6), 515–525.

Talbert, S. (2005). Trauma. In J. Fultz & P. A. Sturt (Eds.), *Mosby's emergency nursing reference* (3rd ed., pp. 682–723). St. Louis: Mosby.

Tamburri, L. M., DiBrienza, R., Zozula, R., & Redeker, N. (2004). Nocturnal care interactions with patients in critical care units. *Am J Crit Care, 13*(2), 102–115.

Tapson, V. F. (2008). Acute pulmonary embolism. *N Engl J Med, 358*(10), 1037–1052.

Teal, J. (2011). Certifiably excellent. *AACN Adv Crit Care, 22*(1), 83–88.

Thachil, J., Fitzmaurice, D. A., & Toh, C. H. (2010). Appropriate use of D-dimer in hospital patients. *Am J Med, 123*(1), 17–19.

Thompson, B. S. (2009). Sudden cardiac death and heart failure. *AACN Adv Crit Care, 20*(4), 356–365.

Thompson, R. (2011). Comprehensive case study: Diabetes ketoacidosis. *MEDSURG Nurs, 20*(6), 338–339.

Tocco, S. B. (2010). Cerebral salt wasting: An overlooked cause of hyponatremia. *American Nurse Today, 5*(3), 34–36.

Tocco, S. B. (2011). Identify the vessel, recognize the stroke. *American Nurse Today, 6*(9), 8–11.

Tomte, O., Draegni, T., Mangschau, A., Jacobsen, D., Auestad, B., & Sunde, K. (2011). A comparison of intravascular and surface cooling techniques in comatose cardiac arrest survivors. *Crit Care Med, 39*(3), 443–449.

Travers, A. H., Rea, T. D., Bobrow, B. J., Edelson, D. P., Berg, R. A., Sayre, M. R., et al. (2010). Part 4: CPR overview. 2010 American Heart Association guidelines for cardiopulmonary resuscitation and emergency cardiovascular care. *Circulation, 122*(18 Suppl 3), S676–S684.

Treece, P. D. (2007). Communication in the intensive care unit about the end of life. *AACN Adv Crit Care, 18*(4), 406–414. doi: 10.1097/01.AACN.0000298633.38029.2d.

Trembly, A. (2010). Stroke care in the 21st century. *Nurs Manage, 41*(6), 30–36; quiz 36-37.

Trevino, C. (2010). Small bowel obstruction: The art of management. *AACN Adv Crit Care, 21*(2), 187–194.

Twedell, D., Lansing, R., McGuire, J., Palmersheim, P., & Baird, G. (2009). Providing holistic care to bariatric patients. *J Contin Educ Nurs, 40*(10), 438–439.

Uchino, S. (2008). Choice of therapy and renal recovery. *Crit Care Med, 36*(4 Suppl), S238–S242.

Unoki, T., Grap, M. J., Sessler, C. N., Best, A. M., Wetzel, P., Hamilton, A., et al. (2009). Autonomic nervous system function and depth of sedation in adults receiving mechanical ventilation. *Am J Crit Care, 18*(1), 42–50; quiz 51.

Urden, L., Stacy, K., & Lough, M. (2010). *Critical care nursing: Diagnosis and management* (6th ed.). St. Louis: Mosby.

U. S. Census Bureau. (2011). Projection of the population by sex, race, and Hispanic origin for the United States: 2010-2050. Retrieved August 12, 2011, from *http://www.census.gov/population/www/projections/reports.html.*

Van den Brink, W. A., Avezaat, C. J. J., & Hogesteeger, C., et al. (1998). Monitoring brain oxygen tension in severe head injury: The Rotterdam experience. *Acta Neurochir, 71*(Suppl), 190–194.

van Es, J., Douma, R. A., Gerdes, V. E. A., Kamphuisen, P. W., & Buller, H. R. (2010). Acute pulmonary embolism. Part 2: Treatment. Retrieved June 26, 2011, from *http://www.medscape.org/viewarticle/728110_print.*

Vanzant, A. M., & Schmelzer, M. (2011). Detecting and treating sepsis in the emergency department. *J Emerg Nurs, 37*(1), 47–54.

Varughese, S. (2007). Management of acute decompensated heart failure. *Crit Care Nurs Q, 30*(2), 94–103.

Vincent, J. L., Pinsky, M. R., Sprung, C. L., Levy, M., Marini, J. J., Payen, D., et al. (2008). The pulmonary artery catheter: In medio virtus. *Crit Care Med, 36*(11), 3093–3096.

Voepel-Lewis, T., Zanotti, J., Dammeyer, J. A., & Merkel, S. (2010). Reliability and validity of the face, legs, activity, cry, consolability behavioral tool in assessing acute pain in critically ill patients. *Am J Crit Care, 19*(1), 55–61; quiz 62.

Vollers, D., Hill, E., Roberts, C., Dambaugh, L., & Brenner, Z. R. (2009). AACN's healthy work environment standards and an empowering nurse advancement system. *Crit Care Nurse, 29*(6), 20–27; quiz 21 p following 27.

Walker, J., Pepa, C., & Gerard, P. (2010). Assessing the health literary levels of patients using selected hospital services. *Clinical Nurse Specialist, 24*(1), 31–37.

Warren, M. L., & Livesay, S. (2006). Taking action against acute COPD. *American Nurse Today, 1*(12), 12–15.

Wavra, T. (2006). *The 4 A's to rise above moral distress handbook.* Aliso Viejo, CA: AACN.

Wavra, T. A., & Bader, M. K. (2009). Bolus cardiac output and accuracy in therapeutic hypothermia. *Crit Care Nurse, 29*(6), 71–73.

Weant, K. A., & Cook, A. M. (2008). Pharmacologic strategies for the treatment of elevated intracranial pressure. Focus on osmotherapy. *Adv Emerg Nurs J, 30*(1), 17–26.

Wells, P. S., & Ginsberg, J. S. (1995). DVT and pulmonary embolism: Choosing the right diagnostic tests for patients at risk. *Geriatrics, 50*(2), 29–32, 35-26.

Wheeler, A. P., Bernard, G. R., Thompson, B. T., Schoenfeld, D., Wiedemann, H. P., deBoisblanc, B., et al. (2006). Pulmonary-artery versus central venous catheter to guide treatment of acute lung injury. *N Engl J Med, 354*(21), 2213–2224.

Whiteside, M., & Fletcher, A. (2010). Anaphylactic shock: No time to think. *J R Coll Physicians Edinb, 40*(2), 145–147; quiz 148.

Whitten, S. E. (2008). Systolic heart failure in a patient with hypertrophic obstructive cardiomyopathy: A potentially life-threatening complication. *Crit Care Nurse, 28*(5), 44–52; quiz 53.

Wiedemann, H. P., Wheeler, A. P., Bernard, G. R., Thompson, B. T., Hayden, D., deBoisblanc, B., et al. (2006). Comparison of two fluid-management strategies in acute lung injury. *N Engl J Med, 354*(24), 2564–2575.

Wiegand, D. L.-M. (Ed.). (2011). *AACN Procedure manual for critical care* (6th ed.). Philadelphia: Saunders.

Wiener, R. S., & Welch, H. G. (2007). Trends in the use of the pulmonary artery catheter in the United States: 1993-2004. *JAMA, 298*, 423–429.

Wieseke, A., Bantz, D., & May, D. (2011). What you need to know about bipolar disorder. *American Nurse Today, 6*(7), 8–12.

Wilkins, R. L., Stoller, J. K., & Kacmarek, R. M. (2009). *Egan's fundamentals of respiratory care* (9th ed.). St. Louis: Mosby.

Wingate, S., & Wiegand, D. L. (2008). End-of-life care in the critical care unit for patients with heart failure. *Crit Care Nurse, 28*(2), 84–95; quiz 96.

Winkelman, C., & Chiang, L. C. (2010). Manual turns in patients receiving mechanical ventilation. *Crit Care Nurse, 30*(4), 36–44.

Winsett, R. P., & Hauck, S. (2011). Implementing relationship-based care. *J Nurs Adm, 41*(6), 285–290.

Wood, G. C., & Swanson, J. M. (2009). Managing ventilator-associated pneumonia. *AACN Adv Crit Care, 20*(4), 309–316; quiz 317-318.

Yang, Y., Salam, Z. H., Ong, B. C., & Yang, K. S. (2011). Respiratory dysfunction in patients with sepsis: Protective effect of diabetes mellitus. *Am J Crit Care, 20*(2), e41–47.

Yantis, M. A., & Velander, R. (2009). Probiotics can thwart antibiotic-associated diarrhea. *Nursing, 39*(3), 58–59.

Yarema, T. C., & Yost, S. (2011). Low-dose corticosteroids to treat septic shock: A critical literature review. *Crit Care Nurse, 31*(6), 16–26.

Yates, W. R. (2009). Anxiety disorders. *Emedicine*, Retrieved on August 29, 2012, from *http://emedicine.medscape.com/article/286227-overview.*

Yeager, S., Doust, C., Epting, S., Iannantuono, B., Indian, C., Lenhart, B., & Thomas, K. (2010). Embrace Hope: an end-of-life intervention to support neurological critical care patients and their families. *Crit Care Nurse, 30*(1), 47–58; quiz 59.

Yoder-Wise, P. (2011). *Leading and managing in nursing* (5th ed.). St. Louis: Mosby.

Young, A. C. (2010). Non-invasive ventilation: Status quo for status asthmaticus? *Respirology, 15*(4), 585–586.

Zannad, F. (2007). Aldosterone antagonist therapy in resistant hypertension. *J Hypertens, 25*(4), 747–750.

Zimmermann, P. G. (2008). Minimally interrupted cardiac resuscitation. *Am J Nurs, 108*(10), 73–74.

Zomorodi, M. (2010). Critical care nurses' values and behaviors with end-of-life care: Perceptions and challenges. *Journal of Hospice and Palliative Nursing, 12*(2), 89–96.

Common Abbreviations and Acronyms Used in Critical Care Nursing

APPENDIX A

2,3-DPG	2,3-diphosphoglyceric acid
A	Alveolar
a	Arterial
a/A	Arterial/alveolar (as in a/A gradient)
A_2	Aortic (first) component of S_2
AAA	Abdominal aortic aneurysm
AACN	American Association of Critical-Care Nurses
AAL	Anterior axillary line
ABG	Arterial blood gas
ABI	Ankle-brachial index
AC	Assist-control
ACC	American College of Cardiology
ACE	Academic Center for Evidence-Based Practice
ACE	Angiotensin converting enzyme
ACLS	Advanced cardiac life support
ACS	Abdominal compartment syndrome
ACS	Acute coronary syndrome
ACT	Activated clotting time
ACTH	Adrenocorticotropic hormone
ADA	American Diabetic Association
ADH	Antidiuretic hormone
ADL	Activities of daily living
ADP	Adenosine diphosphate
AED	Automated external defibrillator
AF	Atrial fibrillation
AGREE	Appraisal of Guidelines for Research and Evaluation
AHA	American Heart Association
AHA	American Hospital Association
AHRQ	Agency for Healthcare Research and Quality
AIDS	Acquired immune deficiency syndrome
AIVR	Accelerated idioventricular rhythm
AKI	Acute kidney injury
ALF	Acute liver failure
ALI	Acute lung injury
ALS	Amyotrophic lateralizing sclerosis

ALT	Alanine aminotransferase
AMP	Applied Measurement Professionals
ANA	American Nurses Association
ANCC	American Nurses Certification Corporation
ANP	Atrial natriuretic peptide
ANS	Autonomic nervous system
AP	Anterior posterior
APA	American Psychiatric Association
APRV	Airway pressure release ventilation
aPTT	Activated partial thromboplastin time
AR	Aortic regurgitation
ARB	Angiotensin receptor blocker
ARDS	Acute respiratory distress syndrome
ARF	Acute respiratory failure
AS	Aortic stenosis
ASA	Acetylsalicylic acid (aspirin)
AST	Aspartate aminotransferase
ATN	Acute tubular necrosis
ATP	Adenosine triphosphate
AV	Arteriovenous
AV	Atrioventricular
AVM	Arteriovenous malformation
BAL	Bronchoalveolar lavage
BBB	Bundle branch block
BE	Base excess
Bi-PAP	Positive airway pressure on both inspiration and expiration
BIS	Bispectral index
Bi-VAD	Biventricular assist device
BLS	Basic life support
BM	Bowel movement
BMI	Body mass index
BNP	Brain-type natriuretic peptide
BP	Blood pressure
BPOC	Bar-code point of care
BSA	Body surface area
BSN	Bachelor of Science in Nursing
BUN	Blood urea nitrogen
C	Celsius (also referred to as centigrade)
CABG	Coronary artery bypass graft
CAD	Coronary artery disease
CaO_2	Oxygen content in arterial blood
CAP	Community-acquired pneumonia
CAPM	Continuous airway pressure monitoring
CAPP	Coronary artery perfusion pressure
CAVH	Continuous arteriovenous hemofiltration
CAVHD	Continuous arteriovenous hemodialysis
CASS	Continuous aspiration of subglottic secretions
CBC	Complete blood count
CBF	Cerebral blood flow
CCO	Continuous cardiac output
CCU	Critical care unit or cardiac care unit

CDC	Centers for Disease Control
CEA	Carcinoembryonic antigen
CHB	Complete heart block
CHO	Carbohydrate
CHP	Capillary hydrostatic pressure
CI	Cardiac index
CINAHL	Cumulative Index of Nursing and Allied Health Literature
CK	Creatine kinase
CKD	Chronic kidney disease
CK-MB	Creatine kinase-myocardial band
CLRT	Continuous lateral rotation therapy
cm	Centimeter
CMV	Cytomegalovirus
CNS	Central nervous system
CO	Cardiac output
CO_2	Carbon dioxide
COLD	Chronic obstructive lung disease
COP	Colloidal oncotic pressure
COPD	Chronic obstructive pulmonary disease
CPAP	Continuous positive airway pressure
CPB	Cardiopulmonary bypass
CPG	Clinical practice guideline
CPOE	Computerized provider order entry
CPP	Cerebral perfusion pressure
CPR	Cardiopulmonary resuscitation
CRH	Corticotropin-releasing hormone
CRRT	Continuous renal replacement therapy
CRT	Cardiac resynchronization therapy
CSF	Cerebrospinal fluid
CSF	Colony-stimulating factor
CSW	Cerebral salt wasting
CT	Computerized tomography
cTnI	Cardiac troponin I
cTnT	Cardiac troponin T
CVA	Cerebrovascular accident
CVA	Costovertebral angle
CvO_2	Oxygen content in venous blood
CVP	Central venous pressure
CVVH	Continuous venovenous hemofiltration
CVVHD	Continuous venovenous hemodialysis
CVVHDF	Continuous venovenous hemodiafiltration
D_5LR	5% dextrose in lactated Ringer's
D_5NS	5% dextrose in normal saline
D_5W	5% dextrose in water
$D_{10}W$	10% dextrose in water
$D_{50}W$	50% dextrose in water
DAI	Diffuse axonal injury
dB	Decibels
DBP	Diastolic blood pressure
DCA	Directional coronary atherectomy
DES	Drug eluting stent

DHA	Docosahexaenoic acid
DI	Diabetes insipidus
DIC	Disseminated intravascular coagulation
DKA	Diabetes ketoacidosis
dL	Deciliter
DM	Diabetes mellitus
DNA	Deoxyribonucleic acid
DNR	Do not resuscitate
DO_2	Oxygen delivery to the tissues
DO_2I	Delivery of oxygen to the tissue index
DPL	Diagnostic peritoneal lavage
dPP	Pulse pressure variation
DT	Delirium tremens
DTBT	Door to balloon time
DTR	Deep tendon reflexes
DVT	Deep vein thrombosis
EAB	Extraanatomical bypass
EBCT	Electron beam computerized tomography
EBP	Evidence-based practice
$ECCO_2OR$	Extracorporeal carbon dioxide removal
ECF	Extracellular fluid
ECF-A	Eosinophil chemotactic factor of anaphylaxis
ECG	Electrocardiogram (may also be abbreviated EKG)
ECMO	Extracorporeal membrane oxygenator
ED	Emergency department
EDH	Epidural hematoma
EEG	Electroencephalogram
EF	Ejection fraction
ELCA	Excimer laser coronary atherectomy
ELISA	Enzyme linked immunosorbent assay
EMG	Electromyogram
EMI	Electromagnetic interference
EMS	Emergency management system
ENG	Electronystagmography
EOM	Extraocular movement
EPA	Eicosapentaenoic acid
EPA	Environmental Protection Agency
EPS	Electrophysiology studies
EPS	Extrapyramidal symptoms
ERCP	Endoscopic retrograde cholangiopancreatography
ERV	Expiratory reserve volume
ESR	Eosinophil sedimentation rate
ET	Endotracheal
ETC	Esophageal tracheal Combitube
ETT	Exercise tolerance test
EVG	Endovascular graft
F	Fahrenheit
f	Frequency of ventilation
FAST	Focused abdominal sonography for trauma
FDA	Food and Drug Administration
FEV	Forced expiratory capacity

FFP	Fresh frozen plasma
FiO_2	Fraction of inspired oxygen
FRC	Functional residual capacity
FSP	Fibrin split products (also referred to as *fibrin degradation products*)
FT_c	Flow time corrected
FTT	Failure to thrive
FVC	Forced vital capacity
g	Gram
GABA	Gamma-aminobutyric acid
GALT	Gut-associated lymphoid tissue
GCS	Glasgow Coma Scale
GERD	Gastroesophageal reflux disease
GFR	Glomerular filtration rate
GGT	Gamma-glutamyl transferase
GI	Gastrointestinal
GP	Glycoprotein
GU	Genitourinary
H^+	Hydrogen ion
H_2O	Water
HAART	Highly active antiretroviral therapy
HAP	Hospital-acquired pneumonia
HAT	Heparin-associated thrombocytopenia
HBV	Hepatitis B virus
HCAP	Healthcare-associated pneumonia
HCl	Hydrochloric
HCO_3	Bicarbonate
Hct	Hematocrit
HDL	High density lipoproteins
HELLP	Hemolysis, elevated liver enzyme levels, and low platelet count (as in HELLP syndrome)
HF	Heart failure
HFJV	High-frequency jet ventilation
HFO	High-frequency oscillation
HFPPV	High-frequency positive-pressure ventilation
HFV	High-frequency ventilation
Hg	Mercury
Hgb	Hemoglobin
HHS	Hyperglycemic hyperosmolar state
HIPAA	Health Insurance Portability and Accountability Act
HIT	Heparin-induced thrombocytopenia
HIV	Human immunodeficiency virus
HLA	Human leukocyte antigen
HME	Heat and moisture exchanger
HOB	Head of bed
HR	Heart rate
HRSA	Health Resources and Services Administration
HRT	Hormone replacement therapy
IABP	Intraaortic balloon pump
IAH	Intraabdominal hypertension
IAP	Intraabdominal pressure
IBW	Ideal body weight
IC	Inspiratory capacity

ICD	Implantable cardiac defibrillator
ICH	Intracranial hematoma
ICOP	Interstitial colloidal oncotic pressure
ICP	Intracranial pressure
ICS	Intercostal space
ICU	Intensive care unit
I : E	Inspiration : expiration
IFD	Intermittent flush device
Ig	Immunoglobulin
IHP	Interstitial hydrostatic pressure
IHSS	Idiopathic hypertrophic subaortic stenosis
IL	Interleukin
ILV	Independent lung ventilation
IM	Intramuscular
IMV	Intermittent mandatory ventilation
INH	Isoniazid
INR	International normalized ratio
INVOS	In-Vivo Optical Spectroscopy
IOM	Institute of Medicine
IPBH	Intraparenchymal brain hemorrhage
IPPB	Intermittent positive-pressure breathing
IRA	Infarct-related artery
IRV	Inspiratory reserve volume
IRV	Inverse ratio ventilation
ISMP	Institute for Safe Medication Practices
ITP	Idiopathic thrombocytopenia purpura
IU	International units
IV	Intravenous
IVP	Intravenous pyelogram
IVUS	Intravascular ultrasound
JCAHO	Joint Commission on Accreditation of Healthcare Organizations
JVD	Jugular venous distention
kg	Kilogram
KUB	Kidneys, ureters, bladder (same as flat plate of abdomen)
KVO	Keep vein open
L	Liter
LA	Left atrium
LAAL	Left anterior axillary line
LAD	Left anterior descending (artery)
LAD	Left axis deviation
LAH	Left anterior hemibundle
LAP	Left atrial pressure
LBB	Left bundle branch
LBBB	Left bundle branch block
LCA	Left circumflex artery
LDH	Lactic dehydrogenase
LDL	Low-density lipoproteins
LES	Lower esophageal sphincter
LICS	Left intercostal space
LLQ	Left lower quadrant
LMA	Laryngeal mask airway

LMAL	Left midaxillary line
LMCL	Left midclavicular line
LMN	Lower motor neuron
LMWH	Low-molecular—weight heparin
LOC	Level of consciousness
LP	Lumbar puncture
LPAL	Left posterior axillary line
LPH	Left posterior hemibundle
LPN	Licensed Practical Nurse (aka, Licensed Vocational Nurse)
LR	Lactated Ringer's
LSB	Left sternal border
LUQ	Left upper quadrant
LV	Left ventricle
LVAD	Left ventricular assist device
LVEDP	Left ventricular end-diastolic pressure
LVEDV	Left ventricular end-diastolic volume
LVF	Left ventricular failure
LVH	Left ventricular hypertrophy
LVMI	Left ventricular myocardial infarction
LVSWI	Left ventricular stroke work index
M_1	Mitral (first) component of S_1
mA	Milliampere (unit of measurement for electrical current)
MAL	Midaxillary line
MALT	Mucosa-associated lymphoid tissues
MAO	Monoamine oxidase (as in MAO inhibitors)
MAP	Mean arterial pressure
MAP	Multidisciplinary action plan
MAST	Military antishock trousers
mcg	Microgram (unit of measurement for weight)
MCH	Mean corpuscular hemoglobin
MCHC	Mean corpuscular hemoglobin concentration
MCL	Midclavicular line
MCT	Medium chain triglycerides
MCV	Mean corpuscular volume
MDF	Myocardial depressant factor
MDMA	Methylenedioxymethamphetamine (i.e., Ecstasy)
M_E	Minute ventilation exhaled
mEq	Milliequivalent (unit of measurement for solutes in solution)
mg	Milligram (unit of measurement for weight)
MI	Myocardial infarction
MIC	Minimum inhibitory concentration
MIDCABG	Minimally invasive coronary artery bypass graft
MIP	Maximal inspiratory pressure (or force) (also referred to as *negative inspiratory pressure* [or *force*])
mL	Milliliter (unit of measurement for volume)
mm	Millimeter (unit of measurement for length)
mm Hg	Millimeters of mercury
MODS	Multiple organ dysfunction syndrome
mOsm/kg	Milliosmoles per kilogram
mOsm/L	Milliosmoles per liter
MR	Mitral regurgitation
MRA	Magnetic resonance angiography

MRI	Magnetic resonance imaging
MRS	Magnetic resonance spectroscopy
MS	Mitral stenosis
MSG	Monosodium glutamate
MSL	Midsternal line
MUGA	Multiple-gated acquisition scan
MV	Mechanical ventilation
MVC	Motor vehicle collision
MVO_2	Myocardial oxygen consumption
MVP	Mitral valve prolapse
MVV	Maximal voluntary ventilation
NAC	N-acetylcysteine
NASPE	North American Society of Pacing and Electrophysiology
NCLEX	National Council Licensure Examination
NCSBN	National Council of State Boards of Nursing
NDE	Near-death experience
NDNQI	National Database of Nursing Quality Indicators
NG	Nasogastric
NIF	Negative inspiratory force
NIH	National Institutes of Health
NIHSS	National Institutes of Health Stroke Scale
NK	Natural killer
NNRTI	Nonnucleoside reverse transcriptase inhibitors
NPO	Nothing by mouth
NPPV	Noninvasive positive-pressure ventilation
NRTI	Nucleoside analog reverse transcriptase inhibitor
NS	Normal saline
NSAID	Nonsteroidal antiinflammatory drug
NSR	Normal sinus rhythm
NTG	Nitroglycerin
NTP	Nitroprusside
NtRTI	Nucleotide reverse transcriptase inhibitor
NYHA	New York Heart Association
O_2	Oxygen
OCD	Obsessive compulsive disorder
O_2EI	Oxygen extraction index
O_2ER	Oxygen extraction ratio
OPB	Ova, parasites, blood
OPCABG	Off-pump coronary artery bypass graft
OPG	Oculoplethysmography
P_2	Pulmonic (second) component of S_2
PA	Posterior anterior
PA	Pulmonary artery
PAC	Premature atrial contraction
PAC	Pulmonary artery catheter
$PaCO_2$	Partial pressure of carbon dioxide in arterial blood
PAd	Pulmonary artery diastolic pressure
PAL	Posterior axillary line
PAm	Pulmonary artery pressure mean
PaO_2	Pressure of oxygen in arterial blood
PAO_2	Pressure of oxygen in alveolar blood

PAOP	Pulmonary artery occlusive pressure (previously referred to as *pulmonary capillary wedge pressure* or *pulmonary artery wedge pressure*)
PAP	Pulmonary artery pressure
PAs	Pulmonary artery systolic pressure
PASG	Pneumatic antishock garments
PAT	Paroxysmal atrial tachycardia
Pb	Barometric pressure
PC/IRV	Pressure-controlled/inverse-ratio ventilation
PCA	Patient-controlled analgesia
PCI	Percutaneous coronary intervention
PCP	Phencyclidine
PCP	*Pneumocystis carinii* pneumonia
PCR	Polymerase chain reaction
PCV	Pressure-controlled ventilation
PD	Postural drainage
PDA	Patent ductus arteriosus
PDE	Phosphodiesterase
PDF	Probability density function
PDSA	Plan-Do-Study-Act
PE	Pulmonary embolism
PEA	Pulseless electrical activity
P_ECO_2	Partial pressure of carbon dioxide in exhaled air
PEEP	Positive end-expiratory pressure
PEFR	Peak expiratory flow rate
PEG	Percutaneous endoscopic gastrostomy
PEJ	Percutaneous endoscopic jejunostomy
PET	Positron emission tomography
$P_{et}CO_2$	Partial pressure of carbon dioxide in end-tidal air
P/F	PaO_2/FiO_2 (as in P/F ratio)
PFT	Pulmonary function tests
pH	Hydrogen ion concentration
pHi	Intramucosal pH
PICC	Percutaneously inserted central catheter
PICOT	Problem, Intervention, Comparison, Outcome, Timing (i.e., format for a clinical question)
PIP	Peak inspiratory pressure
PJC	Premature junctional contraction
PMI	Point of maximal impulse
PML	Progressive multifocal leukoencephalopathy
PMN	Polymorphonuclear leukocytes
PMR	Papillary muscle rupture
PMR	Progressive muscle relaxation
PND	Paroxysmal nocturnal dyspnea
PNS	Parasympathetic nervous system
PO	Oral
PPD	Purified protein derivative
PPF	Plasma protein fraction
PPI	Proton pump inhibitor
PPN	Peripheral parenteral nutrition
PQRST	Provocation, palliation, quality, quantity, region, radiation, severity, timing (i.e., pain description)
PRVC	Pressure-regulated volume-controlled (mode of mechanical ventilation)
PSB	Protected specimen brush
PSV	Pressure support ventilation

PSVT	Paroxysmal supraventricular tachycardia
PT	Physical therapy
PT	Prothrombin time
PTCA	Percutaneous transluminal coronary angioplasty
$P_{tc}O_2$	Transcutaneous partial pressure of oxygen
PTFE	Polytetrafluoroethylene
PTMR	Percutaneous transmyocardial revascularization
PTSD	Posttraumatic stress disorder
PTSMA	Percutaneous transluminal septal myocardial ablation
PTT	Partial prothrombin time
PTU	Propylthiouracil
PV	Peak velocity
PVC	Polyvinyl chloride
PVC	Premature ventricular contraction
PVR	Pulmonary vascular resistance
PVRI	Pulmonary vascular resistance index
Q	Perfusion
QI	Quality improvement
QM	Quality management
QT_c	QT interval corrected for rate
RA	Right atrium
RAA	Renin-angiotensin-aldosterone
RAAL	Right anterior axillary line
RAD	Right axis deviation
RAP	Right atrial pressure
RAS	Reticular activating system
RBB	Right bundle branch
RBBB	Right bundle branch block
RBC	Red blood cell
RCA	Right coronary artery
REF	Right (ventricular) ejection fraction
REM	Rapid eye movement
RHD	Rheumatic heart disease
RICS	Right intercostal space
RIND	Reversible ischemic neurologic deficit
RLQ	Right lower quadrant
RMAL	Right midaxillary line
RMCL	Right midclavicular line
RN	Registered nurse
RNA	Ribonucleic acid
ROM	Range of motion
ROSC	Return of spontaneous circulation
r-PA	Recombinant plasminogen activator
RPAL	Right posterior axillary line
RQ	Respiratory quotient
RR	Respiratory rate
RSB	Right sternal border
RSBI	Rapid shallow breathing index
rSO_2	Regional oxygen saturation index
RSV	Respiratory syncytium virus
rt-PA	Recombinant tissue plasminogen activator

RUQ	Right upper quadrant
RV	Residual volume
RV	Right ventricle
RVAD	Right ventricular assist device
RVEDP	Right ventricular end-diastolic pressure
RVEDV	Right ventricular end-diastolic volume
RVESV	Right ventricular end-systolic volume
RVF	Right ventricular failure
RVH	Right ventricular hypertrophy
RVMI	Right ventricular myocardial infarction
RVSWI	Right ventricular stroke work index
RYGB	Roux-Y gastric bypass
SA	Sinoatrial
SAED	Semiautomatic external defibrillator
SAH	Subarachnoid hemorrhage
SaO_2	Oxygen saturation of arterial blood
SARS	Severe acute respiratory syndrome
SC	Subcutaneous
SCI	Spinal cord injury
SCUF	Slow continuous ultrafiltration
$S_{cv}O_2$	Oxygen saturation of central venous blood
SDH	Subdural hematoma
SIADH	Syndrome of inappropriate antidiuretic hormone
SILV	Synchronized independent lung ventilation
SIMV	Synchronized intermittent mandatory ventilation
SIRS	Systemic inflammatory response syndrome
SjO_2	Oxygen saturation of jugular venous blood
SK	Streptokinase
SLE	Systemic lupus erythematosus
SNS	Sympathetic nervous system
SPECT	Single photon emission computed tomography
SpO_2	Oxygen saturation in plasma (e.g., pulse oximetry)
SRS-A	Slow reacting substance of anaphylaxis
STEMI	ST segment elevation myocardial infarction
STTI	Sigma Theta Tau International
SV	Stroke volume
SVI	Stroke index
SvO_2	Oxygen saturation of mixed venous blood
SVR	Systemic vascular resistance
SVRI	Systemic vascular resistance index
SVT	Supraventricular tachycardia
SVV	Stroke volume variability
T	Temperature
T_1	Tricuspid (second) component of S_1
TAA	Thoracic aortic aneurysm
TB	Tuberculosis
TBI	Toe-brachial index
TCA	Tricyclic antidepressants
$TcPO_2$	Transcutaneous carbon dioxide
TEC	Transluminal extraction catheter
TEE	Transesophageal echocardiography

TENS	Transcutaneous electrical nerve stimulation
TIA	Transient ischemic attack
TIBC	Total iron-binding capacity
TIPS	Transjugular intrahepatic portosystemic shunt
TLC	Total lung capacity
TLC	Total lymphocyte count
TMP-SMX	Trimethoprim-sulfamethoxazole
TNA	Total nutrient admixture
TNF	Tumor necrosis factor
TPN	Total parenteral nutrition
TR	Tricuspid regurgitation
TRH	Thyrotropin-releasing hormone
TSH	Thyroid-stimulating hormone
TTP	Thrombotic thrombocytopenia purpura
UAP	Unlicensed assistive personnel
UES	Upper esophageal sphincter
UFH	Unfractionated heparin
UMN	Upper motor neuron
UTI	Urinary tract infection
V	Ventilation
V_A	Alveolar minute ventilation
VAC	Vacuum-assisted closure
VAD	Ventricular assist device
VAP	Ventilator-associated pneumonia
VAPSV	Volume-assured pressure support ventilation
VBG	Vertical banded gastroplasty
VC	Vital capacity
V_D	Anatomical dead space
V_E	Minute ventilation
VF	Ventricular fibrillation
VILI	Ventilator-induced lung injury
VIP	Volume infusion port
VO_2	Oxygen consumption by the tissues
VO_2I	Consumption of oxygen by the tissues index
VPR	Volume pressure response
V/Q	Ventilation/perfusion ratio
VSD	Ventricular septal defect
VT	Ventricular tachycardia
V_T	Tidal volume
WBC	White blood cell
WPW	Wolff-Parkinson-White syndrome

Normal Laboratory Values

APPENDIX B

Blood Chemistries

Sodium:	136-145 mEq/L
Potassium:	3.5-5.0 mEq/L
Chloride:	96-106 mEq/L
Calcium:	8.5-10.5 mg/dL
Phosphorus:	3.0-4.5 mg/dl
Magnesium:	1.5-2.2 mEq/L or 1.8 to 2.4 mg/dL
CO_2:	23-30 mEq/L
Glucose:	70-110 mEq/L
BUN:	5-20 mg/dL
Creatinine:	0.7-1.5 mg/dL
Uric acid:	3-7 mg/dL
Osmolality:	280-295 mOsm/L
Lactate:	1-2 mmol/L
Ammonia:	15-110 mOsm/dL
Iron:	50-150 mcg/dL
Iron-binding capacity:	250-410 mcg/dL
Carcinoembryonic antigen (CEA):	Less than 2 ng/mL
Homocysteine:	Less than 15 µmol/L
C-reactive protein:	Less than 1 mg/dL
Brain-type natriuretic peptide (BNP):	Less than 100 pg/mL
Bilirubin	
Total:	0.3-1.3 mg/dL
Direct:	0.1-0.3 mg/dL
Indirect:	0.1-1.0 mg/dL

Proteins

Total protein:	6-8 g/dL
C-reactive protein:	Less than 0.8 mg/dL
Albumin:	3.5-4.5 g/dL
Prealbumin:	15-32 mg/dL
Transferrin:	250-300 mg/dL
Globulin:	2.3-3.5 g/dL
Albumin/globulin ratio (A/G):	1.5/1-2.5/1
Fibrinogen:	200-400 mg/dL or 2-4 g/L

Lipids

Cholesterol:	150-200 mg/dL
Triglycerides:	40-150 mg/dL
Lipoprotein-cholesterol fractionation	
HDL:	29-77 mg/dL
LDL:	62-130 mg/dL

Enzymes

Total CK:	55-170 U/L for males; 30-135 U/L for females
CK-MB:	0-4% of total CK
LDH:	90-200 IU/L
LDH-1:	17-25% of total LDH
Alanine aminotransferase (ALT):	5-36 units/mL (formerly called SGPT)
Aspartate aminotransferase (AST):	15-45 units/mL (formerly called SGOT)
Gamma-glutamyl transferase (GGT):	5-38 IU/L
Alkaline phosphatase:	30-85 IU/L
Amylase:	56-190 IU/L
Lipase:	Less than 150 units/L

Muscle Proteins

Myoglobin:	Less than 110 ng/mL
Troponin I:	Less than 1.5 ng/mL
Troponin T:	Less than 0.1 ng/mL

Arterial Blood Gases

pH:	7.35-7.45
$PaCO_2$:	35-45 mm Hg
HCO_3^-:	22-26 mEq/L
Base excess:	−2 to 2
PaO_2:	80-100 mm Hg
SaO_2:	Greater than 95%

Hematology

Red blood cells (RBC):	4.4-5.9 × 10^6/mL for males; 3.8-5.2 × 10^6/mL for females
Red cell indices include the following:	
Mean corpuscular volume (MCV):	80-100 μm^3
Mean corpuscular hemoglobin (MCH):	27-31 pg
Mean corpuscular hemoglobin concentration (MCHC):	32-36 g/dL

Reticulocyte count: 0.5-1.5% of RBC
Erythrocyte sedimentation rate: Up to 15 mm/hr for males; up to 20 mm/hr for females
Hematocrit: 40-52% for males; 35-47% for females
Hemoglobin: 13-18 g/dL for males; 12-16 g/dL for females
White blood cells (WBC): 3,500-11,000 mm^3
Differential
Neutrophils: 40-80%
Eosinophils: 0-5%
Basophils: 0-2%
Monocytes: 3-8%
Lymphocytes: 10-40%
Immune profile
CD4 cell count: 800 cells/mm^3; varies with age
CD4/CD8 ratio: Helper cells: suppressor/cytotoxic cells ratio: 1.8
HIV antibody screening: Negative

Clotting Profile

Prothrombin time (PT): 12-15 seconds
Partial thromboplastin time (PTT): 60-70 seconds
Activated partial thromboplastin time (aPTT): 25-38 seconds
Activated clotting time (ACT): 70-120 seconds
International normalized ratio (INR): Less than 2.0
Thrombin time: 10-15 seconds
Bleeding time: 1-9.5 minutes
Lee White clotting time: 6-12 minutes
Platelets: 150,000-400,000/mm^3
Fibrinogen: 200-400 mg/dL or 2-4 g/L
Fibrin degradation products (FDPs) (also referred to as *fibrin split products* (*FSPs*): 0-10 mcg/dL
D-dimer: Less than 250 ng/mL

Hormones

Triiodothyronine (T_3): 0.2-0.3 mcg/dL
Thyroxine (T_4): 6-12 mcg/dL
ACTH: 15-100 pg/mL in AM, 10-50 pg/mL in PM
Cortisol: 6-28 mcg/dL at 8 AM, 4-12 mcg/dL at 4 PM; 2-12 mcg/dL at 8 PM
ADH: 1-5 pg/mL

Toxicology

Alcohol: 0 mg/dL
Dilantin: Therapeutic 10-20 mcg/mL
Digoxin: Therapeutic 0.5-2.0 ng/mL
Lidocaine: Therapeutic 1.5-5.0 mcg/mL
Phenobarbital: Therapeutic 10-40 mcg/mL
Theophylline: Therapeutic 10-20 ng/dL

Urine

Glucose: Negative
Ketones: Negative
Protein: 0-8 mg/dL; less than 150 mg/24 hr urine output
Amylase: 3-21 IU/hr
Bilirubin: Negative
Urobilinogen: Less than 1 mg/dL
RBCs: 0-2/low power field
WBCs: 0-4/low power field
Hemoglobin/myoglobin: Negative
Specific gravity: 1.005-1.030
Osmolality: 50-1200 mOsm/L
Creatinine clearance: 85-135 mL/min
Culture and sensitivity: No bacteria present; if bacteria are present, appropriate antibiotic therapy is identified
pH: 4.0-8.0 with average of 6.0
Spot urine electrolytes
Sodium: 40-220 mEq/L/day
Potassium: 25-120 mEq/L/day
Chloride: 110-250 mEq/day
Hormone metabolites
17-hydroxycorticosteroids: 4.5-10 mg/24 hr for males; 2.5-10 mg/24 hr for females
17-ketosteroids: 8-15 mg/24 hr for males, 6-12 mg/24 hr for females

Stool

Fecal occult blood test: Negative
Ova, parasites, blood (OPB): Negative
Fecal fat: 5 g/24 hr
Urobilinogen: 0-4 mg/day
Culture: Intestinal flora
Assay for *Clostridium difficile* toxin A or B: Negative; positive if diarrhea is caused by *C. difficile*

NOTE: Values may vary depending on laboratory.

Formulae Significant to Critical Care Nursing

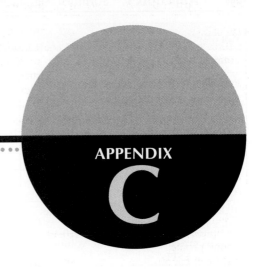

General Conversion

To convert pounds to kilograms	1 lb = 0.45 kg
To convert inches to cm	1 in = 2.54 cm
To convert mm Hg to cm of H_2O	1 mm Hg = 1.36 cm H_2O
To convert Fahrenheit to Celsius	(°F − 32) ÷ 1.8

Drug Administration

To calculate mcg/kg/min if you know the rate of the infusion	$\frac{(\text{mcg/mL}) \times (\text{mL/hr})}{(60\ \text{min/hr}) \times (\text{kg of body weight})}$
To calculate rate in mL/hr if you know the dose in mcg/kg/min	$\frac{(\text{dose in mcg/kg/min}) \times (60\ \text{min/hr}) \times (\text{wt in kg})}{\text{mcg/mL of the solution}}$
To calculate mg/min if you know the rate of the infusion	$\frac{(\text{mg/mL}) \times (\text{mL/hr})}{(60\ \text{min/hr})}$
To calculate rate in mL/hr if you know the dose in mg/min	$\frac{(\text{dose in mg/min}) \times (60\ \text{min/hr})}{\text{mg/mL of the solution}}$
To calculate mcg/min if you know the rate of the infusion	$\frac{(\text{mcg/mL}) \times (\text{mL/hr})}{(60\ \text{min/hr})}$
To calculate rate in mL/hr if you know the dose in mcg/min:	$\frac{(\text{dose in mcg/min}) \times (60\ \text{min/hr})}{\text{mcg/mL of the solution}}$

Cardiovascular

Parameter	Method of Calculation	Normal
Mean arterial pressure (MAP)	[BP systolic + (BP diastolic × 2)] ÷ 3	70-105 mm Hg (Normal systolic BP 90-140 mm Hg; normal diastolic BP 60-90 mm Hg)
Cardiac index (CI)	CO ÷ by body surface area (BSA)	2.5-4.0 L/min/m^2
Stroke volume (SV)	CO ÷ HR	60-120 mL/beat
Stroke index (SI)	SV ÷ BSA	30-65 mL/m^2/beat
Systemic vascular resistance (SVR)	[(MAP − RAP) × 80] ÷ CO	900-1400 dynes/sec/cm^{-5}
Systemic vascular resistance index (SVRI)	[(MAP − RAP) × 80] ÷ CI	1700-2600 dynes/sec/cm^{-5}/m^2

Parameter	Method of Calculation	Normal
Pulmonary vascular resistance (PVR)	$[(PAm - PAOP) \times 80] \div CO$	100-250 dynes/sec/cm^{-5}
Pulmonary vascular resistance index (PVRI)	$[(PAm - PAOP) \times 80] \div CI$	225-315 dynes/sec/cm^{-5}/m^2
Left ventricular stroke work index (LVSWI)	$[SI \times (MAP - PAOP)] \times 0.0136$	45-65 g • m/m^2
Right ventricular stroke work index (RVSWI)	$[SI \times (PAm - RAP)] \times 0.0136$	5-12 g • m/m^2
Coronary artery perfusion pressure (CAPP)	Diastolic BP – PAOP	60-80 mm Hg
Right ventricular end-diastolic volume index (RVEDVI)	RVEDV ÷ BSA	60-100 mL/m^2
Right ventricular end-systolic volume index (RVESVI)	RVESV ÷ BSA	30-60 mL/m^2
Arterial oxygen content (CaO_2)	$1.34 \times Hgb \times SaO_2$	18-20 mL/dL
Venous oxygen content (CvO_2)	$1.34 \times Hgb \times SvO_2$	12-16 mL/dL
Oxygen delivery (DO_2)	$CO \times CaO_2 \times 10$	900-1100 mL/min
Oxygen delivery index (DO_2I)	$CI \times CaO_2 \times 10$	550-650 mL/min/m^2
Oxygen consumption (VO_2)	$CO \times Hgb \times 13.4 \times (SaO_2 - SvO_2)$	200-300 mL/min
Oxygen consumption index (VO_2I)	$CI \times Hgb \times 13.4 \times (SaO_2 - SvO_2)$	110-160 mL/min/m^2
Oxygen extraction ratio (O_2ER)	$CaO_2 - CvO_2/CaO_2$	22%-30%
Oxygen extraction index (O_2EI)	$SaO_2 - SvO_2/SaO_2$	20%-27%
Corrected QT (QT_c)	$QT \div \sqrt{RR}$	0.35-0.43 sec

Pulmonary

Parameter	Method of Calculation	Normal
Static compliance	$\frac{\text{Tidal volume}}{\text{Plateau pressure} - \text{PEEP}}$	50-100 mL/cm H_2O
Dynamic compliance	$\frac{\text{Tidal volume}}{\text{Peak pressure} - \text{PEEP}}$	35-55 mL/cm H_2O
a/A ratio	(PaO_2/PAO_2) NOTE: PAO_2 is calculated as: FiO_2 (760 – 47) – ($PaCO_2$/0.8) NOTE: FiO_2: fraction of inspired oxygen (written as a decimal) Pb: barometric pressure (760 mm Hg at sea level, adjust for higher altitudes) $PaCO_2$: arterial carbon dioxide tension 47 is the pressure of water vapor at sea level and is subtracted from barometric pressure; 0.8 is the usual respiratory quotient	Normal greater than 0.8 Moderately abnormal 0.5-0.8 Significantly abnormal 0.25-0.5 Critically abnormal less than 0.25
A:a gradient	$PAO_2 - PaO_2$	Less than 10 mm Hg NOTE: A:a gradient × 0.05 ≅ % shunt
PaO_2/FiO_2 ratio	$\frac{PaO_2}{FiO_2 \text{ (decimal)}}$	Greater than 300 300 ≅15% shunt 200 ≅20% shunt

Parameter	Method of Calculation	Normal
Respiratory index	$\frac{PAO_2 - PaO_2}{PaO_2}$	Less than 1
Rapid shallow breathing index	f/V_T (in liters) using frequency and average tidal volume for 1 minute	No more than 105 breaths/min/L indicates readiness for weaning

Neurologic

Parameter	Method of Calculation	Normal
Cerebral perfusion pressure (CPP)	$MAP - ICP$	60-100 mm Hg

Nutrition

Parameter	Method of Calculation	Normal
Body mass index (BMI)	$\text{Weight (kg)}/\text{Ht (m)} \times \text{Ht (m)}$	Optimal: 20-25 Obesity: greater than 25 Underweight: less than 20

Fluid, Electrolyte, Acid-Base

Parameter	Method of Calculation	Normal
Serum osmolality	$(2 \times Na) + \frac{BUN}{2.6} + \frac{glucose}{18}$	280-295 mOsm/L
Anion gap	$(Na + K) - (Cl + HCO_3)$	5-15 NOTE: Some formulae omit potassium; if potassium is omitted, normal is 8-12
Corrected serum calcium in hypoalbuminemia	$0.8 \times (4 - \text{serum albumin}) + \text{serum calcium}$	8.5-10.5 mg/dL
Corrected serum potassium in acid-base imbalances	0.1 change in pH (from midline normal of 7.4) causes a change in the potassium level by ~0.5 mEq/L in the opposite direction	3.5-5.0 mEq/L NOTE: This formula is especially helpful to estimate the drop in serum potassium expected with pH correction in diabetic ketoacidosis
Ideal body weight using Devine formula	Ideal Body Weight (men) = 50 kg + 2.3 kg × (Height [in] – 60) Ideal Body Weight (women) = 45.5kg + 2.3kg × (Height [in] – 60)	Varies

INDEX

Note: Page numbers followed by b, f, and t indicate boxes, figures, and tables, respectively.

F

M

O

U